Boyd's
Textbook of Pathology

Boyd's
Textbook of Pathology

A.C. RITCHIE

M.B., Ch.B., D.Phil., F.R.C.P.C., F.R.C.Path., F.R.C.P.A., F.A.C.P.

Professor Emeritus of Pathology, University of Toronto
Consulting Pathologist: Mt. Sinai Hospital; The Hospital for Sick Children;
The Toronto Hospital
Toronto, Canada

Volume II

Ninth Edition

Lea & Febiger
Philadelphia / London
1990

Lea & Febiger
200 Chester Field Parkway
Malvern, Pennsylvania   19355
U.S.A.
1-800-444-1785

Lea & Febiger (UK) Ltd.
145a Croydon Road
Beckenham, Kent BR3 3RB
U.K.

Library of Congress Cataloging-in-Publication Data

Ritchie, A.C.
    Boyd's textbook of pathology.—9th ed. / A.C. Ritchie.
        p.   cm.
    Rev. ed. of: A textbook of pathology / William Boyd. 8th ed. 1970.
    Includes bibliographical references.
    ISBN 0-8121-0726-8
    1. Pathology.   I. Boyd, William, 1885–   Textbook of pathology.
II. Title.   III. Title: Textbook of pathology.
    [DNLM: 1. Pathology.   QZ 4 R599]
    RB111.R57   1990
    616.07—dc20
    for Library of Congress   89-13747
                                                                            CIP

First Edition, 1932
  Reprinted 1933
Second Edition, 1934
  Reprinted 1934, 1935, 1936
Third Edition, 1938
  Reprinted 1938, 1939, 1940, 1941
Fourth Edition, 1943
  Reprinted 1943, 1944, 1945, 1946
Fifth Edition, 1947
  Reprinted 1947, 1948, 1949, 1950, 1951, 1952
  Translated into Portuguese
Sixth Edition, 1953
  Reprinted 1954, 1955, 1956, 1957, 1958
Seventh Edition, 1961
  Reprinted 1961, 1962, 1963, 1964, 1965, 1967
  Translated into Spanish
Eighth Edition, 1970
  Reprinted 1970, 1973, 1975, 1976, 1979, 1980
Ninth Edition, 1990

Print number: 5   4   3   2   1

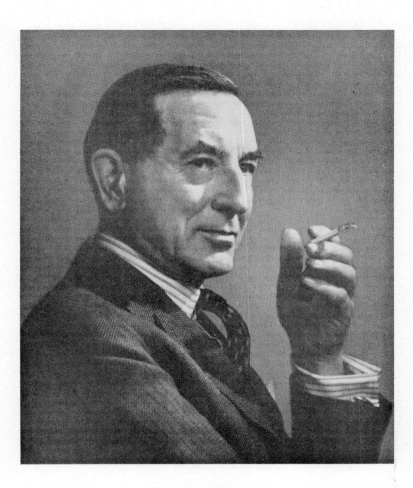

WILLIAM BOYD
M.D., M.R.C.P., F.R.C.P., F.R.C.S.
(1885–1979)

Publisher's Foreword

Dr. William Boyd, whose textbooks enlivened the study of pathology for many a student, was born in Portsoy, Scotland in 1885. He received his M.D. from Edinburgh in 1908. He displayed an early interest in psychiatry, but found his true métier in pathology. Recruited for the University of Manitoba medical faculty, Boyd, after a year of service with a field ambulance in France, took up his chairmanship in pathology in 1915.

Turning away many attractive offers, Boyd stayed in Manitoba until 1937, when he followed his good friend, the anatomist John Grant, to the University of Toronto.

Boyd's greatest achievements as a pathologist were his lucid, highly readable publications. *Surgical Pathology*, later retitled *Pathology for the Surgeon*, was published by W.B. Saunders Co. in 1925. His later books, *Pathology of Internal Diseases*, renamed *Pathology for the Physician* (1st edition, 1931 and 7th edition, 1965), *Textbook of Pathology* (1st edition, 1932 and 8th edition, 1970), and *Introduction to Medical Science*, renamed *Introduction to the Study of Disease* (1st edition, 1937 and 9th edition, 1980) were published by Lea & Febiger.

Boyd was a formidable lecturer, possessing both lucidity and a keen wit. The hematologist, Maxwell Wintrobe, one of Boyd's pupils, wrote that Boyd ". . . was our most stimulating teacher. He was devoted to the development of a museum of pathology and could take a jar containing a preserved specimen and bring the clinical problem to life. For him pathology was fascinating and in his Scottish brogue and, often in flowery language, his lectures always were exciting and memorable."

As a person he was devoid of affectation and ill humor. He was quick to praise those who deserved praise and had a rare ability to rebuke without giving offense. Though relaxed and easily approachable, he liked to maintain a degree of formality in his department.

After retiring from the University of Toronto, he was appointed Professor of Pathology at the University of British Columbia and, thereafter, spent many winters as a visiting professor at the University of Alabama. During the Prohibition days in the United States he often traveled from Canada to lecture; the popularity of his lectures was enhanced by the fact that he always brought Scotch whisky with him carefully hidden under layers of pathologic specimens. That which he did not dispatch was shared with his hosts.

Boyd received many honors in his long life, including honorary degrees from Edinburgh, Saskatchewan, Oslo, Manitoba, Queen's University, and the College of Surgeons of Canada. Especially notable was his award of the gold-headed cane of the American Association of Pathologists and Bacteriologists—he was the only Canadian to be so honored.

Those of us who had the pleasure of working with him shall not forget his unfailing good humor and his courtesy. Nor shall we forget his lovely wife, Enid, whose warm and cheerful nature made her the perfect companion for William Boyd.

R. Kenneth Bussy
for
Lea & Febiger

Preface

Boyd's Textbook of Pathology is concerned with the science of pathology. It describes the cause, development, and lesions of the diseases that afflict us, their effect on the patient, the functional and secondary changes they cause, their course and complications, and the kind of treatment appropriate to overcome them. The practice of pathology, the techniques used, the problems that arise, will not be discussed except insofar as is relevant to our understanding of the disease processes.

The book falls into three parts. First is discussed what is often called general pathology, the processes like inflammation or neoplasia underlying many kinds of disease. Then the infectious diseases are considered, and the diseases caused by other factors that can affect many organs. In the third section of the book are described the diseases of the various organs.

To each chapter is appended a list of references. First comes a list of specialized textbooks that discuss in detail the topics considered in that chapter. If further information is sought, it is usually best to consult first these specialized texts. They review the topics discussed and have long lists of references. Also cited are recent reviews relevant to the matters discussed in each chapter. In general, the most recent review is listed. It is not necessarily the best, but does give entry to the current literature. At the end of Chapter 1 is a list of standard textbooks that discuss matters relevant to many of the chapters.

I would like to thank Sonia Duda, Librarian of the Banting Library, for help with the references. I would also like to thank Richard Leung of the Department of Pathology and Mark Sawyer of the Instructional Media Services of the University of Toronto for help with the illustrations.

Toronto, Ontario   A.C. RITCHIE

Contents

VOLUME I

35

Intestine

THE diseases of the duodenum, small bowel, colon, rectum, and anus are considered together, since many of them affect more than one of these parts of the alimentary tract. The inflammatory diseases of the intestine are considered first and then the ischemic disorders, the conditions that cause malabsorption, the diverticula of the bowel, disorders that cause obstruction, diseases that affect only the anal region, congenital anomalies, other nonneoplastic disorders, and tumors.

INFLAMMATORY DISEASE

Two of the most common forms of inflammatory disease of the intestine have already been discussed, the infections in Chapters 16, 17, 18, 19, 20, and 21 and acute and chronic peptic ulceration in Chapter 34. Of particular importance are the major infections of the intestine such as cholera, bacillary dysentery, typhoid fever, paratyphoid fever, tuberculosis, amebic dysentery, giardiasis, Chagas' disease, and lymphogranuloma venereum; the common bacterial and viral infections that cause diarrhea; the infestations with worms that are a major cause of disease in much of the world; food poisoning caused by salmonellae, staphylococci, and clostridia; and peptic ulceration of the duodenum.

There remain to be discussed ulcerative colitis, Crohn's disease, appendicitis, and the less common forms of intestinal inflammation —eosinophilic enteritis, allergic enteritis, stercoral ulcer, and solitary ulcer of the rectum.

Inflammatory Bowel Disease

Ulcerative colitis and Crohn's disease are disorders of unknown etiology that are at times hard to distinguish clinically or pathologically. They are often grouped together and called inflammatory bowel disease. Some ill-defined conditions closely related to ulcerative colitis or Crohn's disease are sometimes included as forms of inflammatory bowel disease, but appendicitis, diverticulitis, the infectious diseases of the bowel, and other forms of enteritis or colitis are excluded.

ULCERATIVE COLITIS. In Europe and the United States, 1 person in 1000 has ulcerative colitis. About 7 people per 100,000 develop the disease each year. In the tropics, ulcerative colitis is less common. The incidence of ulcerative colitis is three or four times greater in Jews than in the population at large. In the United States, the incidence in white people is three or four times greater than in black people.

Ulcerative colitis may begin at any age, but most patients are between 20 and 40 years old when symptoms first appear. About 60% of the patients are women.

Lesions. Ulcerative colitis probably always begins in the rectum or rectosigmoid region. In 20% of the patients, the disease remains confined to the rectum. In 40%, it extends to involve part or all of the descending colon, and in 40% it involves the whole colon, though the left side of the colon is usually more severely involved than is the right. The disease extends into the distal part of the ileum in from 10 to 20% of the patients in whom the whole colon is involved. The involvement of the ileum rarely extends more than 20 cm from the ileocecal valve.

In most patients, the upper limit of the disease is vague. The inflammation in the colon or ileum gradually lessens and gives way to a normal bowel. Occasionally, the upper limit of the disease is sharp, as in Crohn's disease.

In a few patients, ulcerative colitis appears

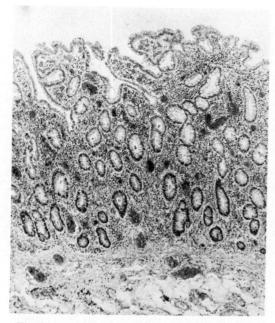

Fig. 35-1. Ulcerative colitis, showing inflammation largely confined to the mucosa.

other conditions. The quantity of mucus in the goblet cells is reduced, or goblet cells are lost altogether, a condition called mucus depletion.

In a mild attack, superficial inflammation may be the extent of the disease. The inflammation persists for several weeks, then subsides.

If the disease is more severe, there is ulceration in the inflamed mucosa. The ulcers vary from tiny erosions to ulcers several centimeters across. Sometimes almost the entire mucosa is denuded. However large the ulcers become, they usually remain superficial and penetrate little beneath the muscularis mucosae. Often, the ulcers tend to line up along the teniae coli. Often they undermine the surrounding mucosa or burrow beneath it, leaving a mucosal bridge between adjacent ulcers.

The inflammatory reaction persists in the mucosa between the ulcers and extends a short way into the underlying tissue at their base. In places, neutrophils are numerous in the exudate; more often lymphocytes, plasma

to be segmental, with segments of diseased colon several centimeters long separated by relatively normal bowel. Close examination shows that the disease is continuous from the rectum to its proximal margin. The alternation is not between diseased and normal segments of colon, as in Crohn's disease, but between more severely and less severely involved segments.

The rectum is nearly always involved. Even if it seems almost normal at proctoscopy, a rectal biopsy can establish the diagnosis in over 95% of patients with ulcerative colitis.

Ulcerative colitis is an inflammation of the mucosa. It begins with congestion and edema in the mucosa of the involved part of the colon, with an exudate predominantly of lymphocytes and plasma cells, though sometimes with many eosinophils. The inflammation may involve the superficial part of the submucosa, but does not often spread more deeply. Emphasis is placed on crypt abscesses. Neutrophils accumulate in some of the mucosal crypts, and as the crypt becomes distended by the neutrophils, it is said to contain a crypt abscess. Crypt abscesses are common in ulcerative colitis, but do occur in

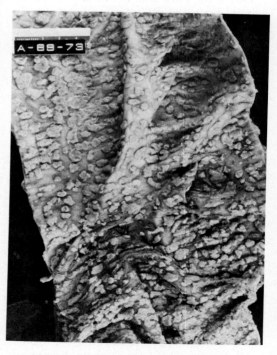

Fig. 35-2. Ulcerative colitis, showing extensive ulceration, leaving only small islands of mucosa.

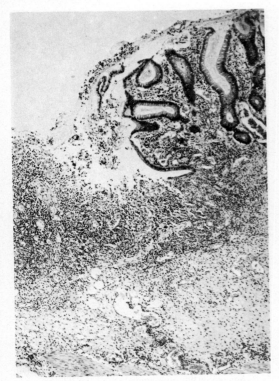

Fig. 35-3. Ulcerative colitis, showing the margin of an ulcer, with edematous mucosa overhanging the inflamed base of the ulcer.

cells, and macrophages are predominant. Especially striking is the congestion and edema in the surviving islands of mucosa.

The edematous mucosa often bulges into the lumen to form pseudopolyps. The pseudopolyps are particularly striking when an island of surviving mucosa is surrounded by ulcers and the swollen mucosa stands high above the bed of the ulcers. The pseudopolyps are not neoplasms, only blobs of edematous mucosa.

In most patients, an attack of ulcerative colitis subsides after several weeks, and the disease becomes quiescent. The neutrophils disappear. The lymphocytes and plasma cells become less numerous. The goblet cells are again distended with mucus. The ulcers heal as epithelial cells slide across the thin layer of granulation tissue in the base of the ulcers and form a simple, mucus-secreting epithelium.

The mucosa rarely returns to normal. It remains thinner than usual, with short, branching glands that are often widely separated. Lymphocytes and plasma cells persist in the lamina propria. Paneth cells and neuroendocrine cells are often numerous in the depths of the crypts. Often the muscularis mucosae is thickened. Occasionally fat ap-

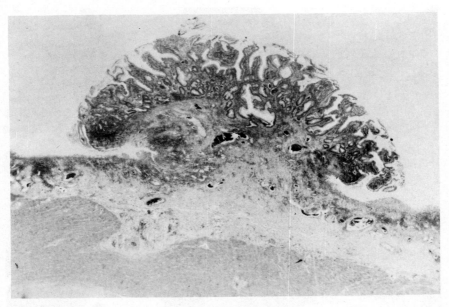

Fig. 35-4. Ulcerative colitis, showing a pseudopolyp of edematous mucosa standing above the surrounding ulceration.

pears in the mucosa. Usually there is no significant fibrosis. When the disease undergoes an exacerbation, the congestion and edema of the early stages of the inflammation reappear, and the whole cycle is repeated.

Foci of dysplasia are evident in the rectal or colonic mucosa in some patients in whom the disease has persisted for several years. The abnormal foci are often small. Several biopsies may be necessary to detect the dysplasia. The dysplastic epithelium is sometimes thrown into fronds like those of a villous adenoma, but more often remains flat and macroscopically is unremarkable. In the affected region, the nucleocytoplasmic ratio is decreased in the epithelial cells, their nuclei are hyperchromatic and often pleomorphic, and the mitotic rate is increased. Sometimes the nuclei of the dysplastic cells are elongated and closely packed together; sometimes the dysplastic cells are cuboidal with a moderate quantity of cytoplasm and spheroidal nuclei. Paneth cells are often prominent in the dysplastic foci. Often goblet cells in the dysplastic foci are distorted and resemble signet ring cells. Similar abnormalities in the epithelium can be caused by severe inflam-

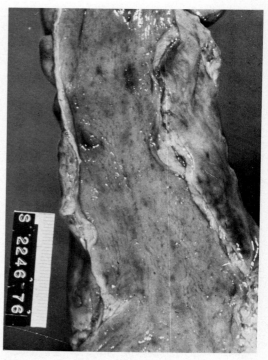

Fig. 35-5. Ulcerative colitis, showing the pale, smooth mucosa of the quiescent stage of the disease.

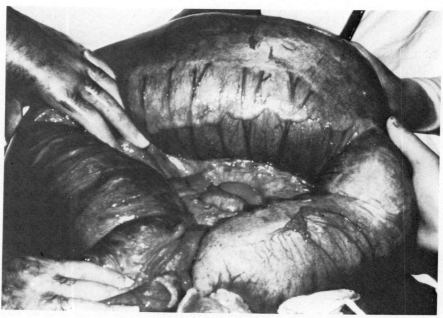

Fig. 35-6. Toxic megacolon, showing the enormously dilated colon found in this form of ulcerative colitis.

mation, sometimes making the diagnosis of dysplasia difficult.

Macroscopically the appearance of the colon reflects the severity of the disease. In the early stages, the mucosa is congested, edematous, and friable. There is hypersecretion of mucus. Often there are petechiae, and swabbing or any sort of trauma brings oozing of blood. Later, ulcers become evident; their base often is covered by mucopurulent exudate. Lines of ulcers often are separated by the ragged remnants of bright red mucosa, with its pseudopolyps. Blood oozes from the tattered mucosa through slimy mucus. At this stage, there is usually considerable muscle spasm, so that the affected part of the colon is narrowed and shortened.

As the disease becomes quiescent, the colon returns more or less to its normal length and diameter. The mucosa sometimes looks fairly normal, but if atrophy of the mucosa is severe, it becomes smooth and pale, without its normal folds. It no longer bleeds easily.

Toxic Megacolon. In 5 to 10% of patients with ulcerative colitis, the disease suddenly becomes much more severe. Perhaps in the initial attack or perhaps after several recurrences part or much of the colon becomes greatly dilated, with extreme toxemia. In the course of a few hours, the patient passes from relative health to the gate of death. The transverse colon is often the most severely affected part of the bowel. The affected part of the colon swells to 10 cm or more in diameter. Its wall becomes thin, with the consistency of wet blotting paper. Perforation is easy, either spontaneously or during operation. Congestion and necrosis in the mucosa are severe. Inflammation extends through the whole thickness of the attenuated colonic wall, often with exudate on the serosa.

Clinical Presentation. In more than 70% of patients with ulcerative colitis, the disease is episodic. An attack lasts a few weeks or a month or two and then resolves. The patient is free of symptoms for months or years, but then the disease recurs, and the cycle is repeated. In some of these people, the disease is mild. In others, the attacks are severe. In 20% of patients the symptoms are continuous. The patient may get somewhat better or somewhat worse, but is never symptom free.

In some people, ulcerative colitis is at first episodic and later becomes continuous. In less than 5% of patients, ulcerative colitis begins as an acute, fulminating disease, with toxic megacolon.

The principal symptom is usually diarrhea. The diarrhea is sometimes mild. The patient may notice that the stool contains bloody mucus. In other patients, bowel movements are frequent and the stool is mushy, mucoid, and bloody. At the extreme, bowel movements are almost continuous. The patient may be incontinent and the stool consists of little but blood, pus, and mucus.

If the disease is severe, there is likely to be abdominal pain, sometimes colic. Tenesmus may be distressing. In the more severe attacks, fever of up to 40°C and leukocytosis are usual. Iron deficiency anemia is common because of the continuous oozing of small quantities of blood. Severe diarrhea may cause alkalosis, hyponatremia, hypochloremia, hypokalemia, hypocalcemia, or hypoalbuminemia. Nearly always there is severe weight loss. Symptoms may begin insidiously, or the attack may start abruptly.

In fulminant ulcerative colitis with toxic megacolon, there is high fever, with crampy abdominal pain, profuse, watery diarrhea, severe bleeding, and severe prostration.

Complications. Some complication develops in more than 50% of patients with ulcerative colitis. The more severe the disease and the longer it persists, the more likely complications become.

About 20% of the patients develop disease in or around the anus. An anal fissure is the most common complication, but there may be an ischiorectal abscess, fistula in ano, a rectovaginal fistula, or a rectovesical fistula.

Massive hemorrhage occurs in about 5% of patients with ulcerative colitis. The bleeding usually is from a multitude of tiny vessels rather than from a single, large artery. Conservative measures can usually control the bleeding.

Perforation occurs in less than 5% of the patients. It is common with toxic megacolon, but can occur in other circumstances, if one of the ulcers penetrates unusually deeply. Generalized peritonitis may follow, or a local pericolic abscess may develop.

The liver is affected in 50% of patients with

ulcerative colitis. Usually the liver disease is mild and causes no dysfunction. A lymphocytic exudate in the portal triads, a condition called pericholangitis or triaditis, or mild fatty liver is the most common finding. Rarely, the pericholangitis causes jaundice or itching. Some 2% of patients with ulcerative colitis develop cirrhosis of the liver. Some develop chronic active hepatitis. Rarely there is sclerosing cholangitis. How the disease in the bowel damages the liver is unknown. Bacteremia in the portal system occurs in 25% of the patients with chronic ulcerative colitis and may damage the liver; lithocholic acid or some other injurious substance may be absorbed from the diseased bowel; or an immunologic attack on the liver may be stimulated.

Fleeting arthritis, affecting now one joint, now another, occurs in 25% of patients with ulcerative colitis. It persists for a week or two, but subsides without residual injury to the joint. In 1% of patients with ulcerative colitis, the injury to the joints is more severe, with lesions like those of rheumatoid arthritis.

About 5% of patients with ulcerative colitis develop ankylosing spondylitis, and up to 20% develop sacroiliitis, with narrowing and sclerosis of one or both sacroiliac joints. From 50 to 90% of the patients with ulcerative colitis who develop ankylosing spondylitis bear the histocompatibility antigen HLA-B27, as do patients with ankylosing spondylitis who do not have ulcerative colitis. The frequency of HLA-B27 in people with ulcerative colitis who do not develop ankylosing spondylitis is less than 10%, as in the general population.

Skin lesions occur in 15% of the patients. There may be any of a variety of urticarial, purpuric, eczematous, or erythematous rashes. About 10% of the patients develop erythema nodosa. Up to 5% suffer the deep, painful ulcers, often several centimeters across, of pyoderma gangrenosum.

About 5% of people with ulcerative colitis have clubbing of the fingers. Conjunctivitis, iritis, or episcleritis develops in up to 10% of the patients. Aphthae often develop in the mouth. Moniliasis can become extensive. About 5% of the patients have clinical evidence of thrombosis of the deep veins of the legs, and up to 40% have thrombi in the deep veins at autopsy. About 3% develop renal stones, usually after colectomy.

Between 3 and 5% of patients with ulcerative colitis develop carcinoma of the colon. The greater the extent of the disease in the colon and the longer its duration, the greater the risk. In patients in whom the whole colon is involved, the risk of carcinoma is more than 10% greater than in the general population when the disease has persisted for 15 years, more than 20% greater when it has continued for 20 years, and over 40% greater when it has lasted for 25 years. The incidence of carcinoma of the biliary tract is also increased in inflammatory bowel disease.

The prognosis is bad in patients with ulcerative colitis who develop carcinoma of the colon. Metastases are often present by the time the tumor is discovered. Several factors combine to cause the bad prognosis. Often the carcinoma is flat and unobtrusive. It causes few symptoms and is not easily detected. The symptoms caused by the carcinoma are masked by those of the colitis. The concentration of the carcinoembryonic antigen in the plasma is increased in patients with active ulcerative colitis and cannot be used to detect carcinoma. The tumor is often unusually anaplastic. There may be more than one carcinoma.

If multiple biopsies are taken, foci of dysplasia are evident in the rectal or colonic mucosa in the majority of patients with ulcerative colitis who have a carcinoma of the colon. Over 50% of the patients who have foci of dysplasia have a carcinoma in some other part of the colon.

Etiology. The etiology of ulcerative colitis is unknown. As is so often the case when the cause of a disease is obscure, theories have proliferated.

In years past, a wide variety of infectious organisms have been proposed as the cause of ulcerative colitis. At present, there is no reason to think that the disease is caused by infection.

It is often suggested that ulcerative colitis results from an immunologic attack on the colon. Abnormal immunologic reactions are common in ulcerative colitis, but it is not clear whether they are the cause of the disease or secondary to it.

Antibodies against colonic epithelium are present in the plasma in 50% of patients with ulcerative colitis. Such antibodies could damage the colon by reacting with the colonic epithelium, but equally could result from the injury to the colon.

Lymphocytes from patients with ulcerative colitis can be activated by colonic epithelium and are cytotoxic to colonic epithelium, but this too could be the result rather than the cause of the disease. There is little reason to think cell-mediated reactions are of importance in the causation of ulcerative colitis.

Some of the colonic bacteria, especially some strains of Esch. coli, have antigens that cross react with colonic epithelium. Antibodies against these antigens could attack the colonic epithelium and so cause colitis, though the presence of these antibodies does not correlate with the severity or activity of the disease.

Another possibility is that hypersensitivity to some food might cause ulcerative colitis. In a few people, milk seems to cause colitis or to exacerbate its severity. In most patients with ulcerative colitis, there is no evidence of any such sensitivity.

Whatever the part played by immunologic mechanisms in the causation of ulcerative colitis, they probably are important in the causation of some of its complications. In particular, the arthralgias and arthritis sometimes prominent in people with ulcerative colitis are like the arthralgias and arthritis found in the collagen diseases and other conditions believed to be immunologically mediated.

Another suggestion is that ulcerative colitis is caused by a Shwartzman-Sanarelli reaction. If the epithelium of the colon were sensitized, exposure to a bacterial product in the colon might initiate the inflammation.

Overproduction of lysozyme or some other damaging enzyme, perhaps by the colonic bacteria, has been proposed as a cause of ulcerative colitis. Proteolytic enzymes can be demonstrated in the stool of patients with ulcerative colitis, but they may be the result of the colitis and not its cause. Others prefer to think that the colitis results from the lack of some protective factor. Vascular, nervous, and motor disturbances have all been proposed, but not proven.

Genetic factors may be important in determining susceptibility to ulcerative colitis. In more than 5% of the patients, some other member of the family has ulcerative colitis, and in 1% of patients with ulcerative colitis some other member of the family has Crohn's disease. Genetic factors may explain the low incidence of ulcerative colitis in some races, for example, in the Maoris in New Zealand.

Pyschologic abnormalities are common in patients with ulcerative colitis. Some of the patients seem overly dependent, unable to meet ordinary demands, beset by hidden hostility. Sometimes a relapse is initiated by psychologic stress. It is not clear how psychologic abnormalities initiate the colitis, if indeed they do. Many patients with ulcerative colitis are well adjusted and have no serious psychologic problems. Ulcerative colitis is an unpleasant disease that continues from year to year and could well cause psychologic strain.

Treatment and Prognosis. During an exacerbation of ulcerative colitis with severe diarrhea, hydration and electrolyte deficiencies must be corrected and nutrition maintained, if necessary, by parenteral alimentation. Adrenocortical steroids or the adrenocorticotropic hormone reduces the severity of the inflammation. The anti-inflammatory drug sulfasalazine releases sulfapyridine and 5-aminosalicylate in the colon. Given during quiescent periods, it reduces the risk of recurrence, probably by impairing the synthesis of prostaglandins. During an attack, it reduces the severity of the inflammation.

Surgical treatment is needed if medical treatment cannot control the disease. Usually a complete colectomy is performed, leaving the patient with an ileostomy, though a variety of methods of ileoanal anastomosis are being developed. Toxic megacolon usually requires immediate colectomy. Because of the risk of carcinoma, some physicians recommend prophylactic colectomy after the disease has persisted for many years, especially when biopsies show epithelial dysplasia.

During the first attack of ulcerative colitis, medical treatment brings remission in 90% of the patients. The mortality is less than 5%. Subsequent attacks require surgical treatment in 20% of the patients. In most of the patients, medical or surgical treatment allows a good and useful life. Less than 10% of the patients die of the disease or the carcinomata that result from it.

CROHN'S DISEASE. Crohn's disease is named after an American physician who described it in 1932. Crohn called the disease terminal ileitis, because in his patients it involved the terminal ileum. Later it was realized that the condition often affected other segments of the small or large bowel, and the disease was called regional enteritis or regional enterocolitis. Granulomata are often present in the lesions and some prefer to call the disorder granulomatous enteritis or granulomatous enterocolitis.

Crohn's disease occurred before 1932. The existence of the condition has been known since 1900, though probably many of the patients were mistakenly diagnosed as intestinal tuberculosis. The earliest report is by Morgagni in 1769.

In northern Europe, the United Kingdom, North America, and Israel, 1 person in 3500 has Crohn's disease and 2 new cases are recognized each year in every 100,000 of the population. The incidence of the disease seems to be increasing, especially in the colon. It is less common in other parts of the world, though its incidence in southern Europe is increasing. In the United States, the incidence of Crohn's disease is three times greater in Jews than in other Caucasians and is three times greater in white than in black people. It is uncommon in North American Indians and in Eskimos.

Crohn's disease can arise at any age, but most patients are between 15 and 30 years old when the disease begins. Men and women are affected equally.

Lesion. Crohn's disease involves one or more clearly defined segments of the bowel, with normal bowel between the affected areas. The involved segments are usually 10 cm or more long and sharply delimited from the adjacent normal bowel.

The terminal ileum is involved in more than 80% of patients with Crohn's disease. In 10% of these patients, there are as well one or more lesions more proximally in the small bowel. Typically, the ileal disease ends sharply at the ileocecal valve, though in more than 10% of the patients the ileal lesion extends to greater or lesser degree into the cecum. Nearly 40% of people with Crohn's disease have lesions in the colon, usually in association with disease in the terminal ileum. In 20% of the patients with Crohn's disease, the colonic lesion is the dominant feature of the disease. Occasionally Crohn's disease involves the esophagus, stomach, or duodenum. Even if proctoscopy reveals no rectal lesion, a biopsy may show the inflammation and granulomata typical of Crohn's disease.

Crohn's disease involves the whole thickness of the bowel wall. Often it involves the mesentery leading to the involved segment of bowel and the lymph nodes that drain it.

In the early stages of Crohn's disease, massive edema thickens the wall of the affected segment or segments of bowel. The lumen is narrowed. Often fat from the mesentery extends beneath the serosa to surround the involved segment of bowel. The lesion feels like a hose pipe or a dead eel.

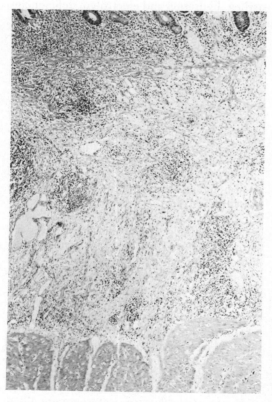

Fig. 35-7. Crohn's disease, showing the greatly thickened submucosa with edema, dilated lymphatics, and scattered clumps of lymphocytes.

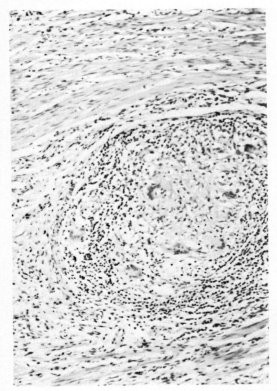

Fig. 35-8. Crohn's disease, showing a well-formed granuloma in the muscularis propria.

Microscopically, the edema thickens all layers of the bowel wall, but is most marked in the submucosa and subserosa. The distention of the tissues pulls the lymphatics widely open. Ill-defined clumps of lymphocytes and plasma cells are scattered in the submucosa and subserosa, but the cellular exudate is not great. Occasionally a germinal center is present in the exudate. Often there is hypertrophy of the muscularis mucosae. Fibrosis of the submucosa and subserosa develops only late in the disease.

Granulomata are present in the lesions in 60% of patients with Crohn's disease. They are often few and inconspicuous. A few macrophages and a few lymphocytes are loosely clumped together in the edematous submucosa or subserosa. Some of the macrophages may be multinucleated. Only occasionally are there well-formed granulomata,

with a core of epithelioid cells and a mantle of lymphocytes, like those of sarcoidosis.

Ulceration of the mucosa is almost universal in the involved segments of bowel. Early in the disease, there may be only tiny erosions, which are easily overlooked. Later, ulceration becomes extensive, with longitudinal chains of ulcers, which undermine the surrounding mucosa. Often the edematous mucosa bulges up between the ulcers, like cobblestones. Most of the ulcers remain superficial, with inflammation, perhaps acute, perhaps chronic, in their base. The mucosa between the ulcers is usually atrophic in Crohn's disease, often with hyperplasia of the mucus secreting cells. Sometimes the distorted mucosa resembles the mucous glands of the gastric antrum or the duodenum.

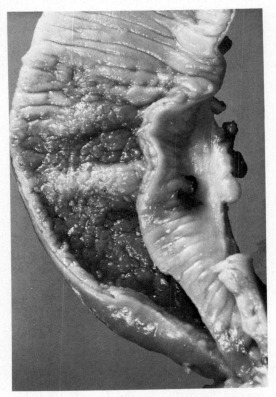

Fig. 35-9. Crohn's disease of the distal ileum, showing the sudden transition from the normal ileum above to the diseased bowel with its stiff, thickened wall and cobblestoned mucosa.

Fissures form in 50% of patients with Crohn's disease. The fissures are deep cracks extending far into the edematous bowel wall. The track of the fissure shows superficial necrosis, surrounded by acute or chronic inflammation. At times fissures extend through the bowel wall, forming the fistulae that are one of the complications of Crohn's disease.

The mesentery leading to the affected segment of bowel is usually edematous, thick, and stiff. Late in the disease it may become fibrosed.

The lymph nodes draining the lesion are often enlarged and edematous. They show chronic lymphadenitis. Granulomata like those in the bowel wall are present in the lymph nodes in 25% of the patients.

Clinical Features. The onset of Crohn's disease is usually insidious. Many of the patients seek medical advice after years of vague symptoms when abdominal pain, often crampy, often in the right lower quadrant, becomes more frequent and more severe, as the obstruction caused by the lesions slowly worsens. Diarrhea, with small, watery stools is common, partially because of excessive secretion of fluid into the dilated bowel proximal to the obstruction, partially because of the loss of absorptive surface, partially because disease in the terminal ileum prevents the absorption of bile salts, which pass into the colon and inhibit the absorption of water there. Usually blood is not evident in the stool, though severe hemorrhage can occur. Appetite declines. The patient loses weight. Sometimes there is a low fever.

From time to time, the patient gets better or worse, but Crohn's disease is not as clearly episodic as is ulcerative colitis. Ileal disease usually advances slowly. Colonic disease may worsen more quickly.

Steatorrhea develops if more than 1 m of the ileum is lost, because absorptive surface is lost, the failure to resorb bile salts depletes the bile salt pool and so interferes with micelle formation in the bowel, and bacteria that proliferate proximal to the obstruction degrade bile salts, again interfering with micelle formation in the bowel. Carbohydrate absorption is usually unaffected unless there are extensive lesions in the jejunum. Occasionally deficiency of intestinal lactase leads to lactose intolerance. Ileal disease may impair the absorption of vitamin B_{12}.

Hypoalbuminemia and hypoprothrombinemia are common as the disease grows severe, though the mechanisms involved are not clear. Iron deficiency anemia is usual, perhaps in part because of malabsorption, probably in large part because of continual, minor loss of blood from the ulcers. There may be hypocalcemia or hypokalemia and, if diarrhea is severe, hyponatremia and hypochloremia.

Complications. Obstruction is the most common complication of Crohn's disease. As the disease grows more severe, the lumen of the affected segment or segments of bowel is increasingly narrowed until it becomes less than 5 mm in diameter. Peristalsis does not occur in the thick, edematous bowel wall.

Adhesions often distort the involved segment or segments of bowel or bind the lesion to adjacent segments of uninvolved bowel. At times adhesions form a matted mass consisting of the lesion and loops of uninvolved bowel bound to it. Kinking caused by the adhesions can add to the obstruction in the lesion or cause obstruction in uninvolved segments of bowel. Adhesions sometimes bind the lesion and other loops of bowel to the abdominal wall or a viscus.

One or more fissures extend through the whole thickness of the bowel wall in 30% of the patients. An extramural abscess walled off by adhesions often results. The abscess is sometimes small and causes no symptoms, but it can cause high fever and leukocytosis. In 10% of the patients, a fissure penetrates into an adherent loop of bowel forming an internal fistula that leads from the lesion into the adherent loop of bowel. Less often a fistula extends onto the skin, usually through the scar of an operation, or into the rectum, urinary bladder, or vagina. Occasionally a fissure forms a sinus that extends beneath the psoas sheath. Because most fistulae in Crohn's disease are narrow and tortuous, there is little leakage through them.

Anal lesions occur in more than 30% of patients with Crohn's disease. More than 70% of the patients with disease in the colon have an anal lesion. Sometimes the anal lesion appears before there is any other evidence of Crohn's disease. Anal fissures are common and may be larger and more indolent than usual. Sometimes biopsy shows a granulomatous reaction like that in the lesions in the intestine. In other patients, fistula in ano develops, there is an ischiorectal abscess or a rectovaginal fistula.

Serious hemorrhage from the lesions occurs in less than 5% of patients. The bleeding usually causes melena.

Changes in the liver like those seen in ulcerative colitis are common in Crohn's disease, especially in patients with involvement of the colon. Over 70% of patients with extensive Crohn's disease show the accumulation of lymphocytes in the portal triads called pericholangitis, and sometimes there is a little fibrosis around the triads. In 10% of the patients, granulomata are present in the portal tracts. Fatty liver is found in about 40% of people with advanced Crohn's disease, but is not usually severe. Cirrhosis is uncommon.

Gallstones occur in 40% of patients with Crohn's disease in whom the function of the terminal part of the ileum is lost. The loss of this part of the bowel impairs the resorption of bile salts. The synthesis of bile salts in the liver is increased, but their concentration in the bile falls, favoring stone formation. Some think that bacterial action in the colon converts some of the unabsorbed bile salts into lithocolic acid and absorption of this acid favors the formation of gallstones.

Renal stones develop in 10% of patients with Crohn's disease. The stones may consist of uric acid, calcium oxalate, or calcium phosphate. Often the urine is acid, because of the loss of bicarbonate into the bowel, and concentrated, because of the loss of water in the diarrhea, factors favoring the precipitation of uric acid stones. Severe disease of the terminal ileum with steatorrhea allows the calcium in the bowel to be bound to unabsorbed fatty acids. Normally the oxalate in the bowel forms insoluble calcium oxalate and is excreted in the feces. If insufficient calcium is available in the bowel, the oxalate is reabsorbed in the colon and excreted by the kidneys, favoring the precipitation of oxalate stones.

About 10% of patients with Crohn's disease develop a fleeting arthritis, 1% have changes indistinguishable from rheumatoid arthritis, 5% develop ankylosing spondylitis, and nearly 20% have sacroiliitis. The majority of people with Crohn's disease who develop ankylosing spondylitis carry the histocompatibility antigen HLA-B27.

The skin may show rashes or erythema nodosum. Pyoderma gangrenosum is uncommon. Indolent ulcers or fissures that may develop near the anus or near an ileostomy or colostomy microscopically show a granulomatous reaction, like that of the lesions in the bowel.

Some 50% of people with Crohn's disease have clubbing of the fingers when the disease is active, but the clubbing often goes when the Crohn's disease becomes inactive. Uveitis occurs in 10% of the patients. Aphthae are common in the mouth.

The risk of developing carcinoma of the small bowel is increased in patients who have Crohn's disease of the small bowel for many years, and the risk of developing a carcinoma of the colon is increased in those with long-standing colonic lesions, though the increase is not great.

Etiology. The etiology of Crohn's disease is unknown. As with ulcerative colitis, theories have proliferated, from infection to pychologic abnormalities.

There is little reason to think Crohn's disease due to infection. Tuberculosis can produce ileocecal lesions like those of Crohn's disease, but neither tubercle bacilli nor any other kind of mycobacterium can be found in the lesions of Crohn's disease. Yersinia pseudotuberculosis causes acute ileitis, but not Crohn's disease. Various kinds of bacterium have been found in macrophages in the colonic lesions of Crohn's disease, but they are probably opportunists taking advantage of the Crohn's disease to invade the weakened colonic wall.

Crohn's disease is not related to sarcoidosis. The two diseases have little in common.

The edema that is so striking a feature of Crohn's disease suggests lymphatic obstruction, but there is no evidence that the lymphatics are obstructed in Crohn's disease. Lesions like those of Crohn's disease occur occasionally in patients with malignant lymphoma of the retroperitoneal lymph nodes, which might, perhaps, cause lymphatic obstruction.

Ingestion of some toxic material may cause Crohn's disease. Beryllium and zirconium cause granulomatous inflammation, but are not the cause of Crohn's disease.

Genetic factors may determine the susceptibility of the patient to Crohn's disease. In 5% of the patients, some other member of the family has Crohn's disease, and in 5%, some other member of the family has ulcerative colitis. Genetic factors may also explain some of the racial differences in the incidence of Crohn's disease.

Immunologic abnormalities are common in Crohn's disease, though as in ulcerative colitis they can well be secondary to the disease rather than its cause. Antibodies against colonic epithelium are present in the plasma in 50% of the patients and often cross react with strains of Escherichia coli. The lymphocytes of patients with the disease are cytotoxic to colonic epithelium. Some think that the inflammatory changes in Crohn's disease suggest a cell-mediated immune reaction.

Psychologic abnormalities have been reported in patients with Crohn's disease, and it has been suggested that they may share in its causation. On the other hand, after years of a long, unpleasant, and incurable disease like Crohn's disease, it is scarcely surprising that the patients come to show some mental imbalance.

Treatment and Prognosis. In patients with Crohn's disease, deficiencies caused by malabsorption or diarrhea must be corrected and nutrition maintained. Sulfasalazine and adrenocortical steroids often improve the patient's condition and ameliorate symptoms, but do not arrest the disease. In over 70% of the patients, obstruction or some other complication necessitates surgical excision of the lesion or an enteroenterostomy to bypass the obstruction. In most patients, the operation brings complete relief from the symptoms.

In over 50% of patients in whom the lesion is excised, the disease recurs, most often immediately proximal to the site of resection, but sometimes in a more distant part of the small or large bowel. Ileal lesions are more likely to recur than are colonic lesions. In

25% of the patients, the recurrence comes within three years. In 50%, the disease recurs within five years. In some, it reappears only many years later. A second operation is needed in 30% of patients with Crohn's disease. About 10% eventually die of the disease.

Other Forms of Enterocolitis

If inflammatory bowel disease and the infectious diseases of the bowel are excluded, inflammation of the small or large bowel is uncommon. Eosinophilic enteritis, inflammatory fibrous polyp, stercoral ulcer, and solitary ulcer of the rectum are discussed here.

EOSINOPHILIC ENTERITIS. Eosinophilic enteritis is a rare condition, which may occur together with eosinophilic gastritis. One or more segments of bowel are thickened and edematous, sometimes sufficiently thickened to cause obstruction. There may be malabsorption or protein-losing enteropathy if the lesion is extensive. Sometimes there is eosinophilia. Microscopically, there is edema, with an exudate containing many eosinophils.

The cause of eosinophilic enteritis is unknown. Sensitivity to onions, chocolate, parasites of herring, and other foodstuffs has been suggested.

INFLAMMATORY FIBROID POLYP. Inflammatory fibroid polyps of the small bowel are uncommon. A submucosal mass usually less than 5 cm in greatest dimension bulges into the lumen. Often the surface of the lesion is ulcerated. Microscopically, the lesion consists of granulation tissue, often with a sparse inflammatory exudate sometimes containing many eosinophils. As the lesion grows older, it becomes increasingly collagenized.

NONSPECIFIC ULCER OF THE COLON. Nonspecific ulcers of the colon are most common on the right side. Usually there is only one, but sometimes a small group of ulcers is present. The lesion is usually on the antimesenteric side of the colon and resembles a small peptic ulcer. The patient may have symptoms like those of acute appendicitis or the lesion can present less acutely. Occasionally a nonspecific ulcer of the colon perforates. The cause of the ulceration is unknown.

STERCORAL ULCER. Stercoral ulcers take their name from the Latin for dung. They usually occur in elderly or feeble patients, in the rectum or sigmoid colon, and result from the irritation of masses of hard and inspissated feces. The ulcers may bleed and are often painful. They are sometimes multiple and may perforate. Microscopically, they show acute inflammation, and overgrowth of bacteria. Ischemia, caused by the pressure of the feces, plays a large part in the pathogenesis of the ulcers.

SOLITARY ULCER OF THE RECTUM. Solitary ulcer of the rectum is most common in young adults and is usually associated with prolapse of the rectal mucosa. One or more shallow ulcers 0.5 to 5.0 cm across are present on the anterior or anterolateral wall of the rectum. The ulcers rarely extend through the muscularis mucosae. Microscopically, the lesions show fibrosis of the lamina propria of the mucosa and extension of bundles of smooth muscle from the muscularis mucosae into the lamina propria. The rectal crypts are distorted. They sometimes extend through the muscularis mucosae, forming cystic dilatations in the submucosa. Bleeding and pain are the usual symptoms. The lesions probably result from ischemia caused by the prolapse.

Appendiceal Inflammation

Any of the inflammatory diseases and infections of the colon can involve the vermiform appendix, though the involvement of the appendix is rarely severe. The threadworm Oxyuris vermicularis commonly infests the appendix. More serious injury to the appendix occurs in acute appendicitis, chronic appendicitis, and mucocele of the appendix.

ACUTE APPENDICITIS. In the Western countries, 1 person in 15 has his or her appendix removed because of acute appendicitis. In other countries, acute appendicitis is less common. In the British Army in India in 1942, the incidence of acute appendicitis was 920 per 100,000 among the British

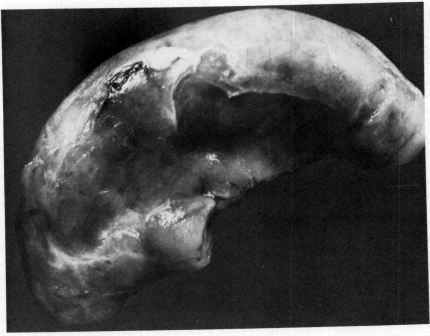

Fig. 35-10. Acute appendicitis. An appendix removed surgically showing a purulent exudate covering the appendix and mesoappendix.

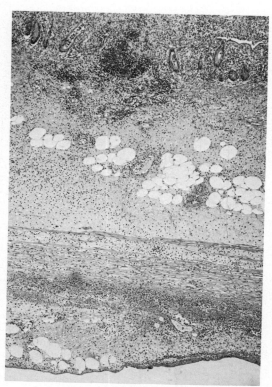

Fig. 35-11. Acute appendicitis, showing all layers of the appendicular wall greatly thickened by edema, from the mucosa at the top to the serosa at the bottom. The cellular exudate is of neutrophils. A little fibrin overlies the serosa.

troops, but only 120 per 100,000 among the Indian soldiers.

Perhaps because of the introduction of antibiotics, the incidence of acute appendicitis in the United States and Europe fell from 1940 to 1955, but has now become constant. In 1941, about 10% of operations in one group of American hospitals were for acute appendicitis. By 1956, the proportion had fallen to 2%.

Appendicitis can develop at any age, but most patients are between 15 and 30 years old. Until the age of 25 years, boys and men are affected rather more commonly than girls and women.

Lesions. Macroscopically, acute appendicitis causes little change in the appearance of the appendix if the organ is removed soon after the onset of symptoms. If the inflammation is more severe, part or all of the appendix is swollen, and its serosa is congest-

ed. If the organ is transected, its lumen is dilated and filled with thin pus. The wall is thickened. As the disease grows more severe, the lumen grows larger and the pus thicker. The appendicular wall becomes increasingly thickened and congested. Often the serosa is covered by a fibrinopurulent exudate. Particularly in the distal part of the appendix, soft, black, or dark green patches of gangrene often appear. In the gangrenous regions the wall is thin, friable, and easily perforated.

In the early stages of acute appendicitis, the mucosa shows microscopically only a small focus of ulceration and acute inflammation. Neutrophils are moderately numerous in the lumen. As the disease worsens, the inflammation becomes more extensive. Edema and a massive exudate of neutrophils thicken the wall of the appendix. Ulceration of the mucosa is often extensive. The lumen is filled with pus. If the disease is severe, thrombosis of vessels in the appendicular wall is prominent and causes ischemic necrosis that becomes the patches of gangrene.

Clinical Presentation. Acute appendicitis usually begins with ill-defined referred pain in the umbilical or epigastric region. Nausea or vomiting develop in over 50% of the patients. After four to six hours, the pain usually moves to the right iliac fossa, becomes more severe, and is aggravated by movement or coughing. The right iliac fossa becomes tender. Guarding is common in the overlying muscles. Pressure on the left colon or flexion of the right hip often increases the pain. Some patients have a fever of up to 38°C. A leukocytosis of 10 to 15 × 10⁹/L (10,000 to 15,000/mm³) is usual.

Especially in young children and the elderly, the disease commonly causes few symptoms and may pass unrecognized until a periappendiceal abscess or some other complication draws attention to it. Occasionally an inflamed appendix is retrocecal or hangs into the pelvic cavity and fails to cause symptoms in the right iliac fossa. Tenderness may be detectable only by rectal or vaginal examination.

Complications. A periappendiceal abscess is the commonest complication of acute appendicitis, especially in children and the elderly. If symptoms persist for more than 24 hours in a young child, 60% of the patients have a periappendiceal abscess. If they persist for more than three days, almost all young children have an abscess. About 30% of elderly people who develop acute appendicitis have a periappendiceal abscess by the time the diagnosis is made.

The abscess sometimes follows perforation of the appendix, often through a patch of gangrene, but can develop around an acutely inflamed appendix that has not perforated. Usually the abscess is walled off by adhesions and confined to the right iliac fossa. Rupture of the appendix often brings temporary relief of symptoms, but the signs of infection soon worsen. Often a mass is palpable in the iliac fossa. Occasionally a periappendiceal abscess ruptures into an adjacent loop of bowel, the urinary bladder, or onto the skin.

Less often, acute appendicitis causes a pelvic abscess, usually when the appendix hangs down into the pelvis. Especially in old people, the infection sometimes spreads up the left paracolic gutter to cause a subdiaphragmatic or subhepatic abscess. Generalized peritonitis is uncommon, but can occur in young children and old people.

Rarely, acute appendicitis is complicated by pylephlebitis, a term derived from the Greek for gate or portal and vien. Infected emboli are carried from the appendix to the liver in the portal veins, causing an abscess or abscesses in the liver.

Pathogenesis. In the majority of patients, acute appendicitis is caused by obstruction. Most often, a fecalith lodges in the proximal part of the appendix and obstructs the lumen. How often this is the case is unknown, for the fecalith is often dislodged or destroyed when the appendix is removed surgically. Less often, the obstruction is caused by the stone of a fruit, a parasite, or some other foreign body lodged in the appendix or by a carcinoma of the cecum or proximal part of the appendix. In children, the lymphoid tissue in the appendix is abundant, and lymphoid hyperplasia may cause obstruction. Kinking of the appendix and spasm of the appendiceal muscle can cause obstruction.

The obstruction prevents the drainage of mucus from the appendix. The pressure in the lumen of the appendix rises to as much as 60 mm of water. Compression of the blood vessels in the mucosa causes ischemia. Small

ulcers develop in the mucosa, with acute inflammation at the base of the ulcers. The bacteria in the lumen of the appendix invade its wall and increase the inflammation.

The initial periumbilical or epigastric pain in acute appendicitis is caused by the distention of the organ or by increased peristalsis in the appendicular muscle. The movement of the pain to the iliac fossa and the other signs that develop at that time are caused by irritation of the parietal peritoneum by the exudate on the serosa of the appendix.

In the minority of patients who do not have obstruction, the cause of acute appendicitis is unknown. A small ulcer in the appendicular mucosa, perhaps caused by a viral infection, could allow the bacteria in the lumen entry to the appendicular wall to augment the inflammation. Small ulcers of this sort are present in 35% of apparently normal appendices removed during an operation for some other disease. In most people they heal. In a few, they may initiate acute appendicitis.

Treatment and Prognosis. Acute appendicitis is treated by appendectomy. If the organ has not ruptured, most patients recover completely within a few days. If the appendix has ruptured, the abscess must be drained. The overall mortality rises to 2%. The very young and the elderly are especially at risk. Many of the patients develop further complications, such as a wound abscess, fistula, or years later suffer intestinal obstruction caused by the adhesions resulting from the appendicitis. Because of the danger of delay, it is wiser to remove a normal appendix when the diagnosis is in doubt than to wait until a complication makes the diagnosis certain. In most hospitals over 20% of appendices removed because acute appendicitis was suspected are normal.

CHRONIC APPENDICITIS. Chronic appendicitis probably does not exist. In the past, it was thought that chronic inflammation of the appendix caused a variety of vague abdominal symptoms. Appendectomy often relieved the symptoms for a few weeks, but then they recurred. There is little reason to think that the appendix had anything to do with the patient's troubles.

In older people, the lumen of the appendix is often partially obliterated by fibrosis, which begins at the tip and gradually extends proximally. Nerves are usually prominent in the fibrosis, so that some call the condition neuroappendicopathy. A few lymphocytes and plasma cells are usually scattered in the fibrosis. The condition causes no symptoms and no dysfunction.

MUCOCELE. In a mucocele of the appendix, the wall of the appendix is thin and its lumen is distended by clear mucus. Usually the appendix is 5 or 10 cm long and 2 or 3 cm in diameter, but it can be much larger. A mucocele is found in 1 appendectomy in 500. Occasionally the patient has periumbilical pain caused by the distention of the appendix, but often there are no symptoms. Two kinds of mucocele are distinguished, a simple mucocele and a neoplastic mucocele.

A simple mucocele of the appendix develops when obstruction fails to cause acute appendicitis. The appendix becomes distended by the mucus secreted by its epithelium. Microscopically, the distended appendix is lined by a flat epithelium of cuboidal and mucus-secreting cells without atypicality.

In a neoplastic mucocele much or all of the appendix is lined by neoplastic epithelium. Usually the tumor forms fronds like those of a villous adenoma of the colon. The epithelium covering the fronds consists in part of closely packed, atypical cells like those of a villous adenoma, in part of mucus-secreting cells. Less often, the distention of the appendix flattens the mucosa, so that the epithelium forms a single layer with many mucus-secreting cells, a form of neoplastic mucocele hard to distinguish from a simple mucocele. Sometimes a neoplastic mucocele is called an adenoma or cystadenoma of the appendix.

Either type of mucocele can rupture, giving rise to a mucinous, periappendiceal abscess walled off by adhesions. Occasionally a mucocele becomes infected, or the wall of a mucocele is calcified.

Pseudomyxoma Peritonei. Rarely, rupture of a mucocele of the appendix or gallbladder gives rise to pseudomyxoma peritonei. More often pseudomyxoma is caused by rupture of a mucinous cystadenoma or cystadenocarcinoma of an ovary.

In pseudomyxoma peritonei, islands of mucus-secreting epithelium are disseminated throughout the peritoneal cavity. The abdomen becomes distended with mucus. Often adhesions between loops of bowel cause intestinal obstruction.

Most consider that only a neoplastic mucocele of the appendix gives rise to pseudomyxoma peritonei and that the islands of mucus-secreting epithelium in the serosa are metastases from the ruptured appendix. It used to be thought that benign epithelium from the appendix might implant on the serosa or that the escape of mucus from the appendix might excite mucinous metaplasia in the peritoneum.

Anal Inflammation

Three kinds of inflammatory lesion occur in the anal region: anal fissure, fistula in ano, and perianal abscesses. Patients with ulcerative colitis or Crohn's disease are particularly likely to develop anal lesions of this sort, though only a small proportion of people with anal inflammation have inflammatory bowel disease.

ANAL FISSURE. Anal fissures are common. An elongated, superficial ulcer that looks macroscopically like a crack or fissure develops in the anal mucosa overlying the internal anal sphincter, nearly always in the midline posteriorly. Often a small projection of mucosa called a sentinel tag marks the lower end of the fissure. Microscopically, the lesion shows chronic inflammation.

An anal fissure causes pain on defecation. If the stool is kept soft, it usually heals, but tends to recur if the patient becomes constipated. If the fissure persists, it causes fibrosis and spasm, narrowing the anal canal. At times, surgical correction is needed.

FISTULA IN ANO. Fistulae in ano are common. The fistula is caused by infection in one of the glands that arise from the anal mucosa in the region of the dentate line and lie between the internal and external anal sphincters. An abscess destroys the gland and burrows through the tissues to form a fistula that leads from the dentate line to the skin or less often the rectum. The opening of the fistula near the dentate line is usually small, consisting only of the duct of the gland.

In 70% of the patients, the fistula tracks between the internal and external anal sphincters to reach the skin close to the anus. Less often, it penetrates the external sphincter and crosses the ischiorectal fossa on its way to the skin or tracks upwards, penetrates the levator ani, and crosses the ischiorectal fossa to reach the skin. Rarely a fistula in ano passes between the internal and external sphincters to open into the rectum or opens both into the rectum and the skin. Occasionally a fistula in ano extends subcutaneously from the dentate line to the skin or beneath the rectal mucosa to open in the rectum. Rarely, a fistula arises high in the rectum and passes through the levator ani and the ischiorectal fossa to reach the skin.

Microscopically, the tract of a fistula in ano shows a mixture of acute and chronic inflammation, with more or less fibrosis. Often, foreign body granulomata are present. Lipophages are sometimes prominent.

A fistula is treated by opening the track widely and allowing it to granulate. Care must be taken to avoid damaging the sphincter.

ABSCESS.   Infection of an anal gland does not always result in a fistula in ano. The abscess may remain localized in the intersphincteric region. More often, it tracks in one direction or another, much as in a fistula in ano, without reaching the skin or rectum. It may extend to give a perianal abscess beneath the skin beside the anus. It may extend through the external sphincter to give an ischirectal abscess or upward to give an abscess beside the rectum.

Wherever the abscess, the patient is likely to develop the fever and malaise usual with abscesses. Often the lesion is painful. Drainage cures.

DIVERTICULA

Diverticula can occur anywhere in the small and large bowel, but are most often detected and most often of clinical significance in the sigmoid colon.

Small Bowel

Three kinds of diverticula occur in the small bowel. The diverticula of the duodenum caused by peptic ulceration are described in Chapter 34. Persistence of part of the vitelline canal gives a Meckel's diverticulum. Wide-mouthed diverticula bulge from the proximal part of the small bowel.

MECKEL'S DIVERTICULUM.   A Meckel's diverticulum, named after a German anatomist (1781–1833), is present in 1 to 3% of people. It is a remnant of the vitelline canal. The diverticulum arises from the antimesenteric border of the ileum, 30 to 90 cm from the ileocecal valve. Usually it is 2 to 8 cm long and looks like the appendix. It usually has a rounded end, which hangs free in the peritoneal cavity, but may be connected to the umbilicus or to a loop of gut by a fibrous cord, representing the remainder of the vitelline canal. Meckel's diverticula are lined for the most part by ileal mucosa. Islands of gastric mucosa are present in 50% of them. Pancreatic rests are present in 10%.

Less than 20% of Meckel's diverticula cause symptoms. Occasionally the gastric mucosa present in some Meckel's diverticula causes peptic ulceration in the diverticulum or adjacent to it, sometimes with hemorrhage or perforation. Occasionally acute diverticulitis develops, with lesions, symptoms, and complications like those of acute appendictis. In children, a Meckel's diverticulum sometimes causes intussusception. Rarely, a volvulus rotates around the fibrous band joining a Meckel's diverticulum to the umbilicus, or the band obstructs a loop of bowel. A stone can form in the diverticulum and escape to obstruct the ileum. A diverticulum can project into a hernial sac. A carcinoid or some other tumor can arise in a Meckel's diverticulum.

Rarely, the whole length of the vitelline canal remains patent, forming a vitellointestinal fistula from the ileum to the umbilicus. Rarely, an isolated segment of the vitelline canal persists to form a cyst somewhere in the length of a fibrous band reaching from a Meckel's diverticulum or from the ileum to the umbilicus.

WIDE-MOUTHED DIVERTICULA.   Widemouthed diverticula of the small bowel can be demonstrated radiologically in 1 to 3% of people. If the small bowel is inflated, diverticula are demonstrable in 10 to 20% of people. The majority of the diverticula are in the duodenum, mostly in the concavity of its second, third, or fourth part. A few occur in

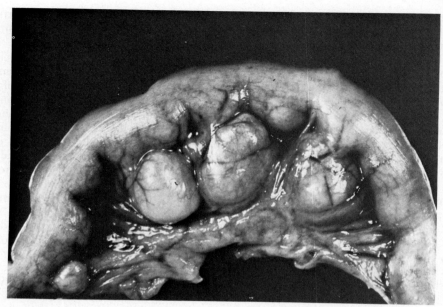

Fig. 35-12. Diverticula of the jejunum, showing the wide-mouthed lesions bulging from the mesenteric side of the bowel.

the jejunum, and very few in the ileum. Most of the diverticula of the small bowel are found in people over 50 years old.

Wide-mouthed diverticula of the small bowel are usually 1 to 3 cm in diameter, though some are larger. They are spheroidal, with a wide mouth. There may be only one or five or more. The whole thickness of the bowel wall bulges out at an area of weakness to form the diverticulum, often at the site of entry of a blood vessel. If the pressure in the lumen increases, the diverticulum bulges out. If pressure in the lumen is reduced, it disappears.

Most wide-mouthed diverticula of the small bowel cause no symptoms. Occasionally, one causes pain, becomes inflamed, or causes malabsorption as in the blind loop syndrome.

Colon

The term *diverticulosis of the colon* means that diverticula are present in the colon. If one or more of the diverticula are inflamed, the lesion is called diverticulitis. The term *diverticular disease* includes both diverticulosis and diverticulitis.

DIVERTICULOSIS. In northern Europe, North America, and Australasia, diverticula of the colon are unusual in people under 40 years old. They are found in 10% of people between 40 and 60 years old and in 30% of people over 60 years old. Diverticulosis of the colon is less common in southern Europe and South America and is still less common in Asia and Africa. In the United States, it is more common in white than in black people.

Lesions. Though any part of the colon or all of it can be involved, colonic diverticula are confined to the sigmoid and descending colon in 90% of the patients.

Colonic diverticula usually project 1 to 2 cm beyond the wall of the colon between the mesenteric and antimesenteric tenia coli. Only in old people with severe diverticulosis do small diverticula sometimes appear between the antimesenteric teniae. Often the diverticula project into an appendix epiploica or into pericolic fat and are not visible from the outer surface of the colon. When a diverticulum is visible, it is often blue because of the fecal matter it contains.

Most colonic diverticula are flask-shaped, with a narrow neck where the diverticulum passes through the muscle of the colonic wall

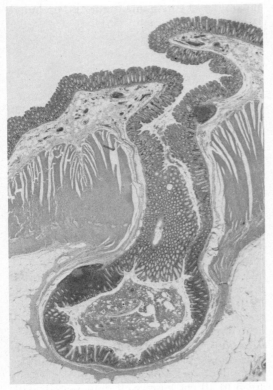

Fig. 35-13. A diverticulum of the sigmoid colon, showing the narrow neck of the diverticulum passing through the muscularis propria and a little fecal material in the lumen of the diverticulum.

and a bulbous body. Microscopically, the diverticula are lined by colonic mucosa. A thin layer of muscle sometimes surrounds a diverticulum, but often its wall consists only of a little collagenous tissue and a few scattered smooth muscle fibers.

In most patients with diverticulosis, the colon is shortened in the region involved. Its circular muscle forms interdigitating, semicircular ridges that bulge into the lumen between the mesenteric and antimesenteric teniae. The teniae are thick. The quantity of elastica in the ridges and teniae is increased. Between the ridges of muscle, the wall of the colon is thin and bulges outward. The diverticula arise from the apex of the thinned zones, often beside an artery that penetrates the muscularis propria. The small orifices of the diverticula are hard to see from within the bowel and are often obscured by the folds

of redundant mucosa that result from the shortening of the colon.

Clinical Presentation. Diverticulosis of the colon causes no symptoms and no dysfunction unless a complication develops. It is sometimes associated with irritable bowel or some other disorder that causes spasm of the colonic mucosa, but the spasm is more likely to be the cause of the diverticulosis than to be caused by it.

Complications. Diverticulitis is the principal complication of diverticulosis. It is discussed in the next section of this chapter.

Sometimes massive hemorrhage occurs from an uninflamed diverticulum, usually on the right side of the colon. Probably a fecalith or a foreign body lodges in the mouth of the diverticulum and erodes the artery often present close to the neck of the diverticulum. In elderly people, hemorrhage from a diverticulum is one of the commoner causes of blood in the stool. If the bleeding does not subside, angiography can often determine the site of the bleeding and allow resection of the diverticulum.

Pathogenesis. Diverticula of the colon develop during adult life when pressure in the colon forces a pouch of mucosa out through a weakness in the colonic wall. Contraction of the ridges of circular muscle often present in patients with diverticulosis could close off segments of the colon and increase the pressure in the closed segments, forcing out a diverticulum from the weakened region between the ridges. The lack of bulk and fiber in the diet in the developed countries may explain why diverticulosis is more common in these countries than in regions in which the fiber content of the diet is high.

Treatment and Prognosis. About 20% of patients with extensive diverticulosis develop diverticulitis or bleed from one of the diverticula. The other patients require no treatment.

DIVERTICULITIS. Inflammation of one or more diverticula is called diverticulitis. In the colon, diverticulitis involves the sigmoid or descending colon in 80% of the patients. It is more common in men than in women. Most of the patients are over 50 years old.

Lesions. Acute diverticulitis causes acute inflammation with congestion, edema, and a neutrophilic exudate in the tissue around the body of the diverticulum involved. If it subsides, little residual injury remains.

Many of the patients have repeated attacks of acute inflammation. The lesion grows larger and shows a mixture of acute and chronic inflammation, sometimes with fibrosis. If the diverticulum ruptures, foreign body granulomata often form around fecal material released into the tissues. Often an abscess develops in the fatty tissue around the diverticulum. Often the inflammation extends to involve several adjacent diverticula.

If diverticulitis of the colon becomes chronic, a mass forms around the colon. The mass often extends for 3 to 5 cm along the length of the colon and completely or largely surrounds it. The mass consists in part of chronically inflamed fibrosis containing one or more abscesses, in part of the thickened wall of the bowel with its ridges of circular muscle.

Macroscopically and clinically, chronic diverticulitis frequently resembles a carcinoma of the colon. Sometimes the nature of the mass can be established only by excision.

Clinical Presentation. Acute diverticulitis usually presents with pain in the lower abdomen on the side involved, sometimes with tenderness, guarding, and other signs of irritation of the parietal peritoneum. Often the patient is feverish, with a leukocytosis. Minor bleeding is evident in the stool in 25% of the patients.

Complications. Obstruction develops in 25% of patients with diverticulitis of the left side of the colon. In 20% of the patients, a large pericolic abscess is found. Occasionally an abscess ruptures into the peritoneal cavity and causes peritonitis; forms a fistula into the urinary bladder, vagina, or some other part of the bowel; or ruptures onto the skin. Major hemorrhage is unusual.

Pathogenesis. Diverticulitis is usually caused by obstruction at the neck of a diverticulum, most often by a fecalith. The pressure in the diverticulum rises as in acute appendicitis, damaging the wall of the diverticulum and allowing the bacteria in the lumen to establish infection.

Treatment and Prognosis. Mild colonic diverticulitis usually subsides if the stool is kept soft and a wide spectrum antibiotic is administered. If the lesion persists, or if the

possibility of carcinoma cannot be excluded, surgical resection is needed.

VASCULAR DISORDERS

Two kinds of ischemic disease are common in the intestine, ischemic enterocolitis and gangrene. The abnormality of the blood vessels called angiodysplasia sometimes causes major hemorrhage. Abdominal angina causes pain in the abdomen. Hemangiomata and lymphangiomata can arise in the bowel. Ischemic enterocolitis, gangrene, abdominal angina, angiodysplasia, and hemorrhoids are considered in this section. Hemangiomata and lymphangiomata are discussed with the tumors of the intestine.

ISCHEMIC ENTEROCOLITIS. Ischemic enterocolitis is common. Probably minor lesions often pass unrecognized. More serious lesions are frequent in patients who are seriously ill or in shock.

Lesions. Ischemic enterocolitis usually causes one or more segmental lesions in the jejunoileum or colon. Most often the lesions are 5 to 10 cm long, well demarcated, with normal bowel between them. They are most common in the left side of the colon. Less often the disease is widespread, involving much of the colon and sometimes the small bowel as well.

Macroscopically the mucosa of the affected segment of bowel is dark, purple, and congested. There may be no ulceration, a few shallow ulcers, or extensive ulceration reaching to the submucosa. The muscularis propria and serosa are unaffected.

Microscopically, the superficial part of the lamina propria of the mucosa is necrotic. Sometimes the basal part of the lamina propria is spared; sometimes it too is necrotic. Hemorrhage into the necrotic mucosa is often striking. The muscularis mucosae is spared. The submucosa is congested and edematous, often with a mild exudate of neutrophils beneath the necrotic lamina propria. The blood vessels and lymphatics in the submucosa are widely dilated. Platelet thrombi are sometimes evident in the blood vessels. Only rarely does necrosis extend into the submucosa or more deeply. The muscularis propria and the serosa are rarely affected.

In a minority of patients, the lesions are covered by a membrane, usually white but sometimes green or yellow. The membrane is firmly attached to the mucosa, which bleeds if the membrane is pulled off. Microscopically, the membrane is composed of fibrin, mixed with mucus and necrotic cells.

Clinical Presentation. If ischemic enterocolitis is mild, it causes no symptoms. If it is more severe, pain and diarrhea are common. Sometimes there is blood or mucus in the stools.

Complications. Complications of ischemic enterocolitis are uncommon. Rarely, the lesion extends deeply enough into the bowel wall to cause peritonitis in the serosa overlying the lesion or perforates. Rarely, healing of a lesion that has damaged the submucosa or the muscularis propria causes a fibrous stricture.

Pathogenesis. Ischemic enterocolitis develops when reduction in the perfusion of the affected segments of the bowel reduces the oxygen tension in the tissues enough to cause necrosis in the mucosa but not sufficiently to damage the submucosa or muscle. Its most common cause is hypotension. Ischemic enterocolitis is common in patients in shock and other conditions that reduce the blood flow to the bowel. Sometimes atherosclerotic narrowing in the artery supplying the part of the bowel involved augments the effect of the hypotension and determines the site of the lesion. Less often the ischemia is caused by vasculitis, the obstruction of blood vessels that occurs in sickle cell disease, intravascular coagulation, or by partial obstruction of the arterial or venous vessels supplying the bowel. Occasionally ischemic enterocolitis develops in a loop of bowel caught in a hernia or twisted by volvulus.

Treatment and Prognosis. Ischemic enterocolitis can be treated only by relieving the condition causing the hypoxia. If this is possible, the mucosa of the affected parts of the intestine regenerates, usually leaving no residual dysfunction.

GANGRENE. Ischemic necrosis of the whole thickness of the wall of the intestine is called gangrene. Lesions intermediate between the full thickness necrosis of gangrene

and the mucosal necrosis or ischemic enterocolitis are unusual.

Lesions. Intestinal gangrene is most common in the small bowel, but can occur in the colon. Occasionally the gangrenous region is only 1 or 2 cm across and does not extend completely around the bowel. More often, it extends round the whole circumference of the bowel and involves a segment of the bowel 1 to 5 cm long. Sometimes almost the whole of the small bowel becomes gangrenous.

The affected segment of bowel is at first dilated and dusky. At this stage, much of the mucosa is necrotic, but the muscularis propria and deeper layers of the bowel wall are still viable. If the ischemia persists longer, the full thickness of the bowel wall becomes necrotic. The affected part of the bowel is

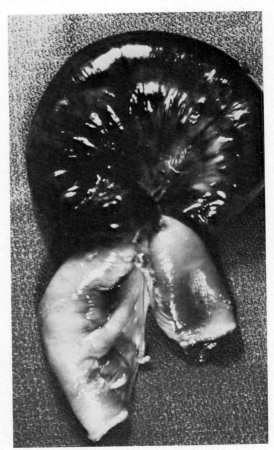

Fig. 35-14.   Gangrene of a loop of strangulated bowel.

dark purple or black. Peristaltic movements stop. The surface of the bowel becomes dull as fibrin is deposited on the serosa.

Clinical Presentation. Pain is usually severe. Its character depends on the site and extent of the gangrene. Often the pain is at first colicky, but later becomes constant. Obstruction is common, with nausea and vomiting. If the gangrene is extensive, abdominal distention is usual and shock is likely.

Complications. Perforation and peritonitis are the principal complications of intestinal gangrene. Both are almost inevitable if a gangrenous segment of bowel remains free in the peritoneal cavity or if a gangrenous segment of bowel that has been incarcerated in a hernia escapes into the peritoneal cavity. Peritonitis can develop without perforation as intestinal bacteria penetrate the necrotic wall of the bowel.

Pathogenesis. Gangrene of the intestine results from complete or almost complete occlusion of the arteries or veins supplying the part involved. The compression of the vessels in a hernia is a common cause of limited gangrene. Volvulus of a loop of bowel sometimes causes gangrene. Occasionally the celiac axis is constricted by the median arcuate ligament of the diaphragm. Lodgement of an embolus in the superior mesenteric artery causes gangrene of the greater part of the small bowel. Rarely, vasculitis causes gangrene of the bowel.

Atherosclerosis of the mesenteric arteries rarely causes intestinal gangrene. The inferior mesenteric artery is commonly occluded by atherosclerosis in elderly people, and the nutrition of the colon is maintained by collateral vessels. Atherosclerosis in the superior mesenteric artery is usually confined to the first 1 to 2 cm of the vessel. Only if sudden thrombosis develops in this part of the artery is gangrene likely.

Treatment and Prognosis. Once gangrene of the bowel is established, the affected intestine must be removed without delay. If the greater part of the small bowel is involved, parenteral nutrition may be needed for the remainder of the patient's life.

ABDOMINAL ANGINA. Abdominal angina is a rare syndrome caused by ischemia in the bowel. Half an hour or so after eating, the patient develops abdominal pain, which persists for an hour or more until the demand for blood in the bowel lessens. Usually abdominal angina results from severe atherosclerosis of the mesenteric arteries. It may be the precursor of more serious ischemic bowel disease.

ANGIODYSPLASIA. Angiodysplasia is the name given to foci of vascular ectasia that develop in the cecum and ascending colon in people over 60 years old and rarely in younger people. Some prefer to call the condition angioectasia, phlebectasia, or an arteriovenous malformation.

Macroscopically, it is difficult or impossible to find the lesions in a resected colon unless the blood vessels are distended by colored material. The lesions are 0.1 to 1.0 cm across and consist only of a tangle of dilated blood vessels. One or more angiodysplastic lesions can be demonstrated in the right

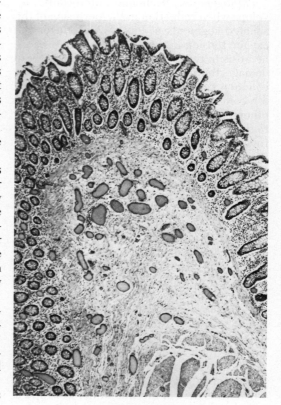

Fig. 35-15. Angiodysplasia of the colon, showing tortuous and dilated veins in the submucosa.

colon in 25% of people over 60 years old. Sometimes there are as many as 50 of them.

Microscopically, early lesions show only mild dilatation and tortuosity of the veins in the submucosa and perhaps slight ectasia of the arteries. In older lesions, the submucosal veins become increasingly dilated and tortuous, and their walls become thin. Thin-walled branches of the dilated veins extend into the mucosa and interconnect to form a mesh of ectatic capillaries. The epithelium overlying the lesions atrophies, so that only a thin layer of endothelium separates the blood in the mucosal capillaries from the lumen of the colon. The arteries in the lesion are slightly ectatic. Rarely, an arteriovenous shunt can be demonstrated.

Angiodysplastic lesions are responsible for 25% of serious hemorrhage into the colon in people over 60 years old. In some patients, the bleeding is massive.

The cause of angiodysplasia is unknown. Possibly the lesions are caused by aging or by the repeated obstruction of the submucosal veins caused by contraction of the muscle of the cecum and ascending colon.

Angiography or colonoscopy performed while the lesion is bleeding can often identify the site of hemorrhage. Endoscopic cauterization can usually control the hemorrhage. If the site of bleeding cannot be identified, colectomy is required.

HEMORRHOIDS. Internal hemorrhoids, or piles, are vascular lesions that occur in the lower rectum or upper part of the anal canal. External hemorrhoids are tags that surround the anus. Both internal and external hemorrhoids are common. Many people have both.

Internal Hemorrhoids. Internal hemorrhoids arise from the cushions of highly vascular tissue present in the lower rectum or anus at 3, 7, and 11 o'clock, looking at the anus from below with 12 o'clock anterior. The cushions are part of the inferior hemorrhoidal venous plexus, but have a rich arterial supply and in some ways resemble erectile tissue.

Lesions. Internal hemorrhoids form soft masses that bulge into the rectum and occasionally prolapse through the anus. Microscopically, they consist of a mesh of large veins usually with thick, muscular walls. If a hemorrhoid prolapses, squamous metaplasia sometimes replaces the rectal mucosa that usually covers an internal hemorrhoid.

Complications. Flecks of red arterial blood in the stool are often the first sign that a patient has internal hemorrhoids. Occasionally the bleeding persists long enough and is severe enough to cause anemia.

In some patients, the hemorrhoids prolapse during defecation, but return spontaneously or are easily replaced. In some, coughing, muscular effort, or anything else that raises intraabdominal pressure causes the hemorrhoids to prolapse. In some, prolapse is permanent. The exposed hemorrhoids cause discomfort and itching. Mucus from the prolapsed rectal mucosa stains the clothes.

Occasionally, the veins in a prolapsed hemorrhoid thrombose. The hemorrhoid becomes dark red, swollen, and painful. It may become necrotic and slough off.

Pathogenesis. Internal hemorrhoids develop in conditions in which the intraabdominal pressure is increased, such as constipation, pregnancy, diarrhea, prostatism, or hard muscular work. Portal hypertension increases the risk of developing internal hemorrhoids. The venous obstruction caused by a carcinoma of the rectum makes internal hemorrhoids more likely.

Treatment and Prognosis. Most internal hemorrhoids can be managed conservatively. If complications develop, injection of a sclerosing solution into the hemorrhoid or surgical excision is needed. If a sclerosing solution is used, the vessels are obliterated by a granulomatous reaction caused by the sclerosing solution. The lesion that remains is called an oleogranuloma.

External Hemorrhoids. Ectasia of the external hemorrhoidal veins causes external hemorrhoids. The dilated veins bulge into tags covered by the stratified squamous epithelium that surround the anus. The lesions are often itchy or uncomfortable. Occasionally the veins in an external hemorrhoid thrombose.

MECHANICAL DISORDERS

Abdominal hernias, volvulus, intussusception, and meconium ileus cause symptoms principally by obstructing the flow of the intestinal content, by obstructing the blood supply to the bowel, or both.

ABDOMINAL HERNIA. An abdominal hernia is the protrusion of a loop of bowel, part of the omentum, or part of some other viscus into an abnormal outpouching from the peritoneal cavity or through a narrow opening within the peritoneal cavity. If the hiatus hernias considered in Chapter 33 are excluded, 1 person in 70 in the United States has an abdominal hernia.

Lesions. The different kinds of abdominal hernia are classified according to the site of the lesion. In most, a hernial sac bulges from the peritoneal cavity through an area of weakness in the peritoneal wall. The sac is lined by mesothelium and has a collagenous wall.

Indirect Inguinal Hernia. More than 50% of abdominal hernias are of the indirect inguinal type. The sac projects through the inguinal ring along the path of the processus vaginalis. In children, the sac is sometimes formed by a processus vaginalis that fails to close. In adults, it is usually a new protrusion along the path of the processus. The neck of the sac is narrow, but its distal part can be large.

Direct Inguinal Hernia. About 25% of abdominal hernias are of the direct inguinal type. The hernia bulges through the transversalis fascia into the floor of the inguinal canal. Its neck is usually large.

Femoral Hernia. Some 6% of abdominal hernias are of the femoral type. The sac extends beneath the inguinal ligament along the femoral vein. The neck of the hernia is small. Over 80% of the patients are women.

Umbilical Hernia. An umbilical hernia is present in 10% of newborn white infants and 50% of black infants. It bulges through the umbilicus and has a wide neck. The hernia usually heals spontaneously within two years. In adults, umbilical hernias are uncommon and have a narrow neck.

Ventral Hernia. A ventral hernia bulges through the scar of an abdominal incision. Ventral hernias are particularly common in the obese. The hernia has a wide neck, but omentum or bowel often becomes attached to the inflamed serosa in the hernial sac.

Epigastric Hernia. Small hernial sacs are present in the midline of the anterior abdominal wall in 5% of people. They are most common in the epigastric region. The sac is too small to permit herniation of more than a small tag of omentum.

Other External Hernias. Occasionally an obturator hernia protrudes into the obturator canal, a sciatic hernia extends through the sciatic foramen, or a perineal hernia bulges through the pelvic floor.

Internal Hernia. Internal hernias are uncommon. A hernial sac sometimes bulges through an area of weakness in the posterior wall of the peritoneal cavity, usually in the vicinity of the duodenum. Occasionally a loop of bowel or a piece of omentum passes through an opening made by an adhesion or through a hole in the omentum.

Sliding Hernia. In most hernial sacs, the sac consists only of serosa and the collagenous tissue that supports it. In a sliding hernia, part of the cecum or colon slides through the opening in the wall of the peritoneal cavity and forms part of the wall of the sac. The hernia is usually of the indirect inguinal type.

Diaphragmatic Hernia. Diaphragmatic hernias have no sac. The abdominal organs pass through a hole in the diaphragm into the thoracic cavity. Often the hole in the diaphragm is large, allowing much of the abdominal content to herniate into one of the pleural cavities. The hernia may be congenital or acquired.

In a congenital diaphragmatic hernia, the hole in the diaphragm is usually on the left, posterolaterally. Stomach, intestine, and spleen easily herniate through the defect. Less often the defect is posterolaterally on the right, allowing the liver and intestines to herniate. Occasionally the hole is beneath the sternum, and liver and gut are likely to herniate.

Acquired diaphragmatic hernias are caused by trauma, either injury to the diaphragm itself, or secondary to greatly increased abdominal pressure. The tear is nearly always on the left and is often large.

Clinical Presentation. An abdominal hernia causes no symptoms and no dysfunction unless some complication develops. If the neck of the hernial sac is large, a loop of bowel or portion of the omentum can easily enter the hernial sac and return to the abdominal cavity without injury.

Complications. Incarceration is the most

common complication of an abdominal hernia. A loop of bowel, portion of omentum, or less often some other abdominal organ is trapped in a hernial sac and cannot return to the general abdominal cavity. Usually incarceration occurs because the neck of the hernial sac is small. Because of the pressure of the neck of the sac, the viscus in the hernial sac become edematous and swollen, too big to escape back into the peritoneal cavity. Incarceration may cause no symptoms, but when a loop of bowel is incarcerated the pressure at the neck of the hernial sac and sometimes twisting or angulation within the sac often cause obstruction.

Strangulation occurs when the blood supply to the herniated viscus, usually small bowel or omentum, is reduced, causing ischemia in the herniated tissue. If a loop of bowel is strangulated, obstruction is almost

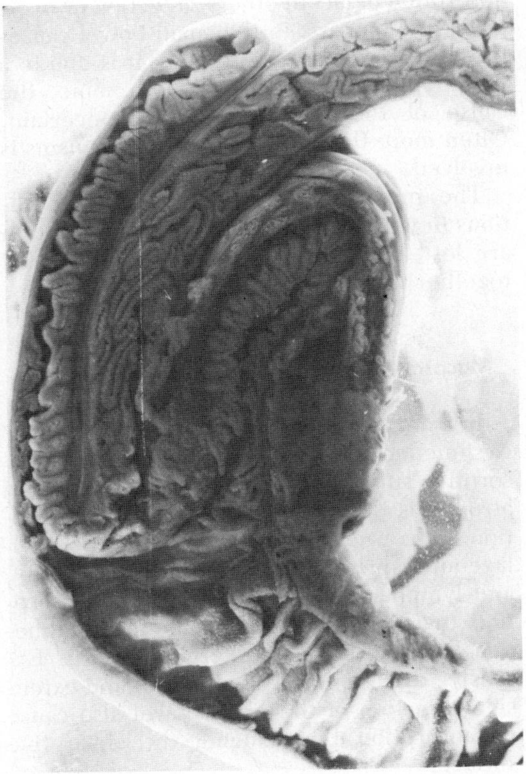

Fig. 35-16. Intussusception, showing the invagination of the proximal part of the bowel into the more distal segment.

invariable and ischemic enteritis or gangrene is likely.

In a Richter's hernia, named after a German surgeon (1742–1812), only part of the circumference of a loop of small bowel is trapped in a hernial sac. Obstruction does not occur, but the portion of bowel in the hernia can become gangrenous. If the gangrenous portion of bowel sloughs, the affected loop can fall back into the peritoneal cavity. The wide perforation caused by the gangrene makes peritonitis inevitable.

Treatment and Prognosis. Once symptoms develop, an abdominal hernia is treated surgically. The herniated viscus is restored to the peritoneal cavity, unless strangulation makes its resection necessary. The hernia sac is excised, and the weakness in the wall of the peritoneal cavity is repaired.

VOLVULUS. Twisting of a loop of bowel or some other structure is called volvulus. It is not common. Any part of the intestine can be affected, but volvulus is most common in the small bowel. Usually both the lumen of the bowel and its blood supply are obstructed. Anything that lengthens the mesentery or narrows its attachment makes volvulus easier. Anything that makes the bowel heavier makes volvulus more likely.

INTUSSUSCEPTION. Intussusception, from the Latin meaning a taking up into the inside, is common only in children under two years old. It may involve any part of the bowel but is most common in the terminal part of the ileum.

In intussusception, the peristaltic movements of the bowel grasp the proximal segment of the affected part of the bowel and pull it into the distal part. The invaginated proximal part of the gut becomes two layers thick as it turns back on itself to meet the distal part, which surrounds the invagination like a sleeve. The invaginated proximal part of the bowel is called the intussusceptum, and the surrounding distal part is called the intussuscipiens.

In young children, there is rarely anything to explain why intussusception occurs. The bowel involved seems normal. In 5% of infants, multiple areas of intussusception are found at autopsy, suggesting that in young children intussusception is common, but transient, and self-curing. In older children and adults, intussusception occurs only if there is a lesion, such as a tumor or Meckel's diverticulum, which can be grasped by the peristaltic waves and which drags the proximal part of the bowel after it to form the intussusceptum.

Usually the invagination of an intussusception extends for 5 or 10 cm. Occasionally it is longer. In an infant, an ileal intussusception may protrude from the anus.

The blood supply to the intussusceptum is precarious. The mesentery of the invaginated part of the bowel is drawn into the intussusception between the two layers of the intussusceptum. The blood vessels in the mesentery are angulated and compressed. If the intussusception is lengthy, the intussusceptum may become ischemic or necrotic.

If an intussusception persists for more than a short time, it causes intestinal obstruction. In infants, a sausage-shaped mass is sometimes palpable in the abdomen. In infants, reduction of the intussusception usually cures. In older children and adults the lesion that caused the intussusception must be resected.

MECONIUM ILEUS. Meconium ileus is a complication of fibrocystic disease of the pancreas, or mucoviscidosis as it is often called. About 10% of infants with fibrocystic disease of the pancreas develop meconium ileus, and about 15% of neonates with intestinal obstruction have meconium ileus.

Infants with meconium ileus pass no meconium. The colon is empty and shrunken. The terminal part of the ileum is beaded by putty-like pellets of meconium in its lumen. The proximal part of the ileum and the jejunum are dilated, hypertrophied and filled with sticky, greenish meconium, which is abnormally tenacious and does not flow from the cut end of the bowel. Volvulus of the heavy proximal loops of the ileum sometimes brings gangrene and perforation. Atresia may result from volvulus in utero. Sometimes necrotic bowel becomes wrapped in a pseudocyst of omentum and adhesions.

Meconium ileus results from the abnormal viscosity of the secretions in fibrocystic disease. Microscopically, the glands in the mucosa of the bowel are dilated and filled with tenacious, inspissated secretion.

MECONIUM PERITONITIS. Meconium peritonitis results from rupture of the bowel in the newborn and is particularly likely in infants with meconium ileus. Meconium is sterile, and infection of the peritoneum does not follow. There is a foreign body reaction, with fibrosis and sometimes calcification.

MECONIUM PLUG SYNDROME. The meconium plug syndrome occurs in neonates who do not have fibrocystic disease of the pancreas. A plug of meconium obstructs the rectum or colon. Remove the plug, and the child is cured.

MALABSORPTION

The disorders that impair the absorption of one or more foodstuffs are called the malabsorption syndromes. In some, the malabsorption is caused by atrophy of the intestinal mucosa or loss of a considerable proportion of the small bowel. In some, it results from lack of one or more of the enzymes needed for absorption, or the bile salts needed for the absorption of fat. In others, infection or overgrowth of bacteria in the small bowel causes the dysfunction. In still others, it is due to a lymphoproliferative disorder. In some, the cause of the malabsorption is uncertain. Often more than one of these mechanisms is involved.

The protein-losing enteropathies, conditions in which excessive quantities of protein are lost from the intestine, are considered together with the malabsorption syndromes.

Mucosal Atrophy and Shortening of the Bowel

In a number of forms of malabsorption, the dysfunction is caused by reduction in the absorptive surface of the small bowel. Mucosal atrophy is the principal cause of malabsorption in celiac disease, tropical sprue, collagenous sprue, idiopathic villous atrophy, and lymphangiectasia and of the malabsorption that complicates hypogammaglobulinemia, kwashiorkor, and allergic enteritis. Extensive disease of the small bowel and extensive resection of the small bowel also cause malabsorption by reducing the absorptive surface.

CELIAC DISEASE. Celiac disease has many names, and the use of the term varies from

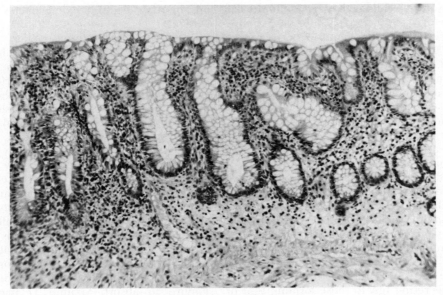

Fig. 35-17. A jejunal biopsy in celiac disease, showing complete villous atrophy, with loss of the jejunal microvilli, and deepening of the jejunal crypts.

one part of the world to another. The word *celiac* comes from the Greek for belly. In this book, the term *celiac disease* will be used to describe the form of malabsorption caused by sensitivity to gluten. Often celiac disease is called nontropical sprue, a name borrowed from Dutch. Sometimes it is called celiac sprue or gluten-induced enteropathy.

Celiac disease is common. In the United Kingdom, 1 person in 3000 suffers from it, and estimates of its prevalence in other countries range from 1 in 6500 in Sweden to 1 in 300 in Eire. About 70% of the patients are women. The disease often becomes apparent in childhood, but it may not become evident until adult life.

Lesions. In celiac disease, the mucosa of the upper part of the small bowel is atrophic. The atrophy is most marked in the duodenum and upper part of the jejunum. It becomes gradually less severe in the lower part of the jejunum. The ileum often is little if at all affected.

Normally, the mucosa of the jejunum consists of a flat base into which the crypts penetrate and on which the villi stand like tiny, crowded skyscrapers. In Caucasians, nearly all the villi are thin and finger-shaped.

In Africans and Asians, some of the villi are broader, like a leaf or the blade of a spade.

In celiac disease, the villi atrophy. At first, they become shorter and broader, so that there are many leaf-shaped or spade-shaped villi. As the atrophy increases, the shortened villi merge into ridges looking like the convolutions of the brain. Finally, the villi disappear altogether. Only the flat base of the mucosa remains, with the regular pattern of the openings of the crypts apparent now that the obscuring villi have gone. Often the flat mucosa is divided by deep clefts into polygonal areas, each containing many crypts. If the villi are completely lost, the patient is said to have complete villous atrophy. If shrunken villi remain, the lesion is called partial villous atrophy.

As the villi atrophy, the crypts become elongated. The basal part of the mucosa becomes thicker. The mitotic rate increases in the depths of the crypts and the interval between mitoses decreases. The rate at which new epithelial cells are produced may increase six times. The Paneth cells and the neuroendocrine cells are not affected.

The new epithelial cells move up the crypts in the usual way, but their maturation into absorptive cells as they turn onto the flat surface of the mucosa or onto the stumps of the surviving villi is imperfect. The microvilli of the absorptive cells are short and ill-formed. The cells have more vacuoles and lysosomes in their cytoplasm than is normal. Their mitochondria are often swollen, or there is an excess of free ribosomes. There is not much room for absorptive cells on the flat surface of a mucosa that shows complete villous atrophy. Their life is short, and they are soon shed.

Villous atrophy reduces enormously the absorptive surface of the bowel. The loss of the villi reduces the number of absorptive cells, and the malformation of their microvilli reduces further the absorptive surface.

Plasma cells and lymphocytes are numerous in the lamina propria. Most of them secrete IgA. Probably the ratio of lymphocytes secreting IgA to those forming IgM or IgG remains normal. Lymphocytes penetrate between the epithelial cells, but opinion differs as to whether they are more or less numerous than in normal intestinal mucosa. Often a few eosinophils are present in the lamina propria. The number of mast cells is increased. Accumulation of lipochrome pigments in the muscle cells sometimes makes the mucosa look brown.

Dysfunction. The atrophy of the intestinal mucosa in celiac disease causes malabsorption of fat. A 24-hour sample of stool contains more than 6 g of fat a day. If the malabsorption of fat is severe, the stools are foul, fatty, frothy, and pale. Deficiency of the fat-soluble vitamins is common.

Absorption of carbohydrate is often less severely depressed, though the D-xylose absorption test is abnormal. Failure to absorb protein sometimes causes hypoproteinemia.

Anemia is common in celiac disease. In children, it is usually caused by malabsorption of iron, in adults by lack of folate. The absorption of vitamin B$_{12}$ is impaired, but not usually sufficiently to cause anemia.

The absorption of calcium is reduced, in part because of poor absorption of vitamin D, in part because calcium forms soaps with the fat in the stool and is excreted in the feces, in part because the diseased jejunum absorbs calcium poorly even if these factors are corrected. Occasionally hypokalemia develops, or other electrolyte deficiencies become evident.

Clinical Presentation. Celiac disease varies considerably in severity. In some patients, it is incapacitating. In some, it is so mild that it is overlooked. The severity of the symptoms depends principally on the extent of the disease. If it is confined to a short segment of the bowel, enough normal mucosa remains to allow normal absorption.

In infants, the disease usually begins abruptly, when the child is a few months old and starts to eat cereals. The child becomes apathetic, anorexic, and miserable. The muscles waste, and become hypotonic and contrast sadly with the swollen and distended abdomen. The child fails to gain weight. Usually there is diarrhea with offensive, soft, pale, bulky stools. Sometimes vomiting is prominent. Anemia is usual. Failure to absorb vitamin D may bring rickets. Hypoproteinemia, edema, and hypoprothrombinemia with easy bruising are common.

As the child ages, the symptoms grow less. By the time the child reaches teen age, he or she can often live normally, eating gluten without provoking symptoms. Nevertheless, celiac disease is never cured. Symptoms may recur during adult life unless the patient persists with a gluten-free diet.

In adults, celiac disease sometimes, begins abruptly as in children, with diarrhea, foul, bulky, pale stools, and weight loss. Sometimes there is vomiting. Usually there is anorexia. Aphthae are common in the mouth. Iron deficiency is usually severe. Hypoproteinemia, edema, and hypocalcemia are common.

More often, celiac disease in adults begins insidiously. The patient is often ill-nourished. Iron deficiency anemia or folate deficiency is sometimes the principal finding. The patient sometimes seeks medical advice because of osteomalacia, edema, bleeding, weight loss, or dermatitis herpetiformis. Diarrhea is often absent, or is mild and episodic, occurring only a few times a year.

Complications. Over 5% of adults with celiac disease develop a malignant tumor, most often a non-Hodgkin's lymphoma involving the bowel and the adjacent lymph nodes. Ulcers sometimes develop in the jejunum or ileum in patients with celiac disease, with sudden worsening of symptoms. Major hemorrhage or perforation can occur. Splenic atrophy, or generalized atrophy of the lymphoid tissues, sometimes develops in adults with celiac disease. There may be hyposplenism or a reduction in the response to antigens. Rarely, a syndrome like subacute combined degeneration of the spinal cord develops, even though there is no deficiency of vitamin B_{12}. A rash sometimes appears in the skin in people with severe celiac disease. The rash usually clears as the patient's condition improves.

Pathogenesis. The villous atrophy in the small bowel and the dysfunction it causes are caused by gluten. If a susceptible person takes gluten in the food, symptoms appear, and villous atrophy develops in the small bowel.

If gluten is removed from the diet, symptoms improve within days or weeks, and the villous atrophy of the mucosa of the small bowel reverts towards normal, though more slowly. Usually the restoration of the structure of the mucosa takes months or years, if indeed it is ever complete. Fortunately, even a minor improvement in the function of the bowel is sufficient to relieve the symptoms. The disaccharidases produced by the mucosa of the small bowel give a useful measure of the function of the mucosa. When gluten is withdrawn from the diet of a patient with celiac disease, the production of disaccharidases increases within a few days or a week and may become normal within a few months.

If gluten is reintroduced into the diet, symptoms usually recur in days or weeks, and the villous atrophy worsens, though it may take months before it is again severe. The production of disaccharidases falls within hours or days of the reintroduction of gluten into the diet of a patient with celiac disease.

Gluten is a mixture of proteins found in wheat, wheat flour, and other products of wheat. The toxic element is believed to be one or more of a group of proteins called gliadins.

Gliadin is directly toxic to the intestinal mucosa in people who have celiac disease, but not in other people. If intestinal mucosa in a person with celiac disease is exposed to gliadin or gluten, the activity of disaccharidase and other enzymes promptly falls. If the exposure continues, villous atrophy develops. The toxicity is probably caused by deficiency of an enzyme needed for the metabolism of fraction 9 of gliadin. The attachment of gluten to the intestinal epithelium by abnormal lectins may be important.

Immunologic abnormalities are common in celiac disease. Antibodies against gluten are present in the plasma in many of the patients. In some patients, gluten causes lymphocytic transformation. The secretion of IgA, IgG, and IgM into the lumen of the bowel is increased in celiac disease. IgA deficiency occurs in 1 person in 70 with celiac disease, as compared with 1 person in 700 in the general population. Whether the abnormalities are important in the causation of the disease or are caused by the disease is uncertain.

Genetic factors are also relevant. As many as 10% of the relatives of patients with celiac disease show abnormalities of the mucosa of their small bowel on biopsy. The HLA antigens B8, DRw3, and DR7 are unduly frequent in patients with celiac disease.

Dermatitis herpetiformis is closely related to celiac disease. About 70% of the patients with dermatitis herpetiformis have a patchy villous atrophy in the small bowel, though it is not often severe enough to cause steatorrhea and other symptoms of celiac disease. A gluten-free diet relieves the intestinal lesion, but not the disease in the skin.

Treatment and Prognosis. A gluten-free diet brings relief to over 80% of patients with celiac disease within a few weeks. In most patients, the diet must be continued for the rest of the patient's life. In a few patients, the benefit does not become evident for some years. In such people, adrenocortical steroids control the symptoms and reduce the villous atrophy.

TROPICAL SPRUE. Tropical sprue occurs in parts of the Far East and in the Caribbean. Usually it affects adults who have lived in the area for many years, though it may attack people who have newly arrived.

Lesions. The small bowel shows partial villous atrophy. The atrophy is usually less complete than in celiac disease and commonly involves the ileum as well as the jejunum.

Clinical Presentation. Tropical sprue begins insidiously, with anorexia, asthenia, and the bulky stools of steatorrhea. After weeks or months, loss of weight becomes striking. Folate deficiency is usually severe, and deficiency of vitamin B_{12} is more severe than is usual in celiac disease. Macrocytic anemia develops in 60% of the patients. Glossitis, cheilosis, iron deficiency, and vitamin deficiencies are common. Calcium deficiency is rare.

Pathogenesis. The cause of tropical sprue is unknown. Antibacterial agents bring prompt relief, suggesting that the malabsorption results from bacterial infection, but no infectious agent able to cause the disease has been discovered. Nutritional deficiency, direct injury to the jejunoileal mucosa caused by bacteria, and mucosal injury caused by a bacterial toxin have all been suggested as possible causes of tropical sprue.

Treatment and Prognosis. Tropical sprue is usually managed by giving a sulfonamide or tetracycline for four weeks. Symptoms are relieved promptly, and in the course of six months the jejunoileal mucosa returns to normal. Treatment with vitamin B_{12} or folate also brings remission.

COLLAGENOUS SPRUE. Collagenous sprue is another rare form of malabsorption. Biopsy shows complete villous atrophy of the jejunal mucosa and a broad band of hyalinized collagen immediately beneath the flattened epithelium. Symptoms are often severe. No treatment is of help. The disease often proves fatal.

HYPOGAMMAGLOBULINEMIA. Malabsorption sometimes develops in patients with congenital or acquired hypogammaglobulinemia or agammaglobulinemia. In some of the patients, villous atrophy is extensive in the small bowel. In some, germinal centers in the mucosa form polypoid lesions in the small bowel. Some patients have both villous atrophy and polypoid lesions. In most of the patients, plasma cells are few or absent in the lesions. The plasma cells that are present form IgG or IgM but not IgA. Infection with Giardia lamblia is common. Other patients have an overgrowth of anaerobic bacteria in the small bowel.

The cause of the mucosal changes and malabsorption in hypogammaglobulinemia is un-

known. In some of the patients, the malabsorption is due to giardiasis, and can be cured by eradicating the infection. In most, antibiotics, a gluten-free diet, and adrenocorticosteroids temporarily improve absorption, but rarely bring cure.

KWASHIORKOR. Villous atrophy often develops in the mucosa of the small bowel in kwashiorkor. The resulting malabsorption worsens the syndrome.

ALLERGIC ENTERITIS. Sometimes allergy to a protein in the diet, such as a milk protein or soy protein causes malabsorption. The mucosa of the bowel becomes edematous. Eosinophils are often numerous in the lamina propria. Partial villous atrophy is common. Exclusion of the allergen cures.

IDIOPATHIC VILLOUS ATROPHY. Some patients have villous atrophy in the upper part of their small bowel, but fail to respond, or respond only temporarily, to the exclusion of gluten from the diet and are not helped by antibiotics, antigiardial therapy, or by folic acid. The cause of the disease in these patients with refractory sprue is unknown. The prognosis is bad.

LYMPHANGIECTASIA. Lymphangiectasia, either primary or secondary to some obstruction, is a rare cause of malabsorption. The villi containing the dilated lymphatics are shortened and distorted.

SHORT BOWEL SYNDROME. To maintain normal absorption, at least 90 cm of jejunum is needed. If more than this is lost because of infarction, Crohn's disease, eosinophilic enteritis, or any other cause, the absorption of fat, calcium, and folic acid is impaired. If much of the terminal ileum is destroyed by disease or is removed, the absorption of vitamin B_{12} and the reabsorption of bile salts is inadequate.

Lack of Enzymes or Bile

If the exocrine pancreatic secretions needed for digestion are deficient, if bile salts are lacking in the bowel, or if one or more of the enzymes needed for the uptake of foodstuffs by the intestinal mucosa are deficient, malabsorption is likely.

PANCREATIC DEFICIENCY. The enzymes secreted by the exocrine pancreas are sometimes deficient in conditions such as pancreatitis, carcinoma of the pancreas, or cystic fibrosis. Because of the lack of lipase in the bowel, much of the triglyceride in the food is lost in the stool, giving the oily stool common in exocrine pancreatic deficiency. Absorption of fat-soluble vitamins is impaired. Hypoprothrombinemia can follow. Hypocholesterolemia sometimes develops. Undigested meat is sometimes evident in the stool. The absorption of vitamin B_{12} is sometimes impaired. Usually D-xylose is absorbed normally.

Similar defects occur in the Zollinger-Ellison syndrome, in part because the low pH in the duodenum caused by the oversecretion of gastric acid inhibits the pancreatic enzymes, in part because the acid precipitates the conjugated bile salts needed for micelle formation in the bowel, in part because the abnormal acidity in the jejunum damages the absorptive cells.

Malabsorption sometimes develops after partial gastrectomy. In some patients, rapid emptying of the stomach dilutes the pancreatic enzymes and jejunal secretions. In some, the lack of gastric secretion in the duodenum reduces the secretion of secretin and cholecystokinin and so impairs exocrine pancreatic secretion. In some, the pancreatic enzymes fail to mix with the bile salts and remain unactivated. In others, bacteria proliferate abnormally in the blind loops of bowel created by the anastomoses.

DEFICIENCY OF BILE SALTS. Biliary obstruction, severe liver disease, and disease of the terminal ileum reduce the concentration of conjugated bile salts in the small bowel. The lack of the bile salts impairs micelle formation in the gut and reduces the absorption of fatty acids and monoglycerides.

EPITHELIAL ENZYME DEFICIENCIES. A congenital deficiency of one of the epithelial enzymes needed for absorption impairs the uptake of the substrate or substrates involved. Macroscopically and microscopically the mucosa of the bowel usually remains normal. Secondary enzyme deficiencies develop when the mucosa of the small bowel is extensively damaged by conditions such as celiac disease, tropical sprue, or Crohn's disease.

Lactase Deficiency. The enzyme lactase, normally found in the microvilli of the epithelial cells of the small intestine, is deficient in 5% of Caucasians and over 50% of Negroes and Orientals. The deficiency is inherited as an autosomal dominant character. Occasionally the defect does not become apparent until adolescence. When a person with lactase deficiency drinks milk, the lactose it contains cannot be absorbed normally. Instead, it is fermented by the intestinal bacteria, causing diarrhea, abdominal cramps, bloating, and flatulence. Avoid milk, and all is well.

Sucrase Deficiency. Sucrase is deficient in 0.2% of people. The deficiency is inherited as an autosomal recessive character. If the deficiency in sucrase is severe, diarrhea and borborygmi develop when sucrose is taken in the diet.

Abetalipoproteinemia. Abetalipoproteinemia is an uncommon defect inherited as an autosomal recessive character. The intestinal epithelium can absorb fat, but is unable to export it into the lacteals or to form chylomicra. The structure of the intestinal mucosa is preserved, but the absorptive cells become distended with fat. The liver fails to synthesize low density and very low density lipoproteins, and the concentrations of β-lipoproteins and pre-β-lipoproteins are low. The severity of the defect varies. In severe cases, steatorrhea begins in childhood. The inability to export lipid from the hepatocytes causes severe fatty change in the liver. Occasionally, cirrhosis follows. Peculiar thorny red cells appear in the blood. Severe neurologic disturbances, with ataxia, nystagmus, muscular weakness, areflexia, and pigmentary degeneration of the retina sometimes develop.

Malabsorption of Vitamin B_{12}. Rarely, the receptor on the ileal epithelial cells necessary for the absorption of vitamin B_{12} is defective. The vitamin cannot be absorbed and is lost into the stool.

Infections

Infection causes malabsorption in Whipple's disease, in bacterial overgrowth in the small bowel, in giardiasis, and sometimes in other forms of enteritis.

WHIPPLE'S DISEASE. Whipple's disease is an uncommon condition named after the

American pathologist who described it in 1907. Before its nature was known, it was often called intestinal lipodystrophy. The patients are usually men over 40 years old.

Lesions. The proximal part of the small bowel is dilated and rigid, with a stiff, edematous wall. Often the serosa is dulled by a fibrinous exudate. The mesentery of the involved segment of bowel is thickened and stiff. Its lymph nodes are often enlarged.

In the involved segment of bowel, the lamina propria is edematous, with widely dilated lacteals. Often there is partial villous atrophy. Large macrophages are numerous in the lamina propria. Most of them contain small, angular bodies that stain strongly with the periodic acid-Schiff reaction. Electron

microscopy shows that these bodies are bacteria about 1 μm long. The bacteria distend the lysosomes in the macrophages and are free in the intercellular fluid.

The edema extends through the whole thickness of the bowel wall and into its mesentery. The enlarged lymph nodes in the mesentery have widely dilated sinusoids, and their macrophages often contain bacteria like those in the bowel. Enlarged lymph nodes in other parts of the body show a similar dilatation of their sinusoids and sometimes have the bacteria in their macrophages. Some of the joints show mild inflammation. Bacteria have not been demonstrated in the inflamed joints.

Clinical Presentation. Whipple's disease

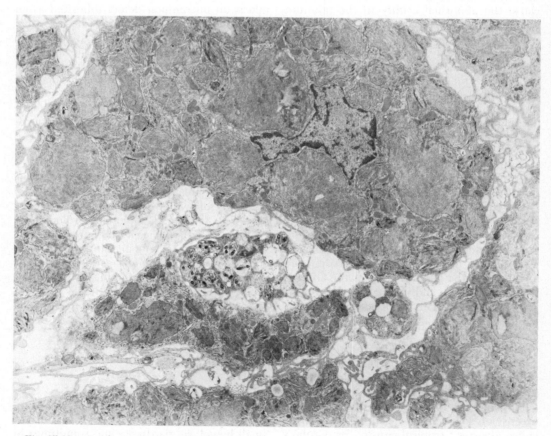

Fig. 35-18. An electron micrograph showing macrophages in the mucosa of a segment of jejunum involved in Whipple's disease. Well-preserved bacteria are present in the cell in the middle of the picture, with partly digested remnants of bacteria distending the lysosomes of the large cell in the upper part of the picture. (Courtesy of Dr. Susan Ritchie)

often begins with migratory polyarthritis. Steatorrhea, weight loss, anemia, and other signs of malabsorption follow. Generalized lymphadenopathy is evident in 50% of the patients. Low fever occurs in 30%. Sometimes there is increased pigmentation of the skin. Some patients have facial palsies or become confused, with loss of memory. Sometimes the indurated segment of bowel is palpable.

Treatment and Prognosis. Treatment with trimethoprim-sulfamethoxazole for a year or more eradicates the bacteria and brings cure. Shorter courses of treatment with tetracycline or penicillin reduce the number of bacteria present and relieve the symptoms, but in 50% of the patients the bacteria and the symptoms return when the drug is withdrawn. The success of the therapy can be monitored by taking a biopsy of the mucosa of the small bowel. If bacteria are present, treatment must be continued.

BACTERIAL OVERGROWTH. Overgrowth of bacteria in the normally sterile proximal part of the small bowel can cause malabsorption. Bacterial overgrowth is likely whenever there is stasis in the small bowel. It can occur in a blind loop of bowel created surgically or in a duodenal or jejunal diverticulum. Scleroderma and other disorders that impair the motility of the bowel sometimes cause bacterial overgrowth in the jejunum. A gastrocolic, gastroileal, jejunocolic, or jejunoileal fistula is sometimes complicated by bacterial overgrowth.

The mucosa of the bowel in the region involved often shows patches of moderate to severe villous atrophy. The patients develop steatorrhea and other signs of malabsorption, nearly always with macrocytic anemia.

The cause of the malabsorption is complex. The damage to the mucosa may be due to proteases elaborated by species of Bacterioides and other bacteria. The malabsorption of fat is due in part to the deconjugation of bile salts by anaerobic bacteria. The lack of conjugated bile salts and the excess of unconjugated bile salts impairs the formation of the micelles needed for the absorption of fats. The overgrowth of bacteria sometimes reduces the absorption of sodium and water. The macrocytic anemia is due mainly to fixation of vitamin B_{12} by the bacteria, reducing the quantity available for absorption.

Treatment with tetracycline, ampicillin, or trimethoprim-sulfamethoxazole usually controls the bacteria and relieves the symptoms.

ENTERITIS. Giardiasis is a fairly common cause of malabsorption, often causing partial villous atrophy. Coccidiosis and strongyloidiasis sometimes cause severe villous atrophy. Capillariasis causes malabsorption, but the intestinal mucosa is usually normal. Occasionally bacterial or viral enteritis causes villous atrophy and malabsorption. Rarely, histoplasmosis or tuberculosis of the bowel does so.

Lymphoproliferative Disorders

Malabsorption is common in alpha heavy chain disease and Mediterranean lymphoma. It occasionally occurs in other forms of lymphoproliferative disease or lymphoma.

ALPHA HEAVY CHAIN DISEASE. Alpha heavy chain disease is most common in the Middle East and around the Mediterranean Sea. The patients are usually from 10 to 30 years old. In most, the disease involves the small bowel. In a few, it affects the respiratory system.

Lesions. The involvement of the small bowel by alpha heavy chain disease is patchy. A single biopsy may fail to show the lesion. In the early stages of the disease, the lamina propria of the mucosa is infiltrated by normal appearing lymphocytes and plasma cells. A similar increase in plasma cells is evident in the lymph nodes draining the affected part of the bowel. Villous atrophy becomes more severe as the infiltrate grows more intense. Alpha heavy chains are present in the plasma.

Later, the infiltrate extends into the submucosa or sometimes into the muscularis propria. Some of the lymphocytes and plasma cells in the bowel wall and the regional lymph nodes are atypical. Immunoblasts are present in the infiltrate.

Finally, the infiltrate becomes malignant. An anaplastic B cell lymphoma usually of the immunoblastic type infiltrates the bowel wall and involves the regional lymph nodes. In a few patients, the lymphoma extends to involve more distant lymph nodes or the bone marrow.

Clinical Presentation. The patients present with severe malabsorption. Weight loss is severe. Protein-losing enteropathy can occur. Abdominal pain is common. Remissions and exacerbations are usual. Late in the disease, obstruction or perforation can complicate the lymphoma.

Pathogenesis. The repeated intestinal infections common in the Middle East may play some part in the pathogenesis of alpha heavy chain disease.

Treatment and Prognosis. Treatment with tetracycline or other antibiotics often brings remission in the early stages of the disease. If lymphoma develops, chemotherapy is necessary, but the prognosis is poor.

MEDITERRANEAN LYMPHOMA. Occasionally a patient from the Middle East or South Africa with malabsorption is found to have lymphoma confined to the small bowel and the lymph nodes that drain it. The lymphoma is usually a poorly differentiated, immunoblastic B cell tumor identical to that which occurs in the late stages of alpha heavy chain disease. It is called a Mediterranean lymphoma, but in most patients is probably the end stage of alpha heavy chain disease.

Protein-Losing Enteropathy

Extensive lesions in the stomach or intestine occasionally cause leakage of large quantities of protein into the lumen of the gastrointestinal tract. In some patients, the loss is sufficient to cause hypoalbuminemia, edema, and ascites. Carcinoma of the stomach, large peptic ulcers, Ménétrier's disease, Crohn's disease, celiac disease, tropical sprue, Whipple's disease, lymphangiectasia of the small bowel, lymphoma of the small bowel, bacterial or parasitic enteritis, ulcerative colitis, and carcinoma of the colon can all cause loss of protein into the bowel, Occasionally protein-losing enteropathy develops in congestive heart failure or renal failure.

CONGENITAL ANOMALIES

The principal congenital anomalies that involve the intestine are Hirschsprung's disease, atresia, imperforate anus, duplication, and malrotation. Often a few rests of misplaced tissue are present in the intestine.

HIRSCHSPRUNG'S DISEASE. Hirschsprung's disease is a congenital disorder named after a Danish pediatrician who reported it in 1888. The disease causes dilatation of the colon and is often called congenital megacolon. It affects 1 child in every 20,000 live-born. Over 90% of the patients are boys.

Lesions. The proximal part of the colon is dilated. If the disease is not treated, the colon can reach 120 cm in diameter and weigh 100 kg. The muscle in the wall of the dilated colon is hypertrophied. Its mucosa is redundant and thrown into folds. At its distal end, the dilated colon funnels smoothly into an apparently normal segment of bowel. Usually, the rectum and lower part of the sigmoid colon appear normal, but occasionally the narrow segment is shorter or extends more proximally.

In the dilated part of the colon, the myenteric plexus and nervous supply of the colon are normal. In the narrow segment, bundles of nerve fibers, principally cholinergic fibers, are prominent in the muscularis propria, but the neurons of Meissner's and Auerbach's plexuses are absent. Usually the aganglionic segment extends to the anus, but rarely a length of normal bowel is present distal to the aganglionic segment.

Clinical Presentation. Hirschsprung's disease usually presents during infancy. The child has no bowel movements. Distention of the proximal colon increasingly distends the abdomen. Malnutrition is inevitable. Less often, the patient passes some feces, and the disease is not discovered until adolescence or adult life.

Pathogenesis. Lack of the neurons prevents peristalsis in the aganglionic segment of bowel. The obstruction causes dilatation of the normal proximal part of the colon.

Treatment and Prognosis. Hirschsprung's disease is diagnosed by a biopsy of the narrow segment of bowel, usually in the rectum. If neurons are absent, the aganglionic segment is resected, or the normally innervated proximal part of the bowel is pulled through the aganglionic segment and anastomosed to the rectal wall just proximal to the anus.

ADYNAMIC BOWEL SYNDROME. Rarely, a

child has megacolon like that of Hirschsprung's disease, but biopsy of the narrow segment of the colon shows a normal complement of neurons or sometimes enlargement of the myenteric ganglia. Probably these children have a more subtle fault in the innervation of the colon.

IDIOPATHIC MEGACOLON.   Idiopathic megacolon is a rare condition more common in boys than in girls in which the whole length of the colon and rectum is dilated, with no narrow segment. The innervation of the colon and rectum is normal. The patients have severe constipation, but in many of them training, enemas, and laxatives eventually achieve more normal function.

ATRESIA AND STENOSIS.   Atresia of some segment of the intestine occurs in 1 live birth in 3000. Stenosis is less common. Atresia, from the Greek for not perforated, means that the bowel is completely occluded. Stenosis, from the Greek for narrowing, means that a segment of the bowel is narrowed, but not totally occluded.

Three kinds of atresia of the intestine occur. A fibrous diaphragm may completely occlude the lumen. A longer or shorter segment of bowel may be reduced to a fibrous cord without a lumen. A segment of the bowel may be absent altogether, with the proximal and distal ends of the surviving bowel smoothly rounded and covered by serosa. When a segment of bowel is absent, the mesentery serving the absent segment is deficient as well. When a segment of intestine is reduced to a fibrous cord, the mesentery serving the cord may or may not be deficient.

Two kinds of stenosis of the intestine are found. A fibrous diaphragm stretched across the lumen may have a hole in it. A segment of bowel may be narrower than normal, though all layers of its wall are more or less normally formed.

In more than 60% of the infants with intestinal atresia the lesion is in the small intestine. In 15% of the infants, more than one segment of bowel is atretic. Proximal to the obstruction, the bowel is dilated and atonic. Distal to the atretic area, the bowel is small and looks hypoplastic. If more than one area is atretic, the intervening segment of bowel is often dilated. In the duodenum, atresia is usually caused by a fibrous diaphragm between the second and third parts of the duodenum. Atresia of the colon is uncommon.

In most patients, intestinal atresia results from an intrauterine catastrophe, rather than from a genetic defect. Ischemia or intussusception causes infarction of a segment of the intestine in utero, and atresia or stenosis follows.

Atresia and severe stenosis of the intestine cause obstruction and require surgical correction within hours of birth.

IMPERFORATE ANUS.   Congenital anomalies in the formation of the rectum and anus occur in 1 live birth in 5000. Traditionally, these anomalies are all called imperforate anus, though this term is far from an accurate description of the lesion in most cases.

In most of these infants, the anus is malplaced and usually ill-formed. In boys, the rectum may open into the bladder, urethra, onto the perineum, or rarely onto the scrotum or penis. In girls, the opening may be into the vagina, onto the perineum, or rarely into the bladder. In girls the rectum and urinary and genital tracts occasionally end in a common cloaca. The cloaca may be wide and functional or tiny and stenotic.

Less often, the rectum ends blindly, 2 or 3 cm from the anus. The anus is formed normally, but is closed by a thin membrane, or there is a zone of stenosis in the anal canal or rectum.

The different kinds of imperforate anus can be divided into those in which the rectum ends above the levator ani, and those in which it extends into or through the levator ani. If the rectum ends above the levator ani, surgical repair is difficult, and it is less likely that the anal musculature and innervation is sufficiently preserved to allow construction of a competent anus.

In over 50% of infants with a congenital anomaly of the rectum or anus, there are serious congenital defects elsewhere. Atresia of the esophagus or intestine, malformation of the urinary tract, or a cardiovascular malformation are common.

DUPLICATION.   Reduplication of the intestine is most common in relation to the ileum, but can involve any part of the small or large bowel. Usually the reduplication lies in the mesentery of the true bowel. Occasionally, it shares the musculature of the true bowel, but more often it is separate with its own muscular wall.

If the reduplication is small, it forms a cyst lined by gastric or intestinal mucosa. If it is larger, a portion of the intestine is duplicated or triplicated. The duplication may be closed at both ends or may open into the true lumen at one or both ends. Many patients with reduplication of the small bowel have malformed vertebrae. Reduplication of the colon is sometimes associated with reduplication of the bladder and genitalia.

Often the reduplication causes no symptoms. Occasionally it acts as a blind loop, allowing bacterial overgrowth that causes malabsorption. Occasionally a reduplication becomes obstructed and acutely inflamed. Occasionally an enteric cyst in the wall of the bowel causes obstruction or intussusception.

MALROTATION AND MALFIXATION. Minor degrees of malrotation of the bowel and minor malfixation of the cecum or colon are common and usually of no significance. Serious malrotation of the bowel and the malfixation of the duodenum or colon that often goes with it are rare.

Occasionally, the cecum is in the epigastrium, and the ileum enters it from below. Sometimes the duodenum and small bowel have a common mesentery with a narrow base. Sometimes the duodenum is compressed by a band leading from the abdominal wall to the cecum.

In other patients, the small bowel is anterior to the colon, which occasionally passes through the mesentery of the small bowel. Sometimes the entire small bowel is on the right side of the abdomen, with the entire large bowel on the left.

SITUS INVERSUS. Situs inversus occurs in 1 live birth in 8000. Usually it involves only the abdominal viscera but sometimes involves the thoracic organs as well. The left and right sides of the body are transposed. The arrangement of the organs is normal, except that everything is on the wrong side. The appendix is in the left iliac fossa. The spleen is on the right, the larger lobe of the liver is on the left. Situs inversus causes no dysfunction, and is usually found by accident, perhaps when the heart is discovered on the wrong side of the body.

Up to 40% of people with situs inversus have chronic sinusitis, and many have bronchiectasis. The combination of situs inversus with sinusitis and bronchiectasis is called Kartagener's syndrome, after the German physician who described it in 1933.

Both the situs inversus and the respiratory disease are due to malformation of the cilia. The peripheral microtubules in the cilia have defective dynein arms, and the cilia are immotile. The direction of the rotation of the internal organs during embryonic life is guided by the beating of the cilia common on embryonic epithelial cells. If the cilia are immotile, chance determines whether the organs rotate to the right or the left.

RESTS. Rests of pancreatic tissue are common in the duodenum. Occasionally an islet cell tumor originates in a rest. Elsewhere in the intestine islands of gastric mucosa are sometimes found, but they are uncommon except in Meckel's diverticulum and in duplications of the intestine.

OTHER NONNEOPLASTIC CONDITIONS

Melanosis coli, cathartic colon, and pneumatosis intestinalis; the involvement of the bowel in scleroderma, endometriosis, and amyloidosis; and the damage to the bowel caused by radiation are discussed in this section.

MELANOSIS COLI. Melanosis coli is more striking than important. The mucosa of the colon turns brown or shiny black. Carcinomata and adenomatous polyps of the colon do not become pigmented and remain pink against the dark mucosa. The whole colon and the appendix may be affected, but often the pigmentation is most intense in the cecum, becoming browner and less intense more distally.

The pigmentation is caused by a pigment related to the lipofuscins that accumulates in the macrophages in the mucosa of the colon. The origin of the pigment is uncertain. The macrophages and epithelial cells of the colon contain many lysosomes, suggesting that there has been some injury to these cells.

Melanosis coli is common in people who take anthracene laxatives such as cascara or senna. It fades or disappears if the drug is discontinued. Presumably the drugs cause some minor derangement of cell metabolism. In 1930, melanosis coli was evident in 10% of autopsies and in 30% of colons resected for carcinoma. Now, it is uncommon, perhaps because anthracene purgatives are used much less widely than in the past.

Melanosis coli causes no symptoms, no dysfunction, and predisposes to no ill. It is a prime example of a disease that causes no illness.

CATHARTIC COLON.   If the intake of anthracene purgatives is prolonged, some people can develop diarrhea, potassium deficiency, malabsorption, or protein-losing enteropathy. The patients have melanosis coli, but in addition the mucosa becomes smooth, looking like the skin of a toad or a snake, and there may be atrophy of the muscularis mucosae or muscularis propria. Eventually, the atrophy of the muscle is so great that the motility of the colon is impaired. Probably cathartic colon results from injury to the myenteric nervous system by the purgatives.

PNEUMATOSIS INTESTINALIS.   Pneumatosis intestinalis is a rare condition that occurs in children and in adults 40 or 50 years old. It may affect the small intestine or the colon, but is more common in the small intestine. Often pneumatosis is secondary to some other disease of the gastrointestinal tract, peptic ulcer, pyloric obstruction, or gastroenteritis. Sometimes it is associated with chronic pulmonary disease.

In pneumatosis intestinalis, the wall of the affected segment of bowel is thickened and distorted by cysts filled with gas. The cysts are usually 0.5 to 2 cm in diameter and do not communicate with one another. If there is no other lesion in the bowel, the cysts are usually in the submucosa. They often bulge into the lumen, so that the mucosa is cobblestoned or polypoid. In adults in whom the pneumatosis is secondary to some other disease of the bowel, the cysts are usually subserosal.

Microscopically, the gas-filled cysts are lined for the most part by a granulomatous reaction, in which macrophages are predominant and often multinucleated. Less often, the cells lining the cysts become flattened. This granulomatous reaction often enables the diagnosis to be made by endoscopic biopsy. A cyst may rupture with a loud plop as it is grasped by the biopsy forceps.

The cause of penumatosis intestinalis is unclear. It may be that gas from the lumen of the intestine is forced into the bowel wall through small cracks in the mucosa and is trapped in the submucosa. It has been suggested that in adults with chronic pulmonary disease air could track down from the lungs. Some have thought that the cysts are dilated lymphatics, but this does not seem to be the case.

Pneumatosis intestinalis usually causes only vague symptoms, but sometimes results in pain, diarrhea, or malabsorption. Occasionally it causes obstruction or pneumoperitoneum. Treatment is symptomatic.

ENDOMETRIOSIS.   Endometriosis is discussed with the diseases of the uterus in Chapter

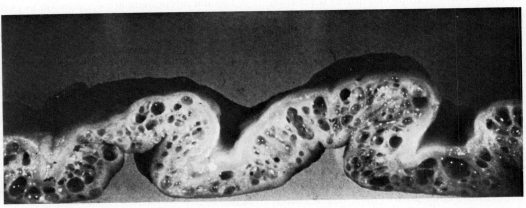

Fig. 35-19.   Pneumatosis intestinalis, showing gas-filled cysts in the wall of the small bowel.

41. In 15 to 20% of the patients, the colon and rectum or, less often, the small bowel, is involved. Small implants of endometrium appear in the subserosa. Rarely, the implants form mass that may mimic a neoplasm or cause obstruction.

SCLERODERMA. Scleroderma occasionally involves the small bowel or less often the colon. The lesions are similar to those of scleroderma of the esophagus, with edema of the submucosa or subserosa in the parts of the gut affected, patchy fibrosis, and sometimes atrophy of the intestinal muscle. There is loss of motility, often with diarrhea or constipation. Partial obstruction may bring distention, vomiting, or pain. Bacterial overgrowth can occur. Malabsorption is sometimes severe. Pneumatosis intestinalis may develop. Wide-mouthed diverticula sometimes develop in the colon.

RADIATION INJURY. Radiation injury is discussed in Chapter 23. The intestine is highly sensitive to radiation. Even a moderate dose of radiation causes extensive mucosal necrosis in the small bowel.

Irradiation of a carcinoma of the endometrium or cervix uteri sometimes causes serious injury to the colon. Symptoms of colonic injury may begin soon after the irradiation, but often are delayed for weeks or months. Occasionally, painful and intractable ulcers develop in the colon, sometimes with obstruction, a fistula to the vagina or bladder, perforation, or hemorrhage. The injury first causes edema and congestion in the involved part of the bowel, with increased secretion of mucus. Later comes increasing fibrosis, with the abnormal fibrocytes and the vascular changes seen in other irradiated tissues.

AMYLOIDOSIS. Amyloidosis rarely causes intestinal symptoms, but it does commonly involve the bowel to a minor degree, lying most often around the small vessels in the submucosa. Rectal biopsy often proves diagnostic in patients with amyloidosis, even though there is no evidence of involvement of the rectum or any other part of the bowel.

PROLAPSE OF THE RECTUM. Prolapse of the rectum occurs in children and in elderly women. In children, the condition usually disappears as the child grows older, but in elderly women it can be distressing, causing fecal incontinence. Surgical correction is needed.

TUMORS

Nonneoplastic conditions that resemble neoplasms will be described in this section together with the true neoplasms.

Benign

Three kinds of benign epithelial proliferation occur in the intestine. Tubular adenomata, villous adenomata, and tubulovillous adenomata are true neoplasms. The polyps of the Peutz-Jeghers syndrome are hamartomata. Juvenile and hyperplastic polyps are hyperplastic or inflammatory lesions. Tubular and tubulovillous adenomata that hang from a stalk are often called adenomatous polyps.

Any kind of benign mesenchymal tumor can occur in the intestine, but only leiomyomata, lipomata, and angiomata are common. Occasionally nodules of lymphoid tissue that resemble a neoplasm are found in the intestine, or a psuedolymphoma like those found in the stomach develops in the intestine.

TUBULAR ADENOMA. One or more tubular adenomata are present in the colon in 50% of patients at autopsy. Over 25% of the patients have more than one. Over 5% have more than five. Most of the adenomata are small, but in 10% of the patients, one or more is big enough to be found easily. In the small bowel, a tubular adenoma is found in 1 autopsy in 2000.

Tubular adenomata are uncommon in people under 30 years old, but grow increasingly common as age increases. They are more common in men than in women. In the United States, they are more frequent in white than in black people. They are more common in North America and Europe than in Japan, Asia, or Africa.

They are evenly distributed throughout the colon. About 20% arise in the cecum, 20% in the ascending or transverse colon, 20% in the sigmoid colon, and 20% in the rectum. The adenomata in the left side of the colon are usually larger than those on the right.

Lesions. Tubular adenomata begin as flat

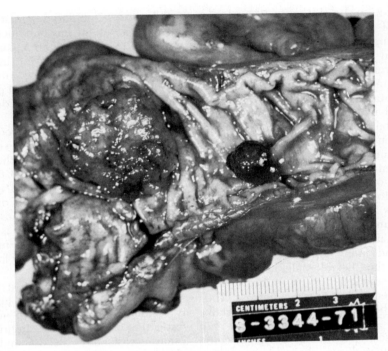

Fig. 35-20. A tubular adenoma of the colon on the right of the picture, showing its dark head and short stalk. The lesion on the left is a carcinoma of the colon.

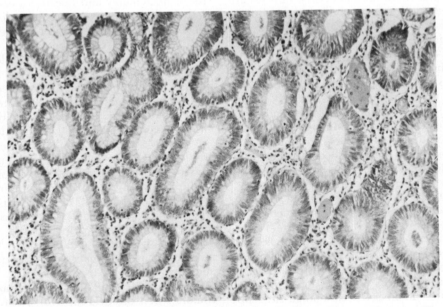

Fig. 35-21. A tubular adenoma of the colon, showing the tubular glands lined by tall, columnar cells cut in cross section.

lesions 1 to 2 mm in diameter. They lie in the plane of the mucosa, without a stalk, and macroscopically or endoscopically can be distinguished from normal mucosa only by minor differences of color or texture. As these tiny tumors enlarge, they are grasped by the peristaltic movements of the bowel and dragged into the lumen of the bowel, pulling a stalk of normal mucosa behind them, to form an adenomatous polyp.

By the time they are discovered, most tubular adenomata are spheroidal tumors. Nearly 75% of them are less than 1 cm in diameter. Most of the rest are 1 to 3 cm across. A few are as much as 10 cm in diameter. The tumor is a darker red than the surrounding mucosa. Its surface is coarsely lobulated and finely granular. The tumor hangs from a thin, flexible stalk, usually 2 to 5 cm long and about 0.5 cm in diameter. The stalk is covered by pale, normal mucosa. The demarcation between the tumor and the stalk is sharp.

Microscopically, a tubular adenoma consists of elongated and branching crypts, which ramify to form the spheroidal mass. The crypts are lined by columnar cells, which are often tall and thin, squeezed together like the fingers of a hand, with basal nuclei and many mitoses. In normal crypts, mitoses are confined to the base of the crypt, but in adenomatous polyps they can be found anywhere in the crypts, even near the surface. Goblet cells are common in the neoplastic epithelium and are sometimes its main feature, especially in the deeper parts of the crypts. Between the crypts is a fine, scanty stroma, with scattered plasma cells and lymphocytes. The junction between the neoplastic epithelium and the surrounding normal epithelium usually occurs where the tumor joins its stalk. The border is sharp. One crypt is neoplastic, the next normal.

About 50% of tubular adenomata show foci of epithelial atypicality. The tumor cells lose their regular arrangement, become larger, with larger more hyperchromatic nuclei and are more pleomorphic. Usually the atypicality is mild. Occasionally, it is sufficient to justify a diagnosis of carcinoma in situ. Sometimes an invasive carcinoma develops in a tubular adenoma, and invades the stalk of the polyp.

Behavior. Tubular adenomata are benign, but once a patient has one adenoma, more are likely to appear. If an apparently single tubular adenoma is removed, in 40% of the patients one or more new tumors appear within a few years. Over 60% of patients with multiple tubular adenomata develop new lesions.

Some tubular adenomata become malignant. A focus of carcinoma develops in the adenoma and extends through the muscularis mucosae to invade the stalk of the polyp or extend further. Fewer than 1% of tubular adenomata less than 1 cm in diameter become malignant, but 10% of those over 2 cm in diameter. Malignant change is more likely when tubular adenomata are multiple and when some of the lesions show foci of severe dysplasia.

Clinical Presentation. Most tubular adenomata cause no symptoms. They are found by accident during a checkup or during investigation of some other condition. A large lesion occasionally bleeds, and rarely an adenomatous polyp of the colon causes pain. A tubular adenoma in the small bowel can cause obstruction or intussusception, like other tumors of the small bowel.

Treatment and Prognosis. Because of the risk of malignancy and because a carcinoma of the colon sometimes masquerades as an adenomatous polyp, most tubular adenomata are removed. Usually the tumor can be removed endoscopically, but if the lesion is large or atypical, surgical resection may be needed. Many physicians recommend that the colon be examined regularly after a tubular adenoma has been removed to detect and remove new adenomata as they develop.

VILLOUS ADENOMA. Villous adenomata are less common than tubular adenomata. About 70% of adenomata of the colon are of the tubular type, 20% are tubulovillous, and 10% are villous. They can arise anywhere in the colon, but are most common in the rectum and lower part of the sigmoid colon. Many of the patients have one or more tubular adenomata as well as a villous adenoma.

Lesions. Most villous adenomata are large tumors when discovered, over 4 cm across, often over 10 cm. They are ovoid, soft, flat, and pliable and lie in the plane of the mucosa

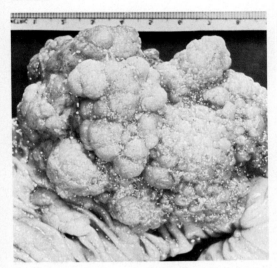

Fig. 35-22. A villous adenoma of the colon, showing the large, granular tumor standing a little above the surface of the mucosa.

without a stalk or stand a few millimeters above it. The surface of the tumor is often covered with fine, villous processes, like velvet, but may be coarser, with thicker papillary bulges. Less often, a villous adenoma is pedunculated, like a tubular adenoma though with a thicker, shorter stalk.

Microscopically, a villous adenoma shows fine fronds, which sometimes branch. The fronds have a delicate core of fibrous tissue and are covered by a single layer of tall, columnar cells, which are squeezed together. Goblet cells may be present. Mitoses are common. Foci of dysplasia and carcinoma in situ are more common than in tubular adenomata.

Behavior. Foci of invasive carcinoma are present in 40% of villous adenomata by the time the tumor is discovered. The foci of invasion are often small. If the tumor is large, even multiple biopsies cannot exclude the possibility of invasion.

Clinical Presentation. Many villous adenomata give no symptoms or cause only a minor feeling of fullness in the rectum. The tumor can be missed on rectal examination, because it is soft and hard to distinguish from the normal mucosa by palpation. Sometimes a villous adenoma secretes large quantities of mucus, as much as 3 or 4 L a day, causing

mucous diarrhea. Sometimes there is considerable loss of sodium chloride and potassium. Hypokalemia may develop, or less often alkalosis and dehydration. Sometimes the symptoms develop suddenly, although the tumor must have been present for years.

Treatment and Prognosis. Villous adenomata should be completely removed. If careful examination shows no evidence of carcinoma, local excision is sufficient. If one or more foci of invasive carcinoma are found, the lesion must be treated as a carcinoma.

TUBULOVILLOUS ADENOMA. Tubulovillous adenomata show a mixture of tubular and villous features. Usually, the tumor resembles a tubular adenoma macroscopically, but microscopically part of the lesion has the structure of a villous adenoma. Dysplasia and carcinoma in situ are more frequent in tubulovillous adenomata than in tubular adenomata, though not as common as in villous adenomata. About 20% of tubulovillous ad-

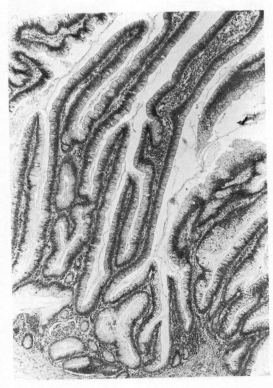

Fig. 35-23. A villous adenoma, showing the long, delicate fronds with a fine, collagenous core lined by narrow, columnar cells.

enomata show foci of invasive carcinoma. The larger the tumor, the more likely it is to show invasion.

FAMILIAL POLYPOSIS. Familial polyposis, or multiple polyposis as it is sometimes called, is a hereditary disorder, in which large numbers of adenomata develop in the colon at an early age. It is inherited as an autosomal dominant character, with reduced penetrance. About 80% of those who carry the abnormal gene manifest the disease. New mutations are common. In 20% of new kindreds with the disease, there is no history of polyposis in the family of the first patient, and it must be assumed that this patient is the first to manifest a new mutation. One child in every 8000 born alive has familial polyposis. Boys and girls are equally affected.

Lesions. A child with multiple polyposis shows no abnormality at birth. Only in late childhood, in adolescence, or as a young adult do adenomata begin to appear in the colon. Within a few years, there are dozens of them, often hundreds, even thousands of them. In some patients, the large bowel is hidden by a cobblestoning of polyps. Most of the tumors are tubular or tubulovillous adenomata. In some patients, there are one or more villous adenomata as well. The small bowel is not affected.

Behavior. From 5 to 20 years after the polyps begin to appear, more than 80% of patients with familial polyposis develop carcinoma of the colon. Often there are multiple primary carcinomata in the large bowel. The patient is often younger than is usual with carcinoma of the colon, perhaps only 30 or 40 years old. In any one kindred, the sequence is usually much the same in all the affected members of the family. The age at which the polyps develop is much the same, and the age at which carcinoma supervenes is much the same.

Clinical Presentation. Patients with familial polyposis often have no symptoms until carcinoma develops. Sometimes the polyps cause bleeding or diarrhea.

Treatment and Prognosis. Familial polyposis requires total colectomy, preferably after patients are full grown, but before the age at which they develop carcinoma. Other members of the patient's family must be examined to see if they too are at risk. Those carrying the abnormal gene should be advised of the nearly 50% risk that they will transmit the disease to their children.

The carcinomata of familial polyposis are like other carcinomata of the colon. They grow, invade, and metastasize in the ordinary way. The prognosis after resection is as for any other carcinoma of the colon of similar character.

MULTIPLE ADENOMATA. Occasionally a patient is found to have between 20 and 100

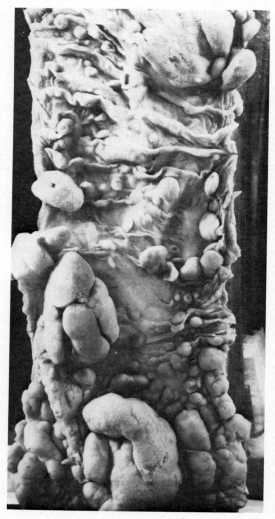

Fig. 35-24. Multiple polyposis, showing numerous polyps in the colon with a carcinoma at the upper edge of the picture.

tubular or tubulovillous adenomata, more than is usual in the general population with sporadic adenomata and fewer than is usual in people with familial polyposis. It has been suggested that these people may be homozygous for a recessive gene which is an allele of the gene causing familial polyposis.

GARDNER'S SYNDROME. Gardner's syndrome, named after the American physician who described it in 1953, is a variant of familial polyposis in which the patients have multiple osteomata of the skeleton, multiple epidermoid cysts in the skin, and multiple lipomata or fibromata in the skin as well as polyposis. Less often a patient has abdominal desmoid tumors, fibrosis of the mesentery and retroperitoneal tissues, dental abnormalities, adenomata in the stomach and small bowel, carcinoma of the ampulla of Vater, carcinoma of the thyroid, hepatoblastoma, or multiple endocrine tumors in addition to the polyposis coli.

TURCOT'S SYNDROME. Turcot's syndrome, named after the Canadian neurosurgeon who reported it in 1959, is rare. The patients have polyposis of the colon and a malignant tumor of the brain. The syndrome is probably inherited as an autosomal recessive character.

PEUTZ-JEGHERS SYNDROME. The rare Peutz-Jeghers syndrome is named after the Dutch physician Peutz who reported it in 1921 and the American physician Jeghers who drew attention to it in 1944. The syndrome is inherited as an autosomal dominant character, with varying expressivity.

In the Peutz-Jeghers syndrome, patchy pigmentation around the mouth, due to the deposition of melanin in the mucosal epithelium and the epidermis, causes freckles and blotches on the lips, the oral mucosa, and circumoral skin. Sometimes there is similar pigmentation around the nose, eyes, or on the fingers. Polyps in the gastrointestinal tract are usually multiple. They are most common in the small bowel, but sometimes develop in the stomach or colon as well. Sometimes there is pigmentation around the mouth but no polyps, or polyps without pigmentation. Usually the pigmentation becomes apparent in childhood or adolescence, and the polyps appear later.

The polyps are hamartomata. Macroscopically, they are sometimes flat, but usually resemble an adenomatous polyp with a thick stalk. Microscopically, there is overgrowth of all elements of the mucosa. Long,

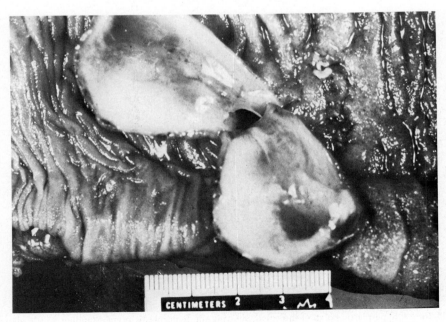

Fig. 35-25.   A juvenile polyp of the colon, showing the mucoid, edematous core of the lesion.

interdigitating crypts lined by normal gastric, intestinal, or colonic epithelium extend deep into the lesion and are separated by bundles of smooth muscle continuous with the muscularis mucosae. At times, the microscopic appearance simulates carcinoma invading the wall of the bowel.

The polyps in the small bowel sometimes cause obstruction, bleeding, or intussusception. They do not become malignant, but the risk of developing carcinoma of the stomach or small bowel may be increased in patients with the Peutz-Jeghers syndrome.

JUVENILE POLYP. Juvenile polyps are common in children between 1 and 5 years old. They are occasionally found in older children and in adults. The polyps may develop anywhere in the colon. Often they are multiple.

Juvenile polyps are usually about 1 cm in diameter, though they may be smaller or much larger. Most have a short stalk, 1 or 2 cm long. The surface of a juvenile polyp is smooth, pale, and rounded. If a juvenile polyp is transected, the cut surface usually shows cysts filled with mucus set in an edematous stroma.

Microscopically, a juvenile polyp is an edematous blob of hyperplastic mucosa. The cysts are dilated crypts, lined by goblet cells and filled with mucus. Inflammation is usually prominent, sometimes acute with neutrophils, sometimes chronic with plasma cells and lymphocytes.

Occasionally a juvenile polyp causes bleeding. Sometimes a polyp protrudes from the anus or is found by an anxious mother in the child's stool.

Some think that juvenile polyps are hamartomatous. Some think that they are inflammatory. They have no relation to cancer. What happens to them as the child ages is unknown. Some slough off. Most just disappear.

JUVENILE POLYPOSIS. In juvenile polyposis the patients develop numerous juvenile polyps in the colon and sometimes in the small bowel and stomach as well. In some patients, the condition occurs during infancy, causing bleeding, diarrhea, and often intussusception. In other patients, the polyps appear later in life. In some kindred the disease is familial, probably inherited as an autosomal dominant character, and is associated with an increased risk of carcinoma of the colon. In other patients, there is no family history and no increased risk of carcinoma.

CRONKHITE-CANADA SYNDROME. The Cronk-

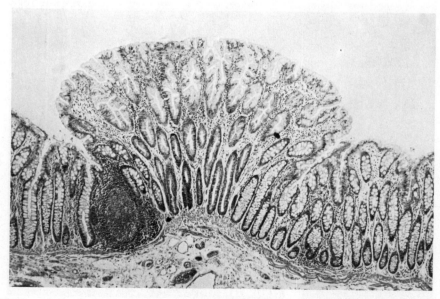

Fig. 35-26. A hyperplastic polyp of the colon, showing the hyperplastic crypts standing a little above the surrounding mucosa.

hite-Canada syndrome is a rare condition in which the patients have multiple juvenile polyps in the stomach and intestine, pigmentation of the skin, alopecia, atrophy of the fingernails and toenails, diarrhea, protein-losing enteropathy, and electrolyte disturbances.

HYPERPLASTIC POLYP. Not uncommonly, small, flat nodules are seen in the rectal or colonic mucosa at endoscopy. The nodules are the same color as the rectal mucosa, a few millimeters in diameter, and are nearly always multiple.

Microscopically, the nodule shows hyperplastic crypts, which are filled with mucus. The epithelium lining the crypts is a little irregular, with a reduction in the number of goblet cells. The lamina propria may be slightly edematous. Some think that the lesion resembles the mucosa of the small bowel and so prefer the term *metaplastic polyp*.

Hyperplastic polyps are the commonest of all the benign tumors and tumor-like lesions of the large intestine. They cause no symptoms. They never grow large. They do not predispose to cancer. They are harmless.

LEIOMYOMA. Leiomyoma is the most common benign mesenchymal tumor of the intestines. In the gastrointestinal tract 65% of leiomyomata occur in the stomach, 5% in the duodenum, 20% in the jejunoileum, 3% in the colon, and 7% in the rectum. The leiomyoma may bulge into the lumen of the bowel, form a mass within the bowel wall, or bulge out into the peritoneal cavity. Sometimes a tumor is dumbbell-shaped, bulging into both the lumen and the celom. Most of the tumors are 1 to 3 cm in diameter, but some grow huge. Microscopically, leiomyomata of the bowel show intertwining bundles of well-differentiated, spindle-shaped leiomyocytes, together with more or less fibrous tissue. The larger tumors often are ulcerated, and the core of the tumor is necrotic, giving a deep ulcer, as in the stomach. Occasionally a leiomyoma of the small bowel causes obstruction, intussusception or hemorrhage.

LIPOMA. Lipomata are fairly common in the small bowel, less frequent in the colon. Most are submucosal. A few are subserosal. Most are 1 to 3 cm in diameter, though larger lipomata can occur. Submucosal lipomata are

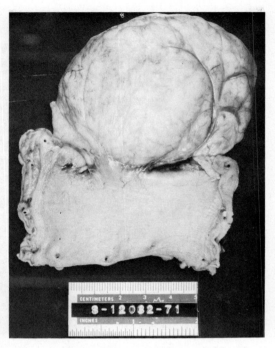

Fig. 35-27. A leiomyoma bulging from the serosal surface of the small bowel.

often polypoid. Sometimes they are numerous. Occasionally a lipoma in the small bowel is large enough to cause obstruction, intussusception, or bleeding.

The ileocecal valve is often enlarged by an excess of fatty tissue. Occasionally the valve is so swollen that it causes obstruction or is mistaken for a tumor.

HEMANGIOMA. A hemangioma of the intestine is found in about 1 autopsy in 14,000. Like other hemangiomata, the lesions are hamartomatous rather than neoplastic. They are most common in the small bowel. A cavernous hemangioma sometimes infiltrates all layers of the bowel wall and thickens and stiffens the bowel wall for 10 cm or more. Other hemangiomata are confined to the submucosa, forming a polypoid mass. Sometimes there is more than one. Hemangiomata of the bowel often are part of one of the syndromes of widespread hemangiomatosis. Rarely, a plexiform angioma occurs in the intestine.

BENIGN LYMPHOID TUMORS. Lymphoid polyps are most common in the rectum,

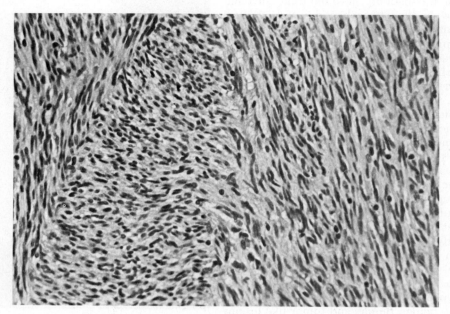

Fig. 35-28. A leiomyoma of the small bowel, showing the intertwining bundles of well-differentiated smooth muscle cells.

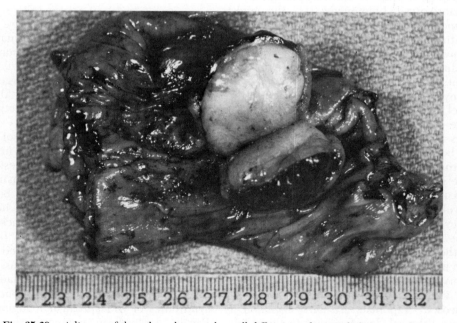

Fig. 35-29. A lipoma of the colon, showing the well-differentiated tumor bulging into the lumen.

usually in people 20 to 40 years old. The lesion may be only 2 or 3 mm across or as much as 3 cm. Occasionally, there is more than one.

The polyp consists of a nodule of lymphoid tissue, lying in the submucosa, covered by intact mucosa. Microscopically, it consists of a clump of lymphocytes, often with prominent germinal centers. The lesion looks much like a little lymph node, except that it has no capsule and no sinusoids.

A lymphoid polyp is sometimes called a benign lymphoma of the rectum, an unfortunate name, for it is not neoplastic and bears no relation to malignant lymphoma. Probably the lesion is inflammatory, a response to minor infection or injury.

Less often, lymphoid polyps like those in the rectum occur in the colon or in the small bowel, usually in children. They are often multiple. Usually the polyps cause no symptoms, but occasionally are associated with intussusception, hypogammaglobulinemia, or malabsorption.

PSEUDOLYMPHOMA. Pseudolymphoma of the intestine is rare. Macroscopically, the lesions are often indistinguishable from a lymphoma or a carcinoma. Microscopically, they show a mixture of different types of well-differentiated inflammatory cell, often with germinal centers in aggregates of lymphocytes. Excision cures.

Malignant

Most primary malignant tumors of the intestine are carcinomata. Carcinoid tumors are most common in the ileum, but occur throughout the intestine. Occasionally a leiomyosarcoma or rarely some other form of malignant mesenchymal tumor arises in the intestine. Sometimes a lymphoma is primary in the small bowel or colon, a mesothelioma arises from the serosa overlying the intestine, or a melanoma takes origin in the anus. Metastases are not uncommon on the serosa of the intestine, but are unusual in the mucosa.

CARCINOMA. The carcinomata of the intestine will be considered in three groups, the carcinoma of the small bowel, carcinoma of the colon and rectum, and carcinoma of the anus.

Small Bowel. Less than 0.2% of malignant tumors and less than 1% of tumors of the intestine arise in the small bowel. About 50% of carcinomata of the small bowel take origin in the duodenum, 75% of them from the ampulla of Vater. Most of the rest develop in the jejunum. Men and women are affected about equally. Most of the patients are over 50 years old.

Lesions. Macroscopically, carcinoma of the ampulla of Vater is often small when obstruction to the bile duct draws attention to the tumor. It sometimes forms a papillary mass, sometimes a small ulcer. Elsewhere in the small bowel, a carcinoma usually thickens and surrounds the bowel wall and extends along its length for 3 to 5 cm. by the time it is discovered. The carcinoma constricts the lumen of the bowel. It is usually ulcerated, with a hard edge that stands above the surrounding mucosa.

Microscopically, the carcinoma of the ampulla of Vater are usually well-differentiated tumors, often with considerable production of mucus. In other parts of the small bowel, the carcinomata form moderately differentiated glands that penetrate the bowel wall, much as do carcinomata of the colon.

Behavior. Carcinoma of the ampulla of Vater invades the biliary and pancreatic ducts and causes obstruction, often drawing attention to the tumor before it has metastasized to the regional lymph nodes. Carcinomata in other parts of the small bowel usually have metastasized to the regional lymph nodes and often by the portal system to the liver before the diagnosis is made.

Clinical Presentation. Obstruction is the principal sign of carcinoma of the small bowel. In most tumors it appears late. The fluid content of the small bowel can easily pass though the segment narrowed by the carcinoma, and symptoms do not develop until the tumor is far advanced. Occasionally a carcinoma of the small bowel bleeds enough to draw attention to it.

Treatment and Prognosis. If possible, a carcinoma of the small bowel is resected. Radiotherapy and chemotherapy are of limited value. Only 25% of the patients survive five years.

Colon and Rectum. In the United States, it is estimated that 15% of all malignant tumors arise in the colon. If carcinoma of the skin is excluded, in men only carcinoma of the lung and carcinoma of the prostate are more common, and in women only carcinoma of the breast and carcinoma of the cervix. It is estimated that in the United States in 1986 140,000 people will develop carcinoma of the colon or rectum. Over 95% of malignant tumors of the intestine arise in the colon. Nearly 70% of carcinomata of the colon arise in women, but 60% of carcinomata of the rectum are in men. The more proximal the tumor, the greater the proportion of colonic carcinomata that arise in women. Most of the patients are over 60 years old.

The incidence of carcinoma of the colon and rectum in Canada, the United Kingdom, northern Europe, and Australasia is similar to that in the United States. In the south of Europe and Japan the incidence is about 50% of that in the United States. In Asia, Africa, and much of South America it is still lower. The reduced incidence in these countries is due principally to a lower incidence of carcinoma of the colon. The incidence of carcinoma of the rectum is little changed.

Lesions. Less than 10% of carcinomata of the large bowel arise in the cecum. About 5% originate in the ascending colon, 2% in the hepatic flexure, 5% in the transverse colon, 3% in the splenic flexure, 5% in the descending colon, 25% in the sigmoid colon, and 45% in the rectum. Carcinoma of the appendix is uncommon.

In the cecum and ascending colon, a carcinoma often forms a fungating mass, from 3 to 10 cm across, which bulges into the lumen with only minor foci of ulceration. The tumors have a broad base, from which the carcinoma invades the bowel wall.

In the transverse colon, descending colon, and sigmoid colon, a carcinoma usually forms a hard mass, which thickens the wall of the bowel and partially or completely encircles it. The carcinoma is usually from 1 to 3 cm thick and extends along the length of the bowel for from 2 to 10 cm. Its hard, raised edge overhangs the adjacent normal mucosa, standing up to 1 cm above it. The center of the carcinoma is ulcerated. The lumen is narrowed. This type of carcinoma is well called a "napkin-ring" tumor.

Napkin ring carcinomata interrupt the peristaltic movements and, particularly in the sigmoid colon where the content of the bowel is becoming thicker, cause obstruction. The bowel proximal to the carcinoma is often dilated, with hypertrophy of its muscle, while the bowel distal to the tumor remains small, with normal musculature.

In the rectum, a carcinoma usually forms a flat ulcer, often 5 to 10 cm across when it is discovered. The ulcer has a hard base and a raised edge that overhangs the surrounding normal mucosa. Occasionally the edge is covered by normal mucosa, so that a biopsy of the edge of the lesion may fail to reach the carcinoma.

Occasionally, a carcinoma of the colon has a stalk and resembles a tubular adenoma. About 10% of carcinomata of the colon are slimy on cross section, because of excessive mucus production by the carcinoma. Rarely, an infiltrating carcinoma like a linitis plastica of the stomach extends for 10 cm or more along a segment of colon.

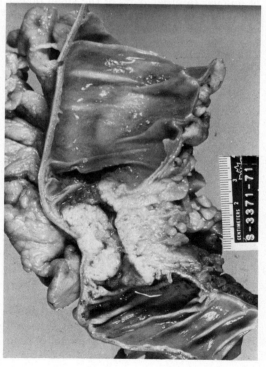

Fig. 35-30. A napkin-ring carcinoma of the sigmoid colon surrounding a narrowing of the lumen of the bowel. The colon proximal to the obstruction is dilated.

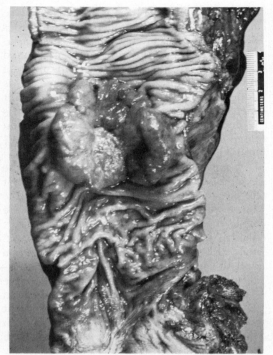

Fig. 35-31. A carcinoma of the rectum, showing the flat, ulcerated tumor close to the anal margin at the bottom of the picture.

Microscopically, more than 80% of carcinomata of the colon and rectum are moderately differentiated adenocarcinomata. The carcinoma forms long, ramifying tubules, which twine through the bowel wall like the roots of a tree. The tubules, or glands as they are usually called, are lined by tall, columnar cells that are moderately pleomorphic. The neoplastic glands are usually supported by an abundant fibrous stroma, explaining the hardness of the carcinoma and the progressive constriction that narrows the lumen in a napkin ring carcinoma. In the ulcerated tumors, secondary infection of the ulcer by the bacteria of the bowel often causes superficial acute and chronic inflammation.

In most carcinomata of the large bowel mucus secretion is not marked. In 10% of the carcinomata, mucus distends the neoplastic tubules in part or most of the tumor. Often the mucus escapes into the stroma to form a colloid carcinoma in which little rafts of carcinoma cells float in pools of mucus.

Occasionally, a carcinoma of the colon consists of sheets of poorly differentiated tumor cells growing with little stroma. Signet-ring cells may be evident. Rarely, an anaplastic carcinoma of the colon has large quantities of collagenous stroma, like linitis plastica of the stomach. Rarely, the stroma of a colonic carcinoma becomes ossified.

Over 4% of the patients develop more than one primary carcinoma of the colon or rectum. In 1%, more than one primary carcinoma is present when the patient is first seen. In the other 3%, the second primary lesion develops later, often five or more years after the first carcinoma has been resected.

Primary malignant tumors in other parts of the body are also common in people with carcinoma of the large bowel. In one series, 8% of patients with carcinoma of the colon or rectum developed a primary malignant tumor in some other part of the body.

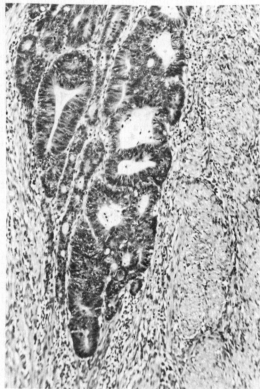

Fig. 35-32. A carcinoma of the colon, showing its tortuous tubules lined by tall, atypical cells extending through the muscularis propria of the sigmoid colon.

Behavior. Carcinomata of the colon and rectum first invade the bowel wall. They extend through the submucosa into the muscularis propria and the subserosa. If the tumor is large, it may extend further, into the mesentery or into adjacent structures.

Sooner or later, the carcinoma gains entry to the regional lymphatics and metastasizes to the regional lymph nodes. The lymph nodes involved can be in or near the bowel wall, at the base of the mesentery, in the para-aortic chain, or in the pelvis. In general, the lymph nodes first involved are those that drain lymph from the tumor. Later, the carcinoma extends to further lymph nodes, up or down the paraaortic chain.

The more extensive the carcinoma, the more likely are lymphatic metastases. With carcinoma of the colon, metastases are found in the regional lymph nodes in less than 50% of the patients in whom the tumor has not extended beyond the colonic wall, but in 90% of those in whom it has invaded the pericolic tissues.

Hematogenous metastases are usually later than is lymphatic extension. Most often, the carcinoma invades small portal veins, and the metastases are confined to the liver. Only late in the course, do carcinomata of the intestine spread more widely. In people dying of carcinoma of the colon, metastases are found in the liver in 75%, in the lungs in 15%, in the bones in 5%, and in the brain in 5%.

Transcelomic spread, with implants on the serosa of the peritoneum is uncommon, but can occur. The ovaries are the most common site of transcelomic extension.

Most carcinomata of the intestine produce the carcinoembryonic antigen. It is detectable in the blood in abnormal quantity in over 90% of people with advanced carcinoma of the colon, though only in 40% of people with small tumors that have not extended beyond the wall of the bowel.

Staging. The classification introduced by the English pathologist Dukes in 1928, or some modification of it, is widely used to measure the extension of carcinoma of the large bowel. In Dukes' classification, carcinomata that have not extended through the muscularis propria are classed as stage A. Carcinomata that have invaded through the whole thickness of the bowel wall but have no metastases in the regional lymph nodes are stage B. Carcinomata that have metastasized to the regional lymph nodes are classed as stage C, irrespective of the depth of direct invasion. Sometimes a fourth stage D is added for those patients with more distant metastases. By the time that a resection is performed, about 15% of carcinomata of the large intestine are stage A, 35% are stage B, and 50% stage C.

Clinical Presentation. Carcinoma of the cecum causes few symptoms until the tumor is far advanced. The fluid content of the bowel flows easily around the tumor in the wide cecum, so that obstruction is unlikely. Pain is unusual until the carcinoma has extended beyond the cecal wall. Often anemia and the weakness it brings are the first indication of the carcinoma. The large, friable carcinoma bleeds easily, oozing blood in multiple, tiny hemorrhages. The blood lost at any one time is not enough to be evident in the stool, but as the oozing continues month after month, it causes iron deficiency anemia.

More distally in the colon, especially in the sigmoid colon, obstruction is often the first sign of carcinoma. The carcinomata are usually of the constricting napkin ring type, and more distally the feces grow thicker and harder to force through the narrow segment. There may be a feeling of fullness in the abdomen or cramping pain as the proximal part of the colon contracts strongly to force the feces past the obstruction. Constipation occurs in 50% of the patients and tends to grow more severe. Sometimes there is diarrhea, sometimes alternating with obstruction. Oversecretion of mucus may be evident in the stool. Often there is blood in the stool, perhaps streaks of red blood, perhaps dark, altered blood mixed with the stool. Pain in the back may develop if the carcinoma extends into the paracolic tissues.

Carcinoma of the rectum often presents with bleeding. The blood may be red or may be dark. There may be streaks of blood on the stool, or more severe bleeding. Iron deficiency anemia can develop. Discomfort on defecation or a feeling of fullness in the rectum are sometimes noted. There may be diarrhea, constipation, or now one, now the other. Pain is unusual, unless the carcinoma has invaded beyond the rectum.

Complications. In 3% of patients with carcinoma of the colon, the bowel perforates through the carcinoma. A pericolic abscess follows or, rarely, peritonitis. If a carcinoma invades a neighboring viscus, a fistula can develop, most often from the colon to the urinary bladder or the vagina. Radiation therapy, by causing necrosis of the tumor, increases the risk of a fistula. Rarely, there is massive hemorrhage from a carcinoma of the intestine.

Etiology. The discovery of remnants of adenoma in 60% of early carcinomata of the colon which have not spread through the submucosa suggests that at least 60% of carcinomata of the colon arise in adenomata. Remnants of adenoma are found in only 20% of carcinomata that have invaded the tunica muscularis propria but have not spread beyond the colon and in 7% of tumors that have invaded the extracolic tissues. Presumably, as the carcinoma grows larger it destroys the adenoma from which it arose.

Also in favor of the theory that most carcinomata of the colon arise from adenomata is the observation that if one or more adenomata are present in the portion of colon resected for carcinoma of the colon, 7% of the patients subsequently develop a second carcinoma of the colon. If no adenomata are found, less than 3% do so.

The relationship between adenomata and carcinoma is not, however, simple. Adenomatous polyps are fairly evenly distributed throughout the colon, but most carcinomata develop in the sigmoid or the rectum. If most carcinomata arise in adenomata, those on the left side of the colon are more likely to become malignant than those on the right, perhaps because dysplasia and villous lesions are more common on the left.

The high rate of carcinoma of the colon in the more developed countries has been related to the low content of fiber in the diet in these countries. The many kinds of fiber in the diet have different properties, and it could be that some kinds of fiber protect the colon aganst carcinoma. There are, of course, other differences between the countries in which carcinoma of the colon is common and those in which it is not.

It has been suggested that bacteria in the colon might make carcinogens from bile acids or some other substrate. Nitrosamines can induce both adenomata and carcinomata in the colon in animals. Exposure to large quantities of asbestos doubles the risk of developing carcinoma of the colon.

It is not known why ulcerative colitis increases the risk of developing carcinoma of the colon. The risk of carcinoma in multiple polyposis probably increases because the adenomata are so numerous, not because an individual adenoma is more likely to become malignant. Carcinoma of the colon sometimes develops when urine is diverted into the colon by a ureterosigmoidostomy, but a ureteroileostomy does not seem to increase the risk of carcinoma in either the small or the large bowel.

Treatment and Prognosis. Carcinomata of the colon and rectum are resected, if this is possible. If not, palliative radiation, chemotherapy, or cauterization of the tumor offers relief for a time. In old people, carcinoma of the rectum often progresses slowly, and cauterization of the tumor may be enough to allow the patient to live in comfort.

If a carcinoma of the colon or rectum is of Dukes' stage A, nearly 100% of the patients are cured. If it is of stage B, the cure rate is about 70%. If the lymph nodes are involved, only 30% of the patients will be alive five years later. Death usually comes from metastases, though in people with carcinoma of the rectum or rectosigmoid local recurrence of the carcinoma can cause death.

The carcinoembryonic antigen is useful to determine whether an extensive carcinoma has been completely removed. If the carcinoma is completely excised, the concentration of the antigen in the blood should fall to normal levels. It is also useful in following patients after resection of a carcinoma of the colon. If the concentration of the carcinoembryonic antigen in the blood begins to rise again after falling to normal, it suggests that the carcinoma has recurred, either locally or in metastases.

Anus. Only 1% of malignant tumors of the intestine develop in the anus. There are two types of anal carcinoma. Carcinomata of the anal margin are squamous cell carcinomata. Carcinomata of the anal canal are

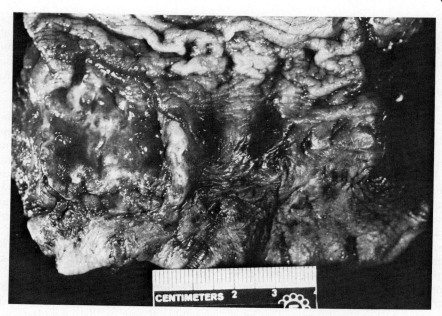

Fig. 35-33.   A carcinoma of the anus, showing an ulcerated tumor at the anal margin.

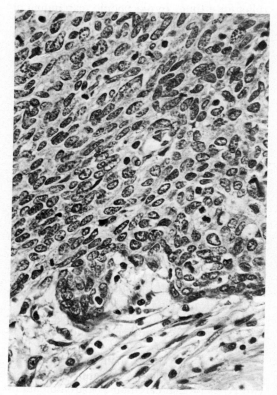

Fig. 35-34.   A basaloid carcinoma of the anus, showing the small, dark cells that make up this form of carcinoma.

basaloid or cloacogenic carcinomata. Some 25% of the anal carcinomata arise in the anal margin; 75% are basaloid carcinomata of the anal canal. About 80% of patients with a squamous cell carcinoma of the anal margin are men; 60% of those with a basaloid carcinoma are women. The patients are usually over 50 years old.

Lesions.   A carcinoma of the anus often forms a small, warty mass, 1 to 2 cm across, but sometimes resembles a fissure of the anus, forms a lump 2 to 3 cm across, which bulges from the anal canal, or a flat ulcer, like a carcinoma of the skin.

The squamous cell carcinomata of the anal margin sometimes resemble moderately differentiated squamous cell carcinomata of the skin, with prickle cells and keratinization. More often, they are less differentiated and resemble carcinomata of the cervix uteri.

The basaloid carcinomata form clumps of tumor cells separated by a collagenous stroma. The tumor cells are usually small and dark, like the cells of a basal cell carcinoma of the skin. The clumps often have a peripheral palisade of tumor cells. Foci of sudden keratinization can often be found in the clumps of tumor cells, sometimes forming keratin pearls. In many basaloid carcinomata, the core of the clumps of tumor cells is necrotic, leaving only a thin margin of viable tumor at the periphery. Occasionally, parts of a basaloid tumor form mucus. Occasionally the tumor cells are more pleomorphic and anaplastic.

Behavior. Squamous cell carcinomata of the anal margin spread to the inguinal lymph nodes. Metastases are present in 40% of the patients by the time the tumor is diagnosed.

Basaloid carcinomata of the anal canal spread both to the pelvic and to the inguinal lymph nodes. Over 40% of the patients have metastases in the pelvic lymph nodes when the tumor is resected, and 30% show involvement of the inguinal lymph nodes. Probably the pelvic lymph nodes are usually involved first.

Clinical Presentation. Carcinoma of the anus causes tenesmus, pain, itching, and bleeding.

Treatment and Prognosis. Carcinoma of the anus is treated surgically, often with resection of the lymph nodes that drain the region. About 50% of the patients with a squamous cell carcinoma of the anal margin survive five years. Some 40% of patients with a basaloid carcinoma of the anus survive five years. If the carcinoma is well differentiated and there are no metastases to the lymph nodes, the cure rate is over 50%. If it is poorly differentiated and lymph nodes are involved, less than 30% of the patients survive five years.

CARCINOID TUMOR. Carcinoid tumors arise from the neuroendocrine cells in the intestine, biliary tract, lungs, and occasionally in an ovary. They are closely related to the islet cell tumors of the pancreas and to neuroendocrine tumors that arise in other organs. In the lungs, some prefer to call these tumors neuroendocrine tumors or neuroendocrine carcinomata, but in the intestine carcinoid tumor is preferred. The term *carcinoid* was coined in 1907 to indicate that these tumors looked like carcinomata microscopically but were benign. Further experience showed that they were malignant, but the name has been preserved to distinguish the carcinoid tumors from the more common form of intestinal adenocarcinoma.

The neuroendocrine cells are so named because at one time they were believed to arise from the neural crest. This is not the case. The neuroendocrine cells in the intestine differentiate from the stem cells in the intestinal crypts, like other epithelial cells in the intestine. The tumors of the intestinal epithelium sometimes show more than one kind of differentiation. In some intestinal tumors of other types, an occasional neuroendocrine cell is present. Some carcinoid tumors produce mucus, like the mucus-secreting cells of the intestinal epithelium.

Occasionally the neuroendocrine cells are called APUD cells, **A**mine **P**recursor **U**ptake and **D**ecarboxylation cells, because some of them take up amines and decarboxylate them. The neuroendocrine tumors are sometimes called apudomata.

Two kinds of carcinoid tumor of the intestine are distinguished. In most, the tumor cells produce predominantly 5-hydroxytryptamine and kallikrein or bradykinin. In others, the production of one or more polypeptide hormones such as gastrin, enteroglucagon, secretin, motilin, vasoactive intestinal peptide, gastrointestinal polypeptide, bombesin, cholecystokinin, or pancreozymin is predominant. Sometimes neuroendocrine tumors that secrete predominantly one of the polypeptide hormones are named after the hormone they produce. A tumor that produces gastrin is called a gastrinoma; one that produces insulin is called an insulinoma.

Over 70% of intestinal carcinoid tumors arise in the appendix and 20% occur in the ileum. Less often a carcinoid tumor is found in the stomach, duodenum, jejunum, colon, or rectum. A carcinoid tumor is found in 1 appendix in every 600 resected. A carcinoid tumor of the gastrointestinal tract is found in 1 autopsy in 500, usually in the ileum. The carcinoid tumors in the appendix and ileum nearly all produce predominantly 5-hydroxytryptamine, while those in other parts of the gastrointestinal tract usually produce mainly one or more of the polypeptide hormones.

In the appendix, 70% of carcinoids arise in women. Elsewhere in the gastrointestinal system, they are equally common in men and women. In the appendix, most carcinoid tumors are found in people 10 to 30 years old, by accident, when the appendix is removed for some other reason. Carcinoid tumors in other parts of the gastrointestinal

polypeptide hormones. They do not stain with the argentaffin, diazo, or chromaffin reactions. The nature of their secretion is best determined by immunohistochemical means. Carcinoids of types C and D produce little or no secretion.

Carcinoid tumors of the appendix and ileum often cause hypertrophy of the muscularis propria as they invade it. The muscle bundles within the tumor are larger and more prominent than normal. Often intimal thickening of the arteries and veins in the uninvolved bowel adjacent to the tumor is sufficient to cause stenosis and ischemia in the adjacent mucosa.

Behavior. Carcinoid tumors grow slowly. Probably most carcinoid tumors have been present for many years before they are detected.

Carcinoids of the appendix rarely metastasize. They often extend through the whole thickness of the appendiceal wall, but go no further.

Over 50% of carcinoid tumors of the ileum have spread to the regional lymph nodes by the time the tumor is discovered. In the rectum, about 10% of the tumors, usually larger tumors, have metastasized by the time the carcinoid is discovered. Carcinoid tumors of the stomach, duodenum and jejunum sometimes metastasize to the regional lymph nodes.

In the lymph nodes, carcinoid tumors continue to grow slowly. They spread from lymph node to lymph node, until the mass of tumor in the lymph nodes becomes large.

Sooner or later, the carcinoid gains entry to the portal venules. Emboli of tumor cells are carried to the liver and establish metastases there. More distant hematogenous dissemination is unusual.

Clinical Presentation. Because of their small size and slow growth, most carcinoid tumors are found by accident. Most are removed because the patient develops appendicitis or an appendix is removed in the course of some other operation. Occasionally, a carcinoid of the small bowel causes obstruction, because of the kinking it produces.

Carcinoid Syndrome. The carcinoid syndrome develops when the mass of a carcinoid tumor that produces 5-hydroxytryptamine grows large. Usually, there are extensive metastases in the retroperitoneal lymph nodes and often metastases in the liver as well.

Episodes of watery diarrhea are the commonest feature of the carcinoid syndrome and often its first sign. Episodes of flushing involve particularly the head and neck. They commonly occur several times a day and often last up to 10 minutes. Patches of cyanosis develop in the flushed skin. Eventually, the patients develop a permanent reddish-purple discoloration of the face, with telangiectasia in the affected skin. In 50% of the patients, the heart valves on the right side of the heart, rarely on the left, are sclerotic. In 30% of the patients, episodes of bronchospasm are troublesome.

The carcinoid syndrome is caused by the presence in the systemic blood of 5-hydroxytryptamine, kinins, and other products released by the tumor. The tumor and its metastases in the abdominal lymph nodes release their secretions into the portal blood. The liver detoxifies 5-hydroxytryptamine and perhaps other products of the tumor. If the tumor and its metastases are not large, no 5-hydroxytryptamine reaches the systemic circulation. The carcinoid syndrome develops only when the bulk of the tumor is so great that it produces more 5-hydroxytryptamine than the liver can detoxify or when metastases in the liver discharge their products into the hepatic veins.

The 5-hydroxyindoleacetic acid produced by the detoxification of 5-hydroxytryptamine is excreted in the urine. If the quantity of 5-hydroxytryptamine produced by a carcinoid tumor and its metastases is sufficiently great, 5-hydroxyindoleacetic acid can be detected in the urine and serves to confirm the diagnosis.

Treatment and Prognosis. The treatment of carcinoid tumors is surgical. Complete excision of the tumor and its metastases cures. If this is not possible, carcinoid tumors grow so slowly that resection of most of the metastases often relieves the patient of symptoms for many years.

LEIOMYOSARCOMA. A leiomyosarcoma of the intestine usually forms a large mass, which becomes attached to neighboring structures. Sometimes the core of the tumor becomes necrotic, and a deep ulcer penetrates far into

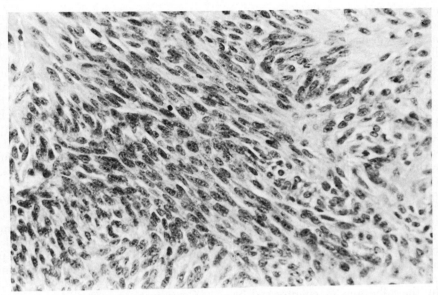

Fig. 35-37. A leiomyosarcoma of the bowel, showing intertwining bundles of moderately atypical cells.

the sarcoma. Hemorrhage may be severe. Microscopically, leiomyosarcomata of the intestine are well differentiated, with the usual intertwining bundles of spindle-shaped leiomyocytes. The tumors grow slowly and metastasize late.

LYMPHOMA. Occasionally, a malignant lymphoma occurs with lesions in the bowel in a person who does not have alpha heavy chain disease, without evidence of involvement of other parts of the body. Usually, the lesion or lesions are in the ileum, though any part of the bowel can be affected. The patient is usually an adult over 40 years old or a child.

The lymphoma most often thickens and surrounds the wall of the bowel, with ulceration of the mucosa, stenosis, and obstruction, producing a lesion much like a napkin ring carcinoma. Less often it is polypoid, with one or more malignant polyps bulging into the lumen of the bowel, or a large, fungating mass projects into the lumen of the bowel. Especially in children, a lymphoma of the small bowel can cause intussusception.

Most lymphomata that present with lesions in the bowel are non-Hodgkin's lymphomata of B cell origin. Often they are poorly differentiated.

The prognosis is bad. The lymphoma soon becomes disseminated. Few patients with a lymphoma arising in the bowel survive more than two years.

METASTASIS. Transcelomic spread of a carcinoma occasionally causes serosal metastases on the intestine. The primary tumor is most often in an ovary or the stomach. Less often a metastasis or metastases develop in the mucosa of the bowel. The primary tumor is most often a small cell carcinoma of a lung, a malignant melanoma, or a lymphoma.

OBSTRUCTION

Intestinal obstruction is common. It may be complete, with total obstruction of the lumen, or partial, allowing a little of the intestinal content to pass. Its causes and effects depend on whether the obstruction is in the small bowel or the colon.

SMALL BOWEL. Obstruction in the small bowel may be due to failure of peristalsis or to mechanical obliteration of the lumen.

Intestinal obstruction resulting from a failure of peristaltic movement is called ileus, from the Greek word meaning colic. Usually the muscle of the affected part of the bowel is flaccid and relaxed, and the condition is called paralytic ileus, or adynamic ileus. Less often, the affected part of the bowel is in spasm, and the condition is called spastic ileus. Ileus is common after surgical procedures and in major illnesses such as pneumonia or myocardial infarction. It is almost universal in peritonitis. It sometimes complicates renal colic or other painful diseases of the abdomen, results from severe hypokalemia, or is caused by drugs and other agents that interfere with the synthesis of acetylcholine. Pseudo-obstruction is the name given a rare syndrome in which repeated episodes of ileus occur as the years pass, without predisposing cause and without significant lesion in the bowel.

Pressure from without is a common cause of obstruction in the small bowel. In over 50% of patients with mechanical obstruction of the small bowel, the obstruction is caused by adhesions. The bowel is angulated or kinked by the adhesions or compressed between them. In 20% of the patients, the obstruction is caused by the narrow neck of a hernia. Sometimes it is due to the pressure of a tumor, an abscess, or some other mass adjacent to the bowel. Volvulus can obstruct the small bowel. Often the external pressure impairs the blood supply to the bowel, adding ischemic enteritis to the injury.

Less often the obstruction results from a lesion in the wall of the bowel. Crohn's disease is the most common cause.

Still less often, obstruction to the small bowel is caused by a foreign body in the lumen, something swallowed, a gallstone that has ulcerated from the gallbladder into the small bowel, or a mass of worms. A polypoid tumor sometimes blocks a narrow intestine. Intussusception is an important cause of obstruction in children.

Ischemia causes obstruction by inhibiting peristalsis, if the ischemic segment of bowel is long enough, and the ischemia involves the muscularis propria.

Clinical Presentation. Mechanical obstruction in the small bowel causes periumbilical colic. The bowel sounds become hyperactive as the intestine struggles to force its content past the obstruction, and the violent contractions cause the pain. Vomiting soon follows. At first the vomitus contains bile and mucus, but later sometimes develops a fecal odor, especially if the obstruction

is low. After a few hours, the obstructed bowel becomes distended, and the lower the obstruction, the greater the distention. As the distention increases, pain becomes less, as the strong contractions of the intestinal muscle weaken. The pain may become constant if the bowel wall becomes inflamed because of ischemia or secondary bacterial infection. The bowel may become tender. At first there is often diarrhea, as the bowel below the obstruction is cleared, but then comes obstipation if the obstruction is complete.

In paralytic ileus, distention and obstipation are the main signs. Vomiting is not usually severe. Pain is absent, as the muscle of the intestine lies still and flaccid. Bowel sounds are absent because of the paralysis of the muscle. The abdomen is ominously silent.

Complications. Fluid loss is considerable when the small bowel is obstructed. Normally, 7 to 10 L of water and electrolytes pour into the small bowel daily, and most of this fluid is resorbed. In obstruction, it collects in the dilating bowel above the obstruction, and even without vomiting can cause major loss of water and electrolytes. There is likely to be dehydration, with hypochloremia and metabolic alkalosis. Hypokalemia can contribute to the weakening of the intestinal muscle. The loss of electrolytes is most severe when the upper small bowel is involved. Renal failure with azotemia may follow, or sometimes there is hypovolemic shock.

Gas accumulates in the distended bowel above the obstruction. Most of it comes from aerophagy, but some is formed by the bacteria that proliferate above the obstruction.

Treatment and Prognosis. Patients with ileus are managed by decompressing the bowel with a nasal tube. Recovery usually comes spontaneously. Mechanical obstruction requires surgical relief after decompressing the bowel and restoring hydration and electrolyte balance. About 10% of the patients die, more if strangulation adds ischemia to obstruction.

LARGE BOWEL. Carcinoma of the colon is the most common cause of obstruction in the large bowel, and together with diverticulitis and volvulus is responsible in 90% of the patients.

Clinical Presentation. Pain is less evident in obstruction of the large bowel than when the small bowel is affected. Elderly patients sometimes make no mention of abdominal discomfort. Vomiting occurs late if at all. Fecal vomiting is unusual. Often the principal sign of the obstruction is gradually worsening constipation leading to obstipation after a week or more.

Complications. If the obstruction is not relieved, increasing distention of the cecum is likely to cause gangrene and perforation if the diameter of the cecum exceeds 10 cm.

Treatment and Prognosis. Obstruction to the large bowel is usually treated by establishing a colostomy proximal to the obstruction to relieve the pressure in the bowel and, if possible, resecting the cause of the obstruction subsequently. The mortality is about 20%.

BIBLIOGRAPHY

General

Brocklehurst, J. C.: Colonic disease in the elderly. Clin. Gastroenterol., *14*:725, 1985.

Cotterill, A. M., and Walker-Smith, J. A.: Gastrointestinal tract. Br. Med. Bull., *42*:176, 1986.

Gray, G. F., Jr., and Wackym, P. A.: Surgical pathology of the vermiform appendix. Pathol. Annu., *21*(Pt 2):111, 1986.

Holt, P. R.: The small intestine. Clin. Gastroenterol., *14*:689, 1985.

James, O. F. W. (Ed.): Gastrointestinal disorders in the elderly. Clin. Gastroenterol., *14*:635, 1986.

Morson, B. C.: The alimentary tract. *In* Systemic Pathology, 3rd ed., vol 3. Edited by W. StC. Symmers. Edinburgh, Churchill Livingstone, 1987.

Morson, B. C., and Dawson, I. M. P.: Gastrointestinal Pathology, 2nd ed. Oxford, Blackwell Scientific Publications, 1979.

Rotterdam, H., and Sommers, S. C.: Biopsy diagnosis of the digestive tract. New York, Raven Press, 1981.

Rotterdam, H., and Sommers, S. C.: Alimentary tract biopsy lesions in the acquired immune deficiency syndrome. Pathology, *17*:181, 1985.

Whitehead, R.: Mucosal Biopsy of the Gastrointestinal Tract, 3rd ed. Philadelphia, W. B. Saunders, 1986.

Inflammatory Disease

Almy, T. P., and Rothstein, R. I.: Irritable bowel syndrome. Annu. Rev. Med., *38*:257, 1987.

Blackshaw, A. J., and Levison, D. A.: Eosinophilic infiltrates of the gastrointestinal tract. J. Clin. Pathol.,
39:1, 1986.

Christophi, C., and Hughes, E. R.: Hepatobiliary disorders in inflammatory bowel disease. Surg. Gynecol. Obstet., *160*:187, 1985.

Clouse, R. E., et al.: Gut and joint disease. Annu. Rev. Med., *37*:283, 1986.

Davidson, A. G., and Bridges, M. A.: Coeliac disease. Clin. Chem. Acta, *163*:1, 1987.

Dobbins, W. O., III.: Dysplasia and malignancy in inflammatory bowel disease. Annu. Rev. Med., *35*:33, 1984.

Dobbins, W. O., III.: Human intestinal intraepithelial lymphocytes. Gut, *27*:972, 1986.

Elson, C. O.: Intestinal immunity and inflammation. Gastroenterology, *91*:746, 1986.

Fazio, V. W.: Complex anal fistulae. Clin. Gastroenterol., *16*:93, 1987.

Gore, A. M., and Ghahremani, G. G.: Crohn's disease of the upper gastrintestinal tract. CRC Crit. Rev. Diagn Imaging, *25*:305, 1986.

Greenstein, A. J.: The surgery of Crohn's disease. Surg. Clin. North Am., *67*:573, 1987.

Hamilton, S. R.: Pathologic features of Crohn's disease associated with recrudescence after resection. Pathol. Annu., *18*(Pt. 1):191, 1983.

Hermanowicz, A., Gibson, P. R., and Jewell, D. P.: The role of phagocytes in inflammatory bowel disease. Clin. Sci., *69*:241, 1985.

Hertzberg, J.: Crohn's disease. Ann. Gastroenterol. Hepatol. (Paris), *21*:227, 1985.

Hodgson, H. J.: Inflammatory bowel disease and food intolerance. J. R. Coll. Physicians Lond., *20*:45, 1986.

Jewell, D. P., and Patel, C.: Immunology of inflammatory bowel disease. Scand. J. Gastroenterol. [Suppl.], *114*:119, 1985.

Kirsner, J. B., and Shorter, R. G. (Eds.): Inflammatory Bowel Disease, 3rd Ed. Philadelphia, Lea & Febiger, 1988.

Lennard-Jones, J. E.: Cancer risk in ulcerative colitis. Br. J. Surg., *72*(Suppl.):S64, 1985.

Lieberman, D. A.: Common anorectal disorders. Ann. Intern. Med., *101*:837, 1984.

MacDermott, R. P.: Cell-mediated immunity in gastrointestinal disease. Hum. Pathol., *17*:219, 1986.

Mackle, E. J., and Parks, T. G.: The pathogenesis and pathophysiology of rectal prolapse and solitary rectal ulcer syndrome. Clin. Gastroenterol., *15*:985, 1986.

Morson, B. C.: Precancer and cancer in inflammatory bowel disease. Pathology, *17*:173, 1985.

Rowland, R., and Pounder, D. J.: Crohn's colitis. Pathol. Annu., *17*(Pt. 1):267, 1982.

Sanderson, I. R.: Chronic inflammatory bowel disease. Clin. Gastroenterol., *15*:71, 1986.

van Spreeuwel, J. P., et al.: Immuno-globulin-containing cells in gastrointestinal pathology. Pathol. Annu., *21*(Pt. 1):295, 1986.

Stenson, W. F., et al.: Immunology in inflammatory bowel disease. Yearbook Immunol., *2*:329, 1986.

Strober, W.: Animal models of inflammatory bowel disease. Dig. Dis. Sci., *30*(12 Suppl.):3S, 1985.

Targan, S. R., et al.: Immunologic mechanisms in intestinal disease. Ann. Intern. Med., *106*:853, 1987.

Whitehead, W. E., et al.: Anorectal physiology and pathophysiology. Am. J. Gasteroenterol., *82*:487, 1987.

Diverticula

Englund, R., and Jensen, M.: Acquired diverticulosis of the small intestine. Aust. N. Z. J. Surg., 56:51, 1986.

Maglinte, D. D., et al.: Acquired jejunoileal diverticular disease. Radiology, 158:577, 1986.

Smith, A. N.: Colonic muscle in diverticular disease. Clin. Gastroeneterol., 15:917, 1986.

Spiller, G. A. (ed.): CRC Handbook of Dietary Fiber in Human Nutrition. Boca Raton, CRC Press, 1986.

Whiteway, J., and Morson, B. C.: Pathology of the ageing—diverticular disease. Clin. Gastroenterol., 14:829, 1985.

Whiteway, J., and Morson, B. C.: Diverticular disease. Clin. Gasroenterol., 14:429, 1986.

Vascular Disorders

Barrett, J. F., and Jamieson, M. H.: Massive lower gastro-intestinal bleeding. S. Afr. J. Surg., 23:110, 1985.

Boley, S. J., Brandt, L. J., and Mitsudo, S. M.: Vascular lesions of the colon. Adv. Intern. Med., 29:301, 1984.

Camilleri, M., Chadwick, V. S., and Hodgson, H. J. F.: Vascular anomalies of the gastrointestinal tract. Hepatogastroenterology, 31:149, 1984.

de Louvois, J.: Necrotizing enterocolitis. J. Hospit. Infect., 7:4, 1986.

Kliegman, R. M.: Necrotizing enterocolitis. N. Engl. J. Med., 310:1093, 1984.

Mitsudo, S. M., et al.: Vascular ectasias of the right colon in the elderly. Hum. Pathol., 10:585, 1979.

Price, A. B., and Day, D. W.: Pseudomembranous and infective colitis. Rec. Adv. Histopathol., 11:99, 1981.

Rees, H. C., and Wright, N. A.: Angiodysplasia of the colon. Rec. Adv. Histopathol., 12:178, 1984.

Smith, L. E.: Hemorrhoids. Clin. Gastroenterol., 16:79, 1987.

Whitehead, R.: The pathology of ischemia of the intestines. Pathol. Annu., 11:1, 1976.

Mechanical Disorders

Cullen, M. L., Klein, M. D., and Philippart, A.: Congenital diaphragmatic hernia. Surg. Clin. North Am., 65:1115, 1985.

Malabsorption

Auricchio, S., De Ritis, G., De Vincenzi, M. D., and Silano, V.: Toxicity mechanisms of wheat and other cereals in celiac disease and related enteropathies. J. Pediatr. Gastroenterol. Nutr., 4:923, 1985.

Butkus, S. N., et al.: Food allergies. J. Am. Diet. Assoc., 86:601, 1986.

Cant, A. J.: Food allergy in childhood. Hum. Nutr. Appl. Nutr., 39:277, 1985.

Feldman, M.: Whipple's disease. Am. J. Med. Sci., 291:56, 1986.

Harty, R. F., and Leirach, J. R.: Immune disorders of the gastrointestinal tract and liver. Med. Clin. North Am., 69:675, 1985.

Kagnoff, M. F.: Coeliac disease: genetic, immunological and environmental factors in disease pathogenesis. Scand. J. Gastroenterol. [Suppl.], 114:45, 1985.

Keusch, G. T., et al.: Microorganisms, malabsorption, diarrhea and dysnutrition. J. Environ. Pathol. Toxicol. Oncol., 5:165, 1985.

MacDermott, R. P.: Cell-mediated immunity in gastrointestinal disease. Hum. Pathol., 17:219, 1986.

Marsh, M. N.: Functional and structural aspects of the epithelial lymphocyte, with implications for coeliac disease and tropical sprue. Scand. J. Gastroenterol. [Suppl.], 114:55, 1986.

Mathias, J. R., and Clench, M. H.: Pathophysiology of diarrhea caused by bacterial overgrowth in the small intestine. Am. J. Med. Sci., 289:243, 1985.

Pearson, D. J., and McKee, A.: Food allergy. Adv. Nutr. Res., 7:1, 1985.

Saavedra-Delgado, A. M., et al.: Interactions between food antigens and the immune system in the pathogenesis of gastrointestinal diseases. Ann. Allergy, 55:694, 1985.

van Spreeuwel, J. P., et al.: Immuno-globulin-containing cells in gastrointestinal pathology. Pathol. Annu., 21(Pt. 1):295, 1986.

Targan, S. R., et al.: Immunologic mechanisms in intestinal disease. Ann. Intern. Med., 106:853, 1987.

Walker-Smith, J. A.: Food sensitive enteropathies. Clin. Gastroenterol., 15:55, 1986.

Walker-Smith, J. A.: Milk intolerance in children. Clin. Allergy, 16:183, 1986.

Weiner, S. R., and Utsinger, P.: Whipple's disease. Semin. Arthritis Rheumatol., 15:157, 1986.

Westergaard, H.: The sprue syndromes. Am. J. Med. Sci., 290:249, 1985.

Ziegler, M. M.: Short bowel syndrome in infancy. Clin. Perinatol., 13:163, 1986.

Other Nonneoplastic Conditions

Berthrong, M.: Pathologic changes secondary to radiation. World J. Surg., 10:155, 1986.

Lewis, J. H.: Gastrointestinal injury due to medicinal agents. Am. J. Gastroenterol., 81:819, 1986.

Mackle, E. J., and Parks, T. G.: The pathogenesis and pathophysiology of rectal prolapse and solitary rectal ulcer syndrome. Clin. Gastroenterol, 15:985, 1986.

Michalowski, A., and Hornsey, S.: Assays of damage to the alimentary canal. Br. J. Cancer, [Suppl.], 7:1, 1986.

Wassef, R., Rothenberger, D. A., and Goldberg, S. M.: Rectal prolapse. Curr. Probl. Surg., 23:397, 1986.

Tumors

Ahlman, H.: Midgut carcinoid tumors. Surg. Annu., 19:65, 1986.

Bruce, W. R.: What chemicals are responsible for colon cancer? J. Cell. Physiol. [Suppl.], 4:47, 1986.

Bussey, H. J. R.: Gastrointestinal polyposis syndromes. Rec. Adv. Histopathol., 12:169, 1984.

Cooper, B. T., and Read, A. E.: Small intestinal lymphoma. World J. Surg., 9:930, 1985.

Dobbins, W. O., III.: Dysplasia and malignancy in inflammatory bowel disease. Annu. Rev. Med., 35:33, 1984.

Floch, M. H.: Fiber, foods, and gastrointestinal microecology. J. Environ. Pathol. Toxicol. Oncol., 5:233, 1985.

Friedman, E. A.: A multistage model for human colon carcinoma development. Cancer Invest., 3:453, 1985.

Gittes, R. F.: Carcinogenesis in ureterosigmoidoscopy. Urol. Clin. North Am., 13:201, 1986.

Greenall, M. J., et al.: Epidermoid carcinoma of the anus. Br. J. Surg., 72(Suppl):S97, 1985.

Ingall, J. R. F., and Mastromarino, A. J.: Carcinoma of the Large Bowel and its Precursors. New York, Alan R. Liss, 1985.

Knudsen, I. (Ed.): Genetic toxicology of the diet. Prog. Clin. Biol. Res., 206:1, 1986.

Lennard-Jones, J. E.: Cancer risk in ulcerative colitis. Br. J. Surg., 72(Suppl.):S64, 1985.

Levine, D. S.: Does asbestos exposure cause gastrointestinal cancer? Dig. Dis. Sci., 30:1189, 1985.

Lewin, K. J.: The endocrine cells of the gastrointestinal tract. The normal cells and their hyperplasias. Part I. Pathol. Annu., 21(Pt. 1):1, 1986.

Lewin, K. J., Ulich, T., Yang, K., and Layfield, L.: The endocrine cells of the gastrointestinal tract. Tumors. Part II. Pathol. Annu., 21(Pt. 2):181, 1986.

Mendelsohn, G.: Vasoactive intestinal peptide (VIP) and the spectrum of tumors producing the watery diarrhea syndrome. Prog. Surg. Pathol., 4:199, 1982.

Mills, S. E., and Cooper, P. H.: Malignant melanoma of the digestive system. Pathol. Annu., 18(Pt. 2):1, 1983.

Morson, B. C. (Ed.): The Pathogenesis of Colorectal Cancer. Philadelphia, W. B. Saunders, 1978.

Morson, B. C.: Precancer and cancer in inflammatory bowel disease. Pathology, 17:173, 1985.

Northover, J. M.: Carcinoembryonic antigen and recurrent colorectal cancer. Br. J. Surg., 72(Suppl.):S44, 1985.

Qizilbash, A. H.: Pathologic studies in colorectal cancer. Pathol. Annu., 17(Pt. 1):1, 1982.

Remmele, W.: Staging, typing and grading of colorectal cancer. Prog. Surg. Pathol., 5:7, 1983.

Richards, M. A.: Lymphoma of the colon and rectum. Postgrad. Med. J., 62:615, 1986.

Shively, J. E., and Beatty, J. D.: CEA-related antigens. CRC Crit. Rev. Oncol. Hematol., 2:355, 1985.

Skinner, J., M.: Gastrointestinal lymphoma. Pathology, 17:193, 1985.

Spiller, G. A. (Ed.): CRC Handbook of Dietary Fiber in Human Nutrition. Boca Raton, CRC Press, 1986.

Stearns, M. J., Jr., et al.: Cancer of the anal canal. Curr. Probl. Cancer, 4(12):1, 1980.

Stevenson, R. J.: Abdominal masses. Surg. Clin. North Am., 65:1481, 1985.

Trump, B. F., et al.: Preneoplasia and neoplasia of the bronchus, esophagus, and colon. Monogr. Pathol., 26:101, 1986.

Watne, A. L.: Syndromes of polyposis coli and cancer. Curr. Probl. Cancer, 7:1, 1982.

Weisburger, J. H.: Role of fat, fiber, nitrate and food additives in carcinogenesis. Nutr. Cancer, 8:47, 1986.

Wilcox, G. M., Anderson. P. B., and Colacchio, T. A.: Early invasive carcinoma in colonic polyps. Cancer, 57:160, 1986.

Wood, D. A.: Tumors of the Intestine. Washington D. C., Armed Forces Institute of Pathology, 1967.

Obstruction

Isaacs, P., and Keshhavarzian, A.: Intestinal pseudo-obstruction. Postgrad. Med. J., 61:1033, 1985.

Milla, P. J.: Intestinal motility and its disorders. Clin. Gastroenterol., 15:121, 1986.

Mucha, P., Jr.: Small intestinal obstruction. Surg. Clin. North Am., 67:597, 1987.

Vantrappen, G., Janssens, J., Coremans, G., and Jian, R.: Gastrointestinal motility disorders. Dig. Dis. Sci., 31(Suppl. 9):5S, 1986.

36

Liver

THE major diseases of the liver are viral hepatitis; the injuries caused by alcohol, drugs, and other chemical agents; cirrhosis and its complications; disorders of hepatic function caused by an inborn error of metabolism; and tumors. Minor abnormalities of hepatic function are almost universal in all severe illnesses.

VIRAL HEPATITIS

The term *viral hepatitis* is used to describe the infections caused by the hepatitis viruses A and B, the viruses that cause non-A, non-B hepatitis, or the delta agent. Sometimes the delta agent is called the hepatitis D virus, and the disease it causes is called hepatitis D. Formerly, hepatitis A was called infectious hepatitis and hepatitis B was named serum hepatitis.

Other viruses can cause similar disease in the liver. The Epstein-Barr virus causes hepatitis in over 90% of patients with infectious mononucleosis. The yellow fever, Lassa, Marburg, and Ebola viruses all cause hepatitis. In infants, Herpesvirus hominis, the cytomegaloviruses, coxsackieviruses of type B and the virus of rubella can all cause liver disease and, except for rubella, occasionally cause hepatitis in adults. Adenoviruses, coxsackieviruses of type A, and echoviruses have been isolated from patients with hepatitis.

Hepatitis A is common. It is usually mild and often passes unrecognized. In the United States, 40% of the population have antibodies against the virus, but only 5% of these people recall an attack of jaundice. The enterovirus that causes the disease is almost always transmitted by the fecal-oral route. The incubation period is 15 to 45 days. The patients are usually children or young adults.

Hepatitis B is less common and tends to cause more severe disease. Less than 0.5% of the population in the United States and northern Europe have antibody against the virus, but in parts of Asia and South Africa over 10% of the population has been infected. The hepadna virus that causes the disease is usually transmitted parenterally by blood or products prepared from blood, though it can pass from mother to child in utero, be transmitted sexually, or spread from one infant to another. The disease is common in promiscuous male homosexuals. It is more common in hospital workers exposed to blood than in the general population. Transmission of hepatitis B by blood transfusion used to be common but in most of the world has become unusual since the introduction of tests to detect HBsAg in the blood. The incubation period is 30 to 180 days. The patient can be of any age.

Non-A, non-B hepatitis usually causes disease of intermediate severity. The infection is most often transmitted parenterally in blood or products prepared from blood, though it can be spread by close contact or the fecal-oral route. In most of the world, 90% of post-transfusion hepatitis is of this type. Hemophiliacs who take products prepared from blood and patients undergoing hemodialysis are particularly at risk. About 20% of patients who seek medical advice because of hepatitis have non-A, non-B infection. The incubation period is 15 to 160 days. The patients are usually adult.

The delta agent often causes severe hepatitis. It is an incomplete RNA virus that competes with the hepatitis B virus for the HBsAg that it needs to become infective. The infection is spread parenterally, as in

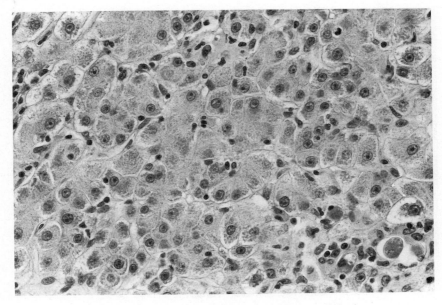

Fig. 36-1.   Acute viral hepatitis, showing mild disarray of the hepatocytes.

hepatitis B, but can occur only in people also infected with the hepatitis B virus or who are carriers of hepatitis B. Hepatitis D is most common in the countries that border the Mediterranean. It has caused small epidemics in South America and the United States.

ACUTE VIRAL HEPATITIS. Acute viral hepatitis is the most common form of the disease. It can be caused by any of the

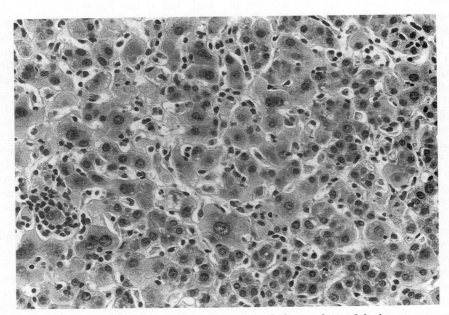

Fig. 36-2.   Acute viral hepatitis, showing greater disarray and pleomorphism of the hepatocytes, with a collection of lymphocytes around a degenerating cell on the left of the picture.

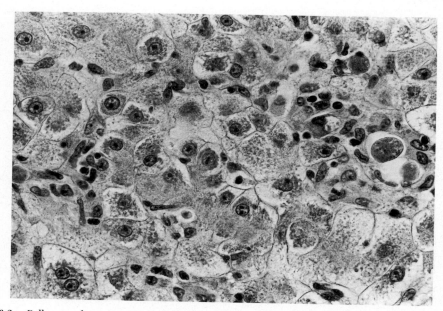

Fig. 36-3. Ballooning degeneration of hepatocytes in viral hepatitis, showing the swollen cells undergoing lysis.

viruses that cause hepatitis, the hepatitis A virus, the hepatitis B virus, the non-A, non-B hepatitis viruses, the delta agent, the Epstein-Barr virus, the cytomegalovirus, or any other of the agents that cause viral hepatitis.

Lesions. In the mildest cases, a biopsy of the liver shows only mild disarray of the liver cells. Normally, the liver cells are all much alike and are arranged in an orderly fashion in plates one cell thick. In viral hepatitis, this careful pattern gets a little disheveled. The hepatocytes vary in size and are not fitted so neatly together. Their nuclei differ in size. Some cells are binucleate. The whole impression is of slight disorder.

Usually, the disease is a little more severe. A few hepatocytes or a few small clumps of hepatocytes scattered at random in the parenchyma degenerate. Two kinds of degeneration are recognized.

The more common form of degeneration is called ballooning. The affected hepatocytes become swollen. By light microscopy they seem distended and empty. Their cell membranes become indistinct. Their nuclei are swollen and often partially lysed. Electron microscopy shows that the swelling is due principally to dilatation of the rough endoplasmic reticulum, which is partially

degranulated. Patchy edema of the hyaloplasm is common. Glycogen is sparse. Sometimes the mitochondria are enlarged, distorted, or contain paracrystalline arrays.

A ballooned hepatocyte can return to normal, but if the injury is severe, derangement of the Na^+, K^+-ATPase ion pump makes it increasingly swollen. The microvilli on the vascular and later on the canalicular pole of the cell are shortened and then lost. The mitochondria become increasingly swollen and distorted. Polyribosomes are lost. The nucleus swells to two or three times its normal size. Nucleoli fragment and disappear. Eventually the cell membrane and the nuclear membrane break, and the debris of the dead cell is phagocytosed by macrophages. Sometimes a hepatocyte or a small group of hepatocytes disappears, leaving no reaction, but often a small accumulation of macrophages, lymphocytes sometimes with a few neutrophils, eosinophils, or plasma cells marks its site.

Less often, a hepatocyte shrinks. Its cytoplasm becomes dark and highly eosinophilic. Its nucleus is pyknotic. The dying cell becomes small and spherical. It is squeezed into the space of Disse, where it lies like a small cannon ball, structureless, hyaline,

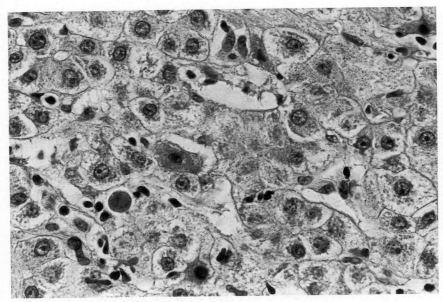

Fig. 36-4.   A Councilman body among the disordered liver plates of a patient with viral hepatitis.

and dense. Often such cells are called acidophilic bodies or Councilman bodies, after the American pathologist (1854–1933) who described them in yellow fever. In the space of Disse, the extruded cell is phagocytosed by the Kupffer cells, broken up, and digested.

Apoptosis is a special form of acidophilic degeneration. As the hepatocyte shrinks, it becomes lobulated and then fragments into several small, spheroidal pieces like little Councilman bodies.

Lymphocytes and a few macrophages accumulate in the portal tracts, sometimes

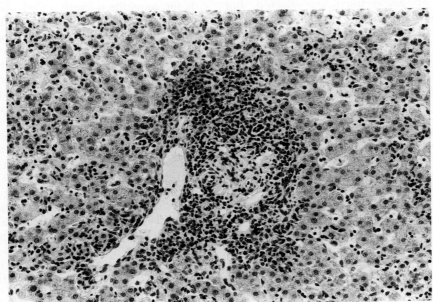

Fig. 36-5.   Triaditis in viral hepatitis, showing the accumulation of lymphocytes in a portal tract.

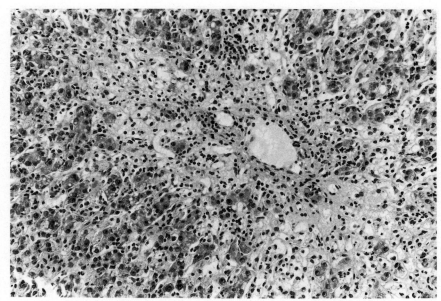

Fig. 36-6. Acute viral hepatitis, showing the accentuation of the injury sometimes evident around the terminal hepatic veins.

with a scattering of eosinophils or neutrophils. The exudate sometimes spills a little into the parenchyma. Occasionally, some of the periportal hepatocytes become necrotic, to give a form of piecemeal necrosis, similar to that seen in chronic active hepatitis. Usually all portal tracts are affected, but sometimes the triaditis is slight or patchy.

Throughout the liver, the Kupffer cells become swollen and perhaps hyperplastic. Their lysosomes are stuffed with golden pigment derived from the debris of the dead cells they have ingested. The big, pigmented phagocytes are called tombstone cells. They mark the tomb of the hepatocytes that perished in the struggle against the virus.

Often the walls of the terminal hepatic veins are inflamed, with edema and an exudate predominantly of lymphocytes and macrophages, perhaps with a few neutrophils and eosinophils. Often the disorder and necroses in the liver cell plates are most marked around the terminal hepatic veins.

Cholestasis is not usually prominent in acute viral hepatitis. Occasionally, a few bile canaliculi contain a plug of bile, especially late in the attack.

Clinical Presentation. Most infections with the virus of hepatitis A and many of those with the hepatitis B virus or the viruses of non-A, non-B hepatitis are mild. The patient feels poorly for a few days and then recovers. There is no jaundice, but there may be a transient rise in aminotransferase activity in the plasma.

If the hepatitis is more severe, as is common in hepatitis B, non-A, non-B hepatitis, and hepatitis D, less often in hepatitis A, prodromal symptoms begin one to two weeks before the patient becomes jaundiced. The patient is tired and run down. Especially in hepatitis A, a fever of 38.5°C often develops. Nausea, vomiting, anorexia, and headache are common. Some patients have coryza or a sore throat. Some have arthralgia or myalgia.

When jaundice appears, the constitutional symptoms often lessen, though the patient frequently continues to lose weight. Bile is usually present in the urine. Sometimes the stool is pale. The liver is usually large and tender. In 50% of the patients, itching complicates the jaundice. In 20%, splenomegaly and enlargement of lymph nodes is evident. In a few, vascular spiders appear in the skin. Depression is common.

The jaundice usually persists from one to four weeks and then slowly wanes. Bile disappears from the urine. The stool darkens.

Weakness and malaise commonly persist. Often it is one to three months before the patient feels fully recovered.

Dysfunction. The damage to the hepatocytes in acute viral hepatitis causes leakage of the intracellular aminotransferases into the blood. Usually, their activity in the plasma begins to rise about a week before symptoms appear and reaches a peak of 500 to 5000 U/L about the time jaundice appears. The magnitude of the elevation in aminotransferase activity gives little guide to the severity of the damage to the liver. As the jaundice fades, the aminotransferase activity in the blood falls to normal in most patients with hepatitis. In some a second rise in aminotransferase activity occurs and persists for weeks or months.

The damage to the hepatocytes impairs both the uptake of unconjugated bilirubin from the blood and the excretion of conjugated bilirubin from the liver. The depth of the jaundice varies a great deal from one patient with hepatitis to another, but usually the concentration of bilirubin in the serum does not exceed 170 µmol/L (10 mg/100 mL). In most patients, both conjugated and unconjugated bilirubin increase about equally, though the concentration of conjugated bilirubin often begins to rise first. Alkaline phosphatase escapes back into the blood with the conjugated bilirubin, but its concentration in the serum does not usually exceed 200 U/L.

Early in the course of viral hepatitis, the renal threshold for conjugated bilirubin is reduced, explaining why bilirubinuria often is evident a few days before there is jaundice. Why the threshold is reduced is unknown. Later in the disease, it returns to its normal level.

The flow of bile to the bowel is often reduced in acute viral hepatitis, though the severity of the impairment varies from one patient to another. Occasionally the lack of bile to form micelles causes steatorrhea. The reduction in bile flow is reflected in the excretion of urobilinogen in the urine. In many patients, urobilinogen disappears from the urine during the prodromal period, and its reappearance is often one of the first signs of recovery.

The blood usually shows neutropenia with a relative lymphocytosis in the early stages of viral hepatitis. The leukocyte count tends to return to normal as jaundice develops. In 25% of the patients, abnormal lymphocytes like those of infectious mononucleosis appear in the blood. The survival of the red cells is reduced, but not sufficiently to cause anemia. In 30% of the patients, there is hypergammaglobulinemia of up to 70 g/L (7 g/100 mL), with increase in both IgG and IgM. With it, there is often mild hypoalbuminemia. Prothrombin and other clotting factors are often deficient, partly because the lack of bile in the bowel prevents the absorption of vitamin K, partly because the damage to the liver cells prevents their manufacture.

Diagnosis. The organism causing viral hepatitis is usually determined by demonstrating viral antigens or antiviral antibodies in the plasma. Less often, the virus is demonstrated by electron microscopy, or its antigens or antibodies are detected in some other secretion or tissue.

Hepatitis A. Hepatitis A is diagnosed by demonstrating antibody against the virus in the plasma. The virus is present in the liver, blood, and feces during the prodrome and for the first week of symptoms, but is not easily demonstrated.

An IgM antibody against the hepatitis A virus appears in the blood towards the end of the prodrome and persists for from six weeks to six months. If it is present in the blood of a patient with hepatitis, it suggests strongly that the patient has hepatitis A.

An IgG antibody against the virus appears later, two to six weeks after the onset of symptoms and reaches a peak after three to 12 months. It persists for years, perhaps for life. The demonstration of the IgG antibody in the blood shows only that the patient has at some time had hepatitis A. Only when there is a fourfold increase in the titer of the IgG antibody in a patient with hepatitis does it suggest that the patient has hepatitis A.

Hepatitis B. Hepatitis B is most often diagnosed by demonstrating the surface antigen of the virus, HBsAg, in the plasma. In acute viral hepatitis B, HBsAg appears in the plasma two to eight weeks before symptoms develop, persists for several weeks, and disappears during convalescence. If the antigen continues to be present in the blood, the infection has become chronic or the patient has become a carrier. The titer of the antigen gives no indication of the severity of acute viral hepatitis.

The e antigen from the core of the hepatitis B virus, HBeAg, appears in the plasma soon after the surface antigen, persists for two to four weeks, and disappears. It shows that the virus is present in the tissues and that the patient's blood and other secretions are infectious. If HBeAg remains in the blood for a longer period, the disease has become chronic and the patient remains infectious. The core antigen of hepatitis B virus, HBeAg, is rarely demonstrable in the blood of patients with acute hepatitis B.

IgM antibody against the core antigen, anti-HBc, appears in the plasma towards the end of the prodrome and persists for a few weeks before it is replaced by an IgG antigen that persists for months. If IgM anti-HBc is present in the plasma, it shows that the patient has had a recent attack of hepatitis B. IgG anti-HBc shows that the patient had hepatitis B some time ago.

Antibody against the e antigen, anti-HBe, in most patients becomes detectable about four weeks after the onset of symptoms, soon after the disappearance of HBeAg from the blood, while the surface antigen is still present in the blood. The antibody is produced earlier, but at first combines with the circulating e antigen, forming immune complexes. Only after the antigen and its complexes are largely cleared from the blood does free antigen become detectable. It persists in the blood for months.

Antibody against the surface antigen, anti-HBs, is first detectable in the plasma some weeks after HBsAg is no longer demonstrable. An IgM antibody appears first, but is soon replaced by IgG antibody. The IgG antibody persists for months or years and shows that the patient is immune to hepatitis B.

If a biopsy is taken during the incubation period of hepatitis B, before symptoms develop, the core antigen of the virus can be demonstrated in the nuclei of many of the hepatocytes, and the surface antigen is present in relation to the cytoplasmic membranes of some of these cells. By the time symptoms develop, only a few hepatocytes in a biopsy show the core antigen in their nuclei, and surface antigen is difficult or impossible to demonstrate.

Hepatitis D. When infection with the delta agent is superimposed on acute hepatitis B and when the agent causes acute hepatitis in a carrier of hepatitis B, the viral antigen, HDAg, is detectable in the plasma only transiently if at all. IgM antibodies against the agent, anti-HD, are present in the plasma for a few weeks, disappearing before HBsAg is cleared from the blood. IgG antibodies against the agent are rarely detectable.

Non-A, non-B Hepatitis. Non-A, non-B hepatitis can be diagnosed only by exclusion of hepatitis A, hepatitis B, and of other forms of viral hepatitis.

Complications. Immune complexes consisting of a viral antigen and the antibody against it circulate in the blood in patients with hepatitis B and probably in those with other forms of viral hepatitis. The complexes may cause the prodromal symptoms common in acute viral hepatitis.

In a small minority of patients with hepatitis B, circulating immune complexes lodge in an extrahepatic organ to cause polyarteritis nodosa, glomerulonephritis, mixed cryoglobulinemia, or less often the Guillain-Barré syndrome, myocarditis, angioedema, rashes in the skin, or the Raynaud phenomenon. The hepatitis is usually mild in patients who develop extrahepatic complications, though a few of the people affected have had chronic persistent hepatitis.

A few patients with hepatitis A or hepatitis B develop pancytopenia, usually about two months after the attack of hepatitis. The bone marrow is aplastic or severely hypoplastic. The cause of the injury to the marrow is unknown.

The relationship of hepatitis B to hepatocellular carcinoma is discussed in the section describing the tumors of the liver.

Pathogenesis. Probably the pathogenesis of hepatitis A and hepatitis B are different. Little is known of the pathogenesis of non-A, non-B hepatitis or of the disease caused by the delta agent.

Hepatitis A. The virus of hepatitis A is cytopathic and probably causes hepatitis by killing or damaging the hepatocytes it infects. The more severe the hepatitis it causes, the greater the shedding of virus into the feces, as would be expected if the virus directly attacked the hepatocytes.

There is nothing to show that the antibodies against the hepatitis A virus increase or prolong the injury to the liver. The concentration of T cells in the blood is reduced in hepatitis A, but a similar reduction in the number of circulating T cells occurs in noninfectious hepatitis induced by chemical injury.

Hepatitis B.   The hepatitis B virus is not cytopathic. It does not damage hepatocytes in vitro or in experimental animals. In man, it can be demonstrated in hepatocytes that show no sign of injury. In carriers of hepatitis B, the virus persists in the liver for years without causing morphologic or functional injury.

The damage to the liver in hepatitis B is probably caused by an immunologic attack on the infected hepatocytes. Both the surface antigen and the core antigen of the hepatitis B virus appear on the surface of the infected hepatocytes. The immunologic attack is probably mediated principally by cytotoxic T cells that react with the HLA antigens and the HBcAg on the surface of the infected hepatocytes. The cytotoxic cells destroy the infected hepatocytes and in most patients eliminate the infection.

It is unlikely that the antibodies against the viral antigens on the surface of the infected cells attack the hepatocytes directly or by activating complement. Most of them appear as the disease is subsiding, and their titer does not bear any relationship to the severity of the hepatic injury. They can rarely be demonstrated in the liver of patients with acute hepatitis B. Nor does it seem likely that immune complexes formed by the circulating viral antigens and the antibodies against them play any part in the pathogenesis of the injury to the liver in hepatitis B.

Treatment and Prognosis. Acute viral hepatitis can be managed only symptomatically. Care should be taken to avoid transmitting the infection. The stool is infectious in hepatitis A, and blood and secretions are infectious in patients with hepatitis B, non-A, non-B hepatitis, or hepatitis D.

Almost all patients with hepatitis A recover completely. Only rarely does a patient

with hepatitis A develop fulminant hepatitis. The chronic forms of the disease do not occur.

In most of the world, 85% of patients with acute hepatitis caused by the hepatitis B virus recover within a few weeks and eliminate the virus from the body. Some become carriers, some develop chronic persistent hepatitis, a few progress to chronic active hepatitis, and a few develop fulminant hepatitis.

About 50% of patients with non-A, non-B hepatitis recover within a few weeks. Most of the rest have signs of continuing infection that persist for more than one year. About 20% of those who contract the disease by blood transfusion progress to chronic active hepatitis, but only 10% of those infected in some other way. Some develop fulminant hepatitis.

Superinfection by the delta agent increases the risk that a patient with hepatitis B will develop fulminant hepatitis, but does not increase the risk that the disease will become chronic.

Prophylaxis. Hepatitis A can be prevented or attenuated by giving immune globulin before infection or early in the incubation period. Immune globulin always contains antibody against the virus. The protection lasts for about three months.

Hepatitis B can be prevented by giving hepatitis B immunoglobulin containing a high titer of antibody against the virus within a few hours of infection. Active immunization using a vaccine containing the surface antigen of the virus gives lasting protection. If it is suspected that a person has been recently infected, both hepatitis B immunoglobulin and active vaccination can be given.

No means of protecting against non-A, non-B hepatitis is known. Infection with the delta agent is prevented by preventing the hepatitis B necessary for the proliferation of the virus.

CHOLESTATIC HEPATITIS.   Cholestatic viral hepatitis is rare. The patient suffers an attack of acute viral hepatitis of the usual type and recovers in the ordinary way, except that jaundice persists, sometimes for as long as eight months.

Lesions.   Biopsy of the liver shows the

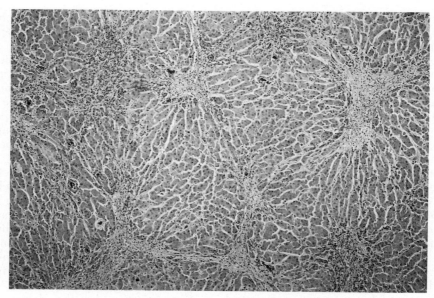

Fig. 36-7. Bridging necrosis, showing passive septa joining terminal hepatic veins and portal triads.

usual changes of acute viral hepatitis, but in addition bile canaliculi throughout the liver are distended, apparently with inspissated bile. The cholestasis may be so striking that the other features of viral hepatitis are obscured. In the portal tracts, neutrophils are sometimes numerous, and there may be some proliferation of bile ductules. In patients in whom cholestatic hepatitis persists for months, fibrosis sometimes develops around portal tracts. A fibrous septum occasionally joins one portal tract to another.

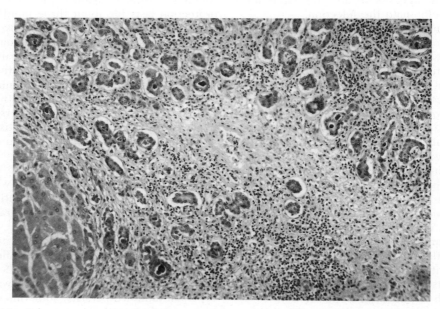

Fig. 36-8. Submassive necrosis in viral hepatitis, showing extensive destruction of the hepatocytes around a terminal hepatic vein.

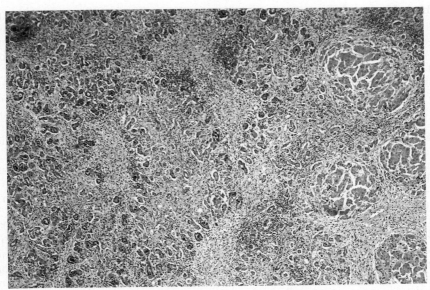

Fig. 36-9.   Massive necrosis in viral hepatitis, showing almost complete destruction of the hepatocytes, with only a few clumps of surviving liver cells on the right of the picture.

Occasionally, a liver biopsy shows the features of cholestatic hepatitis, even though the patient follows the usual clinical course, without unduly prolonged jaundice.

Dsysfunction. The jaundice is often more severe than is usual in viral hepatitis, with a concentration of bilirubin in the plasma of from 150 to 300 μmol/L (10 to 20 mg/100mL). The activity of alkaline phosphatase in the serum is usually greatly increased. There may be hypercholesterolemia. The prothrombin time is usually prolonged. The activity of the aminotransferases in the plasma rises as in the usual type of acute viral hepatitis and may fall to normal at the usual time, even though the jaundice persists. The stools are pale, and bile is excreted in the urine. It may be difficult to distinguish this kind of hepatitis from obstructive jaundice caused by stenosis or occlusion of the common bile duct.

Prognosis. Most patients with cholestatic viral hepatitis recover completely without residual injury to the liver.

BRIDGING NECROSIS. Bridging necrosis is a severe form of acute viral hepatitis in which necrosis of hepatocytes is more extensive than is usual. It is most common in people with hepatitis B, but can occur in

non-A, non-B hepatitis, hepatitis D, or occasionally in hepatitis A. It is more common in women than in men.

Lesions. Bands of necrosis link portal tracts to central hepatic veins or one central hepatic vein to another. Less often, they extend from one portal tract to another. At first, macrophages, lymphocytes, plasma cells, and sometimes neutrophils or eosinophils accumulate around the dying hepatocytes in the bands of necrosis. Later the dead hepatocytes and the inflammatory cells disappear. In the bands of necrosis, the reticulin framework of the liver collapses to form thin bridges called passive septa that join the portal tracts and central hepatic veins. Less involved parts of the liver show the changes seen in the ordinary form of acute viral hepatitis.

Prognosis. Some patients with bridging necrosis recover with little or no residual injury to the liver, but 30% progress to chronic active hepatitis and 20% develop liver failure and die.

FULMINANT HEPATITIS. Fulminant hepatitis is the most severe form of acute viral hepatitis. Much of the hepatic parenchyma is necrotic. Over 50% of the patients have hepatitis B, some with superimposed hepatitis D. Most of the rest have non-A, non-B hepatitis, though a few cases of fulminant hepatitis A have been reported.

Lesions. The liver is small and shrunken, often weighing 500 to 700 g. Its capsule is loose and wrinkled. On section, the liver is usually red and mushy, but occasionally is bright yellow, explaining why extensive necrosis of the liver used to be called acute yellow atrophy. Microscopically, two forms of fulminant hepatitis are distinguished, submassive necrosis and massive necrosis.

In submassive necrosis, most of the hepatocytes around the terminal hepatic veins and in the midzone between the hepatic veins and the portal tracts die. In this zone of devastation, the reticulin framework of the liver collapses. Little remains except a few pigmented Kupffer cells and dilated, hemorrhagic sinusoids engorged with blood. Often the bridges of necrosis called passive septa join one necrotic zone to another. In the surviving parenchyma around the portal tracts, the usual changes of acute viral hepatitis are evident. Often the inflammatory exudate in the parenchyma is unusually extensive. Cholestasis is often severe.

In massive necrosis most of the hepatic parenchyma is necrotic. All that is left in the shrunken, wrinkled liver are the portal tracts and the collapsed desolation that joins them to the hepatic veins. Hepatocytes and Kupffer cells are gone. In the portal tracts, there is often proliferation of bile ductules. Often the ductules are plugged with bile. Often there is moderate acute inflammation.

Clinical Presentation. In the early stages of fulminant hepatitis, there is usually fever, but later hypothermia is common. A leukocytosis with neutrophilia is usual. Jaundice is marked, with a concentration of bilirubin in the plasma of as much as 700 μmol/L (40 mg/100 mL), though a few patients die before jaundice becomes evident. The level of aminotransferases in the plasma is often no greater than in ordinary acute hepatitis and may fall as the liver cells that produce them are destroyed. Bleeding into the bowel, skin, and sometimes the lungs or retroperitoneal tissues is often extensive, because the liver can no longer produce its clotting factors. The sweet, mousey odor of fetor hepaticus becomes evident. Renal fail-

ure is usual. In up to 20% of the patients, bacterial infection such as pneumonia, infection of the urinary tract, or septicemia secondary to infection of intravenous lines complicates the disease.

Hepatic encephalopathy develops as the liver fails. The patient becomes increasingly confused, irritable, perhaps delirious, violent, or antisocial. Increasing obtundation, asterixis, and coma follow. Convulsions may occur, especially in children.

Prognosis. Over 75% of patients with fulminant hepatitis die. Those who survive are left with cirrhosis or some other form of chronic liver disease.

CARRIERS. More than 200,000,000 people are symptomless carriers of the hepatitis B virus. In the United States and northern Europe, less than 0.5% of the population harbor the virus. In the south of Europe and in Japan, 3% of the population are infected. In South Africa, 10% of the population carry the virus; in Hong Kong, Singapore and Taiwan, 15%. Up to 20% of patients with Down syndrome, leprosy, leukemia, Hodgkin's disease, polyarteritis nodosa, or on hemodialysis have HBsAg in the plasma.

Carriers of non-A, non-B hepatitis are also common. Carriers of hepatitis B in the Mediterranean countries often harbor the delta agent. Carriers of hepatitis A do not occur.

The carriers of the hepatitis B virus are divided into two groups. In 60% of the carriers, the activity of the aminotransferases in the plasma is normal. In the other 40%, the activity is increased, at least intermittently.

Biopsy shows that in 96% of carriers of hepatitis B who have normal aminotransferase activity in the plasma the liver is normal histologically, except for the ground glass cells typical of the carrier state, or shows chronic persistent hepatitis. In only 1% does it show chronic active hepatitis or cirrhosis. If the aminotransferase activity is elevated, 75% of the patients have a liver that is normal or shows chronic persistent hepatitis, but 22% have chronic active hepatitis.

Lesions. Ground glass hepatocytes are found only in the liver of people with chronic hepatitis B. They are most common in carriers in whom the liver is otherwise nor-

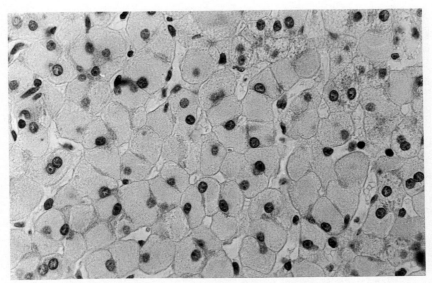

Fig. 36-10. Ground glass hepatocytes in the liver of a carrier of hepatitis B.

mal, but also occur in chronic persistent hepatitis and sometimes in chronic active hepatitis. The ground glass cells are a little bigger than are normal hepatocytes. They may be scattered singly in the parenchyma or grouped into clumps or cords. They may be numerous or only an occasional hepatocyte may be affected. Part or all of the cytoplasm of the ground glass cells is evenly eosinophilic and finely granular, like ground glass. Orcein stains the cytoplasm brown.

Electron microscopy shows that the ground glass cells have dilated rough endoplasmic reticulum filled with the tubular form of HBsAg. The cells stain strongly with labeled antibody against the antigen. Smaller quantities of the surface antigen are sometimes demonstrable on the surface of the cell. Alpha$_1$-antitrypsin and α-fetoprotein are occasionally present in the dilated rough endoplasmic reticulum.

The core of the hepatitis B virus can be demonstrated in the nuclei of some of the hepatocytes in carriers of hepatitis B virus, but is not common. Immunologic staining shows that few of the hepatocytes in carriers contain detectable core antigen. When the core antigen is demonstrable, it is usually in cells that are not producing the surface component of the virus in their cytoplasm.

The liver shows no abnormality in carriers

of non-A, non-B hepatitis. Carriers of the delta agent show only the changes induced by the hepatitis B virus.

Pathogenesis. When hepatitis B becomes chronic, part of much of the viral deoxyribonucleic acid is incorporated into the genome of the cell in some of the hepatocytes. In other hepatocytes, the viral deoxyribonucleic acid remains free in the nucleus. When the viral deoxyribonucleic is incorporated into the genome in the majority of the infected cells, anti-HBe is usually present in the plasma. When the viral deoxyribonucleic acid is free in the nucleus in the majority of the infected hepatocytes, HBeAg is found in the plasma.

In the ground glass cells, the viral deoxyribonucleic acid is incorporated into the nucleus. The cells produce large quantities of HBsAg, but do not form HBcAg. Since the core antigen is not expressed on the surface of the ground glass cells, they are not subject to attack by the cytotoxic lymphocytes. The hepatocytes in which the viral deoxyribonucleic acid is free in the nucleus continue to form HBcAg and to express in the cell membrane. They continue to be destroyed by cytotoxic T cells.

Prognosis. Most carriers of hepatitis B who have no abnormality in the liver other than the presence of ground glass cells con-

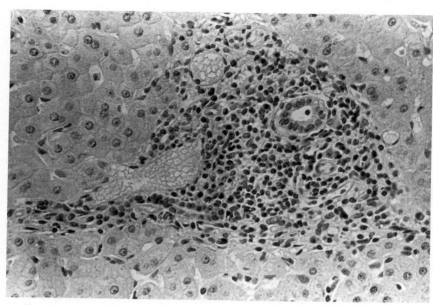

Fig. 36-11. Chronic persistent hepatitis, showing the accumulation of lymphocytes in a portal tract, with little change in the parenchyma of the liver.

tinue with little change for months or years. About 1% per year eliminate the virus, and the liver returns to normal.

CHRONIC PERSISTENT HEPATITIS. Chronic persistent hepatitis develops in 5% of patients with hepatitis B and in 15% of those with non-A, non-B hepatitis. The diagnosis is made when minor changes in hepatic structure and function persist for more than six months after the development of symptoms.

Lesions. In most patients with chronic persistent hepatitis, the principal lesion in the liver is inflammation of most of the portal tracts. The portal tracts are filled with lymphocytes, together with a few plasma cells and perhaps an occasional eosinophil or neutrophil. The exudate does not extend into the parenchyma. The limiting plates of hepatocytes around the tracts are intact.

The parenchyma often shows changes like those seen in acute viral hepatitis, but they are usually slight and easily overlooked. There is only slight disorder in the liver cell plates, with perhaps an occasional necrotic hepatocyte. Only in a few patients with chronic persistent hepatitis are the parenchymal changes more marked, sometimes

overshadowing the inflammation of the triads.

When chronic persistent hepatitis follows hepatitis B, the surface antigen of the virus and antibodies against its core antigen usually persist in the blood. The e antigen can rarely be demonstrated. Occasionally, the surface antigen is not demonstrable in the blood, and instead the patient has circulating antibody against it. In the liver, the surface antigen can be found in the cytoplasm of some of the hepatocytes, but the core antigen is usually hard to demonstrate. Ground glass cells are sometimes demonstrable by light microscopy.

Dysfunction. Aminotransferase activity in the plasma is increased, though it rarely exceeds 400 U/L. Often the activity of the enzymes waxes and wanes. In 10% of the patients, the concentration of bilirubin in the plasma is increased, though rarely to more than 80 μmol/L (5 mg/100 mL). Alkaline phosphatase activity in the serum is usually normal.

Clinical Presentation. Most patients with chronic persistent hepatitis have no symptoms. A few feel tired and feeble and complain of poor appetite or failure to gain weight. Recurrent attacks of acute hepatitis are unusual.

Pathogenesis. The inflammation and continuing destruction of hepatocytes in chronic persistent hepatitis and chronic lobular hepatitis are probably due to the persistence of free viral deoxyribonucleic acid in the nuclei of some of the hepatocytes. The infected cells express the core antigen in their plasma membrane and are destroyed by cytotoxic T cells. In other hepatocytes, the viral genes are incorporated into the genome of the cells, and ground glass cells result.

Treatment and Prognosis. Patients with chronic persistent hepatitis need no treatment. The morphologic and functional changes persist with little change for months or years, but eventually subside without residual injury to the liver.

CHRONIC LOBULAR HEPATITIS. Chronic lobular hepatitis is an uncommon condition in which the changes in the parenchyma similar to those in acute viral hepatitis persist for weeks or months after an attack of hepatitis B or non-A, non-B hepatitis. Recurrent attacks of acute hepatitis are common. Adrenocortical steroids usually bring

remission, leaving the patient with a normal liver.

CHRONIC ACTIVE HEPATITIS. Chronic active hepatitis, sometimes called chronic aggressive hepatitis, develops in 3 to 5% of patients with hepatitis B and in perhaps 30% of patients with non-A, non-B hepatitis. Hepatitis D does not increase the risk that a person with hepatitis B will develop chronic active hepatitis. It rarely if ever complicates hepatitis A. The diagnosis is made when hepatic dysfunction persists for more than six months after the onset of acute hepatitis, and liver biopsy shows the characteristic changes of chronic active hepatitis. Over 80% of the patients are men.

Lesions. Though there is no sharp distinction between them, two kinds of chronic active hepatitis are distinguished morphologically. In the milder form, the disease is largely confined to the portal triads and the parenchyma around them; in the more severe form of the disease, bridging necrosis is added.

When chronic active hepatitis follows non-A, non-B hepatitis, biopsy usually shows the mild form of the disease, without bridging necrosis. When it follows hepatitis

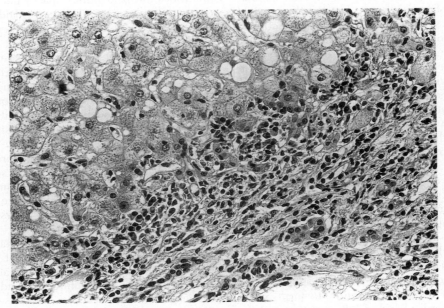

Fig. 36-12. Chronic active hepatitis, showing the erosion of the limiting plate of hepatocytes as the exudate in the portal tract extends irregularly into the parenchyma.

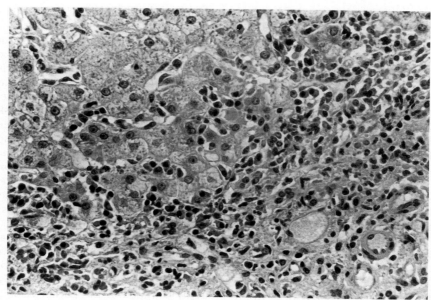

Fig. 36-13. Chronic active hepatitis, showing the destruction of groups of hepatocytes by the exudate spilling from a portal tract.

B, the disease may be mild, or there may be bridging necrosis.

In many patients with chronic active hepatitis, the severity of the injury varies from one part of the liver to another. In some triads, there may be only an exudate mainly of lymphocytes, but in other regions there is severe triaditis, with destruction of the surrounding parenchyma.

In the milder form of chronic active hepatitis, the portal tracts contain an exudate mainly of lymphocytes, with plasma cells and macrophages. The exudate spills out of the tracts, extending irregularly into the parenchyma around the tracts. The limiting plate of hepatocytes around the portal tracts is disrupted and eroded. The exudate surrounds and isolates single hepatocytes or small groups of hepatocytes.

Many of the hepatocytes and small groups of hepatocytes trapped in the inflammation extending out from the portal tracts become necrotic in what is called piecemeal necrosis. The lymphocytes spilling out of the portal tracts seem to gnaw at the parenchyma, killing now a hepatocyte here, now a small group of hepatocytes there, to form a narrow, irregular band of inflammation and destruction around the portal tracts. The dying

hepatocytes often swell in ballooning necrosis but sometimes shrink to small, dense spheroids, like Councilman bodies. In an attempt at regeneration, the surviving hepatocytes at the margin of the portal tracts sometimes forms glandlike spaces lined by a rosette of hepatocytes. Collagen is laid down between the dead and dying hepatocytes at the margin of the portal tracts. First comes the type I collagen stained by reticulin stains; later the type III collagen predominant in the portal triads is laid down.

The hepatocytes more distant from the portal tracts are usually normal, but occasionally show isolated foci of necrosis, like those seen in acute viral hepatitis. Occasionally a few ground glass cells are present.

If chronic active hepatitis is more severe, bridging necrosis is added to the changes in and around the portal tracts. Passive septa form wider or narrower bridges, intersecting the parenchyma and often joining portal tracts to central hepatic veins or portal tract to portal tract. Inflammation like that in the portal tracts is present in the septa and extends out from them into the adjacent parenchyma. Piecemeal necrosis destroys isolated hepatocytes and small groups of hepatocytes at the margins of the septa in the same way that piecemeal necrosis destroys hepatocytes around the portal tracts. New collagen is laid down around the dead and dying hepatocytes at the margins of the septa and extends into the space of Disse around adjacent sinusoids.

As months and years pass, more collagen is deposited around the portal tracts and in the passive septa. In some patients, the condition gradually merges into cirrhosis of the liver.

When chronic active hepatitis is caused by hepatitis B, it is sometimes possible to find the virus in the nucleus of an occasional liver cell or to demonstrate its surface antigen in the rough endoplasmic reticulum in a few of the hepatocytes.

Dysfunction. In the milder forms of chronic active hepatitis, there are only minor abnormalities in hepatic function. The activity of the aminotransferases in the plasma is increased, perhaps to 300 U/L.

If the injury to the liver is greater, the activity of the aminotransferases in the plasma may reach 500 U/L. Often hyperbilirubinemia of up to 80 μmol/L (5 mg/100 mL); increased activity of the alkaline phosphatases in the plasma, usually less than 150 U/L; hypergammaglobulinemia of about 50 g/L (5 g/100 mL); or an abnormal prothrombin time becomes evident.

In the severe forms of chronic active hepatitis, the hepatic dysfunction becomes gradually more severe, as the disease merges into hepatic failure or hepatic cirrhosis.

When chronic active hepatitis follows hepatitis B, antibodies against smooth muscle or antinuclear antibodies can sometimes be found in the blood, though their titer is low. They are rarely demonstrable when chronic active hepatitis follows non-A, non-B hepatitis.

In patients with hepatitis B who develop chronic active hepatitis, the surface antigen of the virus usually persists in the blood, though the more severe and prolonged the hepatitis, the lower the titer of the antigen. Usually the e antigen is demonstrable in the blood, as is antibody against the core antigen. Presence of the IgM antibody against the core antigen suggests continuing replication of the virus in the liver.

Clinical Presentation. In many of the patients with chronic active hepatitis secondary to viral hepatitis, there is a history of a preceding attack of acute viral hepatitis. In some, chronic active hepatitis develops slowly and insidiously, without an acute episode. In these people, the viral etiology of the disease can be established only by demonstrating markers of the hepatitis B virus in the blood or in the liver.

In most patients with chronic active hepatitis secondary to non-A, non-B hepatitis and in 50% of those with chronic active hepatitis secondary to hepatitis B, the patient is asymptomatic or complains only of tiredness. There may be recurrent episodes of mild jaundice, or investigation may show increased activity of the aminotransferases in the plasma, usually of about 300 U/L.

In the other 50% of the patients with chronic active hepatitis secondary to hepatitis B, the patient has more serious injury to the liver by the time the disease is detected. There is likely to be jaundice and hepatomegaly, less often splenomegaly, ascites, or portal hypertension.

Pathogenesis. When chronic active hepatitis complicates hepatitis B, the inflammation and focal necrosis of hepatocytes in regions distant from the portal tracts probably occur because free viral deoxyribonucleic acid persists in the nuclei of some of the hepatocytes. They continue to produce HBcAg and are destroyed by cytotoxic T cells. In other hepatocytes, incorporation of the viral genes into the cell's genome results in the formation of ground glass cells.

The cause of the piecemeal necrosis around the portal tracts is uncertain. The close relationship between the lymphocytes and the cells under attack suggests that it is cell mediated. It does not seem to be a response to any of the viral antigens. It has been suggested that it is an autoimmune reaction, perhaps involving killer cells in an antibody-dependent cell-mediated cytotoxic reaction against the liver surface antigen or the liver membrane antigen, but this has not been proved.

Treatment and Prognosis. The adrenocorticosteroids valuable in treating other forms of chronic active hepatitis are without benefit in patients with chronic active viral hepatitis. In most patients, the lesions persist for months or years without causing symptoms or serious hepatic dysfunction. In some, the disease progresses rapidly to hepatic failure or slowly develops into cirrhosis of the liver. Over 20% of patients with chronic active non-A, non-B hepatitis develop cirrhosis. Nearly 90% of patients with chronic active hepatitis B without cirrhosis live five years, but only 55% of those with cirrhosis.

ALCOHOLIC LIVER DISEASE

Alcohol is one of the commonest causes of hepatic injury. Throughout the world, millions of people drink dangerously large quantities of alcohol. In the United States alone, it is estimated that 7,000,000 people drink so much that they are in grave danger of serious liver disease.

Serious injury to the liver is unlikely unless the daily intake of ethanol is more than 80 g, that is to say 250 mL (8 oz) of whisky, gin, or rum, 750 mL (1 bottle) of wine, or 2 L (8 pints) of beer. As the quantity of alcohol drunk exceeds this limit and as heavy drinking persists for year after year, the chance of serious injury to the liver grows. If a man continues to drink daily more than 500 mL of whisky or more than 1500 mL of wine for more than 10 years, the risk of serious liver disease is high. Women are more susceptible to alcoholic injury to the liver than are men, and a lesser intake of alcohol can cause serious liver disease.

People vary greatly in their susceptibility to alcoholic injury to the liver, perhaps because of inborn variation in the efficiency of the enzyme systems that detoxify ethanol. Some can drink massively for a lifetime without injury, but in others even mild indulgence brings serious trouble. Only 50% of alcoholics develop cirrhosis of the liver.

Alcoholic liver disease is not confined to those we call alcoholics. It can occur in professional men and women, in people who never drink so much that they become drunk.

Alcohol causes three kinds of liver disease. The mildest is fatty liver. Alcoholic hepatitis is more dangerous. Cirrhosis of the liver is considered later in the chapter.

FATTY CHANGE. Even a moderate intake

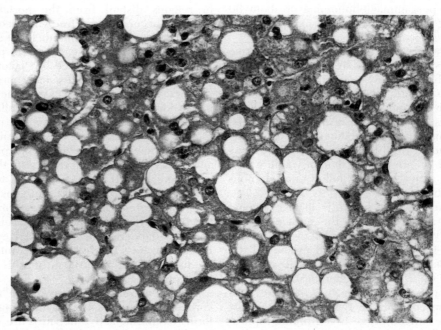

Fig. 36-14. Fatty change in alcoholic liver disease, showing hepatocytes almost entirely filled by a single, large droplet of fat.

of alcohol causes fatty change in the liver. Volunteers drinking the equivalent of 200 to 300 mL (7 to 10 oz) of whisky a day developed fatty change within two days. Because regular intake of alcohol increases the activity of the hepatic enzymes that detoxify ethanol, regular drinkers are less likely to develop fatty change than is a person who drinks only occasionally.

Lesions. Macroscopically, a liver with mild fatty change looks normal. If the steatosis is more severe, the liver is enlarged, pale, or yellowish, and on section feels greasy. When steatosis is severe, the liver weights 6 to 7 kg, is yellow, and on section resembles half frozen butter.

When alcoholic fatty change is mild, fat droplets appear in a minority of the hepatocytes adjacent to the terminal hepatic veins. As it grows more severe, the proportion of hepatocytes involved increases, and cells in the midzone of the liver lobules are involved. In its most severe form, alcoholic fatty change involves all the hepatocytes.

In most patients with alcoholic fatty liver, most of the hepatocytes involved contain a single large droplet of fat. A few contain several smaller droplets. The large droplets fill the cells they occupy, compressing the nucleus and the organelles against the cell membrane. Often the droplets are so large that the cells are two or three times their normal diameter. The enlargement of the hepatocytes is due not only to the increase in the quantity of lipid in the cells but also to the increase in their content of protein and water. If fatty change is severe, a section of liver looks microscopically like wire netting, with the margins of the hepatocytes forming the wire and the fat dissolved out during processing the holes. The smaller droplets are scattered in the cytoplasm. The nucleus remains central.

Electron microscopy shows that the fat droplets lie free in the cell sap without a membrane. Often the mitochondria are dilated and distorted, sometimes containing paracrystalline arrays. Commonly the smooth endoplasmic reticulum is hyperplastic, because of the induction of the microsomal enzymes necessary for the detoxification of ethanol.

Foamy Degeneration. Foamy degeneration is a more severe form of alcoholic fatty change. It is uncommon. The hepatocytes around the terminal hepatic veins and in the midzone of the hepatic lobules contain many small droplets of fat. The hepatocytes around the portal triads are spared. Bile plugs are common between hepatocytes around the hepatic veins. Sometimes there is minor fibrosis around the terminal hepatic veins.

Lipogranuloma. When steatosis is severe, some of the distended hepatocytes rupture. The fat escapes into the tissues and excites a granulomatous reaction with an exudate of macrophages, lymphocytes, and sometimes neutrophils or eosinophils. The macrophages take up the fat and become vacuolated. The lipid that remains free in the center of the lesion is called a fatty lake. Occasionally, fibrosis around the lesion converts it into a fatty cyst. Lipogranulomata and fatty lakes are most common around the terminal hepatic veins, but can occur in other parts of the liver.

Perivenular Fibrosis. In some patients with severe fatty change, fibrosis thickens the wall of some of the central hepatic veins, involving more than 70% of the circumference of the vein and being more than 4 μm thick.

Clinical Presentation. Most patients with alcoholic fatty liver have no symptoms and show little or no evidence of hepatic dysfunction. A few have nausea, vomiting, or epigastric pain. Most have hepatomegaly.

Patients with foamy degeneration usually have jaundice and hepatomegaly. The activity of the aminotransferases in the plasma is increased. The activity of alkaline phosphatase in the plasma is high. Often the presentation suggests extrahepatic obstruction.

Pathogenesis. The fatty change in alcoholic disease is caused by ethanol poisoning. The mechanisms involved are discussed in Chapter 24. Dietary deficiencies sometimes add to the injury, but most people with alcoholic steatosis are well nourished.

Treatment and Prognosis. If patients with alcoholic fatty liver stop drinking, the liver returns to normal within two to four weeks. If the patient continues to drink, alcoholic hepatitis or cirrhosis may follow. Cirrhosis is especially likely in patients who

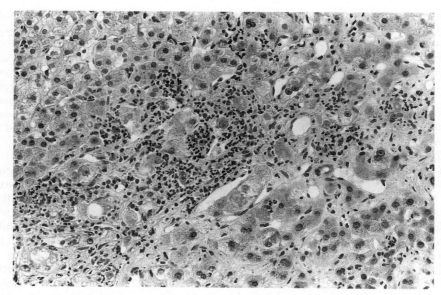

Fig. 36-15. Alcoholic hepatitis, showing the exudate predominantly of neutrophils around the dying hepatocytes.

have perivenular fibrosis. Rarely, a patient with severe alcoholic fatty liver dies suddenly, for reasons unknown.

ALCOHOLIC HEPATITIS. Alcoholic hepatitis is present in 20% of those who seek treat-

ment for alcoholism and can occur in people who are unaware that they are in danger. The patients have necrosis of hepatocytes and a neutrophilic exudate in the liver as well as steatosis.

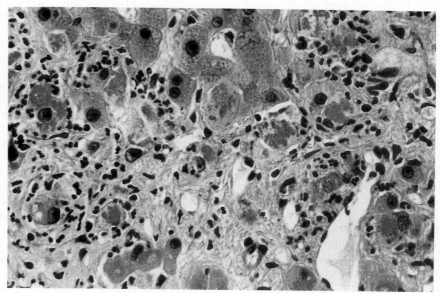

Fig. 36-16. Alcoholic hyaline, forming irregular, darkly stained masses in the cytoplasm of some of the hepatocytes of a patient with alcoholic hepatitis.

Lesion. In alcoholic hepatitis, the liver always shows fatty change, though there is no correlation between the severity of the steatosis and the extent of the hepatocellular necrosis.

The hepatocellular necrosis is patchy, like that in viral hepatitis. It is usually greatest around the terminal hepatic veins, but can be widespread, involving all parts of the parenchyma. The dying hepatocytes sometimes shrink and become hyalinized; sometimes they are ballooned.

Inflammatory cells accumulate around the dead and dying hepatocytes. Usually neutrophils are prominent in the exudate, though lymphocytes and macrophages are also present.

Cholestasis is not usually marked in alcoholic hepatitis. A few bile plugs may be present near the central hepatic veins. Only occasionally is cholestasis severe, with numerous bile plugs, as in cholestatic viral hepatitis.

The organelles are severely damaged in alcoholic hepatitis. The mitochondria are usually swollen and distorted. Their cristae are deranged. Intramitochondrial crystaloids are common. Sometimes a mitochondrion ruptures or is included in an autophagic vacuole. Giant mitochondria are commonly present in the hepatocytes near the central hepatic veins. The smooth endoplasmic reticulum is increased, and the rough endoplasmic reticulum is reduced or degranulated.

Small quantities of iron are present in the hepatocytes and Kuppfer cells in 70% of the patients. The iron can be demonstrated histologically, but is much less than is in the liver in patients with hemochromatosis.

A few patients with alcoholic hepatitis have chronic active hepatitis, in addition to the other lesions of the disease. The terminal plates surrounding the portal triads are eroded by piecemeal necrosis, just as they are in other forms of chronic active hepatitis.

Alcoholic Hyaline. Alcoholic hyaline is usually evident in some of the hepatocytes in alcoholic hepatitis. It may be present in only a few of the cells or prominent in many of them. By light microscopy, alcoholic hyaline is a structureless, hyaline, cytoplasmic mass that is often irregularly shaped. The mass may fill much of the cytoplasm or be confined to a small part of it. The neutrophilic inflammatory reaction usual in alcoholic hepatitis is particularly severe when hepatocytes containing alcoholic hyaline become necrotic.

Alcoholic hyaline consists of a proliferation of filaments of cytokeratin. By electron microscopy, it usually forms of an irregular mesh of fibrils 14 nm in diameter. Sometimes part of the lesion is made of parallel fibrils 7 to 10 nm in diameter that form geometrical patterns or consists of granular, osmophilic material.

Similar hyaline inclusions are found in hepatocytes in other conditions, among them Wilson's disease, primary biliary cirrhosis, Indian childhood cirrhosis, following bypass surgery for obesity, tumors of the liver, drug reactions, ulcerative colitis, diabetes mellitus, obesity, and starvation. Often alcoholic hyaline is called Mallory's hyaline, after the American pathologist who described it in 1911.

Venous Lesions. The adventitia of the terminal hepatic veins is edematous in alcoholic hepatitis. Often fibrosis develops around the terminal hepatic veins and narrows or occludes them. Fine spurs of collagen often extend out from the terminal hepatic veins to surround adjacent hepatocytes or small groups of hepatocytes. Often stellate scars extend out from the terminal hepatic veins towards the portal tracts. Sometimes the fibrosis around the terminal hepatic veins is more extensive, obliterating the parenchyma around the veins, in what is called central hyaline necrosis.

In 10% of patients with alcoholic hepatitis, intimal thickening greatly narrows or obliterates the lumen of the terminal hepatic veins. In 5% of the patients, an exudate of lymphocytes is present in the wall of the central hepatic veins.

Dysfunction. The activity of the aminotransferases in the plasma is increased in alcoholic hepatitis, though rarely to more than 300 U/L. The ratio of the activity of aspartate aminotransferase to that of alanine aminotransferase is usually greater than 2. The concentration of bilirubin in the plasma is normal in mild alcoholic hepatitis and is

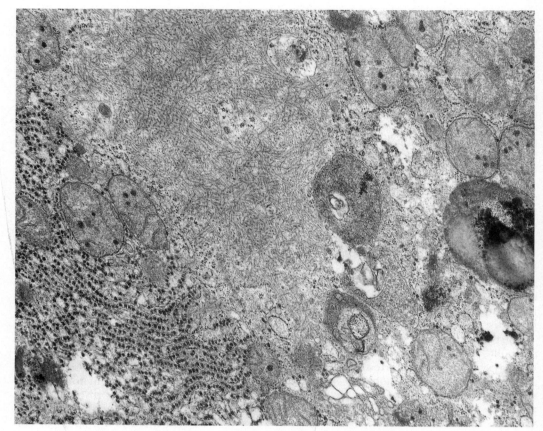

Fig. 36-17. Alcoholic hyaline in a hepatocyte, showing the tangle of filaments of cytokeratin.

not often more than 100 μmol/L (5 mg/100 mL). The activity of alkaline phosphatase in the plasma is often normal and rarely exceeds 300 U/L unless the patient has the rare cholestatic form of alcoholic hepatitis. The concentration of albumin in the plasma falls, sometimes to as little as 10 g/L (1 g/100 mL). As the concentration of albumin falls, the prothrombin time increases. Hypergammaglobulinemia is common, often with high levels of IgA. Anemia and macrocytosis are usual. Patients with severe alcoholic hepatitis often have a leukocytosis, less often leukopenia and thrombocytopenia.

Clinical Presentation. Many patients with alcoholic hepatitis have few or no symptoms. Some complain of anorexia, fatigue, and weight loss. Some have symptoms like those of acute viral hepatitis or of fulmi-

nant hepatic failure. Rarely, the disease mimics extrahepatic biliary obstruction.

The liver is large and tender. The spleen is enlarged in 30% of the patients. Spider nevi are often prominent in the skin. Fever of up to 39.5°C is common. Ascites and edema can accumulate rapidly. Diarrhea, steatorrhea, and gastrointestinal bleeding sometimes complicate the course. Hepatic encephalopathy is likely if the disease is severe.

Pathogenesis. Ethanol poisoning is the major cause of alcoholic hepatitis. Probably the injury is greatest around the terminal hepatic veins because the oxygen tension is least in this part of the liver, and the enzymes that detoxify alcohol are most active in the hepatocytes around the hepatic veins. Malnutrition adds to the injury in some pa-

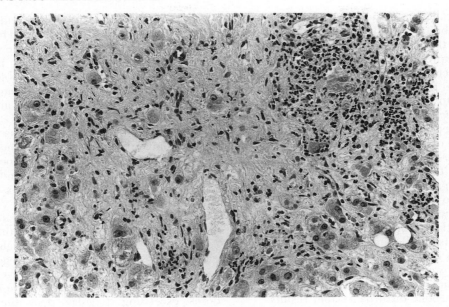

Fig. 36-18. Central hyaline sclerosis in a patient with alcoholic hepatitis, showing the replacement of the perivenular hepatocytes by fine fibrosis.

tients, but many people with alcoholic hepatitis are well nourished.

Antibodies to alcoholic hyaline are present in patients with alcoholic hepatitis, though not in those with fatty liver or alcoholic cirrhosis. The neutrophil reaction prominent in alcoholic hepatitis may be due to the formation of antibody antigen complexes in the liver and the activation of complement, as in an Arthus reaction.

Antibody to the liver specific protein is present in patients with alcoholic hepatitis who have chronic active hepatitis, though not in those who do not, suggesting that an autoimmune reaction against the liver-specific protein is important in these people.

Treatment and Prognosis. Patients with alcoholic hepatitis must give up alcohol. A high protein diet is helpful. Adrenocortical steroids are of no benefit unless the disease is unusually severe. Most patients with alcoholic hepatitis who give up alcohol recover, though recovery is slow, taking from six weeks to six months. In up to 50% of the patients, the hepatic dysfunction worsens when alcohol is withdrawn, and it may be several weeks before improvement is evident. About 20% of the patients die of hepatic failure. About 30% of those who survive

develop cirrhosis. Cirrhosis is especially common in those with extensive fibrosis around the terminal hepatic veins.

TOXIC AND DRUG-INDUCED LIVER DISEASE

Many poisons and drugs damage the liver. Some cause extensive hepatic necrosis. Some cause acute hepatitis, like viral hepatitis. Some cause cholestasis. Some cause chronic hepatitis. Some cause neoplasms. In the United States, 5% of people admitted to a hospital with jaundice have drug-induced disease. Nearly 25% of people with fulminant hepatic failure have drug-induced disease.

The different kinds of hepatotoxic agent will be considered first and then the injury they cause to the liver.

HEPATOTOXIC AGENTS. The poisons and drugs that damage the liver are divided into two groups, the predictable hepatotoxins which inevitably damage the liver if the dose is large enough, and the unpredictable hepatotoxins, which injure the liver in only a small proportion of people exposed to the agent.

The predictable hepatotoxins are sometimes called intrinsic hepatotoxins, because their ability to damage the liver is intrinsic in the nature of the drug or poison. The unpredictable hepatotoxins are called idiosyncratic hepatotoxins, because they damage the liver only in people who respond to the toxin in an unusual way.

Predictable Hepatotoxins. The predictable hepatotoxins are dose-dependent. If enough of the drug or toxin is taken, damage to the liver follows. The larger the dose, the greater the injury to the liver.

The predictable hepatotoxins are divided into two groups, direct hepatotoxins and indirect hepatotoxins. The direct hepatotoxins attack the membranes and other structural elements of the hepatocytes directly. The indirect hepatotoxins poison an enzyme system or some other metabolic process, and the injury to the hepatocytes is caused by the metabolic disturbance that results.

Direct Hepatotoxins. Carbon tetrachloride, chloroform, other halogenated aliphatic hydrocarbons, and phosphorus are the best known direct hepatotoxins. The pathogenesis of the hepatic lesions they cause is discussed in Chapter 24.

If the dose of a direct hepatotoxin is small, the liver is fatty. If the dose is larger, foci of hepatocellular necrosis develop. If it is still larger, massive destruction of the liver follows.

Indirect Hepatotoxins. The list of indirect hepatotoxins is long. Prominent among them are chemotherapeutic agents such as methotrexate, 6-mercaptopurine, or L-asparaginase; antibiotics, such as tetracycline or puromycin; vegetable products such as aflatoxin B_1, the pyrrolizidines present in Jamaican bush tea, the toxins of Amanita phalloides, tannic acid, and the dyes used for cholecystography. The analgesic acetaminophen is an indirect hepatotoxin when taken in a large dose that has become prominent in the United Kingdom because of its popularity among people attempting suicide.

Phalloidin disrupts hepatocellular metabolism by attaching to receptors on the cell surface. The nitrosamines and thioacetamide alkylate molecules in the nucleus and perhaps in the cytoplasm. The tetracyclines and puromycin interfere with transfer ribonucleic acid. Ethionine and orotic acid cause depletion of adenine triphosphate. The dyes used for cholecystography impair the uptake of bilirubin by the hepatocytes. Ethinyl estradiol hampers the excretion of bile into the canaliculi. Other indirect hepatotoxins disturb hepatocellular metabolism in other ways.

Some indirect hepatotoxins cause fatty change. Some cause hepatocellular necrosis. Some cause both steatosis and hepatocellular necrosis. Some cause cholestasis and jaundice. Some injure the hepatic veins or the sinusoids. Some cause cancer.

With most of the therapeutic agents that are indirect hepatotoxins, injury to the liver is important only if the dose is high. Tetracyclines given in the usual dosage may cause minor fatty change in the liver, but only when the drug is given intravenously in doses exceeding 1 g/day does the fatty change become severe.

Unpredictable Hepatotoxins. The unpredictable hepatotoxins are not dose-dependent. Some people can tolerate large and continued exposure to these drugs and poisons without injury to the liver. In other people, even a small dose of the toxin causes major damage to the liver.

Prominent among the unpredictable hepatotoxins are the anesthetics halothane and methoxyflurane; the tranquilizer chlorpromazine and other phenothiazines; the antidepressant iproniazid and other hydrazine amine oxidase inhibitors; phenytoin and other anticonvulsants; cinchophen, gold, indomethacin, salicylates, and other anti-inflammatory drugs; the C-17 alkylated or ethinylated anabolic or contraceptive steroids; chlorpropamide and other oral hypoglycemic drugs; thiourea and related drugs; antibacterial agents such as the sulfonamides, sulfones, para-aminosalicylic acid, isoniazid, rifampicin, and the organic arsenical drugs; the anticoagulant phenindione; α-methyldopa and rarely other antihypertensive or diuretic drugs; antianginal drugs such as perhexiline maleate; nicotinic acid in large dose; antineoplastic agents such as chlorambucil or cyclophosphamide; the laxitive oxyphenisatin; and cimetidine.

The probability that an unpredictable hepatotoxin will cause injury to the liver varies from one toxin to another. Some unpredictable hepatotoxins cause hepatic injury in 1 person in every 50 exposed. Others damage the liver in 1 person in 10,000.

The severity of the hepatic injury caused by the unpredictable hepatotoxins is also unpredictable. Chlorpromazine causes no hepatic injury in 60% of people, minor dysfunction without symptoms in 40%, and serious injury in less than 1%.

Some unpredictable hepatotoxins cause fatty change. Some cause hepatocellular necrosis. Some cause cholestasis. Some damage hepatic veins or sinusoids. Some cause chronic hepatitis. Some cause cancer.

The unpredictable hepatotoxins can be divided into two groups. Some are thought to damage the liver by a hypersensitivity reaction, presumably immunologically mediated. Others produce injury only when an abnormal metabolic pathway in the liver produces toxic metabolites.

The distinction between the two groups is often far from clear. Some of the unpredictable hepatotoxins seem able to produce injury by both mechanisms or by some combination of them.

Hypersensitivity Reactions. With the unpredictable hepatotoxins that are believed to cause injury by a hypersensitivity reaction, damage to the liver usually becomes evident one to four weeks after the first exposure to the toxin, the period required for immunologic sensitization. Often the damage to the liver is accompanied by fever, a rash in the skin, or eosinophilia. If the drug is withdrawn, and later a challenge dose is given, injury to the liver is evident within days.

These features suggest that the damage to the liver is due to an immunologic reaction, but the nature of the reaction has not been elucidated. The antigen inducing the reaction could be the hepatotoxin itself, one of its metabolites, or some alteration in the antigens on the surface of the hepatocytes. Phenytoin, paraaminosalicylic acid, sulfonamides, halothane, chlorpromazine, and phenylbutazone are among the drugs that cause hepatic injury in this way.

Abnormal Metabolism. With the unpredictable hepatotoxins thought to cause injury to the liver only when abnormal metabolites are produced by the hepatocytes, the injury to the liver may be evident within a few days but often is delayed for a year or more. The patients do not develop fever, rash, or other signs suggesting allergy. If the drug is withdrawn and then readministered, injury to the liver may follow quickly or may become evident only after weeks or months.

Isoniazid, iproniazid, valproic acid, and halothane cause injury in this way. In most people, the metabolites of these drugs are harmless. In some, toxic products are produced.

TOXIC HEPATITIS. The hepatic lesions and dysfunction caused by drugs and other hepatotoxins are often similar to those of viral hepatitis or alcoholic liver disease. Table 36-1 lists the kinds of hepatic lesion caused by drugs and other toxic substances and some of the agents that cause them. It is far from complete.

Lesions. The different kinds of lesion caused by hepatotoxins will be discussed separately. Several of the drugs and poisons involved can cause more than one kind of lesion or a combination of lesions.

Fatty Change. Two kinds of fatty change are caused by hepatotoxins. The tetracyclines, sodium valproate, ethionine, phosphorus, and sometimes aflatoxins produce a microvesicular type of fatty change, in which the cytoplasm of the hepatocytes is filled with tiny droplets of fat. The nucleus remains centrally placed. Methotrexate, carbon tetrachloride, and other toxins produce a macrovesicular form of fatty change, in which a single, large droplet of fat fills the hepatocytes, pressing the nucleus against the cell membrane.

Fatty change often co-exists with hepatocellular necrosis. Sometimes the fatty change appears first, and cellular necrosis develops only if the attack is severe. In other cases, necrosis is the principal reaction, with fatty change as a minor accompaniment.

The vasodilator 4, 4'-diethylaminoethoxyhexestrol once used to treat angina pectoris causes the accumulation of phospholipids in the hepatocytes and Kupffer cells in a minority of the patients given the drug. The hepatocytes are swollen,

TABLE 36-1. SOME HEPATOTOXINS

Agent	Predictable/Unpredictable	Steatosis	Necrosis	Cholestasis	Granulomata	Fibrosis	Chronic Active Hepatitis	Biliary Cirrhosis	Cirrhosis	Venooclusive Disease	Peliosis Hepatis	Neoplasia	Frequency
Poisons													
Aflatoxins	P	S	N									T	
Amanita phylloides	P	S	N										
Arsenic, inorganic	P	S	N			f			c				
DDT	P	S	N										
Carbon tetrachloride	P	S	N										
Chlornaphthalenes	P		N										
Paraquat	P		N										
Phosphorus	P	S	N										
Pyrrolizidines	P	S	N							V			
trinitrotoluene	P	S	N										
Vinyl chloride	P					f						T	
Anesthetics													
Chloroform	P	S	N										
Halothane	U		N										0.1%
Methoxyflurane	U		N										
Tribromethanol	P		N										
Trichlorethylene	P	S	N										
Tranquilizers													
Chlorpromazine	U		N	C				B					1%
Other tranquilizers	U		N	C									
Antidepressants													
Iproniazid	U		N						c				1%
Other hydrazines	U		N										1%
Anticonvulsants													
Phenytoin	U		N										R
Sodium valproate	U	S	N										R
Anti-inflammatory Drugs													
Cinchophen	U		N										
Gold salts	U		N										R
Indomethacin	U		N										R
Phenylbutazone	U		N	C	G								0.3%
Salicylates	P		N										
Antimicrobial Drugs													
Arsenicals, organic	U			C				B					R
Chloramphenicol	U		N	C									R
Erythromycin estolate	U		N	C									2%
Ethionamide	U		N										R
Isoniazid	U		N				A		c				3%
Nitrofurantoin	U		N	C			A						R
Novobiocin	P		N	C									
Para-aminosalicylic acid	U		N	C									2%
Penicillins	U			C	G								R
Rifampicin	U		N	C									R
Sulfonamides	U		N	C	G		A						R

TABLE 36-1. (CON'T)

Agent	Predictable/Unpredictable	Steatosis	Necrosis	Cholestasis	Granulomata	Fibrosis	Chronic Active Hepatitis	Biliary Cirrhosis	Cirrhosis	Veno-oclusive Disease	Peliosis Hepatis	Neoplasia	Frequency
Sulphones	U		N	C									5%
Tetracyclines	P	S											
Cardiovascular Drugs													
Ajmaline	U		N	C									R
Aprindine	U		N	C									R
Hydralazine	U		N		G								R
Methyldopa	U		N		G		A						1%
Quinidine	U		N		G								R
Papaverine	U		N										R
Perhexilene maleate	U	S	N				A		c				R
Phenindione	U		N	C									R
Procainamide	U		N	C									R
Antineoplastic Drugs													
Asparaginase	P	S											80%
Azathioprine	U			C									R
Busulfan	U			C									R
Chlorambucil	U		N										R
Chloropurine	P		N										
Cyclophosphamide	U		N										R
Mercaptopurine	P		N										
Methotrexate	P	S				f			c	V			
Mithramycin	P		N										
Puromycin	P	S											
Thioguanine	P		N							V			
Urethane	P		N										
Endocrine Drugs													
Carbutamide	U		N	C	G								1%
Chlorpropamide	U		N	C	G								1%
Metahexamide	U		N	C	G								1%
Propylthiouracil	U		N				A						R
Other thiouracils	U		N	C									R
Tolbutamide	U		N	C			A						R
Other Drugs													
Allopurinol	U		N	C	G								R
Cholecystographic drugs	U			C									R
Cimetidine	U		N	C									R
Dantrolene	U						A						R
Nicotinic acid	P		N	C									
Oxyphenisatin	U		N				A						R
Steriods, anabolic	P			C							p	T	
Steroids, contraceptive										V		T	
Tannic acid	P		N										
Vitamin A	P		N										

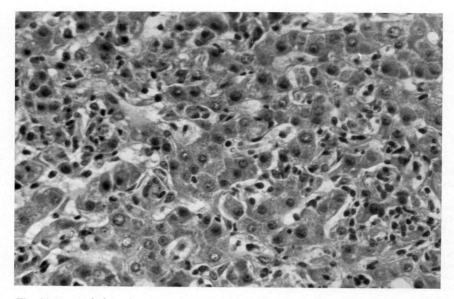

Fig. 36-19.   Halothane hepatitis, showing changes similar to those of acute viral hepatitis.

with foamy cytoplasm. The accumulation of phospholipids develops gradually as the months pass and is probably due to some abnormality in the metabolism of the drug in the people affected. The injury can end in cirrhosis.

Hepatocellular Necrosis. Several of the

hepatotoxic agents cause necrosis of isolated hepatocytes or small groups of hepatocytes. Some cause zonal necrosis, confined to one part of the hepatic lobules. Some cause bridging necrosis or massive necrosis involving much of the liver.

Most of the unpredictable hepatotoxins

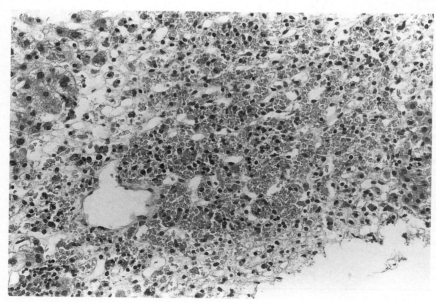

Fig. 36-20.   Acetaminophen poisoning, showing necrosis of the hepatocytes around a terminal hepatic vein and distention of the perivenular sinusoids with blood.

that cause hepatocellular necrosis produce changes like those of acute viral hepatitis. Hepatocytes scattered here and there in the liver degenerate or become necrotic. The dying hepatocytes swell into balloon cells or shrink into acidophilic spheroids like Councilman bodies. The loss of hepatocytes and the proliferation of adjacent hepatocytes causes disorder in the liver cell plates, as in acute viral hepatitis. There are often binucleate hepatocytes or other evidence of regeneration. The inflammatory reaction around the dead and dying hepatocytes and in the portal tracts is usually less than in acute viral hepatitis, though a few drugs such as phenytoin and para-aminosalicylic acid cause a severe inflammatory response, predominantly of lymphocytes and monocytes, but sometimes with eosinophils, that extends diffusely throughout the parenchyma, with accentuation around dying hepatocytes and in the portal tracts. If eosinophils are numerous, it suggests that the injury is a form of hypersensitivity.

Zonal necrosis is characteristic of the predictable hepatotoxins. With carbon tetrachloride, chloroform, tannic acid, pyrrolizidines, the toxins of Amanita phalloides, and acetaminophen, the hepatocytes around the terminal hepatic veins become necrotic. With yellow phosphorus, ferrous sulfate, and other agents the necrotic zone is around the portal tracts. Halothane and a few other of the unpredictable hepatotoxins also cause zonal necrosis, most marked about the terminal hepatic veins.

Occasionally a hepatotoxin causes bridging necrosis or massive necrosis like that of fulminant viral hepatitis. Usually the drug or poison is an unpredictable hepatotoxin, like halothane. Only if the dose is unusually large, does a predictable hepatotoxin cause extensive hepatocellular necrosis.

In some patients treated for a long time with chlorpromazine, barbiturates, azothioprine, phenytoin, and other drugs, some of the hepatocytes are enlarged with a cytoplasm like that of the ground glass cells of chronic hepatitis B. Electron microscopy shows a great increase in smooth endoplasmic reticulum.

Cholestasis. When a hepatotoxin causes cholestasis, the principal finding is bile casts, which distend some or many of the bile canaliculi between the hepatocytes. In addition, there is sometimes mild hepatocellular injury, like that seen in mild, acute viral hepatitis.

Chlorpromazine, erythromycin, and other of the unpredictable hepatotoxins cause both cholestasis and a prominent inflammatory exudate in the portal tracts. The exudate is predominantly of lymphocytes, but often contains many eosinophils. The anabolic steroids and other of the unpredictable hepatotoxins that cause cholestasis induce no such exudate. Hepatocellular injury is more likely with the agents that induce an exudate.

A few predictable, indirect hepatotoxins cause jaundice without cholestasis or any other morphologic change in the liver. The cholecystographic dyes, rifamycin, and novobiocin can act in this way. These agents presumably interfere with the uptake of bilirubin from the blood by the hepatocytes or with the conjugation of bilirubin in the hepatocytes.

Granulomata. Some drugs cause granulomata to appear in the liver. The granulomata sometimes resemble those of sarcoidosis or sometimes are more loosely formed. There may or may not be other evidence of hepatic injury. Allopurinol, hydralazine, α-methyldopa, quinidine, sulfonamides, penicillin, isoniazid, phenylbutazone, oxybutazone, and the derivatives of sulfonylurea used to control diabetes mellitus are among the agents that cause hepatic granulomata. The presence of the granulomata suggests that the lesion is a form of hypersensitivity.

Chronic Active Hepatitis. Chronic, active hepatitis like that caused by hepatitis B can be induced by the laxative oxyphenisatin, α-methyldopa, nitrofurantoin, isoniazid, dantrolene, propylthiouracil, and other unpredictable hepatotoxins.

Fibrosis. Inorganic arsenical drugs, vinyl chloride, methotrexate, and other hepatotoxins sometimes cause periportal fibrosis, sometimes severe enough to cause portal hypertension. Hypervitaminosis A can cause fibrosis around the terminal hepatic veins.

Biliary Cirrhosis. Chlorpromazine and similar drugs, methyltestosterone, organic arsenical drugs, and tolbutamide have been reported occasionally to cause changes in the liver that resemble those of primary biliary cirrhosis, though usually with less prominent destruction of bile ducts.

Cirrhosis. Cirrhosis of the liver sometimes follows drug-induced chronic active hepatitis, extensive, drug-induced hepatocellular necrosis, or drug-induced bridging necrosis. Usually, the cirrhosis is of the irregular, macronodular type. Inorganic arsenical drugs, methotrexate, cinchophen, iproniazid have all been reported to cause cirrhosis.

Veno-Occlusive Disease. The pyrrolizidine alkaloids present in some of the herbal teas drunk in Jamaica and other parts of the world cause obliteration of the terminal hepatic veins, with congestion of the surrounding parenchyma and often extensive hepatocellular necrosis in the congested region. Methotrexate, urethane, and other chemotherapeutic agents can cause similar lesions. Rarely, contraceptive steroids cause thrombosis of the hepatic veins, with congestion and hepatocellular necrosis around the terminal hepatic veins.

Peliosis Hepatis. Peliosis hepatis is a rare condition in which large, blood-filled spaces up to 1 or 2 mm across develop in the parenchyma of the liver. The name comes from the Greek for bruised. Some of the spaces resemble dilated sinusoids. Some have no endothelial lining. In a few of the patients, the condition has followed treatment with androgens or anabolic steroids. More often, these agents cause a dilatation of the sinusoids, without the extreme ectasia of the blood channels called peliosis.

Neoplasia. A number of hepatotoxins cause tumors of the liver. Contraceptive steroids can cause hepatocellular adenomata, focal, nodular hyperplasia of the liver, and rarely hepatocellular carcinoma. Aflatoxins and other mycotoxins cause hepatocellular carcinoma. Exposure to vinyl chloride can cause an angiosarcoma of the liver. Thorotrast lodged in the liver can cause angiosarcoma, hepatocellular carcinoma, or cholangiocarcinoma.

Dysfunction. The kind and severity of the hepatic dysfunction caused by the hepatotoxins depends on the type and severity of the injury they produce in the liver.

In general, fatty change causes little dysfunction. The activity of the aminotransferases in the plasma may rise to 250 U/L, rarely much higher. Sometimes the alkaline phosphatases are slightly elevated, perhaps to 200 U/L.

Hepatocellular necrosis caused by hepatotoxins causes the same kind of dysfunction as is found in acute viral hepatitis, with increase in the aminotransferases in the plasma, hyperbilirubinemia, and some increase in the activity of alkaline phosphatase in the plasma. If the necrosis is extensive, the dysfunction resembles that in fulminant viral hepatitis.

Drug-induced cholestasis is marked principally by hyperbilirubinemia. The severity of the jaundice depends on the degree of cholestasis. The activity of the aminotransferases in the plasma is usually increased, sometimes to as much as 500 U/L. Especially when there is an inflammatory exudate in the portal tracts, the activity of the alkaline phosphatases in the plasma rises, exceptionally to as much as 900 U/L.

The dysfunction caused by the other hepatic lesions induced by hepatotoxins resembles that of similar lesions of different etiology.

Clinical Presentation. The clinical presentation in hepatotoxic liver disease depends on the kind of lesion produced in the liver and, with some hepatotoxins, on the changes caused in other parts of the body.

In general, fatty change causes few if any symptoms. Hepatocellular necrosis similar to that found in viral hepatitis causes symptoms and signs like those of viral hepatitis. Cholestasis caused by hepatotoxins often mimics external biliary obstruction, with itching. The more chronic changes caused by hepatotoxins cause symptoms and signs like those of similar lesions produced in other ways.

The unpredictable hepatotoxins that cause hypersensitivity reactions often cause fever, rashes in the skin, lymphadenopathy, and eosinophilia. Phenytoin, sulfonamides, para-aminosalicylic acid, and other drugs sometimes cause a lymphocytosis, with large, atypical lymphoblasts in the blood, like those in infectious mononucleosis.

Poisoning with carbon tetrachloride, phosphorus, Amanita phalloides, or acetaminophen often causes vomiting and diarrhea, with abdominal pain, bleeding into the gut, and shock. After about 24 hours, the patient often improves, though mild jaundice or signs of injury to the brain or kidneys may be evident. The improvement persists for one to three days, but then the jaundice deepens rapidly, with hepatic failure, often widespread bleeding because of lack of coagulation factors, and often renal failure. Up to 50% of the patients die.

Treatment and Prognosis. Withdrawal of the offending hepatotoxin usually brings recovery within three or four weeks, provided that the injury to the liver is not too severe. Occasionally recovery takes much longer. If the injury caused by the hepatotoxin is more severe, the prognosis is as for similar injury caused by one of the hepatitis viruses.

Identification of the agent causing drug-induced liver injury is not always easy. The list of possible hepatotoxins is long and includes some widely used drugs. If several drugs are being administered, it can be hard to determine the agent at fault. The similarity of the signs and symptoms to those of viral hepatitis or sometimes to obstructive jaundice can make diagnosis difficult.

OTHER FORMS OF CHRONIC HEPATITIS

In this section, three forms of chronic liver disease are discussed: idiopathic chronic active hepatitis, primary biliary cirrhosis, and the hepatic injury common in people with ulcerative colitis or Crohn's disease and in people with fever or toxemia.

IDIOPATHIC CHRONIC ACTIVE HEPATITIS. Chronic active hepatitis can develop in patients with hepatitis B, non-A, non-B hepatitis, or hepatitis D; in patients treated with methyldopa, oxyphenisatin, isoniazid, or other drugs; in people with Wilson's disease; and in alcoholics. Similar changes sometimes occur in cirrhosis. When all these conditions are excluded, there remain a group of patients in whom the cause of the disease is unknown. These patients are said to have idiopathic chronic active hepatitis.

Sometimes the idiopathic chronic active hepatitis is called lupoid hepatitis, because 15% of the patients show a positive LE cell test, or autoimmune chronic active hepatitis, because more than 70% of them have abnormal autoantibodies in the plasma. Nearly 80% of the patients are women. About 50% of them are between 10 and 20 years old.

Lesions. The changes in the liver in idiopathic chronic active hepatitis are indistinguishable from those seen in the chronic active hepatitis that follows viral hepatitis or is induced by a drug, except that the ground glass cells sometimes seen when chronic active hepatitis is caused by the hepatitis B virus are not present.

Clinical Presentation. Idiopathic chronic active hepatitis begins insidiously in 60% of the patients, with fatigue and often recurrent episodes of malaise and anorexia. In 25%, the onset is acute, like that of acute viral hepatitis. In some, the disease only becomes apparent when portal hypertension develops or some extrahepatic complication of the disease brings the patient to a physician.

Jaundice develops in 80% of the patients and often fluctuates in severity. The concentration of bilirubin is rarely over 90 μmol/L (5 mg/100 mL), though severe jaundice resembling cholestatic hepatitis can occur. In 80% of the patients, the liver is enlarged and often tender. The spleen is large in 50%. Recurrent attacks of more acute liver disease with malaise, anorexia, and fever are common.

Diarrhea develops in 30% of the patients. Many of them have ulcerative colitis. Amenorrhea is common. Some patients have abdominal pain, arthralgia, or arthritis. Acne, cutaneous vasculitis, and other skin lesions are common. Spider nevi are usually present in the skin. Livid striae often develop on the thighs or the abdomen. Some patients develop pleurisy, pulmonary infiltrates, the sicca syndrome, or glomerulonephritis. Some develop Hashimoto's thyroiditis, diabetes mellitus, Cushing's syndrome, or autoimmune hemolytic anemia.

Dysfunction. In all patients, the activity of the aminotransferases in the plasma is increased, usually to between 200 and 17,000 U/L. The concentration of albumin in the plasma is often reduced, to less than 30 g/L (3 g/100 mL), and the prothrombin time is lengthened. The activity of the alkaline phosphatases in the plasma is usually slightly increased. Hyperglobulinemia, with a concentration of globulins of about 50 g/L (5 g/100 mL) is evident in most patients. The increase is mainly of IgG, but IgM and IgA are often increased as well.

Abnormal antibodies are present in high titer in the blood of most patients with idiopathic chronic active hepatitis. They are not present or are present only in low titer in people with chronic active hepatitis caused by a hepatitis virus or by a drug. Antinuclear antibodies are present in 80% of the patients, antismooth muscle antibodies in 70%, and antimitochondrial antibodies in 30%. The LE cell phenomenon can be demonstrated in 15% of the patients.

Pathogenesis. Idiopathic chronic active hepatitis is probably immunologically mediated, as the name autoimmune chronic active hepatitis implies. A defect in the regulation of the immune system allows the production of antibodies against hepatic antigens, especially against the liver membrane antigen and the liver surface antigen. Antibody against the liver membrane antigen is present in the plasma in high titer. The piecemeal necrosis is probably due to an antibody-dependent cell-mediated cytotoxic reaction directed against the liver membrane and perhaps the liver surface antigen.

Several observations support the conclusion that idiopathic chronic active hepatitis is immunologically mediated. The nature of the inflammatory response in piecemeal necrosis is similar to that in Hashimoto's disease and other autoimmune disorders. The high incidence of abnormal autoantibodies in the plasma suggests an immunologic derangement. Other disorders believed caused by an autoimmune reaction are common in idiopathic chronic active hepatitis.

The cause of the immunologic derangement is unknown. The HLA antigens B8 and DR3 are unduly common in patients with idiopathic chronic active hepatitis, suggesting that a genetic factor may underlie the immunologic derangement. Genes regulating immunologic reactions are linked to these loci.

Treatment and Prognosis. The course of idiopathic chronic active hepatitis differs from one patient to another. Most often the disease worsens steadily, leading within months to cirrhosis, portal hypertension, and liver failure. In some patients, the course is more benign, with remissions and exacerbations, sometimes remissions lasting months or years.

Without treatment, only 30% of patients with idiopathic chronic active hepatitis live 10 years. The mean survival is three years. Treatment with adrenocortical steroids and, if necessary, azothioprine, increases the 10-year survival to 70% and the mean survival to 12 years.

PRIMARY BILIARY CIRRHOSIS. In primary biliary cirrhosis, there is progressive destruction of the bile ducts in the portal tracts of the liver. Cirrhosis is present only in the late stages of the disease. The condition is also called chronic nonsuppurative destructive cholangitis, Hanot's cirrhosis, after the French physician who described it in 1876, and xanthomatous biliary cirrhosis, because xanthomata are sometimes a prominent feature of the disease.

In the United Kingdom, 4 people per 100,000 have primary biliary cirrhosis. Less than 1 person per 100,000 develops the disease each year. Over 90% of the patients are women. Most are between 40 and 60 years old when the diagnosis is made.

Lesion. In its early stages, primary biliary cirrhosis is patchy. Some of the triads in the liver are severely damaged, but others are spared or almost spared. Some triads show early lesions; in others the disease is far advanced.

First lymphocytes accumulate around the bile ducts in the affected triads. As the exudate increases, it fills and enlarges the triads. The limiting plates of hepatocytes surrounding the triads remain intact. The exudate remains predominantly of lymphocytes, but especially around the bile ducts macrophages and plasma cells are often numerous. Sometimes there are neutrophils or eosinophils. Often the macrophages around the ducts aggregate into granulomata. Some of the granulomata are loose and edematous; some are compact, like the granulomata of sarcoidosis.

The epithelium lining the bile ducts in the inflamed triads becomes irregular and

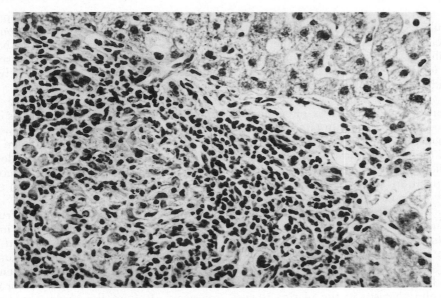

Fig. 36-21. Primary biliary cirrhosis, showing a granuloma in a portal tract.

ragged. Some of the epithelial cells degenerate or become necrotic. Often lymphocytes, plasma cells, or less often neutrophils penetrate between the epithelial cells. Occasionally a few neutrophils are present in the lumen of a duct. Some of the ducts rupture. Eventually, segments of the ducts are destroyed and obliterated. Only the branch of the hepatic artery that accompanies the bile duct remains to show where the duct had been.

At a later stage in the disease, the exudate creeps out from the triads into the surrounding parenchyma, eroding or destroying the limiting plate of hepatocytes. Small bile ducts proliferate at the margin of the triads and together with a few fibrocytes extend out between the hepatocytes. The enlarged triads become irregularly shaped or stellate, perhaps with spurs extending towards neighboring triads. Small groups of hepatocytes at the margin of the triads or the margins of the spurs are trapped in the fibrosis extending from the triads and spurs and become necrotic, much as in the piecemeal necrosis of chronic active hepatitis. Occasionally, some of the macrophages in the triads become filled with lipid and form xanthomatous granulomata.

By this time, most or all of the liver is involved, though different triads often show different stages of the disease. The liver plates, which are normal early in the disease, become irregular and double layered, especially near the terminal hepatic veins. Cholestasis is often evident, usually in periportal biliary canaliculi. Mallory's hyaline, like that of alcoholic hepatitis, appears in the periportal hepatocytes in 25% of the patients. Copper accumulates in the hepatocytes around the triads and along the spurs extending from them. The hepatocytes surrounding the triads are often swollen and vacuolated.

Gradually the inflammation wanes. The ductular proliferation at the margin of the triads disappears. The bile ducts in the triads have gone, leaving only the hepatic arteries and the portal veins in the scarred triads. Fibrosis gradually becomes predominant.

The spurs reaching out from the triads also become fibrotic. Usually they stretch towards an adjacent triad, only rarely towards a terminal hepatic vein. The margins of the spurs are irregular, with small fingers of fibrosis extending out between the adjacent hepatocytes.

At last, true cirrhosis develops, with triad joined to triad by fibrous septa and regeneration nodules in the surviving parenchyma. Mallory's hyaline becomes increasingly prominent in the hepatocytes at the margin of the fibrous septa, and the accumulation of copper in these cells grows. Cholestasis is usual adjacent to the triads and fibrous septa.

Primary biliary cirrhosis is often divided into three or four stages. In one system, the inflammation around the ducts in the portal triads is the main feature in stage I. Ductular proliferation at the margin of the triads is predominant in stage II. Stage III shows fibrosis with septa joining adjacent triads. In stage IV there is true cirrhosis, with regeneration nodules.

Dysfunction. The concentration of bilirubin in the plasma is usually less than 40 μmol/L (2 mg/100 mL) in the early stages of primary biliary cirrhosis. The activity of the alkaline phosphatases in the plasma is over 300 U/L in most patients, sometimes higher. The concentration of cholesterol and phospholipids in the serum is usually increased. If the concentration of cholesterol exceeds 15 mmol/L (500 mg/100 mL) xanthomata and xanthelasmata develop in the skin. Hypergammaglobulinemia is usual. In most patients, the concentration of IgM in the plasma exceeds 2 kg/L (200 mg/100 mL).

Antimitochondrial antibodies are present in the plasma in all patients, though in a few they are not demonstrable by the immunofluorescent methods usually used. Antibody against the M2 antigen present on the inner mitochondrial membrane and associated with ATPase is present in all patients with primary biliary cirrhosis but rarely in other conditions that give rise to antimitochondrial antibodies. When used to stain a rat kidney, it fixes to all renal tubules but most strongly to the distal and collecting tubules. Digestion with trypsin abolishes the staining.

Antibodies against smooth muscle are present in the plasma in 50% of the patients, antinuclear antibodies in 30%, and antithyroid antibodies in 30%. Circulating immune complexes can be demonstrated in the blood in 80% of the patients.

Copper is absorbed normally from the bowel in primary biliary cirrhosis, but is present in the plasma in twice its normal concentration, mainly bound to ceruloplas-

min. Copper is taken up by the hepatocytes in abnormal quantity, in proportion to the increased concentration of copper bound to albumin and amino acids in the plasma. It is not excreted normally into the bile and accumulates in the liver.

Clinical Presentation. Primary biliary cirrhosis is often present for months or years before it produces symptoms. In some series, up to 60% of the patients have been asymptomatic when the diagnosis was made, usually because of some biochemical abnormality discovered during the investigation of some other disease.

Symptoms develop insidiously. Pruritus is often the first symptom. It is often intermittent and may first become evident during pregnancy. Jaundice appears the same time as the pruritus in 25% of the patients, but more often comes later, often not for months or years. It is of the cholestatic type and slowly worsens, though the intensity of the jaundice often fluctuates. Some patients present with tiredness and fatigue. Some seek advice for bleeding esophageal varies, a peptic ulcer, or some other complication of cirrhosis. Some complain of the pigmentation of the skin commonly found in primary biliary cirrhosis. Rarely, a patient presents with xanthomata. On examination, the liver is usually enlarged, and often the spleen is also.

Over 70% of patients with primary biliary cirrhosis show some feature of the sicca or Sjögren's syndrome. They do not show the increased frequency of the HLA antigens B8 and DRW3 seen in the primary form of Sjögren's syndrome. About 5% of the patients have rheumatoid arthritis. Some have scleroderma or the CRST syndrome. Some have autoimmune thyroiditis, renal tubular acidosis, systemic lupus erythematosus, or villous atrophy in the small bowel with malabsorption.

About 40% of the patients have gallstones, as compared with about 10% of the general population. The frequency of gallstones is also increased in other types of cirrhosis.

Pathogenesis. The pathogenesis of primary biliary cirrhosis is unknown, though there is a strong suggestion that the disease is immunologically mediated. The lesions suggest an immunologic attack against the epithelium of the intrahepatic bile ducts.

The association of the disease with conditions considered to be immunologically mediated and the constant presence of abnormal antibodies in the blood suggest an immunologic pathogenesis. The strong association of primary biliary cirrhosis with the Sjögren's syndrome suggests that the immunologic attack is directed not only against the biliary epithelium, but against the epithelia of other kinds of secretory duct.

Treatment and Prognosis. In asymptomatic patients, primary biliary cirrhosis progresses slowly. Some remain asymptomatic for more than 10 years, though in most symptoms begin 2 to 4 years after diagnosis. The inflammatory lesions in the triads can persist for as long as 10 years, and the periferal ductular proliferation for 5 or 10 years more. The death rate in asymptomatic patients in the first 10 years after diagnosis does not differ from that of the general population. Once symptoms develop, life expectancy is about 7 years. Some die within 3 years. Some live for more than 15 years. Death comes from complications of portal hypertension or from liver failure.

Adrenocortical steroids and immunosuppressive agents do little to alter the course. Patients in the late stages of primary biliary cirrhosis treated by liver transplant have a 70% one year survival. A few have developed primary biliary cirrhosis in the transplant.

SECONDARY HEPATITIS. Inflammatory changes are common in the liver in people with ulcerative colitis or Crohn's disease and sometimes occur in people with other kinds of gastrointestinal disease. They are common in severe febrile illnesses and in toxemia.

Lesion. The liver may show any combination of a variety of changes. The nature of the hepatic involvement does not indicate the nature of the underlying illness.

Some of the portal tracts in the liver often contain an exudate of lymphocytes, with a few macrophages and sometimes occasional plasma cells or eosinophils. Germinal centers are sometimes present in the exudate. A few lymphocytes may spill into the adjacent parenchyma, but the limiting plate of hepatocytes remains intact.

In the parenchyma, foci of hepatocellular necrosis are often present. The foci of necrosis are usually small and unobtrusive, but can be large, with a prominent accumulation of lymphocytes and macrophages. Whether or not there is hepatocellular necrosis, the Kupffer cells in the sinusoids are often prominent, especially around the terminal hepatic veins. Foci of fatty change in the hepatocytes are common.

Clinical Presentation. The changes in the liver are usually overshadowed by the underlying disease and pass unnoticed. If the hepatic injury is severe enough, it produces biochemical changes like those of other forms of hepatocellular necrosis.

Treatment and Prognosis. Secondary hepatitis resolves without treatment if the underlying condition is controlled. No residual injury to the liver remains.

CIRRHOSIS OF THE LIVER

The term *cirrhosis of the liver* is used to describe a disease in which fibrous septa divide the hepatic parenchyma into nodules and regenerative nodules develop in the surviving hepatocytes. If there are only fibrous septa without regenerative nodules, the process is called fibrosis of the liver, not cirrhosis. The term *cirrhosis* comes from the Greek for orange or tawny and refers to the tawny color often striking in a cirrhotic liver.

In the United States, cirrhosis of the liver is the fourth most common cause of death. In different countries in Europe, from 3 to 30 people per 100,000 die of cirrhosis. The patients are usually adult, most over 50 years old.

Lesions. Three morphologic types of cirrhosis of the liver are distinguished, micronodular, macronodular, and mixed. Each is further divided into active and inactive forms.

Though the terms are not quite synonymous, micronodular cirrhosis is sometimes called portal cirrhosis, nutritional cirrhosis, or Laennec's cirrhosis, after the French physician who introduced the term *cirrhosis* in 1826. Macronodular cirrhosis is sometimes called postnecrotic cirrhosis or posthepatitic cirrhosis.

Micronodular Cirrhosis. In micronodular cirrhosis, fibrous septa join every portal tract to its neighbors and join the portal

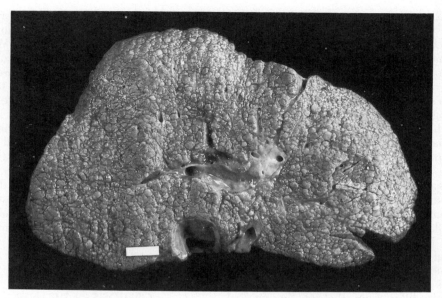

Fig. 36-22. Micronodular cirrhosis, showing the even, small nodules separated by fine scars.

tracts to the terminal hepatic veins. No portal tract and no hepatic vein is spared.

Macroscopically, the liver is often about normal size, weighing 1,500 g or a little more. Occasionally it is large, fatty, and weighs 3,000 or 4,000 g. Late in the disease it sometimes shrinks to less than 1,000 g.

Usually, the liver is the light tan that the word cirrhosis implies. Occasionally its color is normal. A large fatty liver is yellow. A

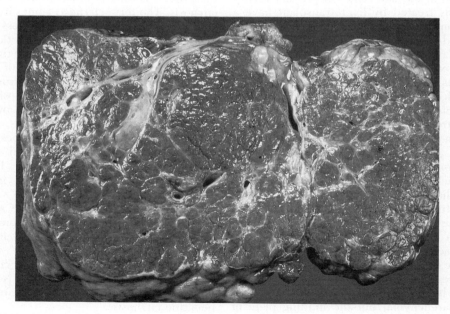

Fig. 36-23. Macronodular cirrhosis, showing the coarse, irregular scarring, with large nodules of surviving parenchyma.

small shrunken liver is gray from the extensive scarring. If jaundice is severe, the liver is green.

The surface of the liver is evenly granular, because the nodules of surviving liver parenchyma bulge above the fibrous septa that separate them and are all much the same size, usually 3 to 5 mm in diameter, though sometimes as much as 1 cm across. A cirrhotic liver of this sort is often called a hobnail liver, because its surface resembles the sole of an old-fashioned boot armed with hobnails.

On cut section, the appearance is similar, with spheroidal or angular nodules of surviving parenchyma separated by the fibrous septa that divide them. Early in the disease, the fibrous septa are fine and delicate, but as the cirrhosis worsens the septa grow thicker and come to occupy an increasing proportion of the hepatic substance, eventually with little nodules of surviving parenchyma isolated by broad scars.

Microscopically, the septa that divide the parenchyma into nodules consist of collagenous tissue, in which the portal tracts and terminal hepatic veins are often recognizable. The septa usually contain a sparse exudate of lymphocytes, with a few macrophages and plasma cells. Occasionally the exudate is marked. Often the bile ducts in the portal tracts proliferate and extend into the fibrous septa.

The hepatocytes in the islands of surviving parenchyma proliferate to form regeneration nodules. At first the nodules are angular, but as the number of hepatocytes in the nodules increases, they become spheroidal. In the nodules, plates of liver cells are separated by sinusoids, much as in normal liver, except that the cell plates in the nodules are usually two cells thick. The hepatocytes in the nodules often vary is size. Cells with two nuclei are common.

Evidence of the disease that caused the cirrhosis sometimes lingers in the liver. In most patients, micronodular cirrhosis is caused by alcohol. Fatty change in the regeneration nodules is almost universal. Less often there is evidence of continuing alcoholic hepatitis.

Macronodular Cirrhosis. In macronodular cirrhosis, collagenous septa join portal tract to portal tract, and portal tracts to terminal hepatic veins, but the pattern is more irregular than in micronodular cirrhosis. Some of the portal tracts and hepatic veins are spared and remain intact within the nodules of surviving parenchyma.

Macroscopically, the liver is usually of normal size or a little smaller. Its color is often unchanged. Most often, the liver is coarsely and irregularly scarred. Often one lobe of the liver is more severely involved than the other. Commonly the bands of scarring vary in thickness. Some are fine and delicate. Others may be up to 5 cm across, replacing large parts of the parenchyma. The nodules on the surface of the liver and those seen when it is sectioned vary in size from 0.5 cm to 5 cm across. They vary in shape and sometimes in color. Some bulge from the surface of the liver. Some are depressed. Only occasionally are the nodules all much the same size, though larger than those of micronodular cirrhosis.

Microscopically, the septa consist of collagenous tissue, usually with a scattering of lymphocytes, plasma cells, and macrophages. Often there is extensive proliferation of bile ducts in the septa. In the large nodules of surviving parenchyma, the structure of the parenchyma and the uninvolved portal tracts and central hepatic veins it contains often remain almost normal. Smaller nodules of surviving parenchyma contain no triads or terminal hepatic veins and develop into spheroidal regeneration nodules like those in micronodular cirrhosis.

In the patients with macronodular cirrhosis in whom all the nodules are about the same size, the surviving parenchyma forms regeneration nodules, differing from micronodular cirrhosis only in that some of the nodules contain intact triads or terminal hepatic veins. Fatty change is common in macronodular cirrhosis, but signs of the disease that caused the cirrhosis are not as often evident as in micronodular cirrhosis.

Mixed Cirrhosis. In mixed cirrhosis part of the liver shows the micronodular pattern, part a macronodular pattern. Often the condition is an incomplete form of micronodular cirrhosis in which some of the portal tracts or terminal hepatic veins are not involved by the fibrosis.

Active and Inactive Cirrhosis. In active cirrhosis, hepatocellular necrosis continues. Most often a process like chronic active hepatitis nibbles at the regeneration nodules where they abut against the fibrous septa. There is similar piecemeal necrosis, similar extension of the fibrosis into the nodules of hepatocytes, and a similar inflammatory reaction.

Less often, alcoholic hepatitis persists in the cirrhotic liver, with foci of necrosis in the regeneration nodules, a neutrophilic reaction, alcoholic hyaline, and all the other features of alcoholic hepatitis. Still less often, some other form of liver disease remains active in the cirrhotic liver.

In inactive cirrhosis, there is no evidence of continuing hepatocellular necrosis. The nodules of surviving parenchyma are sharply defined, with no inflammation and no signs of hepatocellular injury at their margins.

Clinical Presentation. Cirrhosis of the liver often causes no symptoms and no disability. In 30% of the patients the diagnosis is made only at autopsy. In 10%, the disease is discovered when the patient is investigated for some other illness. In only 60% do symptoms of cirrhosis bring the patient to consult a physician.

In some patients, symptoms of cirrhosis develop acutely, with symptoms and signs like those of alcoholic hepatitis. This is particularly likely in patients with alcoholic cirrhosis who continue to drink heavily in spite of previous attacks of liver damage.

More often the onset is insidious. The first sign may be ascites, jaundice, hematemesis, or some other sign of portal hypertension. Muscular wasting, weight loss, weakness, and fatiguability are frequent. Low fever is common, perhaps because of hepatocellular necrosis, perhaps because of some concealed infection. The liver is often enlarged, with a firm, smooth edge, but may be small and impalpable. The spleen is often enlarged.

As cirrhosis grows worse, hepatic failure, portal hypertension, or both are likely to develop. There is usually increasing ascites, and any of the other complications may appear.

Complications. The complications of cirrhosis of the liver develop only when the disease is far advanced, though the correlation between the severity of the cirrhosis, as judged anatomically, and the severity of the dysfunction it causes is not good.

Portal Hypertension. Portal hypertension is present in 60% of patients with symptoms of hepatic cirrhosis. The effects and complications of portal hypertension are discussed later in this chapter. Only its pathogenesis in cirrhosis is considered here.

Obstruction to the portal blood flow is the major cause of portal hypertension in cirrhosis. Many of the smaller intrahepatic branches of the portal vein are lost, and the whole portal blood flow must force its way through the remaining vessels. The portal veins that do persist are often compressed by the enlarging regeneration nodules or narrowed by the fibrosis, further obstructing the portal blood flow. Many of the regeneration nodules lose all or part of their portal blood supply. In those that do receive portal blood, the flow through the sinusoids is impaired by the pressure of the proliferating hepatocytes in the nodule and by the inadequacy of the drainage into the hepatic veins. Anastomoses between the portal and hepatic veins develop in the fibrous septa and carry up to 30% of the portal blood flow, avoiding the obstruction in the sinusoids, but these shunts are thin walled and easily compressed by the regeneration nodules, again obstructing the blood flow. The hepatic veins are also thin walled and are easily obstructed by the enlarging regeneration nodules or distorted by fibrosis, causing further obstruction.

Anastomoses between the intrahepatic branches of the hepatic artery and the portal vessels further increase the intrahepatic portal blood pressure. The hepatic artery supplies the regeneration nodules, emptying blood at high pressure into their sinusoids. Anastomoses between the hepatic artery and the portal veins and between the hepatic artery and the shunts between the portal and hepatic veins develop in the fibrous septa, again bringing blood at arterial pressure into the portal system and increasing the intrahepatic portal blood pressure.

Hepatic Failure. Hepatic failure, which brings death to many people with cirrhosis, results in part from the loss of liver cells, in part from the abnormal circulation in the cirrhotic liver. It is considered further later in the chapter.

In advanced cirrhosis, the number of hepatocytes in the liver is reduced, perhaps to less than 20% of normal. Especially when a person with cirrhosis continues to drink, the function of the hepatocytes is further impaired by the continuing injury induced by the alcohol.

Hepatic function is further compromised by the shunts between the portal and hepatic veins and by the lack of portal blood in some of the regeneration nodules. The shunts mean that much of the portal blood bypasses the liver as effectively as if it passed directly from the portal vein into the vena cava. The lack of portal blood in some of the regeneration nodules means that the value of the hepatocytes in these nodules supplied only by arterial blood is limited.

Ascites. Ascites is common in people with severe cirrhosis of the liver. It becomes evident clinically when 500 mL of fluid have accumulated in the peritoneal cavity, though smaller quantities of fluid can be detected by ultrasonography. Some patients have more than 2 L of fluid in the abdomen. Several factors combine to cause the ascites.

Portal hypertension is an important factor, though ascites can occur in patients with cirrhosis who do not have portal hypertension and is not always present in people with portal hypertension. As the pressure rises in the portal microcirculation with its multitude of capillaries beneath the thin peritoneum, fluid is likely to leak from the blood into the peritoneal cavity.

The hypoproteinemia common in cirrhosis reduces the osmotic pressure that retains fluid in the portal microcirculation and tends to cause ascites. Ascites is more likely if there is both portal hypertension and hypoproteinemia than if there is one or the other.

Because of the obstruction to the portal and hepatic veins common in advanced cirrhosis, the liver becomes edematous. The lymphatics within the liver are dilated and engorged, and the pressure of lymph within them increases. The lymphatics in the capsule share in this distention and hypertension. Lymph leaks from them and oozes from the surface of the liver into the peritoneal cavity.

The kidneys of patients with cirrhosis retain sodium and water. It is not clear whether the retention of sodium is initiated by underfilling of the vasculature caused by pooling of blood in the portal circulation or whether retention of sodium comes first and causes overfilling of the vasculature. The secretion of renin by the kidneys increases, causing hyperaldosteronism. Decreased destruction of aldosterone by the damaged liver increases its activity in the plasma. The production of prostaglandins in the kidneys increases. The kallikrein-kinin system is activated. Formation of natriuretic factor increases. More antidiuretic hormone is released.

Portal Vein Thrombosis. Thrombosis of the portal vein sometimes complicates cirrhosis of the liver. The sudden occlusion of the portal circulation usually causes rapid accumulation of ascites. In some patients, the vein becomes recanalized and a prominent line of anastomoses develops around it, a condition called cavernous transformation of the portal vein.

Spontaneous Bacterial Peritonitis. Patients with cirrhosis of the liver and ascites occasionally develop peritonitis without disease of the bowel or any other apparent cause for the infection. Most often the organism is a gram-negative enteric bacillus, less often a pneumococcus or some other gram-positive bacterium. Some patients with spontaneous bacterial peritonitis have fever, chills, abdominal pain, guarding and other signs of peritonitis, but in some the signs of infection are slight. If the ascitic fluid contains more than 250 neutrophils per mL, the patient probably has bacterial peritonitis.

Alimentary. Bleeding from esophageal varices is the major alimentary complication of hepatic cirrhosis. It is discussed later in the chapter in the section on portal hypertension.

More than 10% of patients with cirrhosis have a peptic ulcer. Gastritis is common, but this may be due to the alcohol rather than to the cirrhosis.

Gallstones are twice as common in people with cirrhosis as in the general population, probably because of impairment of the formation of bile salts. In people with alcoholic cirrhosis, the risk of developing acute or chronic pancreatitis is increased. Diarrhea is common in cirrhosis. Lack of bile salts can cause steatorrhea. Sometimes the parotid glands are enlarged.

Hematologic. The synthesis of the coagulation factors manufactured in the liver is commonly impaired in advanced cirrhosis. The activity of factors V, VII, IX, and XII is reduced, as is the synthesis of prothrombin. There is often an accompanying increase in plasma fibrinolytic activity.

Hypoalbuminemia is common in cirrhosis. Probably it results principally from damage to the hepatocytes, with decreased synthesis. Usually there is hypergammaglobulinemia, with increase in IgG.

Anemia is common in cirrhosis. Blood loss from the alimentary tract often brings iron deficiency anemia. Sometimes there is folate deficiency. Hemolytic anemia can complicate cirrhosis, though it is rarely severe. Hypersplenism sometimes complicates portal hypertension.

Endocrine. Feminization sometimes becomes evident in men with severe cirrhosis. The pubic hair often changes to a female pattern, and axillary hair is lost. Gynecomastia can become prominent. Testicular atrophy and impotence are common. In women, amenorrhea is frequent.

The cause of the feminization is uncertain. The damaged liver fails to detoxify estrogens, but this does not seem to be the only abnormality in estrogen metabolism. The conversion of androgens to estrogens in the tissue may be increased.

Mild, insulin-resistant diabetes mellitus can develop in cirrhosis. Diabetes mellitus is twice as common in people with cirrhosis as in the general population. The diabetes is associated with hyperglucagonemia.

Renal. The hepatorenal syndrome, discussed in Chapter 27, often causes renal failure in the later stages of cirrhosis. Deposition of IgA in the mesangial regions of the renal glomeruli is common.

Fever. A low fever, usually less than 38°C is present in 30% of people with advanced cirrhosis. In some of these people, the fever results from infection. Bacteremia

with gram-negative or gram-positive organisms is common, especially in the end stages of cirrhosis. Some have spontaneous bacterial peritonitis or endocarditis. Occasionally, an inapparent peritonitis or endocarditis is present. In some, the fever seems due to the liver disease itself.

Musculoskeletal. Dupuytren's contracture is more common in people with cirrhosis than in the population at large. Sometimes clubbing of the fingers or hypertrophic osteoarthropathy is evident.

Hepatocellular Carcinoma. The risk of developing hepatocellular carcinoma is increased in people with cirrhosis. Between 5 and 15% of people with cirrhosis develop carcinoma of the liver. In North America, Europe, and Australasia, more than 80% of patients with hepatocellular carcinoma have cirrhosis of the liver.

Pathogenesis. In most forms of cirrhosis, the fibrosis is initiated by hepatocellular necrosis. The continued destruction of small numbers of hepatocytes for months or years releases factors that cause the deposition of collagen. The nature of these factors is unknown. It is not known if the monokines and lymphokines that cause fibrosis are important.

As fibrosis develops in cirrhosis, the Ito cells that lie beneath the sinusoidal epithelium in close apposition to the hepatocytes proliferate and probably become transformed into myofibrocytes and fibrocytes. They deposit collagen and basement membrane at first around the sinusoids and then more widely. As the fibrosis grows more extensive, other fibrocytes proliferate and add to the fibrosis.

The cause of the proliferation of hepatocytes to form the regeneration nodules is obscure. Chalones, growth factors, hormonal imbalance, and other factors may all play a part.

The continuing necrosis of hepatocytes in active cirrhosis often continues long after the agent causing the cirrhosis has been withdrawn, especially in patients with alcoholic cirrhosis. It is often suggested that it is due to an autoimmune reaction like that involved in idiopathic chronic active hepatitis.

Causes. Though alcohol is the major cause of hepatic cirrhosis, many other hepatic injuries can cause cirrhosis. Different agents cause different kinds of cirrhosis.

Alcohol. In North America, Europe, and Australasia, alcohol is the cause of cirrhosis in 90% of the patients. The incidence of cirrhosis in different countries correlates well with the per capita consumption of alcohol. Fewer than 5 people per 100,000 die of cirrhosis in Norway where the consumption of alcohol is low, more than 30 per 100,000 in France where it is high.

Alcohol usually causes micronodular cirrhosis. Less often, it causes either mixed cirrhosis with incomplete fibrous septa in part of the liver or more extensive necrosis and macronodular cirrhosis. Nearly always the liver is fatty. Signs of alcoholic hepatitis are not often evident. In most of the patients, the cirrhosis complicates steatosis and begins with fibrosis around the terminal hepatic veins.

Viral Hepatitis. Hepatitis B, non-A, non-B hepatitis, hepatitis D, and the hepatitis caused by cytomegaloviruses can cause cirrhosis of the liver, usually macronodular cirrhosis. Viruses are a particularly important cause of cirrhosis in Africa and other regions in which viral hepatitis is common.

Biliary Obstruction. Long-standing extrahepatic biliary obstruction is an uncommon cause of cirrhosis. More often biliary obstruction causes fibrosis and enlargement of the biliary tracts in the liver, but does not give rise to fibrous septa that divide the parenchyma.

When extrahepatic obstruction does cause cirrhosis, the cirrhosis is micronodular or mixed. The fibrous septa are usually broad. The proliferation of bile ducts in the septa is extensive. Usually there is little regeneration in the surviving parenchyma. True regeneration nodules are few. Bile plugs are numerous in the canaliculi. Hepatocytes and Kupffer cells are bile stained. Often the liver is bright green because of the obstruction to bile flow. This kind of cirrhosis is often called secondary biliary cirrhosis, or simply biliary cirrhosis.

Hemochromatosis. Hemochromatosis is discussed in Chapter 9. Iron accumulates in the liver, with massive deposits of hemosiderin in Kupffer cells, hepatocytes, macrophages in the portal tracts, and in the epithelium of the bile ducts. Later, fibrous septa extend out from the portal tracts, and eventually a fairly even macronodular or a mixed cirrhosis results. The chocolate brown color of the cirrhotic liver in hemochromatosis is characteristic.

The presence of even large quantities of

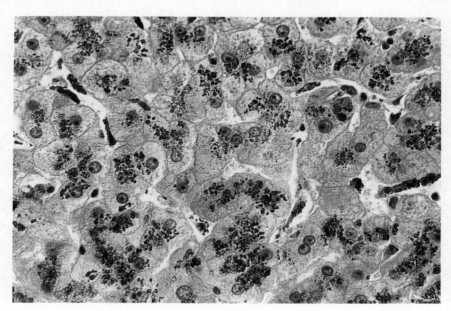

Fig. 36-24. Hemochromatosis, showing the deposition of iron in hepatocytes and Kupffer cells.

iron in the liver does not establish the diagnosis of primary hemochromatosis caused by a genetic defect. Some increase in the quantity of hemosiderin in the Kupffer cells and hepatocytes is common in many kinds of cirrhosis. Occasionally people with cirrhosis who have no other evidence of genetic hemochromatosis have massive deposits of iron in their liver. In such people, the excess of iron probably results from multiple blood transfusions given because of bleeding esophageal varices or for some other cause.

Other Metabolic Diseases. Wilson's disease is discussed in Chapter 9. It may cause chronic active hepatitis or changes like those of alcoholic hepatitis, and eventually macronodular cirrhosis results.

Patients with severe α_1-antitrypsin deficiency often develop micronodular or macronodular cirrhosis. The cirrhosis may become evident during childhood or may appear only in adult life. Galactosemia and type IV glycogen storage disease are unusual causes of macronodular cirrhosis in children.

Fibrocystic disease of the pancreas can cause macronodular cirrhosis. Hereditary fructose intolerance, abetalipoproteinemia, and some of the amino acid disorders are rare causes of cirrhosis.

Drugs and Poisons. Methotrexate, methyldopa, isoniazid, oxyphenisatin, and other drugs that cause hepatocellular necrosis or chronic active hepatitis sometimes cause cirrhosis. If the drug causes submassive necrosis, coarse macronodular cirrhosis will result. If it causes chronic active hepatitis, the cirrhosis is more regular. Pyrrolidizine alkaloids, chemotherapeutic drugs, oral contraceptives, and other agents that cause veno-occlusive disease or the Budd-Chiari syndrome cause scarring and fibrosis of the liver.

Hepatic Congestion. In severe heart failure, congestion of the liver is sometimes followed by fibrosis around the terminal hepatic veins. The fibrosis links vein to vein as it grows more extensive, but rarely involves the portal triads. The fibrosis is often

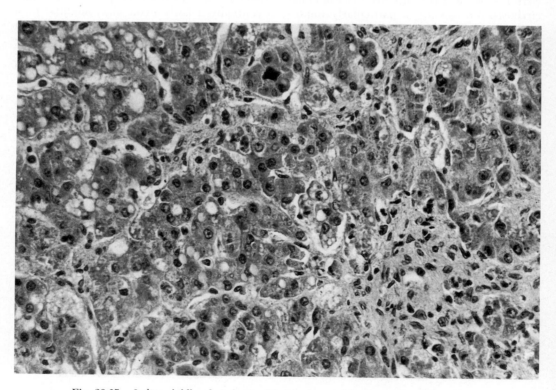

Fig. 36-25. Indian childhood cirrhosis, showing changes like those of viral hepatitis.

called cardiac cirrhosis, though the regeneration nodules required by the definition of cirrhosis are rarely present.

Chronic Active Hepatitis. Viral, drug-induced, and idiopathic chronic active hepatitis all lead to cirrhosis. The similar piecemeal necrosis seen in primary biliary cirrhosis, active cirrhosis, and other conditions causes hepatic fibrosis and leads to or worsens cirrhosis.

Indian Childhood Cirrhosis. Indian childhood cirrhosis is an unusual condition found only in India. Children in the first years of life develop changes in the liver like those of severe alcoholic hepatitis, with Mallory bodies in many of the hepatocytes. Copper accumulates in the liver. The end is cirrhosis, usually of a micronodular pattern. The cause of the disease is unknown.

North American Indian Childhood Cirrhosis. A few North American Indian children have developed severe jaundice and pruritus at birth. The jaundice resolves during the first year, but the activity of alkaline phosphatase in the plasma and the concentration of bile salts remains elevated, and the activity of aminotransferases increases slightly. Periportal fibrosis and cirrhosis follow. At birth, the liver shows giant cell hepatitis and cholestasis. The bile canaliculi are surrounded by an abnormal web of filaments containing actin. The disease is believed to be due to malfunction of the microfilaments necessary for the transport of bile from the liver.

Rare Causes. Occasionally cirrhosis develops in kwashiorkor. It has been reported in patients with an intestinal bypass for obesity. Occasionally cirrhosis has developed in a patient with sarcoidosis, hereditary hemorrhagic telangiectasia, or cystic fibrosis.

Cryptogenic Cirrhosis. When all these possibilities have been considered, there remain patients with cirrhosis of the liver in whom the cause is unknown. The disease in these patients is called cryptogenic cirrhosis, from the Greek for hidden, or secret. About 30% of these patients have circulating antimitochondrial antibodies, and 30% have circulating antibodies against smooth muscle, suggesting a possible relationship to chronic active hepatitis or primary biliary cirrhosis.

Treatment and Prognosis. There is no cure for cirrhosis of the liver. At best, the progress of the disease can be stopped. If alcohol is the cause, the patient must eschew alcohol, preserve a good diet, live reasonably. If so and if there is neither ascites nor jaundice, about 60% of the patients will be alive five years after the diagnosis is made. If ascites, jaundice, or any other serious complication develops, the chance of survival falls progressively.

PORTAL HYPERTENSION

Normally the pressure in the portal veins is 10 to 15 cm of saline. If the pressure exceeds 30 cm, the patient is said to have portal hypertension. Portal hypertension is nearly always caused by obstruction to the portal blood flow. Cirrhosis is its most common cause. The portal veins have no valves, and so obstruction anywhere in the system raises the pressure in all the veins proximal to the obstruction. Rarely, an arteriovenous malformation in the splanchnic region delivers blood at arterial pressure into the portal veins and causes portal hypertension without obstruction.

Causes. The causes of portal hypertension are divided into two groups, presinusoidal and hepatic. In the presinusoidal group, the obstruction causing the hypertension is proximal to the hepatic sinusoids. The parenchyma of the liver and the hepatic veins are normal. The patient may suffer the complications of portal hypertension but will not develop hepatic failure. In the hepatic group, the disease causing the hypertension involves the parenchyma of the liver and often the portal veins leading to the sinusoids and the hepatic veins leading from them as well. The patient is likely to develop both portal hypertension and hepatic failure.

Presinusoidal. In most of the world, thrombosis of the portal vein is the most common cause of presinusoidal portal hypertension. The thrombosis is often secondary to cirrhosis but is sometimes due to infection, pancreatitis, or trauma. In the patients in whom the liver is normal, it causes presinusoidal obstruction. In those with cirrhosis, it worsens the hepatic obstruction.

In India, 30% of patients with portal hypertension have sclerosis and narrowing of the moderate-sized and small portal veins, often with recanalized thrombi in the lumen, a condition called idiopathic portal hypertension. The condition is also common in Japan and does occur in the United States and the United Kingdom.

Other causes of presinusoidal obstruction are uncommon. Occasionally sarcoidosis, a myeloproliferative disorder, congenital hepatic fibrosis, or schistosomiasis obstructs the portal veins within the liver and causes portal hypertension without damaging the parenchyma of the liver. Inorganic arsenical compounds can cause fibrosis of the portal tracts and portal hypertension. Vinyl chloride causes perisinusoidal and portal fibrosis and portal hypertension. Occasionally copper poisoning or hypervitaminosis A does so. Rarely, a tumor compresses extrahepatic or intrahepatic portal veins and causes portal hypertension.

Hepatic. Cirrhosis of the liver is the most common cause of hepatic portal hypertension. The blood flow through the intrahepatic portal veins, the sinusoids, and the hepatic veins is obstructed, and anastomoses with the hepatic artery add to the portal pressure.

Less common causes of hepatic portal hypertension are nodular regenerative hyperplasia and partial nodular transformation.

The obstruction to portal blood flow caused by disease of the hepatic veins is often considered a subtype of hepatic portal hypertension called postsinusoidal portal hypertension. It is uncommon, but occurs in veno-occlusive disease and in the Budd-Chiari syndrome. Occasionally the portal pressure is increased in patients with severe congestive heart failure.

Effects. Portal hypertension raises the venous pressure in the portal vessels. It induces the formation of anastomoses between the portal veins and the systemic veins. It causes enlargement and sometimes dysfunction of the spleen.

Increased Pressure. The increase and pressure in the portal microcirculation tends to cause ascites. The splenic and other large veins of the portal system become dilated and tortuous. The distorted veins often show focal thickening of the intima and fibrosis of the adventitia. Sometimes a vein becomes calcified. The splenic artery may also be tortuous, atherosclerotic, and calcified.

Anastomoses. Anastomoses develop between the portal veins and systemic veins. The best known are the esophageal varices that develop in the cardiac part of the stomach and the lower part of the esophagus, as anastomoses from the left gastric and short gastric veins overtax the radicles of the azygos system in the lower esophagus.

The connections between the portal and caval systems in the hemorrhoidal plexuses of the rectum dilate, causing hemorrhoids. The paraumbilical veins in the falciform ligament carry portal blood to anastomoses with the systemic veins around the umbilicus. Sometimes large, tortuous veins radiate from the umbilicus in the skin, an appearance called a caput medusae, after the snake-haired Medusa.

In the retroperitoneum, innumerable anastomoses between the portal and caval systems develop through the veins of Retzius. The veins of Sappey take portal blood from the liver to the systemic veins in the diaphragm. Adhesions may allow portal blood to find anastomoses in the abdominal wall. Communications between the splenic vein and the left renal vein open and occasionally become enormous.

The anastomoses decompress the portal system. The blood that can no longer pass through the liver finds its way back to the heart by these new routes. Further increase in portal pressure is slowed.

Splenomegaly. The enlargement of the spleen common in portal hypertension is called congestive splenomegaly. It is discussed with the diseases of the spleen in Chapter 54. The spleen is usually from 500 to 1000 g in weight and easily palpable.

Complications. The principal complications of portal hypertension are hemorrhage, hepatic failure, and hypersplenism.

The varices that develop in the esophagus in portal hypertension are described in Chapter 33. Minor trauma easily tears the varices and causes hemorrhage. Increasing intravascular pressure can cause a varix to rupture. The hemorrhage from the varices is sometimes slow and causes melena. Often it is massive, with hematemesis and melena. Commonly the intestine becomes filled with blood.

The shunting of blood away from the liver in portal hypertension tends to cause hepatic encephalopathy, as products normally detoxified in the liver pass directly into the systemic circulation. Hemorrhage from varices increases the likelihood of hepatic failure. The shock and hypotension caused by the bleeding decrease further the perfusion of the failing liver. The blood in the bowel allows the intestinal bacteria to increase the production of the ammonia that is a major factor in the causation of hepatic encephalopathy. The high content of protein in the bowel adds to the risk of encephalopathy.

The enlarged spleen is probably responsible in large part for the shortened life of the red blood cells common in cirrhosis of the liver, but more serious manifestations of hypersplenism, discussed in Chapter 54, are unusual.

Treatment and Prognosis. Portal hypertension is usually managed by treating the complications of the disorder. Bleeding esophageal varices are managed by giving vasopressin to control the bleeding and transfusions to restore the blood volume. If this fails, compression of the varices by an intraesophageal tube, sclerosis of the varices at endoscopy, or surgical interruption of the anastomoses is necessary. Hepatic encephalopathy requires restriction of the protein in the diet and neomycin to prevent the production of ammonia by intestinal bacteria.

The value of propranolol in reducing portal hypertension remains uncertain. Surgery to create shunts between the portal or superior mesenteric vein and the vena cava or between the splenic and renal veins gives relief to some patients, but in 30% causes hepatic encephalopathy because of the diversion of the portal blood directly into the systemic circulation.

Over 70% of patients with portal hypertension who have a plasma bilirubin concentration of less than 35 mmol/L (2 mg/100 mL), a concentration of albumin of over 30 g/L (3 mg/100 mL), little or no ascites, little

or no neurologic dysfunction, and who are well nourished survive more than one year. Less than 30% of those in whom the concentration of bilirubin is greater than 35 g/L, the concentration of albumin less than 30 g/L, in whom ascites or neurologic dysfunction are severe, or who are ill nourished survive one year.

METABOLIC DISORDERS

In the metabolic disorders of the liver, deficiency or abnormality of an enzyme causes hepatic dysfunction. Most of the disorders are genetically determined. Jaundice is the principal sign in jaundice of the newborn, Gilbert's syndrome, the Crigler-Najjar syndromes, the Dubin-Johnson syndrome, the Rotor syndrome, recurrent intrahepatic cholestasis, and progressive intrahepatic cholestasis. In most of these conditions, the liver shows no anatomic abnormality. Other enzymatic disorders that affect primarily the liver include α_1-antitrypsin deficiency, tyrosinemia, abetalipoproteinemia, galactosemia, hereditary fructose deficiency, the glycogen storage diseases, and the disorders of the urea cycle.

Other diseases caused by enzyme deficiency affect the liver but involve more severely organs in other parts of the body. They are discussed with the diseases of those organs. Among them are Gaucher's disease, Niemann-Pick disease, metachromatic leukodystrophy, the gangliosidoses, the mucopolysaccharidoses, Wolman's disease, and cholesterol ester storage disease.

JAUNDICE IN THE NEWBORN. In the newborn, the enzymes needed for the conjugation of bilirubin in the hepatocytes and the Y protein needed for the intercellular transport of bilirubin are often deficient. Unconjugated bilirubin cannot be cleared from the blood adequately, and hyperbilirubinemia with an excess of unconjugated bilirubin occurs. In 50% of the infants born at full term, the bilirubinemia is sufficient to cause mild jaundice during the first week of life. The serum bilirubin concentration rarely exceeds 100 μmol/L (7 mg/100 mL). It falls to normal in seven days or so as the necessary enzymes develop. Often this transient hyperbilirubinema is called physiologic jaundice.

In premature infants, the hepatic enzyme deficiency is sometimes more severe, with serum levels of unconjugated bilirubin of 200 μmol/L (15 mg/100 mL) or more. At times, the bilirubinemia is sufficient to cause kernicterus. In severely jaundiced infants, exposure to blue light of wave length 450 nm causes breakdown of the bilirubin in the tissues, reducing the bilirubinemia. Only in the rare cases in which the concentration of bilirubin in the plasma exceeds 340 mmol/L (20 mg/100 mL) is an exchange transfusion necessary. Phenobarbital administered to the mother induces in the child the microsomal enzymes needed for the conjugation bilirubin and enhances the formation of the Y protein.

GILBERT'S SYNDROME.   Gilbert's syndrome is named after a French physician (1858–1927). It is the commonest of the genetically determined diseases of the liver. About 5% of blood donors have mild hyperbilirubinemia, with serum levels between 20 and 50 μmol/L (1 to 3 mg/100 mL), and probably many of these have Gilbert's disease.

In all probability, Gilbert's syndrome includes more than one condition. In most patients, it is inherited as an autosomal dominant character. The patients develop mild, intermittent hyperbilirubinemia, sometimes enough to cause jaundice. The serum bilirubin level rarely exceeds 50 μmol/L (3 mg/100 mL). The excess bilirubin is unconjugated and results from deficient uptake of bilirubin from the blood. In addition, there may be deficient conjugation of bilirubin in the hepatocytes, and sometimes there is mild hemolysis. Starvation tends to worsen the dysfunction.

The liver shows no morphologic abnormality, though some of the patients feel discomfort over the liver during the attacks of jaundice, with malaise or nausea.

Gilbert's syndrome persists throught the patient's life, but does not impair well being.

CRIGLER-NAJJAR SYNDROME.   The Crigler-Najjar syndrome is named after the American physicians who described it in 1952. There are two forms of this condition. Both are uncommon.

Type I Crigler-Najjar syndrome is inherited as an autosomal recessive character. The enzyme uridine diphosphate glucuronyl transferase is absent in the hepatocytes, and conjugated bilirubin is formed. Unconjugated bilirubin accumulates in the blood. Plasma levels of bilirubin may exceed 700 μmol/L (40 mg/100 mL). The infants born with this defect are deeply jaundiced. Kernicterus is common. No treatment is helpful. Death often comes in the first year of life. The liver shows no anatomic abnormality.

Type II Crigler-Najjar syndrome is inherited as an autosomal dominant character with incomplete penetrance and variable expressivity. Uridine diphosphate glucuronyl transferase is deficient in the hepatocytes, but the deficiency is not complete. Some conjugated bilirubin reaches the bile. Unconjugated bilirubin accumulates in the plasma, to a concentration of between 100 and 300 μmol/L (5 to 20 mg/100 mL). The patient is jaundiced, but otherwise in good health. Kernicterus is exceptional. Phenobarbital and other drugs that induce microsomal enzymes in the liver reduce the jaundice, often lowering the concentration of bilirubin in the plasma to near the normal range. Phototherapy also reduces the jaundice. The liver shows no anatomic abnormality.

DUBIN-JOHNSON SYNDROME.   The Dubin-Johnson syndrome is named after the American pathologists who described it in 1953. It is uncommon. The syndrome is probably inherited as an autosomal recessive character. Bilirubin is normally conjugated, but its excretion from the hepatocytes is impaired.

The patient is mildly jaundiced, and the depth of the jaundice tends to fluctuate. The serum bilirubin concentration is usually about 50 μmol/L (3 mg/100 mL) and rarely over 100 μmol/L (5 mg/100 mL). Over 60% of the bilirubin in the plasma is conjugated, most of it diconjugated. Infection or contraceptive pills augment the jaundice, and sometimes during an exacerbation there is discomfort or tenderness over the liver. The patient cannot secrete sulfobromophthalein (bromsulphalein) or the dyes used for oral cholecystography into the bile. The excretion of coproporphyrin I in the urine is in-

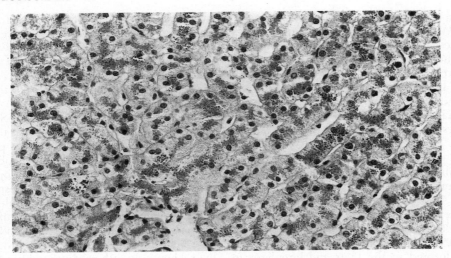

Fig. 36-26. Dubin-Johnson syndrome, showing the accumulation of pigment in the hepatocytes.

creased, and the excretion of coproporphyrin III is decreased. A melanin-like pigment accumulates in the lysosomes of the hepatocytes in such quantity that the liver turns greenish black. The Dubin-Johnson syndrome is benign and does little to interfere with life or longevity.

ROTOR'S SYNDROME. The Rotor syndrome is named after the Filipino physician who described it in 1948. It is inherited as an autosomal recessive character. A defect in the conjugation of bilirubin causes principally conjugated bilirubin to accumulate in the plasma. Most of the bilirubin is monoconjugated. The excretion of sulfobromophthalein and the dyes used in oral cholecystography are more normal than in the Dubin-Johnson syndrome. The total urinary coproporphyrins are increased, but the urinary excretion of coproporphyrin I is not. The liver shows no anatomic abnormality. The disease is mild and compatible with a normal life.

RECURRENT INTRAHEPATIC CHOLESTASIS. Recurrent intrahepatic cholestasis is rare and sometimes familial. The patients suffer repeated attacks of obstructive jaundice, often severe, perhaps with malaise at the onset, with itching. The jaundice lasts for months, with bilirubinuria, steatorrhea, and other signs of obstructive jaundice. Then the attack subsides, and the patient is well until the jaundice recurs weeks or years later.

Biopsy shows severe cholestasis of the kind typical of biliary obstruction during the attacks. Between attacks the liver is normal. The cause of this curious syndrome is unknown. The possibility of a genetic abnormality or an abnormal response to an environmental agent have been suggested.

PROGRESSIVE INTRAHEPATIC CHOLESTASIS. Progressive intrahepatic cholestasis is rare. It is often called Byler disease, after the first patient. Byler disease is transmitted as an autosomal recessive character.

Severe obstructive jaundice develops in infancy and persists. The defect seems to be in the excretion of bile from the hepatocytes. At first, liver biopsy is normal, but cholestasis soon develops around the terminal hepatic veins. The bile canaliculi are dilated, with swollen and blunted microvilli, and the cytoplasm around them is condensed. The bile in the canaliculi is granular. Cirrhosis soon follows. Most patients die of liver failure or hemorrhage from varices within 18 months, though some live a few years.

CHOLESTASIS OF PREGNANCY. Cholestasis of pregnancy occurs in 1 pregnancy in 2000 to 8000. It is most common in Scandinavia and Chile. The patients develop pruritus in the last four months of each pregnancy, and often become jaundiced some two weeks later. The concentration of bilirubin in the plasma rarely exceeds 100 μmol/L (5 mg/100 mL). Women who develop pruritus but not jaundice are said to have pruritus gravidarum. The pruritus and the jaundice disappear a few days after delivery.

The liver shows only cholestasis, with bile plugs in the biliary canaliculi around the terminal hepatic veins. The cholestasis disappears post partum, leaving no permanent injury.

The disease is often familial and results from abnormal sensitivity to the increase in estrogens and progesterones during pregnancy. The women affected are likely to develop cholestasis if given oral contraceptive agents containing these hormones.

α₁-**ANTITRYPSIN DEFICIENCY.** α_1-Antitrypsin is formed in the liver and circulates in the blood. It inhibits proteolytic enzymes. Its production is controlled by 24 alleles that share a single locus on an autosome and are codominant. The alleles are named Pi, for protease inhibitor, followed by a letter indicating the electrophoretic mobility of their product. F means fast, M intermediate, S slow, and Z even slower. Each electrophoretic group is divided into subtypes. Over 80% of the population have

two PiM alleles, a genotype termed PiMM. The plasma contains more than 2.5 g/L (250 mg/100 mL) of antitrypsin. People with the genotype PiZZ or PiSS have little or no antitrypsin in the plasma. Heterozygotes of type PiZM or PiSM have about 50% of the normal activity.

People of genotype PiZZ or PiSS who have little α_1-antitrypsin in the plasma often develop panacinar emphysema. The patients with emphysema commonly have globules of the abnormal antitrypsin in the endoplasmic reticulum of the hepatocytes, especially around the protal tracts. The globules stain strongly with the periodic acid-Schiff reaction, and immunohistologic methods confirm that they consist of antitrypsin. The liver shows no other abnormality. Similar globules are sometimes present in the hepatocytes in people with abnormal antitrypsin who have normal lungs and no other hepatic abnormality.

Infants with the PiZZ genotype often develop severe jaundice soon after birth. Biopsy shows cholestasis of the sort found in extrahepatic obstruction, though giant hepatocytes are not usually prominent. The globules of antitrypsin are not evident in the

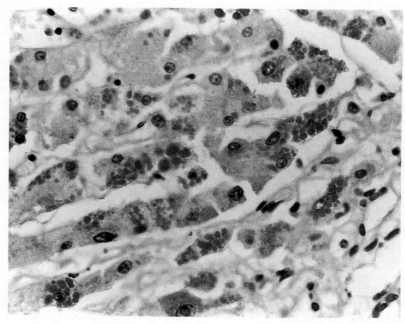

Fig. 36-27. α_1-Antitrypsin deficiency, showing the accumulation of $\alpha_1$antitrypsin in the hepatocytes.

hepatocytes in infants, but become demonstrable as the child ages. The jaundice resolves within a year, but cirrhosis appears a few years later. In some children, the initial cholestatic episode does not occur, and the disease presents with cirrhosis. Patients with liver disease do not develop emphysema, and patients with emphysema do not have cirrhosis.

Over 10% of people of genotype PiZZ who are over 50 years old develop cirrhosis of the liver. The hepatocytes show the globules of antitrypsin. The incidence of hepatocellular carcinoma and perhaps cholangiocarcinoma is increased. Patients treated by transplantation of the liver acquire the Pi genotype of the donor.

TYROSINEMIA. Tyrosinemia is believed due to a deficiency of fumarylacetoacetate hydrolase, though other enzyme deficiences may be also present. It is inherited as an autosomal recessive character.

The disease sometimes presents in infancy with jaundice, acute hepatic failure, vomiting, diarrhea, hepatosplenomegaly, ascites, and hypoprothrombinemia. Such infants have tyrosinemia and methioninemia, with lesser increase in other amino acids in the blood, and aminoaciduria with loss of many amino acids in the urine.

In other children, tyrosinosis is less dramatic, presenting in childhood with cirrhosis and rickets. Such children have an increase in tyrosine and sometimes methionine in the blood, but many amino acids are lost in the urine.

In the infants with acute tyrosinosis, the liver is fatty, with hepatocellular necrosis and cholestasis. In the older children there is macronodular, micronodular or mixed cirrhosis, with regeneration in the nodules of surviving parenchyma. Over 30% of the patients who survive more than two years develop hepatocellular carcinoma.

ABETALIPOPROTEINEMIA. Abetalipoproteinemia is described in Chapter 35. The patients with this defect have severe fatty change in the liver, with hepatocytes distended by large droplets of fat. The inability to synthesize low density and very low density lipoproteins prevents the excretion of triglycerides from the hepatocytes. Sometimes cirrhosis follows.

GALACTOSEMIA. Galactosemia is an inborn error of metabolism in which the enzyme galactose-1-phosphate uridyl transferase is deficient. Similar lesions are caused by deficiency of uridine diphosphate galactose-4-epimerase or galactokinase. One child in every 20,000 live born is affected.

Infants with galactosemia present with vomiting and failure to thrive, beginning a few days after they begin to take milk. Because of the lack of the transferase, the galactose from the milk cannot be metabolized, and galactose-1-phosphate accumulates in cells throughout the body. In the liver, fatty change becomes marked. Cholestasis and jaundice soon develop. Proliferation of bile ductules at the margin of the portal tracts is prominent, often with tubular change in the adjacent parenchyma. Fibrosis may be evident within a few weeks, and if galactose is not avoided, micronodular cirrhosis develops within a few years. Cataracts are apparent in the eyes within a few weeks. Mental retardation and hypotonia become evident within a few months. Often there is aminoaciduria. The galactose spills into the urine and can be detected there.

The diagnosis can be established by demonstrating that the red cells lack galactose-1-phosphate uridyl transferase. Strict avoidance of milk and other foods containing galactose lessens or prevents the injury.

HEREDITARY FRUCTOSE INTOLERANCE. Hereditary fructose intolerance is caused by lack of fructose-1-phosphate aldolase and is inherited as an autosomal recessive character. If infants with this defect are given fructose or sucrose in the diet, they vomit, fail to thrive, and become jaundiced. The liver enlarges. Ascites and edema develop. Fructosemia, fructosuria, and hypophosphatemia are present. Sometimes there are seizures or aminoaciduria. The liver shows fatty change, cholestasis, and proliferation of bile ducts. Abnormal membranes appear in the glycogen zones of the hepatocytes. Unless fructose is avoided, cirrhosis follows.

If an older child with fructose-1-phosphate aldolase deficiency or a child with fructose 1, 6-diphosphatase deficiency is given fructose, hypoglycemia results, but there is little or no injury to the liver.

GLYCOGEN STORAGE DISEASES. The glycogen storage diseases result from a deficiency of one of the enzymes concerned with the metabolism of glycogen. All are genetically determined, usually inherited as an autosomal recessive character. Normal or abnormal glycogen accumulates in one or more organs. The liver and skeletal muscle are the most often involved. Most of the glycogen storage diseases begin during childhood, as glycogen accumulates in the organ or organs affected, often with serious dysfunction.

Type 0. In type 0 glycogen storage disease, glycogen synthetase is deficient. Affected infants are hypoglycemic, fail to grow, and die early in life. The liver is large and fibrotic. The spleen is enlarged.

Type Ia. Type Ia glycogen storage disease is called von Gierke's disease, after a German pathologist (1877–1945). It results from a deficiency of glucose-6-phosphatase and is inherited as an autosomal recessive character. Normal glycogen accumulates principally in the hepatocytes and the renal tubular epithelium. The gastrointestinal epithelium is less severely involved.

Children with von Gierke's disease are short and fat, with a liver three or four times its normal size and large kidneys. The liver and kidneys are smooth and look translucent macroscopically. Microscopically, the hepatocytes and the epithelial cells of the proximal renal tubules are distended with glucose, and there is fatty change as well. Electron microscopy shows glycogen granules crowding around the endoplasmic reticulum. Glycogen is prominent in the nuclei. Fibrosis or cirrhosis of the liver is rare.

The children develop episodes of severe hypoglycemia. Glucagon and adrenalin fail to raise the blood sugar. Chronic lactic acidosis with a fasting plasma lactate concentration of over 3 mmol/L (30 mg/100 mL) is usual. There is sometimes hyperlipidemia, with high triglyceride levels. Hyperuricemia is common. Many of the children die in early childhood, often from infection. Sometimes there is neutropenia or platelet dysfunction. In those who survive, the disease becomes milder after puberty, though the enzyme deficiency persists. Because of the hyperuricemia, gout sometimes develops during adolescence, with gouty nephropathy. Hepatocellular adenomata but rarely hepatocellular carcinomata develop in the survivors.

Type Ib. Type Ib glycogen storage disease is similar to type Ia, but the inactive enzyme is glucose-6-phosphatase.

Type II. Type II glycogen storage results from deficiency of the lysosomal enzyme α-glucosidase. Normal glycogen accumulates in lysosomes in cells throughout the body. The disease is inherited as an autosomal recessive character. The incidence exceeds 1 child in 100,000. Three types of α-glucosidase deficiency are distinguished.

The most common is Pompe's disease, called after the Dutch pathologist who described it in 1932. Symptoms begin in infancy. The heart is greatly enlarged, and there is flaccid weakness of the skeletal muscles. The liver is often slightly enlarged, though there is no hepatic dysfunction. Death usually comes early in childhood from cardiac or respiratory failure.

Less often, the disease first becomes evident later in childhood, with progressive weakness of the skeletal muscles that slowly worsens as years pass. Respiratory failure sometimes develops, but cardiac failure does not. Some of the patients survive for 20 years or more.

Still less severe is the adult form of type II glycogen storage disease. The patients are 20 to 50 years old when symptoms begin. Mild weakness develops in the skeletal muscles. Only occasionally is the disease severe enough to cause respiratory failure.

In all forms of α-glucosidase deficiency, hepatocytes, renal tubular epithelial cells in the loops of Henle and the collecting tubules, other epithelial cells, smooth and striated muscle cells, lymphocytes, neurons, and other cells throughout the body have in their cytoplasm small vacuoles of glycogen in distended lysosomes. Only in the skeletal muscles and the heart does the glycogen cause serious dysfunction, though a few of the patients suffer mental retardation. Alpha-glucosidase deficiency is the only form of glycogen storage disease in which the glycogen is confined in membrane-bound vacuoles. In all others, it is free in the cell sap.

Type III. Type III glycogen storage disease is called Forbes' disease, after the American pediatrician who described it in 1953, or Cori's disease, after an American biochemist. It is one of the more common glycogen storage diseases. The debrancher enzyme amylo-1,6-glucosidase is deficient. The deficiency is inherited as an autosomal recessive character. The liver, heart, and skeletal muscles are principally involved.

Six patterns of type III glycogen storage disease have been distinguished, varying in the extent of the involvement of these organs. There is marked hepatomegaly, with changes in the liver like those of type I glycogen storage disease, though in type III disease the glycogen that accumulates is abnormal. Only the outer part of the branches of the glycogen molecule can be metabolized, and an abnormal stump of the glycogen tree accumulates. The hepatic dysfunction is similar to that of type I disease, but usually less severe. Cirrhosis sometimes results.

Type IV. Type IV glycogen storage disease is called Andersen's disease after the American pathologist who described it in 1956. The brancher enzyme amylo-1,6-transglucosidase is deficient. The deficiency is probably inherited as an autosomal recessive character. The glycogen that accumulates has less branching than normal. In some patients the abnormal glycogen seems to accumulate only in the liver and the heart. In others, the glycogen accumulates in cells throughout the body.

The deposits of glycogen in the cytoplasm fail to stain with hematoxylin and eosin, but are brightly colored by the periodic acid-Schiff reaction. In the liver, they form inclusions that displace the nucleus. In macrophages, they are granular. Electron microscopy show that the abnormal glycogen is in part fibrillar, in part granular.

Some children with type IV disease fail to thrive and develop severe gastroenteritis, hepatosplenomegaly, cirrhosis and ascites. Some have cardiac failure or extreme weakness of the skeletal muscles. Most die within two or three years.

Type V. Type V glycogen storage disease is called McArdle's disease, after the British physician who described it in 1951. The liver is not affected. Phosphorylase in skeletal muscle is deficient, but hepatic phosphorylase is normal. McArdle's disease is inherited as an autosomal recessive character. The abnormal gene is on chromosome eleven. The disorder is uncommon.

As in the other kinds of glycogen storage disease in which skeletal muscle is involved, glycogen accumulates in the skeletal muscle fibers. Vigorous exercise tends to cause weakness and cramps in the muscles used. There is segmental, hyaline necrosis in some of the fibers in the muscles affected, with leakage of glutamic oxaloacetic transaminase, aldolase, creatine phosphokinase, and other muscular enzymes into the plasma, and sometimes leakage of myoglobin and myoglobinuria.

Type VI. In type VI glycogen storage disease, called Hers' disease, hepatic phosphorylase is deficient. It is rare. The patients have hepatomegaly, with liver cells filled with glycogen, but little dysfunction. Microscopically, type VI disease is similar to type I disease. There is the same crowding of the cytoplasm with glycogen granules. Droplets of fat are common. Intranuclear glycogen is uncommon. Often the α-particles of glycogen are fractured in the disorders of the phosphorylase system.

Type VII. Type VII glycogen storage disease is due to deficiency of phosphofructokinase. In one form of the disorder the enzyme is deficient in the muscles and erythrocytes; in another, only in the red cells. The muscular form causes symptoms like those of McArdle's disease. Involvement of the red cells causes mild hemolytic anemia.

Types VIII and IX. Phosphorylase b kinase deficiency was formerly called type VIb, type VIII, and type IX. The most common form of the disorder is inherited as an X-linked character. The enzyme is deficient in the liver, leukocytes, and skin. It is normal in muscle. Boys affected have episodes of hepatomegaly, episodes of hypoglycemia, and some retardation of growth. The abnormalities resolve during adolescence. Heterozygous girls sometimes have mild hepatomegaly.

UREA CYCLE DISORDERS. Rarely, one of the enzymes that forms urea in the liver is deficient. Ornithine transcarbamylase and argininosuccinate synthetase are the most commonly affected. Symptoms often develop soon after birth, but can be delayed for up to two years. Vomiting and failure to thrive are usual. Sometimes there are convulsions. Protein taken in the diet causes an increase in the concentration of ammonia in the plasma and encephalopathy, as in hepatic failure. The liver is normal or shows mild fatty change.

The level of ammonia in the blood is high with deficiency of carbamyl phosphate synthetase and of ornithine transcarbamylase. Lack of ornithine transcarbamylase also causes orotic aciduria. In citrullinemia due to deficiency of arginosuccinic synthetase, arginosuccinic acidura due to deficiency of arginosuccinase, and hyperarginemia due to deficiency of arginase, the ammonia levels in the blood are more moderate.

VASCULAR DISORDERS

The liver is commonly congested in cardiac disease. It is damaged in shock. Venoocclusive disease narrows or occludes the hepatic veins. The Budd-Chiari syndrome results from occlusion of the hepatic veins.

CONGESTION. Congestion of the liver is common and usually results from congestive heart failure. In acute heart failure, the liver can rapidly become congested, swollen, and tender. In tricuspid incompetence, it sometimes pulsates in time with the jugular rhythm. The congestion may be mild and transient or may cause extensive hepatocellular necrosis.

The increased pressure in the vena cava interferes with the flow of blood from the hepatic veins. The sinusoids around the terminal hepatic veins become congested. The compressed hepatocytes in the plates between the swollen sinusoids shrink and atrophy. The atrophy is due mainly to hypoxia. The oxygen tension is always low around the hepatic veins, and the stagnation caused by the congestion lowers it further. If the congestion is severe and continues, many or all the hepatocytes around the terminal hepatic veins disappear. In severe cases, 50% of the hepatic parenchyma is lost.

The congested liver is usually a little enlarged. To the naked eye, the cut section shows innumerable tiny red spots, marking the congestion around the hepatic veins. The intervening parenchyma is usually yellowish. This striking appearance has long been known as a nutmeg liver and does closely resemble the cut surface of a nutmeg.

The congestion causes minor hepatic dysfunction. Sulfobromophthalein (Bromsulphalein) retention is one of its most sensitive measures. If the congestion is severe, there may be hyperbilirubinemia. The serum bilirubin level is rarely over 50 μmol/L (3 mg/100 mL).

In the majority of patients, if the congestion is relieved, regeneration restores the liver perfectly. Only if congestion is severe and long continued, does fibrosis begin around the hepatic veins. Rarely, it extends to join adjacent hepatic veins, and even more rarely true cardiac cirrhosis results.

SHOCK. In shock, congestion of the sinusoids around the terminal hepatic veins, sometimes with atrophy of the hepatocytes in this part of the liver is common. The changes may be indistinguishable from the congestion and atrophy caused by congestive heart failure. No doubt hypoxia caused by the hypotension and failing circulation is the major cause of the hepatic injury, though circulating toxins and other factors also play a part. The damaged hepatocytes sometimes become necrotic, sometimes with an exudate of neutrophils. Mild fatty change is common. Sometimes there is cholestasis and jaundice.

BUDD-CHIARI SYNDROME. The Budd-Chiari syndrome is named after an English physician who mentioned the condition in 1845 and the Austrian pathologist who described it in 1899. The syndrome results from obstruction of the major hepatic veins. It is found in 1 autopsy in 20,000.

Thrombosis is the most common cause of the syndrome. In 70% of the patients, the cause of the thrombosis is unknown. In some it is secondary to a disease that increases the risk of thrombosis, such as polycythemia vera or sickle cell anemia, or occurs in women taking oral contraceptives. Less often the obstruction is caused by a web across the mouth of the veins; the veins are scarred or obliterated, compressed by tumor in the liver, or obstructed by a renal cell carcinoma extending along the inferior vena cava.

The liver is swollen, congested, and purple. Biopsy shows severe congestion around the terminal hepatic veins, with atrophy of the hepatocytes in this part of the liver. Red cells sometimes accumulate between the Kupffer cells and the hepatocytes, leaving the central lumen of the sinusoid empty.

If complete obstruction of the hepatic veins develops quickly, massive necrosis of the liver leads to acute hepatic failure and death. If the occlusion of the hepatic veins comes more slowly, the patient may live for months or years. Fibrosis develops around the hepatic veins and may extend out to link them. True cardiac cirrhosis is unusual.

In the more chronic cases, the patient presents with pain or discomfort from the swollen liver, ascites, and other signs of portal hypertension. There may be jaundice, but the serum bilirubin level is rarely over 30 μmol/L (2 mg/100 mL).

Veno-Occlusive Disease. In veno-occlusive disease, intimal thickening causes stenosis and obliteration of the terminal hepatic and medium-sized hepatic veins. The intimal proliferation is at first loose, but becomes increasingly collagenized. If the cause of the proliferation is removed early in the course, the disease can resolve. If not, the occlusion of the veins is permanent.

The occlusion of the hepatic veins causes congestion around the terminal hepatic veins and necrosis of the hepatocytes in this part of the liver. If the obstruction continues, fibrosis develops around the terminal hepatic veins and links vein to vein. At times, true cirrhosis follows.

Early in the disease, the patients have a swollen, tender liver. As the lesions age, the liver becomes sclerotic. The spleen is enlarged. Portal hypertension and ascites are common. Death is often from hemorrhage from esophageal varices, less often from hepatic failure.

Veno-occlusive disease was first described in Jamaica and was most common in young children. It was caused by the pyrrolizidine alkaloids common in the crotalaria and senicio species used to make the bush teas then widely used. Similar lesions were caused in similar fashion in Africa, India, and elsewhere. More recently, veno-occlusive disease has been caused by the chemotherapeutic agents used to prepare patients for bone marrow transplantation, less often by azothioprine given to patients undergoing renal transplantation or by the chemotherapeutic drugs used to treat malignant tumors. Irradiation of the liver occasionally causes veno-occlusive disease.

Infarction. Infarcts of the liver are uncommon. The double blood supply from the portal vein and hepatic artery and the abundant anastomoses make infarction difficult. If a medium-sized portal vein is occluded, a sharply defined, red zone called an infarct of Zahn after a Swiss pathologist (1845–1904) is likely to appear underneath the capsule. The lesion is not a true infarct, for the hepatic parenchyma is not necrotic, but only a region of severe congestion. True infarcts of the liver are pale, irregularly shaped, and often subcapsular. They nearly always result from occlusion of hepatic artery.

Peliosis Hepatis. Peliosis hepatis is sometimes found at autopsy in patients with no evidence of liver dysfunction, sometimes in those treated with androgens, estrogens, or other drugs. The name comes from the Greek for bruised. To the naked eye, the liver shows on section a few, or sometimes many, bluish dots a millimeter or so across scattered in the parenchyma. Microscopically, the dots are blood-filled spaces, which usually look like dilated sinusoids. Some have a sinusoid lining; some do not. The cause of peliosis hepatis is unknown. It causes no symptoms and no dysfunction.

Cavernous Transformation of the Portal Vein. Cavernous transformation of the portal vein is rare. It is more common in children than adults, but may not become evident until adult life.

The portal vein may be reduced to a fibrous cord or transformed into a maze of cavernous spaces that resemble an extensively recanalized thrombus. To carry the portal blood to the liver, numerous anastomoses develop in the hepatoduodenal and hepatocolic ligaments. If these anastomoses are inadequate, portal hypertension results.

The cause of the occlusion of the portal vein is often not evident. Some cases may result from omphalitis in infancy, with thrombosis extending into the portal vein. In other patients, the condition is due to local injury to the portal vein, with thrombosis.

DISORDERS OF THE INTRAHEPATIC BILIARY SYSTEM

This section discusses the changes that occur in the liver in biliary obstruction, the different kinds of cholangitis, and hepatic abscesses. Primary cirrhosis and secondary biliary cirrhosis are described earlier in the chapter. The diseases of the extrahepatic biliary system are considered in Chapter 37.

CHOLESTASIS. Cholestasis can be caused by extrahepatic obstruction to bile flow or by intrahepatic disease of the liver. Both are common.

Causes. Gallstones are the most common cause of extrahepatic biliary obstruction. The stones lodge in the common bile duct or the major intrahepatic ducts. Carcinoma of the pancreas and carcinoma of the major bile ducts often cause biliary obstruction. Inflammation of the common bile duct sometimes narrows or occludes the duct. Rarely, enlarged lymph nodes compress the common bile duct or the duct is obstructed by parasites, narrowed by a duodenal ulcer, compressed by some other kind of tumor, narrowed by pancreatitis, or obstructed in some other way. In infants, atresia of a major bile duct is an important cause of obstruction.

Intrahepatic cholestasis occurs in many diseases of the liver: viral hepatitis, alcoholic liver disease, drug-induced hepatitis, chronic active hepatitis, primary biliary cirrhosis, cirrhosis, the metabolic disorders of the hepatocytes, sclerosing cholangitis, Caroli's disease, and other conditions. It sometimes complicates disease of other organs, such as sepsis, shock, or cystic fibrosis, or complicates total parenteral nutrition.

Lesions. The changes caused by biliary obstruction are most simple in extrahepatic cholestasis. In intrahepatic cholestasis, the changes caused by obstruction are often obscured by the lesions of the disease causing the cholestasis, and the pathogenesis of the cholestasis is more complicated.

Extrahepatic Cholestasis. In the first days after extrahepatic biliary obstruction becomes severe, with complete or almost complete obstruction to bile flow, bile accumulates in the hepatocytes around the terminal hepatic veins. The hepatocytes and Kupffer cells in this region become stained with bile. Granules of bilirubin accumulate in the cytoplasm of the hepatocytes. Many

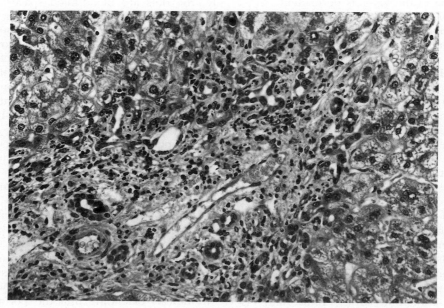

Fig. 36-28. Extrahepatic biliary obstruction, showing inflammation of a portal tract with proliferation of bile ducts at its periphery.

of the bile canaliculi between the hepatocytes are enlarged and plugged with bile. Occasionally a few of the hepatocytes in the region around the terminal hepatic veins become necrotic or hyalinized.

After several days or a few weeks, many of the portal tracts become edematous. They lose their angular shape and become rounded. In some, an exudate mainly of lymphocytes appears. Often a few neutrophils are present in the exudate. The neutrophils are particularly numerous around the bile ducts and can sometimes be found within a duct.

Small bile ducts at the margin of the tracts proliferate. As time passes, they become increasingly numerous. The new ductules are often irregularly shaped, with irregular epithelium. Neutrophils are usually numerous around the new ductules or in their lumina. Because of the neutrophils, the proliferation of ductules is sometimes called cholangiolitis.

If the obstruction continues for several weeks, the accumulation of bile in the hepatocytes and the bile plugs in the canaliculi become more widespread. The midzone of the hepatic lobules is involved and sometimes the periportal regions. Occasionally bile plugs develop in the hepatic ducts in the triads. Some of the canaliculi in the parenchyma enlarge and are surrounded by several hepatocytes. A bile plug may fill the large canaliculus, or it may be empty.

The larger bile ducts are often ectatic and tortuous. Sometimes their epithelium is necrotic or lost. Sometimes the wall of a large duct is inflamed. Concretions sometimes develop in the large ducts if obstruction is prolonged. Occasionally a large duct ruptures, exciting a granulomatous reaction.

Scattered hepatocytes or small groups of hepatocytes undergo feathery degeneration. They become greatly swollen. Their cytoplasm is reduced to a few wisps, often stained with bile. Eventually, the cells lyse. Macrophages and neutrophils accumulate around the dying cells. If a group of feathery hepatocytes becomes necrotic, the lesion is called a bile infarct, though the necrosis is probably caused by the toxicity of the bile salts, not by ischemia. Bile infarcts are rare, except in extrahepatic obstruction.

Occasionally a bile canaliculus ruptures, releasing bile into the parenchyma. The extravasated bile is surrounded by an exudate predominantly of macrophages. Mallory bodies occasionally develop in a few hepatocytes. Copper and occasionally iron accumulate in the hepatocytes.

Eventually, fibrosis begins around the portal tracts. Sometimes the fibrosis is circumferential, and the enlarged triads are round. Sometimes the proliferating ductules form spurs that extend out from the portal tracts and join the tracts together. Collagen is deposited around the ductules. Even if the septa between tracts become broad and heavily collagenized, they rarely involve the terminal hepatic veins. True biliary cirrhosis is uncommon.

Electron microscopy shows that the severity of the cholestasis varies from one part of the liver to another. Even in the most severely involved parts of the liver, some bile canaliculi remain relatively normal, even though neighboring canaliculi are greatly dilated and filled with bile. Even in a single canaliculus, some parts may be dilated and filled with bile, while other parts are almost normal. In the ectatic canaliculi, almost all the microvilli normally present are lost, and the few that remain become bulbous and edematous. Often amorphous debris, membranes, or fat droplets can be seen in the bile filling the dilated canaliculi. The tight junctions that join liver cell to liver cell to close the canaliculi remain intact.

The pericanalicular ectoplasm in the hepatocytes around the dilated canaliculi remains free of organelles, but is often thickened and appears edematous. The Golgi apparatus and smooth endoplasmic reticulum enlarge. The rough endoplasmic reticulum is fragmented. Mitochondrial abnormalities are common, especially lengthening and curling of the cristae. Conjugated bilirubin at first lies free in the cell sap of the hepatocytes, congregated into loose agregates. Later, it sometimes is enclosed in a autophagic vacuole. The bilirubin may be deconjugated by the lysosomal enzymes. Multivescicular bodies are common. Pinocytic vescicles are numerous. Large lobulated vacuoles contain stringy, lamellar material, perhaps a bile salt-phospholipid-cholesterol complex. In hepatocytes showing feathery degeneration, the lobulated vacuoles replace much of the cytoplasm.

As the bile canaliculi and their microvilli become distorted, the Mg^2 adenosine triphosphatase normally present on the microvilli of the canaliculi is lost. 5'-Nucleotidase is normally present in both the canalicular and the sinusoidal cell membranes. In cholestasis, it is lost or reduced in the canaliculi but persists in the sinusoidal membranes. Early in biliary obstruction, alkaline phosphatase activity is increased in all parts of the hepatocellular plasma membrane, but as the canaliculi become distended, it is lost from the canalicular membrane.

Often the space between the hepatocytes in the regions affected widens. Microvilli develop on the lateral wall of the cells. As adenosine triphosphatase is lost from the canaliculi, it appears on the lateral wall of the hepatocytes. The space between the cells is separated from the bile canaliculi by tight junctions, but communicates with the space of Disse.

Macroscopically, as biliary obstruction increases and jaundice grows severe, the liver becomes bright green, as the parenchyma is increasingly stained with bile. The liver remains smooth and of normal consistency, unless fibrosis or cirrhosis develops. If the obstruction is in a major bile duct and is complete, the large ducts proximal to the obstruction become filled with a white, mucoid secretion called white bile. Because of the stasis, water and bile pigments are resorbed from the bile in the large ducts, and the viscid white bile results.

Intrahepatic Cholestasis. The changes in the liver in many types of intrahepatic cholestasis are similar to those in extrahepatic obstruction. Biliary retention and bile plugs appear first in the region around the terminal hepatic veins. The hepatocytes in this region show alterations like those in extrahepatic cholestasis. In many forms of severe intrahepatic cholestasis, small bile ducts proliferate at the margins of the portal tracts, as they do in extrahepatic obstruction. Changes in the larger intrahepatic bile ducts do not occur.

Dysfunction. Increased activity of the alkaline phosphatases is often the first evidence of hepatic dysfunction in cholestasis. Commonly the activity of alkaline phosphatase in the plasma exceeds 300 U/L. The increased activity of the enzyme is caused in part by increased production, in part by reduced secretion into the bile. If there is doubt whether the increased activity of the alkaline phosphatase is caused by liver disease or bone disease, the isoenzymes of alkaline phosphatase can be measured. The activity of gamma-glutamyl transpeptidase is increased in liver disease but not in bone disease.

In extrahepatic obstruction, the concentration of bilirubin in the plasma rises slowly, taking two or three weeks before the level becomes more or less constant. The bilirubin is largely conjugated, though there is an increase in unconjugated bilirubin as well. The slow rise of the concentration of bilirubin in the plasma is probably caused by the leakage of the conjugated bilirubin into the urine, and this leakage helps determine the more or less constant level of bilirubin that is eventually reached. If there is partial obstruction, of the kind commonly caused by a gallstone in the common bile duct, the concentration of bilirubin in the plasma is often between 15 and 150 µmol/L (1 to 10 mg/100 mL) and may fluctuate as the degree of obstruction varies from day to day. If the obstruction is complete, the bilirubinemia may reach 500 µmol/L (30 mg/100 mL), but rarely is higher.

The elevation of the concentration of conjugated bilirubin in the plasma causes bilirubinuria. Sometimes bilirubinuria is noted before jaundice becomes evident. If the obstruction is complete, or nearly so, the stools become colorless, and urobilinogen disappears from the urine.

Bile salts are retained in all types of cholestasis. Their concentration in the plasma may rise to 20 times normal. The proportion of bile salts bound to taurine increases because the conjugated bile salts no longer reach the gut, and their taurine can no longer be split off by bacterial action and lost in the stool. The quantity of taurine available for conjugation increases, and the liver prefers to conjugate bile acids to taurine rather than glycine. The proportion of trihydroxy bile acids increases, because cholic acid can no longer reach the bowel to be converted into deoxycholic acid. Normally little or no bile acid is excreted in the urine, but as the concentration of bile acids in the blood grows high, considerable quantities of bile acids appear in the urine.

The lack of the bile acids in the gut prevents the micelle formation necessary for the absorption of the fat-soluble vitamins and may cause deficiencies of vitamin K, and hypoprothrombinemia; of vitamin D, with osteomalacia; and of vitamin A with night blindness. Osteoporosis is common in patients with chronic biliary obstruction.

The activity of aminotransferases in the plasma is usually little increased. The increase is much less than is seen in viral hepatitis and other conditions in which there is more extensive hepatocellular necrosis. Alanine transferase levels rarely exceed 400 U/L. The injury to the liver cells is not suficient to cause hypoalbuminemia.

The concentration of lipids in the serum is greatly increased. The cholesterol concentration is usually two or three times normal. There is only a slight increase in esterified cholesterol, but the unesterified cholesterol concentration increases five times or so. Phospholipids are increased more than the cholesterol, to three or four times normal, so that the phospholipid-to-cholesterol ratio increases. Neutral fats are little affected. Low density lipoproteins increase, and high density lipoproteins fall. The increase in the concentration of low density lipoproteins in the serum is largely due to the appearance of an abnormal lipoprotein containing a high proportion of unesterified cholesterol and phospholipid. Its origin is unknown. Xanthomata may appear in the skin if the concentration of cholesterol in the plasma remains above 15 mmol/L (600 mg/100 mL) for some months.

Clinical Presentation. The clinical presentation in the diseases that cause intrahepatic cholestasis differs from one disease to another and is described elsewhere in this chapter.

In extrahepatic obstruction, jaundice develops slowly. The patient often feels well, as the color of the skin darkens. Eventually, the skin may acquire a greenish tint as jaundice becomes severe and increase in melanin in the epidermis modifies the coloration.

Pruritus is often severe and is due in part to the increased concentration of bile salts in the blood. The severity of the pruritus does not correlate with the concentration of any

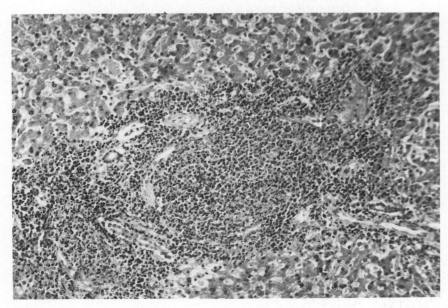

Fig. 36-29. Acute cholangitis, showing severe triaditis with an exudate predominantly of neutrophils.

particular bile salt, and in the late stages of hepatic failure pruritus may disappear, though the concentration of bile salts in the blood remains high.

Treatment and Prognosis. The treatment and prognosis of the conditions that cause intrahepatic cholestasis is discussed in other parts of this chapter. Extrahepatic obstruction is usually treated surgically. If the obstruction is relieved before hepatic fibrosis has become extensive, the structure and function of the liver return almost to normal within several weeks.

CHOLANGITIS. Cholangitis is the term used to describe inflammation of the bile ducts. Three kinds of cholangitis are distinguished, acute cholangitis, recurrent pyogenic cholangitis, and sclerosing cholangitis.

Acute Cholangitis. Acute cholangitis usually is secondary to obstruction of a major bile duct. Bacteria gain entry to the obstructed duct and proliferate in the bile. Infection spreads into the liver along some or many of the branches of the obstructed duct. The infected ducts are acutely inflamed with congestion, edema, and neutrophils. Small abscesses may be beaded along the infected bile ducts, or one or more larger abscesses may develop within the liver. At first the abscesses have a core filled with pus, surrounded by massive acute inflammation, but if the patient survives for a few weeks or months, the abscess becomes enclosed by a fibrous capsule, and the lymphocytes and macrophages replace the neutrophils.

The infection is often mixed. Gram-negative bacilli are usually dominant, Escherichia coli, Proteus, Klebsiella, or Pseudomonas. Staphylococci and streptococci are frequently found. Anaerobic organisms such as Bacteroides, microaerophilic streptococci, or Clostridia are less common. Sometimes Actinomyces is found. Occasionally acute cholangitis is caused by obstruction by liver flukes, Ascaris, or by schistomiasis.

The patient with acute cholangitis has a high, swinging fever, rigors, and sweating. There may be a dull ache over the liver or

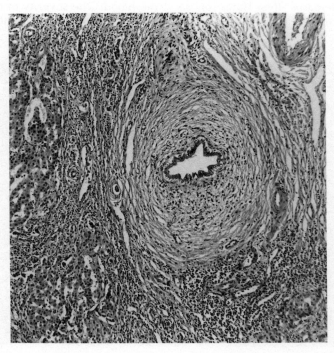

Fig. 36-30. Sclerosing cholangitis, showing massive, concentric fibrosis of an intrahepatic bile duct.

pain if the infection involves the hepatic capsule with peritoneal irritation. Sometimes there is gram-negative shock.

Antibiotics alone are ineffective. If there is a solitary abscess, surgical drainage reduces the mortality to about 40%. If there are multiple abscess, surgical drainage is impossible. Overall, the mortality approaches 90%.

Recurrent Pyogenic Cholangitis. In Hong Kong and the Far East, recurrent pyogenic cholangitis is common. The patients suffer repeated attacks of acute cholangitis, with fever, pain, and jaundice. The first attack usually comes when the patient is between 30 and 40 years old. Death often results from a final attack of cholangitis when the patient is 50 or 60 years old.

In the early stages of the disease, the intrahepatic bile ducts show acute inflammation much as in acute cholangitis. When the patient recovers, the inflammation subsides, only to recur with the next attack. The bile ducts become irregularly ectatic. Increasing fibrosis around the ducts leads to dense periductal scarring. Chronic and recurred acute inflammation persists. Sludge and stones are common in the ectatic ducts.

The cause of recurrent pyogenic cholangitis is unknown. The biliary system is colonized by enormous numbers of intestinal bacteria, often with Escherichia coli predominating, but why the bacteria infect so massively the biliary ducts is obscure.

Sclerosing Cholangitis. Sclerosing cholangitis is a rare condition in which the walls of the intrahepatic and extrahepatic bile ducts become greatly thickened by fibrosis, usually with mild chronic inflammation. The ducts are hard and feel like fibrous cords. Their lumina are narrowed, bringing obstructive jaundice.

In some patients, the sclerosis of the bile ducts is secondary to biliary obstruction. In others, there is no evidence of obstruction, and the cause of the progressive sclerosis is unknown. The idiopathic form of the disease is called primary sclerosing cholangitis.

Some 75% of patients with primary sclerosing cholangitis are 20 to 50 years old. About 70% of the patients are men. Over 50% of the patients have ulcerative colitis, and 5% of patients with ulcerative colitis develop sclerosing cholangitis. A few have Crohn's disease, pancreatits, retroperitoneal fibrosis, or immunodeficiency. Up to 10% of the patients have no symptoms. Most have fatigue, upper abdominal pain, and progressive jaundice. Some have recurrent attacks like those of acute cholangitis.

The disease usually involves the medium-sized and large biliary ducts, intrahepatic and extrahepatic. Occasionally, it is confined to the small ducts. The affected ducts are surrounded by concentric fibrosis, giving them an onion-skinned appearance. The fibrosis causes irregular stenosis and dilation of the ducts. Inflammation is often sparse. Sometimes the biliary tracts are severely inflamed with an exudate mainly of lymphocytes, occasionally with germinal centers. Granulomata do not occur. Eventually, many of the intrahepatic ducts disappear, leaving only a branch of the hepatic artery to mark the site of the duct. Cholestasis grows increasingly extensive as the loss of ducts grows more widespread.

Most of patients with primary biliary sclerosis develop secondary biliary cirrhosis and die of hepatic failure within 7 years. A few have survived as long as 30 years.

OTHER NON-NEOPLASTIC HEPATIC DISEASES

A few non-neoplastic hepatic diseases do not fall into the groups already discussed.

GIANT CELL HEPATITIS. In infants with hepatitis or any other disorder that causes cholestasis, large, multinucleate hepatocytes are often prominent. Because of the histologic appearance, neonatal hepatitis is often called giant cell hepatitis.

Lesions. Macroscopically, the liver is enlarged, firm, and jaundiced. The extrahepatic bile ducts are collapsed and may be difficult to find. The gallbladder is often collapsed and contains only a little mucus.

Microscopically, the liver shows changes like those of viral or drug-induced hepatitis. The liver plates are disordered. Often, scattered hepatocytes are necrotic. A few macrophages, lymphocytes, and plasma cells accumulate around the dead cells. Iron accumulates in the Kupffer cells and hepatocytes. The portal tracts contain an exudate

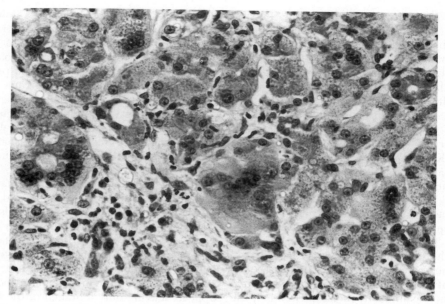

Fig. 36-31. Giant cell hepatitis, showing large, multinucleated hepatocytes.

of lymphocytes, plasma cells, and macrophages, often with a few neutrophils or eosinophils. The bile ducts in the inflamed triads are collapsed. Large multinucleate hepatocytes are present throughout the liver, but are especially numerous around the terminal hepatic veins. Some of them have 20 or 30 nuclei arranged around the periphery of the cell. The cytoplasm of the giant cells is pale and contains much glycogen. Often the cells are bile-stained or contain hemosiderin. If they become necrotic, they excite a neutrophilic reaction.

Clinical Presentation. An infant with giant cell hepatitis usually becomes jaundiced when about a week old. Commonly the concentration of bilirubin in the plasma reaches 200 to 250 μmol/L (10 to 15 mg/100 mL), with bilirubinuria, pale stools, greatly increased activity of alkaline phosphatase in the plasma, and other signs of biliary obstruction.

Pathogenesis. Giant cell hepatitis is often caused by the hepatitis B virus, the viruses that cause non-A, non-B hepatitis, the virus of rubella, Herpes simplex, a coxsackievirus, or an echovirus. Toxoplasmosis and syphilis can cause similar changes. Less often it is due to α_1-antitrypsin deficiency,

galactosemia, or fructose intolerance. Occasionally it is induced by a drug or poison. Giant cell hepatitis is common in the liver of children with biliary atresia.

Treatment and Prognosis. The prognosis depends on the cause of the hepatitis. Over 50% of infants with viral hepatitis recover. Some develop cirrhosis and die during childhood.

REYE'S SYNDROME. Reye's syndrome is named after the Australian pathologist who described it in 1963. It occurs throughout the world, but is uncommon. With few exceptions, the patients are less than 15 years old. Girls and boys are affected equally.

Clinical Presentation. The onset of the syndrome is usually preceded by a viral infection, most often influenza B or varicella. In many but not all patients, large doses of aspirin or other analgesics were given during the infection. From three to seven days after recovery from the infection, the child begins to vomit, becomes lethargic, and suffers progressively more severe neurologic dysfunction. Behavioral changes are usual and are often followed by stupor and coma.

Lesions. The liver is enlarged and orange-yellow. Microscopically, the hepatocytes throughout the liver are swollen. Their cytoplasm is filled with small droplets of neutral fat. The nucleus remains vesicular and centrally placed. Little glycogen remains in the hepatocytes. In some patients, a few cells near the portal tracts show ballooning degeneration or become necrotic. Cholestasis is unusual. Similar fatty change develops in the renal tubular epithelium. The brain shows only edema and sometimes foci necrosis of neurons without inflammatory response.

The mitochondria in the hepatocytes, brain, and muscle are enlarged. Their matrices are rarefied and granular. As the disease grows more severe, they become increasingly distorted. Their cristae are abnormal and often appear to be detached. The space between the inner and outer membranes of the mitochondria is narrowed. Intermitochondrial granules are reduced in size and number. Eventually some of the mitochondria rupture. Other changes in the organelles are less constant. Peroxisomes often increase in number. The smooth endoplasmic reticulum is commonly increased and vacuolated. The fat is free in the cytoplasm.

Dysfunction. The activity of many of the mitochondrial enzymes is reduced. Hypo-glycemia is common. The concentration of ammonia in the plasma rises. Hypoprothrombinemia is usual. The activity of the aminotransferases in the plasma usually exceeds 500 U/L. Metabolic acidosis is frequent. Jaundice is unusual.

Pathogenesis. Reye's syndrome seems to result from mitochondrial dysfunction. The cause of the injury to the mitochondria is unknown. Viral infection, poisoning by some toxin, and the combined action of a viral infection and aspirin or other analgesics have been suggested.

Treatment and Prognosis. Only symptomatic treatment to combat the cerebral edema is available. Patients in whom the disease is mild recover completely, but more than 50% of the children die, and 15% are left with serious neurologic or behavioral defects.

ACUTE FATTY LIVER OF PREGNANCY. Acute fatty liver of pregnancy is a rare disorder that occurs in the last trimester of pregnancy, usually in primipara. The patient presents with acute hepatic failure. Often there is renal failure as well.

Lesions. The liver is smaller than normal and pale yellow. Microscopically, most hepatocytes have numerous small droplets of

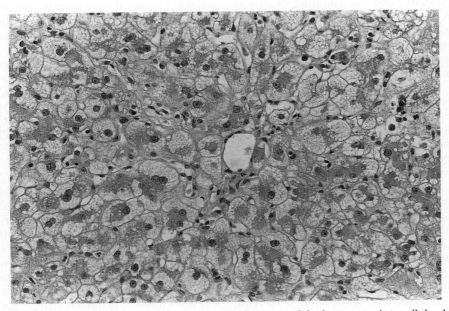

Fig. 36-32. Acute fatty liver of pregnancy, showing the distention of the hepatocytes by small droplets of fat.

neutral lipid in their cytoplasm, though often a rim of hepatocytes around the portal tracts is spared. Mild cholestasis around the terminal hepatic veins is sometimes evident. Hepatocellular necrosis is uncommon. The fetal liver shows similar microvesicular fatty change.

The mitochondria in the hepatocytes are large, irregularly shaped, often with curling or paracrystalline arrangement of their cristae. The rough endoplasmic reticulum is sometimes slightly increased. The smooth endoplasmic reticulum is occasionally dilated. The fat may lie free in the cytoplasm or be surrounded by a single membrane.

Dysfunction. The concentration of bilirubin in the plasma rises to about 100 µmol/ L (6 mg/100 mL). The activity of asparate transferase in the plasma is increased, often to 200 U/L. The prothrombin time is prolonged. Hypoglycemia is often severe. Gamma globulin levels are normal.

Clinical Presentation. The symptoms and signs of patients with acute fatty liver of pregnancy are similar to those of fulminant viral hepatitis.

Pathogenesis. The cause of acute fatty liver of pregnancy is unknown. The similarity of the lesions in the liver to those of Reye's syndrome, tetracycline toxicity, valproate toxicity, and the vomiting disease of Jamaica caused by Ackree poisoning suggest a common mechanism.

Treatment and Prognosis. Only supportive treatment is available. Probably it is wise to perform a caesarian section and terminate the pregnancy without delay. Until recently, over 80% of the mothers and children died. More recently, the maternal mortality has fallen to less than 30% and the fetal mortality to less than 50%.

PARENTERAL NUTRITION. Parenteral nutrition often causes hepatic injury. Infant and adult forms of the disorder are distinguished.

Infants. Infants given parenteral nutrition often become jaundiced three to four weeks after the start of the treatment. First the concentration of bile salts in the plasma rises, then the concentration of conjugated bilirubin. The activity of the aminotransferases and alkaline phosphatases increase little. The liver shows cholestasis around the terminal hepatic veins. In 50% of the infants, there are foci of hepatocellular ballooning or hepatocellular necrosis. After three months, deposition of collagen is evident around the portal tracts and in the spaces of Disse. Bile ducts proliferate in the fibrosis. Occasionally cirrhosis follows. About 40% of the children develop gallstones.

Probably several factors combine to cause the cholestasis. The immaturity of the liver, altered enteric hormone release caused by the lack of food in the alimentary tract, protein toxicity, and lack of essential amino acids all may play a part. The changes are reversible if normal alimentation is resumed before fibrosis develops.

Adults. In adults, parenteral nutrition often causes an increase in the activity of the aminotransferases and alkaline phosphatases in the plasma that starts about 10 days after the start of the artificial alimentation, but hyperbilirubinemia and jaundice are less common than in infants. After a week, the liver shows fatty change in 90% of the patients. After three weeks, some have cholestasis around the terminal hepatic veins and proliferation of bile ducts in the portal triads. Gallstones develop in 40% of the patients. The lesions in the liver tend to subside even if parenteral nutrition is continued and disappear if it is withdrawn. The cause of the hepatic dysfunction is uncertain.

AMYLOIDOSIS. As discussed in Chapter 4, the liver is occasionally massively involved in amyloidosis. The amyloid is deposited in the space of Disse and compresses and destroys a large proportion of the hepatocytes. Liver function is usually little affected, though occasionally there is jaundice.

INFECTION. The infectious diseases are discussed on Chapter 16, 17, 18, 19, 20, and 21. The liver is sometimes seriously involved in leptospirosis, relapsing fever, and syphilis. Tuberculous granulomata are commonly found in the liver in people with pulmonary tuberculosis, but they are usually few and heal without leaving permanent injury. Actinomycosis and histoplasmosis sometimes involve the liver. Amebiasis, schistosomiasis, echinococcosis, and fascioliasis can cause major injury to the liver.

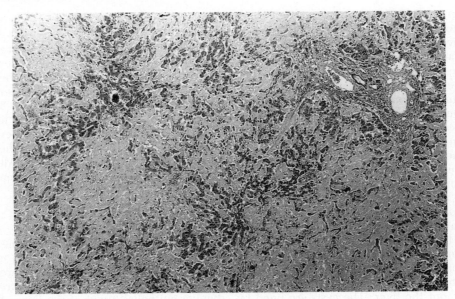

Fig. 36-33. Severe amyloidosis of the liver, with almost complete replacement of the parenchyma by amyloid.

Viral hepatitis is discussed earlier in this chapter.

STRUCTURAL ANOMALIES

The structural anomalies of the liver are mainly congenital, due to a genetic defect. A few are acquired.

ABNORMAL SHAPE OR LOBULATION. Supernumerary lobes of the liver are sometimes seen and are of little significance. Riedel's lobe, named after a German surgeon (1846–1916), is a tongue of normal liver projecting from the right lobe of the liver in the region of the gallbladder. A liver that herniates through a diaphragmatic hernia becomes bizarrely shaped. If the spleen is congenitally absent, the right lobe of the liver enlarges. Sometimes the superior surface of the liver is ridged, to match ridges in the diaphragm. The distortion called corset liver is self-explanatory. Situs inversus has already been mentioned. None of the alterations in shape is of any functional importance.

SIMPLE CYSTS. Simple cysts of the liver are less common than are simple cysts of the kidneys. There may be only one cyst in the liver, but usually there are a few. The hepatic cysts are usually a few centimeters in diameter, but may be smaller or occasionally much larger. The cysts are lined by flattered biliary epithelium and have a thin fibrous wall. They contain mucoid material rather than bile. About 50% of the patients with cysts of the liver have the adult form of polycystic disease of the kidney, and some have cysts in the pancreas or spleen as well. The cysts in the liver are rarely of any functional import.

BILE DUCT HAMARTOMA. Small hamartomata are common in the liver and are believed to be closely related to simple cysts. They are frequent in patients with adult cystic disease of the kidneys, but often occur in people without renal disease. Often the hamartomata are called von Meyenburg complexes.

The hamartomata are usually less than 0.5 cm across. Usually there is only one, but occasionally they are numerous. Macroscopically, they form small, white nodules. Microscopically, the lesions resemble large, ill-formed portal tracts, with irregularly shaped bile ducts separated by collagenous tissue. Often some of the bile ducts in the lesions are ectatic. The lesions cause no symptoms and no dysfunction. At laparotomy, a bile duct hamartoma can be mistaken for metastatic carcinoma.

SOLITARY CYST. Solitary cysts of the liver are uncommon. Over 90% are unilocular. A few are multilocular. Over 80% of the patients are women. Over 70% of the cysts are in the right lobe. The cysts are lined by flattened or cuboidal epithelium that is sometimes ciliated. They have a thin collagenous wall and usually contain clear or opalescent fluid. Most are small, but some contain over 15 L of fluid and fill most of the abdomen. The larger cysts sometimes cause pain, usually when the patient is over 40 years old. Symptoms are unlikely unless the cyst is more than 10 cm in diameter.

Caroli's Disease. Caroli's disease is an unusual condition that usually involves the whole liver, but sometimes is confined to a segment of it. It is named after the French physician who described it in 1964. Segmental ectasia of the bile ducts forms cysts throughout the liver. The cysts are lined by biliary epithelium. They have a thick, collagenous wall, usually with chronic inflammation. Mucous glands are sometimes numerous in the cyst wall. The lumen contains inspissated bile and mucus. The cysts are joined by segments of normal bile duct. Attacks of acute cholangitis sometimes complicate the disease. Occasionally an adenocarcinoma arises in one of the cysts.

CONGENITAL HEPATIC FIBROSIS. Congenital hepatic fibrosis usually occurs in infants, adolescents, or young adults with hepatomegaly and portal hypertension, less often with acute cholangitis, or both cholangitis and portal hypertension. A few patients are discovered while the disease is asymptomatic. The disease is familial, but its pattern of inheritance is uncertain. Patients with infantile cystic disease of the kidneys all have congenital hepatic fibrosis. In many of the patients, the condition is associated with other congenital anomalies.

The liver is enlarged and fibrotic. The portal triads are enlarged by fibrosis. Bands of fibrosis link the portal tracts dividing the parenchyma into islands that often contain several hepatic lobules. Only late in the disease does the fibrosis involve some of the terminal hepatic veins. Small bile ducts are numerous in the septa. Inflammation is sparse.

TUMORS

In the liver, metastatic tumors are more common than primary neoplasms. Less than 1% of cancers arise in the liver, but between 30 and 50% of patients with cancer have metastases in the liver. More than 50% of the tumors arising in the liver are hemangiomata. Carcinomata of the hepatocytes or intrahepatic bile ducts make up another 30% of the tumors primary in the liver. All other primary tumors of the liver are uncommon.

Benign

Except for the hemangioma and the infantile hemangioendiothelioma, benign mesenchymal tumors of the liver are rare. The hepatocellular adenoma is the most frequent benign epithelial tumor of the liver. Adenomata, cystadenomata, and papillomata of the bile ducts are rare. The tumor-like lesions of the liver, focal nodular hyperplasia, nodular regenerative hyperplasia, partial nodular transformation, mesenchymal hamartoma, and inflammatory pseudotumor are considered together with the benign neoplasms.

HEMANGIOMA. A cavernous hemangioma of the liver is found in 1 autopsy in 300. There is usually only one hemangioma, but occasionally there are a few, rarely a large number. Most hemangiomata lie immediately under the capsule and are less than 2 cm across. Rarely, one is much bigger, even enormous, weighing over 2000 g.

The hemangioma is sharply defined and looks purplish black. Microscopically, the tumor consists of large blood spaces, lined by normal endothelium and supported by fibrous septa.

Most hemangiomata of the liver cause no symptoms and no dysfunction. Rarely, one ruptures and hemorrhages into the peritoneal cavity. Occasionally hemangiomata of the liver are associated with hemangiomata in other organs in some of the hemangiomatous syndromes.

INFANTILE HEMANGIOENDOTHELIOMA. An infant with an infantile hemangioendothelioma of the liver has one or more nodules or masses of red or purple tissue in an enlarged liver. Often there are hemangiomata in the skin or other organs.

Microscopically, the lesions in the liver show meshwork of capillaries lined with one or more layers of plump but regular endothelial cells. Between the capillaries is a fine collagenous stroma. Bile ducts are usually present in the stroma and occasionally there are a few clumps of hepatocytes. Clumps of hematopoietic cells are usually prominent in the vessels.

As the child grows, the nodules of tumor enlarge and compress the surrounding parenchyma. High output heart failure often develops the first months of life, because of the massive shunting of blood through the tumor ascites and jaundice are unusual.

Most of the children die of congestive heart failure, less often of hepatic failure, or hemorrhage. In a few the tumor has regressed and disappeared as the child aged. Resection cures, but is not often possible. Ligation of the hepatic artery or radiation may be of help.

HEPATOCELLULAR ADENOMA. Adenomata of the hepatocytes make up less than 1% of primary liver tumors. The patients are nearly all women, usually of child-bearing age.

The adenoma usually forms a well-defined mass, often 10 to 15 cm across. Less often there are several smaller tumors. Microscopically, the lesion consists of well-differentiated hepatocytes, usually a little larger then normal and often with pale, finely vacuolated cytoplasm containing abundant glycogen and sometimes fat. The tumor cells commonly form plates separated by narrow sinusoids. Frequently the plates are two or three cells thick, but the reticulin framework of the liver is preserved. Less often the tumor cells line tubules or form acini. Most hepatocellular adenomata are highly vascular. Some contain dilated blood spaces, like those of peliosis hepatitis. Thrombosis in the abnormal vessels sometimes causes infarction of part of the tumor. Hepatocellular adenomata do not produce α-fetoprotein.

Many hepatocellular adenomata cause no symptoms. Some bleed into the peritoneal cavity. Occasionally an adenoma is large enough to press on an adjacent structure.

Most of the patients with a hepatocellular adenoma have taken oral contraceptives or anabolic steroids. In women taking oral contraceptives, the risk of developing an adenoma increases with the dose of estrogen and the duration of the exposure. The tumors showing peliosis hepatitis are usually induced by anabolic steroids. About 50% of patients with type I glycogen storage disease develop a hepatocellular adenoma.

BILE DUCT TUMORS. Rarely, a small adenoma consisting of acini lined by biliary epithelium or a larger cystadenoma with one or more locules lined by biliary epithelium arises in the liver. The glands and cysts contain mucus but not bile. Also uncommon is multiple papillomatosis of the bile ducts, with numerous papillomata lined by biliary epithelium projecting into the intrahepatic and extrahepatic bile ducts.

FOCAL NODULAR HYPERPLASIA. Focal nodular hyperplasia of the liver is not neoplastic, but closely resembles a neoplasm. Nearly 70% of the patients are women, most 20 to 40 years old.

The patient usually has a well-demarcated mass about 5 cm across beneath the capsule of the liver. Occasionally there is more than one mass, or the lesion is bigger. On section, the mass often has a fibrous center and irregular fibrous septa that radiate from the center towards the periphery.

Microscopically, collagenous septa separate nodules of hepatocytes without portal triads or hepatic veins. The septa contain many small bile ducts and usually a moderate exudate of lymphocytes, plasma cells, and macrophages. Large arteries and veins are often present in the septa.

In most of the patients, the lesion causes no disability and no symptoms. Occasionally it causes discomfort. Rarely, focal nodular hyperplasia causes bleeding into the peritoneal cavity.

The cause of focal nodular hyperplasia is unknown. Though reports differ, it does not seem to be related to contraceptive drugs or to anabolic steroids.

NODULAR REGENERATIVE HYPERPLASIA. Nodular regenerative hyperplasia is an uncommon disorder first described in Felty's syndrome, but also occurring in rheumatoid arthritis, polyarteritis nodosa, diabetes mellitus, inflammatory bowel disease, lympho-

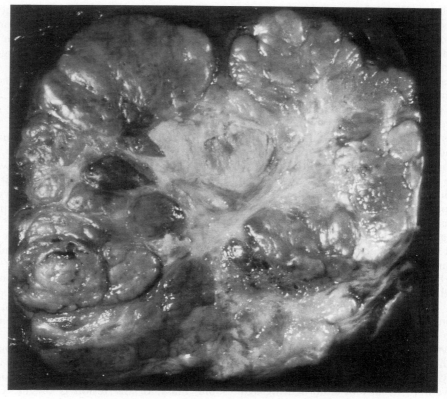

Fig. 36-34. Focal nodular hyperplasia of the liver, showing a lesion excised surgically.

ma, myeloproliferative disorders, in people given anabolic steroids, in patients with a renal transplant, and in other conditions.

Nodules of hyperplastic hepatocytes from 0.1 to 4.0 cm in diameter replace much of the hepatic parenchyma. Within the nodules, the liver plates are two or three cells thick. The nodules compress the surrounding parenchyma, but there is no fibrosis.

Most patients with nodular regenerative hyperplasia have no symptoms and no hepatic dysfunction. A few develop portal hypertension or hepatic failure. The cause of the condition is unknown. Similar changes occur in the liver of animals during hepatocarcinogenesis. Some think the hyperplasia secondary to obstruction to the portal veins.

PARTIAL NODULAR TRANSFORMATION. Partial nodular transformation of the liver is rare. Nodules like those of nodular regenerative hyperplasia develop in the hepatic parenchyma near the hilus of the liver and compress the surrounding liver tissue, causing portal hypertension. There is little or no fibrosis. Biopsy may show only apparently normal parenchyma. The cause of the nodular transformation is unknown.

MESENCHYMAL HAMARTOMA. Mesenchymal hamartomata develop in children. Most patients are less than two years old. Nearly 70% are boys. Abdominal swelling draws attention to a mass in the liver, usually in the right lobe. The mass is soft, fluctuant, and cystic. It usually weighs more than 1 kg. Microscopically, much of the mass consists of loose, edematous collagenous tissue. Dilated lymphatics, blood vessels, and tortuous bile ducts wind through the lesion. Isolated hepatocytes and small clumps of hepatocytes are present in it. Extramedullary hematopoiesis is common. Often portal triads near the mass are enlarged by loose collagenous tissue like that in the hamartoma. Resection or partial resection cures.

INFLAMMATORY PSEUDOTUMOR. Rarely, a

mass in the liver proves microscopically to consist of a dense infiltrate of lymphocytes admixed with plasma cells, macrophages, and often neutrophils and eosinophils. Germinal centers may be present. If the lesion is near the hilus of the liver, it sometimes causes obstructive jaundice or portal hypertension. The lesion is similar to the pseudolymphoma of the lungs or stomach and is inflammatory, not neoplastic.

Malignant

The most common malignant tumors primary in the liver are hepatocellular carcinoma and cholangiocarcinoma. In addition to the usual form of hepatocellular carcinoma, three uncommon types are distinguished, fibrolamellar carcinoma, encapsulated hepatocellular carcinoma, and pedulculated hepatocellular carcinoma. Hemangiosarcoma, epithelioid hemangioendothelioma, and hepatoblastoma are uncommon primary tumors of the liver. Rarely, a malignant tumor of the liver has features of both hepatocellular carcinoma and cholangiocarcinoma; a carcinoid tumor arises in an intrahepatic bile duct; or a malignant lymphoma, teratoma, or some other kind of malignant tumor arises in the liver.

HEPATOCELLULAR CARCINOMA. In North, Central and South America, northern and central Europe, Australasia, India, Pakistan, and in white people in Africa, in any one year less than 5 people in 100,000 develop a hepatocellular carcinoma. In Japan, the Middle East, and southern Europe, and in Indians living in Southeast Asia, each year 5 to 20 people per 100,000 develop hepatocellular carcinoma. In southeast China, Korea, Taiwan, Hong Kong, Vietnam, Singapore, Thailand, and black people in Africa, each year from 20 to 150 people per 100,000 develop hepatocellular carcinoma. In parts of Africa, it is the most common malignant neoplasm.

The tumor is uncommon in white people wherever they live. Chinese who emigrate from a region in which the incidence of hepatocellular carcinoma is high continue to have a high incidence of the tumor. The incidence increases in Indians who move from India to a country in which the incidence of the carcinoma is high. The incidence of the tumor in black people in the United States is similar to that in white Americans.

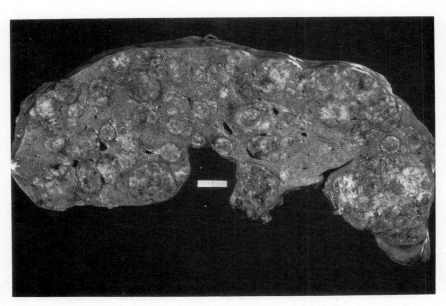

Fig. 36-35. Hepatocellular carcinoma, showing multiple nodules of tumor in the liver.

Nearly 80% of patients with hepatocellular carcinoma are men. In regions in which the incidence of hepatocellular carcinoma is high, many of the patients are under 30 years old. In regions in which the incidence is low, most patients are over 50 years old.

Lesions. A hepatocellular carcinoma usually forms a single large mass, most often in the right lobe of the liver, often with a few smaller satellite nodules of carcinoma adjacent to it. Less often, it forms multiple masses 3 to 5 cm in diameter scattered throughout the liver and all much the same size. Rarely, it infiltrates the liver diffusely without forming a mass. In regions in which the incidence of hepatocellular carcinoma is low and the tumor often develops in a cirrhotic liver, the nodules of tumor can be hard to distinguish from cirrhotic nodules. In regions in which the incidence is high, the involvement of the liver by the carcinoma is usually massive.

The nodules of hepatocellular carcinoma in the liver are usually whitish or yellow, soft, and hemorrhagic. Often some of the nodules or parts of the larger masses are stained green with bile. Commonly parts of a large mass or several of the smaller nodules are necrotic. The blood supply of

the tumor is from the hepatic arteries and is often inadequate.

Invasion of large portal veins within the liver is apparent macroscopically in 60% of the patients. The hepatic veins are invaded in 20%. In 10%, the tumor extends into the inferior vena cava, sometimes extending along the vena cava into the heart. Occasionally a hepatocellular carcinoma extends along the intrahepatic bile ducts.

Microscopically, most hepatocellular carcinomata are pleomorphic, with different patterns of growth in different parts of the tumor. Most commonly the tumor cells form plates separated by sinusoids. In well-differentiated tumors, the plates of tumor cells closely resemble a regeneration nodule or an adenoma. In regeneration nodules and adenomata, the reticulin framework of the liver is normal; in carcinomata it is nearly always distorted. In less well-differentiated tumors, the plates of tumor cells are often several cells thick and disorderly. The sinusoids between the plates are sometimes compressed, so that the tumor appears to consist of solid sheets of cells. Less often the tumor forms glandlike strictures that sometimes resemble bile ducts, sometimes are larger with papillary protrusions of tumor

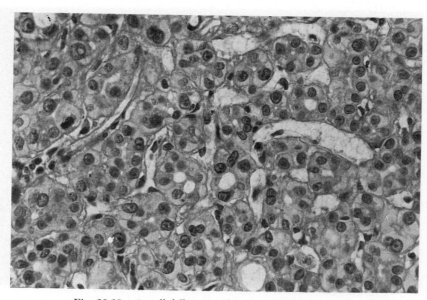

Fig. 36-36. A well-differentiated hepatocellular carcinoma.

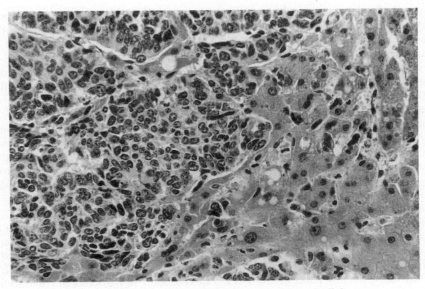

Fig. 36-37. The margin of a less well-differentiated hepatocellular carcinoma.

cells into the lumen. Only occasionally does a hepatocellular carcinoma form sheets of tumor cells without sinusoids or have more than a minimal collagenous stroma.

The tumor cells usually resemble normal hepatocytes and have biliary canaliculi between them. Often some of the canaliculi are distended by bile plugs. Not uncommonly, some of the tumor cells have clear cytoplasm because of large quantities of glycogen in the cytoplasm. Sometimes some of the tumor cells show fatty change. Not uncommonly, some of the tumor cells are anaplastic, often larger than normal hepatocytes with several bizarre nuclei. By electron microscopy, the tumor cells resemble normal hepatocytes, though their content of organelles is reduced and their structure is simplified.

In 15% of the tumors, spheroidal, homogeneous, hyaline bodies are present in the tumor cells or between them. The bodies stain strongly with the periodic acid-Schiff reaction and are acid fast when stained by the Ziehl-Neelsen method. Immunohistologic stains show that the bodies contain α-protein, α_1-antitrypsin, ferritin, and other proteins. Occasionally, a few of the tumor cells contain Mallory's hyalin.

Dysfunction. α_1-Fetoprotein normally appears in the plasma of the fetus about the sixth week of gestation and persists until a few weeks after birth, when it disappears or falls to a concentration of less that 5 μg/L.

In 90% of patients with hepatocellular carcinoma, α_1-fetoprotein reappears in the plasma. In 70% of the patients, the concentration of α_1-fetoprotein in the plasma exceeds 400 μg/L. In many, it exceeds 2000 μg/L. The concentration of fetoprotein is usually higher when the patient has both a hepatocellular carcinoma and cirrhosis. In many hepatocellular carcinomata, α-fetoprotein can be demonstrated in some of the tumor cells by immunohistologic methods.

The concentration of α-fetoprotein in the plasma increases in acute and chronic hepatitis, with metastatic carcinoma of the liver, in pregnancy, and occasionally in a patient with carcinoma of the lung or carcinoma of the stomach, but in these conditions, the concentration rarely exceeds 400 mg/L. Only in patients with a hepatocellular carcinoma and in patients with an embryonic or yolk sac tumor of an ovary or testis is the concentration of α-fetoprotein likely to exceed 2000 μg/L, and only in patients with one of these tumors is the concentration likely to rise rapidly.

The carcinoembryonic antigen is often present in the plasma in patients with hepatocellular carcinoma and can be demonstrated around the bile canaliculi between the tumor cells. It is present in the plasma in higher concentration in most patients with metastatic carcinoma in the liver and is demonstrable in the plasma in low titer in most patients with chronic liver disease.

The activity of γ-glutamyl transpeptidase in the plasma sometimes rises in patients with hepatocellular carcinoma before α-fetoprotein becomes detectable. The concentration of ferritin in the plasma is usually increased. The concentration of the vitamin B_{12} binding protein is often high. Oversecretion of erythropoietin can cause polycythemia.

Behavior. Hepatocellular carcinoma spreads first in the liver, partially by direct extension, but often by invading the blood and lymph vessels and giving rise to emboli that lodge in more distant parts of the liver and establish new nodules of carcinoma. Extension through the capsule of the liver to involve the diaphragm or abdominal wall is uncommon.

Extrahepatic metastases are present in only 50% of the patients at autopsy. The regional lymph nodes are the most common site of extrahepatic extension. In some patients, the portal, paraaortic, peripancreatic, and mediastinal lymph nodes are all involved. Hematogenous metastases are most common in the lungs. Only occasionally are the bones, adrenal glands, or the myocardium involved. Transcelomic spread is rare.

Clinical Presentation. Often a hepatocellular carcinoma causes pain or aching in the liver. Necrosis in the tumor causes fever and leukocytosis. About 50% of the patients have ascites. Occasionally a nodule of tumor ruptures, with massive and often uncontrollable hemorrhage into the peritoneal cavity. Sometimes the only sign of the carcinoma is the decline and wasting seen in many kinds of advanced malignancy. Occasionally the diagnosis is made only at autopsy.

Etiology. Many factors cause or predispose to hepatocellular carcinoma. Prominent among them are chronic hepatitis B, cirrhosis of the liver, and aflatoxin. Alcohol, poisons, drugs, genetically determined disorders, and stenosis of the inferior vena cava are less frequently involved. Liver cell dysplasia may be a precancerous condition.

Occasionally a hepatocellular carcinoma develops in a patient with schistosomiasis or some other parasitic infection, but it is not clear that the infection causes the carcinoma. Usually chronic hepatitis B or other factors that predispose to hepatocellular carcinoma are present.

Hepatitis B. Chronic hepatitis B is intimately related to hepatocellular carcinoma. The association is particularly close in regions in which the incidence of hepatocellular carcinoma is high, but in all parts of the world the incidence of hepatocellular carcinoma correlates closely with the incidence of carriers of hepatitis B. In Taiwan, 89 men in a cohort of 707 followed for nearly five years developed hepatocellular carcinoma. All had evidence of chronic hepatitis B. In Japan, 4 of 3130 men followed for five years developed hepatocellular carcinoma. All were carriers of hepatitis B. In regions where hepatocellular carcinoma is common, chronic hepatitis B is common, and infection occurs in childhood, especially in boys. In regions where hepatocellular carcinoma is uncommon, chronic hepatitis B is less common, and infection usually occurs later in life.

In the regions in which the incidence of hepatocellular carcinoma is high, 80% of the patients have one or more of the genes of the hepatitis B virus incorporated into the genome of the tumor cells and into the genome of some of the nonneoplastic hepatocytes. Unincorporated virus may also be present in the non-neoplastic hepatocytes. The incorporated viral genes in the tumor cells do not produce the viral antigens in vivo, but do produce HBsAg in vitro. In non-neoplastic hepatocytes, they produce the excess of HBsAg present in the ground glass cells of carriers of hepatitis B, but not the other viral antigens. In the regions in which the incidence of hepatocellular carcinoma is low, the proportion of hepatocellular carcinomata with viral genes incorporated into the genome of the tumor cells is lower.

It seems likely that the viral genes cause the carcinoma in the patients in whom they are incorporated into the hepatocellular genome. How they do so is unknown. The virus does have a gene of unknown function that could be oncogenic, or the incorporated virus may activate other genes that are oncogenic. The incorporated viral genes could facilitate the production of a metabolite that is carcinogenic.

Cirrhosis of the Liver. Cirrhosis of the liver is also closely related to hepatocellular carcinoma, especially in regions in which the incidence of hepatocellular carcinoma is low. In the Americas, Europe, and Australasia, over 80% of the patients with hepatocellular carcinoma have cirrhosis of the liver. The cirrhosis is nearly always caused by alcohol and usually precedes the carcinoma by many years. It is usually of the mixed or macronodular type. Cirrhosis is more common than hepatocellular carcinoma. Less than 10% of patients with cirrhosis develop hepatocellular carcinoma.

In regions in which the incidence of hepatocellular carcinoma is high, only 60% of the patients with hepatocellular carcinoma have cirrhosis. The cirrhosis is usually caused by hepatitis B and develops about the same time as the carcinoma. Over 40% of patients with cirrhosis have hepatocellular carcinoma. Hepatocellular carcinoma is probably more common than cirrhosis.

How cirrhosis predisposes to hepatocellular carcinoma is unclear. The hepatocellular proliferation caused by the cirrhosis may potentiate the effect of hepatocarcinogens, as it does in experimental animals. The disordered metabolism in the cirrhotic liver may fail to detoxify carcinogenic substances or may favor the production of carcinogenic metabolites.

Aflatoxin. The aflatoxins are the most important of the carcinogenic substances produced by fungi. In several species of animal, aflatoxin B1 is a highly potent hepatocarcinogen. Food in Africa and Southeast Asia is often contaminated with Aspergillus flavus, the fungus that produces aflatoxins, though it is not clear how often aflatoxins are ingested. Their importance in causing hepatocellular carcinoma in man is uncertain. They may be responsible for some of the tumors in Africa and Southeast Asia that develop in people who are not infected by the hepatitis B virus, or they may potentiate the carcinogenic effect of the virus.

Alcohol. A high intake of alcohol increases the risk of developing hepatocellular carcinoma. In the United States, an intake of more than 80 g of ethanol a day increases the risk four times. The incidence of hepatocellular carcinoma caused by alcohol probably increase not only because it induces cirrhosis. Some product of the disordered metabolism caused by alcohol could be carcinogenic, and alcohol potentiates other agents that cause hepatocellular carcinoma. In the Philippines, a high intake of alcohol doubles the likelihood of hepatocellular carcinoma in people heavily exposed to aflatoxins. Hepatitis B infection is unduly common in patients with alcoholic cirrhosis who develop a hepatocellular carcinoma.

Poisons. Many plants produce substances that cause liver tumors in animals, but it has not been shown that they are carcinogenic in man. Among them are the pyrrolizidine alkaloids that cause veno-occlusive disease, cycasins, safrol, and tannic acid. The nitrosamines that often contaminate foods are hepatocarcinogens in animals. Their importance in man is unknown. Organochlorine pesticides such as DDT, polychlorinated biphenyls, and organic solvents cause liver tumors in animals but are not known to be hepatocarcinogenic in man.

Drugs. Oral contraceptives and anabolic steroids usually produce hepatocellular adenomata, but in a few patients have induced a hepatocellular carcinoma. Occasionally a hepatocellular carcinoma has developed in a patient given thorium dioxide (Thorotrast), a radioactive substance stored in the liver that more often induces a hepatic hemangiosarcoma.

Genetic Disorders. Hepatocellular carcinoma occurs commonly in some genetically determined diseases. Occasionally a patient with type I glycogen storage disease develops a hepatocellular carcinoma. Tyrosinemia, progressive intrahepatic cholestasis, and probably the PIZZ genotype of α_1-antitrypsin deficiency increase the risk of developing hepatocellular carcinoma. Over 20% of patients with the genetically determined form of hemochromatosis develop hepatocellular carcinoma, though it is not known if the carcinoma is caused by the genetic abnormality, the excess of iron in the liver, or the cirrhosis usual in hemochromatosis. Occasionally hepatocellular carcinoma develops in Wilson's disease.

Vena Caval Anomalies. In South Africa, India, and Japan, less often in other parts of the world, a membranous obstruction where the inferior vena cava joins the atrium or a fibrous occlusion lower in the vena cava has been found in many patients with hepatocellular carcinoma. In one series, 20% of patients with hepatocellular carcinoma had caval obstruction, and 50% of patients with caval obstruction had a hepatocellular carcinoma. It is not clear whether the obstruction to the veins is congenital or acquired. The relation between the obstruction and the carcinoma is obscure.

Liver Cell Dysplasia. The presence of clumps of large hepatocytes with bizarre, hyperchromatic nuclei, sometimes with more than one nucleus, is called liver cell dysplasia. In Africa, 1% of people with a normal liver, 5% of patients with hepatocellular carcinoma and an otherwise normal liver, 20% of patients with cirrhosis, and 65% of patients with both cirrhosis and a hepatocellular carcinoma have foci of liver cell dysplasia in the nonneoplastic part of the liver. Many of the patients with liver cell dysplasia have chronic hepatitis B. It is often suggested that liver cell dysplasia is precancerous, but it has not been proved.

Treatment and Prognosis. Resection of a hepatocellular carcinoma is rarely possible. Chemotherapy and radiotherapy are of limited benefit. A few patients have been treated by hepatic transplantation. The mean survival is less than three months from the time of diagnosis. Death usually comes from hemorrhage, hepatic failure, or cachexia. Rarely, a hepatocellular carcinoma regresses and disappears.

Fibrolamellar Carcinoma. Fibrolamellar carcinoma of the liver is an uncommon tumor sometimes called polygonal cell hepatocellular carcinoma, fibrolamellar oncocytoma, fibrolamellar oncocytic hepatoma, and other such names. It occurs in adolescents and young adults. Women are affected a little more often than men.

The carcinoma forms a solitary mass in the liver, most often in the left lobe. The lesion is well demarcated and firm. On section, it is divided into lobules by collagenous septa.

Microscopially, the tumor consists of cords and nodules of tumor cells separated by thin, parallel bands or lamellae of collagenous tissue. The tumor cells are large and polygonal, with a central vesicular nucleus and a single nucleolus. Their cytoplasm is eosinophilic and granular. Mitoses are few. Occasionally some of the tumor cells contain hyaline globules or show fatty change.

Electron microscopy shows that the cytoplasm is crowded with organelles. Mitochondria are especially numerous. They are swollen, with a pale matrix and narrowing of the space between the inner and outer mitochondrial membranes and between the membranes of the cristae. The cristae are often deformed. Smooth endoplasmic reticulum is commonly abundant and sometimes forms fingerprints. Bile canaliculi with microvilli are present between the tumor cells.

The carcinoma sometimes causes pain, but often is detected only when the mass is discovered. The concentration of α-fetoprotein in the plasma is normal or nearly so. The concentration of the vitamin B_{12} binding protein in the plasma is increased. Hypercalcemia is often present. The patients do not have cirrhosis, hepatitis B, or alcoholism.

A lamellar carcinoma grows slowly. It can metastasize, but often it is confined to the liver when discovered. The tumor is treated by surgical excision. Over 80% of the patients are alive two years after resection, and over 60% are alive five years afterwards.

Encapsulated Hepatocellular Carcinoma. Encapsulated hepatocellular carcinomata are most common in Japan and Southeast Asia. In Japan, 10% of malignant hepatocellular tumors are of this type. The tumor is usually 3 to 5 cm in diameter when it is discovered, with a thick collagenous capsule. Microscopically, the carcinoma is similar to a well-differentiated hepatocellular carcinoma of the usual type, except for its capsule. The patients usually have severe cirrhosis and often have chronic hepatitis B. About 50% of the tumors produce α-fetoprotein. If the capsule is intact, the prognosis is good.

Pedunculated Hepatocellular Carcinoma. Pedunculated hepatocellular carcinomata are rare. They usually arise in people over 60

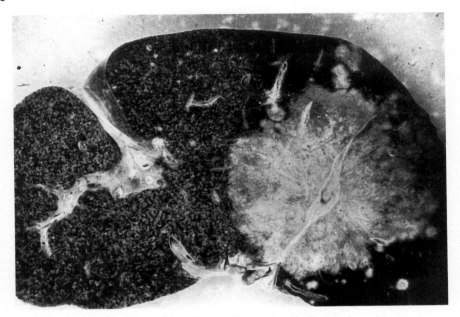

Fig. 36-38. Cholangiocarcinoma of the liver, showing the large mass formed by the tumor.

years old. Nearly 70% of the patients are men. The tumor forms a pedunculated mass 3 to 25 cm across that hangs from the surface of the liver. Microscopically, it resembles the usual form of hepatocellular carcinoma.

Less than 30% of the tumors produce α-fetoprotein. Nearly 70% of the patients have cirrhosis. About 30% have evidence of hepatitis B. Excision usually cures.

CHOLANGIOCARCINOMA. Cholangiocarcino-

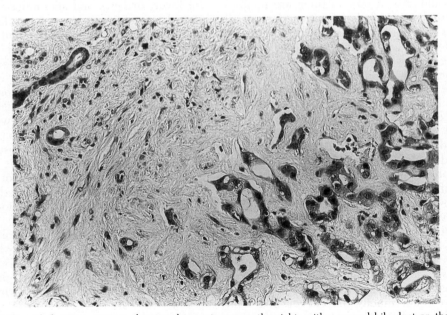

Fig. 36-39. Cholangiocarcinoma, showing the carcinoma on the right, with a normal bile duct on the left.

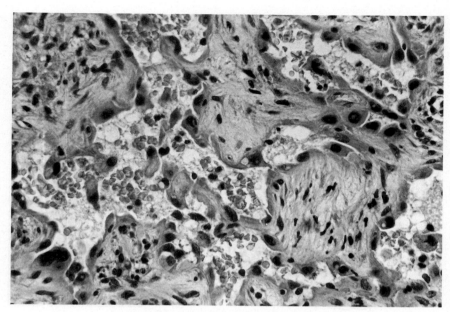

Fig. 36-40.   Hemangiosarcoma of the liver.

mata arise from the bile ducts. The intra-hepatic cholangiocarcinomata are consid-ered here. The extrahepatic tumors are dis-cussed in Chapter 37. About 20% of pri-mary malignant tumors of the liver are of this type. The patients are usually over 50 years old. About 60% of them are men.

Lesions. A cholangiocarcinoma usually forms a single mass in the liver or a large mass with a few satellite nodules. Common-ly the mass is 5 to 10 cm across. Usually it is in the right lobe. Less often the carcinoma forms multiple nodules. The tumor is usual-ly well defined, white, scirrhous, and hard.

Occasionally a cholangiocarcinoma is con-fined to the wall of one or both the major bile ducts at the hilus of the liver, a lesion called a Klatskin tumor after an Ameri-can physician. The carcinoma forms a hard, ill-defined mural thickening that greatly narrows the lumen of the duct or ducts involved.

Microscopically, most cholangiocarcino-mata are well differentiated. They form tu-bules or acini lined by biliary epithelium and set in an abundant and often sclerotic collagenous stroma. The tubules and acini may contain mucus, but never bile. Only rarely is a cholangiocarcinoma poorly differ-entiated and more cellular.

Behavior. Cholangiocarcinomata metas-tasize first to the regional lymph nodes, then to the lungs. Occasionally there are more distant metastases to bone or elsewhere.

Clinical Presentation. Most patients with a cholangiocarcinoma first seek advice for fever, malaise, and abdominal pain. Ob-structive jaundice is apparent in 30% of the patients. The liver is usually about the nor-mal size. Ascites is uncommon. Patients with a Klatskin tumor usually develop se-vere, obstructive jaundice.

Etiology. In China, Hong Kong, Thai-land, and Southeast Asia, cholangiocarcino-ma is often caused by infestation with Chlo-norchis siensis or Opsitorchis viverrini. The incidence of the tumor is increased in in-flammatory bowel disease, cystic fibrosis, and in congenital malformations of the bili-ary system. The radiation emitted by tho-rium dioxide (Thorotrast) occasionally in-duces a cholangiocarcinoma.

Treatment and Prognosis. Cholangiocar-cinomata are treated surgically when it is possible to excise the lesion or bypass the obstruction. Most of the patients die within six months. Few survive more than three years.

HEMANGIOSARCOMA. A hemangiosarcoma of the liver, or malignant hemangioendothelioma as it is sometimes called, develops each year in 1 person in 10,000,000. The patients are usually adults and more often are men than women.

Lesions. The sarcoma forms multiple nodules of soft, hemorrhagic tissue in the liver. Microscopically, it is made of anaplastic, pleomorphic, spindle-shaped cells that sometimes grow in sheets, more often line blood filled spaces supported by a fine collagenous stroma, and particularly at the margins of the tumor nodules often line the walls of sinusoids between plates of normal or compressed hepatocytes. Hemorrhage into the tumor is common. Necrosis is sometimes extensive. Extramedullary hematopoiesis is often evident in the tumor.

Electron microscopy shows little to suggest the origin of the malignant cells. A few of them stain for factor VIII of the clotting system as do endothelial cells, supporting the generally accepted view that the tumor is an angiosarcoma.

Behavior. Hemangiosarcomata of the liver grow rapidly and extend throughout the liver. Metastases in the spleen, bone marrow, lungs, lymph nodes, and implants on the peritoneum are common.

Clinical Presentation. Patients with a hemangiosarcoma of the liver develop rapidly progressive hepatic failure, weight loss, and fever. Bloody ascites and cachexia often follow. Sometimes disseminated intravascular coagulation worsens the course.

Etiology. Thorotrast (thorium dioxide) was used as a contrast medium in radiology up to 1960. About 70% of the dose is stored in the Kupffer cells in the liver, 20% in the spleen, and 10% in the bone marrow. It remains for the rest of the patient's life. Thorotrast emits alpha radiation and has a half life of 400 years. In the liver, it causes fibrosis, portal hypertension, and after 10 or more years hemangiosarcoma, less often hepatocellular carcinoma or cholangiocarcinoma. Occasionally it induces a hemangiosarcoma in the spleen or bone marrow or causes leukemia, lymphoma, or aplastic anemia. Over 50,000 people still have dangerous amounts of Thorotrast in the liver and other organs.

Men exposed to the fumes of vinyl chloride monomer during the manufacture of polyvinyl chloride develop Raynaud's phenomenon, acroosteolysis, hyperplasia of the Kupffer and Ito cells, and peliosis hepatitis. The Kupffer and Ito cells grow increasingly abnormal, and clumps of atypical hepatocytes appear. Reticulin and collagen are deposited in the space of Disse, around portal tracts and beneath the capsule of the liver. Portal hypertension develops and eventually hemangiosarcoma of the liver. The sarcoma appears only many years after the exposure, and though safety measures are now in force to prevent exposure to the monomer, hemangiosarcomata of the liver caused by earlier exposure to vinyl chloride monomer are likely to continue to appear until 2010.

Less often, hemangiosarcoma of the liver has followed exposure to arsenic, either as an arsenical spray used in vineyards and in orchards or as Fowler's solution. In a few patients, the tumor has followed exposure to sprays containing copper or the administration of anabolic or contraceptive steroids.

Treatment and Prognosis. No treatment for hemangiosarcoma of the liver is effective. Most patients die within a few months of diagnosis.

EPITHELIOID HEMANGIOENDOTHELIOMA. An epithelioid hemangioendothelioma of the liver is a rare tumor. The patients are usually about 50 years old. It is more common in women than in men.

The patient usually has several firm, white nodules of tumor in the liver. Microscopically, the tumor at first has clumps of large tumor cells with abundant cytoplasm and vesicular nuclei in sinusoids and veins separated by a fine collagenous stroma. The tumor cells look epithelial, but electron microscopy shows that they have the cell junctions, pinocytic vesicles, and Weibel Palade bodies of endothelial cells. Immunohistologic methods show that they stain for factor VIII, confirming their endothelial nature. As time passes, the tumor becomes increasingly sclerotic. Only narrow strands of endothelial tumor cells remain, separated by abundant, hyalinized collagen.

The tumor grows slowly, but metastasizes. About 30% of the patients are alive five years after diagnosis.

HEPATOBLASTOMA. A hepatoblastoma is a rare tumor. Most of the patients are less than two years old. Nearly 70% are boys. Progressive enlargement of the abdomen

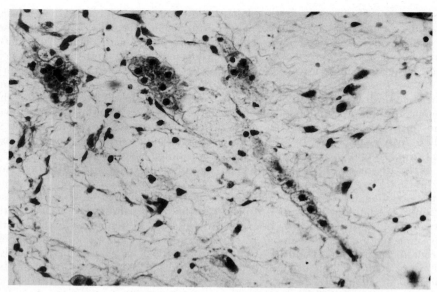

Fig. 36-41. Hepatoblastoma, showing small islands of neoplastic hepatocytes in loose, neoplastic connective tissue.

draws attention to the tumor. The concentration of α-fetoprotein in the plasma is high. Over 30% of the patients have a congenital anomaly in some other part of the body.

The tumor forms a circumscribed, lobulated mass 5 to 25 cm across. Cystic degeneration, necrosis, and hemorrhage are common. Microscopically, it consists of a mixture of malignant epithelial and malignant mesenchymal elements. The epithelial component consists of ribbons or rosettes of small, dark, fusiform embryonal hepatocytes; clumps or plates of larger fetal hepatocytes, often with sinusoids and canaliculi; glandular structures that sometimes resemble bile ducts; and often clumps of squamous epithelium. The mesenchymal component often consists largely of osteoid, but loose connective tissue with spindle cells, cartilage, or occasional muscle cells can sometimes be found.

Hepatoblastomata grow rapidly and untreated bring death by hemorrhage, hepatic failure, or widespread metastases. A combination of surgical excision, chemotherapy, and radiotherapy brings a 25% 10-year survival.

SECONDARY TUMORS. Metastatic tumor in the liver is among the most common of malignant neoplasms. Most often the metastasizing tumor is carried to the liver in the portal blood or by the hepatic artery. Occasionally transcelomic spread of a malignant tumor involves the liver. Sometimes a malignant tumor of the stomach or some other adjacent organ extends into the liver. Rarely, a malignant tumor in the vena cava grows into the hepatic veins.

Most metastatic tumors in the liver are carcinomata. The colon, breast, and lungs are among the most common sites of origin. In 10% of the patients, there is only one metastasis. In most, there are several. Metastatic carcinoma in the liver forms spheroidal masses that vary in size from the microscopic to 20 cm in diameter. The metastases are nearly always well demarcated. They may be firm and white, or soft and hemorrhagic. Particularly with carcinoma of the colon, the center of the metastases is often scarred because of necrosis and hypoxia in the center of the lesion.

Most metastatic carcinomata in the liver reproduce the microscopic structure of the primary tumor. Most probably begin when

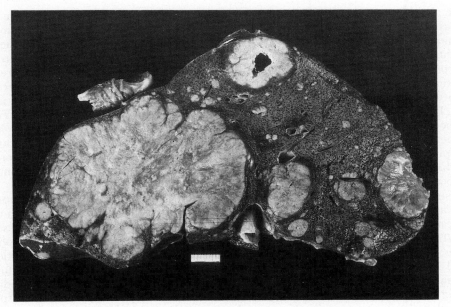

Fig. 36-42. Carcinoma of the breast metastatic in the liver.

an embolus of tumor cells lodges in a portal tract, but as the metastasis grows, its site of origin is destroyed. The metastases draw their blood from the hepatic arteries and push the portal vessels aside.

Even when a liver is largely replaced by metastatic carcinoma and weighs 5000 g or more, there is usually little hepatic dysfunction. The activity of alkaline phosphatases in the plasma is often a little increased, as may be the activity of the aminotransferases. Jaundice is unusual unless one of the metastases obstructs a major bile duct.

Hematopoietic tumors frequently involve the liver. The involvement is often diffuse in leukemia, with involvement of the portal triads predominant in lymphoid leukemia and involvement of the sinusoids in myeloid leukemia. The liver may be twice its normal size, but the infiltrate of leukemic cells is so even that its cut surface often shows little abnormality. Occasionally a pale speckling shows the site of the leukemic deposits. Less often, a lymphoma forms nodular deposits in the liver. Hepatic function is usually little impaired.

Malignant melanoma forms metastases in the liver like those of metastatic carcinoma. Sarcomata rarely metastasize to the liver.

HEPATIC FAILURE

Hepatic failure can result from any form of severe liver disease that causes major loss of hepatocytes or major disruption of the hepatic circulation. Prominent among its causes are cirrhosis, viral and drug-induced hepatitis, mushroom poisoning, fatty liver of pregnancy, sudden occlusion of the hepatic artery near the liver, and occlusion of the hepatic veins. Shock and septicemia can cause hepatic failure. Occasionally massive infiltration of the liver in leukemia does so. Hepatic failure may develop suddenly, as in fulminant hepatitis, or come insidiously, as it often does in cirrhosis.

Two kinds of hepatic failure are distinguished, hepatocellular failure and hepatic encephalopathy. They are closely associated, and often both are present.

HEPATOCELLULAR FAILURE. The first manifestations of hepatocellular failure are often vague: weakness, tiredness, loss of weight. Jaundice is usually marked when hepatocellular failure results from viral or drug-induced hepatitis, but is often absent or slight when it comes slowly in cirrhosis.

Circulatory Changes. The circulation is hyperkinetic in people with hepatic failure. The cardiac output is increased, with tachycardia. Peripheral resistance is reduced, and the blood flow is increased through the skin and the spleen. The skin is flushed. The blood pressure falls.

In the kidneys, vasoconstriction reduces the blood flow to the renal cortices, and the hypotension further reduces renal blood flow. Vasomotor nephropathy commonly follows, causing the hepatorenal syndrome.

In 30% of people with cirrhosis who suffer hepatic failure there is hypoxia, with an arterial PO_2 of between 60 and 70 mm Hg and sometimes cyanosis. It seems due to the opening of shunts within the lungs, giving a right to left shunt. Occasionally there is pulmonary hypertension. In all forms of hepatic failure the diffusing capacity in the lungs is reduced, without a restrictive defect. The oxyhemoglobin dissociation curve shifts to the left, impairing the release of oxygen to the tissues. Clubbing of the fingers is often present if cyanosis is severe.

Vasodilation in the skin causes palmar erythema in some people with hepatocellular failure. The hands are warm. The thenar and hypothenar eminences and the tips of the fingers are particularly flushed.

Vascular spiders of the kind seen also in pregnancy appear on the face, neck, arms, and hands. They are most common in people with cirrhosis, but occur in other forms of hepatic failure. A spider is up to 0.5 cm across and consists of a central arteriole, with numerous small vessels radiating from it, like the legs of a spider. Other forms of vasodilation can also occur in the skin. Occasionally the dilated vessels resemble the silk threads in United States dollar bills, to give the appearance called paper money skin.

Particularly in cirrhosis, the nails of patients with hepatocellular failure are often white, except for a pink zone near the tip.

Metabolic Changes. In hepatocellular failure, the hepatocytes are unable to synthesize proteins normally. The production of albumin falls, bringing hypoalbuminemia.

The more severe the hepatocellular injury, the more severe the hypoalbuminemia.

The production of the clotting factors in the liver fails, bringing prolongation of the prothrombin time. In part this failure is due to poor absorption of vitamin K, because of the lack of bile salts in the intestine, and can be corrected by administering the vitamin. In part it is due to the injury to the hepatocytes and grows increasingly severe as hepatocellular injury increases. Purpura or excessive bleeding from minor wounds sometimes follows.

Fetor hepaticus, a sweet, mouselike smell, is often present on the breath of people with severe hepatocellular disease. It is probably due to abnormal metabolism of methionine in the gut, with production of a mercaptan that is excreted by the lungs.

Endocrine Changes. Hypogonadism is common in hepatocellular failure, especially in cirrhosis, and results principally from abnormal metabolism of estrogens. In men, the testes are small. Impotence is frequent. Unilateral or bilateral gynecomastia occasionally develops. In women, the breasts and uterus atrophy. Menstruation is irregular.

Fever and Infection. About 30% of patients with hepatocellular failure have fever of up to 38°C. It is particularly common in people with active cirrhosis.

Infection is common in people with hepatocellular failure. Most often gram-negative organisms are involved. Over 5% of the patients have bacteremia.

Treatment and Prognosis. Rest and a high protein diet often ameliorate the effects of hepatocellular failure. The prognosis depends on the nature of the underlying disease.

HEPATIC ENCEPHALOPATHY. Hepatic encephalopathy is called hepatic coma or, in its earlier stages, hepatic precoma. Hepatic encephalopathy is a complex syndrome. Different patients have different manifestations of the disorder. Often it varies in severity from day to day. Hepatic encephalopthy may develop rapidly, as in fulminant hepatitis, or slowly over many months, as is often the case in cirrhosis of the liver.

Clinical Presentation. When hepatic encephalopathy develops rapidly, the patient becomes confused, often antisocial, delirious, maniacal, or violent, and soon sinks into decerebrate rigidity and death.

When hepatic encephalopathy develops more slowly, lethargy is often the first sign. The patient becomes dull, apathetic, and tends to sleep a lot. Often the patient becomes childish, irritable, and irresponsible, though jocular, and euphoric when at ease socially. As the disease advances, there is progressive mental deterioration. It may be slight and vary from day to day but can become extreme. The quality of the patient's handwriting is sometimes a good measure. Speech often become slurred and monotonous. As coma approaches, the patient may no longer be able to distinguish between common objects that look more or less alike. The patient becomes stuporous, confused, and often behaves in a grossly inappropriate manner. Fetor hepaticus is often evident, and other signs of hepatocellular failure are likely to be apparent. Towards the end, the muscles may become flaccid. Sometimes there is hyperventilation or hyperpyrexia.

Characteristic of hepatic encephalopathy is the liver flap, or flapping tremor, called asterixis. If the forearm is fixed and the wrist is hyperextended, the hand and fingers flap. The deep tendon reflexes are exaggerated. Muscle tone increases. There may be rigidity. Ankle clonus is sustained.

Before symptoms are marked, the electroencephalograph sometimes shows bursts of slow, symmetrical, synchronous, high voltage waves, 1½ to 3 per second. At first, the abnormal waves occur only in the frontal region, but as the encephalopathy worsens, other parts of the brain are involved. The slow waves persist longer and eventually replace the normal rhythm.

Cerebral Lesions. In the early stages of hepatic encephalopathy, the brain is normal macroscopically and microscopically shows only some increase in astrocytes, usually of the Alzheimer type II type throughout the gray matter of the cerebrum and cerebellum, the putamen, and the globus pallidus.

In the later stages, the brain is edematous. There is widespread but patchy loss of neurons in the cerebral cortex, basal ganglia, cerebellum, and sometimes elsewhere. Particularly in these regions, there is prolif-

eration of Alzheimer type II astrocytes, with large vesicular nuclei, but little cytoplasm. Often there are vacuoles of glycogen in the nuclei of the astrocytes. If the loss of neurons is great, there may be microcavities in the cerebral cortex or basal ganglia.

Pathogenesis. Hepatic encephalopathy develops when much of the portal blood reaches the systemic circulation without having been purified by an active hepatic parenchyma. It occurs when a great part of the hepatic parenchyma is destroyed by fulminant hepatitis or in some other way and when a large proportion of the portal blood is shunted past the hepatocytes, as is often the case in the late stages of cirrhosis and portal hypertension. Probably shunting alone is not sufficient to cause hepatic encephalopathy if the hepatic parenchyma is normal, but precipitates the failure of a liver that would otherwise be adequate.

It seems probable that hepatic encephalopathy results from the absorption of toxic material from the intestine. Normally, toxic substances are carried in the portal blood to the liver, where they are detoxified. In severe hepatic failure, they pass into the systemic circulation and damage the brain. The success of intestinal antibiotics in controlling hepatic encephalopathy suggests that the toxin or toxins are formed in the bowel by bacterial action.

Ammonia is produced in the gut by bacterial action and is absorbed into the portal blood. Normally, it is removed from the blood by the liver and converted into urea. In 90% of patients with hepatic encephalopathy, this conversion fails. The concentration of ammonia in the plasma rises.

It has long been thought that ammonia might be a principal cause of hepatic encephalopathy. In most of the patients, the concentration of ammonia in the plasma correlates roughly with the severity of the encephalopathy. The severity of the encephalopathy usually increases if the production of ammonia in the gut increases and lessens if the production of ammonia is reduced. In the brain, ammonia combines with α-ketoglutarate to form glutamate and glutamine. The concentration of glutamine in the cerebrospinal fluid rises. The lack of α-ketoglutarate needed for Krebs' citric acid cycle impairs oxidative metabolism and can injure the neurons. The consumption of oxygen by the brain falls. The ammonia may damage the membranes of the neurons, adding to the injury.

Against this hypothesis is the lack of hyperammonemia in some patients with hepatic encephalopathy. The clinical findings in children with hyperammonemia caused by a defect in the urea cycle in the liver differ from those of hepatic encephalopathy. In some patients with hepatic encephalopathy, the brain adds ammonia to the blood instead of extracting it. In most patients with liver disease, giving ammonium citrate to increase the concentration of ammonia in the blood does not cause encephalopathy or changes in the electroencephalogram.

The bacteria in the bowel could produce other toxic substances from nitrogenous elements in the food. Some have thought products of tryptophan metabolism might be dangerous. Tryptophan is increased in the brain and cerebrospinal fluid in hepatic encephalopathy. Administration of methionine in the diet increases the severity of hepatic encephalopathy without increasing the ammonia level in the blood. Tetracycline prevents this adverse effect of methionine, suggesting that the intestinal bacteria produce some toxic metabolite from the methionine, perhaps a mercaptan. Toxic factors of this sort could act alone or in combination with ammonia.

Intestinal bacteria produce substances such as octopamine that are normally destroyed in the liver but could serve as false neurotransmitters in the brain. The concentration of octopamine in the plasma is increased in hepatic encephalopathy and correlates with the severity of the encephalopathy. In rats, however, large doses of octopamine failed to induce coma. At autopsy, the concentration of octopamine in the brain is lower in patients with cirrhosis and encephalopathy than in those with normal cerebral function.

The concentration of aromatic amino acids in the plasma increases in hepatic encephalopathy, and the concentration of branched chain amino acids falls. The excess of aromatic amino acids could lead to excessive production of the neurotransmitters serotonin and norepinephrine, but no increase in norepinephrine has been found in the brain of patients with encephalopathy at autopsy, and the increase in aromatic amino acids and the decrease in branched chain amino acids is no greater in patients with cirrhosis who have hepatic encephalopathy than in those who do not.

Gamma aminobutyric acid is the principal inhibitory neurotransmitter in the brain. It is produced in the gut by bacterial action and absorbed into the portal blood. Normally, it is detoxified by the liver. Its concentration in the plasma increases in patients with hepatic encephalopathy. Normally it does not pass the blood barrier, but could do so if the barrier were damaged. Receptors for γ-aminobutyric acid on the postsynaptic membranes of the neurons increase in hepatic encephalopathy. Experimentally, γ-aminobutyric acid causes coma. Many think it the major cause of hepatic encephalopathy.

Treatment and Prognosis. In patients with hepatic encephalopathy, dietary protein is stopped, and antibiotics are given to prevent the formation of toxic products by the bacteria in the gut. Lactulose and lactilol reduce the formation of ammonia in the gut. The patients react excessively to sedatives, which should be avoided. Occasionally levodopa causes temporary benefit by enhancing the content of dopamine in the brain. Bromocriptine reacts with the dopamine receptors in the brain and is sometimes of benefit.

HEPATIC TRANSPLANTATION. Transplantation of the liver is increasingly being used in a variety of end stage diseases of the liver. The transplanted liver does not develop hyperacute rejection of the sort that occasionally occurs in a transplanted kidney, but does suffer acute and chronic rejection.

Acute rejection occurs 5 to 15 days after the operation. The portal tracts are edematous, and an exudate of lymphocytes and macrophages, sometimes with a few eosinophils, collects in the portal tracts and sometimes around the terminal hepatic veins. The inflammatory cells are often most prominent around the blood vessels in the triads. The epithelium of small bile ducts is often irregular and pleomorphic. Hepatocellular necrosis is slight and probably due to operative trauma rather than rejection.

Chronic rejection follows repeated episodes of acute rejection or may develop insidiously without clinically apparent acute rejection. Foamy macrophages accumulate in the intima of portal veins and in sinusoids, narrowing the lumen. Fibrosis develops around the portal triads and the terminal hepatic veins. Septa may extend from portal tract to portal tract. Inflammatory exudate is usually sparse. Small bile ducts show epithelial degeneration and disappear. Cholestasis becomes increasingly prominent.

BIBLIOGRAPHY

General

Denk, H., Lackinger, E., and Venningerholz, F.: Pathology of the cytoskeleton of hepatocytes. Prog. Liver Dis., 8:237, 1986.

Ishak, K. G.: Applications of scanning electron microscopy to the study of liver disease. Prog. Liver Dis., 8:1, 1986.

Ishak, K. G.: New developments in diagnostic liver pathology. Monogr. Pathol., 28:223, 1987.

MacSween, R. N. M., Anthony P. P., and Scheuer, P. J. (Eds.): Pathology of the Liver, 2nd ed. Edinburgh, Churchill Livingstone, 1987.

Paronetto, F.: Cell-mediated immunity in liver disease. Hum. Pathol., 17:168, 1986.

Paronetto, F., Colucci, G., and Columbo, M.: Lymphocytes in liver diseases. Prog. Liver Dis., 8:191, 1986.

Peters, R. L., and Craig, J. R. (Eds.): Liver Pathology. Edinburgh, Churchill Livingstone, 1986.

Phillips, M. J., Poucell, S., Patterson, J., and Valencia, P.: The Liver. New York, Raven Press, 1987.

Reddy, J. K., and Rao, M. S.: Hepatic ultrastructure and adaption. Monogr. Pathol., 28:11, 1987.

Ruebner, B. H., and Montgomery, C. K.: Pathology of the Liver and Biliary Tract. New York, John Wiley & Sons, 1982.

Rushton, D. I.: Fetal and neonatal liver disease. Diag. Histopathol., 4:17, 1981.

Scheuer, P. J.: Liver Biopsy Interpretation, 3rd ed. London, Baillière Tindall, 1980.

Schiff, L. (Ed.): Diseases of the Liver, 5th Ed. Philadelphia, J.B. Lipincott, 1982.

Sherlock, S.: Diseases of the Liver and Biliary System, 7th ed. Oxford, Blackwell Scientific Publications, 1985.

Sherlock, S., Dick, R., and Van Leeuwen D. J.: Liver biopsy today. The Royal Free Hospital experience. J. Hepatol., 1:75, 1985.

Stenger, R. J.: Interpretation of Liver Biopsies. New York, Raven Press, 1984.

Viral Hepatitis

Alter, H. J. (Ed.): Hepatitis B. Semin. Liver Dis., 2:20, 1982.

Balistreri, W. F.: Viral hepatitis: implications to pediatric practice. Adv. Pediatr., 32:287, 1985.

Bernuau, J., Rueff, B., Benhamou, J.-P.: Fulminant and subfulminant liver failure: definitions and causes. Semin. Liver Dis., 6:97, 1986.

Bianchi, L.: Necroinflammatory liver diseases. Semin. Liver Dis., 6:185, 1986.

Blum, H. E., and Vyas, G. N.: Non-A, non-B hepatitis. Haematologica, 15:153, 1982.

Bonino, F., and Smedile, A.: Delta agent (type D) hepatitis. Semin. Liver Dis., 6:28, 1986.

Bradley, D. W., and Maynard, J. E.: Etiology and natural history of post-transfusion and enterically-transmitted non-A, non-B hepatitis. Semin. Liver Dis., 6:56, 1986.

Callea, F., Zorzi, M., and Desmet, V. J. (Eds.): Viral Hepatitis. Berlin, Springer-Verlag, 1986.

Craig, J. R., Govindarajan, S., and DeCock, K. M.: Delta virus hepatitis. Pathol. Annu., 21 (2):1, 1986.

Dienstag, J. L.: Non-A, non-B hepatitis Adv. Intern. Med., 26:187, 1981.

Dienstag, J. L., and Alter, H. J.: Non-A, non-B hepatitis: evolving epidemiologic and clinical perspective. Semin. Liver Dis., 6:67, 1986.

Eder, G., McDonel, J. L., and Dorner, F.: Hepatitis B vaccine. Prog. Liver Dis., 8:367, 1986.

Fagan, E. A., and Williams, R.: Non-A, non-B hepatitis. Semin. Liver Dis., 4:314, 1984.

Fagan, E. A., and Williams, R.: Serological responses to HBV infection. Gut, 27:858, 1986.

Feinstone, S. M.: Hepatitis A. Prog. Liver Dis., 8:299, 1986.

Galambos, J. T.: Transmission of hepatitis B from providers to patients: how big is the risk? Hepatology, 6:320, 1986.

Ganem, D.: Persistent infection of humans with hepatitis B virus. Rev. Infect. Dis., 4:1026, 1982.

Gitnik, G.: Non-A, non-B hepatitis. Annu. Rev. Med., 35:265, 1984.

Gust, I. D., et al.: Taxonomic classification of human hepatitis B virus. Intervirology, 25:14, 1986.

Hellström, U., and Sylvan, S.: Human serum albumin and the enigma of chronic active hepatitis type B. Scand. J. Immunol., 23:523, 1986.

Hollinger, F. B.: Serologic evaluation of viral hepatitis. Hosp. Pract., 22(2):101, 1987.

Hoofnagle, J. H., and Schaffer, D. F.: Serologic markers of hepatitis B virus infection. Semin. Liver Dis., 6:1, 1986.

Howard, C. R.: The biology of hepadnaviruses. J. Gen. Virol., 67:1215, 1986.

Huang, S.-N., and Fisher, M. M.: Pathology of viral hepatitis. Monogr. Pathol., 28:153, 1987.

Jacobson, I. M., and Dienstag, J. L.: Viral hepatitis vaccines. Annu. Rev. Med., 36:241, 1985.

Kelly, D. A., and Tuddenham, E. G. D.: Haemostatic problems in liver disease. Gut, 27:339, 1986.

Koff, R. S.: Fulminant hepatitis due to HBV/HDV coinfection. Hosp. Pract., 22(11):123, 1987.

Larcher, V.: Chronic active hepatitis and related disorders. Clin. Gastroenterol., *15*:173, 1986.

Lefkowitch, J. H.: Liver biopsy interpretation in chronic hepatitis. Prog. Surg. Pathol., *3*:221, 1981.

Lemon, S. M.: Type A viral hepatitis. N. Engl. J. Med., *313*:1059, 1985.

McLean, A. A.: Development of vaccines against hepatitis A and hepatitis B. Rev. Infect. Dis., 8:591, 1986.

Mackinnon, M., Cooksley, W. G. E., and Smallwood, R. A.: Chronic hepatitis: pathogenesis and treatment. Aust. N. Z. J. Med., *16*:101, 1986.

O'Grady, J. G., et al.: Coagulopathy of fulminant hepatic failure. Semin. Liver Dis., *6*:159, 1986.

Phillips, M. J., and Poucell, S.: Modern aspects of the morphology of viral hepatitis. Hum. Pathol., *12*:1060, 1981.

Purcell, R. H., Rizetto, M., and Gerin, J. L.: Hepatitis delta virus infection of the liver. Semin. Liver Dis., *4*:340, 1984.

Rizzetto, M., Verme, G., Gerin, J. L., and Purcell, R. H.: Hepatitis delta virus disease. Prog. Liver Dis., *8*:417, 1986.

Scheuer, P. J.: Viral hepatitis. Rec. Adv. Histopathol., *12*:129, 1984.

Seeff, L. B., and Koff, R. S.: Evolving concepts of the clinical and serologic consequences of hepatitis B virus infection. Semin. Liver Dis., *6*:11, 1986.

Sherlock, S.: Viral hepatitis. Dig. Dis. Sci., *31* (9 Suppl.), 122S, 1986.

Shih, J. W., Mur, J. I. E., and Alter, H. J.: Non-A, non-B hepatitis: advances and unfulfilled expectations of the first decade. Prog. Liver Dis., *8*:433, 1986.

Shorey, J.: The current status of non-A, non-B viral hepatitis. Am. J. Med. Sci., *289*:251, 1985.

Snydman, D. R.: Hepatitis in pregnancy. N. Engl. J. Med., *313*:1398, 1985.

Stevens, C. E., and Taylor, P. E.: Hepatitis B vaccine issues. Semin. Liver Dis., *6*:23, 1986.

Thomas, H. C., Pignatelli. M., and Scully, L. J.: Viruses and immune reactions in the liver. Scand. J. Gastroenterol. [Suppl.], *114*:105, 1985.

Thung, S. N., and Gerber, M. A.: Hepatitis B virus and polyalbumin receptors. Prog. Liver Dis., *8*:335, 1986.

Tiollais, P., Pourcel, C., and Dejean, A.: The hepatitis-B virus. Nature, *317*:489, 1985.

Vogten, A. J.: Hepatitis non-A, non-B. Neth. J. Med., *28*:324, 1985.

White, N. J., and Juel-Jensen, B. E.: Infectious mononucleosis hepatitis. Semin. Liver Dis., *4*:301, 1984.

Alcoholic Liver Disease

Crow, K. E.: Ethanol metabolism by the liver. Rev. Drug Metab. Drug Interact., *5*:113, 1985.

Denk, H., Lackinger, E., and Venningerholz, F.: Pathology of the cytoskeleton of hepatocytes. Prog. Liver Dis., *8*:237, 1986.

Desmet, V. J.: Alcoholic liver disease. Histological features and evolution. Acta Med. Scand. [Suppl], *703*:111, 1985.

French, S. W.: The Mallory body. Hepatology, *1*:76, 1981.

French, S. W., Okanoue, T., Swierenga, S. H. H., and Marceau, N.: The cytoskeleton of hepatocytes in health and disease. Monogr. Pathol., *28*:95, 1987.

Galvaö-Teles, A., Monteiro, E., Gavaler, J. S., and Van Thiel, D. H.: Gonadal consequences of alcohol abuse. Hepatology, *6*:135, 1986.

Hall, P. (Ed.): Alcoholic Liver Disease. London, Edward Arnold, 1985.

Hall, P.de la M.: The pathological spectrum of alcoholic liver disease. Pathology, *17*:209, 1985.

Leevy, C. M., Frank, O., Leevy, C. B., and Baker, H.: Nutritional factors in liver disease in the alcoholic. Acta Med. Scand., [Suppl.] *703*:67, 1985.

Lieber, C. S.: Alcohol and the liver. metabolism of ethanol, metabolic effects and pathogenesis of injury. Acta Med. Scand. [Suppl.], *703*:11, 1985.

Lieber, C. S.: Microsomal ethanol-oxidising system. Enzyme, *37*:45, 1987.

Lieber, C. S., and Leo, M. A.: Interaction of alcohol and nutritional factors with hepatic fibrosis. Prog. Liver Dis., *8*:253, 1986.

MacSween, R. N. M.: Alcoholic liver injury: genetic and immunological factors. Acta Med. Scand., [Suppl.] *703*:57, 1985.

MacSween, R. N. M., and Burt, A. D.: Histologic spectrum of alcoholic liver disease. Semin. Liver Dis., *6*:221, 1986.

Sherlock, S. (Ed.): Alcohol and disease. Br. Med. Bull., *38*:1-, 1982.

Toxic and Drug-Induced Hepatitis

Bernuau, J. Rueff, B., Benhamou, J.-P.: Fulminant and subfulminant liver failure: definitions and causes. Semin. Liver Dis., *6*:97, 1986.

Bianchi, L.: Necroinflammatory liver diseases. Semin. Liver Dis., *6*:185, 1986.

Clissold, S. P.: Paracetamol and phenacetin. Drugs, *32* [Suppl.] *4*:46, 1986.

Davis, M.: Protective agents for acetaminophen overdose. Semin. Liver Dis., *6*:138, 1986.

Døssing, M. J.: Occupational toxic liver damage. J. Hepatol., *3*:131, 1986.

Farber, J. L.: Xenobiotics, drug metabolism, and liver injury. Monogr. Pathol., *28*:43, 1987.

Ishak, K. G., and Zimmerman, H. J.: Hepatic toxicity of drugs used for hematologic neoplasia. Semin. Liver Dis., *7*:237, 1987.

Linden, C. H., and Rumack, B. H.: Acetaminophen overdose. Emerg. Med. Clin. North Am., *2*:103, 1984.

Maddrey, W. C.: Hepatic effects of acetaminophen. Increased toxicity in alcoholics. J. Clin. Gastroenterol., *9*:180, 1987.

Mason, R. P., and Fischer, V.: Free radicals of acetaminophen. Fed. Proc., *45*:2493, 1986.

Popper, H., and Geller, S. A.: Pathogenetic considerations in the histological diagnosis of drug-induced liver injury. Prog. Surg. Pathol., *3*:233, 1981.

Prescott, L. F.: Effects of non-narcotic analgesics on the liver. Drugs, *32* (Suppl. 4):129, 1986.

Schaffner, F., and Thaler, H.: Nonalcoholic fatty liver

disease. Prog. Liver Dis., 8:283, 1986.

Seeff, L. B., et al.: Acetaminophen hepatotoxicity in alcoholics. Ann. Intern. Med., 104:399, 1986.

Sherlock, S.: The spectrum of hepatotoxicity due to drugs. Lancet, 2:440, 1986.

Tucker, R. A.: Drugs and liver disease: a tablular compilation of drugs and the histopathological changes that can occur in the liver. Drug Intell. Clin. Pharmacol., 16:569, 1982.

Zimmerman, H. J. (Ed.): Drug-induced liver disease. Semin. Liver Dis., 1:1, 1982.

Zimmerman, H. J.: Effects of alcohol on other hepatotoxins. Alcoholism, 10:3, 1986.

Zimmerman, H. J.: Hepatotoxic effects of oncotherapeutic agents. Prog. Liver Dis., 8:621, 1986.

Zimmerman, H. J., and Lewis, J. H.: Drug-induced cholestasis. Med. Toxicol., 2:112, 1987.

Other Forms of Chronic Hepatitis

Baum, H., and Palmer, C.: The PBC-specific antigen. Mol. Aspects Med., 8:201, 1985.

Berg, P. A., and Klein, R.: Clinical and prognostic relevance of different mitochondrial antibody profiles in primary biliary cirrhosis. Mol. Aspects Med., 8:235, 1985.

Berg, P. A., Klein, R., and Lindenborn-Fotinos, J.: Antimitochondrial antibodies in primary biliary cirrhosis. J. Hepatol., 2:123, 1986.

Epstein, O.: The pathogenesis of primary biliary cirrhosis. Mol. Aspects Med., 8:293, 1985.

Gerber, M. A.: Immunopathology of chronic hepatitis. Monogr. Pathol., 28:54, 1987.

Jones, E. A. (Ed.): Primary biliary cirrhosis. Semin. Liver Dis., 1:267, 1982.

Larcher, V.: Chronic active hepatitis and related disorders. Clin. Gastroenterol., 15:173, 1986.

Lefkowitch, J. H.: Liver biopsy interpretation in chronic hepatitis. Prog. Surg. Pathol., 3:221, 1981.

McFarlane, I. G.: Autoreactivity against biliary tract antigens in primary biliary cirrhosis. Mol. Aspects Med., 8:249, 1985.

MacSween, R. N. M., and Burt, A. D.: The cellular pathology of primary biliary cirrhosis. Mol. Aspects Med., 8:269, 1985.

MacSween, R. N. M., and Sumithran, E.: Histopathology of primary biliary cirrhosis. Semin. Liver Dis., 1:282, 1981.

Mackinnon, M., Cooksley, W. G. E., and Smallwood, R. A.: Chronic hepatitis: pathogenesis and treatment. Aust. N. Z. J. Med., 16:101, 1986.

Schaffner, F.: Autoimmune chronic active hepatitis. Prog. Liver Dis., 8:485, 1986.

Schrumpf, E., and Gjone, E.: Hepatobiliary disease in ulcerative colitis. Scand. J. Gastroenterol., 17:961, 1982.

Sherlock, S.: Primary biliary cirrhosis. Ann. N. Y. Acad. Sci., 465:378, 1986.

Vento, S., Nouri-Aria, K. T., and Eddleston, A. L. W. F.: Immune mechanisms in autoimmune chronic active hepatitis. Scand. J. Gastroenterol. [Suppl], 114:91, 1985.

Cirrhosis of the Liver

Bassett, M. L., Halliday, J. W., and Powell, L. W.: Genetic hemochromatosis. Semin. Liver Dis., 4:217, 1984.

Crosby, W. H.: Hemochromatosis: current concepts and management. Hosp. Pract., 22(2):173, 1987.

Ring-Larsen, H., and Henriksen, J. H.: Pathogenesis of ascites formation and hepatorenal syndrome. Semin. Liver Dis., 6:341, 1986.

Rocco, V. K., and Ware, A. J.: Cirrhotic ascites. Pathophysiology, diagnosis and management. Ann. Intern. Med., 105:573, 1986.

Ruebner, B. H.: Collagen formation and cirrhosis. Semin. Liver Dis., 6:212, 1986.

Van Thiel, D. H., and Gavalier, J. S.: Hypothalamic-pituitary-gonadal function in liver disease. Prog. Liver Dis., 8:272, 1986.

Walshe, J. M.: Copper: its role in the pathogenesis of liver disease. Semin. Liver Dis., 4:252, 1984.

Portal Hypertension

Benhamou, J.-P., and Lebrec, D. (Eds.): Portal hypertension. Clin. Gastroenterol., 14:1, 1985.

Galambos, J. T.: Portal hypertension. Semin. Liver Dis., 5:277, 1985.

Groszmann, R. J. (Ed.): Portal hypertension. Semin. Liver Dis., 6:277, 1986.

Sherlock, S. (Ed.): Portal hypertension. Semin. Liver Dis., 2:177, 1982.

Metabolic Disorders

Eriksson, S. G.: Liver disease in alpha$_1$-antitrypsin deficiency. Aspects of incidence and prognosis. Scand. J. Gastroenterol., 20:907, 1985.

Freese, D.: Intracellular cholestatic syndromes of infancy. Semin. Liver Dis., 2:255, 1982.

Gollan, J. L., and Knapp, A. B.: Bilirubin metabolism and congenital jaundice. Hosp. Pract., 20(2):83, 1985.

Greene, H. L.: Glycogen storage disease. Semin. Liver Dis., 2:291, 1982.

Hansen, T. W. R., and Bratlid, D.: Bilirubin and brain toxicity. Acta Pediatr. Scand., 75:513, 1986.

Hardwick, D. F., and Dimmick, J. E.: Metabolic cirrhoses of infancy and early childhood. Perspect. Pediatr. Pathol., 3:103, 1976.

Ishak, K. G.: Hepatic morphology in the inherited metabolic diseases. Semin. Liver Dis., 6:246, 1986.

Krejs, G. J.: Jaundice during pregnancy. Semin. Liver Dis., 3:73, 1983.

Mowat, A. P.: Hepatic disorders. Clin. Gastroenterol., 11:171, 1982.

Poulsom, R.: Morphological changes of organs after sucrose or fructose feeding. Prog. Biochem. Pharmacol., 21:104, 1986.

Rolfes, D. B., and Ishak, K. G.: Liver disease in pregnancy. Histopathology, 10:555, 1986.

Sharp, H. L.: Alpha-1-antitrypsin: an ignored protein in

understanding liver disease. Semin. Liver Dis., 2:314, 1982.

Walser, M.: Urea cycle enzymopathies. Semin. Liver Dis., 2:329, 1982.

Wolkoff, A. W. (Ed.): Bilirubin metabolism and hyperbilirubinemia. Semin. Liver Dis., 3:1, 1983.

Vascular Disorders

Ishak, K. G., and Zimmerman, H. J.: Hepatic toxicity of drugs used for hematologic neoplasia. Semin. Liver Dis., 7:237, 1987.

Rollins, B. J.: Hepatic veno-occlusive disease. Am. J. Med., 81:297, 1986.

Disorders of the Intrahepatic Biliary System

Alberti-Flor, J. J., Avant, G. R., and Dunn, G. D.: Primary sclerosing cholangitis. South. Med. J., 78:173, 1985.

Altman, R. P., and Stolar, C. J. H.: Pediatric hepatobiliary disease. Surg. Clin. North Am., 65:1245, 1985.

Balistreri, W. F.: Neonatal jaundice. J. Pediatr., 106:171, 1985.

Balistreri, W. F. (Ed.): Neonatal cholestasis. Semin. Liver Dis., 7:67, 1987.

Chock, E., Wolfe, B., and Matolo, N. M.: Acute suppurative cholangitis. Surg. Clin. North Am., 61:885, 1981.

Denman, S. T.: A review of pruritus. J. Am. Acad. Dermatol., 14:375, 1986.

Desmet, V. J.: Cholestasis. Rec. Adv. Histopathol., 12:146, 1984.

Desmet, V. J.: Current problems in diagnosis of biliary disease and cholestasis. Semin. Liver Dis., 6:233, 1986.

French, S.W.: Role of canalicular contraction in bile flow. Lab. Invest., 53:245, 1985.

Garden, J. M., Ostrow, J. D., and Roenigk, H. H., Jr.: Pruritus in hepatic cholestasis. Arch. Dermatol., 121:1415, 1985.

Griffiths, D. M., and Gough, M. H.: Gas in the hepatic portal veins. Br. J. Surg., 73:172, 1986.

Lefkowitch, J. H., and Martin, E. C.: Primary sclerosing cholangitis. Prog. Liver Dis., 8:557, 1986.

Li, A. K., et al.: Recurrent pyogenic cholangitis. Trop. Gastroenterol., 6:119, 1985.

MacSween, R. N. M.: Primary sclerosing cholangitis. Rec. Adv. Histopathol., 12:158, 1984.

Moinuddin, M.: Pyogenic liver abscess. Compr. Ther., 13:26, 1987.

Moseley, R. H.: Mechanisms of bile formation and cholestasis. Am. J. Gastroenterol., 81:731, 1986.

Mowat. A. P.: Biliary disorders in childhood. Semin. Liver Dis., 2:271, 1982.

Oelberg, D. G., and Lester, R.: Cellular mechanisms in cholestasis. Annu. Rev. Med., 37:297, 1986.

Phillips, M. J., and Poucell, S.: Cholestasis: surgical pathology, mechanisms, and new concepts. Monogr. Pathol., 28:65, 1987.

Phillips, M. J., Poucell, S., and Oda, M.: Mechanisms

of cholestasis. Lab. Invest., 54:593, 1986.

Reichen, J., and Simon, F. R.: Mechanisms of cholestasis. Int. Rev. Exp. Pathol., 26:231, 1984.

Wiesner, R. H., Ludwig, J., LaRusso, N. F., and MacCarthy, R. L.: Diagnosis and treatment of primary sclerosing cholangitis. Semin. Liver Dis., 5:241, 1985.

Williams, L. F., Jr., and Schoetz, D. J.: Primary sclerosing cholangitis. Surg. Clin. North Am., 61:951, 1981.

Other Nonneoplastic Diseases

Crocker, J. F. S.: Reye's syndrome. Semin. Liver Dis., 2:340, 1982.

Farrell, M. K., and Balistreri, W. F.: Parenteral nutrition and hepatobiliary dysfunction. Clin. Perinatol., 13:197, 1986.

Kaplan, M. M.: Acute fatty liver of pregnancy. N. Engl. J. Med., 313:367, 1985.

Krejs, G. J.: Jaundice during pregnancy. Semin. Liver Dis., 3:73, 1983.

Merritt, R. J.: Cholestasis associated with total parenteral nutrition. J. Pediatr. Gastroenterol. Nutr., 5:9, 1986.

Riely, C. A.: Acute fatty liver of pregnancy. Semin. Liver Dis., 7:47, 1987.

Rockoff, M. A., and Pascucci, R. C.: Reye's syndrome. Emerg. Med. Clin. North Am., 1:87, 1983.

Rolfes, D. B., and Ishak, K. G.: Liver disease in pregnancy. Histopathology, 10:555, 1986.

Roy, C. C., and Bell, D. C.: Hepatobiliary complications associated with TPN: an enigma. J. Am. Coll. Nutr., 4:651, 1985.

Schaffner, F., and Thaler, H.: Nonalcoholic fatty liver disease. Prog. Liver Dis., 8:283, 1986.

Wolk, R.: Metabolic complications and deficiencies of parenteral nutrition. Compr. Ther., 11:67, 1985.

Structural Anomalies

Landing, B. H., Wells, T. R., and Claireaux, A. E.: Morphometric analysis of liver lesions in cystic diseases of childhood. Hum. Pathol., 11:549, 1980.

Tumors

Anthony, P. P., and James, K.: Pedunculated carcinoma. Histopathology, 11(4), 1987.

Anthony, P. P., and Telesinghe, P. U.: Inflammatory pseudotumour of the liver. J. Clin. Pathol., 39:761, 1986.

Bassendine, M. F.: Hepatitis B virus and liver cell carcinoma. Rec. Adv. Histopathol., 12:137, 1984.

Bassendine, M. F.: Alcohol—a major risk factor for hepatocellular carcinoma? J. Hepatol., 2:513, 1986.

Berman, M. M., Libbey, N. P., and Foster, J. H.: Hepatocellular carcinoma. Polygonal cell type with fibrous stroma. Cancer, 46:1448, 1980.

Carrasco, D., et al.: Multiple hepatic adenomas after

long-term therapy with testosterone enanthate. J. Hepatol., 1:573, 1985.

Craig, J. R., Peters, R. L., Edmondson, H. A., and Omata, M.: Fibrolamellar carcinoma of the liver. Cancer, 46:372, 1980.

Driver, H. E., and Swann, P. F.: Alcohol and human cancer. Anticancer Res., 7:309, 1987.

Edmondson, H. A.: Tumors of the Liver. Washington DC, Armed Forces Institute of Pathology, 1958.

Greenfield, C., and Fowler, M. J. F.: Hepatitis B virus and primary liver carcinoma. Mol. Biol. Med., 3:301, 1986.

Hanks, J. B., et al.: The pathogenesis, detection, and surgical treatment of hepatic metastases. Curr. Probl. Cancer, 10:217, 1986.

Harrison, T. J., Chen, J.-Y., and Zuckerman, A. J.: Hepatitis B and primary liver cancer. Cancer Treat. Rev., 13:1, 1986.

Hodgson, H. J., and Maton, P. N.: Carcinoid and neuroendocrine tumours of the liver. Baillière's Clin. Gastroenterol., 1:35, 1987.

Huggins, G. R.: Oral contraceptives and neoplasia. Fertil. Steril., 47:733, 1987.

Ishak, K. G., et al. Epithelioid hemangiosarcoma of the liver. Hum. Pathol., 15:839, 1984.

Jaffe, E. S.: Malignant lymphomas: pathology of hepatic involvement. Semin. Liver Dis., 7:257, 1987.

Johnson, P. J., et al.: Cirrhosis and the aetiology of hepatocellular carcinoma. J. Hepatol., 4:140, 1987.

Kondo, Y.: Histologic features of hepatocellular carcinoma and allied disorders. Pathol. Annu., 20(2):405, 1985.

Lack, E. E., Neave, C., Vawter, G. F.: Hepatoblastoma. Am. J. Surg. Pathol., 6:693, 1982.

Lieberman, H. M., and Shafritz, D.: Persistent hepatitis B infection and hepatocellular carcinoma. Prog. Liver Dis., 8:395, 1986.

Liguory, C., and Canard, J. M.: Tumours of the biliary system. Clin. Gastroenterol., 12:269, 1983.

McGlashan, N. D.: Primary liver cancer and food-based toxins. Ecol. Dis., 1:37, 1984.

Malt, R. A.: Surgery for hepatic neoplasms. N. Engl. J. Med., 313:1591, 1985.

Misslbeck, N. G., and Campbell, T. C.: The role of ethanol in the etiology of primary liver cancer. Adv. Nutr. Res., 7:129, 1985.

Nakashima, T., and Kojiro, M.: Pathologic characteristics of hepatocellular carcinoma. Semin. Liver Dis., 6:259, 1986.

Nakashima, T., et al.: Pathology of hepatocellular carcinoma in Japan. Cancer, 51:863, 1983.

Nguyen, G. K.: Fine-needle aspiration biopsy cytology of hepatic tumors in adults. Pathol. Annu., 21(2):321, 1986.

Okuda, K.: Primary liver cancer. Dig. Dis. Sci., 31(9 Suppl.):133S, 1986.

Okuda, K., and McKay, I. (Eds.): Hepatocellular Carcinoma. Geneva, UICC, Technical Report Series, Vol. 74, No 16, 1982.

Pollice, L.: Primary pediatric tumors of the liver. Prog. Surg. Pathol., 3:195, 1981.

Popper, H.: The relation between hepatitis B virus infection and hepatocellular carcinoma. Hepatogastroenterology, 33:2, 1986.

Popper, H., Maltoni, C., and Selikoff, I. J.: Vinyl chloride-induced hepatic lesions in man and rodents. Liver, 1:7, 1981.

Scarpelli, D. G.: Human liver carcinogenesis. Monogr. Pathol., 26:168, 1986.

Schwartz, L. R., and Grim, H.: Environmental chemicals in hepatocarcinogenesis: the mechanism of tumor promoters. Prog. Liver Dis., 8:581, 1986.

van Steenbergen, W., et al.: Carcinoma at the hilus of the liver. Neth. J. Med., 25:344, 1982.

Stocker, J. T., and Ishak, K. G.: Focal nodular hyperplasia of the liver. Cancer, 48:336, 1981.

Stocker, J. T., and Ishak, K. G.: Mesenchymal hamartoma of the liver. Paediatr. Pathol., 1:245, 1983.

Stromeyer, F. W., and Ishak, K. G.: Nodular transformation (nodular 'regenerative' hyperplasia) of the liver. Hum. Pathol., 12:60, 1981.

Weinberg, A. G., and Finegold, M. J.: Primary hepatic tumors of childhood. Hum. Pathol., 14:512, 1983.

Weinbren, K., and Mutum, S. S.: Pathological aspects of cholangiocarcinoma. J. Pathol., 139:217, 1983.

Weinbren, K., and Mutum, S. S.: Pathological aspects of diffuse nodular hyperplasia of the liver. J. Pathol., 143:81, 1984.

Wilson, C. B., and Epenetos, A. A.: Use of monoclonal antibodies for diagnosis and treatment of liver tumors. Baillière's Clin. Gastroenterol., 1:15, 1987.

Zuckerman, A. J.: Prevention of hepatocellular carcinoma by immunization against hepatitis B. Int. Rev. Exp. Pathol., 27:59, 1985.

Hepatic Failure

Bihari, D. J., Gimson, A. E. S., and Williams, W.: Cardiovascular, pulmonary and renal complications of fulminant hepatic failure. Semin. Liver Dis., 6:119, 1986.

Bode, J. C., et al.: Pathophysiology of chronic hepatic encephalopathy. Hepatogastroenterology, 32:259, 1985.

Cuthbert, J. A.: Hepatic transplantation. Am. J. Med. Sci., 291:286, 1986.

Davidson, E. W.: Pathogenesis of the hepatorenal syndrome. Annu. Rev. Med., 38:169, 1987.

Ede, R. J., and Williams, R.: Hepatic encephalopathy and cerebral edema. Semin. Liver Dis., 6:107, 1986.

Fraser, C. L., and Arieff, A. I.: Hepatic encephalopathy. N. Engl. J. Med., 313:865, 1985.

Jones, E. A., and Schafer, D. F.: Hepatic encephalopathy: a neurochemical disorder. Prog. Liver Dis., 8:525, 1986.

MacMath, T. L., and Pons, P. T.: Hepatic encephalopathy. J. Emerg. Med., 3:401, 1985.

Rossi-Fanelli, F., et al.: Amino acids and hepatic encephalopathy. Prog. Neurobiol., 28:277, 1987.

Starzl, T. E. (Ed.): Hepatic transplantation. Semin. Liver Dis., 5:309, 1985.

Zieve, L.: The mechanism of hepatic coma. Hepatology, 1:360, 1981.

Zipser, R. D.: Role of renal prostaglandins and the effects of nonsteroidal anti-inflammatory drugs in patients with liver disease. Am. J. Med., 81(2B):95, 1986.

37

Extrahepatic Biliary System

CHOLELITHIASIS and cholecystitis are common, as are minor anomalies of the extrahepatic bile ducts and the vessels that accompany them. Inflammatory disease of the extrahepatic bile ducts, major congenital anomalies, and neoplasms are uncommon.

CHOLELITHIASIS

In the United States, over 15,000,000 people have gallstones, and 300,000 cholecystectomies are performed annually. Nearly 70% of the patients are women. At autopsy, 10% of men between 50 and 59 years old have gallstones, and 25% of women. In Europe and Australasia their prevalence is similar.

In the United States, 75% of North American Indian women over 25 years old have gallstones and 90% of those over 60 years old. Gallstones are twice as frequent in white Americans as in black Americans. They are uncommon in much of the Far East and in black people in Africa.

The prevalence of gallstones is increased in diabetics, in the obese, and in multipara. About 30% of patients with cirrhosis of the liver have gallstones. Crohn's disease, resection of the terminal ileum, ileostomy, parenteral nutrition, cholestyramine therapy, and chlofibrate therapy increase the risk of developing gallstones. Pigment stones are common in people with hemolytic disorders.

Most gallstones originate in the gallbladder. Often a stone escapes into the cystic duct or the common bile duct. A few develop in the extrahepatic or larger intrahepatic bile ducts. There are four types of gallstone, but in any one patient the stones are nearly always all of the same type.

Types. About 80% of gallstones are of the mixed type, and consist of a mixture of cholesterol, bile pigments, and calcium carbonate. About 10% are pure cholesterol stones. About 10% consist predominantly of bile pigments. Rarely, a gallstone consists only of calcium carbonate.

Less than 30% of gallstones contain enough calcium bilirubinate or calcium carbonate to make them radiopaque, and of these 70% are pigment stones. Ultrasonography can detect gallstones as small as 0.3 cm in diameter. Rarely, a gallstone contains enough gas in its fissures to make it visible radiologically.

Mixed Stones.   Most patients with mixed gallstones have several stones in the gallbladder, and sometimes stones in the bile ducts as well. Most commonly, the gallbladder contains 5 to 20 stones. Occasionally there is only one. In one patient, the gallbladder contained 36,329 stones.

Most mixed stones are between 0.5 and 2 cm across. They are hard, with a polished yellowish-brown surface, and are usually faceted, so that the stones fit together. On section, a mixed stone shows concentric rings, some yellowish, some dark brown, some grayish, indicating how different combinations of cholesterol, bilirubin, and calcium carbonate have been laid down at different times.

Occasionally, the core of a mixed stone is pure cholesterol, suggesting that a pure cholesterol stone formed first and that the other layers were subsequently added to it. Such stones are sometimes called combined gallstones because they have a pure core combined with a mixed shell.

Cholesterol Stones.   Cholesterol stones are usually single. The stone is often large, filling the gallbladder. It is smooth, whitish-yellow, and ovoid. On section, radiating, glistening cholesterol crystals can be seen.

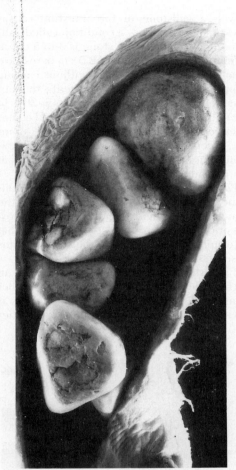

Fig. 37-1. Faceted mixed stones in a gallbladder with its wall thickened by chronic cholecystitis.

The stone is surprisingly light in weight.

Pigment Stones. Pure pigment stones are usually multiple and may be numerous. They are often small, little more than gravel, but can be over 1 cm in greatest dimension. Pigment stones are shiny and intensely black. They are soft and easily crushed. The larger stones are often irregularly shaped, mulberry shaped, or resemble jackstones.

Calcium Carbonate Stones. Calcium carbonate stones are usually multiple, grayish white, faceted, and hard, about 1 cm across. Less often, the stone is soft and mushy, more of a paste than a true stone.

Complications. Of themselves, gallstones cause no symptoms. Over 50% of people with gallstones live out their lives

without any symptoms attributable to the stones. Only if complications develop do symptoms begin.

Cholecystitis. The relationship between gallstones and cholecystitis is complex. Few patients with gallstones do not have some degree of cholecystitis, and 95% of patients with cholecystitis have gallstones. Gallstones tend to cause cholecystitis, and cholecystitis tends to cause gallstones. To debate about which comes first is like the famous question of the chicken and the egg.

In most patients with gallstones and cholecystitis who develop symptoms, the symptoms are probably due to cholecystitis rather than to the cholelithiasis. They are discussed later in the chapter when cholecystitis is considered.

Choledocholithiasis. In 10 to 20% of patients with cholelithiasis, gallstones are found in the common bile duct. In most of these patients, the stones form in the gallbladder and escape down the cystic duct to

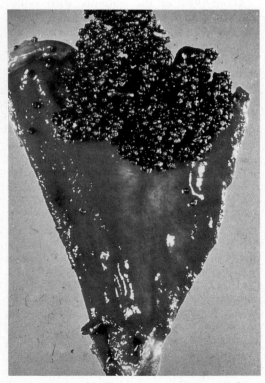

Fig. 37-2. Pigment stones in an otherwise normal gallbladder.

reach the common duct. Less often, the stones form in the common duct or in the hepatic ducts in the liver.

In many people, gallstones in the common bile duct cause no symptoms. We do not know how often small gallstones escape down the bile ducts into the bowel without causing symptoms.

When symptoms develop, there is pain in 75% of people with choledocholithiasis. The pain may be continuous, but is usually a servere, intermittent colic, in the right upper quadrant of the abdomen or in the epigastrium, often radiating to the back. The pain is due principally to the violent muscular contractions in the bile ducts as the duct tries to push the stone along, and its radiation reflects the innervation of the duct.

Jaundice is common in patients with a stone in the common duct and may occur without pain. The jaundice is obstructive and usually not severe. It often varies in severity as the stone moves and the degree of obstruction varies.

About 30% of the patients with symptomatic choledocholithiasis have a fever, suggesting that bacterial cholangitis has developed within the liver.

Biliary Fistula. A fistula between the extrahepatic biliary tract and the bowel or from one part of the biliary system to another develops in less than 1% of patients with gallstones. In 90% of the patients, it is caused by ulceration of a gallstone through the wall of the gallbladder or common duct into an adherent portion of bowel or some other part of the biliary tract. In 5% of the patients, the fistula is caused by a peptic ulcer. In 5%, it results from Crohn's disease or some other disease of the bowel.

In more than 50% of the patients, the fistula is between the gallbladder and the duodenum. Less often the fistula is between the gallbladder and the colon, the gallbladder and the stomach, or involves the gallbladder, duodenum, and colon. In 10% of the patients, the fistula is between the common bile duct and the duodenum and in 1% between the gallbladder and the common bile duct. Rarely, a fistula from the gallbladder opens on the skin.

Gallstone Ileus. In 20% of patients with a fistula between the biliary tract and the bowel, a gallstone in the intestine causes intestinal obstruction, a condition called gallstone ileus. Usually the stone is 3 to 5 cm in diameter. Stones less than 2.5 cm across are usually passed in the feces without causing symptoms. In 70% of the patients the obstruction is in the terminal ileum, in 20% in the jejunum, and in 5% in the sigmoid colon. Occasionally the obstruction is in the stomach, duodenum, or appendix. In some patients, the fistula has closed by the time that the ileus develops.

Pathogenesis. The pathogenesis of gallstones is complex. In most gallstones the principal constituent is cholesterol, and most attention has been given to the factors that determine whether or not cholesterol remains in solution in the bile.

Cholesterol is insoluble in water, but in normal bile it is held in solution by the micelles formed by bile salts and lecithin. If there is too much cholesterol relative to the quantities

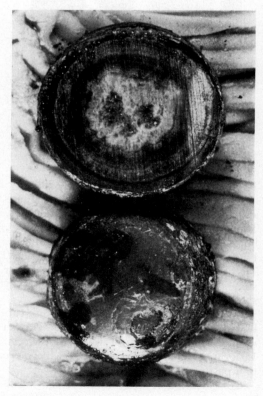

Fig. 37-3. A cross section of a mixed gallstone that lodged in the ileum causing gallstone ileus.

of bile salts and lecithin available, the cholesterol is likely to precipitate. Cholesterol crystals form in the bile. The aggregation of these crystals begins the formation of most mixed and cholesterol gallstones.

In most patients with gallstones, the secretion of bile acids into the bile is inappropriately low, and the secretion of cholesterol is increased. Usually the fault is in the regulation of the synthesis and secretion of bile acids and cholesterol in the liver. Less often the fault is in the bowel. Ileostomy, for example, causes a considerable and continuing loss of bile acids. The bile acid pool is reduced, and the secretion of bile salts into the bile falls. The chance of developing gallstones becomes high.

If the bile reaching the gallbladder is saturated or supersaturated with cholesterol, the risk of developing mixed gallstones or a cholesterol stone is high. Probably the concentration of bile in the gallbladder does little to increase the risk, for it does not alter the balance between the cholesterol and the micelles that solubilize it. Precipitation of cholesterol to begin formation of a stone is probably triggered by droplets of mucus, fragments of desquamated epithelium, or other small bodies in the bile that serve as a nidus around which cholesterol can precipitate.

Pigment gallstones begin in similar fashion. If the concentration of unconjugated bilirubin in the bile is high, calcium and other salts of bilirubin precipitate around a nidus of mucus or some other small body.

The factors that determine the growth of gallstones and determine whether the precipitation of different elements forms a mixed stone or the continued precipitation of a single element forms a pure stone are ill understood. Presumably the nature of the bile determines the type of material that is added to the core of the stone.

Treatment and Prognosis. Gallstones that cause no symptoms need no treatment. If symptoms occur, cholecystectomy is the usual recourse. The gallstones are removed, and though the bile is as lithogenic as ever, they do not often recur in the common duct.

Chenodeoxycholic acid and ursodeoxycholic acid reduce the hepatic secretion of cholesterol and dissolve some uncalcified gallstones. The gallstones disappeared completely in 15% of patients given chenodeoxycholic acid for two years and were reduced in size in 30%. Stones recurred within two years in 30% of those in whom they disappeared in spite of continued administration of chenodeoxycholic acid. Ursodeoxycholic acid dissolves uncalcified stones completely and more quickly than does chenodeoxycholic acid in 30% of the patients treated. In 10% of the patients, the gallstones become calcified.

In the dose needed to dissolve stones, chenodeoxycholic acid often causes diarrhea. In 30% of the patients treated, it causes transient increase in the activity of aminotransferases in the plasma. Electron microscopy often shows intrahepatic cholestasis, probably caused by lithocolic acid, a metabolite of chenodeoxycholic acid. Complications are less prominent with ursodeoxycholic acid.

Gallstones have been dissolved within hours by methyl tertiary butyl ether and other solvents introduced into the gallbladder through a percutaneous catheter.

CHOLECYSTITIS

Acute cholecystitis and chronic cholecystitis caused principally by obstruction to the cystic duct are common. Less often, cholecystitis is caused by primary infection. Also discussed in this section are cholesterolosis of the gallbladder, emphysema of the gallbladder, mucocele of the gallbladder, limey bile, and porcelain gallbladder.

ACUTE CHOLECYSTITIS. Acute cholecystitis is in many ways similar to acute appendicitis. In most of the patients, the inflammation is initiated by obstruction, and infection comes later.

Lesions. Macroscopically, the gallbladder in acute cholecystitis is tense and distended. The organ is congested, red, and often hemorrhagic. Its serosa is often dulled by a fibrinous exudate. When the gallbladder is opened, its mucosa is fiery red. The lumen often contains thin pus mixed with bile. Microscopically, the wall of the gallbladder shows congestion, edema, and an exudate predominantly of neutrophils.

Clinical Presentation. A patient with acute cholecystitis usually develops severe pain in the upper abdomen. Often the pain is slowly episodic, rising to a plateau, persisting 30 to 60 minutes, and then subsiding for a time. The pain sometimes radiates to the right shoulder. Peritoneal irritation may cause guarding and hyperesthesia in the right upper quadrant of the abdomen. The gallbladder is usually tender and may be palpable. Often there is a fever of about 38° C, with a leukocytosis of $12 \times 10^9/L$ (12,000/mm^3) or so. Occasionally, the patient is slightly jaundiced. There may be a history of previous attacks of biliary colic.

Complications. Occasionally, the fundus of the gallbladder becomes gangrenous and may perforate. Usually the perforation is contained by adhesions, but the perforation may open into the general peritoneal cavity or, rarely, into an adherent loop of gut. Bile peritonitis can follow.

Empyema of the gallbladder is uncommon. It occurs when superinfection with a pyogenic organism complicates acute cholecystitis in a patient in whom the cystic duct is obstructed. The gallbladder becomes distended with pus. The patient suffers severe pain in the right upper quadrant, with fever, leukocytosis, and other signs of severe acute inflammation. Bacteremia with Escherichia coli or klebsiella is common.

Pathogenesis. In 95% of the patients, acute cholecystitis is caused by obstruction to the cystic duct by a gallstone. Nearly always the gallstone is wedged into Hartmann's pouch and obstructs the mouth of the cystic duct.

Because of the obstruction, the gallbladder becomes distended. Acute inflammation follows. At this stage, there is usually no infection, and the inflammation is caused chemically. Probably the leakage of the highly irritant bile salts into the wall of the gallbladder does much to establish the inflammation. Within a few days, secondary bacterial infection nearly always occurs. Gram-negative enteric bacilli are the most common invaders, but anaerobic organisms are also common.

Patients with acute cholecystitis in whom no gallstone is found in the pouch of Hartmann or the cystic duct, are said to have acalculous cholecystitis. In a few of these people, the cystic duct is obstructed in some other way, by torsion of the gallbladder, an aberrant cystic artery, or a neoplasm. In a few, the gallstone causing the obstruction may have been dislodged during surgery. In most, no obstruction of the common duct is found. The cause of the cholecystitis in these patients is obscure. The risk of developing acalculous cholecystitis is increased in patients who have suffered severe trauma, extensive burns, or some other condition that causes prolonged immobilization in diabetes mellitus and post partem.

Treatment and Prognosis. Acute cholecystitis is usually treated by cholecystectomy if the diagnosis is made within 72 hours of the onset of symptoms. The mortality is less than 2%, and the risk of perforation, recurrent attacks of cholecystitis, and other complications of cholecystitis and cholelithiasis is avoided.

Medical treatment with rest and antibiotics brings resolution of acute cholecystitis in 75% of the patients. Perforation, a biliary fistula, or some other complication develops in the remainder. Over 25% of the patients in whom medical treatment brings resolution of the inflammation suffer a second attack of acute cholecystitis within a year, and 60% have another attack within six years.

If the gallbladder perforates, surgical drainage is urgent. The mortality exceeds 30% if generalized peritonitis develops.

CHRONIC CHOLECYSTITIS. Chronic cholecystitis and cholelithiasis are almost synonymous. Almost all patients with chronic cholecystitis have cholelithiasis, and almost all patients with cholelithiasis have chronic cholecystitis.

Lesions. In chronic cholecystitis, the wall of the gallbladder is gray, scarred, and often thickened. The gallbladder may be of normal size or may be small and shrunken. Mixed gallstones are almost always present in the gallbladder and often fill it. Sometimes the thick, scarred wall of the shrunken gallbladder squeezes tightly over the stones within it. Occasionally, innumerable tiny stones are sludged in the bile, a condition called biliary mud.

Microscopically, fibrosis is the predominant feature in chronic cholecystitis. Its extent varies. If chronic cholecystitis is severe, the wall of the gallbladder is thickened two or three times by well-formed collagenous

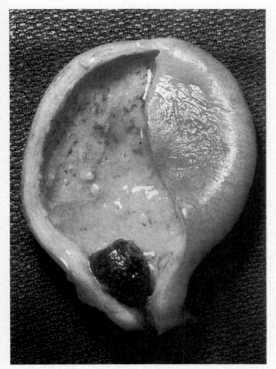

Fig. 37.4. Chronic cholecystitis, showing the thickening of the wall of the gallbladder and a mixed gallstone in Hartmann's pouch.

When symptoms do occur, they are usually vague and ill-defined. The fair, fat, fertile female of forty or fifty with vague postprandial discomfort or intolerance to fatty foods is the model of chronic cholecystitis: fair because cholelithiasis is more common in white than in black people; fat because gallstones are more common in the obese; fertile because gallstones are more common in mulitpara; and female because gallstones are three times as frequent in women as in men. Occasionally there is aching in the region of the gallbladder or tenderness in the right upper quadrant of the abdomen. Sometimes the pain radiates to the right shoulder. Often there is nausea or flatulence. Occasionally acute cholecystitis or biliary colic due to the passage of a stone into the bile ducts complicates chronic cholecystitis. Usually the gallbladder fails to concentrate the media used for cholecystography sufficiently to allow radiologic visualization of the gallbladder.

Pathogenesis. Chronic cholecystitis probably results from numerous attacks of minor tissue. If it is slight, fibrosis is slightly and usually confined to the submucosal region. An exudate of lymphocytes, plasma cells, and macrophages is usually present in the wall of the gallbladder, but it is not always marked. Often small foci of acute inflammation are present. Occasionally a foreign body granuloma containing cholesterol crystals is found, or a small gallstone is imbedded in the wall of the gallbladder.

The mucosa of the gallbladder is usually intact in chronic cholecystitis. Occasionally it is ulcerated with acute inflammation or granulation tissue in the bed of the ulcer. Particularly at the fundus of the gallbladder, the mucosa often dips deep into the wall of the gallbladder, often penetrating its muscular wall, to form Rokitansky-Aschoff sinuses, named after the Austrian pathologist von Rokitansky (1804–1878) and the German pathologist Aschoff (1866–1942).

Clinical Presentation. Most patients with chronic cholecystitis have no symptoms.

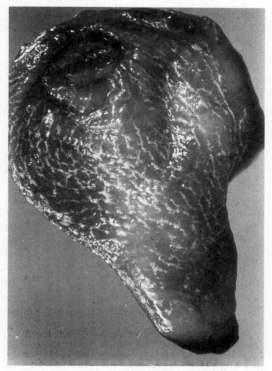

Fig. 37.5. Cholesterolosis of the gallbladder.

inflammation induced by the gallstones in the gallbladder. In some patients, attacks of acute cholecystitis add to the injury.

Treatment and Prognosis. Chronic cholecystitis is usually treated by cholecystectomy, if the symptoms warrant treatment. The mortality is less than 0.1% in people under 50 years old, less than 0.5% in older people. Symptoms clearly caused by cholecystitis or cholelithiasis are cured. If the only symptom is a vague dyspepsia, it recurs after the operation in 50% of the patients.

PRIMARY BACTERIAL CHOLECYSTITIS. Primary bacterial cholecystitis in which the inflammation is initiated by bacterial infection is uncommon. When typhoid fever was more frequent, carriers often had persisting infection in the gallbladder. The infection usually caused little or no inflammation. Similar persistent infection can occur in cholera. Occasionally Giardia lamblia infects the gallbladder. Rarely, candida or some other fungus is found in the gallbladder. Rarely, Ascaris lumbricoides, a trematode, or some other metazoan reaches the gallbladder.

CHOLESTEROLOSIS. Cholesterolosis of the gallbladder is present in between 10 and 30% of gallbladders. When the gallbladder is opened, little yellow flecks are scattered over the scarlet or bile-stained mucosa, like the seeds of a strawberry. The condition has long been called a strawberry gallbladder. Usually, the yellow flecks are less than 1 mm across, but occasionally become larger, forming little polypoid excrescences. In 50% of people with cholesterolosis, there are stones in the gallbladder. In most, the wall of the gallbladder is thin, and the organ functions normally.

Microscopically, the yellow flecks are accumulations of fat-filled macrophages that lie immediately under the epithelium and distend the tips of some of the mucosal folds. Much of the fat in the distended macrophages is cholesterol ester. The source of the cholesterol is uncertain. Some think that the cholesterol is resorbed from the bile. Others think that the cholesterolosis results from the failure to excrete cholesterol formed in the mucosa into the bile.

Cholesterolosis of the gallbladder causes no symptoms and usually is of no clinical significance. Occasionally one of the ex-

crescences it forms is large enough to be mistaken for a tumor of the gallbladder.

EMPHYSEMATOUS CHOLECYSTITIS. Emphysema of the gallbladder is an uncommon type of acute cholecystitis in which the wall of the gallbladder contains gas. In 50% of the patients, the infection is with Clostridium perfringens. In others, gram-negative organisms are found. The patients are usually men and often have diabetes mellitus.

MUCOCELE. Mucocele of the gallbladder, sometimes called hydrops of the gallbladder, is uncommon. It results from obstruction to the cystic duct, nearly always by a gallstone. Instead of the more common acute cholecystitis, the gallbladder becomes distended by its own watery, mucoid secretion. The gallbladder becomes tense, swollen, and white, but its wall shows little or no inflammation. Symptoms like those of chronic cholecystitis may result. Excision cures.

LIMY BILE. Limy bile, also called milk of calcium bile, is an unusual condition in which a high concentration of calcium carbonate and other calcium salts in the bile gives it a creamy appearance. Often the concentration is sufficient to make the gallbladder and bile ducts visible roentgenographically. Limy bile causes no symptoms and no dysfunction, but the patients often have some other form of gallbladder disease.

PORCELAIN GALLBLADDER. Rarely, the gallbladder becomes calcified in a patient with chronic cholecystitis. The organ becomes white and hard, like an egg, and cracks like an eggshell. Up to 20% of the patients have carcinoma of the gallbladder.

DISEASE OF THE EXTRAHEPATIC BILE DUCTS

Choledocholithiasis is the most common nonneoplastic disease of the extrahepatic bile ducts and is discussed earlier in this chapter. Less common are a benign stricture and sclerosing cholangitis.

BENIGN STRICTURE. Benign stricture of the common bile duct or less often of one of the other extrahepatic bile ducts is nearly always due to surgical injury. Rarely, it results from some other kind of trauma. If the duct is damaged at operation or by a T-tube that remains in the duct for a long time, the duct becomes scarred and thickened at the point of injury. As the collagen matures and shortens, the lumen of the duct becomes narrowed, sometimes almost occluded. Usually there is a scattering of lymphocytes, plasma cells, and macrophages in the fibrosis. The submucous glands of the duct persist, distorted and separated by the fibrosis. Proximal to the obstruction, the uninvolved duct is dilated. Often the dilatation extends into the liver.

Obstructive jaundice sometimes develops within a few days of the injury, sometimes not for several months. Often the jaundice is at first variable in intensity, though later it usually becomes constant. Occasionally stones form in the dilated duct proximal to the obstruction. Fever suggests bacterial cholangitis proximal to the obstruction.

Unless the obstruction is relieved, cirrhosis and death are inevitable within 5 to 10 years. The surgical reconstruction needed is often difficult.

When the extrahepatic ducts are involved, they become progressively thickened, fibrotic, and stenotic. At first the wall of the ducts involved is edematous with a sparse exudate of lymphocytes, plasma cells, and macrophages. Increasing quantities of collagen are deposited, forming a cuff that surrounds the duct and narrows it. The glands in the duct wall are trapped in the fibrosis and distorted. Macroscopically and microscopically it is often difficult to distinguish a localized focus of sclerosing cholangitis in an extrahepatic bile duct from carcinoma of the bile duct.

SCLEROSING CHOLANGITIS. Sclerosing cholangitis is an uncommon disorder that usually involves both the extrahepatic and intrahepatic bile ducts. It is discussed in Chapter 36.

When the extrahepatic ducts are involved, they become progressively thickened, fibrotic, and stenotic. At first the wall of the ducts involved is edematous with a sparse exudate of lymphocytes, plasma cells, and macrophages. Increasing quantities of collagen are deposited, forming a cuff that surrounds the duct and narrows it. The glands in the duct wall are trapped in the fibrosis and distorted. Macroscopically and microscopically it is often difficult to distinguish a localized focus of sclerosing cholangitis in an extrahepatic bile duct from carcinoma of the bile duct.

BILIARY ATRESIA. Biliary atresia is found in 1 live birth in 10,000. The extrahepatic bile ducts fail to develop normally. Cholestatic jaundice is present at birth or develops within a few weeks.

Often the whole extrahepatic biliary system is atretic. Less often, the gallbladder persists, with or without a cystic duct. The atretic bile ducts may be reduced to fibrous cords without a lumen. They may contain numerous lumina less than 50 μm in diameter. They may retain a central lumen, often with smaller lumina around the main duct.

The liver enlarges and becomes dark green. Over 15% of the children have giant cell hepatitis. Secondary biliary cirrhosis develops within one to six months. In many of the children, the intrahepatic bile ducts in the fibrosis gradually disappear, even if surgical correction of the anomaly has established good bile drainage.

In some infants with biliary atresia, the defect may be genetically determined, but in most it is probably secondary to infection, most often a viral infection.

If the anomaly cannot be corrected, most of the children die of cirrhosis within two years. Anastomosis of the bile ducts at the hilus of the liver to the bowel has allowed 40% of the children to live for at least five years. Those who do not survive usually die of ascending cholangitis or portal hypertension. Hepatic transplantation may offer a better prognosis.

CONGENITAL ANOMALIES

Congenital anomalies of the gallbladder and extrahepatic bile ducts are common, but except for biliary atresia and occasionally a choledochal cyst rarely cause symptoms or dysfunction. Anomalies in the course of the hepatic artery and its branches are also common and may be important if a surgeon is operating in the region.

GALLBLADDER. In 4% of the population, the fundus of the gallbladder is abnormally mobile, often angulated to give an abnormality called a phrygian cap. Rarely there are 2 or 3 gallbladders, sometimes each with its own cystic duct, sometimes sharing a cystic duct. Rarely the gallbladder is on the left side, transverse, enclosed within the liver, retroperitoneal, above the diaphragm, or in some other abnormal position. Occasionally a septum divides the gallbladder, it is mobile with its own mesentery, or it is hypoplastic or absent.

BILE DUCTS. The cystic duct sometimes is abnormally long or so short that it opens directly into the common duct. The cystic duct may enter the common bile duct abnormally close to the liver or may run beside the common duct to enter it close to the duodenum. Sometimes the cystic duct runs within the wall of the common duct for much or all of its course. It occasionally spirals around the common duct anteriorly or posteriorly to enter the common duct from the left side or enters the right hepatic duct. Sometimes the cystic duct is partially or completely duplicated.

The common bile duct sometimes enters the duodenum unusually high or unusually low, after joining the pancreatic duct, or independently. Rarely, the common duct is completely or partially duplicated.

Accessory hepatic ducts are common, especially on the right. The accessory duct may be tiny or as large as a normal hepatic duct. It often empties into the cystic duct or into the gallbladder. Less often it enters the common bile duct above or below the entry of the cystic duct. Occasionally there are two accessory hepatic ducts, one on each side.

CHOLEDOCHAL CYST. A choledochal cyst is a focal dilatation of the common bile duct. The cyst may occur at any point in the length of the common duct. Sometimes there is more than one. Usually, the cyst is 2 or 3 cm in diameter, but sometimes is enormous. The wall of the cyst is of dense fibrous tissue. It is lined by biliary epithelium, though the epithelium may be lost from part or much of its wall. A choledochal cyst often causes no symptoms, but can cause partial obstruction of the bile duct, become infected, or harbor gallstones.

Carcinoma develops in 15% of the cysts, sometimes in childhood.

HEPATIC AND CYSTIC ARTERIES. The course or origin of the hepatic and cystic arteries is abnormal in 45% of people. The abnormalities rarely cause dysfunction or symptoms, but are important to a surgeon operating in this region.

Origin from the superior mesenteric artery is one of the more common anomalies of the hepatic artery. The two hepatic arteries sometimes arise independently, the right from the superior mesenteric artery and the left from the celiac axis, or the right from the celiac axis and the left from the left gastric artery. When the hepatic arteries arise separately and when a common hepatic artery bifurcates soon after its origin, the gastroduodenal artery arises from the right hepatic artery. Accessary hepatic arteries can arise from the superior mesenteric artery, the left gastric artery, or the right hepatic artery. The right hepatic artery sometimes passes in front of the common bile duct instead of behind it. Sometimes the right hepatic artery adheres to the cystic duct or the neck of the gallbladder.

Instead of passing posterior to the common bile duct, the cystic artery sometimes crosses the common duct anteriorly from left to right. The anteriorly placed artery can arise from the proximal part of the right hepatic artery, the left hepatic artery, the common hepatic artery, an anomalous right hepatic artery, the gastroduodenal artery, or directly from the celiac axis or the superior mesenteric artery.

Sometimes there are two cystic arteries. Both may arise from the right hepatic artery, or one or both can take origin from the gastroduodenal artery, superior mesenteric artery, or elsewhere. One of the arteries may pass in front of the common bile duct, while the other runs behind it.

TUMORS

Benign and malignant tumors of the extrahepatic biliary system are uncommon. The tumor-like lesion called an adenomyoma is the commonest benign lesion. Carcinoma of the gallbladder and carcinoma of the common bile duct are the most common malignant lesions.

Benign

Adenomatous polyps can develop in the gallbladder, but are uncommon. A granular cell myoblastoma sometimes develops in or near the extrahepatic biliary system. Other benign mesenchymal tumors are rare.

ADENOMATOUS POLYP. An adenomatous polyp of the gallbladder is usually pedunculated but can be sessile. Microscopically, it often resembles a villous adenoma of the bowel, but sometimes is similar to a tubular adenoma or tubulovillous adenoma. The risk of malignancy is low. Occasional numerous polyps are present in the gallbladder and in other parts of the extrahepatic and intrahepatic biliary tree.

ADENOMYOMA. An adenomyoma is a malformation of the fundus of the gallbladder. The lesion forms a well-defined nodule, usually about 1 cm in diameter. The nodule consists of exaggerated Rokitansky-Aschoff crypts lined by biliary epithelium extending

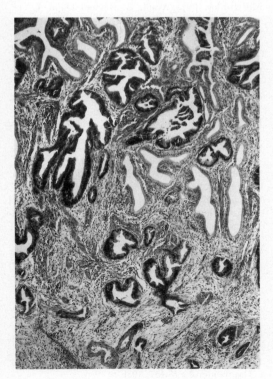

Fig. 37.6. Carcinoma of the gallbladder, showing darkly staining malignant glands infiltrating between the pale normal glands.

into the wall of the gallgladder. The crypts are surrounded by hyperplastic bundles of smooth muscle. An adenomyoma of the gallbladder causes no symptoms and requires no treatment. The lesion is usually discovered when a gallbladder is removed for some other reason.

Malignant

Occasionally an embryonic rhabdomyosarcoma arises in an extrahepatic bile duct in a child. Rarely a sarcoma, carcinosarcoma, carcinoid tumor, or malignant melanoma arises in the extrahepatic biliary system. A secondary tumor is found in the gallbladder in 0.3% of autopsies, but the gallbladder is involved in 5% of patients dying of carcinoma. Only carcinoma of the gallbladder and carcinoma of the bile ducts will be discussed here.

CARCINOMA OF THE GALLBLADDER. Carcinoma of the gallbladder is found in 0.4% of autopsies. The annual incidence is 2.5 per 100,000. Most patients are over 50 years old, and 70% are women. Some 90% have gallstones.

Lesions. The carcinoma sometimes forms a polypoid mass that bulges into the lumen of the gallbladder, sometimes infiltrates the wall of the gallbladder diffusely. Microscopically, 80% of the tumors are adenocarcinomata. Most are moderately differentiated, with glands lined by atypical biliary epithelium in a collagenous stroma. Some are papillary. Some are colloid carcinomata and form mucus lakes. About 10% of the carcinomata are poorly differentiated or anaplastic. About 5% are squamous cell carcinomata. Some show both squamous and adenocarcinomatous differentiation.

Behavior. Carcinoma of the gallbladder causes symptoms only late in the disease. By the time the patient develops pain, has jaundice, or notices a mass, the tumor has usually invaded the liver and often other adjacent organs and has metastasized to the regional lymph nodes, more distant parts of the liver, the lungs, and elsewhere. Implants of carcinoma on the peritoneum are not uncommon.

Etiology. Little is known of the etiology of carcinoma of the gallbladder. Its frequent association with gallstones is striking, and some investigators have been able to induce carcinoma of the gallbladder in animals by implanting artificial stones. Others suggest that degradation of the bile salts may result in the formation of carcinogens.

Treatment and Prognosis. Carcinoma of the gallbladder is treated surgically, but it is rarely possible to extirpate the tumor. Most of the patients die within a year. Only 5% survive five years.

Carcinoma of the Extrahepatic Bile Ducts. Carcinoma of the extrahepatic bile ducts is found in 0.05% of autopsies. It is more common in men. The carcinoma is most frequent in the common duct or at the point at which the hepatic ducts join to form the common duct.

Lesions. A carcinoma of the extrahepatic bile ducts is usually small, extending along the duct for 1 to 2 cm. In the involved segment, the wall of the duct is thickened and fibrotic. Microscopically, the tumor is a well-differentiated adenocarcinoma, with mucus-secreting glands set in an abundant fibrous stroma. Often the carcinoma is so well differentiated that it is difficult to decide at quick section in the course of an operation whether the lesion is a benign stricture or a carcinoma. Sometimes only the presence of perineural invasion shows that the highly differentiated carcinoma is indeed malignant.

Behavior. A carcinoma of the extrahepatic bile ducts causes obstructive jaundice. Metastases are found in the regional lymph nodes in nearly 50% of the patients, but more distant metastases are unusual.

Treatment and Prognosis. Carcinoma of the extrahepatic bile ducts is treated surgically. Death usually comes from local complications rather than from metastases. The mean survival is a little over one year.

BIBLIOGRAPHY

General

MacSween, R. N. M., Anthony, P. P., and Scheuer, P. J. (Eds.): Pathology of the Liver, 2nd ed. Edinburgh, Churchill Livingstone, 1987.

Ruebner, B. H., and Montgomery, C. K.: Pathology of the Liver and Biliary Tract. New York, John Wiley & Sons, 1982.

Schiff, L. (Ed.): Diseases of the Liver, 5th Ed. Philadelphia, J. B. Lipincott, 1982.

Sherlock, S.: Diseases of the Liver and Biliary System, 7th Ed. Oxford, Blackwell Scientific Publications, 1985.

Cholelithiasis

Abate, M. A.: Medical management of cholesterol gallstones. Drug Intell. Clin. Pharm., 20:106, 1986.

Chalmers, T. C. (Ed.): Gallstones. Semin. Liver Dis., 3:87, 1983.

Cholecystitis

Matolo, N. M., LaMorte, W. W., and Wolfe, B. M.: Acute and chronic cholecystitis. Surg. Clin. North Am., 61:875, 1981.

Diseases of the Extrahepatic Ducts

Alberti-Flor, J. J., Avant, G. R., and Dunn, G. D.: Primary sclerosing cholangitis. South. Med. J., 78:173, 1985.

Altman, R. P., and Stolar, C. J. H.: Pediatric hepatobiliary disease. Surg. Clin. North Am., 65:1245, 1985.

Balistreri, W. F.: Neonatal jaundice. J. Pediatr., 106:171, 1985.

Balistreri, W. F. (Ed.): Neonatal cholestasis. Semin. Liver Dis., 7:67, 1987.

Lefkowitch, J. H., and Martin, E. C.: Primary sclerosing cholangitis. Prog. Liver Dis., 8:557, 1986.

MacSween, R. N. M.: Primary sclerosing cholangitis. Rec. Adv. Histopathol., 12:158, 1984.

Mowat, A. P.: Biliary disorders in childhood. Semin. Liver Dis., 2:271, 1982.

Wiesner, R. H., Ludwig, J., LaRusso, N. F., and MacCarthy, R. L.: Diagnosis and treatment of primary sclerosing cholangitis. Semin. Liver Dis., 5:241, 1985.

Williams, L. F., Jr., and Schoetz, D. J.: Primary sclerosing cholangitis. Surg. Clin. North Am., 61:951, 1981.

Congential Anomalies

Gautier, M., and Eliot, N.: Extrahepatic biliary atresia. Arch. Pathol. Lab. Med., 105:397, 1981.

Kamath, K. R.: Abnormalities of the biliary tree. Clin. Gastroenterol., 15:157, 1986.

Puente, S. G., and Bannura, G. C. Radiological anatomy of the biliary tract: variations and congenital anomalies. World J. Surg., 7:721, 1983.

Tumors

Alboref-Saavedra, J., and Henson, D. E.: Tumors of the Gallbladder and Extrahepatic Bile Ducts. Washington, D. C., Armed Forces Institute of Pathology, 1986.

Dunbar, L. L., et al.: Carcinoma of the gallbladder and bile ducts. Am. Surg., 49:94, 1983.

Liguory, C., and Canard, J. M.: Tumours of the biliary system. Clin. Gastroenterol., 12:269, 1983.

van Steenbergen, W., et al.: Carcinoma at the hilus of the liver. Neth. J. Med., 25:344, 1982.

38

Pancreas

THE principal diseases of the pancreas are pancreatitis, diabetes mellitus, cystic fibrosis, and tumors. Other disorders of the pancreas are infrequent or of little importance.

PANCREATITIS

Four kinds of pancreatitis are distinguished. Acute and chronic pancreatitis are of complex pathogenesis. A pseudocyst of the pancreas is a complication of pancreatitis. Occasionally pancreatic inflammation is caused by infection.

ACUTE PANCREATITIS. Acute pancreatitis varies from a minor attack that brings little disability to a major illness that often brings death. Each year, from 5 to 10 people per 100,000 develop acute pancreatitis. About 1% of emergency admissions to the hospital are necessitated by acute pancreatitis. The disease is detected in 1% of autopsies. Men and women are equally affected. Acute pancreatitis can develop at any age, but most patients are between 30 and 70 years old.

Lesions. In mild cases of acute pancreatitis, and early in the disease, the pancreas is edematous. The fibrous planes between the glandular elements are widened. No necrosis and no inflammatory exudate is present. The edema may involve much or all of the gland or be confined to part of it.

If the disease is more severe, foci of necrosis appear in the edematous pancreas after a few days. Often much or all of the pancrease is involved, with small foci of necrosis scattered through its substance. Macroscopically, the foci of necrosis appear as grayish-white flecks. Microscopically, they show coagulation necrosis and dissolution of

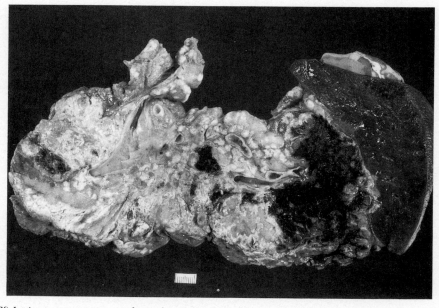

Fig. 38-1. Acute pancreatitis involving the whole gland, with extensive necrosis, fat necrosis, and foci of hemorrhage, especially in the tail adjacent to the spleen.

the parenchyma, sometimes surrounded by a sharply delimited, neutrophilic exudate, sometimes with little inflammatory reaction.

If acute pancreatitis is still more severe, the necrosis becomes extensive, destroying the greater part of the pancreas and extending a little into the neighboring retroperitoneal tissues. Many veins are thrombosed. Often arteries and veins are eroded, with massive but irregular hemorrhage into the necrotic gland. The pancreas is reduced to a hemorrhagic mush, with dark red hemorrhagic blotches alternating with the gray necrosis. Miscroscopically, there is extensive necrosis and hemorrhage, with an intense neutrophilic exudate in the surviving tissue around the necrosis. This severe form of the disease is called acute hemorrhagic pancreatitis.

In the more severe forms of acute pancreatitis, massive edema in the loose retroperitoneal tissues is usual. Often there is ascites, with turbid, sometimes hemorrhagic fluid, perhaps containing globules of fat. Adjacent loops of bowel may be involved, with ileus and dilatation in the duodenum, an adjacent loop of jejunum, or sometimes in the transverse colon. Sometimes the swollen pancreas is big enough to displace the stomach or widen the duodenal loop.

Fat Necrosis. Foci of fat necrosis are common in the peripancreatic fat, mesentery, and omentum in all but the mildest forms of acute pancreatitis and occasionally occur more distantly in the mediastinum, subcutaneous tissue, or bone marrow.

Macroscopically, the foci of fat necrosis are hard, white nodules, usually 0.3 to 1.0 cm across. Often they are calcified. Microscopically, the outline of some of the disrupted fat cells can usually be recognized in the foci of fat necrosis, but most of the nodule is comprised of granular, amorphous material, consisting mainly of fatty acids released from the triglycerides from the necrotic fat cells. At first an intense neutrophilic exudate surrounds the foci of fat necrosis, but as weeks pass the exudate fades. The nodules become increasingly calcified as the fatty acids form calcium soaps. At last, the nodule is hard, calcified, and flaky-white, with little or no reaction round about. It persists as long as the patient lives.

Dysfunction. In acute pancreatitis, amylase from the damaged pancreas leaks into the blood. The activity of the enzyme in the plasma begins to increase within 12 hours of the onset of symptoms, usually reaches a peak after 48 hours or so, and falls to normal within three to four days. The peak activity of amylase in the plasma usually exceeds 800 U/L (400 Somogyi units/100 mL), and often exceeds 2000 U/L. As increased quan-

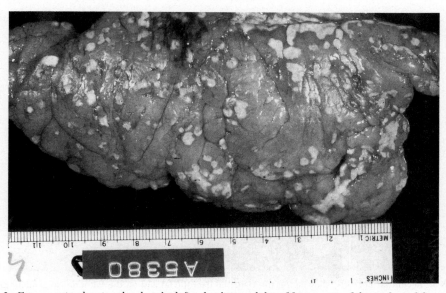

Fig. 38-2. Fat necrosis, showing the sharply defined, white nodules of fat necrosis of the surface of the pancreas.

tities of amylase leak into the blood, the urinary excretion of the enzyme increases. In acute pancreatitis, the urinary excretion of amylase is usually over 1500 U/d (800 Somogyi units/d), and often is much greater. It remains elevated for a week or more after the onset of symptoms. The concentration of amylase in the ascitic fluid of patients with acute pancreatitis is often over 5000 U/L. The magnitude of the increase in activity in the plasma and the urinary excretion of amylase bear little relation to the severity of the underlying pancreatic disease.

Acute pancreatitis is not the only disease that causes hyperamylasemia or hyperamylasuria. Other diseases of the pancreas or salivary glands can do so, as can infarction or perforation of the gut, though the magnitude of the increase is not usually as great as in acute pancreatitis.

Lipase, trypsin, and other enzymes also seep into the blood from the injured pancreas. The activity of lipase in the blood and urine is increased. The increase in the activity of lipase in the plasma tends to occur more slowly than the increase in amylase, with a peak 96 hours after the onset of symptoms.

Complications. Shock is common in patients with severe acute pancreatitis. It is due in part to hypovolemia caused by the loss of fluid into the retroperitoneal space, in part by the release of kinins that cause peripheral vasodilatation and increased vascular permeability, in part by the vascular injury caused by the proteolytic and lipolytic enzymes in the blood, and in part by heart failure caused by the kinins and toxemia. Occasionally disseminated intravascular coagulation complicates acute pancreatitis.

Spread of the inflammation may cause a pleural effusion, usually on the left side, or pneumonia. Mild to moderate respiratory insufficiency with arterial hypoxia and respiratory alkalosis develops in 10% of the patients and at times overshadows the abdominal symptoms.

Hypocalcemia occurs in up to 30% of patients with acute pancreatitis. The concentration of calcium in the plasma falls to about 1.8 mmol/L (0.7 mg/100 mL) and reaches its nadir about one week after the onset of symptoms. The fatty acids released by the hydrolysis of the triglycerides in the patches of fat necrosis fix calcium, but not in sufficient quantity to explain the hypocalcemia. The transient hyperglycemia and glycosuria found in 50% of the patients result from damage to the islets. Jaundice occurs in 15% of the patients, because the swollen pancreas obstructs the common bile duct. Hyperlipemia with chylomicronemia or increase in very low density lipoproteins

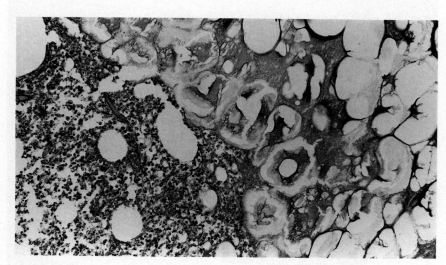

Fig. 38-3. Recent fat necrosis, showing on the right the necrotic fat and on the left a dense exudate mainly of necrotic neutrophils, mixed with remnants of necrotic tissue.

occurs in under 10% of the patients. The risk of thrombophlebitis is increased. Sometimes there is renal failure.

Clinical Presentation. Pain is present in all patients who have signs or symptoms of acute pancreatitis. It may be mild, but when the disease is severe, epigastric pain is excruciating. In 50% of the patients, it radiates to the back, flanks, or substernal region.

The inflamed and swollen pancreas is tender. Peritoneal irritation causes muscular rigidity in the abdomen in 50% of the patients. Leukocytosis of 10 to 20 × 10^9/L (10,000 to 20,000/mm^3) or more is usual. Low fever, nausea and vomiting are common.

Pathogenesis. The edema and necrosis of acute pancreatitis result from the escape of pancreatic enzymes into the tissues. The enzymes damage the blood vessels, causing edema and hemorrhage. They destroy cells, to give foci of necrosis. They are carried in lymphatics or sometimes in the blood to give the foci of fat necrosis.

Normally, the pancreas contains only the inactive precursors of the pancreatic enzymes. The enzymes are activated only when they reach the gut. Inhibitors prevent the premature activation of the enzymes while still in the pancreas. Acute pancreatitis develops when an injury to the pancreas allows the precursors to escape into the tissues and overcomes the inhibitors that normally prevent their activation.

The proteolytic enzymes are particularly important. If a small quantity of trypsin or one of the other proteolytic enzymes is activated, it can activate other enzymes, increasing greatly the likelihood of pancreatitis. Trypsin, chymotrypsin, and elastase are important in causing the initial injury to the cells and blood vessels. The proteolytic enzymes activate kinins, causing increased vascular damage and permeability, the Hageman factor, and the clotting system. The greater the damage to the pancreas, the greater the release and activation of enzymes.

Other enzymes are also important. Phospholipase A attacks cell membranes and forms the toxic lysolecithin from the lecithin in the bile. Lipase splits the triglycerides released from damaged fat cells.

How the many factors that predispose to acute pancreatitis cause the initial injury to the pancreatic acinar cells is not clear. Probably different mechanisms are involved in different patients. Increased pressure in the pancreatic ducts caused by obstruction or hypersecretion may initiate the process. The trauma to the pancreas caused by abdominal operations often causes minor, focal pancreatitis that resolves rapidly, but in most patients with acute pancreatitis there is no history of trauma or infection. Cathepsin B and other lysosomal enzymes can activate trypsinogen suggesting that an intracellular derangement might initiate acute pancreatitis.

The theory that acute pancreatitis is commonly initiated by the reflux of bile into the pancreatic duct and the activation of the pancreatic enzymes by the bile is now discounted. In 80% of people the pancreatic and bile ducts join before entering the duodenum, but the pressure in the pancreatic duct is higher than in the bile duct, and the entry of bile into the pancreatic duct is unlikely.

Predisposing Factors. About 40% of patients with acute pancreatitis have gallstones and 30% are alcoholics. In 20%, no predisposing factor is found. In 10% some other factor is thought to cause the pancreatitis.

Probably gallstones initiate pancreatitis by obstructing the pancreatic duct. In 80% of people, the common bile duct and the pancreatic duct share a common opening into the duodenum, and mechanical obstruction by a gallstone is possible. In the other 20%, perhaps the edema caused by the passage of a stone through the ampulla of Vater is enough to obstruct the pancreatic duct as it enters the duodenum immediately beside the common bile duct.

In alcoholics, several factors probably combine to cause pancreatitis. Alcohol is a potent stimulant to pancreatic secretion and causes constriction of the sphincter of Oddi. Because of the hypersecretion and the obstruction, the pressure in the pancreatic ducts rises, favoring the leakage of enzymes into the tissues. Ethanol may damage pancreatic cells directly. The violent vomiting that accompanies alcoholism can force duodenal content into the pancreatic ducts, where it could activate enzymes and rupture ductules.

Among the uncommon precursors of acute pancreatitis are hyperlipoproteinemia of type

I or type V, diabetic ketosis, acute intermittent porphyria, kwashiorkor, uremia, and hepatic failure. Hypercalcemia may cause pancreatitis, perhaps because the increased concentration of calcium favors the activation of trypsinogen, perhaps because the hypercalcemia tends to cause stones that obstruct the pancreatic ducts. Up to 15% of patients with primary hyperparathyroidism develop pancreatitis.

Infection, especially viral infection, occasionally initiates acute pancreatitis. Rarely, polyarteritis nodosa or some other vascular disease does so. Allergic pancreatitis could do so. A large meal sometimes precipitates acute pancreatitis, probably by causing oversecretion in the pancreas, much as in alcoholism.

Drugs such as azothioprine, sulfonamides, thiazides, furosemide, estrogens, tetracylines, or valproic acid can initiate acute pancreatitis. A scorpion bite may do so.

Trauma, from without or from surgery, can cause leakage from the pancreatic ducts or obstruction to the ducts, and sometimes acute pancreatitis results. Renal transplantation causes acute pancreatitis in 3% of the patients. Obstruction of the pancreatic ducts by carcinoma or a peptic ulcer, occasionally causes acute pancreatitis.

In some patients acute pancreatitis is genetically determined, transmitted as an autosomal dominant with variable penetrance. The pancreatic ducts in patients with genetically determined pancreatitis are often calcified and obstructed, the patients or their relatives often have aminoaciduria. Occasionally carcinoma of the pancreas or thrombosis of the portal or splenic vein develops in these people.

Treatment and Prognosis. Treatment is largely symptomatic, to overcome the pain, to counteract the shock, and to prevent secondary bacterial infection. Food and other agents that stimulate pancreatic secretion should be avoided during the acute stage of the disease. Drugs that reduce pancreatic secretion, such as propantheline, may be useful. If hemorrhagic necrosis is extensive, removal of the necrotic tissue by peritoneal lavage or laparotomy is sometimes beneficial.

In mild cases in which there is edema of the pancreas but not much necrosis, the prognosis is excellent. Recovery usually comes in a week or two and is complete. The edema resolves, and there is no significant residual

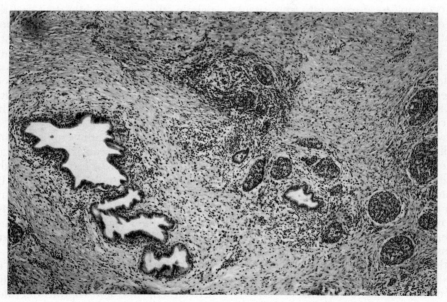

Fig. 38-4. Chronic pancreatitis, showing complete loss of the exocrine parenchyma and its replacement by collagenous tissue containing an exudate mainly of lymphocytes. Only the ducts and the islets survive.

fibrosis. If there is more necrosis, healing can still follow, but the gland will be scarred. If the necrosis becomes widespread and hemorrhagic, the mortality reaches 50%. If the patient does recover, much of the pancreas is scarred and useless. Some exocrine function may be preserved, and usually endocrine function is maintained. Occasionally diabetes mellitus results.

CHRONIC PANCREATITIS. In the United Kingdom, each year 3 people in 100,000 develop chronic pancreatitis. It is found in 0.3% of autopsies. Over 75% of the patients are men. In North America. Europe, and Australasia, most patients are over 40 years old. In Africa and Asia, many are less than 20 years old.

Lesions. The head of the pancreas is often involved more severely than is the body, though as chronic pancreatitis grows severe the whole gland is involved. The part of the pancreas affected is hard, gray, and smooth, usually a little bigger than normal. Usually the fibrosis extends to involve the peripancreatic structures. The main pancreatic duct is often dilated and tortuous. Less often the lateral ducts are ectatic. Calculi consisting mainly of calcium carbonate are common in the dilated ducts. Sometimes dilated ducts from cysts, often true cysts with a lining of ductular epithelium, but sometimes larger false cysts in which the epithelial lining is lost. Calcification is evident in over 40% of the lesions in Europe and more often in Africa and Asia. Foci of fat necrosis are sometimes present in the adjacent fat, but fat necrosis is rarely prominent.

Microscopically, the lesions are lobular in most patients, involving some lobules and sparing others. The exocrine acini atrophy and are replaced by collagenous tissue that extends into the lobules from thickened interlobular septa. A sparse exudate of lymphocytes and plasma cells is present in the fibrosis. The ducts are often filled with proteinaceous casts, which are surrounded by atrophied epithelium. The islets of Langerhans persist with little change for months or years but eventually they too are lost. The fibrosis grows more extensive and destroys the lobular pattern of the gland.

Dysfunction. As chronic pancreatitis grows severe, the patients suffer increasingly severe exocrine and endocrine pancreatic deficiency. The lack of exocrine secretion brings steatorrhea, with foul, bulky stools, and perhaps diarrhoea. With the steatorrhea comes excessive loss of nitrogen in the stool. Usually, a patient with severe chronic pancreatitis loses more than 7 g of fat and more than 2.5 g of nitrogen daily in the feces. A secretin test shows that both the volume and the concentration of bicarbonate in the pancreatic juice are subnormal.

As the islets are destroyed, diabetes mellitus develops. Usually endocrine dysfunction comes later than exocrine dysfunction. Many of the islets are towards the tail of the pancreas and escape if the chronic pancreatitis is predominantly in the head. In the scarred regions, the islets persist long after fibrosis has destroyed the exocrine acini.

Clinical Presentation. About 75% of patients with chronic pancreatitis have recurrent bouts of severe pain, like that of acute pancreatitis. In 10%, the pain is continuous. Some present with steatorrhea, without pain. The patients with repeated attacks of pain are said to have chronic relapsing pancreatitis.

Weight loss is common in the early stages of chronic pancreatitis. Steatorrhea is evident in 35% of the patients. Obstruction of the bile duct causes jaundice in 25%. Over 50% eventually develop diabetes mellitus. Ascites or bleeding from a peptic ulcer can occur. In chronic relapsing pancreatitis, the activity of amylase and lipase in the plasma increases during the attacks, but less so than in acute pancreatitis.

Pathogenesis. In Europe and North America, alcohol is the cause of chronic pancreatitis in over 50% of the patients. About 10% have gallstones. A few have hemochromatosis, stenosis of the sphincter of Oddi, hyperparathyroidism, hyperlipoproteinemia, or carcinoma of the pancreas that obstructs the pancreatic ducts or have had acute pancreatitis. Rarely, chronic relapsing pancreatitis is hereditary. In 30% of the patients, the cause of the pancreatitis is unknown. In Africa and Asia the disease is due principally to malnutrition. In some patients, the diease is caused by eating unripe cassava. The plant contains cyanide, and if the diet is deficient in sulfur-containing amino acids it can damage the pancreas.

Alcohol is thought to cause chronic pancreatitis by inducing the formation of the proteinaceous plugs that obstruct the ducts. In carcinoma, stenosis of the sphincter of Oddi and in patients with gallstones, obstruction is important in the causation of the disease. In most other forms of chronic pancreatitis, the cause of the atrophy and fibrosis is unknown.

Treatment and Prognosis. Replacement therapy does much to control the exocrine and endocrine deficiency common in advanced chronic pancreatitis. If a localized stricture is present in the pancreatic duct, surgical repair sometimes relieves the pain. In some patients, the pain can be controlled only by resecting 50 to 95% of the pancreas.

PSEUDOCYST. A pseudocyst of the pancreas may complicate acute or chronic pancreatitis, trauma to the pancreas, or an operation on the pancreas. If activated pancreatic enzymes leak massively into the tissues, digestion of the tissues forms a cyst. The cyst is filled with murky fluid resulting from the digestion of the tissues and is bounded only by the surrounding connective tissue. The cyst has no epithelial lining. Usually, the fistula from the pancreatic ducts into the cyst persists, and amylase and other pancreatic enzymes are present in high concentration in the fluid within the cyst. When a pseudocyst develops, an elevated level of amylase in the serum persists, instead of falling to normal within a few days, as is usual in acute pancreatitis.

A pseudocyst of the pancreas is sometimes less than 5 cm in diameter, but may be 20 cm or more across, easily felt as a mass in the abdomen. It can develop anywhere in relation to the pancreas. Occasionally, a pseudocyst develops in the mediastinum or some other distant site. If a pseudocyst is large, it often includes the lesser sac of the peritoneal cavity. The lesser sac can be greatly distended, displacing the stomach.

A small pseudocyst may resolve and disappear. Larger cysts persist and must be drained. The presence of high concentrations of pancreatic enzymes within the cyst makes the operation difficult. Usually, the cyst is drained by marsupializing it to the surface of the skin or by establishing good drainage into the stomach or a loop of small bowel.

INFECTIVE PANCREATITIS. Infection of the pancreas is rarely severe enough to cause symptoms. Occasionally a secondary bacterial infection complicates a pseudocyst or acute

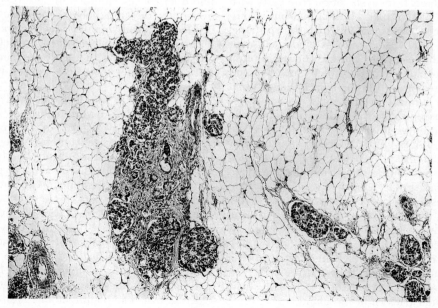

Fig. 38-5. Mucoviscidosis, showing complete loss of the exocrine pancreas and its replacement by fibrofatty tissue, leaving only islets and ducts.

pancreatitis. Rarely, syphilis or tuberculosis involves the pancreas. Mumps sometimes causes pancreatic edema and interstitial inflammation. The importance of viruses in the causation of diabetes mellitus is discussed later in the chapter. Occasionally a hydatid cyst or some other parasitic infestation involves the pancreas.

CYSTIC FIBROSIS

Cystic fibrosis affects cells throughout the body, but involves most severely the exocrine glands. Its name describes the changes it produces in the pancreas. Often cystic fibrosis is called mucoviscidosis, because the mucous glands throughout the body secrete an abnormally thick, viscid, and tenacious mucus.

Cystic fibrosis is inherited as an autosomal recessive character with good penetrance but variable expressivity. The abnormal gene is common in white people, rare in black people, and very rare in orientals. At least 2% of white people are heterozygotes carrying the abnormal gene, though only the homozygotes develop the disease. One white child in every 2000 or 3000 is born with cystic fibrosis.

Lesions. Though the underlying error of metabolism is probably the same in all organs in mucoviscidosis, the lesions are different in different organs.

Pancreas. At birth, the pancreas looks normal macroscopically in most children with cystic fibrosis. As the child ages, the fibrous septa dividing the gland become prominent and progressively thicker. As the years pass, fibrosis of the pancreas becomes ever more extensive, until after several years the pancreas becomes small, shrunken, and scarred. Usually small cysts are easily found in the scarred gland. In the late stages of the disease, the fibrosis may extend beyond the pancreas, into the surrounding tissues. Often nodules of fat necrosis are present in the fat around the pancreas.

Microscopically, the pancreas shows ectasia of its ducts, first the small ducts and then the larger ones. Often a dilated duct is filled with a laminated concretion of inspissated secretion. These concretions sometimes obstruct the duct, causing dilatation of the ducts distal to the obstruction. A concretion may erode a duct, causing periductular fibrosis and perhaps obliteration of the duct.

Probably because of the obstruction, the acini of the exocrine pancreas atrophy. The shrunken acini with flattened epithelium become increasingly separated as collagen is laid down between them. Eventually the acini disappear in much of the pancreas, leaving only islets and ducts separated by collagenous scarring or by fibrofatty tissue.

For many years, the islets remain intact. Eventually, they too are destroyed. All that remains of the pancreas is a few dilated ducts, surrounded by scarring, or fibrofatty tissue.

Intestine. About 10% of children born with cystic fibrosis have meconium ileus. In 50% of the infants with meconium ileus, intrauterine obstruction causes fibrous narrowing or atresia in the small bowel. In some, rupture of the bowel causes meconium peritonitis. The thick, viscid secretions of the intestinal glands result in thick, tenacious meconium, which the infant cannot propel along the intestine. Older children may suffer intermittent intestinal obstruction called the meconium ileus equivalent, because they cannot propel the thick, viscid feces along the intestine. Sometimes a mass of calcified feces obstructs the ileocecal valve. Rectal prolapse is common in children with cystic fibrosis, probably because of the straining necessary to pass the sticky stools.

Microscopically, the mucus-secreting glands throughout the intestine are dilated, often filled with thick, inspissated secretion. Often the epithelium of the glands is atrophic.

Gastric and duodenal peptic ulcers are common in children with cystic fibrosis and in their relatives, perhaps because of the lack of the alkaline pancreatic secretions that usually help neutralize gastric acidity.

Lungs. The lungs are severely injured in most patients with cystic fibrosis who survive for more than a year. The small bronchi and the bronchioles are plugged by the sticky, viscid mucus secreted by the bronchial glands and the goblet cells. An abnormal macroglobulin circulating in the blood impairs ciliary action, making it still more difficult to clear the tenacious mucus from the airways. Because of the obstruction caused by the mucus plugs, parts of the lungs are overinflated, while others collapse.

Bacteria take advantage of the obstruction, and repeated attacks of pulmonary infection follow. In 90% of the patients, the organism is a mucoid strain of Pseudomonas aeruginosa, an organism rarely found in the lungs in any other disease. Less often the bacterium is a staphylococcus, hemophilus, Pseudomonas cepacia or some other bacterium. Many of the infections fail to heal. Once a patient with cystic fibrosis is infected with a mucoid strain of Ps. aeruginosa the bacterium is rarely eradicated from the lungs.

Chronic obstructive pneumonia develops. The upper lobes are often more severely affected than the lower lobes. The lungs become increasingly fibrotic. Small bronchi and bronchioles become dilated. Saccular bronchiectasis may develop in larger airways. Abscesses sometimes develop in the lungs.

Eventually damage to the pulmonary arteries in the lungs brings pulmonary hypertension, cor pulmonale, and heart failure. Clubbing of the fingers is usual.

Nose and Mouth. Sinusitis and nasal polyps are common. The minor salivary glands are distended by sticky mucus in 80% of the patients. The teeth are often discolored by the tetracycline given to combat the infections.

Hepatobiliary System. The biliary secretions are thick and viscid. They commonly obstruct bile ducts within the liver. In 20% of the infants, focal cholangitis develops at the sites of obstruction, with cholestasis proximal to the obstruction. After some years, irregular fibrosis develops in 5% of the infants. At first, the fibrosis is subcapsular and causes no dysfunction. As it extends into the parenchyma, parts of the liver remain fairly normal, while other parts become increasingly scarred. Eventually, irregular, macronodular cirrhosis involves much or all of the liver. The liver becomes increasingly shrunken and scarred. Portal hypertension and the other complications of cirrhosis follow. Jaundice is unusual.

Microscopically, bile ducts proliferate in the scars in the liver. Many of the ducts contain concretions of inspissated secretion. A moderate exudate of lymphocytes and plasma cells persists in the fibrosis.

The gallbladder is involved in 30% of the children. The epithelial cells are distended with mucus. Often the gallbladder atrophies and is filled with colorless secretions.

Skin. The concentrations of sodium, chloride, and potassium in the sweat are abnormally high in children with cystic fibrosis. Normally, the concentrations of sodium and chloride in the sweat are less than 20 mmol/L; in cystic fibrosis they usually exceed 70 mmol/L. The skin appendages show no structural abnormality. If fibrocytes from the skin of a patient with cystic fibrosis or from the skin of a heterozygote carrying the abnormal gene are grown in tissue culture, they accumulate an abnormal mucopolysaccharide in their cytoplasm.

Clinical Presentation. The symptoms and signs of cystic fibrosis depend on the organ or organs involved and the age of the patient when first the disease becomes evident. If the disease is suspected, the demonstration of a high concentration of sodium and chloride in the sweat establishes the diagnosis.

In 10% of infants with cystic fibrosis, meconium ileus, meconium peritonitis, or some other complication of meconium ileus draws attention to the disease. In infancy, maldigestion, distention of the bowels because of meconium ileus equivalent, and rectal prolapse are common. Over 85% of the patients develop almost total pancreatic insufficiency, but diabetes mellitus develops in only 1%. Growth is often impaired.

Pulmonary symptoms usually begin in childhood with cough and often bronchospasm and grow increasingly severe. Respiratory failure and later signs of pulmonary hypertension are common. Signs of biliary cirrhosis develop in 5% of the patients. If the patient survives to adult life, men are usually sterile and women are less fertile than normal. The increased loss of sodium chloride in the sweat increases the risk of developing heat stroke.

Pathogenesis. DNA probes suggest that the gene or genes causing cystic fibrosis are on the long arm of chromosome 7. The nature of the dysfunction causing the secretion of the sticky mucus characteristic of mucoviscidosis remains obscure, though presumably a fault in ion transport across the plasma membrane of the exocrine epithelial cells is involved. The lesions in the many organs involved result from the obstruction caused by the abnormal secretions.

Treatment and Prognosis. Cystic fibrosis is managed by controlling infection, particularly in the lungs, and by replacing the pancreatic enzyme deficiency. The underlying disorder in exocrine secretion cannot be remedied.

Most of the patients die of pulmonary failure in adolescence or as young adults. The average life span is over 20 years, but less than 20% of the patients live past the age of 25 years. About 5% die in infancy from meconium ileus or its complications. A few of the children die of cirrhosis or some other complication of the disease.

DIABETES MELLITUS

The term *diabetes mellitus* is used to describe a group of diseases that have in common hyperglycemia caused by some fault in the production or utilization of insulin. The name *diabetes* comes from the Greek for a siphon and refers to the polyuria common in both diabetes mellitus and in diabetes insipidus. Mellitus is from the Latin, and means sweetened with honey, referring to the sweet taste of glycosuric urine.

It is estimated that in the United States some 2% of the population have diabetes mellitus or will develop it. The prevalence is probably similar in other countries, though juvenile diabetes mellitus is unusual in Africa and in the East, especially in Japan. Throughout the world 30,000,000 people have diabetes mellitus.

As age increases, diabetes mellitus grows more common. Only 0.2% of children have diabetes mellitus, but 40 to 50% of people over 80 years old have the disease. In young people the disease tends to be severe. In the old, it is mild and usually asymptomatic.

The World Health Organization and the American Diabetes Association have suggested criteria for the diagnosis of diabetes mellitus. An adult is considered diabetic if the fasting blood sugar measured in venous plasma exceeds 8 mmol/L (140 mg/100 mL) on more than one occasion. An adult is also considered diabetic, even if the fasting blood sugar is less than 8 mmol/L (140 mg/100 mL),

if on two occasions the concentration of glucose in venous plasma exceeds 11 mmol/L (200 mg/100 mL) 30, 60, or 90 minutes after ingesting 75 g of glucose and remains above this level 2 hours after the ingestion.

In a normal person, the fasting blood sugar measured in venous plasma is below 6 mmol/L (115 mg/100 mL), never exceeds 11 mmol/L (200 mg/100 mL) at any time after the ingestion of 75 g of glucose, and falls to below 8 mmol/L (140 mg/100 mL) within 2 hours of taking the glucose.

In children, a diagnosis of diabetes mellitus is made if the child has symptoms of the disease together with a fasting blood sugar measured in venous plasma in excess of 11 mmol/L (200 mg/100 mL). Normally, a child's blood sugar is less than 7 mmol/L (130 mg/100 mL). The diagnosis is also made if the fasting blood sugar is over 8 mmol/L (140 mg/100 mL) and in addition the child's blood sugar exceeds 11 mmol/L (200 mg/100 mL) 30, 60, or 90 minutes after ingesting 1.75 g/kg of glucose, and is still above this level 2 hours after the ingestion of the glucose.

In pregnancy, a diagnosis of diabetes mellitus is made if the concentration of glucose in venous plasma is excessive on at least two occasions when measured 1, 2, and 3 hours after the ingestion of 100 g of glucose. The concentration should not exceed 11 mmol/L (190 mg/100 mL) 1 hour after taking the glucose, 9 mmol/L (165 mg/100 mL) 2 hours afterwards, or 8 mmol/L (145 mg/100 mL) 3 hours afterwards.

In addition to frank diabetes, a state of impaired glucose tolerance is recognized. In these people, glucose and insulin metabolism are abnormal, but not sufficiently deranged to justify a diagnosis of diabetes mellitus. In adults, a diagnosis of impaired glucose tolerance is made if the fasting blood sugar in venous plasma is below 8 mmol/L (140 mg/100 mL), but exceeds 11 mmol/L 30, 60, or 90 minutes after taking 75 g of glucose by mouth, and falls to between 8 and 11 mmol/L (140 to 200 mg/100 mL) 2 hours after taking the sugar. In children, the diagnosis is made if the fasting blood sugar is below 8 mmol/L (140 mg/100 mL) but exceeds 8 mmol/L (140 mg/100 mL) 2 hours after taking 1.75 g/kg of glucose by mouth.

All values given refer to the concentration

of glucose in venous plasma. The concentration of glucose in whole venous blood is 10 to 15% lower. The concentration of glucose in capillary blood is 7% higher than in venous blood. Care must be taken to avoid stress during a glucose tolerance test. The release of catecholamines caused by stress can cause a diabetic response in a normal person.

Types

Diabetes mellitus is divided into insulin-dependent, noninsulin-dependent, and secondary types, as shown in Table 38-1, though the distinction between the types is not always clear. Impaired glucose tolerance and gestational diabetes are usually considered separately.

The terms *insulin-dependent* and *noninsulin-dependent* are misleading. Patients with insulin-dependent diabetes mellitus must be given insulin to control their disease, but so must many patients with the noninsulin-dependent form of the disease.

INSULIN-DEPENDENT DIABETES MELLITUS. Insulin-dependent diabetes mellitus, also called type I diabetes, was formerly called juvenile diabetes, juvenile-onset diabetes, or ketosis-prone diabetes. The name is often abbreviated to IDDM. About 10% of diabetics have this form of the disease. Insulin-dependent diabetes mellitus usually becomes evident when the patient is less than 40 years

TABLE 38-1.   Types of Diabetes Mellitus

Type I—Insulin-dependent

Type II—Noninsulin-dependent
   In obese people
   In nonobese people
   Maturity-onset diabetes in the young

Secondary
   Pancreatic
   Hormonal
   Drug-induced
   Abnormal insulin receptors
   Genetic disorders

Impaired glucose tolerance

Gestational diabetes

---

old, often in adolescence or childhood. Men and women are affected equally.

Lesions.   At the onset of insulin-dependent diabetes mellitus, the pancreas and its islets are normal morphologically, or nearly so. Within three to four weeks of the onset of the disease, most of the islets lose most of their B cells. Instead of the normal 60 to 85% of B cells, the islets contain less than 10% of B cells. Most of the remaining islet cells are A cells or D cells. The islets are usually irregularly shaped, small, and ill-defined. Their cells are small and dark, with scanty cytoplasm. The cords of islet cells become increasingly separated by fibrovascular connective tissue.

In the first few weeks, a few hyperplastic islets are present. The hyperplastic islets are larger than normal and are sharply demarcated. They consist of large, pale cells, with little stroma between the cords of cells. Most of the cells are degranulated B cells, with smaller numbers of A and D cells.

In the first few weeks, there may be evidence of the formation of new islets from the pancreatic ductules, but this is rare.

The PP islets normally present in the head of the pancreas become more prominent, and perhaps more numerous as the islets containing B cells atrophy and as new PP cells are formed from the pancreatic ductules. They have broad ribbons of columnar cells, though immunologic stains are necessary to identify them with certainty.

Insulitis, as inflammation of the islets is called, from the Latin for an island, usually involves only a few islets and persists only for a few weeks or months. Both atrophic and hyperplastic islets may be affected. An exudate predominantly of lymphocytes, with a few neutrophils and macrophages, is evident in and around the affected islets.

After years of insulin-dependent diabetes mellitus, most of the islets are small and atrophic. Often the islets are surrounded by scar tissue, as the exocrine pancreas undergoes partial atrophy, with fibrosis. Fibrosis within the islets is not severe. Amyloidosis or calcification of islets is uncommon. Hyperplastic islets are not present. New islets are no longer formed from the pancreatic ductules. Insulitis is rare, if present at all.

PP islets grow more prominent. The islet mass shrinks to 10% of normal, and the number of B cells to less than 1% of normal.

Dysfunction. The almost complete lack of insulin caused by the destruction of the B cells in insulin-dependent diabetes mellitus causes a variety of metabolic derangements. Only the more important of them can be described briefly here.

As the concentration of insulin in the plasma falls, the concentration of glucagon rises. In uncontrolled insulin-dependent diabetes, increased secretion of adrenocortical steroids, growth hormone, and catecholamines add to the metabolic derangement. If insulin is given, the secretion of glucagon and the other hormones returns to normal.

The hyperglycemia characteristic of insulin-dependant diabetes results from overproduction of glucose by the liver and inadequate usage by the tissues. As the ratio of insulin to glucagon falls, glycogenogenesis in the hepatocytes is blocked and gluconeogenesis increases. In the peripheral tissues, insulin is necessary for the transport of glucose into the cells.

The excess of glucose in the blood spills into the urine when the renal threshold is passed, causing the glycosuria that gave diabetes mellitus its name. The sugar in the urine carries with it water and electrolytes. If the diabetes is severe, dehydration will reduce the body's store of sodium and potassium.

The lipoprotein lipase in adipose tissue in large part responsible for the breakdown of circulating lipids is insulin-dependent. In insulin-dependent diabetes, failure of the lipoprotein lipase often results in hyperchylomicronemia, hypercholesterolemia, hypertriglyceridemia, or some combination of these abnormalities.

The lack of insulin reduces the uptake of amino acids from the blood by the peripheral tissues, especially in muscle. Synthesis of protein is impaired, and breakdown of protein increases. The wasting common in insulin-dependent diabetes is produced in part by this mechanism.

Lipolysis is enhanced in the adipose tissues, releasing fatty acids into the blood. The free fatty acids are taken up by the hepato-cytes and oxidized to ketones, contributing to the ketoacidosis that develops in uncontrolled insulin-dependent diabetes mellitus.

Clinical Presentation. The onset of insulin-dependent diabetes is often sudden. In the course of a few weeks, the patient develops polydipsia and polyuria, often with an increased appetite and a craving for sweet foods. There is progressive loss of weight and lassitude, perhaps blurred vision or muscular cramps. If treatment is not begun, nausea and vomiting follow. The patient becomes increasingly dehydrated, confused, comatose, and is likely to die. In children, the whole course may take only a few weeks, though more often it extends over several months.

Sometimes the onset of insulin-dependent diabetes mellitus is precipitated by infection, a surgical procedure, or some other stress. Probably the increased secretion of catecholamines caused by the stress inhibits the secretion of insulin, and the patient's failing pancreas cannot compensate. When the patient recovers from the infection or operation, all signs of diabetes may disappear, giving a honeymoon of several months before the symptoms and signs of diabetes mellitus again become evident.

Pathogenesis. Insulin-dependent diabetes mellitus is almost certainly caused by an autoimmune reaction that destroys the B cells. In most patients, a genetic predisposition allows an environmental injury to initiate the immunologic attack.

The predisposition to develop insulin-dependent diabetes mellitus is not inherited as a simple mendelian dominant or recessive character. Probably more than one gene is involved. Only 5% of the siblings of a patient develop the disease and 2% of the offspring. In more than 50% of monozygous twins, only one has the disease.

Over 95% of patients with insulin-dependent diabetes mellitus express the HLA-DR3 antigen, the HLA-DR4 antigen, or both. About 60% of the general population express these antigens. Only 0.3% of people bearing these antigens develop diabetes mellitus, but a person expressing HLA-DR3 is 5 times more likely to develop insulin-dependent diabetes mellitus than is the general population, a person expressing HLA-DR4 is

7 times as likely, and a person expressing both is 14 times more likely. A person expressing HLA-DR2 is less likely to develop insulin-dependent diabetes mellitus than is the general population. Because of linkage disequilibrium between the HLA class II and class I antigens, HLA-B8, and HLA-B15 are more common in people with insulin-dependent diabetes mellitus than in the general population, and HLA-B7 is less frequent.

A viral infection seems to precipitate insulin-dependent diabetes in many of the patients. The onset of the disease is more common in the fall and winter, when viral infections are common. In the United States, 20% of infants with congenital rubella subsequently develop insulin-dependent diabetes mellitus. Coxsackie B viruses, and the viruses of mumps, infections mononucleosis, and viral hepatitis are among organisms associated with insulin-dependent diabetes mellitus, though only a small proportion of people infected with these agents develop diabetes mellitus.

Antibodies against the B cells in the pancreatic islets are demonstrable in 90% of patients with insulin-dependent diabetes mellitus studied within one month of the onset. Some are directed against cytoplasmic components of the B cells, some against surface antigens. Some fix complement and are cytotoxic. Some impair the release of insulin. As months pass and the B cells are destroyed, the antibodies disappear in most of the patients, though in a few they persist for as long as 20 years.

Activated T cells increase in the blood in the first months of insulin-dependent diabetes mellitus and probably are principally responsible for the destruction of the B cells. They disappear as the B cells disappear from the pancreas.

The HLA-DR antigens are present on the surface of the B cells in patients with insulin-dependent diabetes mellitus, but are not present on the other cells of the islets, or on the B cells of normal people. Probably the presence of HLA-DR3 or HLA-DR4 on the surface of the B cells makes autoimmunization easier, while HLA-DR2 makes it more difficult. It could be that autoimmunization is initiated when the plasma membrane of the B cells expresses both a favorable HLA-DR antigen and an abnormal antigen induced by a viral infection or in some other way.

Other autoimmune diseases occur more commonly in patients with insulin-dependent diabetes mellitus than in the general population. They are particularly frequent in patients expressing HLA-DR3 and are often associated with continuing production of antibodies against the B cells.

Antibodies against the B cells of the islets do not necessarily cause diabetes mellitus. They are present in a small proportion of the general population and in 2% of close relatives of patients with insulin-dependent diabetes mellitus. They can remain detectable in the plasma for years in people who never develop diabetes mellitus.

Treatment and Prognosis. Patients with insulin-dependent diabetes mellitus require insulin and a diet adjusted to the dose of insulin taken. If the metabolic fault can be controlled and complications avoided, the patient can live a normal life. Less than 1% of the patients die of ketoacidosis or hypoglycemia. Most die of atherosclerosis or some other late complication of the disease.

NONINSULIN-DEPENDENT DIABETES MELLITUS. Noninsulin-dependent diabetes mellitus, or type 2 diabetes, was formerly called adult-onset diabetes, maturity-onset diabetes, ketosis-resistant diabetes, or stable diabetes. The name is often abbreviated to NIDDM. Over 80% of the patients have this form of the disease.

Most patients with noninsulin-dependent diabetes mellitus are over 40 years old when the disease first becomes evident. As age increases, the likelihood of developing noninsulin-dependent diabetes increases, until 50% of people over 80 years old have diabetes, usually mild diabetes. Maturity onset diabetes in the young (MODY) becomes evident in childhood.

Noninsulin-dependent diabetes mellitus is divided into three types, noninsulin-dependent diabetes in the obese, noninsulin-dependent diabetes in the nonobese and maturity onset diabetes in the young.

Lesions. When noninsulin-dependent diabetes mellitus is first diagnosed, the pancreas is normal macroscopically. The islet cell mass is normal or increased. Microscopically, many of the islets of Langerhans are enlarged. They contain the usual proportion of B cells, many of which show evidence of hyperactivity. Sometimes new islets are being formed from the pancreatic ductules.

As the years pass, there is slow atrophy of both the endocrine and exocrine parts of the pancreas. The atrophy is often patchy and greatest in the peripheral part of the gland. After 10 to 20 years, the parenchyma of the gland is reduced by 10 to 50%. Fatty infiltration of the pancreas increases as its parenchyma atrophies.

Microscopically, the islets gradually grow smaller. Up to 50% of the B cell mass can be lost, but there is a slight increase in A and D cells. In the more atrophic parts of the gland, fibrosis develops in the islands and in and around the lobules of exocrine parenchyma. Arteriolosclerosis and atherosclerosis are usually prominent in and around the pancreas.

Amyloid is present in some of the islets in 10% of patients with noninsulin-dependent diabetes over 50 years old and becomes more common as age increases, being demonstrable in 50% of patients over 70 years old. Similar amyloid is present in from 3 to 20% of elderly people who do not have diabetes mellitus. The amyloid forms irregular or globular masses in the affected islets. It has the usual appearance on electron microscopy, but consists of a polymerization of molecules or parts of molecules of insulin. Amyloid AL and amyloid AA rarely involve the islets.

Dysfunction. The tissues of patients with noninsulin-dependent diabetes mellitus fail to utilize glucose normally. The number of insulin receptors on the cells is reduced, and the metabolism of glucose within the cells is impaired.

The secretion of insulin by the islets is inadequate. The patients often have a normal or increased concentration of insulin in the plasma, but the concentration of insulin is less than would be found in a normal person with a similar concentration of glucose in the plasma.

The secretion of glucagon is increased and cannot be restored to normal except by giving large doses of insulin. The other metabolic abnormalities found in insulin-dependent diabetes mellitus occur in noninsulin-dependent diabetes mellitus only when it is unusually severe.

Clinical Presentation. Noninsulin-dependent diabetes mellitus develops slowly and insidiously. Often the patient has no symptoms when glycosuria or hyperglycemia are found during a physical examination. When there are symptoms, they are often vague and have developed gradually over many months. The patients are well nourished, often overweight, even though many of them have lost weight, sometimes a considerable amount of weight. Nocturnal polyuria is common, with thirst, and some degree of polydipsia. Pruritus vulvae is often troublesome, and occasionally there is balanitis. Cramps in the calves or feet, especially at night, and tingling in the fingers are common. There may be loss of appetitie or a craving for sweet foods. A change in the refraction of the lenses can cause blurred vision.

Pathogenesis. Genetic and environmental factors are both important in the causation of noninsulin-dependent diabetes mellitus. Antibodies against the B cells are present in less than 10% of the patients and are probably secondary to the disease, not its cause.

In the obese and nonobese patients with noninsulin-dependent diabetes, the nature of the genetic factors that govern susceptibility to the disease is obscure. Probably more than one gene is involved. About 20% of close relatives of a patient with noninsulin-dependent diabetes mellitus have the disease. In 90% of monozygous twins involved, both have the disease. The gene for insulin on chromosome 11 is involved only in rare patients who form an abnormal insulin that binds poorly to the insulin receptors in the tissues.

About 80% of patients with noninsulin-dependent diabetes mellitus are overweight. Many are obese. The obesity causes resistance to the action of insulin that can often be corrected if the patient loses weight. Obesity reduces the number of insulin receptors in the peripheral tissues, and losing weight restores the number to normal. The B cells in the islets secrete less insulin than is needed to maintain homeostasis, but it is not clear whether this reduced secretion is due to a primary fault in the islets or is secondary to the insulin resistance and results from exhaustion induced by prolonged overstimulation. Nor is it clear whether the reduction in the number of B cells late in the disease occurs because of a primary fault in the B cells or is secondary to the abnormality in the peripheral tissues.

In nonobese noninsulin-dependent diabetes mellitus the increased resistance to insulin is caused by a fault in the postreceptor stage of insulin metabolism in the peripheral cells, rather than by an abnormality in the number or avidity of the receptors for insulin. Often the increase in resistance is slight, and the disease is due to malfunction of the B cells in the islets. The concentration of insulin in the plasma is often low.

Maturity onset diabetes in the young is inherited as an autosomal dominant character. The B cells fail to respond normally to an increase in the concentration of glucose in the plasma, and there is probably a fault in the utilization of glucose.

Treatment and Prognosis. In many patients, noninsulin-dependent diabetes mellitus can be controlled by diet alone, especially if the patient loses weight. Some need one of the sulfonylureas, oral drugs that control the hyperglycemia principally by increasing the secretion of insulin by the B cells, though there is some enhancement of the utilization of glucose in the tissues. If these measures fail, insulin is needed. The disease causes disability principally by increasing the risk of atherosclerosis and other late complications of diabetes mellitus.

SECONDARY DIABETES MELLITUS. A number of diseases cause diabetes mellitus by reducing the secretion of insulin, reducing the sensitivity of the tissues to insulin, or both. These conditions are discussed in other parts of the book, but some of the more prominent of them are listed in Table 38-2.

In tropical countries, chronic pancreatitis, often with calcification, is a common cause of secondary diabetes. In many of these patients, though not all, there is increased insulin resistance in the peripheral tissues as well as the pancreatic deficiency. In other parts of the world, chronic pancreatitis or cystic fibrosis is only occasionally severe enough to cause diabetes mellitus. Severe stress or a pheochromocytoma can release enough catecholamines to suppress insulin

Table 38-2. Causes of Secondary Diabetes Mellitus

Pancreatic disease
  Hemochromatosis
  Chronic pancreatitis
  Cystic fibrosis
  Total pancreatectomy
  Congenital hypoplasia

Hormonal dysfunction
  Excess of adrenal corticosteroids
  Excess of catecholamines
  Acromegaly
  Glucagonoma
  Somatostatinoma
  Thyrotoxicosis
  Hypopituitarism

Drug toxicity
  Diuretics
    Furosemide
    Thiazides
    etc.

  Psychoactive agents
    Phenothiazines
    Tricyclic antidepressants
    Lithium carbonate
    Diphenylhydantoin
    etc.

  Other
    Isoproterenol
    Levodopa
    Propranolol
    Indomethacin
    L-Asparaginase
    Streptozotocin
    Isoniazid
    Nicotinic Acid
    Oral contraceptives
    etc.

Abnormal insulin receptors
  Congenital lipodystrophy
  Acanthosis nigricans
  Virilism
  Antibody to insulin receptors

Genetic disorders
  Glycogen storage disease type I
  Acute intermittent porphyria
  Ataxia telangiectasia
  Muscular dystrophy
  Huntington's chorea
  Friedreich's ataxia
  Laurence-Moon-Biedl syndrome
  Turner's syndrome
  Klinefelter's syndrome
  Down's Syndrome

secretion and increase glucagon secretion, causing diabetes mellitus. The excess of growth hormone in acromegaly increases resistance to the peripheral action of insulin. The excess of glucocorticoids in Cushing's syndrome causes hyperglycemia by impairing the release of insulin from the B cells of the islets, opposing the peripheral action of insulin, and by stimulating gluconeogenesis in the liver. Thyrotoxicosis may unmask incipient diabetes mellitus, as may oral contraceptives, hyperlipidemia, and hypokalemia.

IMPAIRED GLUCOSE TOLERANCE. People with impaired glucose tolerance have a mild derangement of insulin metabolism like that in diabetes mellitus. Some of these people remain with impaired glucose tolerance for years. Others sooner or later progress to diabetes mellitus. Each year, from 1 to 5% of people with impaired glucose tolerance develop diabetes mellitus.

The severity of atherosclerosis is increased in people with impaired glucose tolerance, as it is in diabetics, but they do not develop the other late complications of diabetes.

GESTATIONAL DIABETES. Pregnancy worsens the metabolic derangements in women with diabetes mellitus and may cause diabetes to appear for the first time. It causes a variety of metabolic changes that increase the severity of diabetes mellitus and make its management more difficult. The concentrations of glucose and amino acids in the plasma fall. At term, the fetus uses from 25 to 30 g of glucose a day. The response to overnight fasting is exaggerated, often bringing concentrations of ketone bodies and free fatty acids in the plasma of the order seen in nonpregnant people in starvation. Probably because of the secretion of human placental lactogen by the placenta, peripheral resistance to insulin rises progressively from the sixteenth week of pregnancy, to return abruptly to normal at delivery. Estrogens and progesterone secreted by the placenta cause exaggerated release of insulin from the islets in response to the usual stimuli.

Most pregnant diabetics have insulin-dependent diabetes. Early in pregnancy, the requirement for insulin may fall because of the hypoglycemia and loss of appetitie caused by the pregnancy. After the sixteenth week of pregnancy, the demand for insulin increases as peripheral resistance to insulin grows. The risk of ketosis increases because of the ketotic diathesis induced by pregnancy.

The risk of death is 10 times greater than in a nondiabetic woman because of ketosis, hypoglycemia, and the increased risk of infection. After delivery, the patient's diabetes returns to its previous state.

The term *gestational diabetes* is used to describe diabetes that develops during pregnancy. Many of these patients do not have glycosuria, and most pregnant women who have glycosuria do not have diabetes. In most pregnant women, the glycosuria is due to impairment of renal reabsorption of glucose, caused by the pregnancy. The diagnosis can be made only by a glucose tolerance test. It is important to make the diagnosis, for gestational diabetes endangers the fetus, as do other forms of diabetes mellitus.

Gestational diabetes is managed by diet and insulin. Sulfonylureas are usually avoided, as they cross the placenta to reach the fetus and can cause serious hypoglycemia in the neonate.

In some patients with gestational diabetes, the glucose tolerance test returns to normal on delivery. Some reserve the term *gestational diabetes* for this group of women. In other women, the pregnancy only serves to unmask diabetes mellitus, usually insulin-dependent, which continues its course after delivery.

Complications

Four types of complication are important in diabetes mellitus: the metabolic complications ketoacidosis and hyperosmolar coma; the complications of therapy, hypoglycemia, insulin resistance, insulin allergy, lipodystrophy, lactic acidosis, and depression of the bone marrow; the late complications that affect organs throughout the body; and the effects of the disease on a child born of a diabetic mother.

KETOACIDOSIS. Ketoacidosis is almost always a complication of insulin-dependent diabetes. It can develop if a patient with insulin-dependent diabetes fails to take insulin or can be precipitated by stress, infection, an operation, or an emotional upset, even though insulin is continued at a dose sufficient to control the diabetes while the patient is healthy.

A failure to take insulin and stress both cause increased secretion of glucagon, with an increase in the concentration of glucagon in the plasma, absolutely and relative to the concentration of insulin. The insulin deficiency and the increased secretion of glucagon combine to cause ketoacidosis.

The lack of insulin and the excess of glucagon cause maximal release of glucose from the liver and impair the utilization of glucose by the peripheral tissues. The concentration of glucose in the plasma rises sharply, to over 15 mmol/L (250 mg/100 mL), often to over 30 mmol/L (500 mg/100 mL). The sugar spills into the urine, causing massive diuresis and dehydration. Potassium and sodium are lost in the urine, though because of the dehydration the concentration of potassium in the plasma remains normal or is increased to 6 mmol/L (6 mEq/L) or so, while the concentration of sodium is only slightly lowered, to about 132 mmol/L (132 mEq/L).

The lack of insulin causes lipolysis in the adipose tissues, releasing free fatty acids into the plasma. Their concentration in the plasma often exceeds 2 mmol/L, the normal being less than 0.7 mmol/L.

The liver takes up the free fatty acids. The excess of glucagon diminishes the activity of malonyl CoA and activates the carnitine system. The carnitine transferases transport the fatty acids into the mitochondria, where they are oxidized to ketone bodies, principally acetoacetate and β-hydroxybutyrate. The ketone bodies escape into the blood, where they cause acidosis. The concentration of ketone bodies in the plasma may exceed 18 mmol/L, as compared with a normal of less than 0.5 mmol/L, and a concentration of about 2 mmol/L in starvation. If the concentration of fatty acids in the plasma is high, there may be fatty liver and hypertriglyceridemia.

Clinically, a patient with ketoacidosis presents with anorexia, nausea, and vomiting. The patient becomes confused, eventually comatose. Respiration is deep and fast. The sickly smell of the ketone bodies on the breath can be recognized by some, but not all, people. Sometimes there is abdominal pain or discomfort. The temperature is normal or low. The blood pressure is normal or low. Often there is a marked leukocytosis.

Insulin must be given in dose adequate to reverse the ketosis and prevent the formation of ketone bodies. The lack of water, sodium, and potassium must be restored intravenously. Bicarbonate is needed only if the acidosis is severe, with a pH of less than 7. The concentration of glucose in the blood falls to normal before the ketone bodies have been cleared from the blood. Glucose must then be given intravenously, while insulin is continued.

Most patients with diabetic ketoacidosis recover. About 10% die, usually from a complication such as myocardial infarction or infection. Occasionally, cerebral edema develops during treatment, perhaps because too rapid a reduction in the plasma glucose concentration causes an osmotic imbalance in the brain.

HYPEROSMOLAR COMA. Hyperosmolar coma usually complicates noninsulin-dependent diabetes mellitus, less often insulin-dependent diabetes. It is caused by severe dehydration. The dehydration is caused by hyperglycemia that continues uncontrolled for a considerable time. The loss of sugar in the urine causes so great a diuresis that the patient cannot drink enough water to maintain hydration. Often the patient is old, perhaps with a stroke, or sick, unable to drink enough.

The blood sugar is high, often about 55 mmol/L (1,000 mg/100 mL). The osmolality of the plasma is high. Often there is prerenal azotemia, with a concentration of creatinine in the plasma of about 450 μmol/L (5.0 mg/100 mL). Starvation may cause mild, metabolic acidosis. Ketoacidosis does not occur, though starvation may cause some production of ketone bodies.

The patient is confused and dull, occasionally in coma. Seizures are common. There may be transient hemiplegia. Infection, especially pneumonia, often with a gram-negative organism, is common. Because of the viscosity of the blood, the risk of thrombosis is high. Bleeding or pancreatitis may occur.

The mortality in hyperosmolar coma is high. Over 50% of the patients die. Rehydration is urgent. Often 10 L or more of fluid are needed. Potassium must be replaced as needed. Often insulin is required to reduce the blood sugar.

HYPOGLYCEMIA. Hypoglycemia can develop rapidly in patients taking insulin after too large a dose, inadequate intake of food, or unusual exertion or stress. It is uncommon in people taking one of the sulfonylureas.

As the supply of glucose to the brain falls, the patient is likely to experience blurring of vision, a growing feeling of uncertainty and confusion, hunger, and headache. The secretion of catecholamines to combat the hypoglycemia brings tingling of the fingers and lips, tremor, sweating, and pallor. The patient can rapidly become stuporous, sometimes comatose.

If recognized early, sugar taken by mouth reverses the hypoglycemia. If the patient becomes stuporous, glucose must be given intravenously.

If hypoglycemia persists, there is danger of cerebral edema. Repeated attacks of hypoglycemia can cause permanent injury to the brain.

INSULIN RESISTANCE. Antibodies against insulin develop within a few weeks in almost all diabetics given the drug. In most people, they do no harm. In 1 diabetic in 1000, they inactivate the insulin, increasing the demand for insulin to over 200 units/day.

Insulin resistance caused by the antibodies can develop suddenly, soon after the start of insulin therapy or not for years, but more often it develops gradually. Sometimes it can be controlled by prednisone. Sometimes it can be avoided by using a different or purer form of insulin.

ALLERGY. Allergy is an uncommon complication of insulin or sulfonylurea therapy. It is usually caused by the development of IgE antibodies to the drug, though IgG antibodies and delayed hypersensitivity reactions can occur. Most often there is pruritus, with an erythematous rash in the skin. Desensitization is usually successful.

LIPODYSTROPHY. Two kinds of local injury occur at a site at which insulin is injected subcutaneously, lipoatrophy and lipohypertrophy.

Lipoatrophy develops at the site of injection in over 25% of diabetics using insulin, especially in young girls. There is loss of adipose tissue in the region, often with considerable disfigurement. It is especially common when one of the less pure insulins is used. Injection of pure insulin into or around the lesion brings regrowth of the fat.

Lipohypertrophy is more common when pure insulins are used, especially in children. There is overgrowth of adipose tissue at the site of injection. If the injections of insulin are given in some other part of the body, the excess of fat gradually disappears.

LACTIC ACIDOSIS. Lactic acidosis is an uncommon complication of therapy with a biguanide, especially with phenethylbiguanide, a drug used in some countries to potentiate a sulfonylurea. It can be precipitated by liver failure, alcoholism, infection, or renal failure, and other conditions that reduce the urinary excretion of the drug.

DEPRESSION OF BONE MARROW. The sulfonylureas are among the drugs able to cause severe depression of the bone marrow, though the complication is rare and usually occurs only when large doses are given.

LATE COMPLICATIONS. The late complications of diabetes mellitus are described in other parts of the book, with the diseases of the organ principally affected. Table 38-3 lists the more important of them.

CHILDREN OF DIABETIC MOTHERS. In newborn children of diabetic mothers, the number and size of the islets of Langerhans are increased. Often new islets are being formed from pancreatic ductules. The islet cell mass may be three times that of a neonate born of a nondiabetic mother. About 50% of the infants have hypoglycemia and hyperinsulinemia, though in only 5% is the hypoglycemia sufficient to cause symptoms.

The hyperplastic islets are surrounded by an inflammatory exudate, with neutrophils, eosinophils, lymphocytes, and macrophages. Often there is edema. The exudate does not extend into the islets. Within a few weeks, the changes in the child's pancreas wane and disappear, leaving no residual injury.

TABLE 38-3. LATE COMPLICATIONS OF DIABETES MELLITUS

Atherosclerosis
Cataract
Diabetic ulcers
Infection
Microangiopathy
Nephropathy
Neuropathy
Retinopathy
Skin lesions

OTHER NON-NEOPLASTIC DISEASES

A few other non-neoplastic diseases of the pancreas deserve brief mention.

HEMOCHROMATOSIS. The pancreas is often involved in hemochromatosis, which is discussed in Chapter 9. Macroscopically the pancreas becomes rusty brown as iron accumulates in the gland. Microscopically there is hemosiderin in the exocrine and endocrine epithelial cells, as well as in macrophages in the fibrous tissue. Fibrosis is sometimes extensive.

FATTY INFILTRATION. In the elderly, the pancreas often appears large and succulent, but on section consists mainly of adipose tissue. Microscopy confirms that there is considerable loss of the exocrine parenchyma, with replacement of the parenchyma by fat. The islets are usually little affected. Fatty infiltration of the pancreas causes no symptoms. Enough exocrine parenchyma remains to permit normal digestion.

HYPERPLASIA OF THE ISLETS. Hyperplasia of the islets of Langerhans occurs in infants born of diabetic mothers, in erythroblastosis fetalis, and in some patients with the Zollinger-Ellison syndrome. These conditions are discussed in other parts of the book.

CALCULI. Except in chronic pancreatitis, pancreatic calculi are rare in people under 70 years old, but one or more pancreatic stones are present in over 5% of older people. The stones consist of calcium carbonate in a protein matrix. They are usually small, but can be up to 2 cm across.

CONGENITAL ANOMALIES

Congenital anomalies of the pancreatic ducts are common, though rarely of much importance. The pancreas is formed by the fusion of two primordia, called the dorsal and the ventral pancreases. Normally the two ducts fuse during embryonic life, so that the whole pancreas drains into the terminal part of the common bile duct through the distal part of the ventral duct. This common pancreatic duct is called the duct of Wirsung.

In 10 to 20% of people, the duct of Wirsung fails to join the common bile duct at or before the ampulla of Vater and drains independently into the duodenum, though in close approximation to the common bile duct. In 20% of people, the main pancreatic duct divides as it approaches the duodenum and drains into the duodenum through both the duct of Wirsung and an accessory duct, called the duct of Santorini, which enters the duodenum cephalad to the ampulla of Vater. In 5% of people, the duct of Wirsung is absent, and the whole pancreas drains into the duodenum cephalad to the ampulla of Vater through the duct of Santorini. In 1% of people, the two duct systems fail to fuse. The ventral pancreatic primordium that forms the uncinate part of the head of the pancreas drains into the common bile duct through the duct of Wirsung, while the dorsal primordium that forms the rest of the head, the body, and the tail of the pancreas drains into the duodenum through the duct of Santorini.

Rarely, malrotation and overgrowth of the ventral primordium of the pancreas results in an annular pancreas, a ring of pancreatic tissue that completely encircles the second part of the duodenum. The anomaly does not affect pancreatic function, but may cause obstruction if the ring of pancreatic tissue constricts the duodenum.

Rarely, the pancreas is mobile, floating at the end of a mesentery or the dorsal pancreas fails to develop, so that the only pancreatic tissue present is a nubbin of ventral pancreas nestled against the duodenum.

Congenital cysts are uncommon in the pancreas. People with a congenital pancreatic cysts usually have cysts in the kidneys and liver. The cysts have a thin, fibrous wall and are lined by flatted ductal epithelium.

PANCREATIC RESTS. Small islands of pancreatic tissue are common in the stomach and duodenum, especially in the submucosa. The rests form small nodules, usually a few millimeters across, but sometimes as much as 3 or 4 cm in diameter.

Microscopically, the rests are made of normal exocrine glands, just like those in the pancreas, together with their ducts. Islets may or may not be present. Often smooth muscle proliferates around the heterotropic elements. Rests rarely produce symptoms, but the larger ones may cause pyloric obstruction or may mimic a neoplasm.

TUMORS

The tumors of the pancreas are nearly all epithelial and nearly all primary. Mesenchymal tumors are uncommon, and the organ rarely harbors metastases, except occasionally by extension from a parapancreatic lymph node involved by metastatic carcinoma.

The primary epithelial tumors of the pancreas form two families, the tumors of the exocrine pancreas and the tumors of the islets.

Exocrine

The tumors of the exocrine pancreas include the benign adenoma, intraductal papilloma, and serous cystadenoma, the borderline cystadenocarcinoma, and the malignant ductal and acinar carcinomata.

ADENOMA. An adenoma of the pancreas is rare. It usually forms a nodule less than 0.1 cm across and microscopically consists of a proliferation of ducts lined by well-differentiated epithelium. Sometimes papillary folds lined by epithelium project into the ducts. Some of the lesions may be neoplastic, but most are probably hyperplastic.

INTRADUCTAL PAPILLOMA. Rarely, the ducts of a pancreas are ectatic and filled with soft, papillary tumor. Microscopically, the tumor has fronds lined by well-differentiated, mucus-secreting epithelium. The tumor obstructs the ducts, causing chronic pancreatitis and fibrosis in the part of the pancreas distal to the obstruction.

SEROUS CYSTADENOMA. About 1% of the exocrine tumors of the pancreas are serous cystadenomata. Nearly 90% of the patients are women, most over 60 years old.

Serous cystadenomata are most common in the tail of the pancreas, but can occur in any part of the gland. They vary from 1 to 25 cm in diameter. The tumor has a thin, tense capsule and often is bosselated. On section, it is multilocular, usually with a multitude of small spaces like a sponge. The cysts contain serous or turbid fluid.

Microscopically, the cysts are lined by well-differentiated flattened or cuboidal epithelium. Often the tumor cells contain much glycogen. Occasionally islets or ducts are trapped within the tumor.

A serous cystadenoma is benign. Most give rise to no symptoms, though occasionally a cystadenoma of the pancreas has obstructed

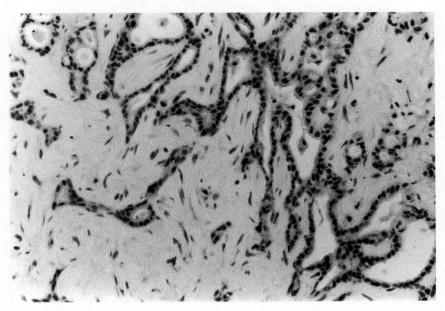

Fig. 38-6. Carcinoma of the pancreas, showing ducts lined by well-differentiated epithelium and separated by an abundant, collagenous stroma.

the pancreatic or a biliary duct. Excision cures.

CYSTADENOCARCINOMA. Some call all the cystic, mucinous tumors of the pancreas cystadenocarcinomata, whether or not they show clear evidence of malignancy. Others call the majority of these tumors mucinous cystadenomata and reserve the term cystadenocarcinoma for those that are frankly malignant.

If the term is used in the broad sense, 1 to 2% of exocrine tumors of the pancreas are of this type. Nearly 80% of the patients are women. Most are between 40 and 60 years old.

The tumor is most common in the tail of the pancreas, but sometimes arises in the body or head. It forms a well-demarcated mass from 1 to 30 cm in diameter. On section, the tumor has a thick, collagenous capsule. It may be unilocular or may contain several large cystic spaces. Often smaller cysts are present near the capsule. The cysts contain mucoid fluid.

Microscopically, the cysts are lined by columnar, mucus-secreting epithelium. Often fronds lined by the neoplastic cells project into the cysts. Most of the epithelium is well differentiated, but foci of atypicality can often be found. Occasionally a tumor seems to be invading its capsule or extends a little way into the adjacent pancreas.

A cystadenocarcinoma of the pancreas grows slowly. Pain is the most common symptom. A tumor in the head of the pancreas can obstruct the pancreatic duct, causing steatorrhea, or obstruct the bile duct. Excision brings cure in 70% of the patients. In 30%, the tumor eventually recurs or metastasizes. The tumor grows so slowly that partial excision has given several years relief.

DUCTAL CARCINOMA. Over 95% of the tumors of the exocrine pancreas are ductal carcinomata. About 3% of all malignant tumors are of this type. Over 60% of the patients are men. Over 60% of the patients are over 60 years old.

The incidence of carcinoma of the pancreas is increasing. In the United States, less than 5 people per 100,000 died of carcinoma of

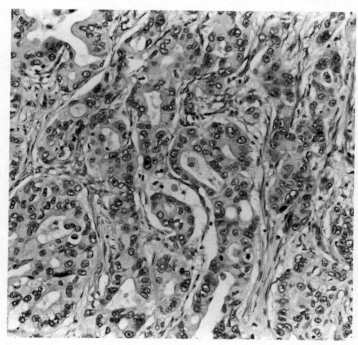

Fig. 38-7. A more anaplastic carcinoma of the pancreas, showing closely packed ducts lined by more poorly differentiated epithelium.

the pancreas in 1930, but more than 10 per 100,000 in 1982. The increase is similar in Europe and Japan.

Lesions. Nearly 70% of ductal carcinomata of the pancreas arise in the head of the gland, about 15% arise in the body, and 15% in the tail. In the head, the carcinoma is usually 5 to 10 cm across when it is discovered. In the body and tail the tumor is often larger. Most of the tumors are hard and sclerotic. A few are soft and mucoid. The carcinoma is ill-defined and invades the surrounding tissues. Small foci of necrosis or small cysts are sometimes visible in the carcinoma.

Carcinoma of the head of the pancreas often obstructs the pancreatic duct, causing chronic pancreatitis in the distal part of the pancreas. At operation, it may be hard to decide if a fibrotic mass in the head of the pancreas is a carcinoma or due to chronic pancreatitis. Foci of fat necrosis are evident in the peripancreatic tissues in 25% of patients with carcinoma of the pancreas.

Microscopically, most ductal carcinomata of the pancreas form irregular ducts separated by an abundant collagenous stroma or grow in solid columns two or three cells thick. In 80% of the tumors, the tumor cells are well differentiated and resemble the cells of the pancreatic ducts. In less than 10%, they are poorly differentiated but preserve the same pattern of growth in an abundant stroma. In 3% of the tumors, foci of squamous differentiation are present. In 1%, mucus secretion is abundant. In 5%, the tumor is plemorphic, with little stroma and bizarre cells.

Behavior. A ductal carcinoma of the pancreas invades slowly but inexorably. Often it causes death by local involvement of the bile ducts, duodenum, and other adjacent structures rather than by metastases.

At autopsy, the regional lymph nodes are involved in over 85% of the patients, and more distal lymph nodes are affected in over 50%. Metastases are present in the liver in 80% of the patients and in the lungs in 30%. Implants are present on the peritoneum in 25%. Less often the adrenal glands, bones, or stomach is involved. In 15% of the patients, no metastases are present.

Clinical Presentation. Carcinoma of the pancreas usually produces symptoms only late, when the tumor is far advanced. Pain is the first symptom in 60% of the patients. At first, there may be only a dull ache in the epigastrium, but as time passes, the pain often becomes severe, unremitting, harrowing. Particularly with tumors of the body and tail of the pancreas the pain often extends through to the back. Often it is relieved if the patient leans forward.

Weight loss is usually striking. The patient often becomes emaciated within a few months.

Jaundice occurs in 75% of patients with carcinoma of the head of the pancreas and in 25% of those with carcinoma of the body or tail. In 25% of people with carcinoma of the head of the pancreas, jaundice is the presenting symptom. Painless jaundice in an elderly person suggests of carcinoma of the pancreas, but more often the jaundice is preceded or soon followed by pain.

Less often, carcinoma of the pancreas presents as acute cholecystitis; acute pancreatitis; with pain that mimics disease of the spine; as a psychiatric disorder, with agitation, anxiety and depression; with symptoms like those of a peptic ulcer; with gastrointestinal hemorrhage; or with diarrhea. About 10% of the patients have diabetes mellitus, and the glucose tolerance test is abnormal in 50%. There may be ascites or evidence of malabsorption.

Thromboses in peripheral veins, sometimes with emboli, occur in 10 to 20% of the patients. Many think that the incidence of thrombosis is increased in patients with carcinoma of the pancreas, especially with carcinoma of the body and tail.

Physical examination often shows little. The carcinoma can rarely be palpated. If there is jaundice, the liver is often enlarged.

In a patient with obstructive jaundice, an enlarged, palpable gallbladder suggests carcinoma of the pancreas. In many patients with carcinoma of the pancreas, the gallbladder is fairly normal and so can dilate as the pressure in the biliary system rises because of the obstruction to the common bile duct caused by the carcinoma. If the jaundice is due to impaction of a gallstone, there is likely to be chronic cholecystitis, with sufficient fibrosis in the gallbladder to prevent its dilatation. The generalization that in obstructive jaundice a large gallbladder suggests carcinoma of the pancreas is often called Courvoisier's law, after a Swiss surgeon (1843–1918).

The distortion caused by the carcinoma may be evident radiologically, or the tumor can be revealed by ultrasonic examination, angiography, or computer assisted x-ray scanning. Cytologic examination of the pancreatic secretions may reveal malignant cells. A skinny needle biopsy can often establish the diagnoses.

Pathogenesis. Smoking cigarettes doubles the risk of developing carcinoma of the pancreas. Alcohol and other dietary factors have not proved important in the pathogenesis of the disease. Pancreatitis and diabetes mellitus do not increase the risk of developing a ductular carcinoma of the pancreas.

Treatment and Prognosis. In 80% of the patients, a ductular carcinoma of the pancreas is too far advanced to permit resection by the time the diagnosis is made, though a bypass to relieve the symptoms temporarily is often possible. Most of the patients die within three to six months. If resection is possible, the operative mortality approaches 20% and the five-year survival in patients with carcinoma of the head of the pancreas is less than 5%. Chemotherapy and radiotherapy are of limited benefit.

ACINAR CARCINOMA. About 1% of exocrine tumors of the pancreas are acinar carcinomata. Most of the patients are over 50 years old. The carcinoma can arise in any part of the pancreas. Usually it forms a soft, yellow, lobulated, well-demarcated mass 2 to 15 cm across. Microscopically, an acinar carcinoma forms small glands lined by cells that resemble those of the pancreatic acini or solid trabeculae of similar cells. Amylase, lipase, and other pancreatic enzymes can be demonstrated in the tumor cells. Electron microscopy shows zymogen granules in their cytoplasm. Some of the patients have extensive fat necrosis in the bone marrow and subcutaneous tissue. Metastases are usually extensive by the time the diagnosis is made. Most patients die within a year.

Endocrine

The endocrine tumors of the pancreas arise from the islets of Langerhans. They are usually called islet cell tumors. At autopsy, an islet cell tumor can be found in 1 person in 100 or 200 if the pancreas is searched carefully. Most of these tumors are small, cause no dysfunction, and cause no symptoms. Less than 1 person in 100,000 has an islet cell tumor that is diagnosed during life.

The features common to all islet cell tumors will be discussed first and then the special features that distinguish the different kinds of islet cell tumor.

Classification. Most islet cell tumors consist predominantly of one of the types of cell found in the islets of Langerhans. The tumor cells secrete the hormone formed by that type of cell, though often in too small a quantity to be evident clinically.

In more than 50% of the tumors, smaller numbers of one or more of the other types of cell found in the islets are also present. These other types of cell can also produce their hormone, though rarely in quantity sufficient to be evident clinically. Occasionally a tumor secretes some other of the polypepticle hormones produced by the neuroendocrine cells.

The islet cell tumors are classified according to the cell type predominant in the tumor and the secretion it produces (Table 38-4). An A cell tumor secretes glucagon and is called a glucagonoma; a B cell tumor secretes insulin and is called an insulinoma; a D cell tumor secretes somatostatin and is called a somatostatinoma; a G cell tumor secretes gastrin and is called a gastrinoma, or Zollinger-

TABLE 38-4. ISLET CELL TUMORS

Cell of Origin	Name	Major Secretion
A cell	Glugagonoma	Glucagon
B cell	Insulinoma	Insulin
D cell	Somatostatinoma	Somatostatin
G cell	Gastrinoma	Gastrin
?	Vipoma	Vasoactive intestinal polypeptide
PP cell	PP-oma	Pancreatic polypeptide
?	Mixed islet cell tumor	More than one hormone

Ellison tumor; a tumor that secretes the vasoactive intestinal polypeptide VIP, is called a vipoma; a tumor that secretes the pancreatic polypeptide PP is called a PP-oma. In some islet cell tumors, more than one hormone is produced in significant quantity. Such tumors are called mixed islet cell tumors.

In practice, it is often impossible to determine the nature of an islet tumor. Especially when the tumor is found only at autopsy, the tissue is often too poorly preserved to permit identification of the cell type by electron microscopy or the nature of the secretion of the tumor cells by immunologic techniques.

Lesions. The different types of islet cell tumor are indistinguishable macroscopically and to light microscopy, except when special stains are used to show the nature of the secretion in the tumor cells. The tumor is usually well demarcated macroscopically, often encapsulated. Most are less than 2 cm across and spheroidal, though an islet cell tumor can be larger. Some are so small they are difficult or impossible to find at operation. About 30% of the tumors arise in the head, 30% in the body, and 30% in the tail. Gastrinomata and the tumors of multiple en-

docrine neoplasia type I are usually multiple, but 85% of the other types of islet cell tumor are solitary.

Microscopically, the tumors often consist of well-differentiated islet cells arranged in anastomosing cords separated by a vascular stroma, much as are normal islet cells. Indeed, the tumor may look like a big islet.

Other tumors or other parts of a single tumor consist of solid clumps of cells, with a sparse, collagenous stroma between the clumps. Small acini may be present within the clumps. There may be central necrosis in the larger clumps. The cells at the margin of the clumps sometimes form a palisade around the clump.

Still other islet cell tumors or other parts of a single tumor consist of well-formed acini, with microvilli on the acinar surface of the tumor cells and tight junctions.

As in other endocrine tumors, occasional tumor cells are large, with large nuclei, but there is little other evidence of anaplasia. Most of the tumors are well demarcated microscopically, like normal islets. Some are encapsulated.

In 20 to 30% of the tumors, the tumor cells

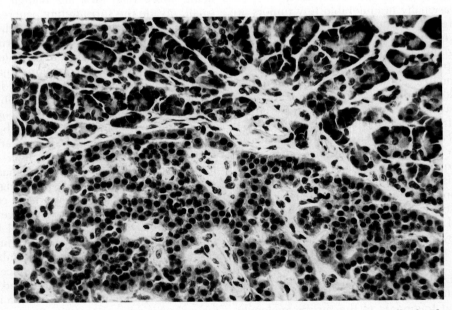

Fig. 38-8. An islet cell tumor showing the anastomosing cords of well-differentiated tumor cells often found in this sort of tumor. The tumor is well defined, but no capsule separates it from the normal pancreatic acini in the upper part of the picture.

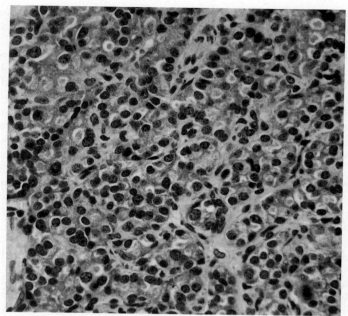

Fig. 38-9. A less well-differentiated islet cell tumor with the tumor cells growing in large sheets, with little stroma.

invade the capsule of the tumor or extend a little way into the adjacent pancreas. In some, the mitotic rate is increased.

Occasionally innumerable tiny tumors are scattered throughout the gland. Sometimes there is a general hyperplasia of the islets throughout the pancreas, rather than discrete tumors or hyperplasia of the islets in addition to a tumor. When there is more than one islet cell tumor, the predominant type of cell may be the same in all the tumors or may differ from tumor to tumor.

Special stains can often identify the nature of the tumor cells. Immunohistochemical techniques are more accurate, and in well-fixed tissue can demonstrate the hormone or hormones produced by the tumor. Electron microscopy shows granules like those seen in normal neuroendocrine cells, though in the tumors the granules are often sparse, smaller than normal and atypical.

The stroma of islet cell tumors is often hyalinized. In insulinomata, amyloid is often deposited in the stroma and consists of polymerized fragments of the insulin molecule. Amyloid is only occasionally seen in other kinds of islet cell tumor.

Behavior. The distinction between benign and malignant islet cell tumors is difficult. More than 90% are benign, remain small, invade the surrounding pancreas little if at all, and are discovered only if they produce a significant excess of their hormone.

The 10% that are malignant are sometimes larger, more invasive, or more anaplastic than the benign islet cell tumors, but are often indistinguishable from the benign tumors, macroscopically or microscopically. The malignant nature of the tumor becomes evident only when metastases appear in the regional lymph nodes or the liver, rarely more distantly. Most of the malignant islet cell tumors grow slowly. Even though they are often unresectable, the patients can survive in good health for 10 or more years.

About 60% of malignant islet cell tumors secrete human chorionic gonadotropin or its alpha or beta subunits. The alpha subunit is the most frequently detected. Since these substances are rarely if ever produced by benign islet cell tumors, they serve as a marker for malignancy.

GLUCAGONOMA. About 1% of active islet cell tumors secrete glucagon. These tumors are white or pink, 2 to 30 cm across. About 60% are malignant. Electron microscopy of the tumor cells shows granules about 350 nm across with a dense core and a gray halo. PP cells are sometimes numerous.

Patients with high levels of glucagon in the blood develop a crusting, necrotizing, migratory erythema in the skin. Intraepidermal bullae that develop in the erythematous regions and rupture, to give the crusting. The dermis shows chronic inflammation and edema. The lesions heal after one to three weeks, but new lesions appear elsewhere. Impaired glucose tolerence or mild diabetes mellitus and anemia is common. There may be alopecia, stomatitis, or diarrhea. Severe infections sometimes occur. Venous thromboses develop in 30% of the patients. Removal of the tumor cures.

Rarely, a glucagonoma arises in a lung, a kidney, or the duodenum.

INSULINOMA.   Over 70% of functioning islet cell tumors arise from the B cells, and most of the islet cell tumors found at autopsy, that produced no symptoms during life are B cell tumors. The tumors that cause no symptoms are often called nonfunctional, but probably most of them secrete a little insulin.

In 90% of patients with a functioning B cell tumor, the insulinoma is single and benign. Occasionally, there is more than one tumor, sometimes many, In 5% of the patients with a functioning tumor, the insulinoma is malignant, as shown by the development of metastases. The patient is usually 35 to 60 years old when symptoms first become evident, though a functioning insulinoma can develop at any age.

Nonfunctional B cell tumors are usually 1 to 2 cm in diameter, but may be as much as 15 cm across or may be tiny. Most functioning tumors are over 2 cm across, but even a small tumor can cause serious hyperinsulinism. Malignant tumors are usually large.

Microscopically, B cell tumors can show any of the patterns of growth seen in islet cell tumors. If there are sufficient secretory granules in the tumor cells, they can be stained for light microscopy with the aldehydefuchsin stain. By electron microscopy, the granules of the tumor cells are vacuoles about 300 nm in diameter, which contain irregular, angular,

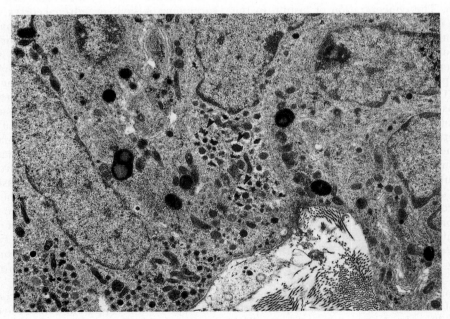

Fig. 38-10. An electron micrograph of an insulinoma, showing well-differentiated tumor cells limited by a basement membrane. The arrowheads point to secretory granules containing the irregular bodies characteristic of the B cells of the islets. (Courtesy of Dr. K. Kovacs)

paracrystalline bodies similar to those seen in normal B cells. Immunohistologic methods can demonstrate insulin in almost all B cell tumors.

Functioning B cell tumors secrete a mixture of insulin and proinsulin. Sometimes as much as 20% of the secretion is proinsulin. The tumors often secrete only intermittently, but when a tumor is secreting, the plasma contains an inappropriately high concentration of insulin and an abnormally high concentration of proinsulin.

In normal people, the concentration of insulin in the plasma rises when the concentration of glucose rises, but the ratio between the concentration of insulin and the concentration of glucose is below 50, when insulin is measured in pmol/L and glucose in mmol/L, and below 0.4 when insulin is measured in μU-100 mL and glucose in mg/100 mL. In patients with an insulinoma, the ratios are usually above 130 when the measurements are in pmol and mmol and above 1 when they are in U and mg.

In normal people, the secretion of insulin ceases if the concentration of glucose in the plasma falls below 2.7 mmol/L (50 mg/100 mL) in men or 2.2 mmol/L (40 mg/100 mL) in women. The concentration of insulin in the plasma is less than 35 pmol/L (5 μU/100 mL). In patients with a functioning insulinoma, secretion usually continues despite the hypoglycemia, and the concentration of insulin in the plasma is much higher.

The C peptide cleaved from proinsulin to free insulin is released into the plasma in equimolecular quantities with insulin, and its concentration in the plasma rises in parallel with the concentration of insulin.

Other kinds of secretion can be produced by insulinomata: gastrin, glucagon, somatostatin, or the pancreatic polypeptide. They are rarely in sufficient quantity to produce symptoms.

Because of the excessive secretion of insulin from the tumor, patients with a functioning insulinoma tend to become hypoglycemic. Typically, the hypoglycemia develops in the morning. The blood sugar falls to below 3 mmol/L (50 mg/100 mL), but symptoms can be rapidly relieved by giving glucose. The symptoms result in part from the hypoglycemia, in part from the secretion of catecholamines that it stimulates. There may be rest-lessness, muscle spasms, convulsions, or coma. Often there is sweating, flushing, nausea, weakness, sometimes epigastric pain, or hunger. There may be emotional lability or confusion. The diagnosis can be confirmed by giving tolbutamide, leucine, or glucagon. In most patients with a functioning insulinoma, these secretagogues cause excessive secretion of insulin, with profound and prolonged hypoglycemia.

In over 80% of the patients, the tumor or tumors can be found and removed surgically. The patient is cured. Even if the tumor cannot be identified, resection of the body and tail of the pancreas offers a good chance of cure. If the tumor cannot be removed or has metastasized, diazoxide may depress insulin secretion and relieve symptoms. The antibiotic streptozotocin can destroy B cells, but it and other chemotherapeutic drugs have proved of limited value in the control of B cell tumors.

Rarely, a B cell tumor arises in a pancreatic rest outside the pancreas.

Other Tumors Causing Hypoglycemia. Hypoglycemia similar to that caused by an insulinoma can be caused by a retroperitoneal sarcoma; less often by a sarcoma elsewhere, carcinoma of the liver, adrenal cortex, gut, or elsewhere; or rarely by a lymphoma. How these tumors cause hypoglycemia is uncertain. They do not secrete insulin. They may secrete some other substance that causes hypoglycemia, or in some cases the tumor may utilize excessive quantities of glucose, overwhelming the body's homeostatic mechanisms.

Nesidioblastosis. A rare cause of hypoglycemia and hyperinsulinism in infancy is hyperplasia of the islets of Langerhans and continuing formation of new islets from the pancreatic ductules. The hyperplasia and formation of new islets may involve the whole of the pancreas or may be confined to part of it. B cells are prominent in the hyperplastic islets and in the new islets, but all types of islet cell are present in both. The condition has been called nesidioblastosis, from the Greek for an islet and a bud.

The hyperinsulinemia causes hypoglycemia that becomes apparent before the child is two years old. The syndrome is called persistent hypoglycemia of infancy, for the hyperinsulinism and hypoglycemia continue as the child ages. The hyperinsulinism is not caused by increase of the B cell mass, but because the B cells are abnormal or the factors that control the secretion of insulin are disrupted. Often the hypoglycemia causes cerebral damage and mental retardation. Drugs such as diazoxide sometimes control the hyperinsulinism, but frequently subtotal or almost total pancreatectomy is necessary.

SOMATOSTATINOMA. Only a few D cell tumors have been reported. Most have been malignant. One arose in the duodenum. The tumors secrete somatostatin, and some of them have also secreted calcitonin or the adrenocorticotropic hormone. The patients have diabetes mellitus, cholelithiasis, steatorrhea, and perhaps hypochlorhydria or anemia. The tumor may be painful. Electron microscopy shows granules with a gray core, which fills the vacuole, leaving no halo between the core and the limiting membrane. The granules resemble those of normal D cells, though they are about 300 nm across, a little smaller than normal.

GASTRINOMA. About 25% of islet cell tumors arise from G cells. They secrete gastrin. They are most common in people 30 to 50 years old. About 60% of the patients are men.

Gastrinomata are most common in the body and tail of the pancreas, but 10% of them arise in the duodenum. Rarely, a gastrinoma has arisen in the stomach, a parathyroid gland, or an ovary.

In 70% of the patients, there is more than one tumor. In 60% of the patients, one or more of the tumors is malignant. In 10% of the patients, no tumor can be found. Instead, there is generalized hyperplasia of the islets. In some, there is both hyperplasia of the islets and one or more tumors.

G cell tumors are usually less than 10 cm across. Many are only a few mm across. Even small tumors can produce abnormal quantities of gastrin.

Microscopically, the tumors can show any of the patterns seen in islet cell tumors. Many of them resemble the carcinoid tumors of the ileum. Electron microscopy shows in the tumor cells granules like those of the antral G cells, about 275 nm across, membrane bound, with ill-defined content that varies in or smaller granules 170 to 190 nm across, electron density from one granule to another; with an electron-dense core, sometimes with a narrow halo between it and the limiting membrane of the granule, like the granules of the gastrin-secreting cell found in the intestine. Cells with these types of granule are not found in a normal pancreas. A normal pancreas secretes little or no gastrin.

Gastrin has not been identified in the hyperplastic islands found in some of the patients with hypersecretion of gastrin from the pancreas, suggesting that the hyperplasia might be secondary to the hypersecretion and that these people have a gastrin-secreting tumor in the pancreas or elsewhere. If so, the tumor is so small that it escapes detection.

The concentration of gastrin in the plasma is less than 50 ng/L (50 pg/100 mL) in normal people. In patients with a gastrinoma, it is usually over 200 ng/L (200 pg/100 mL) and can exceed 400,000 ng/L (400,000 pg/100 mL). If the diagnosis is in doubt, intravenous secretin increases the concentration of gastrin in the plasma by at least 200 ng/L (200 pg/100 mL) in patients with a gastrinoma. In normal people and in patients with a peptic ulcer, secretin causes no change in the gastrin level or reduces it. An intravenous infusion of calcium gluconate increases the concentration of gastrin in the plasma in people with a gastrinoma, more than 50% or more than 400 ng/L (400 pg/100 mL). Calcium gluconate causes a smaller rise in people with a peptic ulcer. A test meal causes no increase in the concentration of gastrin in the serum in people with a G cell tumor, but a moderate increase in people with a peptic ulcer.

In the tumor, over 90% of the gastrin is little gastrin, G-17. In the plasma, over 70% of the gastrin is big gastrin, G-34. Most of the rest of the circulating gastrin is little gastrin, but large forms of gastrin and small fragments of the molecule are also present in the plasma.

In 3% of patients with a gastrinoma, the tumor produces other hormones as well as gastrin: the adrenocorticotropic hormone, insulin, glucagon, parathormone, the melanocyte-stimulating hormone, secretin, the vasoactive intestinal peptide, or the pancreatic polypeptide. The concentration of the pancreatic polypeptide in the plasma is increased in 30% of the patients.

Zollinger-Ellison Syndrome. The hypersecretion of gastrin produces the Zollinger-Ellison syndrome, named after the American surgeons who described it in 1955. The patients have peptic ulceration, gastric hypersecretion, and a tumor in the pancreas. They are usually between 30 and 60 years old when symptoms begin. The syndrome is not common. Less than 1% of peptic ulcers are caused by a gastrinoma.

In most patients with a gastrinoma, the excess of gastrin in the blood causes gastric hypersecretion. In 70% of them, the basal output of acid is in excess of 10 mmol/h (10 meq/h), as compared with less than 3 mmol/h (3 meq/h) in normal people. Though it varies from person to person, the basal acid output in a patient with a gastrinoma is often over 60% of the maximal output; in normal people and in patients with a peptic ulcer it is usually less than 60% of the maximum.

Over 90% of the patients with a gastrinoma develop one or more peptic ulcers. In 75% of the patients, the ulcer is in the first part of the duodenum or in the stomach. Often there is only one. The ulcer may behave as do peptic ulcers in other people or may be more fulminant and more agressive. If the ulcers are multiple, they often involve the second and third parts of the duodenum or the jejunum, as well as the first part of the duodenum and stomach. Ulcers develop in the distal parts of the duodenum in 15% of the patients and in the jejunum in 10%. The excess of gastric secretion acidifies the distal part of the duodenum and the jejunum, in spite of an attempt by the exocrine pancreas to compensate by increasing the flow of the alkaline pancreatic juice.

Watery diarrhea develops in 40% of patients with the Zollinger-Ellison syndrome. The patients with diarrhea all have hypersecretion of gastric juice. The large volume of gastric secretion washing into the intestine contributes to the causation of the diarrhea, but it is not the only factor. In some patients with a gastrinoma and diarrhea, the gastric hypersecretion is no greater than in patients with a duodenal ulcer who do not have a tumor and do not develop diarrhea. Probably the other hormones secreted by the tumor are important. Several of the enteric hormones can cause watery diarrhea.

Less often there is steatorrhea, probably because the excess of gastric acid in the duodenum inhibits pancreatic lipase and precipitates bile salts. Impairment of micelle formation in the gut caused by the lack of bile salts can reduce the absorption of fatty acids and monoglycerides. Occasionally the increased acidity in the bowel reduces the absorption of vitamin B_{12}.

Cimetidine, an H_2 receptor antagonist, reduces gastric secretion and brings healing of the peptic ulcers in over 80% of patients with a gastrinoma. Other medical means of treating people with a peptic ulcer have usually proved ineffective. Total gastrectomy has also proved effective in relieving the symptoms of the Zollinger-Ellison syndrome, by ending gastric secretion. A subtotal gastrectomy is usually followed by prompt recurrence of the ulcer or ulcers.

Attempts to remove the tumor or tumors in the pancreas, together with their metastases, have succeeded in only 10% of the patients. Fortunately, most G cell tumors grow slowly and spread sluggishly. Nearly 50% of patients treated by total gastrectomy are alive and well 10 years later, even though the tumor was not removed. Chemotherapy can slow the growth of some G cell tumors and reduce the secretion of gastrin.

Antral G Cell Hyperplasia. In 1% of patients with the Zollinger-Ellison syndrome, the hypergastrinemia is caused by hyperplasia of the G cells in the gastric antrum, not by a tumor. Hypergastrinemia caused by antral hyperplasia can be distinguished from that caused by a gastrinoma by giving a test meal. If the hypergastrinemia is caused by a tumor, the concentration of gastrin in the plasma will increase by less than 50%. If it is caused by antral hyperplasia, in will increase by over 300%. Injection of secretin increases the concentration of gastrin in the plasma if hypergastrinemia is caused by a tumor, but causes a decrease if it is caused by hyperplasia of the G cells in the antrum.

VIPOMA. About 4% of islet cell tumors cause profuse, watery diarrhea, hypokalemia, and achlorhydria or hypochlorhydria. About 70% of the patients are hypercalcemic, and 50% have hyperglycemia. The gallbladder is often dilated. The diarrhea and hypokalemia can be severe, even threatening life. The condition has been called pancreatic cholera or the WDHA syndrome, for Watery Diarrhea, Hypokalemia, Achlorhydria.

Most of these tumors secrete the vasoactive intestinal peptide, VIP, and are called vipomata. Often the tumor secretes secretin, glucagon, or the pancreatic polypeptide as well as the vasoactive peptide. Some secrete predominantly the pancreatic polypeptide; some secrete other hormones. Over 50% of the tumors are malignant.

If the tumor is benign, resection cures. If it is malignant, metastases are often present by the time the diagnosis is made.

PP-OMA. A few islet cell tumors consist entirely of PP cells and secrete only the pancreatic polypeptide. This type of tumor is sometimes called a PP-oma. The excess of the peptide causes no symptoms or dysfunction. The tumors are benign.

OTHER ISLET CELL TUMORS. Occasionally an islet cell tumor secretes 5-hydroxytryptamine and causes the carcinoid syndrome. A few secrete a substance like the adrenocorticotropic hormone and cause Cushing's syndrome. Rarely, an islet cell tumor produces significant quantities of the melanocyte-stimulating hormone, vasopressin, parathormone, or calcitonin.

MULTIPLE ENDOCRINE NEOPLASIA. Islet cell tumors are one element in the syndrome of multiple endocrine neoplasia type I, sometimes called the Wermer syndrome, after the American physician who described it in 1954. In the multiple endocrine neoplasia syndromes, hyperplasia or a neoplasm develops in at least two endocrine organs. In type I, the islets of Langerhans, parathyroid glands, adrenal cortices, anterior pituitary gland, or the parafollicular cells of the thyroid are involved. The neoplasms in the parathyroid and pituitary glands are usually benign, but those in the pancreas, adrenal cortex, and thyroid are commonly malignant. In addition, there are often multiple lipomata in the skin and elsewhere, and sometimes carcinoid tumors in the gut. About 70% of the patients show lesions in two of the organs; 20% have lesions in three. Sometimes an islet cell tumor appears months or years before lesions in other endocrine organs become evident.

Multiple endocrine neoplasia is inherited as an autosomal dominant character with variable penetrance. Symptoms can develop at any age. Men and women are affected equally. The pancreas is involved in 70% of the patients, the parathyroid glands in 90%, the pituitary in 50%, the adrenal glands in 40%, and the thyroid in 20%.

In 50% of patients with Wermer's syndrome, the tumor in the pancreas is a gastrinoma, though only 20% of patients with a gastrinoma have Wermer's syndrome. In 75% of the patients with multiple endocrine neoplasia who have a gastrinoma, the tumors are multiple. Often the pancreas is studded with tiny tumors or shows widespread hyperplasia of the islets and the formation of new islets from the ductules. Most gastrinomata in multiple endocrine neoplasia are malignant.

In 30% of patients with multiple endocrine neoplasia, the islet cell tumor is an insulinoma, but only 5% of patients with an insulinoma have Wermer's syndrome. Many of the patients have more than one insulinoma. In 85% of the patients, the tumors are benign. In 10% of the patients, the islet cell tumor is a vipoma. Rarely, it is a glucagonoma or some other form of islet cell tumor.

Many of the islet cell tumors in multiple endocrine neoplasia secrete more than one hormone. Sometimes more than one kind of islet cell tumor is found in the pancreas. Occasionally another kind of islet cell tumor develops years after the excision of an insulinoma.

BIBLIOGRAPHY

General

Bloodworth, J. M. B., and Grieder, M.: Endocrine pancreas and diabetes mellitus. *In* Endocrine Pathology, 2nd ed. Edited by J. M. B. Bloodworth. Baltimore, Williams & Wilkins, 1982.

Cooperstein, S. J., and Watkins, D. (Eds.): The Islets of Langerhans. New York, Academic Press, 1981.

Cruickshank, A. H.: Pathology of the Pancreas. Berlin, Springer-Verlag, 1986.

Klöppel, G., and Heitz, P. U.: Pancreatic Pathology. Edinburgh, Churchill Livingstone, 1984.

Longnecker, D. S.: Pathology and pathogenesis of diseases of the pancreas. Am. J. Pathol., *107*:102, 1982.

Pancreatitis

Aho, H. J., et al.: Human acute pancreatitis. A light and electron microscopic study. Acta Pathol. Microbiol. Immunol. Scand., Sect A, *90*:367, 1982.

Baker, R. J., and Duarte, B.: The current status of recognition and treatment of severe necrotizing pancreatitis. Surg. Annu., *18*:129, 1986.

Bank, S.: Chronic pancreatitis: clinical features and medical management. Am. J. Gastroenterol., 81:153, 1986.

Bess, M. A., Edis, A. J., and van Heerden, J. A.: Hyperparathyroidism and pancreatitis. JAMA, 243:246, 1980.

Carey, L. C.: Pathophysiologic factors in recurrent acute pancreatitis. Jpn. J. Surg., 15:333, 1985.

Foulis, A. K.: Histological evidence of initiating factors in acute necrotizing pancreatitis. J. Clin. Pathol., 33: 1125, 1980.

Foulis, A. K.: Acute pancreatitis. Rec. Adv. Histopathol., 12:188, 1984.

Glazer, G., Gilliland, E. L., and Aldridge, M. A.: The role of prostaglandins in acute pancreatitis. Surg. Annu., 19:175, 1987.

Greenberger, N. J.: Etiology and pathogenesis of chronic pancreatitis. Hosp. Pract., 20(9):83 1985.

Helin, H., Mero, M., Helin, M., and Markkula, H.: Elastic tissue and injury in human pancreatitis. Pathol. Res. Pract., 172:170, 1981.

Hollender, L. F., Lehnert, P., and Wanke, M.: Acute Pancreatitis. Munich, Urban and Schwartzenberg, 1983.

Isolauri, J., Teerenhovi, O., Lehmusto, P., and Auvinen, O.: Surgical treatment of pancreatic pseudocysts. Ann. Chir. Gynaecol., 74:270, 1985.

Kane, M. G., and Krejs, G. J.: Pancreatic pseudocyst. Adv. Intern. Med., 29:271, 1984.

Lake-Bakaar, G.: Alcohol and the pancreas. Br. Med. Bull., 38:57, 1982.

Lott, J. A.: Inflammatory disease of the pancreas. CRC Crit. Rev. Clin. Lab. Sci., 17:201, 1982.

Malagelada, J. R.: The pathophysiology of alcoholic pancreatitis. Pancreas, 1:270, 1986.

Reynolds, J. C., et al.: Acute pancreatitis in systemic lupus erythematosus. Medicine, 61:25, 1982.

Sanfrey, H., Sarr, M. G., Buckley, G. B., and Cameron, J. L.: Oxygen-derived free radicals and acute pancreatitis. Acta Physiol. Scand. (Suppl), 548:109, 1986.

Sarles, H.: Alcohol and the pancreas. Acta Med. Scand. (Suppl), 703:235, 1985.

Sarles, H.: Etiopathogenesis and definition of chronic pancreatitis. Dig. Dis. Sci., 31(9 Suppl):91S, 1986.

Sarles, H., and Sahel, J.: Pathology of chronic calcifying pancreatitis. Am. J. Gasteroenterol., 66:117, 1976.

Steinberg, W.M.: Acute drug and toxin induced pancreatitis. Hosp. Pract., 20(5):95, 1985.

Volkholz, H., Stolte, M., and Becker, V.: Epithelial dysplasias in chronic pancreatitis. Virchow's Arch., [A], 396:331, 1982.

Cystic Fibrosis

Abramowsky, C. R., and Swinehart, G. L.: The nephropathy of cystic fibrosis. Hum. Pathol., 13:934, 1982.

Adrian, T. E., et al.: Pancreatic gut hormone abnormalities in cystic fibrosis. Gut, 21:A 448, 1980.

David, T. J.: Nasal polyposis, opaque paranasal sinuses and usually normal hearing: the otorhinolaryngological features of cystic fibrosis. J. R. Soc. Med., 79(Suppl 12):23, 1986.

David, T. J. (Ed.): Current clinical management of cystic fibrosis. J. R. Soc. Med., 79(Suppl 12):1, 1986.

Fiegal, R. J., et al.: Cystic fibrosis. Ann. N. Y. Acad. Sci., 488:82, 1986.

Friend, P. A.: Pulmonary infection in cystic fibrosis. J. Infect., 13:55, 1986.

Holsclaw, D. S.: Cystic fibrosis. Clin. Chest Med., 1: 407, 1980.

Iannucci, A., Mukai, K., Johnson, D., and Burke, B.: Endocrine pancreas in cystic fibrosis. Hum. Pathol., 15:278, 1984.

Park, R. W., and Grand, R. J.: Gastro-intestinal manifestations of cystic fibrosis. Gastroenterology, 81:1143, 1981.

Phillips, B. M., and David, T. J.: Pathogenesis and management of arthropathy in cystic fibrosis. J. R. Soc. Med., 79(Suppl 12):44, 1986.

Pier, G. B.: Pulmonary disease associated with Pseudomonas aeruginosa in cystic fibrosis. J. Infect. Dis., 151:575, 1985.

Rubio, T. T.: Infection in patients with cystic fibrosis. Am. J. Med., 81(1A):73, 1986.

Sant'Agnese, P. R., and Davis. P. B.: Cystic fibrosis in adults. Am. J. Med., 66:121, 1979.

Diabetes Mellitus

Ahmad, A., and Abraham, A. A.: Pancreatic isletitis with coxsackie virus B5 infection. Hum. Pathol., 13:661, 1982.

Bennett, P. H.: The diagnosis of diabetes mellitus: new international classification. Annu. Rev. Med., 34:295, 1983.

Boitard, C., Debray-Sachs, M., and Bach, J. F.: Autoimmune disorders in diabetes. Adv. Nephrol., 15:281, 1986.

Bottazzo, G. F., et al.: In situ characterization of autoimmune phenomena and expression of HLA moleules in the pancreas in diabetes mellitus. N. Engl. J. Med., 313:353, 1985.

Buse, J. B., and Eisenbarth, G. S.: Autoimmune endocrine disease. Vitam. Horm., 42:253, 1985.

DeFronzo, R. A., and Ferrannini, E.: The pathogenesis of non-insulin-dependent diabetes mellitus. Medicine, 61:125, 1982.

Doniach, D., Bottazzo, G. F., and Cudworth, A. G.: Etiology of type I diabetes mellitus. Annu. Rev. Med., 34:13, 1983.

Dunger, D. B., and Grant, D. B.: Endocrine disorders: diabetes mellitus, congenital hypothyroidism, and congenital adrenal hyperplasia. Br. Med. Bull., 42: 187, 1986.

Eisenbarth, G. S.: Type I diabetes mellitus. A chronic autoimmune disease. N. Engl. J. Med., 314:1360, 1986.

Ekoe, J. M.: Recent trends in the prevalence and incidence of diabetes mellitus. Diabetes Res. Clin. Pract., 1:249, 1985.

Ferrannini, E.: Insulin resistance, insulin deficiency and the pathogenesis of diabetes mellitus. Clin. Physiol., 6:311, 1986.

Gerich, J. E.: Insulin-dependent diabetes mellitus:

pathophysiology. Mayo Clin. Proc., *61*:787, 1986.

Grammer, L.: Insulin allergy. Clin. Rev. Allergy, *4*:189, 1986.

Grundfest-Broniatowski, S., and Novick, A.: Pancreas transplantation — 1985. Transplant. Proc., *18*(3 Suppl 2):31, 1986.

Henson, V., et al.: Molecular genetics of insulin-dependent diabetes mellitus. Mol. Biol. Med., 3:129, 1986.

Klöppel, G., et al.: Ultrastructure and immunocytochemistry of the endocrine pancreas in diabetes. Medicina, 2:299, 1982.

Lacey, P. E., and Sharp, D. W.: Transplantation of pancreatic islets. Annu. Rev. Med., 37:33, 1986.

Maloy, A. L., Longnecker, D. S., and Greenberg, E. R.: The relation of islet amyloid to the clinical type of diabetes. Hum. Pathol., *12*:917, 1981.

Marble, A. M. (Ed.): Joslin's Diabetes Mellitus. 12th Ed. Philadelphia, Lea & Febiger, 1985.

Mukai, K.: Functional pathology of pancreatic islets. Pathol. Annu., *18*(Pt 2):87, 1983.

National Diabetes Group: Classification and diagnosis of diabetes mellitus and other categories of glucose intolerance. Diabetes, 28:1039, 1979.

Neumer, C., Brandt, R., and Zühlke, H.: The human insulin gene and diabetes mellitus. Exp. Clin. Endocrinol., *87*:89, 1986.

Powers, A. C., and Eisenbarth, G. S.: Autoimmunity to islet cells in diabetes mellitus. Annu. Rev. Med., 36: 533, 1985.

Rabinowe, S. L., and Eisenbarth, G. S.: Polyglandular antoimmunity. Adv. Intern. Med., *31*:293, 1986.

Raskin, P., and Rosenstock, J.: Blood glucose control and diabetic complictions. Ann. Intern. Med., 105: 254, 1986.

Reaven, G. M. (Ed.): The role of insulin resistance in the pathogenesis and treatment of non-insulin-dependent diabetes mellitus. Am. J. Med., *74*(1A):1, 1983.

Rose, N. R., and Mackay, I. R. (Eds.): The Autoimmune Diseases. New York, Academic Press, 1985.

Rossini, A. A., Mordes, J. P., and Like, A. A.: Immunology of insulin-dependent diabetes mellitus. Annu. Rev. Immunol., 3:289, 1985.

Schneider, H. M., Störkel, F. S., and Will, W.: The influence of insulin on local amyloidosis of the islets of Langerhans and insulinoma. Pathol. Res. Pract., *170*: 180, 1980.

Stefan, Y., et al.: Quantitation of endocrine cell content in the pancreas of nondiabetic and diabetic humans. Diabetes, *31*:694, 1982.

Ungar, R. H.: Glucagon physiology and pathophysiology in the light of new advances. Diabetologia, 28:574, 1985.

Ward, W. K., Beard, J. C., and Porte, D. Jr.: Clinical aspects of islet B-cell function in non-insulin-dependent diabetes mellitus. Diabetes Metab. Rev., 2:297, 1986.

Weir, G. C., et al. Experimental reduction of B cell mass: implications for the pathogenesis of diabetes. Diabetes Metab. Rev., 2:125, 1986.

Westbroek, D. L.: Pancreas tissue transplantation. Neth. J. Surg., 39:4, 1987.

Zimmet, P.: Type 2 (non-insulin-dependent) diabetes — an immunological overview. Diabetologia, 22:399, 1982.

Other Non-Neoplastic Diseases

Nagai, H., and Ohtsubo, K.: Pancreatic lithiasis in the aged. Gastroenterology, *86*:331, 1984.

Tumors

Akagi, T., and Fujii, Y.: Hitology, ultrastructure, and tissue culture of human insulinomas. Cancer, 47:417, 1981.

Allen-Mersh, T. G.: Significance of the site of origin of pancreatic exocrine adenocarcinoma. J. Clin. Pathol., 35:544, 1982.

Andrén-Sandberg, Å.: Estrogens and pancreatic cancer. Scand. J. Gastroenterol., 21:129, 1986.

Benarde, M. A., and Weiss, W.: Coffee consumption and pancreatic cancer. Br. Med. J., *1*:400, 1982.

Berger, M., et al.: Functional and morphologic characterization of human insulinomas. Diabetes, 32:921, 1983.

Blackman, M. R., et al.: Human placental and pituitary glycoprotein hormones and their subunits as tumor markers. J. Nat. Cancer. Inst., 65:81, 1981.

Bloom, S. R., et al.: Diarrhoea in vipoma patients. Lancet, 2:1163, 1983.

Bloom, S. R., and Polak, J. M.: Glucagonomas, VIPomas, and somatostatinomas. Clin. Endocrinol., 9:285, 1980.

Bogomoletz, W. V., et al.: Cystadenoma of the pancreas. Histopathology, *4*:309, 1980.

Bombi, J. A., et al.: Papillary-cystic neoplasm of the pancreas. Cancer, 58:780, 1984.

Cantrell, B. B., et al.: Acinar cell cystadenocarcinoma of the human pancreas. Cancer, 47:410, 1981.

Capella, C., et al.: Morphological patterns and diagnostic criteria of VIP-producing endocrine cell tumors of the pancreas and gut. Cancer, 52:1860, 1983.

Chen, J., and Baithun, S. I.: Morphological study of 391 cases of exocrine pancreatic tumours. J. Pathol., *146*: 17, 1985.

Chen, J., Baithun, S. I., and Ramsay, M. A.: Histogenesis of pancreatic carcinomas. J. Pathol., *146*:65, 1985.

Corrente, R. F.: Cystadenocarcinoma of the pancreas. Am. J. Surg., *139*:265, 1980.

D'Arcangues, C. M., Awoke, S., and Lawrence, G. D.: Metastatic insulinoma with long survivial and glucagonoma syndrome. Ann. Intern. Med., *100*:233, 1984.

DeLellis, R. A., et al.: Multiple endocrine neoplasia (MEN) syndromes. Int. Rev. Exp. Pathol., 28:163, 1986.

Frantz, V. K.: Tumors of the Pancreas. Washington D. C., Armed Forces Institute of Pathology, 1959.

Friesen, S. R.: Tumors of the endocrine pancreas. N. Engl. J. Med., *306*:580, 1982.

Gould, V. E., Memoli, V. A., Dardi, L. E., and Gould, N. S.: Nesidiodysplasia and nesidioblastosis of infancy. Pediatr. Pathol., *1*:7, 1983.

Heitz, P. U., Kasper, M., Polak, J. M., and Klöppel, G.: Pancreatic endocrine tumors. Hum. Pathol., *13*:263, 1982.

Heuch, I., Kva(v)le, G., Jacobsen, B. K., and Bjelke,

E.: Use of alcohol, tobacco and coffee, and risk of pancreatic cancer. Br. J. Cancer, 48:637, 1983.

Kameya, T., Shimosato, Y., Abe, K., and Takeuchi, T.: Morphologic and functional aspects of hormone-producing tumors. Pathol. Annu., 15(Pt 1):351, 1980.

Kaplan, E. L., and Michelassi, F.: Endocrine tumors of the pancreas and their clinical syndromes. Surg. Annu., 18:181, 1986.

Karnauchow, P. N.: Nesidioblastosis in adults without insular hyperfunction. Am. J. Clin. Pathol., 78:511, 1982.

Kinlen, L., Goldblatt, P., Fox, J., Yudkin, J.: Coffee and pancreas carcinoma. Lancet, 1:282, 1984.

Learmouth, G. M., Price, S. K., Visser, A. E., and Emms, M.: Papillary and cystic neoplasm of the pancreas — an acinic cell tumor? Histopathology, 9:63, 1985.

Levin, D. L., Connelly, R. R., Devesa, S. S.: Demographic characteristics of cancer of the pancreas. Cancer, 47:1456, 1981.

Longnecker, D. S., Wiebkin, P., Schaeffer, B. K., and Roebuck, B. D.: Experimental carcinogenesis in the pancreas. Int. Rev. Exp. Pathol., 26:177, 1984.

McCarthy, P. H.: The Zollinger-Ellison syndrome. Annu. Rev. Med., 33:197, 1982.

Mendelsohn, G.: Vasoactive intestinal peptide (VIP) and the spectrum of tumors producing the watery diarrhea syndrome. Prog. Surg. Pathol., 4:199, 1982.

Moosa, A. R. (Ed.): Tumors of the Pancreas. Baltimore, Williams & Wilkins, 1980.

Moosa, A. R., and Dawson, P. J.: The diagnosis of pancreatic cancer. Pathobiol. Annu, 11:299, 1981.

Morohoshi, T., Held, G., and Klöppel, G.: Exocrine pancreatic tumours and their histological classification. Histopathology, 7:645, 1983.

Norbin, A., et al.: Pancreatic polypeptide-producing tumors. Cancer, 53:2688, 1984.

Pour, P. M., Sayed, S., and Sayed, G.: Hyperplastic, preneoplastic and neoplastic lesions found in 83 human pancreases. Am. J. Clin. Pathol., 77:137, 1982.

Scarpelli, D. G., Reddy, J. K., and Longnecker, D. S. (Eds.): Experimental pancreatic carcinogenesis. Boca Raton, CRC Press, 1987.

Schimke, R. N.: Genetic aspects of multiple endocrine neoplasia. Annu. Rev. Med., 35:25, 1984.

Yamaguchi, K., Kameya, T., and Abe, K.: Multiple endocrine neoplasia type 1. Clin. Endocrinol., 9:261, 1980.

39

Urinary Tract

THE urinary tract consists of the renal pelvis, ureters, urinary bladder, and urethra. Infection, obstruction, stones, and tumors are its major disorders, though neuromuscular dysfunction, congenital anomalies, and a variety of other conditions can involve the urinary system.

INFECTION

Infection of the urinary tract is common, especially in girls and women. Most of the people infected have bacteriuria, with an excess of bacteria in the urine, but no other sign of urinary infection. Less often, inflammation of the tissues of some part of the urinary tract is evident.

Pathogenesis. Urinary tract infection is usually caused by the entry of bacteria into the urethra. The bacteria multiply in the urine in the urethra and often the bladder. Less often the urine in the ureters, renal pelves, or kidneys is infected. Occasionally the bacteria are carried to the urinary tract in the blood or spread into the tract from some neighboring infection.

Infection is easier in girls and women because the short female urethra makes it easier for the bacteria to reach the relatively stagnant urine in the bladder, where they can multiply more easily. In boys and men, the bacteria are likely to be flushed out of the urethra by micturition before they reach the bladder.

Obstruction increases the risk of urinary infection. The frequent flushing of the urinary tract as the urine passes down the ureters and is expelled from the bladder and urethra during micturition is one of the tract's major defenses against infection. Bacteria can proliferate more easily in the stagnant urine proximal to an obstruction.

Instrumentation easily carries bacteria into the urinary bladder or beyond an obstruction. If an indwelling catheter remains in place for more than a short time, urinary infection is almost inevitable.

The ureterovesical sphincters normally prevent the ascent of infection from the bladder into the ureters. The ureters pass obliquely through the bladder wall and are squeezed shut during micturition. If the sphicters are incompetent, reflux of urine into the ureters readily causes infection of the urine in the ureters, renal pelves, and kidneys.

The urothelium lining the urinary tract usually prevents infection of the tissues lining the urinary tract. Few bacteria can penetrate the epithelium, and except in the urethra there are no glands to facilitate the entry of the bacteria into the tissues.

BACTERIURIA. The urine is infected in between 1 and 10% of girls and women, but is usually sterile in boys and men unless there is obstruction or some other factor that favors urinary infection. Only the infections of the tissues of the urinary tract are discussed here. Bacteriuria without evidence of infection of the tissues is considered in Chapter 27 with the diseases of the kidneys.

PYELITIS. Inflammation of a renal pelvis is called pyelitis, from the Greek for a trough. It is often, perhaps always, associated with infection of the kidney. Usually the infection of the kidney overshadows the infection of its pelvis.

Acute. Probably acute pyelitis is common when an ascending urinary infection reaches one or both renal pelves. It is invariably present in acute pyelonephritis. The pelvis is congested and edematous with an exudate predominantly of neutrophils. In most people, the inflammation in the pelvis resolves with little residual injury.

Chronic. Chronic pyelitis probably results from repeated attacks of mild acute

1235

pyelitis. The wall of one or both renal pelves is thickened and fibrotic, usually with a moderate exudate of lymphocytes, plasma cells, and macrophages. Sometimes nodules of lymphocytes are present in the wall of the inflamed pelvis. Chronic pyelitis is present in all patients with chronic pyelonephritis and is sometimes found in people without evidence of renal inflammation.

URETERITIS. Infection of the ureter is almost always secondary to pyelitis or cystitis. In pyelitis, the proximal part of the ureter often shows acute or chronic inflammation, similar to that in the renal pelvis. In cystitis, infection and inflammation sometimes spread into the distal part of the ureter. Infection confined to the ureter is rare. The inflammation of the ureter is usually mild, but occasionally acute ureteritis causes ulceration or bleeding.

CYSTITIS. Inflammation of the urinary bladder is called cystitis, from the Greek for a bladder. Infection usually follows obstruction or instrumentation and is caused by bacteria that ascend the urethra in the urine.

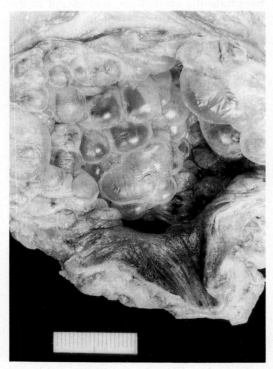

Fig. 39-1. Bullous cystitis, showing edematous blebs of mucosa bulging into the urinary bladder.

Escherichia coli is the most common invader, though Proteus, Klebsiella, Aerobacter, Pseudomonas, Serratia, and other gram-negative bacteria are frequently found, alone or in combination. Staphylococci and other gram-positive organisms are less common. Occasionally cystitis is caused by extension of infection from diverticulitis or some other pelvic infection. Occasionally diverticulitis causes a fistula between the colon and the bladder.

Acute. In acute cystitis, the infection may range from mild edema and congestion of the mucosa, with an exudate of a few neutrophils, to massive edema and congestion, with an intense exudate of neutrophils, often with lymphocytes and macrophages as well. If the inflammation is severe, ulceration is common. Pus escapes in large quantity into the urine. Hemorrhage into the inflamed mucosa often causes leakage of blood into the urine. Fibrin sometimes forms a membrane over the ulcers and surrounding mucosa. Particularly when infection complicates irradiation or trauma, part of the wall of the bladder may become necrotic and gangrenous.

Acute cystitis causes frequency and urgency of urination and often burning pain when water is passed. The urine may be cloudy, malodorous, or bloody. Discomfort or tenderness is sometimes evident over the bladder. Fever and leukocytosis are usually slight or absent if the infection is confined to the bladder.

Chronic. Chronic cystitis usually results from repeated attacks of acute cystitis and is often complicated by recurrent bouts of acute cystitis. Chronic cystitis varies greatly in severity. There may be only a mild exudate predominantly of lymphocytes and macrophages in the subepithelial tissues, or the inflammation may involve the whole thickness of the bladder wall, with an extensive exudate of lymphocytes, macrophages, and plasma cells. Occasionally fibrosis is severe enough to make the bladder small and shrunken.

Not uncommonly, Esch. coli or other bacteria split the urea present in the urine, forming ammonia and rendering the urine in the bladder alkaline. Because of the alkalinity, calcium carbonate, calcium magnesium carbonate, and other salts precipitate in the inflamed mucosa, forming hard, gray, calcareous patches, which appear to overlie the mucosa, a condition called encrusted cystitis, or calcareous cystitis. The calcareous patches are most common at the base of the bladder, over the trigone or around the ureteric orifices. The salts are deposited in the inflamed tissue, so that if the plaque is pulled off, a raw, bleeding surface is left.

In other patients with chronic cystitis, edematous masses of mucosa bulge into the lumen in polypoid fashion, a condition called bullous cystitis. The inflammatory exudate may form discrete nodules in the submucosa, perhaps with germinal centers in the nodules, a variant called follicular cystitis. Sometimes the nodules are large enough to make the mucosa granular, especially over the trigone. Uncommonly, most often in diabetics, the bacteria form bubbles of gas in the tissues, a condition called emphysematous cystitis.

URETHRITIS. The most common infections of the urethra are gonorrhea, discussed in Chapter 16, and the nonspecific urethritis caused by chlamydial or mycoplasmal infection and discussed in Chapter 17. The infections with gram-negative bacilli common in the urinary tract rarely involve the tissues of the urethra, though the organisms are present in the urine.

TUBERCULOSIS. The renal pelves, ureters, and bladder are often involved in renal tuberculosis, as discussed in Chapter 27. The usual tuberculous granulomata appear in the submucosa. The granulomata are usually few but may become confluent, with caseous necrosis and ulceration. If the ureters are severely involved, their wall becomes thick and fibrotic. The scarring sometimes causes stenosis; sometimes the ureter becomes widely dilated and ectatic. In the bladder, the tubercles appear first around the ureteric orifices and on the trigone. They may coalesce to cause ulceration and, occasionally, scarring. In most patients, the ureteric and vesical disease resolves if the infected kidney is removed.

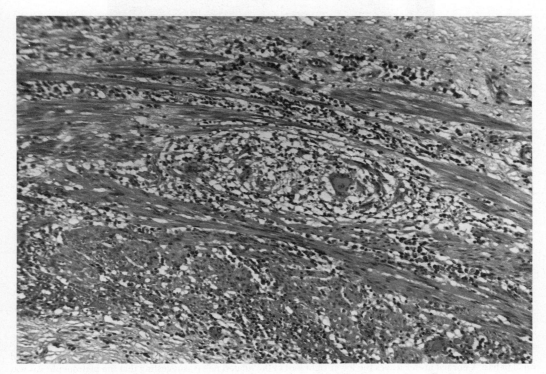

Fig. 39-2. Tuberculous ureteritis, showing a tuberculous granuloma in the wall of a ureter.

OTHER KINDS OF INFECTION. Mycotic infections of the bladder are rare, except for candidiasis in the debilitated. Schistosomiasis is important in much of the world. The lesions it causes in the urinary tract are discussed in Chapter 21. The bladder may be involved in lymphogranuloma venereum, as described in Chapter 17. Trichomonal infection of the urethra is discussed in Chapter 20.

OBSTRUCTION

Obstruction in the urinary tract is common and may occur at any age, from infancy to old age. Hydronephrosis is found in over 3% of autopsies. Obstruction can occur in any part of the urinary tract. It can cause dilatation and hypertrophy of the bladder, the dilatation of one or both ureters called hydroureter,

or the dilatation of one or both renal pelves called hydronephrosis.

In children, congenital defects such as malformation of a ureter, valves in the urethra, or a disturbance in the innervation of the ureters are the commonest causes of urinary obstruction. In women, a gravid uterus can compress the ureters causing obstruction, a calculus can obstruct a ureter, or carcinoma of the cervix uteri can occlude a ureter as it spreads across the pelvic brim. Radiation or surgery used to treat the carcinoma can damage a ureter. In men, enlargement of the prostate is the most frequent cause of urinary obstruction, with calculi, strictures, and spinal injuries less common causes. In both sexes and at all ages obstruction often occurs at the ureteropelvic junction, sometimes because the ureter is compressed by a blood vessel or is kinked,

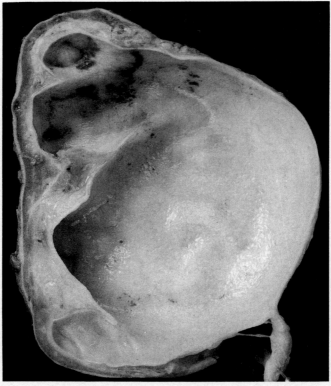

Fig. 39-3. A massive hydronephrosis, showing the remnant of the kidney stretched around the greatly dilated renal pelvis. A normal ureter leaves the lower right part of the dilated pelvis, suggesting that the hydronephrosis was caused by a kink, or some other lesion at the ureteropelvic junction.

but commonly without obvious cause. Occasionally a congenital anomaly in a ureter, phimosis, a sloughed renal papilla, blood clot, trauma, carcinoma of the bladder, or some other neoplasm, an aortic aneurysm, retroperitoneal fibrosis, or a foreign body causes urinary obstruction.

HYDRONEPHROSIS. Obstruction at any level in the urinary tract can cause hydronephrosis, though if the obstruction is distal to the ureteropelvic junctions, hydronephrosis develops only if one or both the ureteropelvic sphincters are incompetent. If the sphincters are competent, obstruction in the urethra causes dilatation and hypertrophy of the bladder, but not hydronephrosis.

Lesions. If the obstruction is sudden and complete, the renal pelvis dilates only slightly before the pressure in the glomeruli of the affected kidney or kidneys becomes so great that glomerular filtration ceases. The obstructed kidney slowly atrophies as weeks pass. If the obstruction is not relieved, the kidney will be destroyed.

More often, the obstruction is incomplete or intermittent. The renal pelvis slowly dilates as weeks pass. The increased pressure in the pelvis blunts the renal papillae, which become progressively shrunken and flattened. First the collecting tubules and then the convoluted tubules in the kidney atrophy. An increase in interstitial tissue separates the atrophic tubules, but the glomeruli remain normal for a long time.

In some patients with incomplete obstruction, the condition becomes stable and remains so for years. The renal pelvis is dilated, and the kidney shows moderate tubular atrophy, but sufficient renal parenchyma remains to preserve normal renal function. In other patients, the hydronephrosis enlarges progressively, and the kidney becomes increasingly atrophic, until all that remains is a thin remnant of the kidney stretched around the circumference of a sac of urine perhaps 20 cm across.

Microscopically, the wall of a hydronephrotic sac is scarred and often shows chronic inflammation.

Dysfunction. The urine in a hydronephrotic sac is not stagnant. Water, electrolytes, and easily diffusible molecules like urea escape from the pelvis into the blood and from the blood into the pelvis. The exchange takes place both in the wall of the renal pelvis and in the renal medulla. Lymph flow from the obstructed kidney is increased.

At first the increased intratubular pressure in the affected kidney causes an increase in renal blood flow, though the glomerular filtration rate and the medullary blood flow fall. Later, the renal blood flow falls, and the glomerular filtration rate is further reduced. At first sodium and water are retained, but as tubular injury becomes more severe, the concentrating power of the kidney and the transport of sodium, potassium, and hydrogen ions are impaired. The synthesis of prostaglandins and later the release of renin increase. Azotemia and hypertension are common. Sometimes there is hyperchloremic hyperkalemic acidosis. If the obstruction is bilateral, oliguria is usual in the early stages of the disease, but later there is often polyuria and nocturia.

Clinical Presentation. Hydronephrosis often causes no symptoms. If the disease is unilateral, and the distention of the pelvis develops slowly, the kidney may have been destroyed before the hydronephrosis is discovered. If the distention develops more rapidly, pain in the region of the affected kidney is common. Particularly in children, a hydronephrosis may present as an abdominal mass.

Treatment and Prognosis. If useful renal function remains in the obstructed kidney, the obstruction should be relieved as soon as possible. If not, slow erosion of the function of the kidney is likely to continue. Sometimes the relief of bilateral obstruction is followed by a massive diuresis, with serious loss of water and electrolytes. The prognosis depends on the degree of renal injury, but usually relief of the obstruction brings some improvement in renal function.

Pyonephrosis. The relatively stagnant urine in hydronephrosis is easily infected. Many of the patients with chronic hydronephrosis have repeated attacks of pyelitis. In some, the infection is more severe and the dilated pelvis becomes filled with pus, a condition called pyonephrosis. The pelvic wall shows the fibrosis caused by the preceding hydronephrosis with superimposed acute inflammation.

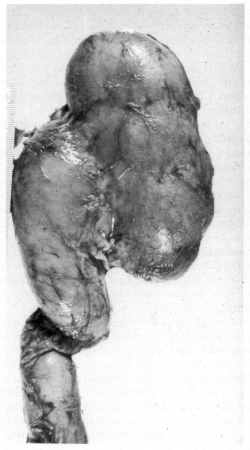

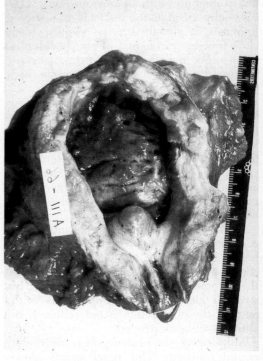

Fig. 39-5. Hypertrophy of the urinary bladder caused by a enlarged prostate gland, showing thickening of the bladder wall and trabeculation of the mucosa.

Fig. 39-4. Hydroureter, showing a considerably dilated ureter in a patient with ureteric obstruction at the pelvic brim.

HYDROURETER. Hydroureter is nearly always associated with hydronephrosis and is overshadowed by the pelvic lesion. The obstruction is often at the ureterovesical junction or in the urethra. The affected ureter or ureters become greatly dilated, perhaps 2 or 3 cm in diameter, elongated, and tortuous. The wall of the ectatic ureter is fibrotic, with chronic inflammation. It can no longer move the urine down into the bladder by peristalsis.

HYPERTROPHY OF THE BLADDER. Obstruction at the bladder neck or in the urethra causes hypertrophy and dilatation of the bladder. Enlargement of the prostate gland is its most common cause.

The bladder is often dilated to several times its normal volume. Its muscle is hypertrophied. At first, the bladder wall is thickened, but as the dilatation increases, the bladder wall becomes thin, in spite of the hypertrophy. The inner aspect of the bladder becomes strikingly trabeculated, as hypertrophic bundles of muscle crisscross beneath the mucosa. Sometimes diverticula bulge through the thin parts of the vesical wall between the trabeculae. The bladder can no longer empty completely. Infection is commonly superimposed on the obstruction.

Normally, the ureters run obliquely through the vesical wall and are compressed and occluded by the contracting vesical muscle during micturition. As the bladder becomes dilated and its wall is thinned, the ureters pass more directly into the bladder, and the ureterovesical sphincters often become incompetent. When they do, the increased pressure in the bladder is transmitted to the ureters and renal pelves, and hydroureter and hydronephrosis are added into the dilatation and hypertrophy of the bladder.

NEUROMUSCULAR DYSFUNCTION

The neurologic mechanisms that govern the peristaltic movements of the ureters and the contraction and relaxation of the urinary bladder can be disrupted by injury to the central or peripheral nervous system. The injury is caused by disease or trauma or a congenital defect.

NEUROGENIC BLADDER. In an infant, when the bladder fills, the distention excites a reflex though the spinal cord that causes complete and efficient emptying of the bladder. Older people control this reflex and voluntarily relax or contract the urinary sphincters by neurologic stimuli that originate in the cerebral cortex.

If the cerebral cortex or the pathways leading from it to the spinal cord are damaged by infarction, tumor, multiple sclerosis, or in some other way, voluntary control of the urinary sphincters is sometimes impaired. The patients suffer frequency, urgency, and enuresis. When the bladder fills, it must be emptied. The most the patient can do is to contract the urinary sphincters for a few moments. The capacity of the bladder is less than normal, but it empties completely, with no increase in the quantity of residual urine.

If there is more serious injury to the brain, transection of the spinal cord, or serious injury to the cord, all voluntary control of urination may be lost, but the spinal reflex that governs micturition remains intact. The patient loses all sensation from the bladder, and micturates automatically whenever the bladder is full. In many of these patients the bladder is spastic. The bladder wall is thick and trabeculated. The capacity of the bladder is reduced, so that urination is frequent. The bladder often fails to empty completely. In other patients, the tone of the bladder and its capacity remain more normal. Urination is less frequent and more complete.

If there is injury to the conus or cauda equina, the neurons governing the spinal reflex controlling micturition may be lost.

Efficient automatic micturition is no longer possible, and micturition cannot be initiated voluntarily. All that remains to control the action of the bladder is its intrinsic nervous system. Urination is irregular and incomplete. In some patients the bladder is atonic and becomes greatly dilated, with overflow incontinence and little ability to contract. In other patients, the bladder retains a better tone, and the dilatation is less. Sometimes reasonable function can be maintained if the patient learns to empty the bladder by increasing abdominal pressure or by manual compression.

If the sensory nerves from the bladder are interrupted by disease of the dorsal columns of the spinal cord, the patient no longer has any sensation from the bladder and no longer knows when the bladder is full. Automatic urination does not occur, because the afferent arm of the spinal reflex governing micturition has been destroyed. The patient can urinate voluntarily, but only too often, does not remember to do so. The bladder becomes greatly overdistended. Overflow incontinence occurs. If overdistention of this sort is allowed to continue, the overstretched muscle of the bladder atrophies, and the bladder can no longer contract. It becomes a great flaccid bag. The internal sphincter is atonic and wide open. Only the external sphincter remains to retain the urine.

If the motor side of the reflex governing micturition is destroyed by poliomyelitis or in some other way, both the automatic emptying of the bladder and the power to initiate urination voluntarily are lost. The bladder becomes dilated, with overflow incontinence. The distention of the bladder is painful, because the sensory innervation remains intact.

BLADDER NECK OBSTRUCTION. Especially in infants, obstruction may occur at the bladder neck, in the absence of any mechanical lesion. The cause of this obstruction is uncertain, but it seems likely that at least some cases are due to a neuromuscular disturbance.

URETERAL REFLUX. Reflux of urine from the bladder into the ureters sometimes occurs in the absence of any deformity of the ureteric orifices or any lesion in them and in the absence of any increase in intravesical pressure. In some of these patients, the reflux probably results from malfunction of the muscle in this region.

STONE

In most of the world, most urinary stones originate in a kidney or a renal pelvis. In the United States, each year 120 men and 40 women in every 100,000 develop symptoms caused by a renal or ureteric stone. A renal or ureteric calculus is found in 1% of autopsies. Renal calculi are particularly common in the southeastern part of the United States, in South Africa, in parts of India, and in Southeast Asia. Most of the patients are young adults when a renal stone first becomes evident.

Stones in the bladder used to be common. At the end of the eighteenth century, 1 patient in every 38 admitted to the hospital in Norwich, England, had a bladder stone. Now bladder stones are uncommon except in Thailand, India, and Turkey. In these areas, they are found mainly in young boys. In one hospital in Thailand, 1 boy in every 3 admitted had a bladder stone. The stone may form in the bladder itself, or in a diverticulum bulging from the bladder wall.

Often a familial predisposition to urinary stones is evident, though the nature of the defect in most of these people and the manner of its inheritance are uncertain.

Types. All urinary stones consist of crystals of one or more kinds, bound together by a scant matrix of mucoprotein. The matrix is similar in all urinary stones, but makes up only about 2.5% of the dry weight of the stone.

Must urinary stones consist of salts of calcium. Nearly 40% are a mixture of calcium oxalate and calcium phosphate, nearly 30% of calcium oxalate alone, and under 10% of calcium phosphate alone. Another 15% are made principally of magnesium ammonium phosphate, often called struvite. Less than 5% are made of uric acid, and less than 2% of cystine. Rarely, a stone is made of xanthine.

Morphology. Calcium stones are usually ovoid and small, a centimeter or less in greatest dimension. They are hard and often dark brown. Their surface may be smooth, but often is granular, like a mulberry. Oc-

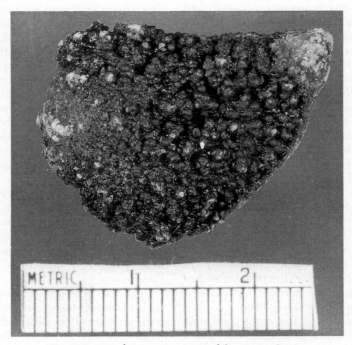

Fig. 39-6. A calcium stone removed from a renal pelvis.

casionally they have long spikes, like a jack-stone. When fractured, calcium stones are usually laminated.

Struvite stones are yellowish white or gray. They may be hard, but often are soft and friable. They tend to be irregularly shaped and large, often filling the renal pelvis and adopting its shape, to form what is called a staghorn calculus.

Uric acid stones are smooth, yellowish brown, and fairly hard. They may be as much as 2 cm in greatest dimension, and are often multiple. On section, the stone is laminated.

Cystine stones are yellowish and waxy. They are small, rounded, smooth, and usually multiple.

Clinical Presentation. Most urinary calculi pass unnoticed. They are small, easily washed down the ureter, and are passed when the bladder is emptied. With uric acid stones and occasionally with calcium oxalate stones, the patient sometimes becomes aware of fine gravel in the urine.

Small renal calculi cause renal colic. As they pass along the ureter, the stone excites violent muscular contractions, to give the excruciating episodic pain typical of renal colic, with its radiation to the lower abdomen, genitalia, or thigh. The pain may persist only a few minutes or may continue for hours. Larger stones in the renal pelvis give few symptoms, perhaps only a dull ache in the loin.

Most renal stones, even asymptomatic ones, damage the urinary tract, causing proteinuria and microscopic hematuria. More severe injury can cause macroscopic, even massive, hematuria. At times a stone in a ureter causes obstruction and hydronephrosis.

The symptoms and signs of stones in the bladder are like those of cystitis and are often associated with infection. Pain aggravated by movement, hematuria, and dysuria are common. Sometimes a stone causes a ball valve obstruction at the bladder neck. Bladder stones may be of the jackstone type, but often become large and spheroidal, filling the bladder or the diverticulum in which they form.

Pathogenesis. Urinary stones form when one or more of the crystalloids that form stones can no longer be held in solution. The concentration of the crystalloid in the urine may be abnormally great, or the factors that normally hold the crystalloids in the urine in solution may be deficient.

If the urine is supersaturated with the ions that form a stone, the ions tend to cluster together. If more than 100 ions form a cluster, it becomes stable and can serve as the nucleus of a stone. Once nucleation has occurred, the stone will continue to grow even if the concentration of the ions in the urine falls.

If the core of the stone and the ions that are subsequently added to it are the same, the process is called homogeneous nucleation. If the ions in the core are different from those subsequently added, the process is called heterogeneous nucleation or epitaxy. Heterogeneous nucleation can occur only if the shape of the ions in the core and those subsequently added are sufficiently alike to enable them to bind together. Inhibitors that prevent nucleation prevent the formation of calcium stones and slow their growth, but have little part in controlling the formation of other kinds of stone.

Calcium Stones. Calcium stones develop when the urine is supersaturated with the ions forming the stone. Often, the stone begins in a renal papilla. Crystals of calcium oxalate or calcium phosphate are precipitated on some irregularity in the tubular lining or around some fragment of debris that serves as a nidus for crystallization. The stone grows as more crystals of calcium oxalate or phosphate are added. Eventually the stone escapes, to lie free in the renal pelvis or to pass into the ureter.

Over 50% of patients with a calcium stone have idiopathic hypercalciuria. The concentration of calcium in the plasma is normal, but excessive amounts of calcium are excreted in the urine. Its cause is unknown. The underlying defect could be in the bowel or in the kidneys. Excessive absorption of calcium from the gut would tend to cause hypercalcemia, reducing the secretion of parathormone and so increasing the excretion of calcium in the urine, to maintain homeostasis. Alternatively, a fault in the renal tubules could cause increased excretion of calcium, tending to cause hypocalcemia, increasing the secretion of the parathyroid hormone, increasing the activation of vitamin

D in the kidneys, and so increasing the absorption of calcium from the gut, again to maintain homeostasis. Whatever the mechanism, the high concentration of calcium in the urine favors the precipitation of calcium crystals and the formation of calcium stones.

Not all people with idiopathic hypercalciuria develop stones. About 5% of the population have idiopathic hypercalciuria, but less than 0.5% develop a urinary stone.

Other causes of hypercalciuria also favor the formation of calcium stones. About 5% of patients with nephrolithiasis have hyperparathyroidism. Under 5% have renal tubular acidosis. Some have sarcoidosis or some other cause of hypercalcemia.

Another 30% of people with calcium stones have hyperuricuria. A high concentration of uric acid in the urine favors the formation of calcium stones because the crystals of uric acid are sufficiently similar to those of calcium oxalate to allow them to serve as a nidus for a calcium stone.

About 15% of people with a calcium stone have hyperuricuria, with a normal concentration of urate in the plasma and with no abnormality of calcium metabolism. These patients are usually men, with a high intake of purines from a diet predominantly of meat. They usually form calcium oxalate stones. Another 10% of people with calcium stones have both hyperuricuria and hypercalciuria, though they are normouricemic and normocalcemic. They tend to develop stones late in life and to form calcium phosphate stones. Some 5% of people with calcium stones have hyperuricemia, with consequent hyperuricuria, from gout or some other cause.

Excess of oxalate in the urine is an uncommon cause of calcium stones. Renal stones are common in oxalosis, as discussed in Chapter 27. Steatorrhea, Crohn's disease, and resection of the ileum, can cause hyperoxaluria, probably because the binding of calcium to fatty acids prevents the formation of calcium oxalate in the bowel, allowing increased absorption of free oxalate. Only rarely does excess ingestion of oxalate, as in rhubarb gluttony, or the ingestion of excessive quantities of precursors of oxalate cause hyperoxaluria. Rarely, it results from pyridoxine deficiency.

The pyrophosphates present in the urine are the principal inhibitors that prevent the formation of calcium oxalate and calcium phosphate stones and slow their growth. Mucopolysaccharides and perhaps citrates in the urine act in similar fashion. In most people with calcium stones, the concentration of the inhibitors in the urine is reduced.

In 20% of patients with calcium stones, the cause of the stone is unknown. There is no abnormality in the urinary excretion of calcium, uric acid, or oxalate or in any other factor known to favor lithiasis.

Struvite Stones. Magnesium ammonium phosphate precipitates in the renal pelvis only if the urine is alkaline and the concentrations of phosphate and of ammonium in the urine are high. Normally, this does not occur. If the urine is alkaline, the concentration of phosphate is high, but the concentration of ammonium is low. Only if the urine is infected with bacteria that form a urease able to split urea to give ammonia can struvite stones develop. The ammonia hydrolyzes to ammonium hydroxide, making the urine alkaline and increasing the concentration of phosphate and of ammonium. Bicarbonate is also ionized in the alkaline urine, and most struvite stones contain calcium apatite as well as struvite.

Infection with one of the species of Proteus is the usual cause of struvite stones, though occasionally a Klebsiella, Pseudomonas, or Enterobacterium is responsible. Esch. coli does not form urease.

Uric Acid Stones. Urates are soluble in urine, but undissociated uric acid is poorly soluble. As the urine grows more acid, the proportion of undissociated uric acid increases, and the risk of stone grows. A low urinary volume increases the risk by increasing the concentration of uric acid. If the pH of the urine is below 6 and the concentration of undissociated uric acid is above 100 mg/L, precipitation of uric acid crystals is likely. This limit can be trangressed even in normal people.

The risk of uric acid stone becomes great if there is hyperuricemia and hyperuricuria, as in gout, or sometimes in leukemia, especially after chemotherapy.

Not all patients with uric acid stones have hyperuricuria. In some the concentrations of uric acid in the plasma and urine are normal, and the cause of the stones is unknown. In some of these people the disease is familial.

Other Stones. The factors leading to the formation of cystine stones are discussed in Chapter 27.

Xanthinuria is a rare congenital anomaly, in which there is deficiency of the enzyme xanthine oxidase, which catalyzes the oxidation of hypoxanthine to xanthine and xanthine to uric acid. Xanthine stones may form in the kidneys in these people.

Treatment and Prognosis. Once urinary stones have begun to form, they are likely to continue to do so throughout the patient's life, unless treatment is instituted. In many patients, symptoms develop every few years. Some of the stones that cause symptoms pass in the urine; others must be removed surgically or be fragmented by lithotripsy.

In people with idiopathic hypercalciuria, thiazide diuretics stimulate the resorption of calcium in the renal tubules and bring relief, reducing the risk of recurrence by more than 90%. In people with hyperuricuria, allopurinol brings relief, both to those forming calcium stones and to those with uric acid stones. Often uric acid stones can be prevented more simply, by increasing the urinary volume and giving citrate to keep the urine alkaline. Large struvite stones are difficult to control and often must be removed before antibiotics can control the infection. Methenamine mandelate (Mandelamine) reduces the alkalinity of the urine and helps control the infection.

OTHER NON-NEOPLASTIC LESIONS

A variety of other non-neoplastic lesions develop in the lower urinary tract. Some are common but of little or no clinical significance. Others are rare but unpleasant.

BRUNN'S NESTS. Brunn's nests, named after the German anatomist von Brunn (1849–1895), are common in the urinary tract. They can be found in the renal pelves; ureters; urinary bladder, especially in the trigone; and sometimes in the urethra. Nearly 90% of people have lesions of this sort somewhere in

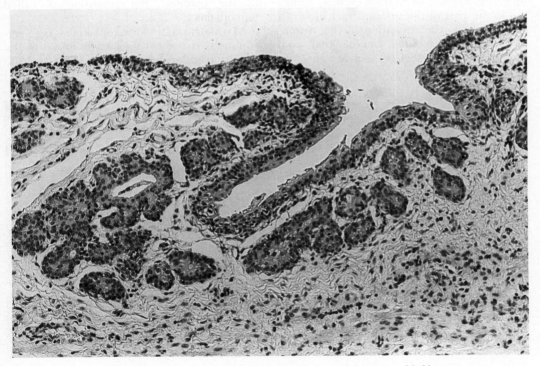

Fig. 39-7. Brunn's nests beneath the epithelium of the urinary bladder.

the lower urinary tract, though they are rarely big enough to be visible to the naked eye.

Brunn's nests begin as a local proliferation of the epithelium in a few or many foci in the urinary tract. The epithelial cells form downgrowths, which bulge into the underlying connective tissue and in cross section appear as isolated nodules of epithelial cells in the connective tissue. Usually, Brunn's nests are solid, but occasionally they contain a small lumen extending down from the surface. The epithelial cells in the nests are fully differentiated and show no abnormality. The epithelial proliferation never extends more than a short distance into the underlying tissue.

In some people, Brunn's nests become cystic. Lumina appear in the center of the clumps of epithelial cells and form small cysts, lined by mucus-secreting epithelium or by low cuboidal epithelium. The cysts may be a millimeter or two in diameter and sometimes bulge up beneath the epithelium or give the epithelium a granular appearance. Lesions of this sort are called pyelitis cystica, ureteritis cystica, or cystitis cystica, according to the part of the urinary tract involved.

Less often, the cavitation of the Brunn's nests forms branching lumina that communicate with the surface, to give a structure that mimics a gland. This kind of lesion is called pyelitis glandularis, ureteritis glandularis, or cystitis glandularis.

The pathogenesis of Brunn's nests is uncertain. If they are sufficiently developed to be apparent macroscopically, they are often associated with chronic inflammation, and many assume that the chronic inflammation causes the epithelial proliferation.

Brunn's nests are almost never of any clinical importance. Rarely is one of the cysts of ureteritis cystica big enough to cause obstruction.

SQUAMOUS METAPLASIA. Squamous metaplasia sometimes complicates inflammation or irritation of the lower urinary tract. Stratified, squamous epithelium, sometimes with keratinization, replaces the transitional epithelium normal in the urinary tract.

Squamous metaplasia of the urinary tract is most common in the urinary bladder; in people with a bladder stone, but it also occurs in conditions like exstrophy of the bladder, in which there is repeated injury to the bladder wall. If the thick, opaque squamous epithelium forms a white plaque in the bladder, the condition is called leukoplakia.

MALAKOPLAKIA. Malakoplakia is uncommon. It is most frequently found in the urinary bladder, but can occur in a testis, the

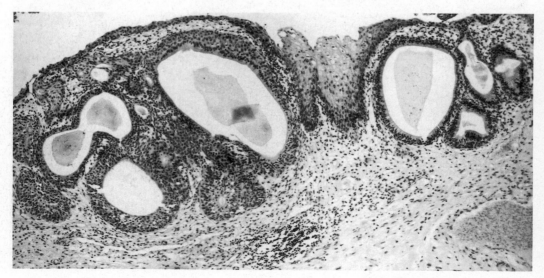

Fig. 39-8. Cystitis cystica, showing the cystic spaces lying beneath the epithelium of the urinary bladder.

prostate, a ureter, or a kidney and occasionally is found in the colon, a lung, a bone, or some other organ. The name comes from the Greek words for soft and flat. In the bladder, soft, flat, yellow or brown plaques form in the mucosa. They are from 0.5 to 5.0 cm across and are slightly elevated above the adjacent epithelium. In other organs, the disease causes similar soft, yellow or brown lesions.

Microscopically, the lesions consist of a massive accumulation of macrophages, a few of which are multinucleated, together with a few lymphocytes and plasma cells. The cytoplasm of the macrophages is finely vacuolated. A few or many of the macrophages contain cytoplasmic inclusions called Michaelis-Gutmann bodies, after the German physicians who described them in 1902. The Michaelis-Gutmann bodies are about the size of a nucleus, spheroidal, and laminated. They stain well with the periodic acid-Schiff reaction and often for iron or calcium. Electron microscopy shows that the bodies are lysosomes filled with debris, consisting principally of the partly digested bodies of Esch. coli and other bacteria.

The cause of this unusual reaction is unknown. In most patients, the disease complicates persistent chronic inflammation. The macrophages phagocytose the bacteria, but are unable to digest them fully.

INTERSTITIAL CYSTITIS. Interstitial cystitis is an uncommon condition, sometimes called Hunner's ulcer after the American surgeon who described it in 1915. The patients are nearly all middle-aged women. Frequency of urination, dysuria, urgency, and abdominal pain are distressing and intractable.

In the early stages of the disease, patches of edema thicken the wall of the vault of the bladder, usually sparing the trigone. Ulcers are not always present. As the lesions age, they become increasingly fibrotic, and fibrosis extends out from the lesions in stellate fashion. As more and more of the bladder is involved, the whole thickness of the bladder wall becomes scarred. The bladder becomes small and shrunken. If it is dilated forcibly, the mucosa splits, giving rise to linear ulcers.

Microscopically, the bladder shows edema with an exudate of lymphocytes, plasma cells, and macrophages and sometimes a few

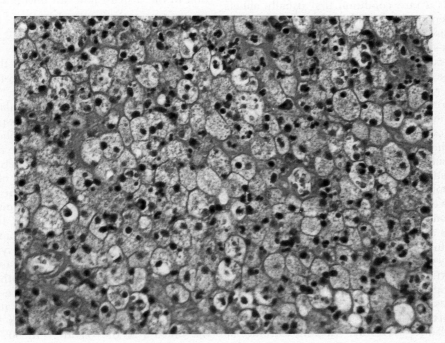

Fig. 39-9. Malakoplakia, showing the massive accumulation of foamy macrophages seen in this condition.

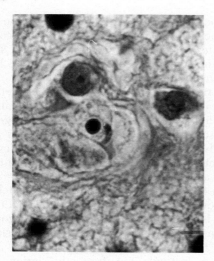

Fig. 39-10.   A high power view of a portion of Fig. 39-9, showing a Michaelis-Gutmann body.

neutrophils or eosinophils. The number of mast cells in the bladder wall increases. If there are ulcers, the inflammation is accentuated in the bed of the ulcer.

The cause of interstitial cystitis is unknown. Treatment is difficult.

EOSINOPHILIC CYSTITIS. Eosinophilic cystitis is a rare condition that usually affects children or young adults. In some patients, it is diffuse, involves much of the bladder, and causes symptoms like those of other kinds of cystitis. In some, it forms one or more tumor-like masses that bulge into the lumen of the bladder. Some of the patients have a history of allergy or asthma. Some have eosinophilia. The tumor-like form of the disease is sometimes called an eosinophilic granuloma.

In the diffuse form of eosinophilic cystitis, the bladder wall is thickened by edema and congestion, with an exudate containing many eosinophils. In the tumor-like form, the masses consist of edematous granulation tissue with an exudate containing many macrophages and eosinophils.

Eosinophilic cystitis resolves, leaving no serious injury. Its cause is unknown.

REITER'S SYNDROME. Reiter's syndrome, the triad of urethritis, conjunctivitis, and arthritis, is discussed in Chapter 60.

RADIATION. Radiation therapy may injure the bladder severely, causing chronic or bullous cystitis that persists for months.

Vesicorectal or vesicovaginal fistulae may develop. Microscopically, there is edema with the atypical fibrocytes and vascular changes usual in radiation injury.

CHEMOTHERAPY. Cyclophosphamide, busulfan, and other chemotherapeutic agents injure the epithelium of the bladder and sometimes the muscle and connective tissues as well. Atypical cells like those shed by carcinomata may be desquamated into the urine and can easily be mistaken for malignant cells.

AMYLOIDOSIS. One or more nodules of amyloid are sometimes found in the bladder in people who have no other evidence of amyloidosis. The nodules lie beneath the mucosa and are up to 3 cm across. Occasionally giant cells are present around the amyloid. The nodules may mimic a neoplasm or cause hematuria.

CONGENITAL ANOMALIES

Congenital anomalies that cause little or no dysfunction are common in the urinary tract, but malformations that cause serious obstruction to the urinary flow are uncommon.

Renal Pelvis and Ureter

The principal abnormalities of the renal pelvis and ureter are duplication, ureterocele, retrocaval ureter, ureteric valves, ureteric stenosis, aperistalsis, and diverticula.

DUPLICATION. In 5% of the population, the renal pelvis and ureter are duplicated on one or both sides. Most often, there is a small upper pelvis and a larger lower pelvis, each leading to its own ureter. In 80% of people with such a duplication, only one side is affected. In 70%, the two ureters join before entering the bladder. Occasionally, the junction of the two ureters is stenotic, but usually ureteropelvic duplication causes no symptoms and no dysfunction. Rarely, there are three, or even four, ureters on one or both sides.

URETEROCELE. Ureteroceles are uncommon. The terminal part of the ureter is dilated and forms a cyst that lies beneath the mucosa of the bladder. In 80% of the patients, the ureterocele drains a duplicated ureter, though only 0.5% of duplicated ureters lead to a ureterocele. There are two kinds of ureterocele.

In one type, the ureteric orifice is in the normal position, but is stenotic. In the other, the ureter runs beneath the mucosa of the bladder to open in an abnormal site, usually in the urethra but sometimes in the vagina, rectum, or a seminal vesicle. The second type of ureterocele is most common in girls. The ureter is often compressed as it runs beneath the bladder mucosa, causing obstruction, but its orifice is widely patent so that the patient commonly has dribbling incontinence.

RETROCAVAL URETER. Rarely, the right ureter passes behind the vena cava, to descend into the pelvis medial to the vena cava. The ureter is sometimes obstructed as it passes behind the vein.

VALVES AND STENOSES. Congenital valves are rare in the ureters, but may cause obstruction. Congenital stenosis of the ureter is also uncommon, though it can occur at the ureteropelvic junction or less often at the ureterovesical junction. More often, an abnormal position of a kidney or unusual motility of a kidney results in kinking of the ureter, usually near the ureteropelvic junction, and causes obstruction. Occasionally an

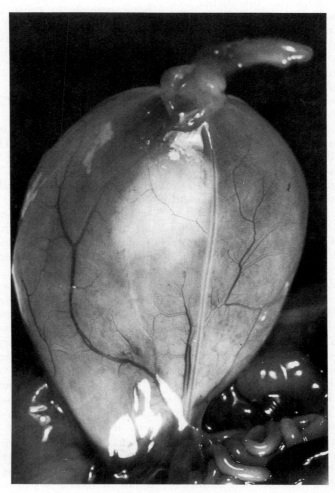

Fig. 39-11. A urachal cyst, showing massive dilatation of the urachus in a stillborn infant. Note the size of the loops of bowel in the lower part of the picture.

aberrant renal artery compresses the ureter near the ureteropelvic junction.

APERISTALSIS. Rarely, peristalsis in the lower part of the ureter fails, impairing the flow of urine and causing megaureter. Probably the dysfunction is caused by an aganglionic segment in the ureter, in the same way as megacolon is caused by an aganglionic segment in the colon.

Diverticula. Diverticula of the ureter are rare, but when they do occur they are congenital.

Bladder

Duplication, agenesis, diverticula, exstrophy, and malformations of the urachus are the main congenital anomalies of the urinary bladder.

DUPLICATION, AGENESIS, DIVERTICULA. Rarely, the urinary bladder is absent, duplicated, or completely or partly divided by a septum. Congenital diverticula of the bladder are uncommon and usually occur in relation to the ureteric orifice. Much more common are the diverticula that develop in elderly men as the vesical mucosa bulges out through the bladder muscle as the bladder hypertrophies in an attempt to overcome the obstruction caused by prostatic enlargement.

EXSTROPHY. Exstrophy of the bladder occurs in 1 birth in 30,000. More than 70% of the infants affected are boys. The ventral part of the bladder and the overlying part of the ventral abdominal wall fail to form properly. The abdominal wall may have only a small orifice through which the trigone sometimes prolapses or a major defect that exposes the whole posterior wall of the bladder. Unless the defect can be repaired, infection is inevitable, with cystitis cystica, cystitis glandularis, often extensive squamous metaplasia. Only about 30% of the infants survive to adult life, but if they do, carcinoma of the bladder is common. Often the symphysis pubis fails to form in infants with exstrophy of the bladder. In boys, epispadias is almost universal.

URACHAL ANOMALIES. Complete involution of the urachus with complete closure of its canal rarely occurs. Some remnant of its canal can be found in a high proportion of the population, and remnants of urachal mucosa can often be found at the apex of the bladder. Major defects of the urachus, a vesicoumbilical fistula, an umbilical or vesical sinus, of a urachal cyst somewhere between the bladder and the umbilicus are uncommon.

Urethra

Duplication of the urethra is usually associated with duplication of the bladder and of the distal part of the intestine. Atresia of the urethra is rare. Occasionally meatal stenosis, valves at the verumontanum or elsewhere, or a diaphragm at the bladder neck causes obstruction. Rarely, the verumontanum is large enough to cause obstruction. Congenital diverticula of the urethra are rare, almost always extend dorsal to the urethra, and sometimes cause dysuria.

TUMORS

The neoplasms arising in the urinary tract are nearly all epithelial. They arise from the urinary epithelium, but are often called transitional cell tumors, because the urothelium is sometimes called a transitional epithelium.

Many of the epithelial tumors of the urinary tract are small, sharply demarcated, well differentiated, and do not invade. Some call these well-differentiated tumors papillomata, but most prefer to call them carcinomata. They cannot be clearly separated from more anaplastic tumors of the urinary tract, and many of the patients with a well-differentiated tumor subsequently develop other tumors in the urinary tract, sometimes a more anaplastic tumor that invades the wall of the viscus.

If all the epithelial tumors of the urinary tract are called carcinomata, nearly 10% of malignant tumors in men and 5% in women arise in the urinary tract. Over 70% of the patients are men. Most are over 50 years old.

Most carcinomata of the urinary system arise in the bladder. Less than 1 malignant tumor in 1000 arises in a renal pelvis. Carcinoma of a ureter is still less common. Carcinoma of the urethra is rare.

Bladder

Over 95% of carcinomata of the bladder are transitional cell carcinomata. A few are squamous cell carcinoma or adenocarcinoma. Foci of carcinoma in situ are often present in the epithelium of the bladder of patients with a vesical tumor and are sometimes found in people without a tumor. Occasionally a lymphoma, botryoid sarcoma, mixed mesodermal tumor, mesenchymal tumor, or secondary tumor develops in the bladder.

TRANSITIONAL CELL CARCINOMA. In this section, all the transitional cell tumors of the bladder are considered to be malignant. About 90% of the tumors are papillary; 10% are flat and indurated.

Lesions. Macroscopically, the papillary tumors of the bladder are coral colored, with fronds floating like the tentacles of a sea anemone. Some of the tumors arise from a broad base; some have only a narrow pedicle. Most are a centimeter or more across. The tumors are most common in the trigone, around the ureteric orifices, and on the lateral walls of the bladder, but can arise anywhere in the bladder. About 20% infiltrate the bladder wall.

The nonpapillary tumors form bulky plaques, with a rough, irregular surface, often ulcerated, and extend deeply into the bladder wall, which is thickened and stiffened by the carcinoma.

Microscopically, the fronds of a papillary

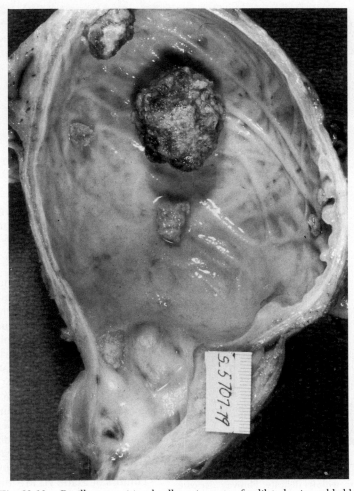

Fig. 39-12. Papillary transitional cell carcinomata of a dilated urinary bladder.

tumor have a thin core of fibrovascular tissue covered by a uniform layer of thickened urinary epithelium. In 80% of them, there is no evidence of invasion of the underlying tissue. In the other 20%, columns of tumor cells like those lining the fronds extend into the subepithelial connective tissue. With papillary carcinomata, the extent of the invasion is often limited. The carcinoma invades the subepithelial tissue, but extends little, if at all, into the muscularis of the bladder.

The nonpapillary carcinomata usually invade extensively, into or through the wall of

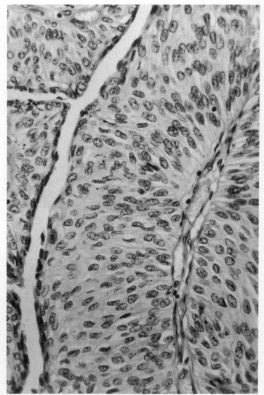

Fig. 39-14.   A grade I papillary, transitional cell carcinoma of the urinary bladder.

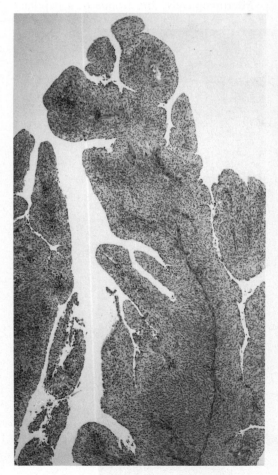

Fig. 39-13.   A well-differentiated, papillary transitional cell carcinoma of a urinary bladder, showing a frond of the tumor, with its delicate, fibrovascular core and thick covering of neoplastic epithelium.

the bladder. Columns of invading transitional cells supported by their stroma wind through the bladder wall and destroy it. In 20% of the tumors, droplets of mucus are present in some of the tumor cells.

Transitional cell carcinomata of the urinary bladder are often divided into three grades.

Tumors of grade I are almost all papillary. The neoplastic epithelium lining the fronds is thickened, but the nuclei of the tumor cells are regular, only slightly larger than normal, and are rarely hyperchromatic.

Tumors of grade II may be papillary or invasive. The nuclei of the tumor cells are larger, and the arrangement of the cells is less regular. From 25 to 50% of the nuclei are hyperchromatic. Occasionally some of the cells of grade II tumors are small and spindle-shaped or large with clear cytoplasm.

Tumors of grade III are almost all invasive, extending deep into the vesical wall, though

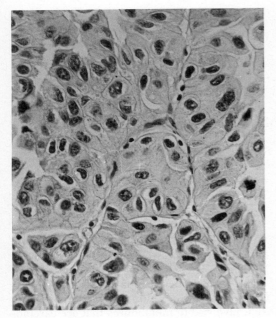

Fig. 39-15. A less well-differentiated, papillary transitional cell carcinoma of the urinary bladder.

papillary fronds. They are large and pleomorphic, with hyperchromatism evident in over 50% of their nuclei. There may be foci of squamous differentiation. Occasionally much or all of a tumor consists of small cells, like those of an oat cell carcinoma of the lung.

The TNM system developed by the International Union against Cancer is used to record the extent of the invasion of bladder tumors. The extent of the tumor as gauged by clinical examination is recorded by T categories, and its extent as judged by pathologic examination by P categories. If a tumor seems to be carcinoma in situ to clinical examination, it is classed as TIS. If it is carcinoma in situ by pathologic examination, it is classed as PIS. If the tumor extends into but not beyond the lamina propria, it is classed as T1 or P1. If it extends into the muscle of the bladder wall, but not more than half way through it, the tumor is T2 or P2. If the carcinoma extends into the outer half of the bladder muscle or into the perivesical tissue, it is classed as T3 or P3. If the carcinoma invades the prostate or other extravesical tissues, it is considered T4 or P4. If there is no evidence of involvement of lymph nodes, the tumor is recorded as N0.

some remnant of papillary structure often remains. The tumor cells are irregularly arranged in the invading columns or on the

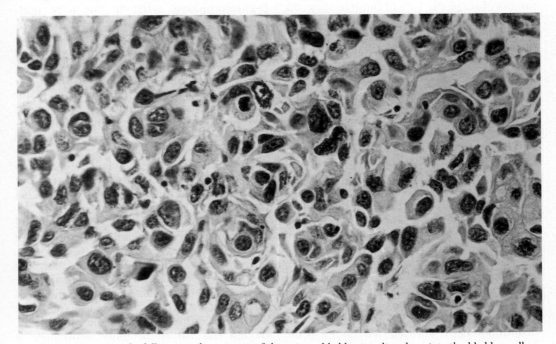

Fig. 39-16. A poorly differentiated carcinoma of the urinary bladder invading deep into the bladder wall.

If a single homolateral node is involved, it is N1. If there is more extensive involvement of the regional lymph nodes, the tumor is graded as N2. If the regional nodes are fixed to the pelvic wall, the tumor is N3. If more distant lymph nodes are involved, it is graded as N4. If no more distant metastases are evident, the tumor is considered M0. If distant metastases are evident, it is classed as M1. If there is insufficient information to judge the extent to the carcinoma, it is called TX, PX, NX, or MX.

Behavior. Transitional cell carcinomata of the urinary tract are often multiple. About 25% of patients with transitional cell carcinoma of the bladder have more than one carcinoma in the bladder when first seen, and over 50% of them will develop one or more new tumors in the bladder or some other part of the urinary tract within five years.

Most of the papillary carcinomata of grade I remain localized and do not invade. The more anaplastic carcinomata of the bladder usually invade slowly, but sometimes involve the perivesical tissues massively by the time the tumor is discovered. Metastases in the regional lymph nodes are found in 5% of tumors of stage P1, 15% of those of stage P2, 20% of those of stage P3, and 45% of those of stage P4. Distant metastases are most common in the liver, lungs, and bones and sometimes develop without involvement of the lymph nodes. They are present in 85% of patients who die of carcinoma of the bladder.

Clinical Presentation. In 70% of patients with carcinoma of the bladder, hematuria is the first sign of the carcinoma. The patient seeks advice when the hematuria becomes massive enough to be obvious. Less often, there is urgency, frequency, or dysuria. Diagnosis is established by cystoscopy and biopsy. Cytologic examination of the urine is often of considerable value, especially in demonstrating the presence of lesions not evident on cystoscopy. The larger tumors are apparent as a filling defect on cystography.

Etiology and Pathogenesis. The multiple tumors common in carcinoma of the bladder were once thought to be secondary tumors from a single primary tumor. It was thought that tumor cells were carried in the urine from the primary tumor to other parts of the urinary tract and implanted to give multiple secondary tumors. This is no longer believed. Tumor cells are commonly shed into the urine, but cannot penetrate the strong urothelium to establish a metastasis.

Nor can the multiple tumors be lymphatic metastases from a single primary tumor. In many of the patients, the tumors are all papillary carcinomata of grade I that do not invade and do not reach the lymphatics.

It is now believed that the multiple tumors are all primary carcinomata. It is thought that the tumors are caused by carcinogens in the urine that bathe the whole of the urinary tract. The carcinogens induce a tumor now in one part of the tract, now in another.

Workers in industries that produce aniline, fuchsin dyes, rubber, or leather goods have long been known to have a high incidence of transitional cell carcinoma of the bladder. These and other industries use chemicals that give rise to metabolites that are carcinogenic when excreted in the urine. Prominent among them are benzidine, 2-naphthylamine, 4-aminobiphenyl, and 4-4'-diaminobiphenyl. Usually the metabolite is excreted into the urine in inactive form, conjugated to glucuronic or sulfuric acid. It is only when the β-glucuoronidase active in the urine splits off the glucuronic acid that the active carcinogen is released. In most workmen exposed to agents of this sort, 20 or more years pass before the tumors begin to appear.

The incidence of transitional cell carcinoma is increased in patients treated for long periods with cyclophosphamide, which gives rise to carcinogenic metabolites excreted in the urine, such as acrolein and phosphoramide mustard. The drug chlornaphazine used to treat polycythemia rubra vera and Hodgkin's disease increases the risk of developing a transitional cell carcinoma of the bladder. Phenacetin increases the incidence of carcinoma of the renal pelvis, and to a lesser degree of transitional carcinoma of the bladder. Irradiation increases the risk of developing transitional cell carcinoma of the bladder. Smoking cigarettes doubles or trebles the risk of developing carcinoma of the bladder, probably by increasing the urinary excretion of carcinogenic substances, though the nature of these substances is uncertain.

Dietary factors may be of importance. Tryptophan could give rise to carcinogenic metabolites that are excreted in the urine, though it has not been proved that it does so. The artificial sweeteners cyclamate and saccharin cause bladder tumors in animals, but have not been proved to do so in man. There is no evidence that coffee or caffeine cause carcinoma of the bladder. Certain brackens cause carcinoma of the bladder in cattle, but do not seem to do so in man.

Infection with Schistosoma haematobium increases the risk of developing transitional cell carcinoma of the bladder, though more often patients with bilharziasis develop a squamous cell carcinoma of the bladder. The incidence of urothelial carcinoma is high in patients with Balkan nephropathy.

In spite of this long list of possible etiologic agents, the cause of transitional cell carcinoma of the bladder is obscure in most patients. If a carcinogen is excreted in the urine, its nature is unknown. Nitrosamines are powerful urinary carcinogens, but their importance in man is unknown.

Treatment and Prognosis. Superficial papillary carcinomata of the bladder are treated endoscopically by excision and fulguration. If the tumor recurs, intravesical chemotherapeutic agents such as thiotepa, doxorubicin, or mitomycin C are sometimes added. The patient must be examined cystoscopically at regular intervals to detect new tumors. Invasive carcinoma requires partial or total cystectomy. If the tumor is inoperable, chemotherapy or radiation gives temporary relief.

The prognosis in a patient with a transition cell carcinoma of the bladder depends on the degree of differentiation and the extent of invasion. These are not independent variables, because well-differentiated tumors usually do not invade, and anaplastic tumors commonly invade extensively. Cure of a superficial, well-differentiated papillary carcinoma does not mean that a more dangerous carcinoma will not develop subsequently.

In one series of over 2000 patients, 60% of patients with a carcinoma of grade I without invasion were alive 12 years after treatment, 32% of those with a carcinoma of grade II without invasion, 24% of those with a carcinoma of grade II with superficial invasion, 15% of those with a carcinoma of grade III with superficial invasion, and 9% of those with tumors of grade II or III that invaded deeply. About 70% of people of similar age without carcinoma of the bladder survived 12 years.

SQUAMOUS CELL CARCINOMA. In most of the world, less than 5% of bladder carcinomata are predominantly squamous in differentiation. Most of these patients have a bladder stone, exstrophy of the bladder, or some other condition that induces squamous metaplasia, and the squamous cell carcinoma seems a complication of the metaplasia. In Egypt and other countries in which infection with Schistosoma haematobium is common, more than 50% of carcinomata of the bladder are of the squamous cell type. The schistosomes induce squamous metaplasia in the bladder, and again the carcinoma seems a complication of the metaplasia.

Squamous cell carcinomata of the bladder are usually flat, invasive tumors, often ulcerated. The carcinoma may be well differentiated, with keratin pearls, or may be more anaplastic. Occasionally a squamous cell carcinoma of the bladder has bizarre, pleomorphic giant cells or spindle cells that mimic a sarcoma. Usually foci of squamous metaplasia are present in other parts of the bladder, and often squamous metaplasia is extensive. Sometimes there is dysplasia in the metaplastic foci or carcinoma in situ.

Squamous cell carcinomata of the bladder behave much as do transitional cell carcinomata, but the prognosis is worse. Over 60% of the patients die within a year.

ADENOCARCINOMA. Adenocarcinoma of the bladder is rare. The adenocarcinomata usually form flat, invasive tumors and microscopically resemble the adenocarcinomata of the gut. Often there is mucus production, and at times it is so abundant that the tumor cells float in a sea of mucus, as in other colloid carcinomata. Some adenocarcinomata are more scirrhous, with signet-ring cells or massive fibroplasia like linitis plastica.

Some of the adenocarcinomata of the bladder arise from the remnants of urachal epithelium often present at the apex of the bladder. Similar adenocarcinomata can arise in a urachal cyst or elsewhere along the course of the urachus. Other adenocarcinomata of the bladder originate from the paraprostatic glands or the paraurethral glands. A few arise by metaplasia of the urinary epithelium. Adenocarcinoma sometimes complicates exstrophy of the urinary bladder.

Adenocarcinomata of the bladder behave like transitional carcinomata of the bladder, except that the prognosis is bad in tumors of the urachus or its remnants.

CARCINOMA IN SITU. Foci of epithelial dysplasia or carcinoma in situ are present in other parts of the bladder in 40% of patients with a noninvasive, papillary, transitional cell carcinoma and in 60% of patients with an invasive transitional cell carcinoma. The foci of dysplasia or carcinoma in situ are most frequent near the tumor, but can occur in distant parts of the bladder. They are particularly common in patients with recurrent or multiple tumors. Similar foci of dysplasia or carcinoma in situ are present in the ureters in 30% of patients with a transitional cell carcinoma of the bladder and less frequently in the renal pelves or urethra. Sometimes carcinoma in situ precedes the development of a transitional cell carcinoma.

Patients with a squamous cell carcinoma of the bladder commonly have foci of carcinoma in situ and epithelial dysplasia in the metaplastic squamous epithelium in the bladder. Carcinoma in situ in the metaplastic squamous epithelium sometimes precedes the development of invasive carcinoma.

Dysplasia and carcinoma in situ of transitional urothelium are not usually evident macroscopically, though occasionally the affected part of the mucosa looks reddish, yellowish, or granular. Microscopically, the cells in the affected regions are hyperchromatic, with prominent nuclei. The nucleocytoplasmic ratio is increased. The arrangement of the abnormal cells is disorderly. Sometimes the abnormal cells resemble one another closely; sometimes they are pleomorphic. Mitoses are common and sometimes atypical. The foci of dysplasia and carcinoma in situ are not well demarcated, but merge gradually into the surrounding urothelium.

Carcinoma in situ of the bladder causes no symptoms, but is sometimes discovered in patients with frequency, dysuria, urgency, or hematuria who have no tumor. The diagnosis can be established by cytologic examination of the urine or by taking random biopsies of the vesical mucosa.

In one series of patients with carcinoma in situ of the bladder without tumor, treated by resection or fulguration of the lesions, 60% of the patients subsequently developed invasive carcinoma of the bladder and 5% had persistent carcinoma in situ. Patients with carcinoma in situ of the bladder treated by total cystectomy have subsequently developed carcinoma of a renal pelvis or a ureter.

SARCOMA BOTRYOIDES. In infants or rarely in older children or adults, a botryoid embryonic rhabdomyosarcoma can arise in the bladder, usually from the trigone. It sometimes involves the proximal part of the urethra and the prostate gland or extends into a ureter. The tumor forms edematous, polypoid masses that sometimes fill the bladder. Microscopically, the tumor is like the embryonic rhabdomyosarcomata that involve the cervix uteri and vagina in female infants.

The prognosis is bad. If the sarcoma is incompletely removed, it recurs promptly. Death usually comes from urinary obstruction or some local complication.

LYMPHOMA. In adults, a lymphoma occasionally arises in the bladder, and for a considerable time remains confined to the bladder. The lymphoma forms a rounded mass in the bladder wall and may ulcerate. Microscopically, the tumor is usually a non-Hodgkin's lymphoma. If the disease is localized, radiotherapy offers a 50% five-year survival.

MIXED MESODERMAL TUMOR. Rarely, a mixed mesodermal tumor arises in the bladder. It forms a bulky, infiltrative tumor that microscopically shows carcinomatous elements set in a sarcomatous stroma. The carcinomatous part of the tumor may be transitional, squamous, or adenocarcinomatous. The sarcomatous part is made principally of nondescript spindle cells, but foci of osteogenic sarcoma or chondrosarcoma may be found. Rarely, the tumor is almost entirely osteogenic sarcoma or chrondrosarcoma.

MESENCHYMAL TUMORS. Nonepithelial tumors of the urinary bladder are rare. Leiomyomata and other benign mesenchymal tumors are extremely uncommon, but a few pheochromocytomata have arisen in the bladder from an adrenal rest. A leiomyosarcoma or an rhabdomyosarcoma of the adult type occasionally arises in the urinary bladder. Rarely, a pheochromocytomata arises in the bladder.

SECONDARY TUMORS. Serosal implants of carcinoma sometimes develop on the outer surface of the bladder in carcinomatosis peritonei, and the bladder can be invaded by extension from a neighboring organ. Hematogenous metastases are rare.

Renal Pelvis

Over 90% of the tumors that involves the kidneys and renal pelves are renal cell carcinomata. Most of the rest are carcinomata of the renal pelvis. Hemangioma, lymphangioma, fibroma, and other benign tumors of the renal pelvis are rare.

CARCINOMA. Nearly all carcinomata of the renal pelvis are transitional cell carcinomata. Occasionally the tumor is a squamous cell carcinoma or an adenocarcinoma. Foci of epithelial dysplasia or carcinoma in situ are sometimes found in a renal pelvis.

Lesions. The carcinomata of the renal pelves are like those of the bladder. Most are papillary transitional cell tumors that are often big enough to fill the pelvis by the time the carcinoma is discovered. Superficial invasion is present in 50% of the tumors. Less often a carcinoma of the renal pelvis is flat and invasive, like the less well-differentiated tumors of the bladder.

Nearly 50% of patients with a transitional cell carcinoma of a renal pelvis have more than one carcinoma in the pelvis or have as well a carcinoma in the ipselateral ureter or the bladder. Involvement of the pelvis or ureter on the other side is unusual.

Behavior. Carcinoma of the renal pelvis is often followed months or years later by transitional cell carcinomata in the bladder or other parts of the urinary tract. The carcinomata of the renal pelvis usually metastasize first to the regional lymph nodes and later more distantly, most often to the liver, lungs, and bones.

Clinical Presentation. Hematuria is the presenting sign in 90% of patients with a

carcinoma of a renal pelvis. In 50%, it is the only sign; in 40%, there is also pain in the loin. In most of the patients, dilatation or deformity of the renal pelvis can be demonstrated radiologically.

Etiology. The misuse of analgesics, in particular the misuse of phenacetin, is a well-known cause of carcinoma of the renal pelvis, but as in the urinary bladder most carcinomata of the renal pelvis are probably caused by carcinogens present in the urine.

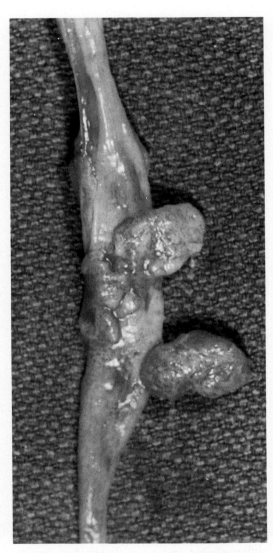

Fig. 39-17. Two papillary, transitional cell carcinomata of a ureter, showing how the tumors bulge into the lumen.

Treatment and Prognosis. If a transitional cell carcinoma of the renal pelvis is well differentiated and has not invaded the wall of the pelvis, and there are no lesions in the ureter, local resection usually controls the lesion. If it has invaded the wall of the renal pelvis, a radical nephroureterectomy is needed. If the lymph nodes are not involved, 50% of the patients survive five years. If there is tumor in the lymph nodes, less than 15% live for five years.

Ureter

Most primary tumors of the ureters are well-differentiated transitional cell carcinomata, though anaplastic transitional cell carcinoma, squamous cell carcinoma, and adenocarcinoma can occur. Often the carcinoma extends along the ureter for several centimeters, projecting into the lumen and thickening the wall. Sometimes there is more than one carcinoma.

The ureters are often surrounded and invaded by carcinoma of the cervix uteri as it extends across the pelvic brim, less often by a carcinoma of some other organ. Commonly the ureter is obstructed by the carcinoma or by the radiation used to treat it.

Urethra

Except for the urethral caruncle, tumors of the urethra are rare. Carcinoma can occur in the proximal or the distal part of the urethra. Occasionally one or many squamous cell papillomata develop in the distal part of the urethra, usually near the meatus.

CARCINOMA. Carcinoma of the urethra is most common in the distal urethra, near the meatus, in both men and women. The carcinoma is nearly always a squamous cell carcinoma, though transitional cell carcinoma can occur and adenocarcinoma can arise from a periurethral gland. In men, the carcinoma sometimes develops at the site of a gonococcal stricture. Squamous cell carcinomata of the distal urethra usually form an indurated mass that is commonly ulcerated. Most are well differentiated and grow slowly, but eventually metastasize to the regional lymph nodes.

Rarely, a transitional cell carcinoma develops in the proximal urethra. More often, the proximal urethra is involved by extension of a vesical carcinoma. Foci of epithelial dysplasia or carcinoma in situ are sometimes present in the proximal urethra.

CARUNCLE. Urethral caruncles occur only in women. They are not uncommon. Most are found in older women, though a caruncle can develop at any age. The name comes from the diminutive of the Latin for flesh.

A caruncle is a pink or red mass that bulges into the urethra or protrudes from the meatus. Most are about 1 cm across, though some are larger. Usually the lesion bleeds easily. Microscopically, a caruncle is often polypoid with thick fronds covered by squamous or transitional epithelium. The underlying tissue resembles a pyogenic granuloma. Young blood vessels proliferate and are accompanied by proliferating fibrocytes. Acute inflammation, chronic inflammation, or both are usually present. Sometimes the blood vessels are greatly dilated so that the lesion is telangiectatic. Skene's glands are sometimes included in the lesion. The glands can be hypertrophic or can undergo squamous metaplasia.

Many urethral caruncles cause no symptoms. Some cause pain or itching. Often micturition, coitus, or movement increases the pain. Sometimes there is bleeding, frequency, or deflection of the urinary stream. Excision cures.

Probably urethral caruncles are not neoplastic, but are inflammatory lesions that result from some injury to the part.

BIBLIOGRAPHY

General

Ahmed, M. N. (Ed.): Urinary Tract Cytology. New York, Thieme Medical Publishers, 1987.

Brawn, P. N.: Interpretation of Bladder Biopsies. New York, Raven Press, 1984.

Infection

Bowie, W. R.: Nongonococcal urethritis. Urol. Clin. North Am., *11*:55, 1984.

Britigan, B. E., Cohen, M. S., and Sparling, P. F.: Gonococcal infection. N. Engl. J. Med., *312*:1683, 1985.

McCutchan, J. A.: Epidemiology of venereal urethritis: comparison of gonorrhea and nongonococcal urethritis. Rev. Infect. Dis., 6:669, 1984.

Michaeli, J., et al.: Emphysematous pyelonephritis. J. Urol., 131:203, 1984.

ørskov, I., and ørskov, F.: Escherichia coli in extraintestinal infections. J. Hyg., 95:551, 1985.

Roberts, J. A.: Reflux nephropathy follows obstruction or infection. Semin. Urol., 4:70, 1986.

Roy, J. B., Goyer, J. R., and Mohr, J. A.: Urinary tract candidiasis. Urol., 23:533, 1984.

Sobel, J. D.: New aspects of pathogenesis of lower urinary tract infections. Urology, 26(5 Suppl):11, 1985.

Turner, J. W., Jr.: Reflux. Semin. Urol., 4:63, 1986.

Watson, R. A.: Gardnerella vaginalis: genitourinary pathogen in men. Urology, 25:217, 1985.

Stone

Andriani, R. T., and Carson, C. C., III: Urolithiasis. Clin. Symp., 38:3, 1986.

Baumann, J. M.: Can the formation of calcium oxalate stones be explained by crystallization processes in the urine? Urol. Res., 13:267, 1985.

Goldwasser, B., Weinerth, J. L., and Carson C. C., III: Calcium stone disease. J. Urol., 135:1, 1986.

Osborne, C. A., et al.: Struvite urolithiasis in animals and man: formation, detection, and dissolution. Adv. Vet. Sci. Comp. Med., 29:1, 1985.

Rosenstein, I. J. M.: Urinary claculi: microbiological and crystallographic studies. CRC Rev. Clin. Lab. Sci., 23:245, 1986.

Scott, R.: Epidemiology of stone disease. Br. J. Urol., 57:491, 1985.

Spirnak, J. P., and Resnick, M. I.: Urinary stones. Primary Care, 12:735, 1985.

Zerwekh, J. E., and Pak, C. Y. C.: Mechanisms of hypercalcuria. Pathobiol. Annu., 12:185, 1982.

Other Non-Neoplastic Diseases

Chasko, S. B., Gray, G. F., and McCarron, G. F., Jr.: Urothelial neoplasia. Pathol. Annu., 16(Pt 2):127, 1981.

Damjanov, I., and Katz, S. M.: Malakoplakia. Pathol. Annu., 16(Pt. 2):103, 1981.

Stewart, F. A.: Mechanism of bladder damage and repair after treatment with radiation and cytostatic drugs. Br. J. Cancer (Suppl), 7:280, 1986.

Tauscher, J. W., and Shaw, D. C.: Eosinophilic cystitis. Clin. Pediatr., 20:741, 1981.

Congenital Malformations

Berry, A. C., and Chantler, C.: Urogenital malformations and disease. Br. Med. Bull., 42:181, 1986.

Cladamone, A. A.: Duplication anomalies of the upper tract in infants and children. Urol. Clin. North Am., 12:75, 1985.

Young, D. W., and Lebowitz, R. L.: Congenital abnormalities of the ureter. Semin. Roentgenol., 21:172, 1986.

Tumors

Bach, P. H., and Bridges, J. W.: Chemically induced renal papillary necrosis and upper urothelial carcinoma. Part 1, CRC Crit. Rev. Toxicol., 15:216, 1985.

Bennington, J. L., and Beckwith, J. B.: Tumors of the Kidney, Renal Pelvis, and Ureter. Washington, D.C., Armed Forces Institute of Pathology, 1975.

Buerton, D., et al.: Bladder tumours in children. Prog. Clin. Biol. Res., 162B:289, 1984.

Cangir, A.: Malignant genital tract tumors in children. Curr. Probl. Cancer, 10:301, 1986.

Chasko, S. B., Gray, G. F., and McCarron, G. F., Jr.: Urothelial neoplasia. Pathol. Annu., 16(Pt 2):127, 1981.

Cohen, S. M., Greenfield, R. E., and Friedell, G. H.: Urinary bladder carcinogenesis. Pathobiol. Annu., 12: 267, 1982.

Connolly, J. G. (Ed.): Carcinoma of the bladder. Prog. Cancer Res., 18:1, 1981.

Gentile, J. M.: Schistosome related cancers. Environ. Mutagen., 7:775, 1986.

Gittes, R. F.: Carcinogenesis in ureterosigmoidoscopy. Urol. Clin. North Am., 13:201, 1986.

Hanash, K. A.: Carcinoma of the bilharzial bladder. Prog. Clin. Biol. Res., 162B:249, 1984.

Ibrahim, N. B. N., Briggs, J. C., and Corbishley, C. M.: Extrapulmonary oat cell carcinoma. Cancer, 54:1645, 1984.

Khoury, S., et al.: Nontransitional cell carcinomas of the bladder in adults. Prog. Clin. Biol. Res., 162B:275, 1984.

Koss, L. G.: Tumors of the Urinary Bladder. Washington, D.C., Armed Forces Institute of Pathology, 1974.

Koss, L. G.: Evaluation of patients with carcinoma in situ of the bladder. Pathol. Annu., 17(Pt 2):353, 1982.

Kramer, S. A.: Pediatric urologic oncology. Urol. Clin. North Am., 12:31, 1985.

Küss, R., et al. (Eds.): Bladder cancer. Prog. Clin. Biol. Res., 162A:1, 162B:1, 1984.

Morgan, R. W., et al.: Epidemiological studies on artificial sweeteners and bladder cancer. Food Chem. Toxicol., 23:529, 1985.

Murphy, W. M.: Current topics in the pathology of bladder cancer. Pathol. Annu., 18(Pt 1):1, 1983.

Murphy, W. M., and Soloway, M. S.: Developing carcinoma (dysplasia) of the urinary bladder. Pathol. Annu., 17(Pt 1):197, 1982.

Nagy, G. K., Frable, W. J., and Murphy, W. M.: Classification of premalignant urothelial abnormalities. Pathol. Annu., 17(Pt 1):219, 1982.

Peehl, D. M., and Stamey, T. A.: Oncogenes: a review with relevance to cancers of the urogenital tract. J. Urol., 135:897, 1986.

Ramaekers, F. C., et al.: Intermediate filament proteins in the study of tumor heterogeneity. Ann. N.Y. Acad. Sc., 544:614, 1985.

Ray, P., Sharifi, R., Ortolano, V., and Guinan, P.:
    Involvement of the genitourinary tract in multiple
    malignant neoplasms. J. Clin. Oncol., *1*:574, 1983.
Schulte, P. A., et al.: Risk assessment of a cohort
    exposed to aromatic amines. J. Occup. Med., *27*:115,
    1985.

Walther, M., O'Brien, D. P., and Birch, H. W.:
    Condylomata acuminata and verrucous carcinoma of
    the bladder. J. Urol., *135*:362, 1986.
Weinstein, R. S., et al.: Pathology of superficial bladder
    cancer with emphasis on carcinoma in situ. Urology,
    26(4 Suppl):2, 1985.

40

Male Reproductive System

THE male reproductive system consists of the testes, epididymides, vasa deferentia, seminal vesicles, prostate gland, scrotum and penis. Pathologically, these structures do not have a great deal in common, in spite of their functional interaction.

INFLAMMATION

Most of the infections involving the male reproductive system have been discussed in earlier chapters and will be mentioned only briefly here. Inflammation of the testis is called orchitis, from the Greek for a testicle. Inflammation of the glans penis is called balanitis, from the Greek for an acorn, and inflammation of the prepuce is called posthitis, from the Greek for the prepuce.

Specific Infections

The term *specific infection* is used to describe infections caused by a single organism. In the male reproductive tract, tuberculosis, gonorrhea, syphilis, chancroid, granuloma inguinale, lymphogranuloma venereum, and trichomoniasis are important causes of specific infection, and occasionally other organisms infect some part of the tract. These conditions are discussed in Chapters 16 to 20. Only gonorrhea, tuberculosis, and syphilis will be discussed in this chapter.

GONORRHEA. In men, gonorrhea begins as an acute inflammation in the anterior part of the urethra. If the infection is allowed to persist, involvement of the posterior urethra becomes likely, often with infection of the urethral glands and the prostate. The prostate becomes acutely inflamed, swollen, edematous, and congested, with an exudate of neutrophils, sometimes with abscesses. To the dysuria, urgency, frequency, and hematuria caused by the urethritis is added perineal pain. The swollen, tender prostate can be palpated by rectal examination.

The infection can spread along the ejaculatory ducts to involve the seminal vesicles, epididymides or testes. The organs affected show diffuse acute inflammation. Sometimes abscesses develop and destroy much of the inflamed tissue. If treatment is inadequate, foci of gonococcal infection can persist in the prostate or epididymides, causing chronic prostatitis or chronic epididymitis.

SYPHILIS. The chancre of syphilis common on the penis is discussed in Chapter 16. Only the lesions in the testes and epididymides are considered here. Many think that the testes are involved in almost every man with syphilis, but if so, the injury is usually slight.

Testicular injury most often becomes evident in the tertiary stage of the disease

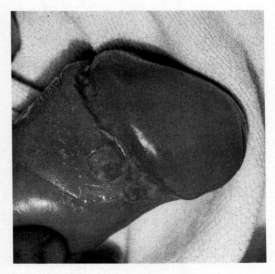

Fig. 40-1. A chancre of the penis. (St. Michael's Hospital, Toronto, Medical Art and Photography Department)

and in patients with congenital syphilis. Usually there is diffuse orchitis in one or both testes, with an exudate of lymphocytes and plasma cells greatest around the blood vessels. The intima of the vessels is often thickened. As time passes, the seminiferous tubules gradually atrophy, and fibrosis increases, until the testis is converted into a smooth, round, hard ball. The Leydig cells are usually preserved.

Syphilitic orchitis usually causes no symptoms and may well pass unnoticed. No doubt the epididymides are often involved as well, but the lesions in the epididymis are rarely severe enough to attract notice.

Less often, one or more gummata form in a testis, and may destroy the organ as they slowly enlarge. Occasionally a testicular gumma ulcerates through the skin. Still more rarely, the testis and epididymis are involved in the secondary stage of syphilis, with acute edema, swelling, and pain.

TUBERCULOSIS.   Tuberculosis of the geni-
tal tract is evident clinically in less than 10% of men with active tuberculosis. It is always secondary to infection in some other organ. Over 90% of the patients have renal tuberculosis and 75% have pulmonary tuberculosis.

In 60% of men with genital tuberculosis, the disease affects the prostate, one or both seminal vesicles, and one or both epididymides. In most of the rest, it is confined to the prostate or to the prostate and seminal vesicles.

Probably the infection of the genital organs usually begins in the prostate gland and results from the bacilluria caused by renal tuberculosis. The seminal vesicles are also easily infected from the urine. The epididymitis could be caused by mycobacteria that ascend the vas deferens from the urine or from a tuberculous lesion in the prostate or a seminal vesicle, or by lymphatic extension from a tuberculosis lesion in the prostate or a seminal vesicle. Less often, genital tuberculosis is caused by hematogenous carriage of

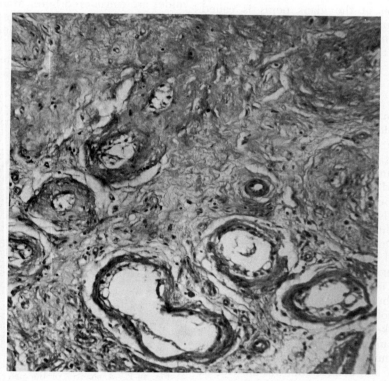

Fig. 40-2.   Syphilitic orchitis, showing almost complete replacement of the testis by scar, with only a few remnants of tubules at the bottom of the picture.

tubercle bacilli from a lesion in a lung or elsewhere.

Granulomata develop in the organs involved and slowly cause increasing necrosis until in the late stages of the disease the tissue is largely destroyed by caseous abscesses and the scarring that surrounds them. Tuberculous epididymitis sometimes extends into the testis, but the injury to the testis is never great. Occasionally tuberculous epididymitis causes a cutaneous sinus.

Genital tuberculosis in men causes few symptoms. Painless swelling of the epididymis is the usual sign, or nodular swelling of a seminal vesicle may be felt on rectal examination. Only occasionally is tuberculous prostatitis sufficient to cause pain, discomfort, or dysuria. Chemotherapy usually controls the disease.

Nonspecific Inflammation

The term *nonspecific inflammation* is used when the cause of the inflammation is not apparent. Probably nonspecific inflammation of the male genital tract is most often caused by Escherichia coli or other of the gram-negative bacteria common in the urine. Less often the inflammation is caused by hematogenous or lymphogenous infection or by direction extension of infection from some neighboring organ. Sometimes it is caused by the escape of secretions into the tissues.

ACUTE PROSTATITIS. Small foci of acute inflammation are probably common in the prostate gland, but soon subside. They cause no symptoms and pass unnoticed.

Severe acute prostatitis is uncommon.

The prostate is swollen and tense. An exudate mainly of neutrophils is prominent. Often the prostatic acini are dilated and filled with neutrophils. Sometimes abscesses form within the gland. Nearly always the seminal vesicles are also inflamed, sometimes severely.

In the more severe cases, there are malaise and leukocytosis. Aching or heaviness in the perineum is common. Sometimes pain in the perineum, rectum, or groin is severe. Defecation may be painful. Nearly always there are dysuria, frequency, and pyuria from an associated urinary infection. Rectal examination shows the enlarged and tender prostate gland, and the swollen, tender seminal vesicles.

Rest, antibiotics, and local application of heat cure most cases, but at times it is necessary to drain an abscess.

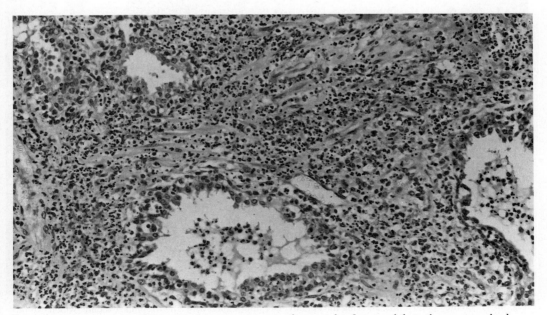

Fig. 40-3.   Acute prostatitis, showing a prominent exudate mainly of neutrophils in the prostate gland.

CHRONIC PROSTATITIS. Foci of chronic inflammation are common in the prostate gland in men over the age of 40 years and grow increasingly common and increasingly extensive as age increases. Often, there is chronic inflammation of the seminal vesicles as well. In the inflamed regions, lymphocytes, plasma cells, or macrophages lie between the prostatic acini. At times, occasional acini contain neutrophils. The prostatic secretion contains increased numbers of inflammatory cells. Often cocci or coliform bacilli can be cultured from the fluid.

Chronic prostatitis usually causes no symptoms, but at times vague pains or urinary symptoms are attributed to it. Some think the chronic infection in the prostate may lead to allergic reactions, iritis, neuritis, or arthritis, much as it is thought dental infections may do.

GRANULOMATOUS PROSTATITIS. Granulomatous prostatitis is not common. Macroscopically, the affected part of the gland may be indurated. Microscopically, a prominent exudate of macrophages lies in the fibro-

muscular tissue between the prostatic acini, often with lymphocytes, plasma cells, and sometimes a few neutrophils. Multinucleated giant cells are sometimes present. There is no necrosis. The lesions seem to heal by scarring.

Some think that granulomatous prostatitis is caused by leakage of prostatic secretions into the tissues. Others consider it of autoimmune origin. The inflammation causes few if any symptoms, but microscopically can closely mimic an infiltrating carcinoma of the prostate.

POSTPROSTATECTOMY GRANULOMA. Granulomata sometimes develop in a prostate gland after prostatectomy. The granulomata resemble rheumatoid nodules. They have a cord of fibrinoid necrosis surrounded by a palisade of macrophages. The cause of the lesions is unknown.

EPIDIDYMITIS. Minor acute or chronic epididymitis is probably not uncommon. More severe acute epididymitis is usually unilateral. In younger men it is usually caused by Chlamydia trachomatis or Neisseria go-

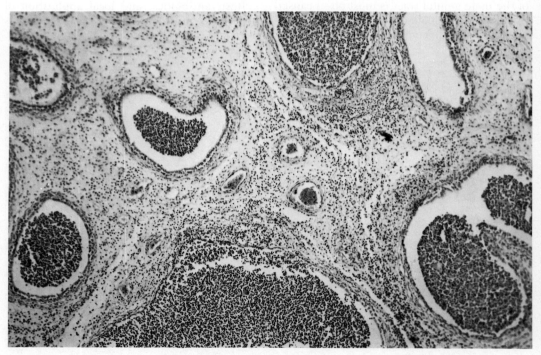

Fig. 40-4. Acute epididymitis, showing the epididymal tubules filled with a neutrophilic exudate, which extends into the connective tissue between them.

norrhoeae. In older men, infection with a gram-negative organism sometimes follows instrumentation or prostatectomy.

GRANULOMATOUS ORCHITIS. Granulomatous orchitis is an unusual condition in which the testis is slightly enlarged and becomes firm. Granulomata from adjacent to the seminiferous tubules. The granulomata consist of macrophages, some of which are multinucleate, together with lymphocytes, plasma cells, and a few neutrophils. They heal by scarring. Often the tunica albuginea is thickened.

Probably granulomatous orchitis results from leakage from the seminiferous tubules. In some patients, there is a history of trauma that supports this hypothesis. Some prefer to call the condition traumatic orchitis.

SPERMATIC GRANULOMA. Spermatic granulomata are most common in the epididymides but can occur at the end of a divided vas deferens. The lesions are white, yellow, or brown and usually from 0.5 to 3 cm across. Microscopically, large numbers of sper-

matozoa are free in the tissues where they excite an inflammatory reaction. At first there is acute inflammation with an exudate predominantly of neutrophils, but this is soon replaced by granulomatous inflammation with macrophages, some of which are multinucleate, lymphocytes, and plasma cells. Eventually the lesion heals by scarring.

Inflammatory Skin Diseases

Many of the inflammatory skin diseases discussed in Chapter 62 can occur in the skin of the penis or scrotum. Scabies, pediculosis, herpes simplex, eczema, psoriasis, erythema multiforme, fungal infections, contact dermatitis, and intertrigo are among the more common. Microaerophilic streptococci and other bacteria, extravasation of urine, and Rocky Mountain spotted fever can cause gangrene of the scrotum. Elephantiasis sometimes causes gross distortion of the genitalia.

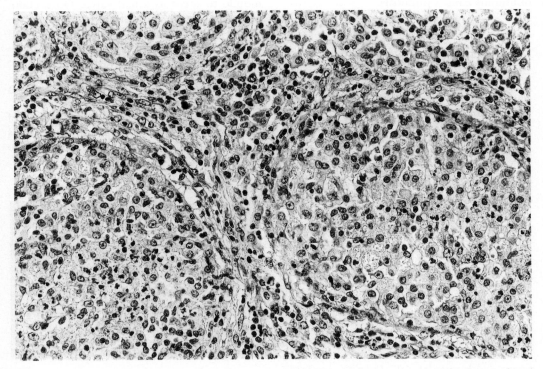

Fig. 40-5. Granulomatous orchitis, showing portions of large granulomata consisting predominantly of macrophages, with chronic inflammation between them.

BALANITIS. Balanitis and balanoposthitis usually reflect a lack of cleanliness. Phimosis makes cleaning the glans difficult and favors infection. The retained smegma encourages bacterial growth. Any of a variety of organisms can be found: staphylococci, streptococci, coliform bacilli, or gonococci. There may be acute or chronic inflammation, sometimes with ulceration. Infection or superinfection with fusospirochetal organisms derived from the sputum can cause severe erosive or gangrenous balanitis.

Occasionally balanitis forms part of the Stevens-Johnson syndrome, Behçet's syndrome, or one of the other syndromes in which there is some combination of balanitis, urethritis, stomatitis, conjunctivitis, uveitis, arthritis, and dermatitis.

BALANITIS XEROTICA OBLITERANS. In balanitis xerotica obliterans, white, atrophic lesions appear on the glans penis and the prepuce. Microscopically, the lesions are identical to those of the lichen sclerosus et atrophicus seen on the vulva and described in Chapter 41. Occasionally balanitis xerotica obliterans causes phimosis.

PROSTATIC HYPERPLASIA

Prostatic hyperplasia is so common that some consider it a normal part of aging, rather than a disease. Prostatic hyperplasia is rarely evident in men under 50 years old, but in older men it becomes increasingly common as age increases, until 80% of men 80 years old have an enlarged prostate. In 90% of the men affected, the hyperplasia causes no symptoms and no dysfunction.

Prostatic hyperplasia is often called prostatic hypertrophy, an unfortunate usage, for the enlargement is due to hyperplasia of both the epithelial and mesenchymal elements of the prostate gland. Sometimes terms such as benign prostatic hyperplasia or nodular prostatic hyperplasia are used, to emphasize that the condition is not neoplastic or to emphasize its nodular character.

Lesions. In embryonic life, the prostate gland has five lobes: anterior, middle, posterior, and two lateral. Late in fetal life, the lobes fuse and can no longer be distinguished, though the terms are often used to describe the location of lesions in the gland.

Functionally, the prostate can be divided into two parts, an inner portion around the urethra and an outer part, which is thickest posteriorly and forms a horseshoe-shaped sheath around the inner part. The inner part of the gland is responsive to both estrogens and androgens, but the outer part responds only to androgens. It is the inner part of the prostate that becomes hyperplastic, and as it enlarges, the outer part of the gland is stretched and compressed.

Usually a hyperplastic prostate is two to four times its normal size, weighing 40 to 80 g, though occasionally it is 200 g or more. The enlarged gland is smooth and nodular, sometimes firm, sometimes rubbery. The hyperplasia is usually greatest in the lateral and middle lobes, with compression of the posterior part of the gland. Sometimes a hyperplastic middle lobe bulges up into the bladder, forming a mass 1 to 2 cm across, often called a median bar. Sometimes the protrusion into the bladder is sufficiently mobile to serve as a ball valve. On section, the hyperplastic part of the gland is comprised of nodules 0.5 to 2 cm in diameter that compress the surrounding tissue. The nodules are sometimes firm and white, but usually are spongy and exude glairy fluid. Occasionally a nodule is cystic or contains a calculus.

Microscopically, the hyperplastic part of the prostate shows hyperplasia of both its glands and the fibromuscular stroma. The lobular structure of the gland is accentuated.

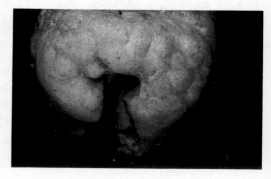

Fig. 40-6. Hyperplasia of the prostate, showing the nodularity of the cut surface of the transected gland.

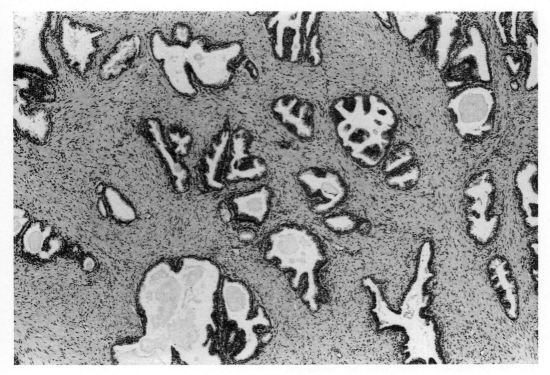

Fig. 40-7. Hyperplasia of the prostate, showing hyperplasia of both glands and connective tissue.

Most of the nodules seen macroscopically consist of hyperplastic glands separated by a sparse fibromuscular stroma. The glands are grouped closely together and form a well-demarcated, spheroidal nodule. The stroma of the nodule is continuous with the hyperplastic stromal tissue between the lobules.

In most of the nodules, the glands form large acini, often with papillary infoldings. Less often, the acini are small and round. The acini are nearly always lined by a double layer of epithelial cells. In the large acini, the epithelial cells in the surface layer are usually pale and columnar while the cells in the deeper layer are small and dark. In small acini, both the surface and the deeper cells are cuboidal. The nuclei of the epithelial cells are regular with fine chromatin. Nucleoli are absent or inconspicuous. Corpora amylacea are often present in the lumen of the glands.

The epithelial cells contain many lysosomes, moderate numbers of mitochondria, and a little endoplasmic reticulum. Alkaline and acid phosphatase are usually present in the luminal part of the cells. Often acid phosphatase is abundant in the lumen of the acini.

Occasionally the glands are atypical in some of the hyperplastic nodules and mimic a prostatic carcinoma. Some of the glands may be lined by a single layer of epithelium, rather than the double layer usual in prostatic hyperplasia. In these glands, the epithelial cells are cuboidal, with pale cytoplasm. Their nuclei are small, without nucleoli. In some cells they are basal; in some they are in the midpart of the cell.

In basal cell hyperplasia, some of the prostatic ducts are filled or nearly filled by a proliferation of small, dark basal cells.

In clear cell cribriform hyperplasia, some of the acini are filled or partially filled by a cribriform proliferation of the pale, superficial cells that line the acini. The nuclei of the hyperplastic cells are regular, with inconspicuous or no nucleoli. The epithelium remains two layered, with small, dark cells at the periphery of the glands.

In all kinds of prostatic hyperplasia, the quantity of stromal tissue between the glandular nodules is increased. The stromal cells are often arranged in a swirling pattern. Sometimes they form a well-defined nodule that resembles a leiomyoma. Often a few lymphocytes are scattered in the stroma. The peripheral part of the prostate gland, which does not share in the hyperplasia, is compressed, has flattened glands, often with atrophic epithelium, and often is fibrotic.

Complications. When a hyperplastic prostate becomes large, it obstructs the urethra. Hypertrophy and dilatation of the bladder follow. Less often, incompetence of one or both ureterovesical valves leads to hydronephrosis and hydroureter on one or both sides. Often the patient cannot empty the bladder completely. Perhaps because hyperplasia of the middle lobe of the prostate elevates the vesicourethral orifice above the floor of the bladder, 100 or 200 mL of residual urine may remain in the bladder after micturition. In part because of the stagnant urine in the bladder, urinary infection is common. Sometimes an enlarged prostate interferes with the vesicourethral sphincters, causing dribbling incontinence.

Clinical Presentation. As a hyperplastic prostate becomes large, the patient usually notices decreasing force in his urinary stream. Frequency and nocturia are common. Often the patient has difficulty in starting or stopping micturition. Sometimes there is intermittency or hesitancy in the urinary stream. If the volume of residual urine left in the bladder after urination is large, dribbling overflow incontinence is common. Bleeding from the veins in the prostatic urethra sometimes causes hematuria.

Occasionally an old man with a large prostate has an abdominal tumor that turns out to be a greatly dilated bladder. Sometimes a patient with a hyperplastic prostate seeks medical advice only when uremia develops. Sometimes an enlarged prostate causes sudden urinary obstruction. Sometimes cystitis draws attention to an enlarged prostate.

Pathogenesis. Prostatic hyperplasia is probably caused by imbalance between estrogen and androgen secretion. As a man ages, the level of estrogen in the blood increases, both absolutely and in relation to testosterone levels. The part of the prostate gland that responds to estrogens becomes hyperplastic. The mechanisms involved are not understood, but experimental evidence suggests that increased estrogen levels increase the receptors for androgens in the periurethral part of the prostate, increasing the effect of the dihydrotestosterone formed from testosterone in the prostate. As this theory suggests, orchidectomy prevents prostatic hyperplasia.

Treatment and Prognosis. If the degree of obstruction warrants it, the treatment of prostatic hyperplasia is surgical. Often the gland can be reduced by partial resection through a cystoscope, though 10% of these patients will require a further resection later. A more extensive prostatectomy can be performed by open operation, enucleating the hyperplastic part of the prostate through the compressed peripheral and posterior part of the gland. Unless some major complication has developed, normal urinary function is restored.

OTHER NON-NEOPLASTIC DISEASES

A number of other non-neoplastic diseases involve the male reproductive tract. Many are rare or of little clinical importance, but some are common or cause serious dysfunction.

THROMBOSIS OF PROSTATIC VEINS. Thrombosis of the veins of the periprostatic plexus is common in patients long bedridden with debilitating disease. Probably the thrombosis is of little clinical importance. The veins are too small to give rise to significant emboli. Sometimes the thrombi become calcified, forming phleboliths that are visible radiologically.

PROSTATIC INFARCTS. One or more infarcts are present in 25% of prostate glands resected for hyperplasia. They are particularly common in chronic prostatitis and after instrumentation.

A prostatic infarct is usually less than 1 cm across. It shows coagulation necrosis, often with ghosts of the dead tissue. A little acute or chronic inflammation is sometimes present around the infarct, but inflammation is slight. Squamous metaplasia is often prominent in the acini adjacent to the infarct.

PROSTATIC CALCULI. Calculi are present in the prostate gland in 30% of men over 50 years old, but are uncommon in younger people. Rarely, a stone develops in a seminal vesicle.

Prostatic calculi form in the prostatic acini or ducts. There may be only a few, or there may be hundreds. The calculi are 0.1 to 5 cm across. Most are hard and ovoid. Some are triangular or faceted. The stones have a core of organic material but consist mainly of calcium phosphate and carbonate. They are radiopaque. An acinus or duct that harbors a stone is usually dilated. Chronic inflammation is common in the adjacent tissue. The calculi are rarely of clinical significance, but occasionally infection develops in a lobule obstructed by a calculus.

HYPERTROPHY OF THE VERUMONTANUM. Hypertrophy of the verumontanum is an unusual cause of urethral obstruction in young boys. Some think it results from hyperestrinism.

TORSION. Normally, the testis and epididymis are so firmly fixed that they cannot rotate. Only if the mesorchium is abnormally mobile, or if the tunica vaginalis extends up around the spermatic cord, can the testis and epididymis twist on the spermatic cord, cutting off their arterial and venous blood supply. Torsion of this sort can occur at any age, but is most common in boys before puberty, especially in those with undescended testes.

The twist is usually in the spermatic cord high in the tunica vaginalis. The direction of the turn is usually from out in, as seen from the front. It may vary from half a turn to two or more complete rotations. In young boys, the twisting occasionally takes place between the testis and the epididymis.

The result is sudden, severe pain in the testis, with extreme tenderness. The scrotum soon becomes swollen and hyperemic. Fluid accumulates in the tunica vaginalis. If nothing is done to relieve the torsion, the pain subsides after three or four days. If the twisted testis is unwound, symptoms are promptly relieved. Sometimes torsion causes less complete vascular obstruction, and the patient experiences repeated, short-lived

episodes of partial vascular obstruction. Torsion may be precipitated by violent muscular effort or may occur when the patient is at rest or asleep.

The outcome depends on the completeness of the obstruction to the blood supply and on its duration. If the obstruction is complete and persists for six hours or more, hemorrhagic infarction of the testis and epididymis and often of the parietal part of the tunica vaginalis is usual. If the obstruction persists for more than 1 hour but less than 6 hours, the testis is likely to become shrunken and fibrotic, with severe impairment or loss of spermatogenesis. The blood supply must be restored within an hour if serious dysfunction is to be avoided. If episodes of incomplete obstruction are repeated, the testis is likely to become atrophic and fibrotic, with severe reduction in spermatogenesis.

Treatment is surgical, to reduce the torsion and fix the testis, so that the twisting cannot occur again.

The appendix testis, or hydatid of Morgagni, is a pedunculated remnant of the müllerian duct attached to the tunica albuginea in one man in three. It is usually less than 1 cm in diameter. The hydatid can twist on its stalk, giving symptoms like those of torsion of the testis.

HYDROCELE. A hydrocele is an accumulation of serous fluid in the tunica vaginalis. About 1% of men admitted to hospital have a hydrocele. In tropical countries in which parasitic diseases are prevalent, they are more frequent. Hydroceles occur in people of all ages, but 90% of the patients are over 21 years old.

Most of the patients have a simple hydrocele, with the fluid in a normally formed tunica vaginalis. In a congenital hydrocele the funicular process remains patent, so that there is communication between the tunica vaginalis and the peritoneal cavity. In an infantile hydrocele, a finger-like projection of the tunica vaginalis extends along the spermatic cord, but does not communicate with the peritoneal cavity. A hydrocele of the cord occurs when a remnant of serosa forms a cyst somewhere along the length of the spermatic cord. In an encysted hydrocele adhesions confine the fluid to a small area posteriorly, behind the testis or epididymis. Sometimes an inguinal hernia is associated with a hydrocele.

By the time it is discovered, a hydrocele usually contains about 100 mL of fluid, though some are larger. The fluid is clear and amber, like plasma. It contains from 4 to 6% of protein. Occasionally free bodies comprised largely of fibrin float in the fluid. The wall of the hydrocele usually shows little abnormality, though there is a minor accumulation of lymphocytes and macrophages in the tunica albuginea.

If the hydrocele is allowed to persist for months or years, the wall of the cavity becomes thickened and fibrotic, perhaps in plaques, perhaps diffusely. Sometimes the thickening is so extensive that the characteristic translucency of a hydrocele is no longer evident. In long-standing cases, the wall of the hydrocele may become calcified. The testis remains unharmed for a long time, but eventually becomes atrophic, perhaps because of compression by the thickened tunica albuginea.

If a hydrocele becomes infected, organisms and pus cells appear in the fluid. If the tunica vaginalis is filled with pus, the lesion is called a pyocele.

In most hydroceles, the cause of the lesion is uncertain. They develop slowly, without evidence of any other disease of the genital tract. Probably in many of these men the hydrocele is due to mild, repetitive trauma. Surgical procedures in the region can cause a hydrocele. Less often, a hydrocele develops acutely, sometimes from trauma, sometimes secondary to epididymitis or orchitis. Lymphatic obstruction, as in filariasis, can cause a hydrocele.

Hydroceles cause few symptoms. The patient may notice the enlargement or feel a dragging pain. In children and in adults with small hydroceles, no treatment is needed. In children, the hydrocele is likely to resolve in a year or two. In adults with larger hydroceles, drainage of the sac into the loose scrotal tissues by incision or excision of part of the parietal wall of the sac is usually required, though some prefer to aspirate the fluid and inject a sclerosing fluid.

HEMATOCELE.   The accumulation of blood in the tunica vaginalis is called a hematocele. It may result from trauma or may complicate the introduction of a needle for diagnostic or therapeutic purposes.

CHYLOCELE.   A chylocele usually results from filarial infection and is like a hydrocele except that the leakage of the obstructed lymphatics into the tunica vaginalis fills it with milky chyle. Sometimes in filariasis the lymphatic distention makes lymph ooze through the epidermis of the scrotum.

SPERMATOCELE.   A spermatocele is a cyst that bulges from the epididymis, usually into the tunica vaginalis, but sometimes into the scrotal wall. The cyst has a thick fibrous wall and is lined by pseudostratified epithelium. The fluid within the cyst is milky and contains large numbers of spermatazoa and fat droplets, with a few epithelial and inflammatory cells. The cyst is usually 1 or 2 cm in diameter and feels like a little third testis. If treatment is needed, the cyst can be excised.

VARICOCELE.   A varicocele is caused by dilatation, elongation, and increased tortuosity of the veins of the pampiniform plexus around the spermatic cord. Varicoceles are common in unmarried men from 15 to 25 years old. In the army, more than 10% of young men are affected. When the patient stands, the dilated veins can be felt like a bag of worms around the cord. When he lies down, the veins collapse, and the varicocele disappears.

Most varicoceles are idiopathic, nearly always on the left, and tend to grow less evident as the patient grows older. Only 1% of idiopathic varicoceles are bilateral.

Less often, a varicocele is secondary to pressure on the spermatic veins by a renal tumor, an enlarged liver, a big spleen, or some other intra-abdominal mass. If a varicocele appears in a man over 30 years old, is on the right side, or does not disappear when the patient lies down, it is probably secondary.

Most varicoceles need no treatment. Some patients complain of pain or dragging, and in such people the condition can be relieved surgically.

FIBROMATOUS PERIORCHITIS.   Fibromatous periorchitis, sometimes called chronic vaginalitis, affects men 20 to 40 years old. The tunica vaginalis becomes thickened by multiple fibrous nodules, especially along the epididymis. The nodules are from 0.1 to 2 cm in diameter. On section, they resemble a fibroid of the uterus, though microscopically they consist mainly of fibrous tissue. A few lymphocytes or plasma cells are often scattered in the fibrosis. The cause of fibromatous periorchitis is unknown, though some cases seem related to trauma.

RADIATION. As discussed in Chapter 23, radiation damages or destroys the spermatogonia, though sparing the well-differentiated spermatozoa. Aspermia becomes evident after a few weeks and persists for years, though if the dose of radiation is not too large at least partial recovery may eventually follow. The hormone-producing Sertoli and Leydig cells are spared. The size or texture of the testis and its hormonal activity do not change. Radiation can produce sterility without the man being aware that he has been injured.

PRIAPISM. Persistent and usually painful erection of the penis is called priapism, after the god of procreation and gardens. Lesions of the pelvic nervous system, local irritation in the urinary tract, thrombosis of the penile veins, leukemia, and sickle cell anemia can all cause priapism. In many patients, no such cause is evident, and the disease is considered idiopathic.

Treatment should not be delayed if impotence is to be avoided. The erection will nearly always subside, but injury to the corpora cavernosa brings fibrosis and impotence. If the cause of the priapism is known, it should be controlled. Idiopathic priapism can be relieved by sedation or anesthesia. Sometimes aspiration of the corpora cavernosa is effective. Sometimes a vein graft is needed to drain the corpora cavernosa.

PEYRONIE'S DISEASE. Peyronie's disease is named after the French surgeon de la Peyronie (1678–1747). It usually becomes evident in men 40 to 50 years old.

In Peyronie's disease, diffuse or nodular fibrosis in the intercavernal septum of the penis or in the sheath of the corpora cavernosa makes the penis curve on erection. Often erection is painful. Microscopically, the lesion shows compact fibrosis, similar to that of Dupuytren's contracture. Indeed, 25% of men with Peyronie's disease have Dupuytren's contracture.

Usually Peyronie's disease is mild, and treatment is not needed. If it is more severe, radiation may help or perhaps large doses of vitamin E. Steroids have proved of little value. The disease usually recurs after surgical repair.

CONGENITAL ANOMALIES

The congenital anomalies of the male reproductive system fall into two groups: those that affect principally the penis— phimosis, hypospadias, and epispadias—and those that involve mainly the testes— cryptorchism, Klinefleter's syndrome, and intersexuality.

Other congenital malformations of the penis, scrotum, and testes are rare. The penis can be too small or too large. Occasionally it is in the wrong place or duplicated. The scrotum is sometimes bifid. One or both testes may be absent. Sometimes there is a supernumerary testis, or the testes are fused. Occasionally a testis is ectopic, lying in the perineum, the inner aspect of the thigh, or over the pubis. In germinal aplasia, the testes are normally formed except that their tubules lack germinal cells and are lined only by Sertoli cells.

PHIMOSIS. Phimosis is the commonest of penile anomalies. The name comes from the Greek for muzzling and is used to describe any condition in which the prepuce cannot be returned over the glans.

Some degree of phimosis is common in infant boys. Often complete separation between the glans and the prepuce is not achieved until some weeks or months after birth, because the ingrowth of epithelium that separates them is slow to divide into the epithelia lining the glans and the inner surface of the prepuce.

If the opening of the prepuce is too small in an infant, the condition is called congenital phimosis. Commonly the opening of the meatus is also small. Congenital phimosis can cause urinary obstruction, even uremia. More often, it impairs the drainage of smegma, increasing the risk of infection. Preputial stones sometimes develop. The risk of carcinoma of the penis later in life increases. Congenital phimosis is treated by dividing the prepuce or circumcision.

Acquired phimosis develops in adult life and results from infection, trauma, or edema of the penis.

PARAPHIMOSIS. If the retracted prepuce cannot be reduced, the condition is called paraphimosis. Paraphimosis usually results from infection. It is sometimes painful. Occasionally paraphimosis causes urinary obstruction by constricting the urethra. Treatment is surgical.

HYPOSPADIAS. If the urethra opens on the under surface of the penis, between the glans and the perineum, the condition is called hypospadias, from the Greek words for under and a rent. Hypospadias is present in 1 boy in every 500 live born. In 25% of the children, the condition is inherited as an autosomal recessive character.

Nearly always in hypospadias the penis is curved downwards, a condition called chordee, the French word meaning bound with a cord. The cause of the chordee is in dispute, but most think it is due to a fibrous cord that runs along the urethral surface of the penis.

Other anomalies are commonly found. About 50% of the children with hypospadias have a stricture of the urethral meatus. Sometimes part of the urethra persists distal to the opening, forming a blind sac. The scrotum may be bifid, the testis undescended or anomalous. Repair is surgical.

EPISPADIAS. If the urethra opens on the upper surface of the penis, the condition is called epispadias, from the Greek for upon and a rent. Epispadias is found in 1 birth in 50,000. It is commonly associated with cryptorchidism, exstrophy of the bladder, or absence of the prostate gland. Correction is surgical.

CRYPTORCHIDISM. Cryptorchidism is the term used to describe the failure of one or both testes to descend into the scrotum. The name is from the Greek for hidden and testicle.

At birth, 1 boy in 50 is cryptorchid, usually on both sides. In most of these children, the testes descend spontaneously within the first year, so that only 1 boy in 250 is cryptorchid at the age of 15 years. Spontaneous descent of the testes can occur at puberty, and only

1 man in 500 is cryptorchid. In adults, cryptorchidism is unilateral in 80% of the patients. It is bilateral in 75% of children, with the two sides being affected equally.

In 70% of the patients, the undescended testes are in the inguinal canal. In 25%, they are in the abdomen. In the other 5%, the testes are in the perineum, pubic region, or some other abnormal site.

Until puberty, cryptorchidism does not harm the undescended testes. The undescended testis is indistinguishable from a normally descended organ in the scrotum.

After puberty, undescended testes begin to atrophy. As years pass, the germinal cells gradually disappear, until the testicular tubules are lined only by Sertoli cells. The basement membranes of the atrophying tubules thicken, and the wall of the tubules becomes hyalinized. The Leydig cells persist and form prominent clumps in the interstitium between the atrophic tubules. Eventually, the shrunken testis consists mainly of Leydig cells, set in a scant fibrous stroma, with only an occasionally fibrotic tubule here and there. In extreme cases, the Leydig cells are also lost, and only a fibrotic remnant of the testis remains.

The cause of the maldescent of the testes is not usually clear. Mechanical factors such as a short spermatic cord or malformation of the inguinal canal may sometimes be to blame. In other patients, the maldescent results from deficient androgenic secretion. The atrophy that follows puberty is due to suppression of spermatogenesis by the high temperature within the body. It is only when the testis is kept cool in the scrotum that spermatogenesis can proceed normally.

In 70% of the patients, the processus vaginalis remains patent, so that there is a congenital inguinal hernia, usually of the indirect type. Hydrocele or torsion of the spermatic cord may occur in the inguinal canal. The epididymis is sometimes separated from the testis, or its attachment to the testis is abnormal.

Cryptorchidism increases the risk of developing testicular cancer 10 to 50 times. The risk of cancer is greater with an intra-abdominal testis than with a testis in the inguinal canal.

Because of the danger of sterility and the

risk of cancer if the testes do not reach the scrotum by puberty, undescended testes should be brought down into the scrotum when the patient is about five years old. If there is no mechanical obstacle to descent, giving chorionic gonadotropins may bring the testes into the scortum. If not, surgical correction is required.

KLINEFELTER'S SYNDROME. Klinefelter's syndrome and the related conditions in which chromosomal abnormalities cause maldevelopment of the testes are discussed in Chapter 11. Patients with these syndromes have an excess of X chromosomes in their cells, and after puberty spermatogenesis fails to develop normally. The testes remain small. Their seminiferous tubules are atrophic, with thick hyalinized walls, and are lined mainly by Sertoli cells. The Leydig cells are normal or hyperplastic and form prominent clumps between the wasted tubules.

INTERSEXUALITY. A person who has some combination of male and female sexual organs is said to be intersexual. Such people are often called hermaphrodites, after Hermaphroditus, the son of Hermes and Aphrodite who became bisexual after the nymph Salmacis became merged into his body. True hermaphrodites have both an ovary and a testis; pseudohermaphrodites have either ovaries or testes, but have sexual organs inappropriate for their gonadal sex.

Male Pseudohermaphroditism. Male pseudohermaphrodite usually have a normal male chromosomal pattern but show feminization of the genitalia. The extent of the feminization varies and can vary from hypospadias to so complete a mimicry of the female genitalia that the child is brought up as a girl. The penis is small. The urethra opens on the perineum. The testes fail to descend. The scrotum is split and looks more like labia than a scrotum. Sometimes a vagina is present, though it is usually ill-formed. It may open on the perineum or into the urethra at the verumontanum. Müllerian derivatives are rarely more than vestigial. Rarely, an otherwise normal man has müllerian derivatives in the sac of an inguinal hernia.

Testicular Feminization. Testicular feminization is a form of male pseudohermaphroditism in which the external genitalia are female,

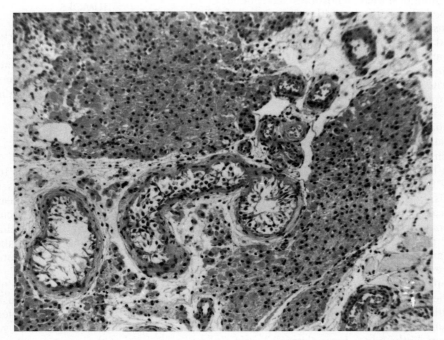

Fig. 40-8. Klinefelter's syndrome, showing the atrophy of the seminiferous tubules, their thick walls, and the large masses of Leydig cells.

with a short vagina, but no uterus or other evidence of müllerian differentiation. At puberty, the breasts develop in normal female fashion. The hair is of female distribution. The patient looks and acts like a woman. The testes are usually intra-abdominal, but may be inguinal. They are atrophic as in other forms of cryptorchidism but often have hyperplastic Sertoli cells.

The fault in these patients seems to be a lack of the receptor for androgen on the surface of the cells that normally react to androgen. During organogenesis, the tissues that normally respond to androgen fail to do so. The penis and wolffian derivatives fail to develop. The genital swellings do not fuse to form the scrotum. Androgen is not necessary for the regression of the müllerian structures, and these regress normally.

The patient usually consults a physician because of amenorrhea at puberty. Orchidectomy is often performed because of the danger of cancer, as in other kinds of cryptorchidism, and the female habitus is maintained with estrogens.

Gonadal Dysgenesis. In gonadal dysgenesis, the chromosomal sex is usually male, though similar syndromes have been described in patients with a variety of chromosomal abnormalities. The patients are tall and eunuchoid. They have female external and internal genitalia, but these fail to develop at puberty and remain infantile. True gonads are absent. Instead, there are fibrous streaks on the posterior surface of the broad ligaments. Rarely, a patient has gonadal dysgenesis on one side, with müllerian differentiation on that side and a testis on the other, with wolffian differentiation on that side.

True Hermaphroditism. True hermaphriditism, or ambisexuality as it is sometimes called, is rare. The people affected have both ovaries and testes. Most have a female complement of chromosomes, but some have male chromosomes or are mosaics.

Three types of true hermaphroditism are distinguished. In bilateral hermaphroditism, the patient has both an ovary and a testis on both sides of the body or has an ovotestis containing both ovarian and testicular elements on both sides. In unilateral hermaphroditism, the patient has an ovotestis or both an ovary and a testis on one side, but a normal testis or ovary on the other. In lateral hermaphroditism, there is an ovary on one side and a testis on the other.

The testes and ovaries in true hermaphrodites are usually well formed and normally placed. The ovarian and testicular elements in an ovotestis are well formed but the organ rarely has an epididymis or vas deferens. It is usually more or less in the position of an ovary. An ovary or an ovotestis induces the formation of a uterus and its adnexa on its side of the body, though with an ovotestis the uterus usually remains infantile. A testis induces the formation of an epididymis and vas deferens on its side, but an ovotestis rarely does so.

The patients usually have a small penis and are brought up as boys. The genital swellings develop into a scrotum if they contain testes and into labia if the gonads are intra-abdominal. The vagina may open onto the perineum or into the urethra at the verumontanum. The breasts usually show female development.

TUMORS

The tumors of the different parts of the male reproductive system have little in common. The tumors of the prostate gland will be discussed first and then the tumors of the seminal vesicles, testes, penis, and scrotum.

Prostate Gland

Carcinoma is the only common tumor of the prostate gland. Benign tumors are uncommon and rarely of clinical significance. An embryonal rhabdomyosarcoma occasionally arises in the prostate in a young child, and rarely a leiomyosarcoma or a rhabdomyosarcoma takes origin in the prostate in an old man.

CARCINOMA. Carcinoma of the prostate gland is uncommon in men less than 50 years old, but after that age its prevalence increases rapidly until 80% of men 80 years old have carcinoma of the prostate. Many of the carcinomata are small and are found only at autopsy or at resection of part of a prostate gland because of prostatic hyperplasia. Some invade and metastasize.

It is estimated that in 1986 in the United States carcinoma of the prostate caused 10% of deaths from cancer, that 90,000 men developed the disease, and over 25,000 died of it. In North America, most of Europe, and Australasia, each year from 15 to 25 men in every 100,000 die of carcinoma of the prostate. In Greece, Israel, and the Middle East, fewer than 10 men in 100,000 die of it; in Japan, Hong Kong, Singapore, and Thailand, fewer than 5; in South America, from 5 to 15.

Small carcinomata of the prostate that cause no symptoms and are found only when the gland is examined microscopically at autopsy or when a prostatectomy is performed for prostatic hyperplasia are called latent, incidental, or occult tumors. If a carcinoma causes urinary obstruction or other local symptoms, it is said to be clinically evident. The term *occult carcinoma* is also used to describe carcinomata of the prostate

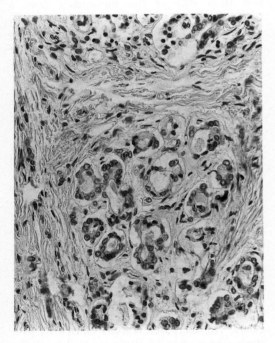

Fig. 40-9. Carcinoma of the prostate, showing the small, closely clumped tubules often seen in this kind of carcinoma.

in which metastases are evident, but there is no clinical evidence of a tumor in the prostate.

Lesion. Most carcinomata of the prostate arise in the posterior and lateral part of the gland, which is responsive to androgens but not to estrogens. Only as the carcinoma grows bigger, does it involve the inner estrogen-sensitive part of the gland. In one series, the carcinoma was confined to the outer zone in 46% of the patients, involved both the outer and the inner zones in 53%, and was confined to the inner zone in less than 1%.

Small carcinomata of the prostate cannot be detected clinically and are not apparent when a resected gland is examined macroscopically. Larger carcinomata form one or more nodules of firm, yellowish-white tissue and usually lie immediately under the capsule of the gland. As a carcinoma grows, it replaces more of the gland. The tumor is usually scirrhous and hard and often is gray, perhaps flecked with yellow. Only occasionally is a carcinoma of the prostate soft with hemorrhage and necrosis in the tumor.

Microscopically, most carcinomata of the prostate are well-differentiated adenocarcinomata. The neoplastic glands disrupt the normal pattern of the prostate. Instead of the radiating glands of a normal prostate or the swirl of glands common in the nodules of prostatic hyperplasia, the malignant glands grow in no logical pattern. They sometimes form a well-demarcated nodule, but often extend into the adjacent tissue without a clear margin.

Most well-differentiated carcinomata of the prostate form small acini or tubules. The tubules sometimes wind through the tissue, sometimes are closely clumped together. Less often a carcinoma forms large acini, like those of prostatic hyperplasia, though usually without papillary infoldings. Occasionally the tumor cells grow in a cribriform pattern and fill the glands. Occasionally the tumor cells grow in sold columns or form broad sheets of well-differentiated neoplastic cells. Often a carcinoma shows more than one of these patterns of growth.

The acini and solid columns of tumor cells are supported by a fibromuscular stroma like that of a normal prostate. In most tumors, the stroma is moderately abundant, explaining the hardness of the tumor.

In the well-differentiated carcinomata of the prostate, the neoplastic acini are lined by a single layer of tumor cells rather than by the two layers of epithelial cells usual in normal and hyperplastic prostate glands. The tumor cells are well differentiated, uniform, cuboidal, or columnar, with well-defined cytoplasm. Their nuclei are regular and spheroidal, with even chromatin. Many of them contain nucleoli. Mitoses are usually absent. Often the tumor cells in a carcinoma of the prostate are so well differentiated that it is easier to make the diagnosis of carcinoma by using a low power of the microscope to observe the tumor's abnormal pattern of growth than by using a high power to study the tumor cells.

Anaplastic tumors of the prostate gland are less common. The tumor cells are large, pleomorphic, perhaps multinucleate, often with many mitoses. They sometimes form glands, but more often grow in sheets. Necrosis and hemorrhage are common.

Occasionally a few of the tumor cells in a carcinoma of the prostate secrete mucus, but tumors that are predominantly mucus-secreting are rare. Rarely a carcinoma of the prostate is a transitional cell or squamous cell tumor.

Behavior. As a carcinoma of the prostate grows, it invades the inner part of the prostate to surround the urethra or bulge into the bladder from beneath the trigone. The carcinoma rarely breaches the vesical or urethral mucosa. It extends into or through the capsule posteriorly only after some delay. By the time the patient comes to surgery, the carcinoma has reached but not penetrated the capsule in 20% of the patients, has extended partially through it in 35%; and has reached the periprostatic tissue in 15%. The carcinoma may invade a seminal vesicle but rarely involves the rectum.

Most carcinomata of the prostate grow slowly and metastasize only after a delay of months or years. Only the anaplastic tumors grow rapidly and metastasize early. Carcinomata that produce no symptoms do not often give rise to metastases, but metastases become evident sooner or later in 80% of the patients in whom the tumor causes urinary obstruction. Many of the patients with carcinoma of the prostate are old and die of some other cause.

At autopsy, the lymph nodes in the pelvis are almost always involved in patients dying of carcinoma of the prostate, and often the carcinoma has extended to involve the para-aortic or more distant lymph nodes. Metastases are evident in the sacrum and pelvis in 60% of men dying with a carcinoma of the prostate that caused symptoms, in the lumbar spine in 40%, in the femora in 25%, the doral spine in 15%, and the ribs in 15%. Up to 20% of the patients have metastases in the lungs, liver, adrenal glands, kidneys, or some other organ. Metastases in the sacrum, pelvis, and lower part of the spine are frequent because the carcinoma travels from the prostate to this part of the skeleton in Batson's paravertebral plexus of veins.

Over 90% of the bony metastases of carcinoma of the prostate are sclerotic. The metastasis causes thickening of the bony trabeculae until only small spaces filled with tumor cells are left in the sclerotic bone. In less than 10% of the metastases does a carcinoma of the prostate cause lysis of the bone in the way usual in bony metastases from most other kinds of tumor. In other groups, the metastases usually reproduce the structure of the tumor in the prostate.

Dysfunction. Well-differentiated carcinomata of the prostate produce acid phosphatase, as does normal and hyperplastic prostatic epithelium. If the quantity of tumor in the body is large enough, the activity of the enzyme in the plasma rises. Small carcinomata that cause no symptoms rarely increase the activity of acid phosphate in the plasma, but increased activity of the enzyme in the plasma is evident in 60% of patients in whom the tumor causes urinary obstruction and in 80% of those with evidence of metastases.

Hyperparathyroidism, multiple myeloma, Paget's disease, and other diseases of bone also increase the activity of acid phosphatase in the plasma, as does trauma to the prostate gland. The increased activity caused by prostatic disease can be distinguished from the increase caused by disease of bone by esti-

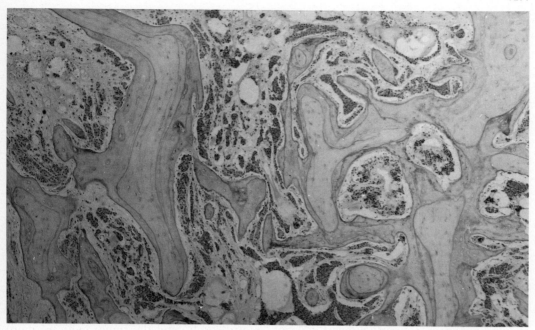

Fig. 40-10.   A metastasis of carcinoma of the prostate in a vertebra, showing the massive deposition of new bone induced by the dark islands of carcinoma in the fibrotic marrow.

mating the prostatic fraction of acid phosphatase rather than the total activity.

Lactic acid dehydrogenase, especially its isoenzymes IV and V, is produced by many carcinoma of the prostate in sufficient quantity to increase its activity in the plasma when metastases develop. In 10% of the patients, the carcinoma produces enough plasminogen to cause increased fibrinolytic activity in the plasma.

Clinical Presentation. Carcinoma of the prostate causes symptoms only late in the disease. Urinary obstruction with dysuria, slowing of the urinary stream, frequency, and retention are usually the first signs of the tumor. In 10% of the patients, pain in the back from metastases or hematuria draws attention to the disease.

By the time symptoms are evident, the carcinoma is usually palpable by rectal examination. If the tumor is localized, there is a single, hard nodule in the gland. If it is larger, the gland is nodular, hard, and fixed to the surrounding tissues. A rectal or perineal needle biopsy can usually establish the

diagnosis. Ultrasonic examination is valuable to locate the carcinoma and guide the biopsy. Tumor cells are present in the urine in 60% of the patients with advanced disease.

Etiology. The cause of carcinoma of the prostate is unknown. Probably prostatic hyperplasia plays no part in causing the carcinoma, though both are common in elderly men.

Treatment and Prognosis. The carcinoma in the prostate gland is usually treated surgically, by transurethral resection or radical prostatectomy. External radiation or the implantation of I^{131} can also control the primary tumor in the gland.

The metastases of the well-differentiated carcinomata of the prostate require androgen for continued growth. Bilateral orchidectomy reduces the concentration of testosterone in the plasma to less than 10% of normal and can often relieve symptoms caused by the metastases, though it does not increase the longevity of the patients. Diethyl stilbesterol and other estrogens give similar relief by reducing the secretion of luteinizing hormone by the pituitary gland and the secretion of androgen by the testes and adrenal glands. Other drugs that impair the release of the luteinizing hormone act similarly. Chemotherapeutic agents are of limited value.

The altered hormonal balance caused by orchidectomy and the administration of stilbesterol cause vacuolation and atrophy of some of the tumor cells in the metastases. Usually the damage to the tumor cells is sufficient to cause a reduction in the activity of acid phosphatase in the plasma. The success of the treatment can be judged by the extent of the reduction. If the carcinoma escapes from the hormonal control, the activity of acid phosphatase in the plasma will again rise.

The altered hormonal balance also causes atrophy of the normal prostatic tissue and often squamous metaplasia of the urethra and prostatic ducts. Sometimes the patient develops gynecomastia, or the retention of sodium enhances congestive heart failure. The risk of developing carcinoma of the breast increases.

The prognosis in carcinoma of the prostate worsens as the carcinoma becomes more extensive. The carcinoma is often divided into four stages. In stage A, there are no symptoms of carcinoma. In stage A1, the tumor is of microscopic size and confined to a single focus. In stage A2, it involves the prostate more widely. In stage B, there is a single nodule in the prostate. In stage B1, it is less than 2 cm in diameter. In stage B2 it is larger. In stage C, the carcinoma has extended beyond the prostate, and in stage D metastases are present. Over 90% of patients with symptoms caused by carcinoma of the prostate are in stage C or D.

Most patients in stage A1 are cured by a transurethral prostatectomy, though some do develop recurrent tumor or metastases. More than 10% of those in stage A2 develop recurrent or metastatic carcinoma. Over 85% of those in stage B1 live for 5 years, and 50% live for 15 years. Only 20% of those in stage B2 live 5 years, and 1% survive for 15 years. If the carcinoma has extended beyond the prostate, 40% of patients in stage C but less than 20% of those in stage D live for 5 years.

The pattern of growth of the carcinoma also affects the prognosis. In the system of grading named after the M. D. Anderson Hospital in Houston, four histologic grades are distinguished. In grade 1, over 75% of the tumor forms glands and a cribriform pattern of growth is not present. In grade 2, from 50 to 75% of the tumor forms glands, or some glands show a cribriform pattern. In grade 3, from 25 to 50% of the tumor forms glands. In grade 4, less than 25% forms glands. Over 90% of patients with a tumor of grade 1 survive 5 years, 60% of those in grade 2, 50% of those in grade 3, and 15% of those in grade 4.

In the Gleason system of grading named after the American pathologist who reported it in 1967, the tumors are divided into five patterns. In pattern 1, the tumor consists of well-differentiated, small, closely packed, uniform glands in circumscribed masses. Pattern 2 is similar but the size and shape of the glands vary more, they are arranged more loosely, and the tumor cells are more atypical. A cribriform pattern of growth is sometimes present. In pattern 3, the glands are still more irregular, the tumor extends into the surrounding tissue, or solid cords of tumor cells are present. In pattern 4, the tumor consists of large clear cells like those of a renal cell carcinoma that grows in sheets or form glands. In pattern 5, the tumor is poorly differentiated and shows no differentiation into glands. As some tumors show more than one of these patterns, the numerical value of the predominant and second most predominant grades are added to give 9 grades numbered from 2 to 10. If a tumor shows only one pattern of growth, the number assigned to that pattern is doubled. With this system, over 90% of patients with tumors of grade 2 to 4, 70% of those with tumors of grades 5 to 7, but less than 50% of those with tumors of grades 8 to 10 live over 30 months.

Seminal Vesicles

Primary tumors of the seminal vesicle are rare. The most common is a papillary adenocarcinoma with cells containing the brown pigment typical of the seminal vesicle. The carcinoma behaves much as do prostatic carcinomata, but few patients survive a year.

Testes

Over 90% of testicular tumors arise from the germ cells. About 5% are tumors of the sex cord-stromal type. A gonadoblastoma and the mixed germ cell sex cord-stromal tumor combine germ cell and sex cord-stromal elements. Occasionally a non-Hodgkin's lymphoma arises in the testes. Rarely, a benign mesenchymal tumor or an adenocarcinoma develops in a rete testis, or a mesothelioma involves the serosa covering a testis.

GERM CELL TUMORS. The germ cell tumors of the testes are almost all malignant. Most of the patients are between 20 and 45 years old. Only 0.5% of malignant tumors are of this type, but over 10% of men 20 to 30 years old dying of cancer die of a germ cell tumor.

In North America, most of Europe, and Australasia, 3 to 5 men per 100,000 develop a germ cell tumor. In South America, Africa, and Asia, the incidence is less than 1.5 per 100,000. In the United States, the incidence in white men is three times that in black men. In many of the countries in which the incidence of germ cell tumors is high, the incidence has nearly doubled in the last 20 years.

The germ cell tumors of the testes originate from the germ cells in the seminiferous tubules or from some precursor of these cells. Except for the spermatocytic seminoma, which is found only in the testes, similar tumors arise in the ovaries and occasionally in the mediastinum and elsewhere in the midline of the body.

Lesions. There has been much debate about the classification and terminology of the germ cell tumors of the testes, but in 1978 the World Health Organization divided them into seven types—seminoma, spermatocytic seminoma, embryonal carcinoma, endodermal sinus tumor, polyembryoma, choriocarcinoma, and teratoma—and this classification or some modification of it has been widely accepted (Table 40-1).

In 50% of the germ cell tumors of the testes more than one pattern of differentiation is evident. The more malignant the tumor, the more likely it is to show more than one form of differentiation. Only the

TABLE 40-1.   TYPES OF TESTICULAR NEOPLASM

Tumors of the germ cells
 Seminoma
 Embryonal carcinoma
 Infantile embryonal carcinoma
 Teratoma
 Choriocarcinoma
 Mixed germ cell tumors

Tumors of the gonadal stroma
 Leydig cell tumor
 Sertoli cell tumor
 Granulosa-theca cell tumor
 Mixed tumors of the gonadal stroma.

Gonadoblastoma

Tumors of the supporting mesenchyme and the ducts
 Benign mesenchymal tumors
 Adenocarcinoma of the rete testis

Lymphoma

Metastatic tumors

spermatocytic seminoma is never mixed with another form of germ cell tumor. Germ cell tumors that show only one pattern of differentiation are called pure. Those showing more than one pattern are called mixed germ cell tumors.

Seminoma. About 40% of germ cell tumors are pure seminomata. In another 15%, seminoma is a major component of the tumor. In others, small foci of seminomatous differentiation are sometimes present, often at the edge of the tumor. In 2% of the patients, the tumor is bilateral.

A testis containing a seminoma is usually enlarged, sometimes to 10 times its normal size. When the testis is sectioned, a well-defined, homogeneous, grayish-white tumor is found within it. Necrosis and hemorrhage into the tumor are uncommon, unless the seminoma is large. In 10% of the patients, the seminoma extends into the epididymis, spermatic cord, or into the scrotum.

Microscopically, a seminoma consists of clumps of tumor cells separated by a collagenous stroma. In 90% of the tumors, the tumor cells are well demarcated. Their cytoplasm is sometimes clear, sometimes eosinophilic and granular. The nuclei are round or ovoid. They sometimes have granular

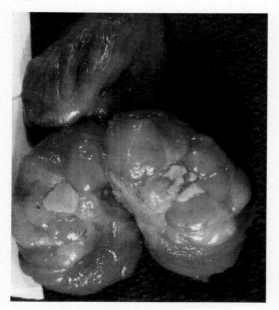

Fig. 40-11. A testis largely replaced by a seminoma. The necrosis present in the center of the tumor is unusual in this kind of neoplasm.

chromatin and one or more nucleoli; sometimes they are pyknotic. Mitoses are often present.

Electron microscopy usually shows abundant glycogen in the cytoplasm of the tumor cells. Desmosomes and other intercellular attachments are absent or small and ill-developed. The nucleoli have a skein-like nucleolonema.

The septa that separate the clumps of tumor cells are usually fine, but can be thick with hyaline collagen. In parts of some seminomata, only thin columns of tumor cells remain in a dense collagenous stroma. Lymphocytes are almost always abundant in the septa, though the density of the lymphocytic exudate varies from tumor to tumor and from one part of a tumor to another. The lymphocytes are often accompanied by smaller numbers of plasma cells, macrophages, and eosinophils.

In some seminomata, tumor cells are present in the seminiferous tubules at the

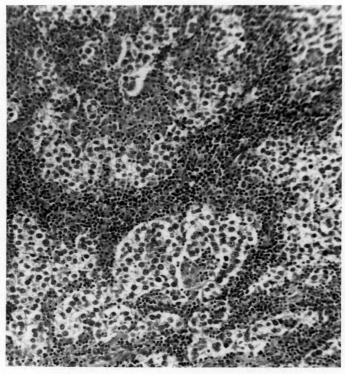

Fig. 40-12.   A seminoma, showing clumps of tumor cells with clear cytoplasm, even, round nuclei, and extensive infiltration of the stroma with lymphocytes.

edge of the tumor and sometimes extend into the rete testis. Tubules more distant from the tumor often contain occasional atypical cells that resemble the tumor cells.

In 10% of seminomata, a few large, multinucleated syncytiotrophoblastic cells are scattered among the tumor cells. Often the cytoplasm of the trophoblastic cells is vacuolated. Immunologic stains show that they contain human chorionic gonadotropin and its β subunit.

Granulomata are present in the stroma of the tumor in 50% of seminomata and are numerous in 25%. They consist of large, multinucleate macrophages surrounded by lymphocytes and plasma cells. Hyperplasia of the Leydig cells is prominent in 80% of the patients.

About 10% of seminomata are anaplastic. The pattern of the tumor is preserved, though lymphocytes in the stroma are not numerous. Granulomata are usually absent. The nuclei of the tumor cells are large, with coarse, irregular chromatin. Mitoses are numerous and may be atypical. The cytoplasm of the cells is ill-defined and usually is granular and eosinophilic. Electron microscopy shows the simplification common in anaplastic tumors.

Spermatocytic Seminoma. Less than 2% of germ cell tumors are spermatocytic seminomata. The patients are usually over 40 years old. The tumor is bilateral in 10% of the patients.

Macroscopically, a spermatocytic seminoma is well-defined and forms a mass from 3 to 15 cm in diameter. The tumor is homogeneous, gray, and friable. Usually it is edematous, gelatinous, or mucoid, sometimes with small cysts.

Microscopically, the tumor consists of clumps of cells set in a scanty, edematous stroma. Lymphocytes and granulomata are not found. Three kinds of tumor cell are present. Most common are cells 15 to 29 μm in diameter with a rim of eosinophilic cytoplasm and a spheroidal nucleus with fine, granular chromatin. Intermixed with them

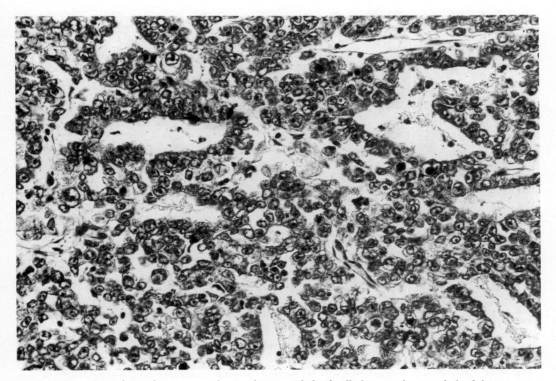

Fig. 40-13. An embryonal carcinoma, showing large, epithelioid cells forming sheets and glandular spaces.

are small cells 6 to 8 μm in diameter that resemble lymphocytes. They have scant cytoplasm and a hyperchromatic nucleus. Less common are mononuclear or multinuclear cells 50 to 100 μm across. They have abundant cytoplasm and nuclei that are sometimes fine and granular, sometimes consists of filamentous strands of chromatin. Mitoses are usually evident. Pools of eosinophilic material sometimes lie between the tumor cells. Extension along the seminiferous tubules or between them is common at the margins of the tumor.

Electron microscopy shows that the chromatin is arranged in a meiotic pattern in some of the tumor cells. Zonulae adherentes and intercellular cytoplasmic bridges like those between spermatocytes and spermatids join some of the cells. Fragments of basement membrane are often present between the tumor cells.

Embryonal Carcinoma. Embryonal carcinoma is a major constituent of 40% of germ cell tumors of the testes, though tumors consisting only of embryonal carcinoma are uncommon. Most often it is combined with a teratoma, sometimes with an endodermal sinus tumor, seminoma, or choriocarcinoma, or some combination of these tumors.

An embryonal carcinoma is usually under 5 cm in diameter. The tumor is spheroidal, ill-defined and yellowish-white, with extensive necrosis and hemorrhage. In 10 to 20% of the patients, invasion of the epididymis or spermatic cord is evident. In 30%, there is clinical evidence of intra-abdominal metastases.

Microscopically, an embryonal cell carcinoma consists of sheets of tumor cells separated by a sparse stroma. Often clefts or acini are present in the sheets. Sometimes papillary processes bulge into a cystic space in a sheet of tumor cells.

The tumor cells are large and resemble epithelial cells. Their margins are ill-defined. They have a moderate quantity of cytoplasm. Their nuclei are large with irregular chromatin. Mitoses are numerous and often

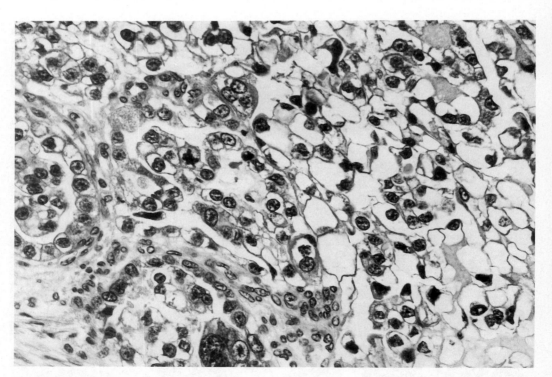

Fig. 40-14. An endodermal sinus tumor, showing the large, irregular, sometimes vacuolated tumor cells forming sheets and glands.

atypical. Immunohistochemically, some of the tumor cells stain for α-fetoprotein. Some stain for isoenzyme 1 of lactic dehydrogenase, some for the carcinoembryonic antigen. Multinucleated syncytiotrophoblastic cells like those sometimes seen in seminomata are often present in the tumor and stain for human chorionic gonadotropin.

Electron microscopy shows that the clumps of tumor cells are often surrounded by a basement membrane. Desmosomes frequently link adjacent cells. Tight junctions surround acini. The tumor cells lining the acini often have microvilli on their surface.

Endodermal Sinus Tumor. The endodermal sinus tumor is also called an infantile embryonal carcinoma and a yolk sac tumor. In infants and young children a pure endodermal sinus tumor without admixture of other types of germ cell tumor is the commonest testicular neoplasm. In adults, endodermal sinus tumor makes part of 40% of germ cell tumors if pure seminomas are excluded, but pure endodermal sinus tumors are rare.

In infants, the tumor is 2 to 6 cm across. It has usually replaced the testis and invaded the epididymis and other structures. The mass is ill-defined, soft, and yellow-white.

In adults, the macroscopic appearance of the lesion depends on the other elements present in the tumor. If endodermal sinus tumor is a major part of the lesion, the mass is often soft and mucoid, with extensive hemorrhage and necrosis.

Microscopically, an endodermal sinus tumur can show any combination of a variety of patterns of growth. The tumor cells often form solid sheets. In the sheets, the tumor cells are sometimes well-defined with pale cytoplasm; sometimes they resemble hepatocytes. Often microcysts a little bigger than a cell are numerous between the tumor cells. Sometimes larger cysts form. Occasionally the tumor is myxomatous. Sometimes the tumor forms branching ducts separated by a loose stroma. Papillary projections with a collagenous core covered by one or more layers of tumor cells sometimes bulge into cystic spaces. Not uncommonly a fold containing a blood vessel is covered by cuboidal or columnar tumor cells and projects into a space lined by flattened epithelium to form

a structure that resembles the endodermal sinus of rodents. Many of the tumor cells stain for α-fetoprotein. Some stain for α-antitrypsin.

In most endodermal sinus tumors, spheroidal, hyaline bodies 5 to 15 μm in diameter are present in or between the tumor cells. The bodies stain brightly with the periodic acid-Schiff reaction. Many of them contain α-fetoprotein. Some contain α-antitrypsin.

Electron microscopy shows that the tumor cells are joined by desmosomes. Cells lining glandular spaces have microvilli. The nucleoli are often threadlike, as in a seminoma. The hyaline bodies seen by light microscopy form in the endoplasmic reticulum and are condensed in the cytoplasm of the cells. Those containing α-fetoprotein are homogeneous and electron dense. Those that do not are filamentous and less electron dense.

Polyembryoma. A pure polyembryoma has not been reported, but embryoid bodies are sometimes found in germ cell tumors. They resemble an 18-day embryo. A plaque one or two cells thick lies between a space lined by flattened cells like the endoderm of the amniotic sac and a smaller space lined by cuboidal cells like the ectoderm of the yolk sac. Less well-formed embryoid bodies show some modification of this structure.

Choriocarcinoma. Pure choriocarcinoma of the testis is rare, but not uncommonly choriocarcinoma forms part of a testicular germ cell tumor. If choriocarcinoma is a major part of the tumor, the patient is usually under 30 years old.

If choriocarcinoma makes up a considerable part of a germ cell tumor, the tumor is soft and hemorrhagic. When choriocarcinoma predominates in a tumor, it is usually small.

Microscopically, a tumor is not called a choriocarcinoma unless it shows both cytotrophoblast and syncytiotrophoblast. Germ cell tumors that show only scattered syncytiotrophoblastic cells are not considered to contain choriocarcinoma. The cytotrophoblastic cells are cuboidal and well-defined. They have clear cytoplasm and centrally placed, spheroidal nuclei with prominent nucleoli. Mitoses are common. They occur in clumps, often surrounded by the syncytiotrophoblastic cells, which are large and irregular, with abundant often vacuolated cytoplasm and several nuclei. Often the tumor cells lie in large blood spaces. Necrosis and hemorrhage are extensive. Human chorionic gonadotropin and its β subunit are demonstrable immunohistochemically in the syncytiotrophoblast, but not in the cytotrophoblast.

Electron microscopy shows that the cyto-trophoblastic cells have few organelles but are sometimes joined by desmosomes. The syncytiotrophoblast has dilated endoplasmic reticulum, often swollen mitochondria, and microvilli that project into the blood spaces.

Teratoma. Less than 10% of germ cell tumors of the testes are pure teratomata. Most of them arise in infants and young children or in young adults. Teratoma is often present in mixed germ cell tumors in adults. Tumors containing embryonal carcinoma mixed with teratoma are particularly common and are sometimes called teratocarcinomata.

Teratomata of the testes are divided into mature and immature forms. The mature forms show a mixture of well-differentiated tissues; in the immature teratomata the tissues making up the tumor are poorly differentiated. Almost all teratomata in infants and young childern are mature, but in adults most tumors show a mixture of mature and immature tissues or are entirely immature. Sometimes mature teratomata of the testes are called benign teratomata and immature teratomata are called malignant, but since apparently mature testicular teratomata can metastasize, this usage is undesirable.

If a germ cell tumor consists entirely or largely of teratoma, it is often cystic, with cysts filled with clear, gelatinous or mucinous material. Between the cysts, the tumor is solid, sometimes cartilaginous. Necrosis and hemorrhage are rare in the mature tumors, but occur in the immature forms. In 10% of the patients, the tumor has extended beyond the testis.

Microscopically, a mature teratoma shows a mixture of well-differentiated tissues of all three germ layers. Commonly the tumor forms organoid structures, islands of neural cells; tubules lined by gastrointestinal, res-

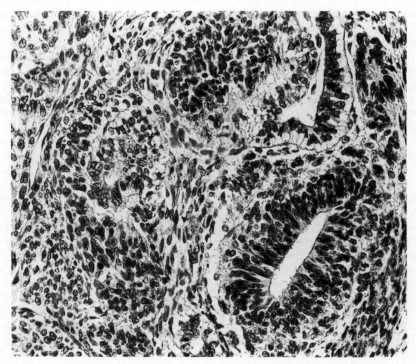

Fig. 40-15. A moderately differentiated testicular teratoma, showing spaces lined by epithelium.

piratory or squamous epithelium; fragments of liver, pancreas, or bone marrow; and often cartilage, bone, fat, and smooth or striated muscle. An immature teratoma shows a similar mixture of tissues from different germ layers, but the tissues are ill-formed with poorly differentiated cells and are often hard to recognize. In 30% of teratomata, some of the tumor cells stain for α-fetoprotein.

The chromosomal abnormalities in teratomata of the testis are discussed in Chapter 13.

Rarely, a carcinoid tumor, a cyst lined by keratinizing stratified squamous epithelium without appendages or other evidence of a teratoma, or a retinal anlage tumor like those found in the mouth arises in a testis. The origin of these tumors is unknown, but it is often suggested that they may be an unusual form of teratoma that shows only one pattern of differentiation.

Mixed Germ Cell Tumors.   The frequency with which the germ cell tumors of the testes are mixed has already been emphasized. The more carefully a germ cell tumor of a testis is examined microscopically, the more likely it is to show more than one pattern of differentiation.

Even if a primary germ cell tumor seems to show only one pattern of differentiation, its metastases are sometimes mixed. In 25% of patients with an apparently pure seminoma who develop metastases, the metastases consist entirely or partially of embryonal carcinoma, less often of choriocarcinoma or teratoma. Tumors that seem entirely embryonal carcinoma can show foci of choriocarcinoma, endodermal sinus tumor, or teratoma in their metastases. Tumors that are predominantly teratoma often show embryonal carcinoma, endodermal sinus tumor, or choriocarcinoma in some of their metastases.

Burnt Out Tumors.   Occasionally no primary tumor can be found in a man with metastatic germ cell tumor. The testes seem normal and no primary tumor is present in the mediastinum or any other site.

In some of these patients, a small scar is

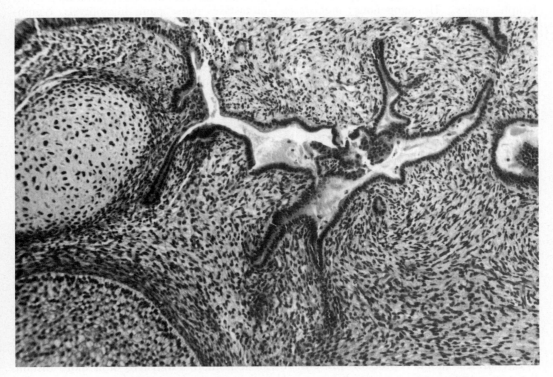

Fig. 40-16.   A poorly differentiated testicular teratoma, showing ill-defined spaces lined by epithelium, that is not clearly demarcated from the mesenchymal part of the tumor.

present in one of the testes. Often hemosiderin in the scar suggests old hemorrhage. Ovoid, amorphous, or granular masses that stain strongly with hematoxylin frequently lie among the bundles of collagen. Occasionally remnants of a teratoma or seminoma are present in the scar. Probably these scars are the remains of a primary germ cell tumor that was destroyed by hemorrhage or infarction. Similar scars are sometime present in testicular germ cell tumors and probably are caused in similar fashion.

Behavior. Seminomata metastasize predominantly by the lymphatic system. The testicular lymphatics accompany the testicular arteries and drain into the paraaortic lymph nodes near the renal arteries. The first metastases usually appear in this region. In 20% of the patients, both sides are involved. If the tumor involves the scrotum, the iliac nodes are often affected.

If the tumor is not eradicated, involvement of the lymph nodes becomes extensive as the seminoma spreads along the paraaortic chain, often involving mediastinal or supraclavicular lymph nodes. Hematogenous metastases develop late in the course of the disease. They are found at autopsy in only 50% of people dying of seminoma.

Embryonal carcinomata, endodermal sinus tumors, choriocarcinomata, and teratomata of the testes metastasize to the lymph nodes as do seminomata, but in most patients the metastases in the lymph nodes are overshadowed by hematogenous metastases, to the liver, lungs, kidneys, gut, or bone. In over 30% of the patients, metastases are evident clinically at the time the diagnosis is made. Especially in patients with choriocarcinoma, the hematogenous metastases often develop rapidly and are widespread.

Dysfunction. The syncytiotrophoblast secretes human chorionic gonadotropin or its β subunit in sufficient quantity to increase the concentration of the hormone in the plasma in all patients with a testicular germ cell tumor containing choriocarcinoma, in 5% of those with a pure seminoma, and in 70% of those with tumors containing embryonal carcinoma. If the concentration is over 100,000 U/L, choriocarcinoma is probably present. If the concentration is lower, the hormone is probably produced by the syncytiotrophoblastic cells scattered in the tumor.

α-Fetoprotein is synthesized by the cells of the endodermal sinus tumors and by some of the tumor cells in an embryonal carcinoma or teratoma. Its concentration in the plasma is increased in all patients with a testicular germ cell tumor containing endodermal sinus tumor, in 75% of those with a tumor predominantly of embryonal carcinoma, and less markedly in 50% of patients with a tumor containing teratoma.

Ferritin is present in the plasma in increased concentration in 90% of patients with a germ cell tumor. The activity of placental alkaline phosphatase is increased in 60% of patients with seminoma. The activity of isoenzyme 1 of lactic dehydrogenase in the plasma is raised in most patients with a germ cell tumor. In many patients with a seminoma production of the follicle-stimulating enzyme by the pituitary gland is increased.

Clinical Presentation. In most patients, a testicular germ cell tumor is discovered only when it is large enough to cause discomfort or dragging in the testis. In over 10% of the patients, the tumor is discovered only when metastases cause pain, hemoptysis, lymphadenopathy, or urinary obstruction.

Etiology. Uncorrected maldescent of the testes increases the risk of developing a germ cell tumor up to 50 times. The tumor is most often a seminoma, but any kind of germ cell tumor can develop. Genetic factors are important in a few kindred in which the incidence of testicular germ cell tumors is high. Endocrine imbalance and trauma are often proposed as causes of testicular tumors, but their importance seems slight. In animals, testicular tumors can be induced by injecting zinc chloride, copper sulfate, or a carcinogenic hydrocarbon into the testes.

Treatment and Prognosis. A seminoma is treated by orchidectomy followed by abdominal irradiation. A seminoma is highly radiosensitive, and the radiation usually destroys any tumor in the abdomen. If there is no evidence of intra-abdominal involvement, over 95% of the patients are cured. If computerized tomography shows only lymph nodes less than 5 cm across, over 85% of the patients are cured. If the abdominal involvement is more extensive, or if more distant metastases are present, the patients are also given cisplatin and other chemotherapeutic agents. About 80% are cured.

Other types of testicular germ cell tumor are not radiosensitive and are treated by orchidectomy and dissection of the abdominal lymph nodes. If the lymph nodes are not involved. 90% of the patients are cured. If microscopic metastases are present in fewer than five lymph nodes, 60% are cured. If combination chemotherapy including cisplatin is added, 85% of the patients are cured, even if the metastatic disease is massive and distant metastases are present. When a tumor recurs, it usually does so within two years. The residual tumor that remains in patients not cured by chemotherapy is often teratoma, probably because the teratomatous element in the tumor is less sensitive to the chemotherapeutic drugs than are other kinds of germ cell tumor.

Infertility often complicates the chemotherapy, radiotherapy, and lymph nodes dissection used to treat a testicular germ cell tumor. The chemotherapeutic drugs used commonly cause nausea and vomiting, alopecia, or neuropathy or damage the ears, lungs, or kidneys.

SEX CORD-STROMAL TUMORS. The sex cord-stromal tumors make up less than 5% of testicular tumors. Most of them arise from the Leydig cells and some from Sertoli cells. The tumor-like masses that develop in the testes in the adrenogenital syndrome resemble Leydig cell tumors. Rarely, a granulosa cell tumor similar to the granulosa cell tumors of the ovaries develops in a testis, or a sex cord-stromal tumor shows some combination of these kinds of differentiation.

Leydig Cell Tumor. Most Leydig cell tumors arise in men 20 to 50 years old, but they can arise in children and in older men. In 3% of the patients, the tumor is bilateral.

Macroscopically, the tumor is usually 3 to 5 cm in diameter, well demarcated and often lobulated. It may be yellow, tan, brown, or gray. Foci of hemorrhage are evident in 25% of the tumors. In 10%, the tumor extends beyond the testis.

Microscopically, the tumor usually consists of sheets or cords of tumor cells that resemble normal Leydig cells. They have abundant eosinophilic cytoplasm and small pyknotic nuclei. Occasionally the cytoplasm is vacuolated or foamy because of fat in the cells. Mitoses are few. Crystalloids of Reinke are evident in 30% of the tumors and lipochrome pigment is present in 10%. The stroma is usually sparse, but can be hyalinized. Less often, a Leydig cell tumor consists of small spindle-shaped cells or is anaplastic with a high mitotic rate. Electron microscopy shows abundant smooth endoplasmic reticulum and tubular mitochondrial cristae.

The tumor cells secrete testosterone in most of the patients, often together with estrogens and progesterone. Less often, corticosteroids are formed.

In a child, a Leydig cell tumor nearly always causes sexual precocity. The penis enlarges, pubic hair takes an adult pattern, the voice deepens, facial hair appears, and acne is common. In 85% of adults with a Leydig cell tumor, the tumor causes no hormonal dysfunction and is detected only when a mass in found in the testis. In 15% of adults, it causes gynecomastia.

A Leydig cell tumor is treated by orchidectomy. In children, the tumors are benign. In adults, 10% of them metastasize, but usually only to the regional lymph nodes in the abdomen. Leydig cell tumors are radioresistant, but grow slowly. Resection of the metastases may bring cure.

Adrenogenital Tumor. The bilateral tumors that arise in the testes in the adrenogenital syndrome may be as much as 10 cm in diameter. Microscopically, they resemble a Leydig cell tumor, though Reinke crystalloids are not present. The tumors secrete cortisol and testosterone. Probably they are not neoplasms, but a hyperplastic response induced by the excess of the adrenocorticotropic hormone. If the concentration of the hormone in the plasma is reduced, the lesions regress.

Sertoli Cell Tumor. Sertoli cell tumors usually form a well-circumscribed, white, yellow, or tan mass in a testis. Microscopically, the tumor usually consists of sheets or cords of cuboidal or columnar cells with clear cytoplasm and spheroidal, vesicular nuclei. Less often, the tumor forms tubules that resemble seminiferous tubules. In the large cell calcifying Sertoli cell tumor the tumor cells are large, and foci of calcification are prominent in the tumor. Sertoli cell tumors usually have no hormonal activity, but a few have caused gynecomastia in an adult or precocious sexual development in a child. Most Sertoli tumors are benign. A few have metastasized, usually only to the regional lymph nodes in the abdomen.

TUMORS CONTAINING GERM CELL AND SEX CORD-STROMAL ELEMENTS. Two tumors of the testes show a mixture of germ cell and sex cord-stromal elements, the gonadoblastoma and the mixed germ cell sex cord-stromal tumor.

Gonadoblastoma. Gonadoblastomata are rare. The patients are almost all intersexual. Nearly 80% of them are of female habitus. About 50% have a normal male chromosomal pattern. Most of the rest are mosaics, most commonly 45,X/46,XY. In 30% of the patients, the tumor is bilateral.

A gonadoblastoma usually arises in the pelvis from a testis or a streak of the kind seen in gonadal dysplasia. The tumor is from 0.5 to 10 cm in diameter. It may be white, yellow, or brown, soft or firm. Often the lesion is partially or largely calcified.

Microscopically, a gonadoblastoma consists of clumps of tumor cells separated by a collagenous stroma. In the clumps, cells like those of a seminoma are mixed with smaller, darker cells like those of a granulosa cell tumor or a Sertoli cell tumor. Often the seminoma cells are in the center of the clumps and are surrounded by the sex cord-stromal cells. Sometimes the sex cord-stromal cells surround individual seminoma cells or small clumps of seminoma cells. Sometimes the sex cord-stromal cells form structures like the Call-Exner bodies of a granulosa cell tumor, with granulosa or Sertoli cells surrounding a small lumen filled with amorphous material that stains strongly with the periodic acid-Schiff reaction. Sometimes these structures are confluent and replace much of the tumor.

Often the stroma between the clumps of tumor cells contains Leydig cells or cells that resemble the luteinized cells of ovarian stroma. Calcification is evident in 80% of the tumors. It begins in the structures resembling Call-Exner bodies and forms spheroidal, laminated structures like psammoma bodies. In many of the tumors, calcification becomes extensive and replaces much of the lesion.

In 50% of the patients, part of the tumor

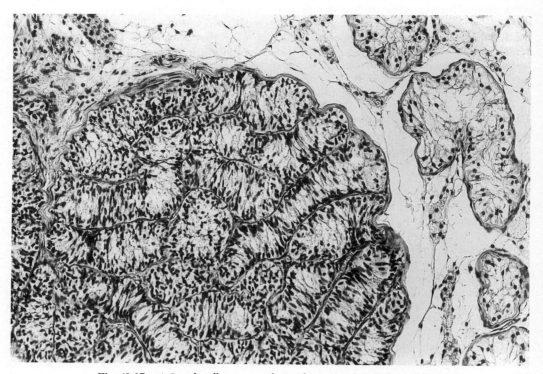

Fig. 40-17. A Sertoli cell tumor, with neoplastic Sertoli cells lining tubules.

consists only of seminoma. In 10%, foci of embryonal carcinoma, endodermal sinus tumor, or teratoma are present.

About 50% of gonadoblastomata secrete androgens, in sufficient quantity to cause virilization in patients of female habitus. Some secrete estrogens.

A gonadoblastoma is usually treated by the excision of both gonads, because of the risk that the contralateral gonad will harbor a small tumor. If the tumor contains no admixture of a germ cell tumor other than seminoma, the prognosis is excellent. Excision usually cures, though metastases of the seminomatous element can occur. If a gonadoblastoma is mixed with a more malignant germ cell tumor, the prognosis is poor, though chemotherapy has improved the outlook.

Mixed Germ Cell Sex Cord-Stromal Tumor. The mixed germ cell sex cord-stromal tumor is an uncommon neoplasm most often found in a normal ovary in a child, but can arise in a normal testis in an adult. The tumor is often large, replacing the testis and invading the epididymis. It is firm, white, and well demarcated. Microscopically, the tumor cells form anastomosing cords separated by a collagenous stroma or tubules without a lumen or grow in large sheets. In the cords and clumps of tumor cells, large, pale germ cells are intermixed with small, dark sex cord-stromal cells that resemble granulosa or Sertoli cells. Orchidectomy cures, though a few of the ovarian tumors have metastasized.

Epididymis and Spermatic Cord

Tumors of the epididymis and spermatic cord are uncommon. A lipoma of the spermatic cord is the most common tumor in adults but rarely is large enough to cause symptoms. In children, an embryonal rhabdomyosarcoma sometimes arises in a spermatic cord. Only the adenomatoid tumor and cystadenoma of the epididymis are discussed.

ADENOMATOID TUMOR. Adenomatoid tumors are uncommon. They arise in relation to the epididymis and the adjacent parts of the tunica vaginalis and spermatic cord, in relation to the uterus, fallopian tubes, and ovaries, and occasionally in or near an adrenal gland.

In the epididymis, an adenomatoid tumor forms a white nodule or plaque from 0.5 to 5.0 cm across. Microscopically, the tumor consists of tubules lined by cuboidal or flattened cells or forms solid cords of similar cells. Often the tumor cells contain vacuoles that seem to coalesce to form the lumen. The tubules and cords are supported by a fibromuscular stroma. Electron microscopy shows that the tumor cells are mesothelial, with the long microvilli and intercellular filaments typical of mesothelial cells.

Adenomatoid tumors are benign. They grow slowly if at all.

CYSTADENOMA OF THE EPIDIDYMIS. Cystadenomata of the epididymis are uncommon. They may be bilateral, and in several patients have been associated with von Hippel-Lindau disease. The cystadenoma forms a cystic mass up to 5 cm in diameter in one or both epididymides. Microscopically, the tumor consists of ectatic ducts lined by cuboidal cells with clear, vacuolated cytoplasm. Often the epithelium of the ducts is thrown into papillary folds. The lesion is benign.

Penis

The penis is covered by skin and mucosa and develops tumors like those of the skin and mucosa in other parts of the body. Condylomata are the most common benign tumors of the surface of the penis. Eyrthroplasia of Queyrat and Bowen's disease are forms of carcinoma in situ. Squamous cell carcinoma is the principal malignant tumor. Rarely, a basal cell carcinoma, malignant melanoma, Kaposi's sarcoma, a benign or malignant mesenchymal tumor, or a metastases involves the penis. The tumors of the penile urethra are considered in Chapter 39.

CONDYLOMA. Condylomata occur in the preputial sac or, less often, on the shaft of the penis. They are caused by human papilloma viruses. Most of the lesions are condylomata acuminata, with coarse fronds covered by hyperplastic epithelium, and are benign. Koilocytotic cells with empty cytoplasm and pyknotic nuclei are common in the superficial part of the epithelium, as in other tumors caused by human papilloma viruses.

The giant condylomata caused by human papilloma viruses are large, warty lesions that arise in the preputial sac of uncircumcised men. Grotesque, warty masses extend widely and slowly erode into the underlying tissues. Ulceration and infection are common. The prepuce may be perforated. Microscopically, the lesions show broad, papillary fronds covered by hyperplastic epithelium. The bases of the fronds are smooth and rounded. They push into the underlying tissues, rather like a verrucous carcinoma. Indeed, some consider the lesion to be a verrucous carcinoma. Some of the giant condylomata progress to invasive squamous cell carcinoma.

Also caused by the human papilloma virus are flat condylomata called bowenoid papulosis. Microscopically, the lesions resemble

Bowen's disease. Some of the lesions regress spontaneously; some persist. Some are caused by human papilloma viruses of type 16 or 18, the types associated with carcinoma of the cervix, but bowenoid papulosis does not progress to invasive carcinoma.

ERYTHROPLASIA OF QUEYRAT. Erythroplasia of Queyrat is named after a French dermatologist born in 1872. The patients are from 20 to 90 years old. A velvety plaque about 1 cm across develops on the glans of the penis or the inner surface of the prepuce. About 10% of the patients progress to invasive squamous cell carcinoma.

Microscopically, the epithelium shows carcinoma in situ. Keratinization is slight, but often there is parakeratosis. The underlying connective tissue is congested with a dense exudate containing many plasma cells.

BOWEN'S DISEASE.   Carcinoma in situ of

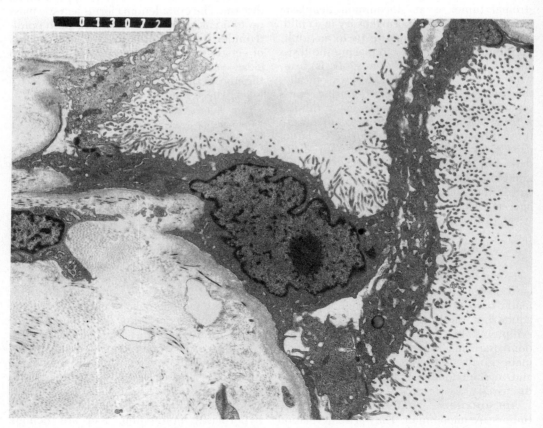

Fig. 40-18.   An electron micrograph of an adenomatoid tumor, showing the long microvilli of the flattened tumor cells lining the tubules (Courtesy of Dr. Y. Bédard)

the shaft of the penis is called Bowen's disease and is similar to Bowen's disease in other parts of the skin. About 5% of the patients develop invasive squamous cell carcinoma.

CARCINOMA. About 1% of cancers in men arise on the penis. Most of the patients are over 50 years old. Carcinoma of the penis is more common in Africa, Asia, and South America than in Europe or North America.

Carcinoma of the penis usually begins on the glans or inner surface of the prepuce. The carcinoma may form an ulcer, like the ulcer of a squamous cell carcinoma of the lip, a verrucous nodule, or a large fungating mass. If the carcinoma becomes infected, ulceration and a foul, blood-stained exudate are common.

Microscopically, a carcinoma of the penis is nearly always a squamous cell carcinoma, usually moderately or well differentiated. The surface of the tumor is often verrucous, with hyperkeratosis and parakeratosis. Metastases are usually confined to the regional lymph nodes. Hematogenous metastases occur in less than 10% of the patients.

Carcinoma of the penis is treated surgically, by excision of the primary tumor and, if necessary, dissection of the inguinal lymph nodes. If the tumor has not metastasized, excision cures. If the inguinal lymph nodes are involvled, 50% of the patients are cured.

Circumcision in infancy almost entirely prevents carcinoma of the penis. In Africa, carcinoma of the penis is unknown in a tribe that practices circumcision in infancy, but is common in a neighboring tribe in which the men remain uncircumcised. Probably the retention of smegma causes the carcinoma, though whether the smegma itself is at fault, or the organisms that grow in it, is unknown.

Scrotum

Tumors of the scrotum are uncommon. Multiple sebaceous cysts sometimes develop in the scrotum and cause striking deformity. Occasionally multiple leiomyomata develop in the scrotum. Squamous cell carcinoma of the scrotum is rare, but is one of the first tumors proved to be caused by the patient's

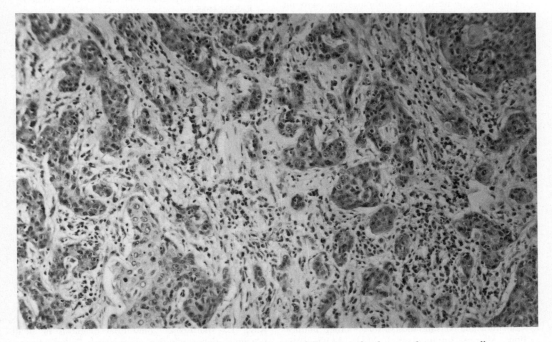

Fig. 40-19. A carcinoma of the penis, showing moderately differentiated columns of squamous cell carcinoma invading the underlying tissues.

occupation. The high incidence of carcinoma of the scrotum in chimney sweeps was noted in 1775, and later a high incidence of carcinoma of the scrotum was observed in mule skinners and paraffin workers whose clothes were saturated with carcinogenic oils.

BIBLIOGRAPHY

General

Nistal, M., and Paniagua, R.: Testicular and Epididymal Pathology. New York, Thieme Medical Publishers, 1984.

Talerman, A., and Roth, L. M.: Pathology of the Testis and Its Adnexa. New York, Churchill Livingstone, 1986.

Tannenbaum, M.: Urologic Pathology: The Prostate. Philadelphia, Lea & Febiger, 1977.

Inflammation

Corey, L., and Spear, P. G.: Infections with herpes simplex viruses. N. Engl. J. Med., 314:686, 749, 1986.

Gorse, G. J., and Belshe, R. B.: Male genital tuberculosis. Rev. Infect. Dis., 7:511, 1985.

Mikuz, G., and Damjanov, I.: Inflammation of the testis, epididymis, peritesticular membranes, and scrotum. Pathol. Annu., 17(Pt 1):101, 1982.

Nilsen, A.: Herpes genitalis. Scand. J. Infect. Dis. (Suppl), 47:51057, 1985.

Swenson, R. M.: Herpes simplex virus genital infections. Clin. Ther., 8:145, 1986.

Wildy, P.: Herpes viruses. Br. Med. Bull., 41:339, 1985.

Prostatic Hyperplasia

Ablin, R. J., and Gonder, M. J.: Immunological aspects of benign and malignant tumors of the prostate. Contrib. Gynecol. Obstet., 14:185, 1985.

Ayala, A. G., et al.: Clear cell cribriform hyperplasia of prostate. Am. J. Surg. Pathol., 10:665, 1986.

Brawn, P. N.: Interpretation of Prostate Biopsies. New York, Raven Press, 1983.

Kovi, J.: Microscopic differential diagnosis of small acinar adenocarcinoma of prostate. Pathol. Annu., 20(Pt 1):157, 1985.

Other Non-Neoplastic Diseases

Blaustein, D., et al.: Immunological consequences of vasectomy and consideration of some of their implications. Allergol. Immunopathol. (Madr), 14:95, 1986.

Galvaö-Teles, A., Monteiro, E., Gavaler, J. S., and Van

Thiel, D. H.: Gonadal consequences of alcohol abuse. Hepatology, 6:135, 1986.

Gondos, B., and Riddick, D. H.: Pathology of Infertility. New York, Thieme Medical Publications, 1987.

Klimas, R., Bennett, B., and Gardner, W. A. Jr.: Prostatic calculi. Prostate, 7:91, 1985.

Lennox, B.: The infertile testis. Rec. Adv. Hisopathol., 11:135, 1981.

Schellhammer, P. F., Jordan, G. H., and El-Mahdi, A. M.: Pelvic complications after interstitial and external beam irradiation of urologic and gynecologic malignancy. World J. Surg., 10:259, 1986.

Sheldon, C. A.: Undescended testis and testicular torsion. Surg. Clin. North Am., 65:1303, 1985.

Congenital Anomalies

Chilvers, C., et al.: Undescended testis: the effect of treatment on subsequent subfertility and malignancy. J. Pediatr. Surg., 21:691, 1986.

Sheldon, C. A.: Undescended testis and testicular torsion. Surg. Clin. North Am., 65:1303, 1985.

Siebermann, R. E.: The pathology of the gonads and adrenal cortex in intersex. Prog. Pediatr. Surg., 16:149, 1983.

Sultan, C.: Androgen receptors and partial androgen insensitivity in male pseudohermaphroditism. Ann. Genet., 29:5, 1986.

Troche, V., and Hernandez, E.: Neoplasia arising in dysgenetic gonads. Obstet. Gynecol. Surv., 41:74, 1986.

Wu, F. C.: Male hypogonadism. Clin. Obstet. Gynaecol., 12:531, 1985.

Tumors

Ablin, R. J., and Gonder, M. J.: Immunological aspects of benign and malignant tumors of the prostate. Contrib. Gynecol. Obstet., 14:185, 1985.

Brawn, P. N.: Interpretation of Prostate Biopsies. New York, Raven Press, 1983.

Brawn, P. N., et al.: Histologic grading of prostate adenocarcinoma. Cancer, 49:535, 1982.

Cangir, A.: Malignant genital tract tumors in children. Curr. Probl. Cancer, 10:301, 1986.

Chilvers, C., et al.: Undescended testis: the effect of treatment on subsequent subfertility and malignancy. J. Pediatr. Surg., 21:691, 1986.

Chu, T. M., and Murphy, G. P.: What's new in markers for prostate cancer? Urology, 27:487, 1986.

Doll, D. C., and Weiss, R. B.: Malignant lymphoma of the testis. Am. J. Med., 8:515, 1986.

Einhorn, L. H.: Cancer of the testis. Hosp. Pract., 21(4):175, 1986.

Hays, D. M.: Malignant solid tumors of childhood. Curr. Probl. Surg., 23:161, 1986.

Khoury, S., et al. (Eds.): Testicular cancer. Prog. Clin. Biol. Res., 203:1, 1985.

Kovi, J.: Microscopic differential diagnosis of small acinar adenocarcinoma of prostate. Pathol. Annu., 20(Pt 1):157, 1985.

Kramer, S. A.: Pediatric urologic oncology. Urol. Clin. North Am., *12*:31, 1985.

Loehrer, P. J., Sr., Sledge, G. W., Jr., and Einhorn, L. H.: Heterogeneity among germ cell tumors of the testis. Semin. Oncol., *12*:304, 1985.

Miller, G. J.: The use of histochemistry and immunohistochemistry in evaluating prostatic neoplasia. Prog. Surg. Pathol., 5:115, 1983.

Mostofi, F. K., and Price, E. B., Jr.: Tumors of the Male Genital System. Washington, D.C., Armed Forces Institute of Pathology, 1973.

Murphy, G. P., et al. (Eds.): Prostatic Cancer. New York, Alan R. Liss, 1987.

Powell, B. L., Craig, J. B., and Muss, H. B.: Secondary

malignancies of the penis and epididymis. J. Clin. Oncol., 3:110, 1985.

Sawczuk, I.: Primary transitional cell carcinoma of the prostatic periurethral ducts. Urology, 25:339, 1985.

Talerman, A.: Germ cell tumours. Ann. Pathol., 5:145, 1985.

Troche, V., and Hernandez, E.: Neoplasia arising in dysgenetic gonads. Obstet. Gynecol. Surv., *41*:74, 1986.

Truong, L. D., et al.: Endodermal sinus tumor of the mediastinum. Cancer, 58:730, 1986.

Valadez, R. A., and Watters, W. B.: Leiomyosarcoma of the penis. Urology, 27:265, 1986.

41

Female Reproductive System

THE female reproductive tract consists of the ovaries, fallopian tubes, uterus, vagina, and vulva. As with the male reproductive tract, there is little similarity between the disease of the various parts of the female genital system, but because of their close functional interaction it is desirable to consider them together.

INFLAMMATION

Inflammation of the ovaries is called oophoritis, from the Greek for egg-bearing. Inflammation of the fallopian tubes is called salpingitis, from the Greek for trumpet, because of the shape of the tubes. Inflammation of the uterus is called metritis, or more often endometritis, myometritis, or perimetritis from the Greek for womb. Inflammation of the cervix uteri is called cervicitis, from the Latin for neck; inflammation of the vagina vaginitis, from the Latin for a sheath; and inflammation of the vulva vulvitis, from the Latin for womb.

Ovaries

Inflammation of the ovaries often begins in the fallopian tubes and sometimes by extension of infection from some other organ. Inflammatory lesions confined to the ovaries are uncommon.

Fallopian Tubes

The term *pelvic inflammatory disease* is used to describe acute and chronic inflammation of the fallopian tubes and adjacent structures. Less often the fallopian tubes develop granulomatous salpingitis or salpingitis isthmica nodosa.

PELVIC INFLAMMATORY DISEASE. Each year 850,000 women in the United States develop pelvic inflammatory disease. Almost all the patients are sexually active. A sexually active person 15 to 16 years old is more likely to develop the disease than is an older women. An intrauterine contraceptive device increases the risk of developing salpingitis 3 times. Having multiple sexual partners increases the risk of developing pelvic inflammatory disease. Oral contraceptives reduce the risk.

In the United States, Neisseria gonorrhoeae and Chlamydia trachomatis are the principal causes of tubal inflammation. N. gonorrhoeae alone is isolated in 25% of the patients, C. trachomatis alone in 25%, and both in 25%. In Scandinavia where gonorrhea is less prevalent, N. gonorrhoeae is found in only 20% of the patients. Bacterioides, Escherichia coli, streptococci, Mycoplasma hominis, or Ureaplasma urealyticum are frequently isolated, both in patients with neisserian or chlamydial infection and those without. Especially in chronic cases, more than one organism is often present.

The gonococci and chlamydiae that cause salpingitis ascend from the vagina through the uterus, often during menstruation. Inflammation of the endometrium is usually slight, but endometritis is present in 50% of women with a chlamydial infection of the endocervix, less often in women with gonorrhea. The other organisms that cause or complicate pelvic inflammatory disease probably reach the region in the blood.

Lesions. The lesions of pelvic inflammatory disease form a continuum, beginning with acute salpingitis and progressing to chronic salpingitis, a tuboovarian abscess, hydrosalpinx, or pyosalpinx unless the infection is controlled. One or both tubes may be involved.

Acute Salpingitis. In gonococcal salpingitis, the gonococci attach to the nonciliated cells in the fallopian epithelium and penetrate into and between the cells. Focal necrosis of the epithelium with acute inflammation follows. C. trachomatis causes similar epithelial necrosis and inflammation. The infected tube becomes congested and edematous. Pus is often present in the lumen of the tube and oozes from its fimbriated end. Microscopically an exudate mainly of neutrophils is most intense in the submucosa but often extends through the whole thickness of the wall. Sometimes a fibrinous exudate roughens the peritoneal surface of the tube.

Chronic Salpingitis. If acute salpingitis fails to resolve, chronic salpingitis follows. Often the tube is distorted, with fine adhesions between the tube and adjacent structures. Less often, adhesions are massive, filling much of the pelvis. The mucosal folds in the tube are low, and the collagenous tissue in the subepithelial tissue is increased. Sometimes adjacent folds of mucosa adhere together. Occasionally the bridges between the folds are so numerous that the lumen of the tube is divided into multiple channels, and on section the lumen of the tube seems replaced by gland-like spaces, a condition called salpingitis follicularis. Often the lumen of the tube is obliterated in one or more places.

Hydrosalpinx. Occasionally the fimbrial end of a tube is obliterated, and the tube becomes greatly distended by clear, serous fluid, a condition called hydrosalpinx. Usually the fimbrial end of the tube is markedly dilated and the uterine end remains thin, giving the tube the appearance of an old-fashioned retort. The dilated fimbrial end of the tube is sometimes 10 cm across. The wall of the tube shows fibrosis and chronic inflammation.

Pyosalpinx. If the tube is distended with pus, the condition is called a pyosalpinx. The wall of the tube is fibrotic and shows a mixture of acute and chronic inflammation.

Tubo-Ovarian Abscess. Salpingitis often causes adhesions between the fimbriated end of the tube and the ovary. A tubo-ovarian abscess results if the infection spreads into this space. The ovary is in the wall of the abscess but is little involved by the infection. For the most part, the abscess is bounded by adhesions.

Complications. In 25% of women with acute pelvic inflammatory disease, laparoscopy shows inflammation of the capsule of the liver, a condition called perihepatitis. In 10% of the patients, the perihepatitis is severe enough to cause upper abdominal

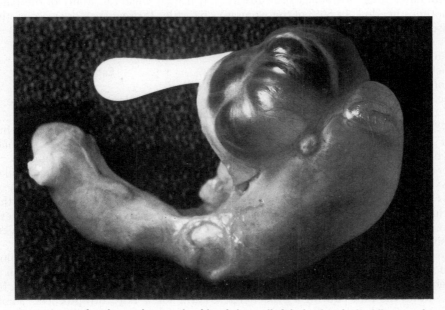

Fig. 41-1. Hydrosalpinx, showing the dilated thin-walled fimbrial end of a fallopian tube.

pain and tenderness. The inflammation of the liver usually resolves but sometimes causes perihepatic adhesions.

Periappendicitis is present in many patients with pelvic inflammatory disease. The serosa of the appendix is inflamed, but the inflammation does not involve the mucosa.

Rarely, a tubo-ovarian abscess ruptures causing generalized peritonitis, or peritonitis complicates acute salpingitis. Rarely, a patient develops a fistula into the vagina, bladder, or rectum.

Clinical Presentation. Patients with pelvic inflammatory disease usually have a history of vaginal discharge or other symptoms of cervicitis. Some patients have no other symptoms, but in most, signs of pelvic inflammation develop gradually. Pain in the lower abdomen develops in 70% of the patients, menorrhagia in 40%, urethritis in 20%, and proctitis in 10%. A mass is palpable in 50% of the patients. Often the lesions are tender, or movement of the uterus causes pain. Only 30% of the patients have a fever of more than 38°C, but the level of C-reactive protein is almost always increased; 75% of the patients have an increased erythrocyte sedimentation rate, and 60% have a leukocytosis.

Treatment and Prognosis. Pelvic inflammatory disease is usually treated by antibiotic therapy. Surgical drainage of an abscess is sometimes needed. In 80% of the women, the disease is controlled. In 20%, repeated attacks of pelvic inflammation follow.

Even if the disease is promptly controlled, obstruction to the tubes causes infertility in 20% of women with pelvic inflammatory disease. In 5% of those who become pregnant, the pregnancy is ectopic, because chronic salpingitis impairs the movement of the ovum through the tube. The risk of developing a tubal pregnancy is 7 times greater than in a healthy woman.

GRANULOMATOUS SALPINGITIS. Granulomatous salpingitis is often caused by Mycobacterium tuberculosis, but occasionally is due to actinomycosis, enterobiasis, schistosomiasis, echinococcosis, or some other disease. Sometimes it is caused by talc, lubricant jelly, the oily solutions used for salpingography, or other foreign material introduced into the tubes during a gynecologic examination. Rarely, the fallopian tubes are involved in Crohn's disease or sarcoidosis.

Tuberculosis. Tuberculous salpingitis is the commonest form of genital tuberculosis in women. It is usually secondary to pulmonary tuberculosis, but can complicate a primary lesion in the gut. About 10% of women dying of tuberculosis have lesions in the fallopian tubes. Nearly always, both tubes are involved.

Early in the disease, granulomata are numerous in the mucosa of the tubes. As the infection progresses, the tubes become increasingly fibrotic, and granulomata become few. Caseous abscesses sometimes develop. Calcification of some of the granulomata is common. The tubes are usually ectatic and surrounded by dense adhesions. In 50% of the patients, the fimbrated ends of the tubes remain widely patent.

Pain and menstrual irregularity are the most common symptoms of tuberculous salpingitis. Because of the scarring and distortion of the fallopian tubes, most of the patients are infertile.

SALPINGITIS ISTHMICA NODOSA. Salpingitis isthmica nodosa is uncommon. It occurs in adults. Its pathogenesis is unknown. Diverticula surrounded by a proliferation of smooth muscle bulge from the wall of the isthmus of the fallopian tubes, forming nodules 1 to 2 cm in diameter. Salpingitis isthmica nodosa is usually bilateral. Many of the patients are infertile. If pregnancy does occur, the risk of an ectopic gestation is high.

Endometrium

Endometritis is divided into acute, chronic, and granulomatous forms.

ACUTE ENDOMETRITIS. Acute inflammation of the endometrium is normal during menstruation and after pregnancy. The inflammation is caused by the breakdown of the tissues, not by infection. Rarely, a uterus obstructed by a carcinoma or by the occlusion of the cervix that sometimes develops in old age becomes filled with pus, a condition called pyometra.

Puerperal Endometritis. Infection of the endometrium after pregnancy or an abortion is called puerperal endometritis, from the Latin for a boy. Streptococci, staphylococci, gram-negative bacilli, clostridia, and occasionally fungi can cause massive infection of the raw endometrium if they gain entry to the uterine cavity. Puerperal fever used to be common and lethal, but has become uncommon since the introduction of antibiotics.

If the infection is severe, acute inflammation extends deep into the myometrium, sometimes into the periuterine tissues. Thrombosis of the pelvic veins or generalized peritonitis can complicate the infection. Often the patient is in shock, with severe toxemia.

CHRONIC ENDOMETRITIS. Chronic endometritis is present in 5% of women with menstrual irregularity. The cause of the inflammation is often not apparent, and the patients are said to have nonspecific endometritis. In 50% of these people, Chlamydia trachomatis or Neisseria gonorrhoeae can be isolated from the endocervix and may be responsible for the endometritis. In other patients, Mycoplasma hominis, Mycoplasma fermentans, or Ureaplasma urealyticum is responsible for the inflammation. Patients with a ureaplasmal or mycoplasmal infection are often infertile. Occasionally a cytomegaloviral or some other viral infection involves the endometrium.

Ill-defined clumps of lymphocytes are normally present in the endometrium, but plasma cells are not. If more than a rare plasma cell is present in the endometrium, the patient has chronic endometritis. Often the maturation of the epithelium in the endometrial glands is irregular in chronic endometritis, or spindle-shaped stromal cells swirl round the glands.

GRANULOMATOUS ENDOMETRITIS. Tuberculosis is the major cause of granulomatous endometritis. Less often a fungal or parasitic infection causes endometrial granulomata, or talc excites foreign body granulomata in the endometrium.

Tuberculosis endometritis develops in 50% of patients with tuberculous salpingitis. The endometrium may show either granulomata like those of miliary tuberculosis or only chronic endometritis. The tubercles are found in the superficial part of the endometrium and are shed with the endometrium at menstruation.

Cervix Uteri

Inflammation of the cervix uteri can be acute or chronic. Acute inflammation is not often severe enough to be important clinically, but chronic inflammation is frequent in women of reproductive age. Cervicovaginitis emphysematosa is an unusual condition in which blebs of gas appear beneath the mucosa of the cervix and vagina.

A number of infections cause inflammation in the cervix uteri. About 10% of women have antibodies against Herpesvirus hominis 2, often because of cervical infection. Candidiasis and less often other fungal infections sometimes involve the cervix. Tuberculous granulomata are present in the cervix in 5% of women with tuberculous salpingitis, and occasionally more massive tuberculous lesions develop in the cervix. Syphilis, actinomycosis, schistosomiasis, amebiasis, and other infections sometimes involve the cervix uteri.

In most patients, acute or chronic cervicitis causes no symptoms. In some, they cause a mucopurulent discharge from the endocervix. In a few, cervicitis causes backache, pain in the lower abdomen, dyspareunia, menorrhagia, or dysmenorrhea.

ACUTE CERVICITIS. Acute cervicitis is often caused by trauma, douching, or deodorants, but can be due to infection. The cervix is swollen, reddened, and edematous. Microscopy shows acute inflammation with an exudate of neutrophils.

CHRONIC CERVICITIS. Infection is a common cause of chronic cervicitis. Chlamydia trachomatis can be isolated from the cervix in 2% of women in the United States, 10% of pregnant women, 40% of those attending clinics for sexually transmitted disease, and in 60% of those with chronic cervicitis severe enough to cause a mucopurulent exudate. Neisseria gonorrhoeae, group B streptococci, Gardnerella vaginalis, Mycoplasma hominis, Ureaplasma urealyticum, and Trichomonas vaginalis are less common causes of chronic cervicitis. Often more than one organism is involved. Occasionally chronic cervicitis is caused by trauma or chemical irritation.

The subepithelial tissue in the endocervix shows an increased number of lymphocytes together with plasma cells and macrophages. Occasionally the exudate contains germinal centers, a condition called follicular cervicitis. If chronic cervicitis is severe, the inflammatory cells form a dense infiltrate beneath the epithelium of the endocervix. Especially when there is squamous metaplasia of the endocervix, the infiltrate sometimes extends into the epithelium, and the epithelium is atypical, showing changes like those of epithelial dysplasia. If the cervicitis is caused by Chlamydia trachomatis, the organism can be demonstrated in the epithelial cells by immunohistochemical techniques.

Squamous metaplasia is common in the endocervix in chronic cervicitis. Often some of the mucous glands are obstructed and dilate to form mucus-filled cysts up to 1 cm in diameter, which are called nabothian cysts after the German anatomist Naboth (1675–1721).

CERVICOVAGINITIS EMPHYSEMATOSA. In cervicovaginitis emphysematosa subepithelial blebs filled with air appear in the cervix and vagina. In some of the lesions, multinucleate macrophages are prominent at the margin of the bleb. The cause of cervicovaginitis emphysematosa is unknown, but many of the patients have trichomoniasis.

Vagina

Vaginitis is common. Gardnerella vaginalis, Trichomonas vaginalis, Neisseria gonorrhoeae, Candida albicans, Mycoplasma hominis, and Ureaplasma urealyticum are among its more frequent causes, and often other organisms are present. Often the vaginitis caused by Gardnerella vaginalis and other organisms is called bacterial vaginosis, because more than one organism is active, and inflammatory changes in the vaginal wall are slight.

Less often inflammation in the vagina is caused by syphilis, amebiasis, or some other infection or results from trauma caused by a tampon or in some other way.

Vulva

Infections of the vulva include herpes genitalis, molluscum contagiosum, syphilis, chancroid, granuloma inguinale, lymphogranuloma venereum, and tuberculosis. Diseases of the skin that involve the vulva are discussed in Chapter 62. Among them are hidradenitis, pyoderma gangrenosum, Fox-Fordyce disease, pemphigoid, Darier's disease, Hailey-Hailey disease, and psoriasis.

ENDOMETRIOSIS, ADENOMYOSIS, AND ENDOSALPINGOSIS

If islands of endometrium are found outside the uterus, the condition is called endometriosis. If they are present within the myometrium, the disorder is called adenomyosis. Occasionally adenomyosis causes a tumor-like mass in the myometrium, a condition called an adenomyoma. In endosalpingosis, glands lined by epithelium like that of the fallopian tubes are present beneath the serosa or in some other site outside the fallopian tubes. During pregnancy, foci of ectopic decidua are common beneath the pelvic serosa and elsewhere.

Endometriosis

Over 20% of women have endometriosis, though in many it remains asymptomatic. The disease is more common in those who are childless or have only one or two children. It is more common in women in the higher economic levels of society. Over 80% of the patients who develop symptoms are 25 to 40 years old. About 10% are adolescents, and 5% are postmenopausal.

Lesions. The lesions in endometriosis are usually multiple. They are most common in the pelvis. One or both ovaries are involved in 40% of the patients, and lesions are common in the serosa lining the pelvic cavity. The pouch of Douglas, rectovaginal septum and the serosa covering the fallopian tubes, uterine ligaments, uterus, urinary bladder, and sigmoid colon are often involved.

Less often, lesions are found in the wall of the cervix or vagina; in the wall of the sigmoid colon, appendix, bladder, or ureter; in the omentum or umbilicus; in the vulval, perineal, or inguinal skin; in a surgical scar; or in the inguinal lymph nodes. Rarely, an endometriotic lesion is found in the lungs; in the wall of the stomach or small intestine; the pancreas or kidneys; the diaphragm; breasts; subarachnoid space; skeletal muscles; or bones.

Many of the lesions appear macroscopically as reddish purple specks 0.1 to 0.5 cm across. Some are larger and form a firm mass or a cyst up to 15 cm across. The small lesions are in the serosa, but the larger lesions often extend more deeply into the tissues. Sometimes a large lesion is called an endometrioma. Endometriotic cysts are most common in the ovaries. When the cyst is opened, brown or chocolate-colored altered blood escapes. Often an endometriotic cyst is called a chocolate cyst.

Microscopically, the small lesions and the larger solid masses consist of glands and stroma like those of the endometrium in the uterus. In 80% of the lesions, the endometrium undergoes cyclic changes and bleeds at menstruation, though often the hormonal response is irregular or atypical. The epithelial cells in endometriosis have estrogen and progesterone receptors, but in lower concentration than in normal endometrium. Often macrophages containing hemosiderin and ceroid are present around the lesions. In other lesions, the endometrium is inactive, and there is no evidence of past bleeding. Dense adhesions are common around endometriotic lesions and probably result from the irritation caused by the bleeding at the time of menstruation.

When endometriosis develops in the muscular wall of a viscus, the smooth muscle around the lesion is often hyperplastic. The smooth muscle cells surround the lesion and form a small nodule. In the gut, the hyperplasia of the smooth muscle sometimes causes kinking of the bowel and obstruction. Less often smooth muscle develops around lesions in a site where muscle is not normally present.

Endometriotic cysts are usually lined by a single layer of cuboidal epithelium. Often the nuclei in some of the epithelial cells are large and irregular with prominent nucleoli. In many endometriotic cysts, the attenuated endometrial stroma is no longer evident at the margin of the cyst. Instead, the cyst is surrounded by granulation tissue or by a broad band of macrophages filled with lipid and hemosiderin.

Clinical Presentation. Many women with endometriosis have no symptoms. In 50% of those with symptoms attributed to endometriosis, swelling of the foci of ectopic endometrium causes dysmenorrhea, with pain in the lower abdomen or back that begins a little before the menstrual period and persists for some time afterwards.

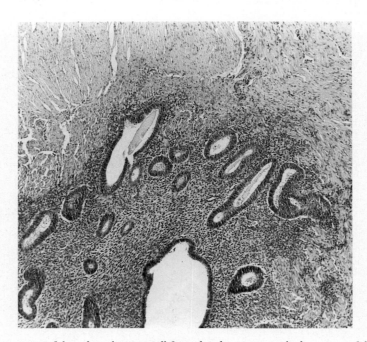

Fig. 41-2. Endometriosis of the colon, showing well-formed endometrium in the lower part of the picture, with the wall of the colon in the upper part.

Menorrhagia develops in 60% of the patients. About 30% are infertile, perhaps because of ovarian dysfunction, perhaps because anti-endometrial antibodies prevent implantation of the ovum. Abnormal ovulation is more common in women with endometriosis than in other women. Antibodies against the endometrium are present in 85% of patients with endometriosis, but only 2% of normal women. Occasionally there is dyspareunia, pain on defecation, or the patient notices a mass.

Pathogenesis. Some think that endometriosis is caused by the metastasis of endometrium shed from the uterus. Some think that it results from metaplasia. The theories are not incompatible. Both could be true.

In 90% of women, fragments of endometrium pass through the fallopian tubes into the peritoneal cavity during menstruation. The metastatic theory postulates that most endometriosis is caused by the implantation of these fragments of endometrium on the ovaries or the serosa. The endometrium that passes through the tubes is viable and grows when implanted subcutaneously. The theory well explains the frequency of lesions in the pelvis and why they appear only after puberty.

The more distant lesions in endometriosis are thought to be due to the carriage of fragments of endometrium in the blood or lymph. Fragments of endometrium do enter the myometrial blood and lymph vessels during menstruation and could establish lesions in other organs. The lesions in surgical scars might result from implantation of fragments of endometrium by the surgeon or from fragments of endometrium in the blood that find it easy to colonize a healing wound.

The metaplastic theory suggests that endometriosis results from metaplasia of the peritoneum caused by some form of irritation, perhaps the retrograde passage of menstrual blood through the fallopian tubes. Endometriosis sometimes occurs in people in whom the metastasis of endometrium seems unlikely, women who are amenorrheic or who have aplastic endometrium. It has been reported in men. In animals, endometriosis can be induced in the serosa under conditions that make metastasis impossible. In a few kindred, endometriosis is familial

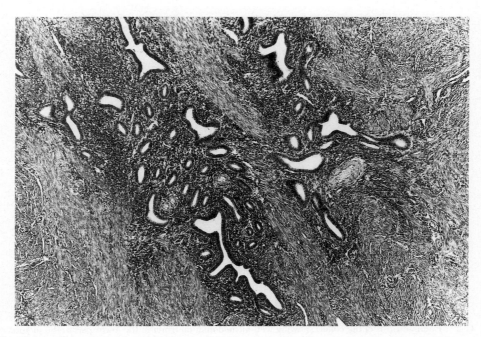

Fig. 41-3. Adenomyosis, showing columns of endometrium cut in cross section in the wall of the uterus.

and seems to be inherited by a polygenic mechanism.

Treatment and Prognosis. Endometriosis often needs no treatment or requires only symptomatic care. If the symptoms are more severe, or if infertility develops, hormonal treatment often can bring relief. If the lesions are large, surgical excision is required.

ADENOMYOSIS. Adenomyosis is present in 25% of uteri removed during the reproductive years. It is not found before puberty, and after the menopause the islands of endometrium in the myometrium become inconspicuous. About 20% of the patients have endometriosis.

Lesions. In adenomyosis, tortuous columns of endometrium extend down from the endometrium lining the uterus, and wind between the bundles of muscle in the myometrium. The columns may extend only a few millimeters from the cavity of the uterus or may extend far into the myometrium, even to the serosa. They may be few or numerous. Most of the infiltrating columns are too small to be seen with the naked eye, but some of them are over 0.1 cm across. When the columns of adenomyosis are numerous, the surrounding myometrium becomes hyperplastic.

If adenomyosis is not extensive, the uterus is normal macroscopically. If adenomyosis is severe, the myometrium is two or three times its normal thickness. The posterior wall is often more thickened than the anterior wall. On section, the thickened muscle is whorled and trabeculated. The thickening is due mainly to muscular hypertrophy, but sometimes tiny red or brown spots of endometrium can be seen. Sometimes dense adhesions surround the uterus, especially if there is associated endometriosis.

Microscopically, the columns of endometrium in the myometrium are cut in cross section and appear to be islands of endometrium surrounded by smooth muscle. Both glands and stroma are present. The glands often show proliferative changes in the early part of the menstrual cycle, but rarely show evidence of secretion.

Clinical Presentation. Often adenomyosis causes no symptoms. Occasionally it causes pain at the time of menstruation or menorrhagia.

Pathogenesis. Normally, the endometrial glands extend a little way into the myometrium. The cause of the exaggeration of this process in adenomyosis is unknown.

Treatment and Prognosis. Adenomyosis usually needs no treatment. If the symptoms are severe, hysterectomy is needed.

ADENOMYOMA. An adenomyoma is an uncommon lesion of the myometrium in which proliferation of smooth muscle around a focus of adenomyosis forms a mass resembling a fibroid of the uterus.

ENDOSALPINGOSIS. Endosalpingosis develops in over 10% of women during the reproductive years. Glands lined by epithelium like that of the fallopian tubes develop in the serosa covering the ovaries, tubes, or uterus, less often in other parts of the peritoneum, rarely in a scar or a lymph node. The epithelium shows the mixture of ciliated, secretory, and small dark cells seen in normal tubular epithelium. Endometrial stroma is not present. Psammoma bodies are frequently numerous in the lesions.

In most women, the lesions of endosalpingosis are small and cause no symptoms. They are probably caused by the implantation of tubular epithelium that escapes from the tubes during pregnancy or by metaplasia of the serosa. The lesions regress at the menopause and are rarely evident in postmenopausal women.

ECTOPIC DECIDUA. Foci of decidua develop on the surface of the ovaries and beneath the serosa covering the uterus and tubes in 90% of pregnant women. They are less common elsewhere in the peritoneum. Rarely, decidua is found in a pelvic lymph node. The lesions are usually too small to be visible macroscopically. In most women, they cause no symptoms and regress after delivery.

OTHER NON-NEOPLASTIC DISEASES

A number of noninflammatory, nonneoplastic diseases involve the female reproductive tract. The lesions of the ovaries will be discussed first, then the disorders involving the fallopian tubes, endometrium, myometrium, cervix, vagina, and vulva.

Ovaries

Cysts are common in the ovaries. They may arise from the follicles, corpora lutea, or surface epithelium. They may be solitary or multiple. In polycystic disease of the ovaries, numerous cysts are present. Sometimes the stroma of the ovaries is hyperplastic. Occasionally one or both ovaries are edematous or fibrotic. Occasionally torsion causes ischemia in an ovary.

FOLLICLE CYSTS. Follicle cysts are common in the ovaries in children, adolescents, and adults of reproductive age. They are unusual after the menopause. Most are less than 1 cm in diameter and are found only when an ovary is examined for some other reason. A few become as much as 10 cm across. The cysts are thin walled and are filled with serous fluid, sometimes tinged with blood. Microscopically, the smaller cysts are lined by granulosa cells supported by a theca interna. Either or both layers of the wall may be luteinized. The larger cysts are often lined only by a single layer of cuboidal cells.

Most patients with a few small follicle cysts or a solitary larger cyst have no symptoms attributable to the cyst. A few have hyperestrinism. Rarely, a cyst ruptures, causing hemoperitoneum.

The cause of solitary follicle cysts is not apparent, but probably some fault in the hormonal mechanisms governs the growth and regression of the cyst. In most patients, the cyst shrinks and disappears within two months.

Patients with a high level of gonadotropins in the plasma often have numerous follicle cysts. The ovaries are enlarged and their cortex seems filled with cysts 0.5 to 3 cm in diameter. Luteinization is prominent in the theca interna and sometimes in the granulosa cells lining the cysts. Most of the patients have one of the trophoblastic diseases of pregnancy: hydatid mole, choriocarcinoma, or fetal hydrops caused by Rh incompatibility. The cysts usually regress when the level of gonadotropins falls after the uterus is emptied. Juvenile hypothyroidism, prematurity, and deficiency of the 17-hydroxylase needed for the synthesis of cortisol and estrogens are less common causes of the excess of gonadotropins that induces multiple follicle cysts.

LUTEIN CYSTS. Cysts of the corpus lu-

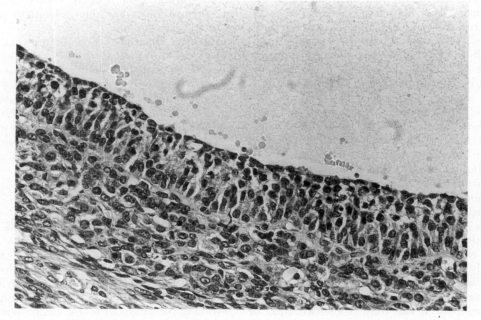

Fig. 41-4. A follicle cyst of an ovary, showing the lining of granulosa cells supported by theca interna.

teum are less common than follicle cysts of the ovary. Usually the cyst results from bleeding into a corpus leutum. The cyst is up to 5 cm across, with a hemorrhagic center bordered by the bright yellow wall of the corpus luteum. Less often, a lutein cyst is filled with serous fluid.

Microscopically, the wall of a lutein cyst consists of luteinized granulosa cells and theca interna supported by a fibrous theca externa. The rich vascularization of a corpus luteum is evident in the cyst wall.

Lutein cysts cause no dysfunction in most patients. They resolve within two months. Occasionally, a corpus albicans cyst results, or a corpus luteum cyst delays the next menstrual period or causes continued bleeding.

Rarely, a corpus luteum cyst 20 to 50 cm across develops during pregnancy, sometimes in a patient with a trophoblastic lesion that produces an excess of gonadotropins. The cyst is often multiloculated. Granulosa cells are not prominent in the wall of the cyst, which consists mainly of luteinized theca interna. When the uterus is emptied, the cyst resolves, but often takes several months to do so.

GERMINAL INCLUSION CYSTS. Germinal inclusion cysts become common after the menopause. In older women, the surface of the ovaries becomes irregular and corrugated. Invaginations of the germinal epithelium are nipped off to form small cysts near the surface of the ovary. The cysts are lined

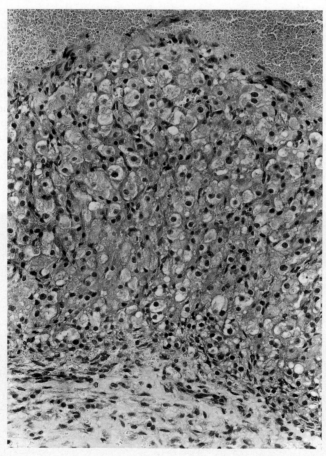

Fig. 41-5. A lutein cyst of an ovary, showing blood in the cavity at the top of the picture and a wall consisting mainly of large, luteinized granulosa cells.

by cuboidal germinal epithelium or less often by epithelium like that of the tubes or the endometrium. Germinal inclusion cysts are less than 1 cm across and are of no clinical importance.

POLYCYSTIC OVARIAN DISEASE. Polycystic ovarian disease affects 1 woman in 1500. Most of those affected are 20 to 40 years old. In some kindred, the disease is inherited as an autosomal dominant or X-linked character.

Lesions. In polycystic ovarian disease, both ovaries are about twice their normal size, grayish white, smooth, and firm. Small, bluish follicle cysts stud their surface. Corpora lutea and corpora albincantia are present in less than 30% of the patients and are never numerous. If the ovary is hemisected, the outer part of the cortex often forms a thick, hard rind, with the follicle cysts lined up beneath it.

Microscopically, the outer part of the cortex is collagenized and sometimes hyalinized. The follicle cysts are lined by granulosa cells and often have a prominent theca interna around them. The stroma in the deeper part of the ovaries is increased and sometimes luteinized.

In polycystic ovarian disease, oversecretion of the luteinizing hormone releasing factor in the hypothalamus causes increased secretion of the luteinizing hormone by the pituitary gland. The luteinizing hormone stimulates the ovarian stroma to secrete androstenedione, which is converted into estrone in the fatty tissues. The excess of estrone suppresses the secretion of the follicle-stimulating hormone and sensitizes the pituitary to the luteinizing hormone releasing factor, increasing the secretion of the luteinizing hormone. Inhibin-F, a polypeptide secreted by the granulosa cells in the ovaries, may reduce further the secretion of the follicle-stimulating hormone. The increase in the ratio of luteinizing to follicle-stimulating hormone in the plasma is characteristic of polycystic ovarian disease.

The imbalance between the luteinizing and follicle-stimulating hormones becomes self-perpetuating. Increased secretion of the luteinizing hormone increases the concentration of estrone in the plasma, increasing further the secretion of luteinizing hormone and depressing the secretion of follicle-stimulating hormone.

Androstenedione is also converted to testosterone, but the concentration of testosterone is the plasma usually remains in the high normal range. The formation of estrogens by the ovaries is reduced. The obesity common in the patients with polycystic ovarian disease worsens the endocrine imbalance by increasing the conversion of androstenedione to estrone and reducing the synthesis of the steroid hormone binding globulin, increas-

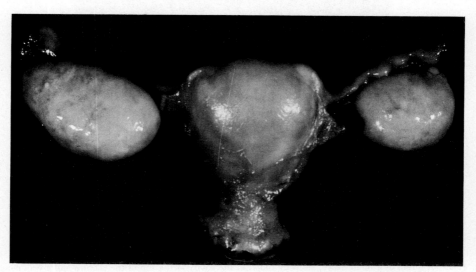

Fig. 41-6.   Polycystic ovarian disease, showing considerably enlarged ovaries.

ing the concentration of free testosterone in the plasma.

Dysfunction. Patients with polycystic ovarian disease fail to ovulate and are infertile. The primordial follicles are normal, but almost all develop into cysts that atrophy without releasing the ovum or forming a corpus luteum.

Clinical Presentation. Many of the patients with polycystic ovarian disease have the Stein-Leventhal syndrome, named after the American gynecologists who drew attention to it in 1935. The patients are infertile, have oligomenorrhea that usually progresses to amenorrhea, become hirsute after the menarche, and are obese. Other patients with polycystic ovarian disease are infertile and have oligomenorrhea or amenorrhea but maintain a normal body habitus. Some develop hyperestrinism. A few show other signs of virilization. A few have insulin-resistant diabetes mellitus and acanthosis nigricans.

Treatment and Prognosis. In most patients with polycystic ovarian disease, ovulation and pregnancy can be induced by correcting the hormonal imbalance. The synthesis of androstenedione by the ovaries can be reduced by wedge resection of the ovaries or by giving oral contraceptives. The secretion of the follicle-stimulating hormone can be enhanced by giving human placental gonadotropin, gonadorelin, or clomiphene. In some patients, loss of weight restores ovulation.

STROMAL HYPERPLASIA. In stromal hyperplasia, the stroma of the ovaries is hyperplastic. Often foci of luteinization are present in the stroma, a condition called stromal hyperthecosis. Over 30% of women between 50 and 70 years old have ovarian stromal hyperplasia, but symptoms develop in only a small minority of the people affected.

Lesions. The ovaries are usually enlarged, sometimes up to 7 cm in length. Their surface is smooth. On section, the ovaries are firm, homogeneous, and yellowish. Occasionally a few cysts like those of polycystic ovarian stromal disease are present.

Microscopically, the ovarian cortex is thickened and stromal cells replace part or most of the medulla. The stromal cells are plump, with oval, vesicular nuclei. Small clumps of cuboidal, luteinized cells are common, especially in the medulla.

Dysfunction. The production of testosterone, dihydrotestosterone, and androstenedione by the ovaries is increased. In some patients, their concentration in the plasma is in the male range. The estrogen in the blood is predominantly estrone, formed by the aromatization of androstenedione in the tissues. The ratio of estradiol to estrone in the plasma is low. The production of gonadotrophins is normal.

Clinical Presentation. If symptoms develop in a patient with ovarian stromal hyperplasia, virilization, obesity, and hypertension are usual. Patients with extensive stromal hyperthecosis sometimes develop hyperestrinism.

Treatment and Prognosis. If treatment is needed, bilateral oophorectomy reverses the virilization and commonly relieves the other symptoms of stromal hyperplasia.

HAIR-AN Syndrome. Some patients with stromal hyperthecosis have hyperandrogenism (HA), insulin resistance (IR) and acanthosis nigricans (AN). Less often the syndrome develops in patients with polycystic ovarian disease.

Probably the ovarian dysfunction is caused by the insulin resistance. A reduction in the number of insulin receptors in the tissues, a reduction in their affinity for insulin, or a fault in the postreceptor response to insulin causes hyperinsulinemia. The insulin binds to receptors in the ovaries, increasing the production of androgens. Insulin can also increase the secretion of the luteinizing hormone by the pituitary gland, explaining the increased secretion of the hormone seen in some of these patients.

Bilateral oophorectomy corrects the hyperandrogenemia and often causes regression of the acanthosis nigricans but does not ameliorate the insulin resistance.

MASSIVE OVARIAN EDEMA. Massive ovarian edema is uncommon. It usually involves one ovary, but in 20% of the patients both are affected. The patients are from 5 to 35 years old.

The ovary affected is 5 to 35 cm across, with a smooth, white surface and feels soft. On section, it has a fibrous capsule around a tan, gelatinous interior. A few follicle cysts may be present. Sometimes the fallopian tube on the affected side is also edematous.

Microscopically, edema separates the ovarian structures except in the superficial part of the cortex, which is often fibrotic. Small foci of luteinized cells are present in 40% of the patients.

The edema causes abdominal pain and menstrual irregularity. In 20% of the patients, hirsutism or other signs of virilization develop.

Massive ovarian edema probably is caused by torsion of the ovary, with secondary changes in ovarian function. Oophorectomy cures.

OVARIAN FIBROMATOSIS. Ovarian fibromatosis is similar to massive ovarian edema, except that the affected ovary or ovaries become fibrotic. It is probably caused in similar fashion and causes similar dysfunction.

TORSION. Torsion of an ovary is uncommon and usually affects an ovary enlarged by a tumor or some other condition. The patients develop abdominal pain and tenderness. Often a mass is palpable. At laparotomy, the ovary and tube are usually twisted, swollen, edematous, and hemorrhagic. Occasion-

ally they are infarcted. Only in a few patients does massive ovarian edema or ovarian fibromatosis develop.

WALTHARD'S RESTS. Walthard's rests, named after a Swiss gynecologist (1867–1933), are common in the hilus of the ovary and beneath the serosa of the broad ligaments and tubes. Usually they are too small to be seen by the naked eye. The rests consist of one or more well-defined clumps of epithelial cells. The cells sometimes form solid masses, sometimes are arranged around a small, central lumen. The epithelial cells are well-defined, large, and polyhedral, with pale, agranular cytoplasm. Their nuclei are uniform and ovoid, often with a longitudinal fold along their long axis. The origin of the Walthard's rests is in doubt. Probably they arise from the germinal epithelium of the ovary or the mesothelium, like the Brenner tumors that closely resemble them.

Endometrium

This section considers endometrial hyperplasia, and the endometrial abnormalities caused by hormonal imbalance and by drugs.

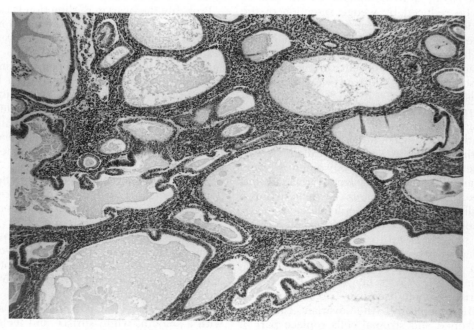

Fig. 41-7. Simple hyperplasia of the endometrium, showing dilated endometrial glands lined by low columnar epithelium separated by endometrial stroma.

HYPERPLASIA. Endometrial hyperplasia is divided into three types, simple hyperplasia, complex hyperplasia, and atypical hyperplasia. Formerly simple hyperplasia was often called cystic hyperplasia, and complex and atypical hyperplasia were called adenomatous hyperplasia. Endometrial hyperplasia can occur at any age, but is most common after the menopause and soon after the start of menstruation.

Lesions. Macroscopically, hyperplastic endometrium often looks normal. It is usually 0.5 to 1 cm thick. The surface is commonly smooth and velvety, but may be irregular and polypoid. Only microscopy can distinguish the different types of hyperplasia.

Simple Hyperplasia. In simple hyperplasia, the endometrial glands extend down from the surface like normal glands, but often run obliquely rather than perpendicular to the surface as do normal glands. Usually the glands are separated by abundant stroma, but occasionally they are crowded more closely together. When cut in cross section, the glands vary in size and shape. Some are small like the glands of proliferative endometrium; some are large or cystic. Some are round; some are irregularly shaped. Many of the glands are lined by a single layer of cuboidal or columnar epithelium, but especially in the regions in which the glands are close together the epithelium is often pseudostratified. The nuclei of the epithelial cells are uniform and resemble those of proliferative endometrium. They remain at the base of the epithelial cells. Mitoses are often present. Secretory activity is unusual. Often the pattern differs from one part of the endometrium to another.

The stromal cells are small, plump, and closely packed, with dark even nuclei. Mitoses are sometimes evident in the stroma. In the superficial part of the endometrium, the stromal cells sometimes swirl around spiral arterioles. Small clumps of stromal cells distended with fat are present in 30% of the patients. The lipid-laden cells have pyknotic nuclei and abundant, foamy cytoplasm.

Complex Hyperplasia. In complex hyperplasia, the endometrial glands are closely grouped together with little stroma between them. In cross section, they are irregularly shaped. Often folds of stroma covered by

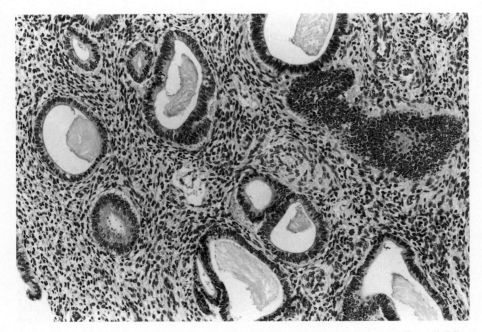

Fig. 41-8. A higher power view of simple hyperplasia of the endometrium showing the well-differentiated epithelium and normal stroma.

epithelium project into the lumina, or buds of epithelium bulge into the stroma. The epithelium lining the glands is usually pseudostratified, with two to four layers of basal nuclei. The nuclei remain vesicular and uniform. Mitoses in the epithelial cells may be few but are often numerous.

The stromal cells are like those of simple hyperplasia but are often compressed between the glands and become spindle shaped. Clumps of fat-filled stromal cells are present in 30% of the patients.

Atypical Hyperplasia. In atypical hyperplasia, the epithelial cells are atypical in part or all of the lesion. The pattern of growth may resemble simple hyperplasia, but more often it is similar to complex hyperplasia. The atypical cells are larger than those in the other forms of hyperplasia, with an increased nucleocytoplasmic ratio. The nuclei lose their basal position and move towards the surface of the cells. They are usually spheroidal, with coarse chromatin and prominent nucleoli. Mitoses are usually numerous, but may be few.

The stromal cells are like those in simple and complex hyperplasia. Groups of fat-filled cells are evident in 50% of the patients.

Metaplasia. Metaplasia is common in endometrial hyperplasia, and sometimes occurs in endometritis, inactive postmenopausal endometrium, endometrial polyps, and endometrial carcinoma. Sometimes more than one kind of metaplasia is present in a hyperplastic endometrium.

Foci of squamous metaplasia are present in 5% of simple and complex hyperplasias and 25% of atypical hyperplasias. The metaplasia is sometimes called acanthosis. Most often the glandular mucosa in the regions involved is partially replaced by well-differentiated squamous epithelium. Less often, the squamous cells are smaller, spindle-shaped, and form a spheroidal nodule called a morule or morula within the lumen of a gland. Keratinization is uncommon. Mitoses are rare in the foci of squamous metaplasia.

In ciliated or tubal metaplasia, some of the glands are lined by ciliated cells that resemble tubal epithelium. It is most frequent in simple hyperplasia.

Less common is mucinous metaplasia, in which some of the glands in a hyperplastic endometrium are lined by mucus-secreting cells like those of the endocervix.

Especially in atypical hyperplasia, some of

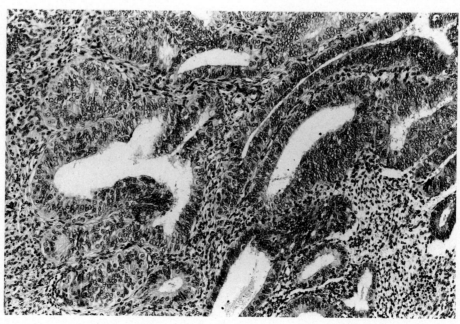

Fig. 41-9. Atypical hyperplasia of the endometrium, showing closely packed glands lined by multilayered epithelium showing mild disorder.

the glands are sometimes lined by large cells with abundant, eosinophilic cytoplasm. Rarely, the cells lining some of the glands have clear cytoplasm. Rarely, papillary processes covered by cuboidal epithelium project from the surface of hyperplastic endometrium or into the lumina of some of its glands.

Behavior. In most patients, endometrial hyperplasia regresses, and the endometrium returns to normal. In some, it persists with little change. In some, it progresses to carcinoma of the endometrium. The more atypical the hyperplasia, the greater the risk of carcinoma. The presence of foci of metaplasia does not alter the risk of carcinoma.

In one series, simple endometrial hyperplasia regressed in 80% of the patients, persisted in 19%, and progressed to carcinoma in 1%. Complex hyperplasia regressed in 80% of the patients, persisted in 17%, and progressed to carcinoma in 3%. Atypical hyperplasia of the simple pattern regressed in 70%, persisted in 23%, and became malignant in 8%. Atypical hyperplasia of the complex pattern regressed in 60%, persisted in 10%, and became malignant in 30%.

Clinical Presentation. Many patients with endometrial hyperplasia have no symptoms. Some have menorrhagia or metrorrhagia.

Pathogenesis. Endometrial hyperplasia is caused by an excess of estrogen. In the reproductive years, it is often due to an estrogen-secreting tumor, polycystic ovarian disease, or some other condition causing hyperestrinism. At the menarche and after the menopause, it is commonly due to temporary imbalance in the secretion of estrogen and progesterone.

Treatment and Prognosis. Women less than 40 years old who have simple or complex hyperplasia and wish to have children can be treated conservatively. The risk of carcinoma is low. Carcinoma rarely develops until the hyperplasia has persisted for 10 years. Commonly atypical hyperplasia becomes evident before the carcinoma develops.

Young women who have atypical hyperplasia and wish to have children can also be treated medically, though the risk is greater, and careful surveillance is necessary. In most older women with simple or complex hyperplasia, the hyperplasia regresses. In 30%,

curettage eliminates the lesion. Hysterectomy is indicated if symptoms persist or if atypical hyperplasia is present.

ANOVULATORY CYCLE. Anovulatory cycles are common at the menarche and the menopause but can occur at any time during the reproductive years. About 60% of the cycles in the first year of menstruation are anovulatory. The graafian follicle develops in the usual way, but the ovum is not shed. No corpus luteum develops, and no progesterone is produced. Estrogen remains dominant throughout the cycle.

The endometrium remains in the proliferative phase. The spiral arterioles of secretory endometrium do not develop. Instead ectatic venous sinuses, often thrombosed, are present in the superficial part of the endometrium. The ischemia causes focal necrosis and irregular shedding of the endometrium. When the time of menstruation comes, the level of estrogen falls. The endometrium fragments. The stromal cells form dense clumps. The glands are crowded together.

If anovulatory cycles are numerous, the continued excess of estrogen often causes endometrial hyperplasia, commonly with squamous metaplasia. Patients with anovulatory cycles often experience irregular bleeding because of the irregular shedding of the endometrium. Menses are irregular and vary in duration. In young women, oral contraceptives containing progesterone often control the bleeding. In older women and in young women who continue to bleed, an endometrial biopsy is necessary to exclude atypical hyperplasia or carcinoma.

INADEQUATE LUTEAL PHASE. An inadequate luteal phase is found in less than 5% of women who are infertile. The corpus luteum fails to produce enough progesterone to induce fully the secretory phase of the endometrial cycle, or the endometrium lacks progesterone receptors and fails to respond fully to progesterone. The development of secretory changes in the endometrium are delayed, so that an endometrial biopsy shows a histologic pattern that would have been expected two or more days earlier in the cycle. Sometimes the development of the glands and the stroma are discordant.

IRREGULAR SHEDDING. Irregular shedding is an uncommon cause of prolonged and heavy menstrual bleeding. A biopsy taken five or more days after the onset of bleeding shows both proliferative and secretory patterns. In some patients, only one cycle is affected. In others, the abnormality occurs repeatedly.

ORAL CONTRACEPTIVES. If an oral contraceptive containing both estrogen and progestin is taken from the fifth to the twenty-fifth day of the cycle, the proliferative stage of the endometrial cycle is shortened. The glands remain straight and are lined by a single layer of cuboidal or columnar epithelium. Irregularly distributed secretory granules appear about the eighth day of the cycle, but disappear a few days later as the glands atrophy. Stromal edema is often prominent early in the cycle and is followed by decidual changes with many endometrial granulocytes. If the dose of progestin is high, the stromal cells become spindle-shaped and resemble the cells of an endometrial stromal sarcoma.

If a contraceptive containing estrogen and progestin is continued for a long time, endometrial glands become few. Many of those that remain are lined by flattened epithelium and resemble capillaries. No secretory changes occur. No decidual changes are evident. The endometrial stroma consists mainly of collagen. The spiral arterioles disappear and are replaced by large venous sinusoids. Often some of the sinusoids become thrombosed, causing irregular bleeding.

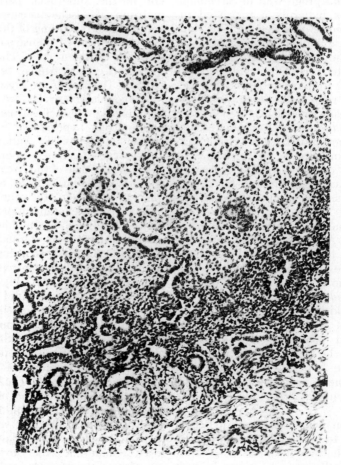

Fig. 41-10. An endometrial biopsy taken on the 20th day of the cycle in a woman taking contraceptive pills containing estrogen and progesterone, showing premature decidualization in the superficial part of the endometrium.

If estrogen only is taken from day five of the cycle until day 18, and then both estrogen and progesterone are taken for 6 days, the endometrium remains in the proliferative phase until the twentieth day of the cycle. Subnuclear vacuoles of secretion appear about the twenty-second day of the cycle, and the development of a secretory endometrium follows, though five to seven days later than is normal. Bleeding comes before decidual changes develop or spiral arterioles appear.

Myometrium

Abnormalities of the myometrium include hypertrophy, prolapse, and various types of malposition.

HYPERTROPHY. Hypertrophy of the smooth muscle fibers of the myometrium sometimes causes diffuse enlargement of the uterus. Except for the increased size, the organ is normal.

The weight of the uterus depends on the age and parity of the woman. A nulliparous uterus in a young woman weighs 45 to 55 g, but the weight of the organ increases with age and with every pregnancy until the menopause. After the menopause, the myometrium atrophies and the weight of the uterus falls. A nulliparous uterus is considered to be hypertrophied if it weighs more than 130 g. After one to three children, a weight of over 210 g is abnormal. In a woman with four or more children, the uterus should not weigh more than 250 g.

PROLAPSE. Prolapse of the uterus into the vagina is common, particularly in elderly women. Sometimes the condition is called procidentia, from the Latin for to fall. As a woman ages, the ligaments and fasciae supporting the uterus weaken. The stretching of childbirth often damages or weakens the ligaments and fasciae. Anything that increases intra-abdominal pressure favors prolapse or accentuates it.

The uterus becomes retroverted to lie in the axis of the vagina and slides down into the vagina. Three degrees of procidentia are distinguished. In the first degree, the cervix remains within the vagina. In the second degree, the cervix protrudes from the vulva when the patient strains or stands. In the third degree, or complete procidentia, the vagina is inverted, and the uterus is outside the vulva. Complete procidentia is uncommon, but the milder forms of prolapse of the uterus are frequent.

If the cervix protrudes through the vulva, it is exposed to trauma and irritation, and often its epithelium becomes thick, white, and keratinized. Sometimes the prolapse becomes ulcerated. If the lower part of the cervix descends while the upper part remains well supported, the cervix becomes elongated, sometimes as much as 15 cm long. Often the prolapsed cervix is congested. Sometimes the endocervical mucosa becomes hyperplastic.

Prolapse of the uterus often can be prevented with a pessary. If not, surgical intervention is necessary to repair the weakened supports.

MALPOSITION. In anteversion, the uterus is tilted unusually far forward. It rarely causes symptoms or dysfunction.

Anteflexion of the uterus means that the body of the uterus is bent sharply forward at the junction between the body and the cervix, so that the organ becomes C-shaped. A uterus of this kind is called cochleate, from the Greek for a snail or spiral screw. Cochleate uteri are common in young nulliparous women. The abnormality causes no symptoms and is usually corrected by pregnancy.

Retroversion means that the whole uterus is tilted backwards. The cervix points downwards or anteriorly, instead of posteriorly, and the fundus of the uterus lies against the sacrum or in the pouch of Douglas. Retroversion may be congenital or acquired. Pregnancy, inflammation, neoplasia, and trauma can all displace a normal uterus backwards. Retroversion of the uterus usually causes no symptoms, though backache and dysmenorrhea are sometimes attributed to it. A pessary can be used to determine if the symptoms are due to the retroversion. If necessary, retroversion can be corrected surgically.

Retroflexion of the uterus means that the body of the uterus is bent backwards in relation to the cervix. If retroflexion is great, the uterus is C-shaped, a mirror image of the cochleate uterus of anteflexion.

Inversion of the uterus occasionally occurs

at the time of delivery but may not be discovered for weeks or months. Less often it occurs in the old or is caused by a tumor bulging into the uterine cavity. The uterus turns inside out and bulges into the vagina. The exposed endometrium soon becomes infected and ulcerated. Treatment is surgical.

Cervix Uteri

Cervical erosions and squamous metaplasia are the principal non-neoplastic, noninflammatory diseases of the cervix uteri. The polyps common in the cervix are considered together with the neoplasms.

EROSION. The presence of glandular endocervical mucosa on the portio of the cervix uteri is called a cervical erosion, or cervical ectropion. Cervical erosions are common during the reproductive years. The anterior lip of the cervix is involved more frequently than the posterior lip, but often both lips are eroded.

Macroscopically, a cervical erosion is bright red, continuous with the endocervical mucosa, and sharply defined. Its surface may be smooth or granular. By colposcopy, the surface often appears papillary or cystic. Microscopically, the erosion is covered by intact endocervical mucosa. The lesion is red because the blood vessels show through the thin endocervical mucosa. It bleeds easily because the thin endocervical mucosa is easily torn.

The term *erosion* is misleading. There is no erosion. The endocervical mucosa is present on the portio because the squamous epithelium has not completed its normal progression upwards to the external cervical os. As the patient ages, most cervical erosions are replaced by squamous epithelium.

SQUAMOUS METAPLASIA. Squamous metaplasia is common in the cervix uteri. It

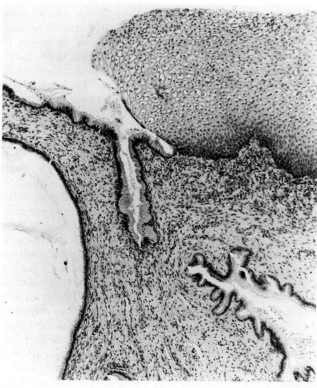

Fig. 41-11.   Squamous metaplasia of the endocervix, showing squamous epithelium replacing the original columnar epithelium. Part of a nabothian cyst is on the left.

gradually replaces the endocervical mucosa in cervical erosions and often extends into the endocervix. Two types of squamous metaplasia occur in the cervix uteri.

At the margin of an erosion, less commonly at the squamocolumnar junction in the endocervix, tongues of squamous cells from the basal layers of the squamous epithelium extend beneath the columnar endocervical epithelium, between the endocervical cells and their basement membrane. The squamous cells multiply and become multilayered, pushing up the endocervical cells. Eventually the endocervical cells are lost and replaced by the squamous cells.

Within an erosion and often within the endocervix, islands of squamous epithelium develop in the glandular epithelium. Small basal cells appear between the columnar cells of the endocervix and their basement membrane. The basal cells proliferate and differentiate into squamous cells. As the squamous cells become more numerous, they push up the columnar cells of the endocervical epithelium and replace them, forming a small island of squamous epithelium.

As the extension of squamous epithelium in from the squamocolumnar junction progresses and the islands of squamous epithelium within the endocervical epithelium enlarge, more and more of the glandular mucosa is replaced. Often there is a sharp, oblique line between the pre-existing squamous epithelium and the less completely differentiated squamous epithelium that has replaced the endocervical epithelium. Often the new squamous epithelium is thinner than mature squamous epithelium and contains less glycogen.

The squamous epithelium often obstructs the ducts of some of the endocervical glands. The glands become dilated to form nabothian cysts. Often the squamous epithelium extends into some of the cervical glands, filling or partially filling them.

Vagina

Herniation of neighboring organs into the vagina is common. Vaginal abnormalities develop in a high proportion of women whose mothers were given diethylstilbestrol or a similar estrogen during pregnancy.

HERNIATION. Pregnancy and age often weaken the vaginal wall. If the weakness is high in the anterior vaginal wall, the urinary bladder bulges into the vagina and forms a cystocele. Weakness lower in the anterior wall permits herniation of the urethra to form a urethrocele. If the fault is high in the posterior wall of the vagina, an enterocele containing loops of bowel may form. If the weakness is low and posterior, a rectocele develops. If the lesions cause symptoms, surgical correction is needed.

DIETHYLSTILBESTROL-INDUCED LESIONS. Structural abnormalities and adenosis are common in the vagina in young women whose mothers were treated with diethylstilbestrol or another estrogen during pregnancy. Nearly all the patients have cervical erosions. Some develop adenocarcinoma of the vagina.

In 20% of the daughters, the cervix uteri or vagina is malformed or hypoplastic. The cervix is often distorted by concentric rings or constrictions. The vaginal fornices are sometimes obliterated. Sometimes a transverse septum partially obstructs the vagina. In many of the patients, the abnormalities lessen or disappear as the patient ages.

In 30% of the daughters, adenosis is evident in the upper third of the vagina, and in some it is more extensive. Macroscopically, the lesions appear as red dots in the mucosa. Microscopically, mucus-secreting columnar cells like those of the endocervix replace the vaginal epithelium and form small glands like those of the endocervix. Ciliated cells like those of the fallopian tubes are present in the glands in 20% of the patients. As the patient ages, the adenosis is often replaced partly or wholly by squamous metaplasia in the same way as a cervical erosion is replaced by squamous metaplasia.

Vulva

Lichen sclerosus and epithelial hyperplasia are the principal non-neoplastic, noninflammatory lesions of the vulva. Sometimes the term *dystrophy* is used to include both lesions. Patients who have both lichen sclerosus and epithelial hyperplasia are said to have mixed dystrophy.

LICHEN SCLEROSUS. Lichen sclerosus of the vulva was formerly called lichen sclerosus et atrophicus. The term *kraurosis vulvae* was used to describe a similar condition. Lichen sclerosus affects more than 100 women in 100,000. Most of the patients are postmenopausal, but the disease can arise at any age. A similar condition in men is called balanitis xerotica obliterans.

Macroscopically, the lesion is well demarcated. It often involves much or all of the vulva and sometimes the adjacent inguinal or perianal skin. The affected skin is shrunken and seems tight. Often it is scaly or fissured.

Microscopically, the epidermis is thin. Often its basal cells are swollen and hydropic. Melanocytes are absent. The rete ridges of the epidermis are lost, but sometimes irregular extensions of epidermis project into the dermis. Hyperkeratosis is often prominent, with keratotic plugs in hair follicles and in the mouths of glands. Mitoses are few or absent.

A band of homogeneous dermis is present immediately beneath the epidermis. Its thickness varies but tends to increase as the lesion ages. In the homogeneous band, cells are few. The collagen bundles are degenerate and often hyalinized. Elastic fibers are sparse. Usually a band of lymphocytes is present deep to the homogenized zone.

Fibrin is demonstrable immunohistochemically along the epidermodermal junction in 75% of the patients. IgM and C3 are commonly present in the basement membrane. In many of the patients, the concen-

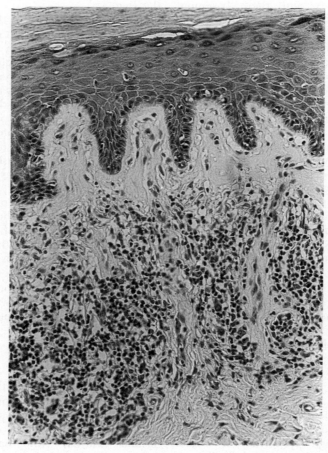

Fig. 41-12. Lichen sclerosus of the vulva, showing thin epidermis with prominent hyperkeratosis, a narrow band of hyalinization in the superficial dermis, and an exudate of lymphocytes and macrophages more deeply.

tration of dihydrotestosterone in the plasma is low, but the concentration of free testosterone is increased.

Lichen sclerosus does not increase the risk of developing carcinoma of the vulva. It is managed by the topical application of testosterone and progesterone.

EPIDERMAL HYPERPLASIA. Epidermal hyperplasia of the vulva is most frequent in women 30 to 60 years old. The lesion is like that of lichen sclerosus macroscopically, but is usually pink or red. Microscopically, the epidermis is thickened. The rete pegs are elongated. Hyperkeratosis is usual. Mitoses are often numerous, but the normal pattern of epidermal differentiation is not disturbed. The dermis commonly contains an inflammatory exudate mainly of lymphocytes, but is otherwise normal.

CONGENITAL ANOMALIES

Most of the congenital abnormalities in the female reproductive tract result from maldevelopment of the müllerian ducts that form the fallopian tubes, uterus, and upper part of the vagina. Rests are also common. Congenital malformations of the ovaries, lower vagina, or vulva are less frequent.

MÜLLERIAN ANOMALIES. In 1 woman in 10, the müllerian ducts fail to fuse normally to form the uterus. In most of these women the abnormality is minor and causes no dysfunction, but in 1 woman in 1000 it is severe enough to cause difficulty during pregnancy.

If the defect in the fusion of the müllerian ducts is minor, the fundus of the uterus bulges downward into the cavity of the uterus more than is normal, separating the cornua of the uterine cavity more clearly than is usual, but the uterus is otherwise normal. If the failure of fusion is more extensive, a septum extends downward from the fundus in the midline, dividing the upper part of the endometrial cavity in two. Such a uterus is called septate, or if the septum is short, subseptate. The outer surface of the uterus usually maintains its normal shape, but sometimes the fundus of a septate uterus is flattened or concave, forming what is called an anvil uterus.

If the failure of the fusion of the müllerian ducts is more complete, the uterus has two horns, each with its own endometrial cavity and myometrial wall. Such a uterus is called bicornuate, from the Latin for two-horned. Usually the two horns merge into a single uterine cavity somewhere in the body of the uterus, but sometimes they share only a common cervix. The cervix may open into a normal vagina or into a vagina divided by a midline septum in its upper part.

Occasionally, there are two uteri, each with its own fallopian tube and cervix, joined only by merging of the cervical muscle. Usually the upper vagina is divided by a midline septum, and each uterus opens into its own vagina. Such a uterus is called a uterus didelphys, from the Greek for twice and uterus.

In 1 woman in 25,000, the two müllerian ducts remain entirely independent. There are two reproductive systems, each with its own fallopian tube, uterus, and vagina.

If only one müllerian tube develops, the uterus is asymmetrical and has only one tube. Such a uterus is called unicornuate. Occasionally, one müllerian tube forms a unicornuate uterus, while the other forms a tube and a malformed uterus, which ends blindly, without communication to the vagina or to the better formed uterus on the other side. This kind of malformation is called a uterus bicornis unicollis, because the two horns of the uterus are present, though there is only one cervix. Unicollis is from the Latin for one and neck. Because there is no egress from the malformed uterus, except through the tube, it gradually becomes distended with blood when menstruation starts, forming an abdominal mass and causing increasing dysmenorrhea. Pelvic endometriosis is common in women with this kind of hematometra, as distention of the uterus with blood is called, and doubtless results from the escape of fragments of endometrium through the tube.

Occasionally the fallopian tubes are present, but the uterus and upper part of the vagina are absent, or the tubes and a hypoplastic uterus are present, but no vagina. Rarely, the tubes, uterus, and upper part of the vagina are all absent.

Congenital atresia or stenosis can obstruct

one or both fallopian tubes. Occasionally the uterus is rudimentary and lacks a cavity. Atresia of the cervix is sometimes present in a uterus that is otherwise normal. Occasionally the upper part of the vagina is reduced to a solid, fibrous cord.

Duplication of the organs formed from the müllerian ducts is rare. Women with two uteri and four tubes have been reported. Occasionally an accessory fallopian tube is present on one or both sides. Partial duplication sometimes forms a diverticulum in a tube or the uterus or gives rise to an accessary ostium in a tube.

Because of the close relationship between the müllerian and wolffian ducts during organogenesis, abnormalities of the kidneys and ureters are common in women with maldevelopment of the müllerian system. If the müllerian abnormality is predominantly on one side, the renal malformation is on the same side. The development of the ovaries is not related to the development of the müllerian ducts, and the ovaries are nearly always normal in women with müllerian defects.

RESTS. Rests are common in the female reproductive tract. Usually they are tiny and

of no significance, found only by microscopy. If they become evident clinically, it is usually because the rest has formed a cyst. Rarely, a rest gives rise to a tumor.

Tubular or cystic rests are common in the vicinity of the ovaries or tubes, less often in relation to the uterus or vagina. Some are remnants of the müllerian or paramesonephric ducts; some are derived from the wolffian or mesonephric ducts. Inclusions of mesothelium sometimes cause similar small cysts. If a rest or mesothelial inclusion forms a cyst, it is called a parovarian cyst if it is near an ovary, a paratubal cyst if it is close to a tube.

Over 80% of the parovarian cysts large enough to be visible macroscopically and most paratubal cysts that can be seen with the naked eye are derived from the müllerian ducts. They have a lining of ciliated cells and contain clear, serous fluid. The wall of the cyst is thin. The hydatid of Morgagni, named after the Italian pathologist who was one of the principal founders of modern pathology, is the most commonly recognized paratubal cyst. It hangs by a pedicle from the fimbriated end of a tube and is usually 1 to 3 cm in diameter.

Most other parovarian cysts big enough to

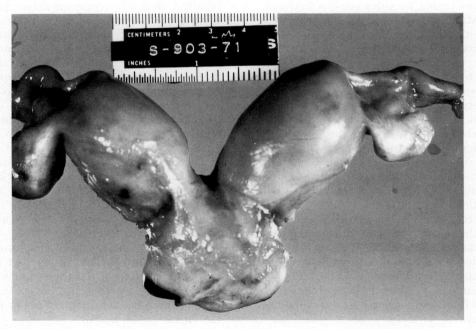

Fig. 41-13.   A bicornuate uterus, showing the two horns merging to share a common cervix.

be seen with the naked eye are mesothelial cysts. They are not congenital, but result from some minor injury. They have a lining of flat or cuboidal mesothelial cells and a thin wall. They lie immediately beneath the serosa.

Remnants of the wolffian ducts are common in the hilus of the ovaries and in the broad ligaments and are sometimes present in the serosa of the uterus, the muscle of the cervix, or the wall of the vagina. In the hilus of the ovaries, they often form tubes or small cysts that resemble the rete testis and are called the rete ovarii. In the broad ligaments, wolffian rests are usually too small to be visible macroscopically. They are lined by cuboidal epithelium with occasional clear cells and often have a muscular wall. In the parametric region, the cervix uteri, and vagina, wolffian rests sometimes form multilocular cysts 1 to 3 cm across with a similar lining. The cysts are often called Gartner's cysts after the Danish surgeon (1785–1827) who studied this part of the mesonephric apparatus.

Small clumps of hilar cells are nearly always present in the hilus of the ovaries, usually near nerves. They resemble the Leydig cells of the testes and contain similar crystalloids. Occasionally an adrenal rest made of adrenocortical cells is present in the hilus of an ovary.

OVARIAN ANOMALIES. The ovarian abnormalities that occur in intersexuality are discussed in Chapter 40. Less than 5% of women have a tiny, supernumerary ovary, usually in the hilus of an otherwise normal ovary. The supernumerary ovary is rarely large enough to be evident clinically. Rarely, the spleen and an ovary are fused, or one or both ovaries are absent.

LOWER VAGINAL ANOMALIES. Not uncommonly, a transverse septum obstructs the vagina. The membrane is sometimes complete, sometimes has a small opening. Occasionally the membrane is close to the cervix uteri, a condition called cervical phimosis, but more often it is lower in the vagina, sometimes just above the hymen. The upper surface of the septum is covered by endocervical epithelium, and the lower surface by squamous epithelium. Rarely, the hymen is imperforate.

Occasionally, the part of the vagina above the septum becomes distended by mucus, a condition called mucocolpos. More often the septum is discovered only when menstruation begins and the upper part of the vagina and sometimes the endometrial cavity become filled with blood. At times, the distention of the vagina is so great that it reaches the umbilicus, or the tense septum bulges from the introitus. Symptoms are few, unless the endometrial cavity is distended and causes pain. Surgical incision of the septum allows normal function.

In 1 woman in 5000, the lower vagina is absent or hypoplastic. The uterus and upper vagina may or may not be formed normally. If the uterus is functional, the upper vagina and sometimes the endometrial cavity fill with blood when menstruation begins. Surgical correction is needed.

VULVAR ANOMALIES. The vulva is sometimes hypoplastic if the müllerian part of the genital tract is hypoplastic and may be duplicated when the uterus and vagina are duplicated. Occasionally the clitoris is bifid, most often in patients with exstrophy of the bladder or an open symphysis pubis. The labia minora are sometimes partially fused, though the fusion may be due to vulvitis in infancy, rather than a congenital defect. Sometimes the labia minora are annoyingly large.

Rarely, there is a persistent cloaca, with a common opening for vagina, bowel, and bladder. More often there is a vaginal anus, usually low in the vagina, or a perineal anus. Sometimes a ureter or an accessory ureter opens into the uterus, the vagina, or the vulva.

TUMORS

The tumors of the different organs in the female reproductive system bear little relationship one to another. The cysts and other lesions that mimic neoplasms are described with the neoplasms.

Ovaries

In the United States, nearly 5% of tumors of clinical importance in women arise in an

TABLE 41-1.   CLASSIFICATION OF OVARIAN TUMORS

Common "Epithelial" Tumors

  Serous tumors
    Benign
      Serous cystadenoma
      Serous adenofibroma
      Serous cystadenofibroma
      Papilloma
    Borderline
      Serous cystadenoma
      Serous adenofibroma
      Serous cystadenofibroma
      Papilloma
    Malignant
      Serous cystadenocarcinoma
      Serous carcinoma
      Malignant serous adenofibroma

  Mucinous tumors
    Benign
      Mucinous cystadenoma
      Mucinous adenofibroma
      Mucinous cystadenofibroma
    Borderline
      Mucinous cystadenoma
      Mucinous adenofibroma
      Mucinous cystadenofibroma
    Malignant
      Mucinous cystadenocarcinoma
      Mucinous carcinoma
      Malignant mucinous adenofibroma

  Endometrioid tumors
    Benign
      Endometrioid cystadenoma
      Endometrioid adenofibroma
      Endometrioid cystadenofibroma
    Borderline
      Endometrioid cystadenoma
      Endometrioid adenofibroma
      Endometrioid cystadenofibroma
    Malignant
      Endometrioid carcinoma
      Malignant endometrioid adenofibroma
      Mixed müllerian tumor
      Endometrioid stromal sarcoma

  Clear cell tumors
    Benign
      Clear cell adenofibroma
    Borderline
      Clear cell adenofibroma
    Malignant
      Clear cell carcinoma

  Brenner tumor
    Benign
    Borderline
    Malignant

  Mixed "epithelial" tumors

Unclassified "epithelial" tumors

Sex Cord-Stromal Tumors

  Granulosa cell tumor
    Adult type
    Juvenile type

  Thecoma-fibroma tumors
    Thecoma
    Fibroma
    Fibrosarcoma
    Sclerosing stromal tumor

  Sertoli-stromal tumors
    Sertoli-Leydig cell tumor
    Sertoli cell tumor

  Gynandroblastoma

  Sex cord tumor with annular tubules

  Unclassified sex cord-stromal tumors

Lipid Cell Tumors

  Stromal luteoma

  Leydig cell tumor

  Adrenocortical tumor

  Unclassified lipid cell tumors

Germ Cell Tumors

  Dysgerminoma

  Endodermal sinus tumor

  Embryonal carcinoma

  Polyembryoma

  Choriocarcinoma

  Teratoma
    Immature
    Mature solid
    Mature cystic
    Mature cystic with malignant change
    Specialized
      Struma ovarii
      Carcinoid tumor
      Strumal carcinoid tumor

Tumors Containing Germ Cell and Sex Cord-Stromal Elements

  Gonadoblastoma

  Mixed germ cell-sex cord-stromal tumor

Other Primary Tumors

Secondary Tumors
  Krukenberg tumor

ovary. Nearly 50% of deaths from cancer in women result from a tumor of an ovary. Each year, ovarian cancer develops in 20,000 women.

In North America, northern Europe, and Australasia up to 15 women in every 100,000 develop ovarian cancer. In South America, southern Europe, Africa, and Asia, the incidence is less than 5 per 100,000; in Japan, it is less than 3 per 100,000. The low incidence in Africa and Asia is due principally to the low incidence of the common "epithelial" tumors in these countries. In the United States, ovarian cancer is more common in white people than in black people or orientals.

The classification of ovarian tumors proposed by the World Health Organization in 1973 has been widely adopted. Table 41-1 shows a modification of this classification.

Clinical Presentation. Ovarian tumors often produce no symptoms until the tumor has grown large. In over 50% of the patients, the tumor is discovered only when it causes abdominal distention. The tumor itself may be so big that it bulges up into the abdomen, where it lies in the midline and causes abdominal swelling, or the swelling may be due to the ascites often caused by ovarian tumors. The abdominal distention often causes dyspepsia, with loss of appetite, nausea, constipation, or diarrhea. Often there is abdominal discomfort or abdominal pain. Pressure of the tumor on the bladder causes dysuria or urinary retention in 10% of the patients. Pressure on the pelvic veins can cause edema of the legs or the vulva.

The menstrual cycle is usually unaffected in premenopausal women with an ovarian tumor, though occasionally there is irregularity, menorrhagia, or amenorrhea. In postmenopausal women, there may be slight, irregular uterine bleeding. The menstrual changes are usually due to the distortion and congestion caused by the tumor, rather than to hormonal activity.

Ascites is common in patients with an ovarian tumor, benign or malignant. It may be due to leakage of fluid from the tumor itself or to metastatic implants on the peritoneum. The ascites resolves within a few weeks if the tumor is removed and the im-plants on the peritoneum are controlled by chemotherapy or radiotherapy.

Hypersecretion of Hormones. Only a minority of ovarian tumors secrete estrogens, androgens, or gonadotropin in quantity large enough to be important clinically.

Estrogen. About 75% of granulosa cell tumors arising before puberty and most of those in older people produce excessive estrogens. Almost all thecomata secrete an excess of estrogens. Occasionally, a Sertoli-Leydig cell tumor or a lipid cell tumor does so. The stroma of one of the common "epithelial" tumors of an ovary, a germ cell tumor, or a carcinoma metastatic to the ovaries sometimes produces estrogens or androgens that are converted to estrogens in the peripheral tissues. The effect of the hyperestrinism depends on the age of the patient.

In girls before puberty, an excess of estrogens produced by an ovarian tumor causes precocious puberty. The breasts enlarge. The pubic and axillary hair takes an adult configuration. The internal and external sex organs enlarge and develop. Later comes irregular uterine bleeding and a white, endocervical discharge. The development of the bones is accelerated.

In women of the reproductive years, the excess of estrogens usually causes irregular uterine bleeding or, less often, amenorrhea. There may be swelling of the breasts, with pain or tenderness. The endometrium is often hyperplastic. The hyperplasia may be simple, but it can be complex or atypical. Rarely, it shows evidence of secretion, sometimes with a decidual reaction in the stroma. The risk of developing carcinoma of the endometrium increases. If the contralateral ovary is not involved by the tumor, it is small, with the collagenization of the outer part of the cortex seen in polycystic ovarian disease.

In postmenopausal women, a tumor secreting estrogens usually causes uterine bleeding, with endometrial hyperplasia and perhaps changes in the breasts. Carcinoma of the endometrium develops in about 5% of the patients. Cytologic examination of vaginal cells shows the differentiation and keratinization induced by the hyperestrinism.

Androgen. About 80% of Sertoli-Leydig cell tumors and almost all lipid tumors and Leydig cell tumors secrete androgens in sufficient quantity to cause virilization. Occasionally a granulosa cell tumor or a thecoma causes virilization rather than hyperestrinism. Rarely, the stroma of one of the common "epithelial" tumors, a germ cell tumor, or a carcinoma metastatic to the ovaries produces enough androgen to cause virilization.

First comes oligomenorrhea and then anmenorrhea. The breasts atrophy, and the body loses its feminine shape. Acne and hirsutism are likely, and the voice deepens as the larynx enlarges. The clitoris increases in size. The hair recedes. There may be erythrocytosis, obesity, hypertension, impaired glucose tolerance, or diabetes mellitus.

If the tumor is removed, the menses return within a few weeks. Some excess hair may be lost, but the enlargement of the clitoris and the deepening of the voice usually persist.

Most ovarian tumors causing virilization secrete testosterone, androstenedione, or both. In contrast to adrenal virilization in which the excretion of 17-ketosteroids in the urine is usually greater than 30 mg/day, the excretion of 17-ketosteroids is usually normal or only slightly raised.

Gonadotropin. Ovarian choriocarcinomata produce human chorionic gonadotropin in sufficient quantity to cause precocious puberty in 50% of children with the tumor. The concentration of the gonadotropin or its β subunit in the plasma can be used to monitor the progress of the tumor. Smaller quantities of gonadotropin are sometimes produced by embryonal carcinomata or other types of ovarian germ cell tumor.

Complications. Torsion sometimes causes hemorrhage or infarction in an ovarian tumor. It is particularly common in patients with a dermoid cyst. Up to 15% of these tumors become twisted.

In 10% of patients with a granulosa cell tumor, rupture of one or more of the cysts in the tumor causes intraperitoneal hemorrhage. The bleeding is usually slight, but it can be massive. About 2% of dermoid cysts leak into the peritoneal cavity. Usually the leak is slow, and the irritant content of the cyst causes a foreign body reaction. Occasionally

the rupture is massive, causing acute peritonitis and shock. Rarely, a dermoid cyst ruptures in the bladder, vagina, or bowel, and the content of the cyst is passed in the urine, stool, or per vaginam. Rupture of other kinds of ovarian tumor is uncommon.

Rarely, a dermoid cyst, or some other kind of ovarian tumor, causes hemolytic anemia,

TABLE 41-2. STAGING OVARIAN TUMORS

Stage	Extent
I	GROWTH LIMITED TO OVARIES
Ia	Growth limited to one ovary No ascites No malignant cells in peritoneal washings
Ia 1	No tumor on external surface Capsule intact
Ia 2	Tumor on external surface and/or capsule ruptured
Ib	Growth in both ovaries but limited to the ovaries No ascites No malignant cells in peritoneal washings
Ib 1	No tumor on external surface Capsule intact
Ib 2	Tumor on one or both external surfaces and/or one or both capsules ruptured
Ic	Growth in one or both ovaries Ascites present and/or malignant cells in peritoneal washings
II	GROWTH IN ONE OR BOTH OVARIES WITH PELVIC EXTENSION
IIa	Extension and/or metastases only to uterus or tubes No ascites No malignant cells in peritoneal washings
IIb	Extension and/or metastases to other pelvic tissue No ascites No malignant cells in peritoneal washings
IIc	Extension and/or metastases to some pelvic structure Ascites and/or malignant cells in peritoneal washings
III	GROWTH IN ONE OR BOTH OVARIES WITH INTRAPERITONEAL EXTENSION BEYOND THE PELVIS Implants on the extrapelvic peritoneal serosa and/or involvement of retroperitoneal lymph nodes
IV	GROWTH IN ONE OR BOTH OVARIES WITH DISTANT METASTASES Metastases to extraperitoneal organs and/or hepatic metastases.

cured by resection of the tumor. Occasionally, an ovarian carcinoma causes hypercalcemia.

Staging. The most widely used system for estimating the extent of an ovarian tumor is that of the International Federation of Gynecology and Obstetrics, commonly called FIGO. In this system, the extent of the tumor is judged after laparotomy and pathologic examination of any tissue removed. Table 41-2 shows a modification of this method of staging.

COMMON "EPITHELIAL" TUMORS. About 70% of ovarian tumors and 90% of malignant ovarian tumors are of the common "epithelial" type. Most of these tumors arise from the germinal epithelium covering the ovaries. A few arise from a focus of endometriosis, and a few are associated with a teratoma of the ovary and may be part of the teratoma.

The common "epithelial" tumors are divided into three groups: benign, borderline and malignant. The borderline lesions are tumors of low malignancy that metastasize or recur only occasionally. Some prefer to consider them a form of malignant tumor.

Serous Tumors. Over 30% of ovarian tumors and 40% of malignant ovarian tumors are of the serous type. About 60% of the serous tumors are benign, 10% are border-line, and 30% are malignant. Benign serous tumors are most common in people 20 to 40 years old, and borderline lesions in women 30 to 60 years old. Most patients with a serous carcinoma are over 40 years old.

Lesions. Most serous tumors of the ovaries are cystic or predominantly cystic. A few are solid. A few form papillary projections on the surface of an ovary. The benign forms are termed serous cystadenoma, serous adenofibroma, serous cystadenofibroma, or serous papilloma. The malignant tumors are called a serous cyst of borderline malignancy, serous carcinoma, or serous cystadenocarcinoma.

Serous Cystadenoma. About 20% of benign ovarian tumors are serous cystadenomata. In 10% of the patients, the tumor is bilateral.

A serous cystadenoma is usually 5 to 10 cm in diameter. The distinction between the germinal inclusion cysts common in the ovaries and serous cystadenomata is not clear. If the lesion is less than 1 cm in diameter, it is usually called an inclusion cyst. If it is larger, it is considered to be a cystadenoma. Most serous cystadenomata are unilocular; a few are multilocular.

A serous cystadenoma bulges from the

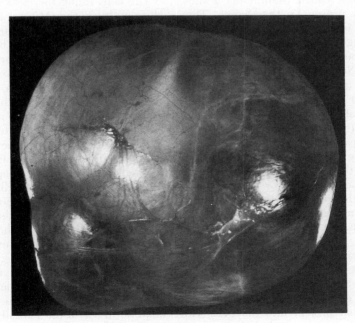

Fig. 41-14.   A serous cystadenoma of an ovary.

surface of the ovary. Its outer surface is smooth and glistening, often with prominent blood vessels beneath the serosa. The cyst wall is thin and fibrous. Most serous cystadenomata contain serous fluid, but in some the content is mucoid. Part or all of the inner lining of the cyst is smooth and shiny. Part may show papillary excrescences that bulge into the lumen. The excrescences are sometimes hard, like cartilage; sometimes they are soft and edematous.

Microscopically, serous cystadenomata are lined for the most part by cuboidal epithelium, like the germinal epithelium of the ovaries. In many of the tumors, in some regions the cuboidal cells are replaced by columnar, mucus-secreting cells, ciliated cells, clear cells, hobnail cells, or some combination of these cell types. The tumor cells have regular, spheroidal, basal nuclei without atypicality. Mitoses are rare. Electron microscopy shows well-formed cilia on the luminal surface of the ciliated cells, tight junctions, and prominent intercellular interdigitations. The epithelium is supported by a collagenous tissue or by ovarian stroma. Occasionally clumps of luteinized cells are present in the stroma.

Calcified, laminated spheroids up to 50 μm in diameter, called psammoma bodies, are commonly present in the stroma. They consist of calcium apatite deposited on the debris of degenerating cells. The name comes from the Greek for sand.

Borderline Serous Cyst.   Borderline serous cysts are sometimes called borderline cystadenomata or serous cystadenocarcinomata of low malignancy. They are bilateral in 40% of the patients.

Macroscopically, serous cysts of borderline malignancy are like the benign serous cystadenomata. If the papillae that bulge into the cyst are fine and delicate or cover a great proportion of the interior of the cyst, the risk of borderline malignancy is high. Often the fluid in a serous cyst of borderline malignancy is mucoid.

Microscopically, the epithelium lining borderline serous cysts is pseudostratified or multilayered. Solid clumps of tumor cells bulge into the cyst, particularly at the tips of the papillae that project into the cyst. The tumor cells are often atypical. A few mitoses

are usually evident. In some of the tumors, much or all the epithelium is of borderline malignancy. In others, much of the epithelium is benign, with only small foci of borderline character. Electron microscopy shows prominent infolding of the nuclei and simplification of the intercellular interdigitations, but cilia are still present on the luminal surfaces of the ciliated cells. The basement membrane is intact.

Borderline serous tumors do not invade the adjacent tissues, but often small locules lined by tumor cells bulge into the surrounding tissue. Psammoma bodies are present in the stroma in 25% of the patients.

Serous Carcinoma.   Serous carcinoma is the commonest malignant tumor of the ovaries. These tumors are usually cystic and are commonly called cystadenocarcinomata. The tumor is bilateral in over 50% of the patients.

Serous carcinomata are more than 5 cm across in 95% of the patients and over 15 cm across in 50%. They are usually multiloculated, with extensive and prominent papillae bulging into the cysts. The outer surface may be smooth or may show warty projections of the carcinoma. Often part of the tumor is solid and clearly invading the ovary.

The cells lining the cysts are atypical and often multilayered. Mitoses are present. The papillary fronds projecting into the cysts are often crowded together. They have only a fine core of collagenous tissue and are lined by atypical perhaps multilayered cells. In the solid parts of the carcinoma, the tumor cells are often more anaplastic than are the cells lining the cysts. The tumor may form glands lined by atypical cells but often grows in solid sheets. Invasion of the adjacent tissues by the carcinoma is usually clear. Electron microscopy shows irregularly shaped nuclei and simplification of the intercellular interdigitations. Only a few cilia remain.

Psammoma bodies are present in over 30% of serous carcinomata of the ovaries. They can be sufficiently numerous to be evident radiologically.

Serous Adenofibroma.   Over 40% of benign ovarian tumors are cystadenofibromata or adenofibromata. The tumor is bilateral in 5% of the patients.

Adenofibromata and cystadenofibromata

range from 1 to 15 cm across. An adenofibroma forms a hard, white, fibrous mass. A
cystadenofibroma is similar, but scattered
in the fibrosis are small cysts, usually with
prominent, rounded papillae protruding into
their lumina.

Microscopically, the greater part of a
cystadenofibroma or adenofibroma consists
of collagenous tissue, sometimes arranged
in a storiform pattern. Often the collagenous
tissue is edematous, but sometimes it is hyalinized and sclerotic. Occasionally it is highly
cellular. Scattered in the collagenous tissue
are glands or cysts lined by epithelium like
that of a serous cystadenoma. Usually cuboidal cells are predominant, but foci of ciliated, mucus-secreting, clear, or hobnail cells
are common. Often a narrow band of acellular collagenous tissue lies immediately under
the epithelium. An occasional psammoma
body is often present.

Occasionally the epithelium lining the
cysts or glands in a serous adenofibroma or
serous cystadenofibroma shows borderline
changes, like those in a borderline serous
cystadenoma. Rarely, the epithelial element
in the tumor is malignant.

Serous Papilloma. Papillary projections
on the surface of the ovaries lined by epithelium like that of a serous tumor are called papillomata. Most are benign, but occasionally
the epithelium of one of the larger papillomata shows borderline changes.

Extraovarian Serous Tumors. Occasionally a serous carcinoma arises from in the pelvic peritoneum without a lesion in an ovary.
Probably these tumors result from metaplasia of the mesothelium.

Behavior. Benign serous cystadenomata,
benign serous adenofibromata, and benign
serous cystadenofibromata grow slowly and
remain confined to the ovaries. In the rare
patients with a benign serous cystadenoma in
which implants of tumor develop on the
peritoneum, there is, presumably, an undetected focus of borderline malignancy or of
invasive carcinoma somewhere in the tumor.

Serous tumors of borderline malignancy
give rise to implants on the peritoneum in
from 20 to 50% of the patients. Metastases to
lymph nodes or more distantly are rare. The
peritoneal implants often grow sluggishly and
may regress, though some invade deeply.
Sometimes peritoneal implants appear long
after the primary tumor or tumors are removed, sometimes as long as 20 years after
the original operation.

Serous cystadenocarcinomata and solid

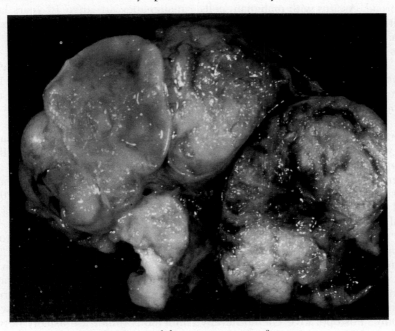

Fig. 41-15.   A solid serous carcinoma of an ovary.

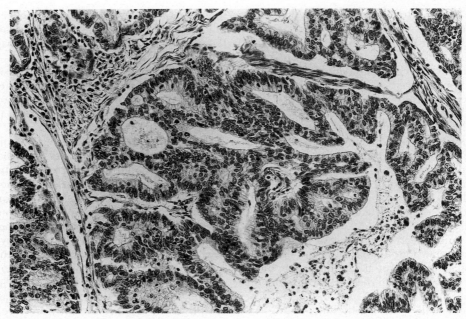

Fig. 41-16. A serous cystadenocarcinoma of an ovary, showing papillary fronds projecting into cyst spaces. The fronds have a fine collagenous core and are lined by moderately atypical tumor cells.

serous carcinomata invade extensively around the ovary or ovaries involved. Peritoneal implants are usual and often are numerous and widespread. Ascites with malignant cells in the ascitic fluid is common. Often there is a malignant effusion in one or both pleural cavities. Metastases in the pelvic and abdominal lymph nodes are common. Hematogenous metastases to distant organs are not frequent.

Treatment and Prognosis. Benign serous tumors of the ovaries are usually treated by unilateral salpingo-oophorectomy if the patient is young. In older women and for bilateral tumor, salpingo-oophorectomy and hysterectomy are preferred.

Serous tumors of borderline malignancy are treated like benign lesions if there is no evidence of extension beyond the ovaries. If metastases are present, bilateral salpingo-oophorectomy and hysterectomy are needed. Postoperative chemotherapy is of limited value.

Malignant serous tumors require a radical hysterectomy and bilateral salpingo-oophorectomy. Postoperative chemotherapy has proved valuable in controlling metastases.

If there is no evidence of extension beyond the ovaries at the time of operation, 80% of patients with a serous cyst of borderline malignancy are alive 10 years later. Even if there are implants on the peritoneum when the diagnosis is made, 75% of the patients live more than 10 years.

Only 20% of the patients with a serous carcinoma survive 10 years. If there are peritoneal implants at the time of operation, under 10% live 10 years. The presence of psammoma bodies improves the prognosis. If none are found in the carcinoma, under 20% of the patients live five years. If psammoma bodies are present, nearly 40% are alive five years after removal of the tumor.

Mucinous Tumors. About 20% of ovarian tumors are mucinous. Over 85% of them are benign, 5% are of borderline malignancy, and 10% are malignant. Teratomatous elements are present in 5% of the tumors, suggesting that the tumor arises in a teratoma, but most mucinous tumors contain no teratomatous tissues and probably arise from the germinal epithelium. Patients with a benign mucinous tumor are usually between 20 and 50 years old, though some are younger.

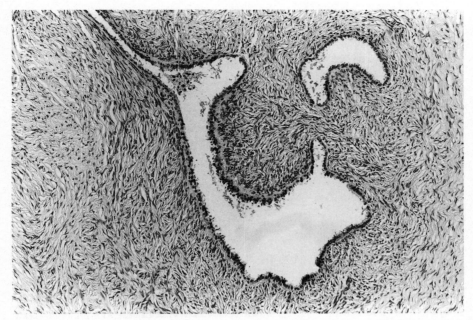

Fig. 41-17. A serous adenofibroma, showing glandular spaces lined by cuboidal epithelium separated by the fibrous component of the tumor.

Mucinous carcinomata usually develop in women over 40 years old.

Lesions. Most mucinous tumors of the ovaries are cystic, forming a mucinous cystadenoma, a mucinous cyst of borderline malignancy, or a cystadenocarcinoma. Some are mainly solid and are classed as adenofibromata, cystadenofibromata, or solid carcinomata.

Mucinous Cystadenoma. About 20% of benign ovarian tumors are mucinous cystadenomata. The tumor is bilateral in 5% of the patients.

Mucinous cystadenomata of the ovaries are usually multilocular, with a smooth outer surface. The cysts have thin walls and contain mucinous fluid, sometimes thick and viscous, sometimes thin and watery. The inner surface of the cysts is usually smooth. Most mucinous cystadenomata are 15 to 30 cm across when discovered. A few weigh over 5 kg. A mucinous cyst weighing 150 kg has been reported.

Microscopically, the cysts are usually lined by a single layer of tall, columnar, mucus secreting cells with basal nuclei. Less often, the epithelium lining the cysts resembles that of the gut, with goblet cells set among cells that do not secrete mucus, perhaps with Paneth cells and neuroendocrine cells like those of the gut. Rarely, there is squamous metaplasia. Electron microscopy shows that the tumor cells resemble endocervical cells in most patients, but resemble the epithelium of the gut in others.

The wall of the cysts consists of collagenous or ovarian stromal tissue, occasionally with bundles of smooth muscle adjacent to the cysts. Rarely, a giant cell reaction is evident in the stroma. Occasionally, mucus escapes from the cysts into the stroma, forming pools of mucus in the stroma, a condition called pseudomyxoma ovarii.

Borderline Mucinous Cysts. Borderline mucinous cysts are bilateral in 10% of the patients. Macroscopically, they are similar to benign mucinous cystadenomata, except that in 50% of the patients papillary excrescences are present on the inner surface of the cysts. Microscopically, the epithelium lining the cysts is stratified, atypical, with hyperchromatic nuclei and nucleoli. Mitoses are present. Sometimes clumps of tumor cells bulge into the lumen of a cyst. Invasion is not present.

Mucinous Carcinoma. Less than 10% of

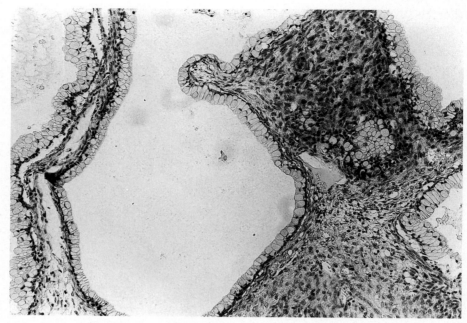

Fig. 41-18.   A mucinous cystadenoma of an ovary, showing cysts lined by a single layer of mucus-secreting epithelium.

malignant ovarian tumors are mucinous carcinomata. About 25% of the tumors are bilateral. The tumor is nearly always multicystic and is often called a mucinous cystadenocarcinoma.

Most mucinous carcinomata are 5 to 50 cm across. Usually part of the tumor is solid, partly cystic. Papillary projections into the cysts are often numerous. Some of the tumors are anaplastic, with columns of tumor cells invading the surrounding tissues. Some are well differentiated and hard to distinguish from borderline malignancies. Some suggest that mucinous tumors of the ovaries should be considered to be malignant if the epithelium lining the cysts is more than 4 cells thick, of borderline malignancy if it is 2 or 3 cells thick, and benign if it is 1 cell thick.

Mucinous Adenofibroma. Mucinous adenofibroma and cystadenofibroma are rare. Occasionally a tumor of this type is of borderline malignancy or malignant. The tumors resemble a serous adenofibroma or cystadenofibroma, except that the cysts are lined by mucinous epithelium.

Behavior.   Benign mucinous tumors remain confined to the ovary and rarely cause other than mechanical trouble, even if they grow gigantic. Rarely, pseudomyxoma peritonei develops in a patient with an apparently benign mucinous cystadenoma, perhaps because it contains a focus of borderline malignancy that is not discovered.

About 15% of mucinous tumors of borderline malignancy have extended beyond the ovary by the time the diagnosis is made. They may recur after excision, but rarely extend beyond the pelvis, except when associated with pseudomyxoma peritonei.

Mucinous carcinomata also tend to remain confined to the pelvis, with implants of carcinoma in the general abdominal cavity in only 20% of the patients. Late in the disease, metastases may appear in the lymph nodes and more distantly.

Pseudomyxoma Peritonei. Pseudomyxoma peritonei develops in 5% of women with mucinous ovarian tumors, usually in association with a tumor of borderline malignancy. Islands of well-differentiated mucus-producing epithelium are scattered throughout the abdominal cavity. Massive, mucinous ascites develops. Sooner or later, though perhaps not for years, the dense adhesions that develop around the pools of mucus cause intestinal obstruction, sepsis develops in one of the pools of mucinous ascites loculated by the adhesions, or the patient becomes weak and cachectic. Occasionally, a patient with pseudomyxoma peritonei has both a mucinous tumor and a mucocele of the appendix. The islands of mucinous epithelium in the peritoneal cavity are believed to be metastases from the ovary.

Treatment and Prognosis. A unilateral benign or mucinous cystadenoma in a young woman is treated by unilateral salpingo-oophorectomy. Borderline tumors are treated similarly, unless there is evidence of extension. Bilateral tumors, malignant tumors, and mucinous tumors in older women require hysterectomy and bilateral salpingo-oophorectomy.

More than 80% of patients with a borderline malignancy of the mucinous type and over 30% of those with a mucinous cystadenocarcinoma are alive 10 years after surgical treatment. Nearly 50% of patients with pseudomyxoma peritonei are alive five years after the diagnosis.

Endometrioid Tumors. About 5% of ovarian tumors are endometrioid. They have epithelium that resembles endometrial epithelium. Most are malignant. Some arise in a focus of ovarian endometriosis, but in most there is no evidence of endometriosis and the tumor probably arises from the germinal epithelium. Most of the patients are between 40 and 60 years old, though the tumors can arise at any age.

Lesions. Benign endometrioid tumors of the ovary are divided into adenomata, cystadenomata, adenofibromata, and cystadenofibromata. Borderline endometrioid tumors are rare. The malignant endometrioid tumors are called endometrioid carcinomata.

Classified with the endometrioid tumors are two rare ovarian tumors, sarcoma of endometrioid stroma and mixed müllerian tumor. They resemble the stromal sarcomata and mixed müllerian tumors of the uterus.

Benign. The benign endometrioid tumors are similar to the similarly named serous tumors. Adenofibromata and cystadenofibromata are the most common. The epithelium lining the glands and cysts resembles endometrium, but the collagenous stroma of the tumors is the same. Foci of squamous

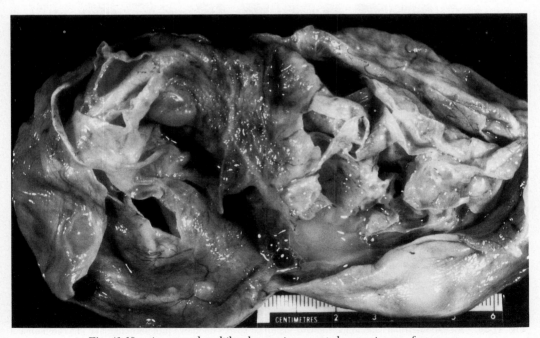

Fig. 41-19. An opened multilocular mucinous cystadenocarcinoma of an ovary.

metaplasia are often present. In a few of the adenofibromata, the glands are closely packed and resemble atypical endometrial hyperplasia.

Endometrioid Carcinoma. About 20% of malignant ovarian tumors are endometrioid carcinomata. The tumor is bilateral in 30% of the patients.

Most endometrioid carcinomata are cystic, though often with regions in which the tumor forms a solid mass. Occasionally, an endometrioid carcinoma of an ovary is entirely solid. Often papillary fronds and projections bulge into the lumina of the cysts. The fluid in the cysts may be clear, but often is mucoid, or dark and bloody. The solid part of the carcinoma may be soft and mushy or hard and fibrous. Foci of necrosis or hemorrhage are common.

Microscopically, an endometrioid carcinoma of an ovary resembles a carcinoma of the endometrium. It grows in a similar fashion and shows a similar range of differentiation. It differs from an endometrial carcinoma principally in its greater tendency to become cystic and to form papillae that project into the cysts. In nearly 50% of the

patients, the tumor contains islands of well-differentiated squamous epithelium, like that present in an adenoacanthoma of the endometrium. Less often, both the glandular and squamous parts of an endometrioid carcinoma are anaplastic, as in an adenosquamous carcinoma of the endometrium. Occasionally, the tumor cells contain basal vacuoles, like those of a secretory carcinoma of the endometrium. Foci of clear cell carcinoma, mucinous carcinoma, serous carcinoma or some other kind of common "epithelial" tumor are present in 10% of endometrioid carcinomata. Mucus is often abundant in the lumina of an endometrioid tumor, even when the epithelium of the tumor is all of the endometrial type. The stroma of the tumor is usually collagenous, perhaps with some admixture of ovarian cortical stroma. A few psammoma bodies are sometimes present.

Mixed Müllerian Tumor. A mixed müllerian tumor of an ovary usually forms a mass, which is partially cystic, partially solid, often with foci of necrosis and hemorrhage. About 10% of the tumors are bilateral.

Microscopically, the tumor resembles a

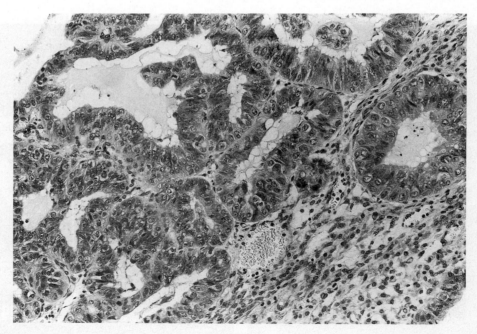

Fig. 41-20.   An endometrioid carcinoma, showing glandular spaces lined by epithelium like that of a carcinoma of the endometrium.

mixed müllerian tumor of the endometrium, showing the glands of an adenocarcinoma separated by a malignant stroma. The carcinoma usually resembles an endometrioid or serous carcinoma, but can be mucinous, or may show some other form of common "epithelial" differentiation. The malignant stroma consists mainly of small, spindle cells, but may contain foci of malignant cartilage or cells showing rhabdomyomatous differentiation.

Behavior. Endometrioid carcinomata of the ovaries are usually confined to the pelvis when diagnosed. Only 20% of them show extension into the general abdominal cavity. Metastases to lymph nodes and by the blood stream come late.

In 20% of patients with an endometrioid carcinoma of an ovary, there is also an endometrial carcinoma. Usually the structures of the endometrial and endometrioid tumors are the same. The endometrial carcinoma is often small. It is usually assumed that the two carcinomata are both primary, though in some patients it does seem more probable that one is a metastasis from the other.

Mixed müllerian tumors grow rapidly and metastasize. Most patients die within one or two years.

Treatment and Prognosis. Endometrioid tumors of the ovaries are usually treated by bilateral salpingo-oophorectomy and hysterectomy. About 40% of patients with an endometrioid carcinoma are alive 10 years after the diagnosis. The prognosis depends principally on the stage of the tumor. If it is confined to the ovaries, over 90% of the patients are alive five years later. If it has extended to involve other pelvic structures, 30% survive for five years. If there are implants of tumor in the general peritoneal cavity or involvement of the para-aortic lymph nodes, under 5% live five years. If there are distant metastases, few if any of the patients live five years. The presence of a carcinoma in the endometrium does little to alter the prognosis.

Clear Cell Tumors. Clear cell tumors of the ovaries are almost all malignant. Most are found in women between 40 and 70 years old.

Lesions. Benign clear cell tumors of the ovaries are called adenofibromata. Borderline lesions are rare and resemble an adenofibroma macroscopically. The malignant lesions are termed clear cell carcinomata.

Benign. Clear cell adenofibromata are

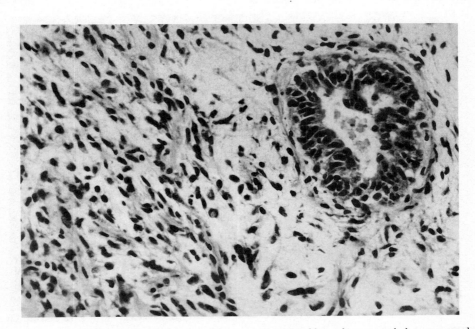

Fig. 41-21. A mixed müllerian tumor of an ovary, showing a gland lined by malignant epithelium surrounded by the spindle cells of the malignant stroma.

similar to other ovarian adenofibromata, except that the glands are lined by clear cells, hobnail cells, or low cuboidal cells. The rare borderline clear cell tumors are similar to the adenofibromata, but have atypical epithelium with mitoses.

Clear Cell Carcinoma.   About 5% of malignant ovarian tumors are clear cell carcinomata. The tumor is bilateral in 40% of the patients.

Most clear cell tumors of an ovary are cystic, usually unilocular, sometimes multilocular. Most are 5 to 25 cm across. Often solid nodules of tumor bulge into the cyst or cysts. Sometimes part or all of the tumor is solid, resembling an adenofibroma. The solid parts of the tumor may be white, yellow, or brown.

Microscopically, clear cell carcinomata of the ovaries consist of tubules, cysts, and solid sheets of tumor cells separated by collagenous tissue or ovarian cortical stroma. The clear cells, which give the tumor its name, resemble those of a clear cell carcinoma of a kidney. They have well-defined cell borders, abundant clear cytoplasm rich in glycogen and often containing fat, and small, often eccentric nuclei. The clear cells may grow in solid sheets, line tubules, or line cysts. Hobnail cells are apparent in parts of most clear cell tumors. They line tubules or cysts and have prominent nuclei bulging from the luminal surface of the cell. Sometimes cells with abundant eosinophilic cytoplasm line tubules in part of a clear cell tumor or grow in solid sheets. Sometimes small cystic spaces are lined by flattened epithelium. Often the tubules or spaces contain mucus. Often papillary structures bulge into the lumen of some of the cysts, at times suggesting vaguely the structure of a renal glomerulus or the Arias-Stella phenomenon in the endometrium. Sometimes an excess of basement membrane forms hyaline masses in the papillae. Over 10% of the tumors contain areas indistinguishable from an endometrioid carcinoma or foci that show some other form of common "epithelial" differentiation.

Behavior.   Most clear cell tumors of the ovaries remain confined to the pelvis. Over 60% of them do not extend beyond the ovaries, and in another 20% the extension is confined to the pelvis.

Treatment and Prognosis.   Clear cell

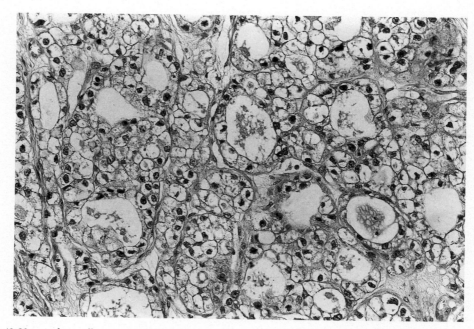

Fig. 41-22.   A clear cell carcinoma of an ovary, showing tumor cells with clear cytoplasm lining glandular spaces or growing in solid sheets.

tumors of the ovaries are treated by bilateral oophorectomy, bilateral salpingectomy, and hysterectomy, perhaps with chemotherapy or radiotherapy.

About 40% of patients with a clear cell carcinoma of an ovary survive for five years. If the tumor is confined to one ovary, 80% of the patients will be alive five years after the resection. If it has extended further, only 10% live five years.

Brenner Tumor. The Brenner tumor is named after the German pathologist who described it in 1907. About 3% of ovarian tumors are of this type. Less than 2% of them show borderline changes or are malignant, though the risk of malignancy is greater in the larger tumors. Most Brenner tumors are found in women over 40 years old, though they can occur in younger women and in children.

Lesions. Most Brenner tumors are small. About 30% of them are so small that they are found only by microscopy. Nearly 60% are under 2 cm across. Only occasionally is a Brenner tumor over 5 cm in diameter. Most develop in an otherwise normal ovary, but 20% of them develop in the wall of a mucinous cystadenoma, less often in the wall of a serous cystadenoma, a dermoid cyst, or a mucinous cystadenocarcinoma.

Most Brenner tumors are well circumscribed and solid. On section, they are grayish or yellowish. Often the cut surface is gritty from foci of calcification. Less often, but especially in the tumors of borderline malignancy or true malignancy, the tumor is multicystic, with papillae projecting into the cysts. Under 10% of Brenner tumors are bilateral.

Microscopically, Brenner tumors consist of anastomosing columns of epithelial cells that wind down from the surface of the ovary. In section, the columns appear as well-defined clumps of epithelial cells, often with a small, central lumen. The cells in the clumps are polygonal, with pale cytoplasm and oval, vesicular nuclei. Some of the nuclei show a prominent longitudinal fold. The cells lining the lumina may be flattened or columnar. They often contain mucus or are ciliated. Mucus is often present in the lumina. Occasionally small cysts lined by epithelium like that of a mucinous cystadenoma are present. The columns of epithelial cells are separated

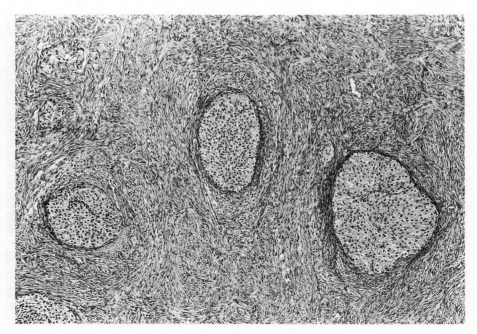

Fig. 41-23. A Brenner tumor of an ovary, showing islands of epithelial cells separated by an abundant collagenous stroma.

by an abundant stroma, usually collagenous, but sometimes of ovarian cortical stroma. There may be foci of hyalinization in the stroma. Foci of calcification are common in and around the columns of epithelial cells.

Brenner tumors of borderline malignancy show cysts containing papillary infoldings and lined by epithelium like that of the urinary bladder. The epithelium is moderately atypical. A few mitoses are usually present. Sometimes, mucus-secreting cells are present.

Malignant Brenner tumors show cysts lined by atypical epithelium or clumps of atypical epithelial cells. The epithelium usually is like that of a carcinoma of the urinary bladder, but occasionally is squamous. There may be an admixture of mucous cells.

Behavior. Most of the few Brenner tumors of borderline malignancy have behaved as benign tumors. Malignant Brenner tumors usually remain confined to the pelvis, though distant metastases have occurred.

Treatment and Prognosis. Brenner tumors are usually treated by unilateral or bilateral salpingo-oophorectomy, though if the tumor

is malignant a hysterectomy should be performed.

The prognosis in Brenner tumors of borderline malignancy is excellent, with 95% of the patients apparently cured. If the tumor is malignant, 30% or more of the patients die within a few years.

Mixed "Epithelial" Tumor. Any of the common "epithelial" tumors of the ovaries may show a minor admixture of some other type or types of common "epithelial" tumor. Such tumors should be classified according to their predominant structure. Only if two or more of the forms of common epithelial tumor are prominent should it be classified as a mixed "epithelial" tumor.

Undifferentiated Carcinoma. Carcinomata so anaplastic that their nature is uncertain make up about 5% of malignant ovarian tumors. The patients are usually over 40 years old.

The poorly differentiated carcinomata usually form solid masses in the ovaries, but may be cystic. Necrosis and hemorrhage are common. The tumor is bilateral in 50% of the patients.

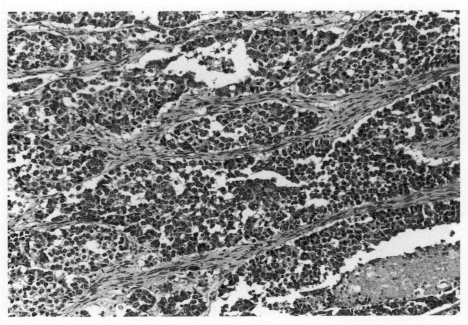

Fig. 41-24.   An undifferentiated carcinoma of an ovary, showing poorly differentiated tumor cells growing in sold sheets.

Microscopically, the tumor may form glands or grow as a carcinoma simplex, with solid columns of tumor cells winding through a collagenous stroma. The tumor cells are usually large, pleomorphic, and much simplified, with nothing to suggest their nature.

Probably most of the anaplastic tumors of the ovaries are poorly differentiated forms of one of the common "epithelial" tumors, though some arise from germ cells or the sex cords. Probably most are anaplastic variants of a serous carcinoma or an endometrioid carcinoma.

The prognosis is bad. Only 10% of the patients survive for 10 years.

SEX CORD-STROMAL TUMORS. The sex cord-stromal tumors of the ovaries arise from cells derived from the sex cords of the developing gonads or the stroma between them. They include the granulosa cell tumor, thecoma, fibroma, sclerosing stromal tumor, Sertoli-Leydig cell tumor, Sertoli cell tumor, gynandroblastoma, tumors that combine more than one of these elements, and rare tumors whose nature is uncertain. Together, the sex cord-stromal tumors make up 8% of primary ovarian neoplasms. Many of them occur in the testes as well as in the ovaries.

Granulosa Cell Tumor. All granulosa cell tumors are considered to be malignant. They make up less than 2% of ovarian tumors and less than 10% of ovarian cancers. About 5% of them arise before puberty, with the rest evenly distributed through the reproductive and postmenopausal years.

Lesions. Two kinds of granulosa cell tumor are distinguished: adult and juvenile. About 95% of them are of the adult type. Tumors of the adult type can develop at any age, but the juvenile type is uncommon in women over 30 years old. Most of the tumors in children are of the juvenile type.

Adult Type. Adult granulosa cell tumors may be a few millimeters in diameter to 40 cm or more across. The largest on record weighed nearly 70 kg. They show some combination of solid and cystic growth. Most are polycystic, with clear fluid or clotted blood in the cysts. Occasionally a granulosa cell tumor is unilocular and resembles a serous cystadenoma. The solid part of the tumor is yellow, white, or gray. It may be soft or hard. Often there are foci of necrosis or hemorrhage. About 5% of the tumors are bilateral.

Microscopically, the tumors can show any of a variety of patterns of growth. Often a

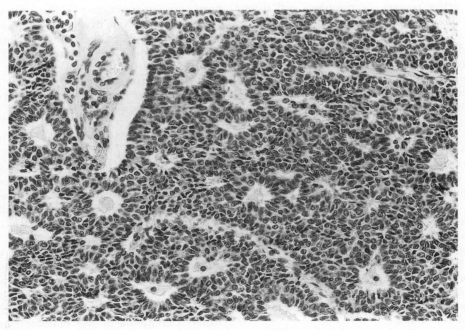

Fig. 41-25.   A microfollicular granulosa cell tumor, showing Call-Exner bodies in a clump of granulosa cells.

single tumor shows more than one of these patterns.

In the microfollicular pattern of growth, the tumor consists of well-defined clumps of granulosa cells separated by ovarian cortical stroma. The granulosa cells usually are small with little cytoplasm. Occasionally some of them are large with eosinophilic, vacuolated cytoplasm. Their nuclei are ovoid or angular, vesicular, and often folded or grooved. Call-Exner bodies like those of the graafian follicles are numerous within the clumps. The Call-Exner bodies have a small, central cavity containing eosinophilic fluid, hyalinized basement membrane, or a few pyknotic nuclei. A prominent palisade of granulosa cells surrounds the cavity. A similar palisade of granulosa cells is often present at the margin of the clumps. Betwen the Call-Exner bodies, the granulosa cells are jumbled in disorderly fashion. Mitoses are sometimes numerous.

In macrofollicular regions, granulosa cell tumors form cysts, lined by granulosa cells supported by the thecal cells of the ovarian cortical stroma. The thecal cells, the granulosa cells, or both may be luteinized. Often the tumor is so well differentiated that the wall of the cyst is indistinguishable from that of a graafian follicle or a follicle cyst.

In other regions, a granulosa cell tumor may show a trabecular or insular pattern, with anastomosing cords of granulosa cells or islands of granulosa cells separated by ovarian cortical stroma. Sometimes the thecal cells around the columns of granulosa cells are luteinized.

Sometimes the granulosa cells grow in narrow, sinuous columns resembling watered silk. Occasionally, a granulosa cell tumor forms tubules or large sheets of small, closely packed granulosa cells.

In some granulosa cell tumors, the stroma is abundant, sometimes even the predominant feature of the tumor. It is usually considered that the stromal element in the granulosa cell tumors develops in response to the neoplastic granulosa cells and is not itself neoplastic. It may be, however, that in tumors in which the stromal element is unusually abundant the stroma too is neoplastic and the lesion is a mixed granulosa-thecal cell tumor.

If it is difficult to distinguish between granulosa cells and thecal cells, a reticulin stain is useful. Reticulin fibers surround each thecal cell, but are not found between granulosa cells, except when the granulosa cells are adjacent to a blood vessel.

Juvenile Type. Macroscopically, juvenile granulosa cell tumors resemble the adult type. In 10% of the patients, the tumor appears to be ruptured when the abdomen is opened. Jueuvenile granulosa cell tumors are bilateral in 2% of the patients.

Microscopically, the granulosa cells form clumps separated by a collagenous stroma, grow in large sheets, or line irregular spaces. The spaces often contain mucus. Occasionally granulosa and thecal cells are mixed together. The granulosa cells are large, with abundant, eosinophilic cytoplasm. Their nuclei are small, round, and hyperchromatic. They are rarely folded or grooved. In some tumors, the nuclei are pleomorphic and atypical. Mitoses are usually numerous. Luteinization of the granulosa cells and the adjacent thecal cells is common.

Behavior. Granulosa cell tumors invade locally, but rarely spread beyond the pelvis. In 90% of the patients with an adult granulosa cell tumor, the tumor is discovered before it has spread beyond the ovary. Distant metastases are uncommon. If the tumor has spread beyond the ovary, recurrence after surgical removal of the tumor is common. Juvenile granulosa cell tumors usually recur in less than three years and often the recurrent tumor grows rapidly. In tumors of the adult type, recurrence is often delayed for many years, sometimes for as long as 30 years.

Dysfunction. Many granulosa cell tumors secrete estrogen probably produced mainly by the thecal cells in the tumor. The granulosa cells usually lack the enzymes needed to synthesize steroids and ultrastructurally do not have the abundant smooth endoplasmic reticulum or the tubular mitochondrial cristae usual in cells synthesizing estrogen.

In adults, the excess of estrogen causes endometrial hyperplasia, often with atypicality. In women of reproductive age, irregular, excessive menstrual bleeding is common. In older women, postmenopausal bleeding is usual. Carcinoma of the endometrium develops in 5% of the patients.

Sexual precocity develops in 80% of children with a granulosa cell tumor. The breasts enlarge. Pubic and axillary hair take an adult pattern. Enlargement of the genitalia follows, often with irregular endometrial bleeding and a whitish vaginal discharge. Skeletal growth is accelerated.

Less often, an adult granulosa cell tumor secretes androgens and causes hirsutism or virilization. Most of the androgenic tumors are of the macrocystic type.

Treatment and Prognosis. Granulosa cell tumors are usually treated by bilateral oophorectomy, bilateral salpingectomy, and hysterectomy, though in young women wishing children a unilateral oophorectomy is sufficient if there is no evidence of spread. Recurrences are treated by operation, radiation, chemotherapy, or some combination of these means.

If an adult granulosa cell tumor is confined to the ovary, 90% of the patients survive more than 10 years. If it extends beyond the ovaries, 40% are alive after 10 years. Rupture of the tumor worsens the prognosis. The larger and more anaplastic tumors tend to have extended beyond the ovaries and to have a poor prognosis. Juvenile granulosa cell tumors confined to the ovary have an excellent prognosis, but the prognosis is poor if the tumor has extended beyond the ovary.

Thecoma. With a few exceptions, thecomata are benign. They make up less than 1% of ovarian tumors. Most patients are menopausal or postmenopausal. Fewer than 10% are under 30 years old.

Lesions. A thecoma is usually 5 to 10 cm across. The tumor is firm and well defined. On section, it is usually yellowish or orange and solid. Only occasionally are a few cysts evident in the tumor. Less than 3% of the tumors are bilateral.

Microscopically, a thecoma consists of spindle-shaped cells like the thecal cells of a normal ovary. The cells usually have pale, vacuolated cytoplasm containing large quantities of lipid. Their nuclei are round. Occasionally, mitoses are evident. In parts of the tumor, collagen is formed by cells like those of an ovarian fibroma. Occasionally the collagen is hyalinized. Clumps of luteinized cells are often present. Exceptionally, a small clump of granulosa cells is present in the tumor.

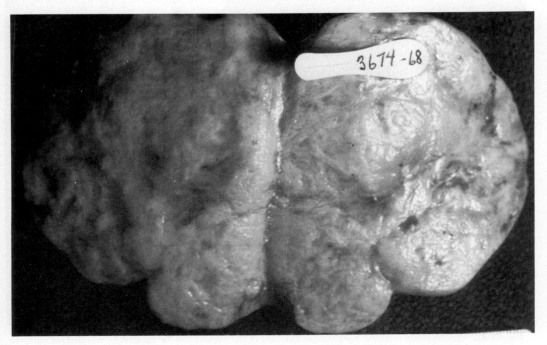

Fig. 41-26. A thecoma of an ovary, showing the cut surface of the well-defined, hard, fibrous tumor.

Dysfunction. Most thecomata secrete estrogens. Endometrial hyperplasia causes postmenopausal bleeding in 60% of the patients. About 20% of the patients develop an endometrial carcinoma. Occasionally, a luteinized thecoma secretes androgens and causes virilization.

Treatment and Prognosis. Thecomata are benign. Oophorectomy cures, though hysterectomy and bilateral salpingo-oophorectomy are often preferred.

Fibroma. Fibromata of the ovary are benign. They constitute 4% of ovarian tumors. A fibroma of an ovary can arise at any age, but most are found in women 30 to 60 years old. Rarely, a fibrosarcoma arises in an ovary.

Lesions. A fibroma of an ovary forms a well-defined, hard, white mass. Occasionally, the tumor contains softer, edematous areas, small cysts, or partially calcified areas. Some fibromata are less than 1 cm across; some are more than 20 cm in diameter. The tumor is bilateral in fewer than 10% of the patients.

There may be more than one fibroma in an ovary.

Microscopically, a fibroma of an ovary consists of swirling bundles of spindle-shaped cells separated by the collagen they produce. Usually the collagen is fine, but in places it may be thick and hyalinized. Occasionally the tumor has a myxoid appearance. Plaques or spherules of calcification are sometimes present. Some tumors show a few mitoses.

Complications. Sometimes a patient with an ovarian fibroma develops Meigs' syndrome or has the hereditary basal nevus syndrome.

Meigs' Syndrome. Meigs' syndrome, named after the American gynecologist who described it in 1954, develops in 1% of patients with an ovarian fibroma and can occur in patients with other kinds of ovarian tumor. The patient has ascites and a pleural effusion that disappear after the tumor is removed. The effusion is on the right in 70% of the patients, on the left in 10%, and is bilateral in 20%.

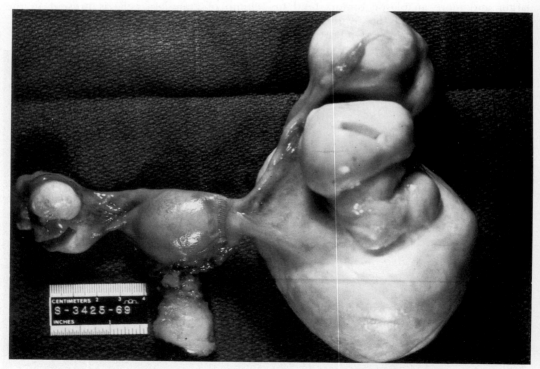

Fig. 41-27. Bilateral fibromata of the ovaries. The size of the tumors can be gauged by comparison with the uterus.

About 15% of women with an ovarian fibroma develop ascites that disappears when the tumor is removed, but not a pleural effusion. The larger the tumor, the more likely is ascites to develop. If an ovarian fibroma is over 10 cm across, 40% of the patients have ascites. Fibromata that are myxoid microscopically are particularly likely to cause ascites. Nearly 70% of patients with a myxoid fibroma over 10 cm across have ascites. About 10% of women with a granulosa cell tumor develop similar ascites that resorbs when the tumor is removed.

Hereditary Basal Nevus Syndrome. Patients with the hereditary basal nevus syndrome usually have multiple calcified fibromata in both ovaries. They develop basal cell carcinomata in the skin at an early age and often have cysts in the jaws and mesentery, calcification of the dura, and other abnormalities.

Treatment and Prognosis. Excision of a fibroma of an ovary cures.

Sclerosing Stromal Tumor. Sclerosing stromal tumors are uncommon. Over 80% of the patients are 10 to 30 years old. The tumor is unilateral and forms a well-defined mass.

On section, it is white, often with small cysts or foci of edema. Microscopically, cellular nodules are separated by more edematous, less cellular collagenous tissue. In the cellular nodules, fibrocytes are mixed with larger vacuolated cells that contain lipid. Thin-walled blood vessels are often prominent in the nodules, and sometimes the collagenous tissue is sclerotic. A few of the sclerosing stromal tumors have secreted estrogen or androgen. All are benign.

Sertoli-Leydig Cell Tumor. An ovarian tumor made of cells that resemble the Sertoli and Leydig cells of the testes is called a Sertoli-Leydig cell tumor, or sometimes an androblastoma, from the Greek for man, or an arrhenoblastoma, from the Greek for male. Less than 0.2% of ovarian tumors are of this type. Most arise in young women, but 5% appear before puberty and 10% after the menopause.

Lesions. Macroscopically, a Sertoli-Leydig cell tumor looks like a granulosa cell tumor. Most are 5 to 15 cm across. The tumor may be solid or cystic. In its solid regions, it may be gray, white, or yellow. Foci of necrosis or hemorrhage are some-

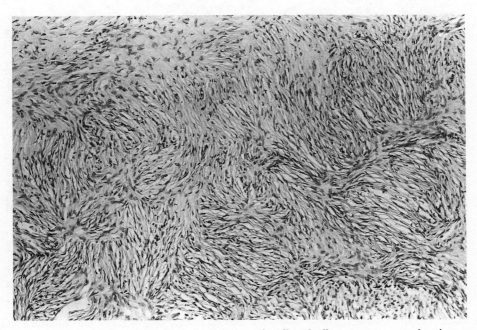

Fig. 41-28.   A fibroma of an ovary, showing the interwoven bundles of collagenous tissue usual in these tumors.

times present. The cysts may be large and full of blood. Sertoli-Leydig cell tumors are bilateral in less than 5% of patients.

Microscopically, well-differentiated Sertoli-Leydig cell tumors are usually lobulated, with islands of tumor cells separated by collagenous septa. The islands of tumor cells contain tubules lined by columnar or cuboidal Sertoli cells with regular spheroidal or ovoid nuclei or solid columns made of similar cells. Leydig cells are usually numerous in the collagenous stroma between the tubules and columns of Sertoli cells. Mitoses are few.

Less well-differentiated Sertoli-Leydig tumors can show any of a variety of patterns of growth. Often parts of the tumor are better differentiated than others. The Sertoli cells are small, with spheroidal or angular nuclei. They may form tubules or solid columns, but often grow in large sheets. Occasionally they line microcysts filled with eosinophilic material. In 15% of the tumors, they form tubules like those of the rete testis except that papillary excrescences covered by Sertoli cells commonly bulge into the spaces.

The columns and sheets of Sertoli cells are separated by a collagenous stroma containing clumps of Leydig cells. The stroma is sometimes loose and edematous. Sometimes it is highly cellular and consists of small, poorly differentiated spindle cells. Occasionally it resembles a fibrosarcoma. Often droplets of fat are present in the Sertoli cells, the Leydig cells, or both.

Glands or cysts lined by intestinal epithelium containing neuroendocrine cells, and sometimes Paneth cells are present in 20% of Sertoli-Leydig tumors. In 15%, microscopic foci of carcinoid tumor are present. In 5%, the stroma contains foci of cartilage or of striped muscle.

Behavior. In 95% of the patients, a Sertoli-Leydig tumor is confined to the ovary. In 10%, the tumor has ruptured. Extension beyond the ovaries is usually confined to the pelvis. Distant metastases are rare.

Dysfunction. In 30% of patients with a Sertoli-Leydig cell tumor, the concentrations of testosterone, androstenedione, and other androgens in the plasma are increased. The urinary secretion of 17-ketosteroids is usually normal. Oligomenorrhea is followed by amenorrhea. The breasts atrophy; the contour of the body changes; acne, hirsutism, balding,

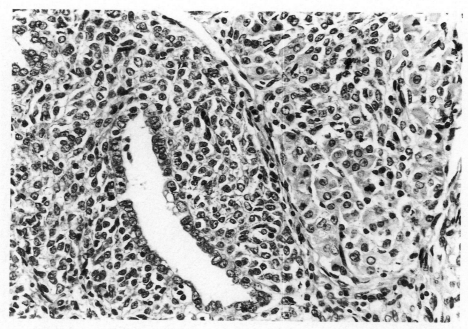

Fig. 41-29.   A Sertoli-Leydig cell tumor of an ovary, showing a tubule lined by Sertoli cell surrounded by a sheet of poorly differentiated cells. A clump of Leydig cells is on the right.

deepening of the voice, and enlargement of the clitoris follow. Occasionally there is erhtyocytosis or an increase in the concentration of α-fetoprotein in the plasma.

Treatment and Prognosis. Sertoli-Leydig cell tumors are treated by oophorectomy if the patient is young and the tumor is localized to one ovary or by hysterectomy and bilateral salpingo-oophorectomy if the tumor is more extensive or the patient is older. If the tumor has extended beyond the ovary, chemotherapy or radiotherapy is added. In the virilized patients, menstruation begins after four weeks. The hirsuitism lessens, but the deep voice and clitoromegaly persist.

If the tumor is confined to the ovary, almost all patients with well-differentiated tumors are cured, but in 10% with those of moderately differentiated tumors and 60% of those with poorly differentiated lesions the tumor recurs and the prognosis is poor.

Sertoli Cell Tumor. Rarely, an ovarian tumor consists of tubules or columns of Sertoli cells, but does not have Leydig cells in the stroma. In some of the tumors, fat is abundant in the cytoplasm of the tumor cells. Some have caused sexual preciosity in children. The tumors are well differentiated. Oophorectomy cures.

Gynandroblastoma. A gynandroblastoma is an extremely rare tumor that is in part a Sertoli-Leydig cell tumor, in part a granulosa cell tumor. The name comes from the Greek words for woman and man. The diagnosis should not be made unless the smaller component makes up at least 10% of the lesion. Sertoli-Leydig tumors often contain a few clumps of cells that resemble granulosa cells, and granulosa cell tumors commonly contain a few cells resembling Leydig cells.

Sex Cord Tumor with Annular Tubules. The sex cord tumor with annular tubules consists of tubules in which one or more masses of basement membrane are surrounded by tall, columnar cells with clear cytoplasm and basal nuclei. Some think the tumor cells are Sertoli cells; some think they are granulosa cells. In some patients, the tumor has been partly a sex cord tumor with annular tubules, and partly a Sertoli-Leydig cell tumor. In some, the tumor is partially annular tubules and partially a granulosa cell tumor. By electron microscopy, some of the tumor cells contain the Charcot-Böttcher filaments found in Sertoli cells.

Most women with the Peutz-Jeghers syndrome have sex cord tumors with annular tubules. In 70% of the patients, the tumors are bilateral, multifocal, and of microscopic size. They are often calcified. All are benign. In other women, the tumor is usually unilateral, single, and large enough to be palpable. The tumor extends beyond the ovary in 20% of the patients. In 20% of the patients with a solitary tumor and in some of those with the Peutz-Jeghers syndrome, the tumor secretes enough estrogen to cause sexual precocity or other signs of hyperestrinism.

Unclassified Sex Cord-Stromal Tumors. About 10% of the sex cord-stromal tumors of the ovaries are poorly differentiated and cannot be further classified.

LIPID CELL TUMORS. Ovarian tumors that consist entirely of cells secreting steroid hormones, lutein cells, Leydig cells, or adrenocortical cells are called lipid cell tumors, lipoid cell tumors or steroid cell tumors.

Stromal Luteoma. Occasionally a nodule of luteinized or partially luteinized stromal cells large enough to be visible macroscopically is found in an ovary. Stromal cortical hyperplasia and hyperthecosis are usually evident elsewhere in the ovary. Most stromal luteomata secrete estrogen; some secrete androgen; some secrete both estrogen and androgen. The tumors are benign.

Leydig Cell Tumor. Ovarian tumors composed only of Leydig cells are rare. They are sometimes called hilus cell tumors. Leydig cell tumors can arise in women at any age, but most develop after the menopause.

Ovarian Leydig cell tumors usually arise in the hilus of an ovary. The tumor is rarely bilateral. It is usually less than 5 cm in diameter, and on section is yellow, orange, or brown.

Microscopically, the tumors consist of well-differentiated Leydig cells. The eosinophilic, rod-shaped crystalloids of Reinke must be demonstrated in some of the tumor cells to establish that they are Leydig cells, rather than one of the other types of cell that can closely resemble them.

In 75% of the patients, an ovarian Leydig

cell tumor causes hirsutism or virilization. Less often, it secretes an excess of estrogen. The tumor is benign. Excision cures.

Adrenocortical Tumor. Rarely, an ovarian tumor consists of adrenocortical cells. It secretes 17-ketosteroids like other adrenocortical tumors and responds to the adrenocorticotropic hormone and other stimuli that regulate adrenocortical activity. Some of the tumors are malignant.

Unclassified Lipid Cell Tumors. In most lipid cell tumors, the origin of the tumor cells cannot be established. Such lesions are called a lipid cell tumor or steroid cell tumor of uncertain origin. Less than 0.1% of ovarian tumors are of this type. The tumor can arise at any age. Most are virilizing. A few are estrogenic. A few produce no hormonal effects.

Lipid cell tumors can be large or small. They are solid but may show areas of cystic degeneration. On section, the tumor may be yellow, orange, reddish brown, or dark greenish brown. They are rarely bilateral.

Microscopically, the tumor resembles the adrenal cortex. Columns or clumps of the large tumor cells are separated by vascular sinusoids. The cytoplasm of the tumor cells sometimes contains lipid, lipochrome granules, or glycogen. Moderate atypicality and mitoses are evident in malignant tumors.

Over 20% of the lipid cell tumors have proved to be malignant. Distant metastases can occur, but more often the tumor remains confined to the abdominal cavity. Almost all the malignant tumors are over 7 cm across.

GERM CELL TUMORS. Over 20% of ovarian tumors arise from the germ cells. Nearly 98% of them are benign; nearly all the benign tumors form of teratoma called a dermoid cyst. In Caucasians, 30% of benign ovarian tumors arise from the germ cells, but only 2% of malignant ones. In oriental and black people, the proportion of malignant ovarian tumors arising from the germ cells rises to 10%, because the serous and endometrioid carcinomata common in white people are unusual in oriental and black people.

Germ cell tumors make up 70% of ovarian tumors found in people under 21 years old. Unfortunately, nearly 30% of the germ cell tumors in younger people are malignant.

Most germ cell tumors of the ovaries also arise in the testes and sometimes in the mediastinum or elsewhere in the midline of

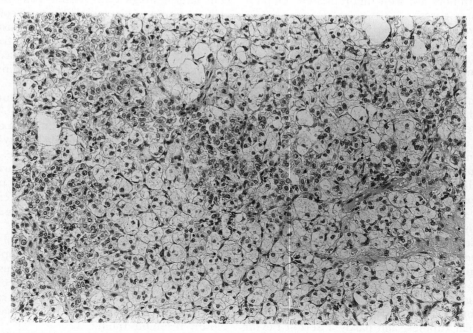

Fig. 41-30. A lipid cell tumor of an ovary, showing its similarity to a tumor of the adrenal cortex.

the body. The frequency of the different kinds of germ cell tumor differs from one site to another. The benign dermoid cysts so common in the ovaries are rare in the testes.

Ovarian germ cell tumors often show more than one pattern of differentiation. Lesions that show only one form of germ cell tumor are called pure. Those that show more than one kind of germ cell tumor are said to be mixed.

Dysgerminoma. The tumor called a seminoma when it arises in a testis is called a dysgerminoma when it originates in an ovary, and a germinoma when it arises in some other part of the body. The name *dysgerminoma* comes from the Greek for wrong and the Latin to bud or sprout. In the United States and Europe, 1% of ovarian tumors are of this type. In Japan and other parts of Asia, 10% of malignant ovarian tumors are dysgerminomata, probably because other kinds of malignant ovarian tumor are less common than in Caucasians.

About 80% of patients with a dysgerminoma are between 10 and 30 years of age, and 5% are between 5 and 10 years old. The tumor is rare in girls under 5 years old and in women over 50 years old. Because of its frequency in young women, 25% of ovarian tumors found during pregnancy are dysgerminomata.

Lesions. A dysgerminoma forms a solid mass in an ovary. The tumor may be small, but can be up to 50 cm across. Its surface is often bosselated, but is sometimes smooth. On section, the tumor is lobulated, cream-colored, tan, or pink. Cysts are not usually present. The tumor is bilateral in 15% of the patients.

Microscopically, a dysgerminoma resembles a seminoma. It has the same clumps of cells with clear cytoplasm and rounded nuclei and the same stroma usually infiltrated with lymphocytes. Granulomata are evident in the stroma in 20% of the tumors and sometimes are prominent. Occasionally, a dysgerminoma is less well differentiated, resembling an anaplastic seminoma. Scattered syncytiotrophoblastic cells are present in 10% of the tumors.

Behavior. Over 70% of dysgerminomata are confined to the ovaries at the time of operation. Extension is first to the regional lymph nodes in the pelvis and sometimes to the abdominal nodes. Hematogenous metastases are usually late.

Dysfunction. About 10% of patients with a pure dysgerminoma have a moderate in-

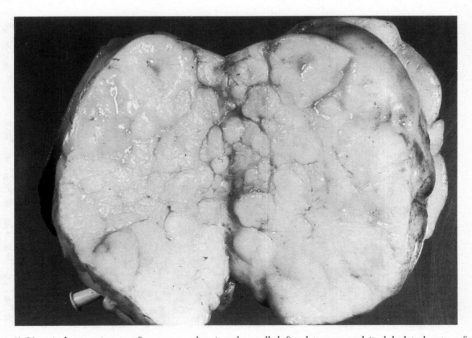

Fig. 41-31.   A dysgerminoma of an ovary, showing the well-defined tumor, and its lobulated cut surface.

crease in human chorionic gonadotropin in the plasma. Most have an increase in the isoenzyme 1 of lactic dehydrogenase and an increase in placental alkaline phosphatase.

Treatment and Prognosis. A dysgerminoma is treated by oophorectomy. Some clinicians irradiate the pelvis while shielding the other ovary. Some prefer to reserve irradiation until the tumor recurs. If the tumor is confined to one ovary, over 90% of the patients survive 10 years and are probably cured. If it extends beyond the pelvis, radiation and chemotherapy can often control the metastases.

Endodermal Sinus Tumor. The endodermal sinus tumor, or yolk sac tumor as it is sometimes called, takes its name from its similarity to the endodermal sinus of the yolk sac in rodents. In the past, it was sometimes called a mesonephroma. Pure endodermal sinus tumors are uncommon. Most patients are between 10 and 30 years old.

Lesions. Endodermal sinus tumors are solid, but often show foci of cystic degeneration. The tumor is soft and friable, gray or yellowish, often with foci of necrosis or hemorrhage. It varies from 3 to 30 cm across.

The tumor is usually unilateral, but may metastasize to the other ovary.

Microscopically, an endodermal sinus tumor may show any or all of a variety of patterns. Often the tumor forms a mesh of small cysts lined by flattened epithelium. The cysts may be closely packed together or may be separated by larger or smaller sheets of pale, cuboidal cells with indistinct cytoplasm. Sometimes mitoses are numerous. In other regions, the tumor may form anastomosing columns of cuboidal cells or branching glands lined by cuboidal cells, sometimes separated by a myxomatous tissue containing fine, stellate cells. Sometimes part or much of an endodermal sinus tumor consists of small cysts or vesicles separated by a poorly differentiated connective tissue. The cysts are lined by columnar or cuboidal cells, often with vacuoles in their cytoplasm, and by flattened epithelium. At times part of a tumor consists of solid sheets of epithelial cells, sometimes with clear cytoplasm or darker, eosinophilic cytoplasm. Sometimes the cells resemble hepatocytes.

In 70% of the tumors, some structures resemble the endodermal sinuses of the

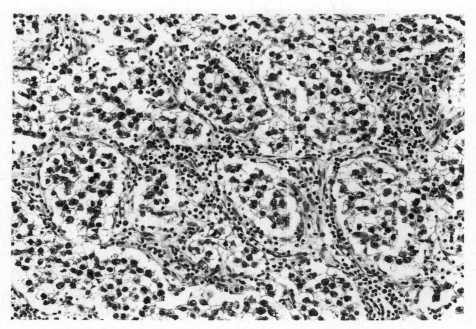

Fig. 41-32.   A dysgerminoma of an ovary, showing its similarity to a seminoma.

rodents. In these structures, a fold projects into a small space lined by flattened epithelium. As seen in cross section, the folds have a central blood vessel supported by a little connective tissue and are covered by cuboidal epithelium.

Often small, eosinophilic globules are present in the tumor cells and between them. The globules stain brightly with the periodic acid-Schiff reaction and resist digestion with diastase. They contain α-fetoprotein and $α_1$-antitrypsin. Some of the tumor cells stain for α-fetoprotein.

Behavior. Endodermal sinus tumors of the ovaries invade extensively and rapidly. Implants on the abdominal peritoneum are common. Metastases in the pelvic and abdominal lymph nodes appear early and may extend to involve the lymph nodes in the mediastinum and neck. Hematogenous metastases come later, with spread to the lungs and liver and often to other organs.

Dysfunction. Endodermal sinus tumors release α-fetoprotein into the blood. Often the concentration of α-fetoprotein in the serum is high, over 10,000 mg/L (10,000 ng/ 100 mL). If the tumor is completely removed, the concentration of α-fetoprotein in the serum falls to its normal level of under 20 mg/L (20 ng/100 mL) within six weeks. If the tumor recurs, the concentration of α-fetoprotein will rise again.

Treatment and Prognosis. Endodermal sinus tumors are treated by local excision of the tumor followed by chemotherapy. The tumor is radioresistant, and radiotherapy is of little help.

When treated by surgical excision alone, few patients with an endodermal sinus tumor live more than a year. Chemotherapy and the use of α-fetoprotein to detect recurrence of the tumor have greatly improved the outlook. Over 40% of the patients are alive two years after diagnosis, and some have lived for 10 or more years.

Embryonal Carcinoma. An ovarian embryonal carcinoma is similar to the embryonal carcinomata of the testis. Usually it is mixed with some other kind of germ cell tumor. The patients are nearly all under 30 years old.

Ovarian tumors that are predominantly embryonal carcinoma form a solid mass. Necrosis and hemorrhage are common. Microscopically, the tumor forms sheets of epithelial cells, as in the testis. Some of the tumor cells stain for α-fetoprotein, isoenzyme

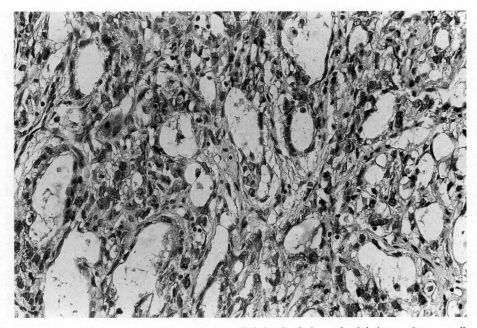

Fig. 41-33. An endodermal sinus tumor, showing ill-defined tubules and solid sheets of tumor cells.

1 of lactic dehydrogenase, or the carcinoembryonic antigen. Syncytiotrophoblastic cells that stain for human chorionic gonadotropin are often scattered in the tumor.

Ovarian embryonal carcinomata grow rapidly and spread extensively in the pelvis. Metastases to the regional lymph nodes or more distantly are common. Radical excision and chemotherapy allow a 40% five-year survival.

Polyembryoma. A tumor consisting predominantly of embryoid bodies is rare, though embryoid bodies are sometimes found in lesions that consist predominantly of some other type or types of germ cell tumor. An embryoid body resembles an 18-day embryo. It consists of a cellular plate that separates one or more yolk sacs from one or more amniotic cavities. The yolk sacs are lined by columnar epithelium and the amniotic cavities by cuboidal or flattened epithelium.

Choriocarcinoma. A pure choriocarcinoma of an ovary is rare. The patients are usually under 20 years old. When choriocarcinoma is present in an ovarian tumor, it is nearly always mixed with some other kind or kinds of germ cell tumor.

The tumor is usually unilateral, solid, and hemorrhagic. Microscopically, it resembles a choriocarcinoma of the placenta. A mixture of cytotrophoblastic and syncytiotrophoblastic cells line or grow between dilated sinusoids filled with blood. The tumor cells synthesize human chorionic gonadotropin. The level of gonadotropin in the plasma is high.

The prognosis is bad. The tumor grows rapidly and metastasizes widely. It does not respond to methatrexate, as do placental choriocarcinomata, but other forms of chemotherapy are of help.

Teratoma. The teratomata of the ovaries are divided into immature, mature, and specialized forms. The immature teratomata are malignant. Less than 1% of malignant ovarian tumors are of this type. The mature teratomata are benign and are divided into solid and cystic forms. Solid mature teratomata are uncommon, but the cystic tumors, called dermoid cysts, are one of the most common tumors of the ovaries. Over 99% of ovarian teratomata, 20% of ovarian tumors, and 30% of benign ovarian tumors are of this type. Most dermoid cysts remain benign, but occasionally one of the tissues in a benign cystic teratoma becomes malignant. The

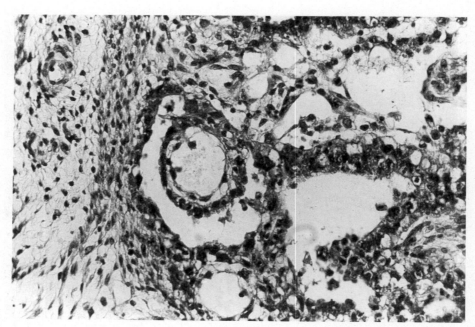

Fig. 41-34.   An endodermal sinus tumor, showing structures resembling the endodermal sinus of a rodent.

specialized teratomata of the ovaries form only one kind of tissue, most often thyroid. The carcinoid tumors of the ovaries are considered to be a form of specialized teratoma.

Over 80% of dermoid cysts of the ovaries arise during the reproductive years, though they can occur at any age. Malignant teratomata of the ovaries are most common in patients under 20 years old, comprising 15% of malignant ovarian tumors of girls under 20 years old. Patients with a solid, benign teratoma are usually young, but those with a teratoma consisting principally of a single element are usually 40 or more years old.

Lesions. The mature, cystic teratomata of the ovaries will be described before the less common kinds of ovarian teratoma.

Dermoid Cyst. The dermoid cysts of the ovaries take their name from the Greek for skin, because the cyst formed by the tumor is usually lined by skin. Most dermoid cysts of an ovary are 10 to 15 cm in diameter when discovered, though the tumor can be from 0.5 cm to 40 cm across. The tumor forms a smooth, rounded cyst covered by glistening mesothelium. At body temperature, it is fluctuant, but the content of the cyst often solidifies when the cyst is removed from the body. The tumor is bilateral in 10% of the patients. Occasionally there is more than one dermoid cyst in an ovary.

On section, the tumor is usually unilocular, but occasionally is polycystic. The cyst has a thin, tough wall. It is usually filled with a tangled mass of hair, matted in a thick, sebacious secretion. Less often, the cyst contains mucoid material or thin watery fluid like the cerebrospinal fluid. One or more solid masses of tissue bulge into the cyst, forming a little hump or humps, sometimes called a dermoid nipple or nipples. In 30% of the tumors, one or more teeth project into the cyst, usually from a dermoid nipple. Occasionally, a well-formed finger or some other organoid form projects into the cyst.

Microscopically, the cyst is nearly always lined by well-differentiated skin, with keratinizing epithelium, sebaceous glands, and

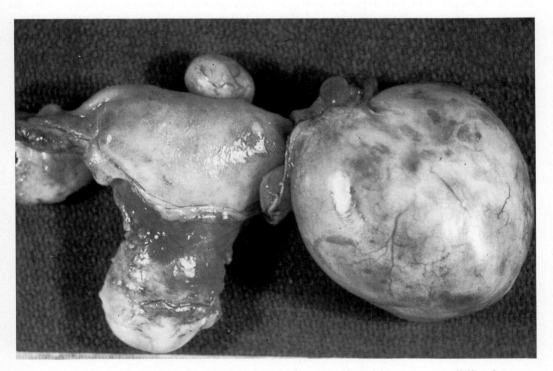

Fig. 41-35.   A dermoid cyst of an ovary, showing the smooth outer surface of the tumor. A small fibroid projects from the fundus of the uterus.

hair follicles. Occasionally, the lining is in part or mostly of well-differentiated bronchial epithelium or gastrointestinal epithelium.

In the dermoid nipple or nipples, there is a muddle of well-differentiated tissues jumbled together. In 60% of the tumors, the adipose tissue and bundles of smooth muscle look normal. In 30%, tubes or cysts are lined in whole or in part by respiratory epithelium, sometimes with supporting cartilages to mimic a bronchus. More than 30% of the tumors contain nodules of well-differentiated brain, choroid plexus, bone, or cartilage. Often there are well-formed apocrine glands. Less often there are clumps of thyroid acini, pieces of salivary gland, or tubes and cysts lined in whole or part by intestinal epithelium. Occasionally, pancreas, thymus, adrenal tissue, renal tissue, pulmonary alveoli, or mammary tissue can be identified. If a dermoid cyst ruptures, the keratin, sebaceous secretion, and hair in the cyst escape into the surrounding tissue and excite a foreign body reaction.

Malignant Change in a Dermoid Cyst.   In 2% of patients with a dermoid cyst, a malignant tumor develops from one of the elements in the cyst. In over 70% of these patients, the malignant tumor is a squamous cell carcinoma. Less often, it is a poorly differentiated carcinoma, an adenocarcinoma, a sarcoma, or a melanoma. Most of the patients are over 40 years old, though a malignant tumor can develop in a dermoid cyst in younger people.

Macroscopically, the malignancy sometimes forms a warty mass projecting into the cyst or causes diffuse thickening of the wall of the cyst, occasionally with necrosis and hemorrhage. Microscopically, the malignant element is like the tumors that arise from normal adult tissues.

Immature Teratoma.   An immature teratoma is usually solid, but commonly contains many small cysts. Occasionally, one is predominantly cystic, with one or more large cysts. The tumor is bilateral in less than 5% of the patients. In another 5%, the contralateral ovary contains a benign, dermoid cyst.

Microscopically, parts of an immature teratoma may be well differentiated, like the tissues in a dermoid cyst, but in part or most of the tumor the tissues are poorly differentiated and resemble embryonic tissue. Often

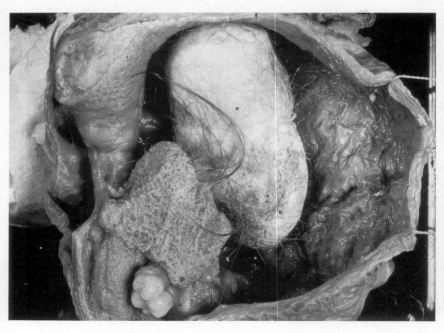

Fig. 41-36.   A dermoid cyst of an ovary, showing the hair and inspissated sebaceous material in the cyst. A well-formed tooth projects into the cyst (lower parpt of picture).

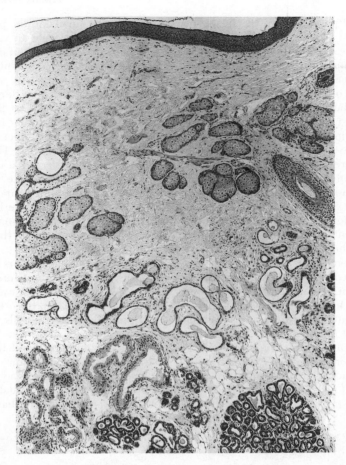

Fig. 41-37. A dermoid cyst of an ovary, showing the epidermis lining the cyst and the jumble of well-formed structures in the underlying tissue.

neural tissue is predominant in an immature ovarian teratoma, but usually there are also foci of immature cartilage or muscle and tubules lined by undifferentiated cells.

Mature Solid Teratoma. The rare mature solid teratomata of the ovaries form a solid mass, but microscopically show only fully differentiated tissues, like those in the solid regions of a dermoid cyst. If any immature tissue is present, the tumor is classed as an immature teratoma.

Struma Ovarii. Less than 3% of ovarian teratomata consist largely or entirely of thyroid tissue. Such a tumor is called a struma ovarii. *Struma* is from the Latin word meaning a mass in the neck caused by scrofula, and, by extension, a goiter.

Microscopically, the tumor usually consists of well-formed thyroid acini. Occasionally, an adenoma develops in the lesion. Thyrotoxicosis has been caused by a struma ovarii.

Most strumata ovarii are benign. Rarely, a struma ovarii is malignant, giving rise to peritoneal implants of thyroid tissue, to metastases in the pelvic and abdominal lymph nodes, or occasionally to more distant metastases.

Carcinoid Tumor. A carcinoid tumor is primary in an ovary and usually resembles the carcinoid tumors of the ileum microscopically, forming clumps of tumor cells with occasional acini. Neurosecretory granules are prominent in the cells. Less often a primary ovarian carcinoid tumor forms ribbons of tumor cells or secretes considerable quantities of mucus. The carcinoid syndrome develops in 30% of patients with the ileal type of tumor.

Rarely, an ovarian tumor consists of a mixture of carcinoid tumor and struma ovarii. Occasionally a carcinoid tumor is a minor element in some other kind of ovarian tumor.

Behavior. Mature ovarian teratomata remain confined to the ovary. If a malignant tumor develops in a dermoid cyst, it invades locally, but metastases to the lymph nodes or more distantly are uncommon.

Immature teratomata of the ovaries grow rapidly, invade adjacent structures, and give rise to implants on the peritoneum. At the time of operation, extension beyond the ovary is apparent in 30% of the patients. Metastases to the lymph nodes and more distant organs come later. The implants and metastases may consist of a mixture of tissues like that in the primary tumor or of only one element of the teratoma. Occasionally, the peritoneal implants of an immature teratoma consist mainly of glial tissue.

Most ovarian carcinoids remain confined to the ovaries. Even in patients who develop the carcinoid syndrome, metastases are rare.

Treatment and Prognosis. Dermoid cysts are usually removed by oophorectomy, though if the tumor is small and the patient is young, it is sometims possible to conserve part of the ovary. If the cyst contains a malignant tumor, hysterectomy and bilateral salpingo-oophorectomy are usually advised. When malignancy develops in a dermoid cyst, only 20% of the patients survive five years.

An immature teratoma is excised, and chemotherapy is given. Recurrence within a few months is common. The greater the proportion of the tumor that is immature and the higher the mitotic rate, the worse the prognosis. If foci of immature tissue are few, 80% of the patients are alive 10 years later. If much of the tumor is immature and the mitotic rate is high, less than 20% of the patients survive five years.

Primary carcinoid tumors in the ovaries are excised. Most patients are cured.

TUMORS CONTAINING GERM CELL AND SEX CORD-STROMAL ELEMENTS. Ovarian tumors containing both germ cells and sex cord-stromal elements are rare. There are two kinds, gonadoblastoma and the mixed germ cell-sex cord-stromal tumor.

Gonadoblastoma. A gonadoblastoma nearly always arises from a malformed gonad. Some 80% of the patients have a female ha-

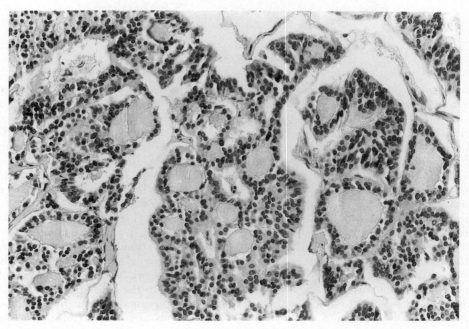

Fig. 41-38. Struma ovarii, showing the well-differentiated thyroid follicles that make up the tumor.

bitus, but over 90% have a male chromosomal pattern or are mosaics with a Y chromosome in some of their cells. The tumor is discussed with the tumors of the male genital system in Chapter 40.

Mixed Germ Cell-Sex Cord-Stromal Tumor. The mixed germ cell-sex cord-stromal tumor is rare. It can arise in a normal ovary or a normal testis. The tumor shows a mixture of cells like those of a dysgerminoma or seminoma with cords, tubules, or sheets or cells like those of a sex cord tumor. It is discussed in Chapter 40.

OTHER PRIMARY TUMORS. Other primary tumors of the ovaries are rare. Occasionally the ovary is the site of a leiomyoma, an angioma, or some other type of benign mesenchymal or a leiomyosarcoma, an angiosarcoma, or some other malignant mesenchymal tumor. In a few patients, a lymphoma, usually a poorly differentiated B cell lymphoma, has arisen in an ovary. In a few, a mesothelioma has involved an ovary.

SECONDARY TUMORS. Metastatic carcinoma is common in the ovaries. In over 5% of patients with an ovarian mass who undergo laparotomy, the tumor proves to be metastatic. In Brazil, nearly 30% of women dying with a malignant tumor had metastases in the ovaries, but in the United States only 5% of women with a malignant tumor were found to have ovarian metastases at autopsy. The primary tumor is most often in the endometrium, the gastrointestinal tract, or the breast. In over 70% of the patients, both ovaries are involved. In patients with carcinoma in the endometrium and the ovaries, it is sometimes hard to decide if the tumor is an endometrial carcinoma with metastases in the ovaries or an endometrioid carcinoma of an ovary with metastases in the endometrium.

Ovarian metastases are found at autopsy in 25% of patients with disseminated non-Hodgkin's lymphoma, but rarely in people with Hodgkin's disease. Burkitt's lymphoma frequently involves the ovaries. In 40% of the

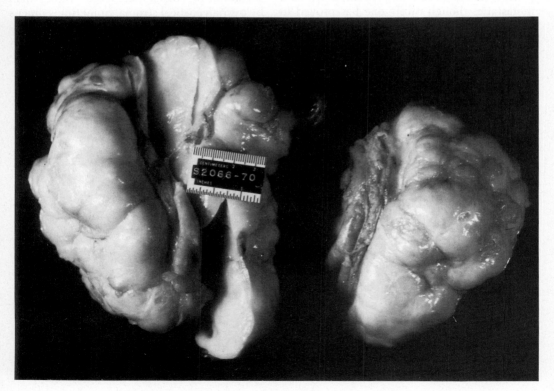

Fig. 41-39. Bilateral Krukenberg tumors of the ovaries, showing the white, bosselated surface usual in these tumors.

patients, an ovarian mass is the principal sign of the disease. The ovaries are involved in 40% of patients with leukemia, though the infiltrate in the ovaries is often slight.

A malignant tumor can reach the ovaries in several ways. A tumor of a contiguous organ can invade an ovary directly. Fragments of a tumor of the endometrium can pass through the fallopian tubes to reach the ovaries. Tumor cells released into the peritoneal cavity can be carried in the peritoneal fluid to implant on an ovary. Tumor emboli can reach an ovary in the lymph or in the blood.

Ovarian metastases may be large and obvious or small, found only by microscopy. Their structure is usually similar to that of the primary tumor.

Krukenberg Tumor. Krukenberg tumors of the ovaries are named after the German pathologist who described them in 1896. Microscopically, they show signet-ring cells filled with mucus singly or in small clumps in hyperplastic ovarian cortical stroma.

Most Krukenberg tumors of the ovaries are metastatic, though rarely one has proved to be primary in the ovary, probably a variant of a mucinous carcinoma. In over 70% of the patients, the primary tumor is in the stomach. About 15% of Krukenberg tumors are metastatic from the colon, and 5% from a breast. Nearly 30% of clinically apparent ovarian metastases are of this type.

Krukenberg tumors usually form firm, grayish-white masses from 5 to 10 cm across. The mass may be spheroidal or kidney-shaped. Often its surface is lobulated. Less often a Krukenberg tumor is cystic or gelatinous. On section, the tumor sometimes shows areas of necrosis or hemorrhage.

Microscopically, all Krukenberg tumors show regions in which the tumor consists of small clumps or columns of mucus-filled, signet-ring cells separated by hyperplastic cortical stromal cells. Other parts of the tumor may show acini lined by tumor cells, which may or may not secrete mucus, or cysts lined by mucus-secreting cells. Sometimes parts of the tumor consist of solid sheets of tumor cells producing little or no mucus. In places, the tumor cells may be separated by collagenous tissue, rather than by ovarian cortical stroma. Sometimes mucus escapes into the stroma as in a colloid carcinoma, or the stroma is loose and edematous.

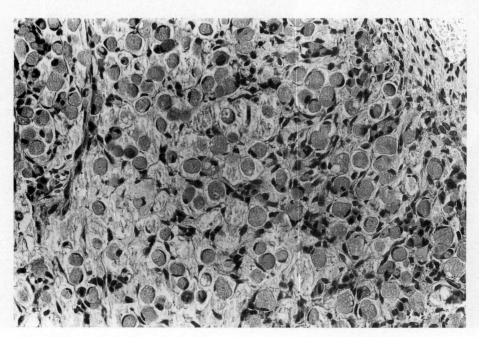

Fig. 41-40. A Krukenberg tumor of an ovary, showing large tumor cells filled with mucus.

Fallopian Tubes

Tumors of the fallopian tubes large enough to be important clinically are uncommon. An adenomatoid tumor is present in the serosa of a tube or in the broad ligament in 1 woman in 2500, but is rarely as much as 1 cm in diameter. The tumor is similar to those that develop in relation to the testes. Occasionally a leiomyoma or some other mesenchymal tumor develops in a tube. A hydatidiform mole complicates 1 tubal pregnancy in 5000. Rarely, a wolffian remnant near a tube gives rise to an adenoma. Metastatic carcinoma sometimes involves the serosa of the tubes in patients with a tumor that is seeding the peritoneum. Only primary carcinoma of the fallopian tubes is discussed in this section.

Carcinoma. Less than 0.5% of malignant tumors of the female reproductive tract arise in a fallopian tube. The patient is usually over 50 years old.

Lesions. The affected tube or tubes are usually enlarged by the time the carcinoma is discovered and look like a hydrosalpinx or a tuboovarian abscess. On section, the dilated tube or tubes are filled with fungating, friable, partially necrotic tumor. The fimbriated end of the tube is occluded in 50% of the patients. Occasionally a hydrosalpinx or hematosalpinx caused by the tumor adds to the distention of the tube.

The carcinoma is bilateral in less than 10% of women with an early carcinoma that has not breached the serosa, but involves both tubes in 30% of women with a more advanced tumor. It is not known whether the tumor metastasizes from one tube to the other or whether both carcinomata are primary.

Microscopically, most carcinomata of a fallopian tube are papillary, with complex fronds bulging into the lumen of the tube. The fronds have a core of collagenous tissue and are covered by one or more layers of cuboidal or columnar cells, with atypical nuclei and mitoses. Sometimes the fronds fuse, so that the carcinoma bulging into the lumen of the tube looks like an adenocarcinoma. Occasionally, a tubal carcinoma is more anaplastic, forming solid sheets of poorly differentiated tumor cells. The wall of the tube is stretched and thinned by the carcinoma, but invasion of the wall usually comes late.

TABLE 41-3.   CLASSIFICATION OF TUMORS OF THE UTERUS

Myometrium
  Leiomyoma
  Diffuse leiomyomatosis
  Intravenous leiomyomatosis
  Benign metastasizing leiomyoma
  Disseminated intraperitoneal leiomyomatosis
  Leiomyosarcoma
  Adenomatoid tumor

Endometrium
  Endometrial polyp
  Atypical polypoid adenomyoma
  Carcinoma
    Endometrioid
    Carcinoma with squamous metaplasia
    Adenosquamous carcinoma
    Mucinous carcinoma
    Serous carcinoma
    Clear cell tumor
    Squamous cell carcinoma
    Undifferentiated carcinoma
  Endometrial stromal nodule
  Endometrial stromal sarcoma
  Adenofibroma
  Adenosarcoma
  Mixed müllerian tumor

Cervix uteri
  Endocervical polyp
  Endocervical microglandular hyperplasia
  Condyloma
  Cervical intraepithelial neoplasia
    Dysplasia
    Carcinoma in situ
  Microinvasive carcinoma
  Invasive squamous cell carcinoma
  Adenocarcinoma
  Mucoepidermoid carcinoma
  Adenoid cystic carcinoma
  Carcinoid tumor
  Anaplastic neuroendocrine carcinoma

Secondary Tumors

If the carcinoma has spread beyond the tube through its fimbriated end and involves the ovary, a carcinoma of a tube may be impossible to distinguish from a serous cystadenocarcinoma of the ovary. In such cases, the carcinoma is usually assumed to arise in the ovary.

Behavior. Carcinoma of the fallopian tubes spreads to the regional lymph nodes in the pelvis, less often to the inguinal lymph nodes. Hematogenous metastases to the liver, the lungs, and elsewhere may occur before there is significant invasion of the tubal wall. If the fimbriated end of the tube remains open, the carcinoma may implant on the peritoneal serosa.

Clinical Presentation. The tumor usually causes irregular endometrial bleeding, a vaginal discharge, an abdominal mass, or abdominal pain.

Treatment and Prognosis. Carcinoma of a fallopian tube is treated by bilateral salpingo-oophorectomy and hysterectomy, radiation, and chemotherapy. The prognosis is poor. In 70% of the patients, the carcinoma has spread beyond the tube by the time the diagnosis is made. Less than 20% are alive and free of tumor five years after the diagnosis is made, with another 20% living with tumor.

Uterus

Table 41-3 shows a classification of the tumors of the uterus. The polyps are not neoplastic, but are included because they resemble neoplasms.

MYOMETRIUM. Leiomyoma of the myometrium is one of the commonest of tumors. Occasionally a leiomyosarcoma develops in the myometrium. Less often, diffuse leiomyomatosis, intravenous leiomyomatosis, a benign metastasizing leiomyoma, or diffuse peritoneal leiomyomatosis occurs. A small adenomatoid tumor is found in 1% of uteri, but the lesion is rarely large enough to be evident clinically. Exceptionally, an angioma, angiosarcoma, or pericytoma arises in the myometrium.

Leiomyoma. A leiomyoma of the uterus is usually called a fibroid. The name, though widely used, is inaccurate, for the tumor is comprised mainly of smooth muscle. About

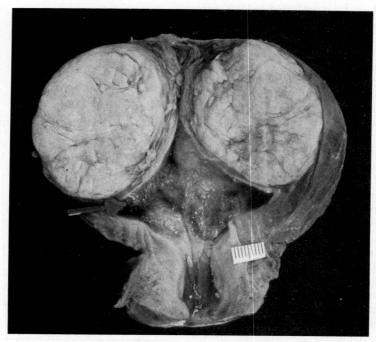

Fig. 41-41. A leiomyoma of the myometrium. The tumor was bisected when the uterus was opened.

20% of white women 35 years old and 40% of white women over 50 years old have fibroids in their uterus. In black people fibroids are even more common. They are rare in girls under 20 years old.

Lesions. Fibroids form hard, spheroidal tumors in the myometrium. In 70% of the patients, fibroids are multiple. There are commonly 10 or 20 in a uterus, and occasionally there are hundreds. Most are 2 to 10 cm in diameter, but they may be microscopic or huge masses weighing 200 or 300 g. Fibroids can arise anywhere in the myometrium, but are most common in the posterior wall of the body of the uterus.

Most fibroids develop within the myometrium and are called intramural. Some bulge from the serosal surface of the uterus and are called subserosal. About 5% bulge into the cavity of the uterus and are called submucosal. Sometimes a subserosal fibroid becomes pedunculated and hangs into the peritoneal cavity or burrows into the broad ligament. Occasionally such a fibroid loses its attachment to the uterus and becomes attached to some other structure, to give what is called a parasitic fibroid. Less often a submucosal fibroid becomes pedunculated and hangs into the endometrial cavity. Rarely, a submucosal fibroid protrudes through the cervix.

On section, a fibroid shows macroscopically a firm, white surface, with a swirling pattern, like watered silk. Microscopically, it consists of intertwining bundles of well-differentiated smooth muscle cells, with collagenous tissue between the bundles. Blood vessels are usually few. The tumor compresses the surrounding myometrium, but is not encapsulated. Mitoses are not present.

In 60% of uterine leiomyomata, the collagen in part of the tumor is hyalinized. In 50%, foci of edema are present within the tumor. In 10%, there is hemorrhage into the tumor. In 5%, small cysts containing gelatinous material are present. In 5%, the tumor is partially calcified. Hemorrhage and edema are particularly common in women who are pregnant or are taking progestins. Especially in pregnancy, part of a fibroid can become necrotic. Occasionally a pedunculated fibroid undergoes torsion and is infarcted.

Several special types of fibroid are distinguished. None is common. Some can be mistaken for a leiomyosarcoma.

Cellular Leiomyoma. In some leiomyomata or parts of a leiomyoma, the tumor consists of highly cellular bundles of leiomyocytes with little or no collagenous tissue between the bundles. The tumor cells are well differentiated and show no atypicality. Mitoses may be present, but there are not more than 5 in 10 high-power fields. If there are 5 to 10 mitoses in 10 high-power fields, the nature of the tumor is in doubt. If there are more than 10, it is malignant.

Occasionally the cells in a cellular leiomyoma are small and resemble those of an endometrial stromal tumor. A reticulin stain distinguishes between the two types of tumor. Reticulin fibers outline bundles of cells in a leiomyoma. They surround each tumor cell in an endometrial stromal tumor.

Atypical Leiomyoma. In an atypical leiomyoma, the nuclei in part or all of the tumor are large, irregular, and hyperchromatic. Cytoplasmic inclusions in the nuclei are common. If there are less than 5 mitoses in 10 high-power fields, the tumor is benign. If there are more than 10, it is considered malignant. If there are between 5 and 10, its nature is uncertain.

Epithelioid Leiomyoma. An epithelioid leiomyoma is sometimes called a leiomyoblastoma, plexiform leiomyoma, or clear cell leiomyoma. The tumor cells form clumps or cords. They are usually large and polygonal. In some of the tumors, they have dark, eosinophilic cytoplasm. In some, the tumor cells are well demarcated with clear cytoplasm. In some tumors, both types of tumor cell are present. The nuclei are spheroidal and usually in the center of the tumor cells. Mitoses are often present, but if there are more than 5 in 10 high-power fields, the tumor should be considered malignant.

Myxoid Leiomyoma. Occasionally the collagenous tissue between the bundles of smooth muscle in a leiomyoma is myxoid. The margins of the tumor remain well demarcated, and the tumor cells show no atypicality and no mitoses.

Vascular Leiomyoma. Rarely, large, thick-walled blood vessels are numerous in a fibroid.

Lipoleiomyoma. Occasionally a leiomyoma of the myometrium contains adipose tissue between the bundles of muscle.

Clinical Presentation. Many leiomyomata of the uterus cause no symptoms and no dysfunction. Some cause pain or a feeling of fullness. Abnormal endometrial bleeding is common, probably because of the distortion and congestion of the endometrium caused by the tumors. Occasionally a large fibroid presses on the bladder, causing urinary frequency, or compresses the pelvic veins, causing edema of the legs. Rarely, leakage of fluid from a fibroid causes ascites or Meigs' syndrome. Rarely, a fibroid secretes erythropoietin and causes erythrocytosis or secretes an insulin-like substance and causes hypoglycemia.

If fibroids are large and numerous, they sometimes cause infertility. Large fibroids can obstruct delivery. The ratio of estrogen receptors to progestin receptors is higher in fibroids than in the surrounding myometrium. Fibroids often enlarge during pregnancy and in women treated with estrogens or progestins they sometimes shrink if the activity of the luteinizing hormone is reduced.

Treatment and Prognosis. If symptoms warrant it, leiomyomata of the uterus are removed by hysterectomy or local excision. With the exception of the rare metastasizing leiomyoma, fibroids of the uterus are benign, and excision cures.

Diffuse Leiomyomatosis. Rarely, the myometrium is greatly thickened by ill-defined nodules of smooth muscle. All parts of the myometrium are involved, and the enlargement is symmetrical. The uterus may weigh over 1000 g. Microscopically the nodules consist of smooth muscle with little collagen. They are not well defined, but merge with one another and with the intervening myometrium.

Intravenous Leiomyomatosis. Occasionally proliferations of smooth muscle bulge into the veins in the myometrium. Arteries are not involved. Sometimes the tumor arises from the media of the veins, and there are no fibroids in the uterus. Sometimes the lesions seem due to venous permeation by an otherwise benign leiomyoma.

Macroscopically, the lesions form nodules or coiled, worm-like masses that extend along the veins. The veins in the broad ligaments are often involved. In 10% of the patients, the tumor reaches the vena cava. Microscopically, the tumor lies free within the veins. It may show any of the patterns seen in fibroids, but usually is sclerotic with much collagen and few muscle cells.

Intravenous leiomyomatosis is treated by hysterectomy, bilateral salpingo-oophorectomy, and excision of any tumor that extends beyond the uterus. Even if complete eradication of the tumor is impossible, it often remains confined to the pelvis for many years. Metastases in the lungs develop in a minority of the patients. In some, excision of the pulmonary metastases has given long-term survival.

Benign Metastasizing Leiomyoma. Metastases rarely develop in the lungs in a patient with apparently benign uterine fibroids. The metastases, which are similar to the leiomyomata in the uterus, show no sign of malignancy. Such patients are said to have a benign metastasizing leiomyoma.

In most of the patients, the metastases appear after the patient has undergone uterine surgery. It is possible that the operation allowed fragments of a benign leiomyoma to enter the venous blood and reach the lungs to establish the metastases. In other patients, the metastases are probably from an undetected leiomyosarcoma of the uterus.

The metastases in the lungs grow slowly. Resection of the metastases sometimes eradicates the disease.

Disseminated Peritoneal Leiomyomatosis. Disseminated peritoneal leiomyomatosis is an uncommon condition that occasionally develops during pregnancy, in women taking oral contraceptives, or in patients with a tumor that secretes estrogens. Multiple nodules less than 1 cm across appear in the serosa of the peritoneal cavity. They consist of well-differentiated leiomyocytes, fibrocytes or myofibrocytes, collagen, and often decidua. Presumably the nodules result from metaplasia of the serosa induced by the estrogens. Estrogens can induce similar peritoneal nodules in animals. The nodules regress when the level of estrogens in the plasma falls after delivery, withdrawal of the contraceptive, or control of the tumor.

Leiomyosarcoma. About 1% of malignant

tumors of the uterus and 25% of sarcomata of the uterus are leiomyosarcomata. About 0.1% of smooth muscle tumors of the myometrium are malignant. Less than 1 woman in every 100,000 over 20 years old develops a leiomyosarcoma of the uterus. Most patients are over 50 years old.

Lesions. Leiomyosarcomata of the uterus are usually 5 to 15 cm across. Most are soft, yellowish or pink, and ill demarcated. Foci of necrosis and hemorrhage are common. In 60% of the patients, sarcoma is the only lesion in the myometrium. Less often, the sarcoma resembles a fibroid or develops in a uterus that also contains fibroids.

Microscopically, leiomyosarcomata of the myometrium consist of bundles of spindle-shaped cells. In some tumors, the cells are well differentiated and the tumor resembles a cellular leiomyoma. In some, the tumor cells are more anaplastic, with atypical nuclei and ill-defined cytoplasm. Multinucleated tumor cells are present in 50% of the tumors. A few show the atypical or epithelioid pattern sometimes seen in a leiomyoma.

In most leiomyosarcomata, little collagen is present between the tumor cells. In some, the tissue between the tumor cells is loose and myxoid. In some of the more anaplastic tumors, the myxoid stroma is abundant. Vascular invasion is evident in 20% of the tumors. Infiltration of the myometrium at the margin of the tumor is sometimes, but not always, apparent.

If a leiomyosarcoma is well differentiated or shows an atypical or epithelioid pattern of growth, it can be distinguished from a leiomyoma only by the mitotic rate. Tumors with more than 10 mitoses in 10 high-power fields are considered to be malignant. Those with 5 to 10 mitoses in 10 high-power fields are of borderline malignancy. All tumors in which the tumor cells are atypical and all tumors with abundant myxoid stroma are considered to be malignant, regardless of the mitotic rate.

Behavior. Most leiomyosarcomata of the uterus grow rapidly and invade adjacent structures. A few remain quiescent like a fibroid. Metastases are most often to the lungs.

Treatment and Prognosis. Leiomyosarcomata of the uterus are treated by hyster-ectomy and bilateral oopherosalpingectomy. The tumors are likely to recur and to metastasize. Only 30% of the patients survive free of tumor. Radiation and chemotherapy are of limited value.

ENDOMETRIUM. Non-neoplastic polyps that resemble neoplasms are common in the endometrium. Occasionally an atypical polypoid adenomyoma protrudes into the endometrial cavity. Endometrial carcinoma is one of the most frequent neoplasms in women. Three kinds of tumor with both neoplastic epithelial and neoplastic mesenchymal elements arise in the endometrium: adenofibroma, adenosarcoma, and the mixed müllerian tumor. Less frequently, an endometrial stromal nodule or an endometrial stromal sarcoma arises in the endometrium.

The histogenesis of these different kinds of endometrial tumor has been much debated, but all are now believed to arise from the cells that form the endometrium.

Endometrial Polyp. Endometrial polyps are most common in women 40 to 50 years

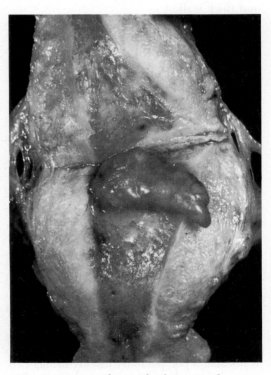

Fig. 41-42. An endometrial polyp arising from near the fundus of the opened uterus.

old. They are rare before the menarche but are not uncommon after the menopause.

Lesions.   A polyp can arise from any part of the endometrium but is most frequent in the fundus and cornua. The polyp may form a flat plaque, but more often it is pedunculated. It may be only a few millimeters across or may fill and distend the uterine cavity. In 20% of the patients, there is more than one.

Microscopically, endometrial polyps consist of endometrial glands and stroma. In the reproductive years, the glands and stroma in most polyps are like those of proliferative or hyperplastic endometrium. Only exceptionally do the glands and stroma in a polyp show the cyclic changes that continue normally in the rest of the endometrium. After the menopause, the glands are often dilated and lined by cuboidal or columnar epithelium, and the stroma is loose and edematous. Foci of squamous metaplasia are sometimes present in a polyp or, less often, some other form of metaplasia. Occasionally smooth muscle fibers are present in its stroma. The blood vessels in the polyp are often tortuous and thick walled.

Clinical Presentation.   Endometrial polyps often cause abnormal uterine bleeding. In women in the reproductive years, intermenstrual bleeding or menometrorrhagia is the most common symptom.

Relation to Carcinoma.   The risk of developing endometrial carcinoma is probably increased in women with an endometrial polyp. Endometrial polyps do not often become malignant, but the proliferative stimulus that causes the polyp may also increase the risk of developing endometrial carcinoma. Carcinoma is found in less than 0.5% of polyps removed surgically. Polyps are present in 20% of uteri removed for carcinoma. In one series, 3% of women with polyps eventually developed endometrial carcinoma, but many of these patients had been treated by radiation. The likelihood that a woman with an endometrial polyp who has not been irradiated will develop carcinoma is not known.

Treatment and Prognosis.   In young women in whom the rest of the endometrium is normal, a polypectomy usually brings cure even if the polyp shows atypical hyperplasia or a carcinoma confined to the polyp. In women past the menopause who have a polyp showing foci of atypicality, a hysterectomy is indicated.

Atypical Polypoid Adenomyoma.   An atypical polypoid adenomyoma resembles an endometrial polyp macroscopically. It is most frequent in the lower uterine segment. Microscopically the lesion consists of irregularly shaped endometrial glands separated by well-differentiated smooth muscle. The epithelium lining the glands is hyperplastic and atypical. Squamous metaplasia is common. An occasional mitosis is sometimes present in the smooth muscle. If more than 2 mitoses in 10 high-power fields are found, the lesion is probably a mixed müllerian tumor.

Carcinoma.   In the United States, each year nearly 40,000 women develop carcinoma of the endometrium and 3000 die of it. Nearly 10% of malignant tumors in women arise in the endometrium. The incidence is similar in Europe and Australasia, but is lower in South America, Asia, and Africa. In

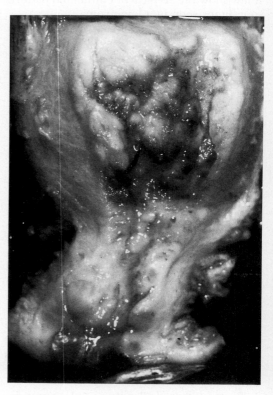

Fig. 41-43.   A carcinoma of the endometrium, showing the polypoid tumor invading the myometrium.

North America and Europe, the incidence is rising. Over 75% of the patients are over 50 years old.

Lesions. In the diffuse form of endometrial carcinoma much or all of the endometrium is replaced by carcinoma. The involved part of the endometrium is thickened, irregular and often polypoid. It is friable and sometimes ulcerated or hemorrhagic. Occasionally the carcinoma extends into the endocervix. Invasion of the myometrium is evident in 70% of the patients. In some, the carcinoma remains superficial, with little or no invasion of the myometrium. Some carcinomata reach the serosa by direct invasion through the uterine wall or by lymphatic extension with metastases beneath the serosa.

A localized endometrial carcinoma can arise anywhere in the endometrium, from the lower uterine segment to the cornua. The carcinoma may be polypoid, indistinguishable macroscopically from an endometrial polyp. It sometimes forms an irregular plaque of endometrial thickening. It may be ulcerated. Invasion of the myometrium is usually obvious and sometimes is extensive.

Microscopically, a number of different types of endometrial carcinoma are distinguished. About 80% of the tumors are of the typical or endometrioid pattern. In some, foci of benign squamous metaplasia are present in the tumor. In a few, there are both malignant glands and malignant squamous epithelium. Occasionally a mucinous, serous, or clear cell carcinoma arises in the endometrium. Rarely, a carcinoma shows only squamous differentiation. A few endometrial

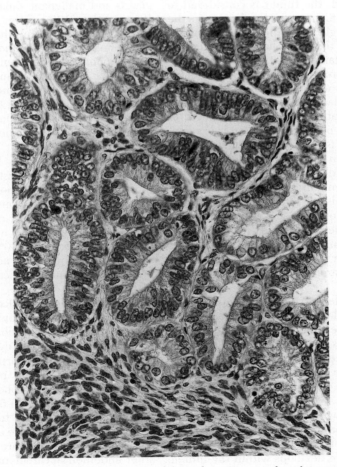

Fig. 41-44.   An endometrioid carcinoma of the endometrium invading the myometrium.

carcinomata are anaplastic, without evidence of glandular or squamous differentiation. Sometimes a carcinoma shows more than one of these patterns of differentiation.

Endometrioid Carcinoma. Most endometrioid carcinomata of the endometrium are well differentiated. They form glands like those of hyperplastic endometrium. Usually the epithelial cells are pseudostratified, but often they show little atypicality. The basement membrane around the glands is usually intact. The distinction from hyperplastic endometrium can be difficult. Several criteria have been found valuable in distinguishing between carcinoma and hyperplasia when only endometrial curettings are available for histologic examination.

If the glands are packed closely together without intervening stroma for at least half a low-power field, the tumor is considered to be malignant. Sometimes the lumen in the closely packed glands is filled by a cribriform proliferation of the epithelial cells. If glandular lumina containing multiple thin, branching papillary projections with a collagenous core covered with neoplastic epithelium occupy more than half a low-power field, the tumor is probably malignant. If sheets of squamous cells occupy more than half a low-power field, it is probably malignant. If the stroma between the glands is collagenous, the tumor is probably malignant.

In papillary endometrioid carcinomata, the neoplastic glands are filled with fine papillae with a collagenous core covered by pseudostratified epithelium. In a secretory carcinoma, the tumor cells contain subnuclear or supranuclear secretory vacuoles. In the rare ciliated carcinomata, the tumor cells have cilia.

In poorly differentiated endometrioid carcinomata, the glandular pattern is partially or largely lost. The tumor cells fill many of the glandular spaces and extend beyond them, to form solid sheets of poorly differentiated tumor cells. The basement membrane around the sheets of neoplastic cells is usually disrupted.

Carcinoma with Squamous Metaplasia. Foci of squamous metaplasia are present in 40% of endometrial carcinomata. The squamous epithelium develops within the lumen of the neoplastic glands, partially or com-

pletely replacing the glandular endometrium. It is well differentiated and shows no sign of malignancy. Keratinization is common. Occasionally the squamous cells form the spheroidal nodules of spindle cells called morules.

The term *carcinoma with squamous metaplasia* is used only if squamous epithelium makes up more than 10% of the tumor. If the squamous metaplasia is less extensive, it is disregarded. Sometimes an endometrial carcinoma with squamous cell metaplasia is called an adenoacanthoma. Acanthoma is from the Greek for thorn and refers to the prickle cells of the squamous epithelium. Most carcinomata with squamous metaplasia are well differentiated.

Adenosquamous Carcinoma. Some endometrial carcinomata contain both malignant glands and malignant squamous epithelium. If more than 10% of the tumor consists of malignant squamous epithelium, it is called an adenosquamous carcinoma. If the malignant squamous epithelium is less extensive, the tumor is classed as an adenocarcinoma. Less than 10% of endometrial carcinomata are of the adenosquamous type. Usually both the glandular and the squamous elements in the carcinoma are moderately or poorly differentiated.

Mucinous Carcinoma. If most of an endometrial carcinoma consists of glands like those of an ovarian mucinous carcinoma, the tumor is called a mucinous carcinoma. Less than 10% of endometrial carcinomata are of this type, though foci of mucinous differentiation are present in 40% of endometrial carcinomata. Squamous metaplasia is often prominent in mucinous carcinomata of the endometrium.

Serous Carcinoma. Occasionally a papillary carcinoma of the endometrium has fronds lined by stratified epithelium like that of a serous carcinoma of the ovaries. The tumor cells are usually pleomorphic and atypical. Multinucleated cells are present in 50% of the tumors. Psammoma bodies occur in 30%.

Clear Cell Tumor. In 5% of endometrial tumors, much or all the tumor resembles a clear cell carcinoma of the ovaries. Small foci of clear cell carcinoma are often present in other endometrial carcinomata, but the term *clear cell carcinoma* is not used unless the major portion of the tumor is of the clear cell type.

Squamous Cell Carcinoma. Endometrial carcinomata that are purely squamous are rare. Most arise in patients with pyometra or chronic endometritis.

Undifferentiated Carcinoma. A few endometrial carcinomata show no evidence of glandular or squamous differentiation. Such tumors are called undifferentiated carcinomata. They usually form sheets of poorly differentiated cells.

Behavior. Most endometrial carcinomata grow slowly and slowly invade the myometrium. Often the carcinoma remains confined to the uterus for months or years. At the time of operation, carcinoma is confined to the endometrium in 25% of the patients, has reached the inner third of the myometrium in 50%, and the middle or outer third in 25%.

A carcinoma of the endometrium usually metastases first to the lymph nodes in the pelvis and around the lower part of the aorta. As months pass, more lymph nodes are involved as the carcinoma spreads up the para-aortic chain. If the carcinoma involves the cornua of the uterus, extension along the lymphatics that accompany the round ligaments can give rise to metastases in the inguinal lymph nodes. At the time of surgical excision, lymph nodes are involved in less than 20% of the patients. In women dying of carcinoma of the endometrium, the para-aortic lymph nodes are involved in 60% of the patients, the hypogastric nodes in 60%, the external iliac nodes in 50%, the common iliac nodes in 40%, the obturator nodes in 40%, the mediastinal nodes in 20%, the inguinal nodes in 15%, and the nodes in the neck in 10%.

Fragments of carcinoma can pass through the fallopian tubes to establish metastases in the ovaries or on the peritoneum. Carcinomata extending through the whole thickness of the myometrium can release tumor cells into the peritoneum more directly. At autopsy, 30% of patients with endometrial carcinoma have metastases in the ovaries, and 40% have implants on the peritoneum. Implants of carcinoma in the vagina are present in 20% of the patients.

Hematogenous extension of an endometrial carcinoma usually comes late and is less common. At autopsy, 40% of the patients have metastases in the lungs, 30% in the liver, and 20% in the spine.

About 30% of endometrial carcinomata produce the carcinoembryonic antigen in sufficient quantity to raise the concentration of the antigen in the plasma. The concentration of α-fetoprotein in the plasma is increased in 50% of the patients. In 20%, the concentration of the β fragment of human chorionic gonadotropin in the plasma is increased.

Staging. The International Federation of Gynecology and Obstetrics (FIGO) has divided carcinoma of the endometrium into four stages. In stage I, the carcinoma is confined to the body of the uterus. In stage II, it involves the body of the uterus and the cervix. In stage III, it extends beyond the uterus but is confined to the pelvis and does not involve the urinary bladder or the rectum. In stage IV, it extends outside the pelvis or involves the urinary bladder or the rectum.

Clinical Presentation. Carcinoma of the endometrium often produces few symptoms. Abnormal uterine bleeding and spotting are its most frequent manifestations. In premenopausal women, the menses may become irregular or diminished.

Pathogenesis. Prolonged stimulation by estrogens increases the risk of developing carcinoma of the uterus. Over 5% of patients with a granulosa cell tumor of the ovaries develop a carcinoma of the endometrium. The risk of endometrial carcinoma is increased in other conditions that cause increased secretion of estrogens. It is increased in women treated with estrogens.

There are probably two types of endometrial carcinoma. Type I is associated with prolonged exposure to estrogens. Type II is not.

Type I carcinoma is most common before or about the menopause. The patients often have been treated with estrogens or have an estrogen-secreting tumor. The endometrium is often hyperplastic. The carcinoma is usually well differentiated, often with squamous metaplasia. It grows slowly and has an excellent prognosis. In the United States, this type of carcinoma is more common in white than in black women.

Type II carcinoma is most common in post-menopausal women. There is usually no history of estrogen excess. Endometrial hyperplasia is unusual. The carcinoma is often poorly differentiated, grows rapidly, and has a poor prognosis. In the United States, type II carcinoma is more common in black than in white women.

About 20% of women with atypical endometrial hyperplasia have or will develop carcinoma of the endometrium. The more atypical the endometrium, the greater the risk. The carcinomata are usually well differentiated and slow growing. The endometrium is usually atrophic in women with the more anaplastic endometrial carcinomata.

Over 80% of women with endometrial carcinoma are obese. About 50% are nulliparous. Some have diabetes mellitus or an abnormal glucose tolerance curve. Some are hypertensive. The relation of these factors to hormonal imbalance is complex and not fully understood.

In some kindred, the incidence of carcinoma of the endometrium and carcinoma of the breast is increased, probably because of a genetic predisposition to these tumors. In Israel, 3% of patients with endometrial carcinoma have had a carcinoma of the breast.

Treatment and Prognosis. Endometrial carcinoma is treated by hysterectomy and bilateral oophorosalpingectomy, sometimes with postoperative irradiation to the pelvis or chemotherapy. Progestins help control metastatic disease and relieve its symptoms.

The extent of the tumor determines the prognosis. In 80% of the patients, the tumor is clinically in stage I, confined to the body of the uterus. About 80% of these patients survive five years, and 65% are alive 10 years later. If the carcinoma involves the cervix, 40% survive five years, and 30% live 10 years. If it is clinically in stage III, involving extrauterine structures in the pelvis, 40% live five years, and 25% 10 years. Only 10% of patients with a carcinoma that has spread beyond the pelvis live five years, and few survive 10 years.

If the carcinoma is confined to the endometrium, 80% of the patients survive five years. If it extends deep into the myometrium, 60% live five years. The lymph nodes are involved in 5% of carcinomata that involve only the inner third of the myometrium, 20% of those that involve the middle third, and 30% of those that involve the outer third.

The more anaplastic tumors invade more extensively and metastasize more rapidly. Over 80% of patients with a well-differentiated carcinoma of the endometrium live five years, but only 30% of those with an anaplastic tumor. Metastases in the lymph nodes are found in 5% of patients with a well-differentiated tumor, but in 30% of those with a poorly differentiated carcinoma.

Nearly 90% of patients with a carcinoma with squamous metaplasia survive five years, probably because these tumors are usually well differentiated and slow growing. About 80% of patients with an endometrioid or mucinous carcinoma survive five years, and 70% of those with a serous carcinoma. Adenosquamous and clear cell carcinomata are usually poorly differentiated. Only 50% of patients with an adenosquamous carcinoma live five years, and 40% of those with a clear cell carcinoma.

Estrogen and progesterone receptors are both present in 70% of well-differentiated carcinomata of the endometrium but in only 40% of poorly differentiated tumors. Both are absent in 10% of well-differentiated carcinomata and 30% of poorly differentiated tumors. Some tumors have one receptor but not the other. Though the data are not clear, probably the presence of the receptors improves the prognosis.

Endometrial Stromal Nodule. Endometrial stromal nodules are rare. About 25% of endometrial stromal neoplasms are of this type. The patients range from 20 to 75 years old.

Endometrial stromal nodules develop in the myometrium or bulge from it. They are 1 to 15 cm across, soft, gray, yellow, or orange, and well defined. Occasionally the tumor is cystic. Sometimes it is polypoid and projects into the endometrial cavity. In 5% of patients, there is more than one.

Microscopically, the lesions consist of cells like those of the stroma of proliferative endometrium. The cells are uniform in size and shape and show no atypicality. Mitoses are usually few, but there can be as many as 15 in 10 high-power fields in parts of the tumor.

Occasionally the tumor cells form cords or trabeculae, or a few smooth muscle cells are present in the tumor. The margin of the lesion is well defined. The surrounding myometrium is compressed, but there is no capsule.

Most patients with an endometrial stromal nodule have abnormal uterine bleeding. Some have pelvic discomfort or pain. About 10% have no symptoms. Removal of the tumor by local excision or hysterectomy cures.

Endometrial Stromal Sarcoma. Endometrial stromal sarcomata are uncommon. About 25% of uterine sarcomata are of this type. Most of the patients are between 40 and 60 years old, but the sarcoma can occur in young people.

Lesions. The tumor usually forms a smooth mass or masses that bulge into the uterine cavity. It infiltrates the myometrium extensively. Most often the sarcoma forms poorly demarcated cords 2 to 15 mm across that wind through the myometrium. Often the cords extend out into the broad ligament. Less often the tumor forms an ill-defined, bosselated mass or masses in the myometrium or causes diffuse thickening of the myometrium. On section, the nodules of tumor are soft, yellowish or tan, and in the more

anaplastic tumors show foci of hemorrhage and necrosis.

Microscopically, the well-differentiated stromal sarcomata resemble the stroma of proliferative endometrium. The cells are uniform and show little atypicality. Mitoses are few, never more than 10 in 10 high-power fields. Reticulin fibers surround each tumor cells. Blood vessels are often prominent. The poorly differentiated sarcomata are usually more atypical and have more than 10 mitoses in 10 high-power fields. The reticulin mesh around the tumor cells is often imperfect.

Especially in the well-differentiated tumors, the tumor cells often fill the lymphatic and blood vessels in the myometrium with little or no invasion of the tissues. The more anaplastic tumors also permeate lymph and blood vessels but usually invade the myometrium extensively.

Rarely, the stromal cells of an endometrial stromal sarcoma are intermixed with smooth muscle cells, like those of a leiomyoma. Such a tumor is called a stromomyoma. Rarely, tubules like those of an ovarian sex cord tumor are found in a stromal sarcoma.

Behavior. Well-differentiated endometrial stromal sarcomata grow slowly. As they

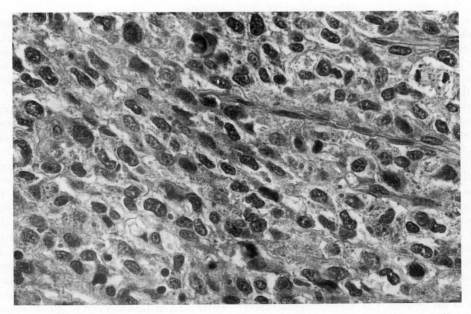

Fig. 41-45. An endometrial stromal sarcoma, showing moderately differentiated tumor cells.

extend beyond the uterus they often involve the bladder, rectum, ureters, or bowel. Implants on the peritoneum are not uncommon. Metastases in the lungs develop in a minority of the patients. Poorly differentiated stromal sarcomata grow rapidly and often metastasize to the peritoneum or lungs.

Clinical Presentation. Endometrial stromal sarcomata cause irregular uterine bleeding and often pain. The enlargement of the uterus can be detected by palpation.

Treatment and Prognosis. Radical hysterectomy eradicates the tumor in 50% of patients with a well-differentiated stromal sarcoma. In the others, the tumor recurs, most often in the pelvis or from implants on the peritoneum, but it may be more than 20 years before the recurrence becomes evident. Pulmonary metastases develop in 10% of patients with recurrent tumor. Progestins cause regression of the tumor in many patients, especially in those with a high concentration of progestin receptors on the tumor cells.

Poorly differentiated endometrial stromal sarcomata are treated by radical hysterectomy and pelvic irradiation. Progestins and chemotherapy are of limited value. The tumor usually recurs within two years. Metastases in the peritoneum or lungs are common. Less than 50% of the patients survive five years.

Adenofibroma. Adenofibromata of the uterus are uncommon. They are most common in patients over 60 years old, but can occur in younger people. Both the epithelium and the mesenchymal tissue in the tumor are neoplastic. Both are benign.

The tumor can arise from any part of the endometrium. It is usually polypoid or papillary, but can be sessile. Often the tumor is 2 to 10 cm across and fills the uterine cavity. Small cysts are often present within the lesion.

Microscopically, broad papillae extend from the surface of the tumor and project into the cysts. The papillae and cysts are lined by well-differentiated cuboidal or columnar epithelium. Most of the epithelium resembles endometrial epithelium, but other kinds of müllerian differentiation are often evident in parts of the tumor. The mesenchymal tissue consists of well-differentiated collagenous tissue often with some admixture of endometrial stroma. A few mitoses are sometimes present in the stroma, but never more than 5 in 10 high-power fields.

The tumor usually causes irregular bleeding, but sometimes causes pain or protrudes from the cervix. An adenofibroma of the endometrium should be removed by hysterectomy. Local removal is often followed by recurrence.

Adenosarcoma. An adenosarcoma of the uterus is an unusual tumor consisting of benign epithelium and malignant mesenchymal tissue. It can occur at any age. One or more polypoid tumors fill the uterine cavity and enlarge the uterus. Hemorrhage or necrosis are evident in 25% of the lesions. Cysts are present in 20%.

Microscopically, an adenosarcoma consists of cysts and papillae, like those of an adenofibroma, lined by inactive, well-differentiated epithelium. Often glands and clefts lined by similar cells are intermixed with the cysts. The epithelium is most often endometrial, but can be mucinous or squamous. The tumor differs from an adenofibroma in that the stroma is less well-differentiated, resembling a fibrosarcoma or an endometrial stromal sarcoma. In 25% of the tumors, cartilage, striated muscle, or fat is present in the stroma.

Adenosarcomata are malignant. They invade the underlying myometrium, with both the sarcomatous mesenchymal tissue and the benign-looking epithelium present in the invading tumor. Metastases sometimes develop if the tumor is not eradicated.

The tumor causes irregular bleeding and often pain. Sometimes there are urinary symptoms or a vaginal discharge, or the tumor protrudes from the vagina.

The tumors are treated by hysterectomy with bilateral salpingo-oophorectomy and radiation. In 40% of the patients, the tumor recurs in the pelvis, though often not for five or more years. Occasionally, more distant metastases develop. The recurrences and metastases may consist only of the sarcomatous mesenchymal part of the tumor, but often contain the epithelial element as well. Often the recurrences and metastases are more anaplastic than the original tumor.

Mixed Müllerian Tumor. A mixed müllerian tumor of the endometrium contains both neoplastic epithelium and neoplastic mesenchymal tissue. Less than 2% of malignant tumors of the uterus are of this type. The patients are usually over 50 years old.

Lesions. A soft, polypoid mass often fills the uterine cavity and may protrude through the cervix. Necrosis and hemorrhage are often evident in the tumor. Foci of calcification may be evident. Invasion of the myometrium is usually obvious.

Microscopically, the epithelial element in the tumor usually resembles an endometrioid carcinoma of the endometrium, less often a mucinous carcinoma, serous carcinoma, or clear cell carcinoma. In 5% of the tumors, the epithelial element is a squamous cell carcinoma.

The mesenchymal element in the tumor usually resembles a fibrosarcoma or an endometrial stromal sarcoma. Less often it is like a leiomyosarcoma or shows some combination of these types of differentiation. Often the mesenchymal tissue in part of the tumor is poorly differentiated and consists of small, closely packed spindle cells. Especially in the poorly differentiated regions, occasional cells sometimes show the cross striations of rhabdomyocytes, the tumor forms islands of cartilage or, less often, fragments of osteoid or fat.

If the mesenchymal part of the lesion consists only of fibrosarcomatous, stromal sarcomatous, or leiomyosarcomatous tissue, the tumor is called a homologous mixed müllerian tumor. If rhabdomyocytes or cartilage is present, it is called a heterologous tumor. Some reserve the term *mixed müllerian tumor* for the heterologous lesions and call a homologous tumor a carcinosarcoma.

Behavior. Mixed müllerian tumors grow rapidly and invade the myometrium. Metastases in the pelvic lymph nodes are present in 30% of the patients in whom the tumor has extended more than halfway through the myometrium. In 30% of the patients the tumor has extended beyond the uterus by the time the diagnosis is made. Implants on the peritoneum and hematogenous metastases can be extensive.

Clinical Presentation. Pain, abdominal swelling, and irregular vaginal bleeding are often the first signs of a mixed müllerian tumor. Frequently a mass in the pelvis is evident. Sometimes gastrointestinal dysfunction caused by peritoneal implants is the first sign of the tumor. Sometimes the tumor protrudes from the vagina.

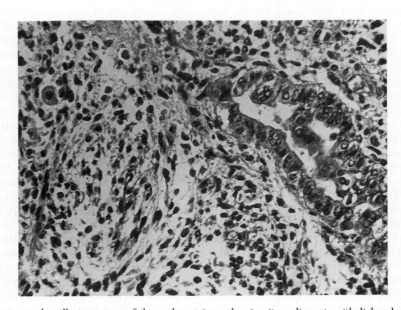

Fig. 41-46. A mixed müllerian tumor of the endometrium, showing its malignant epithelial and mesenchymal tissues.

Treatment and Prognosis. A mixed müllerian tumor is treated by radical hysterectomy and radiation. Chemotherapy has proved of little help. Few if any of the patients in whom the tumor has extended beyond the uterus live more than two or three years. Even if the tumor seems confined to the uterus, recurrences and metastases are common. Less than 30% of the patients live five years.

CERVIX UTERI. Non-neoplastic endocervical polyps are common in the cervix uteri. Sometimes microglandular endocervical hyperplasia causes a polypoid lesion. Infection with the human papilloma virus is the principal cause of the condylomata, dysplasia, carcinoma in situ, and microinvasive and invasive squamous cell carcinomata common in the cervix. Adenocarcinoma can arise in the cervix. Rarely, a mucoepidermoid tumor, carcinoma adenoides cysticum, carcinoid tumor, or an anaplastic neuroendocrine tumor like an oat cell carcinoma of a lung takes origin in the cervix. The clear cell carcinomata of the cervix are considered with the tumors of the vagina.

Endocervical Polyp. Endocervical polyps are common, especially in multipara 40 to 60 years old.

Lesions. Endocervical polyps are usually single. Most are less than 3 cm across, but occasionally a polyp is large enough to protrude from the vagina. They are red, fragile, pedunculated, and often irregularly shaped. They may become ulcerated or infected.

Microscopically, most cervical polyps are made of endocervical mucosa. Some are lined in part by the squamous epithelium of the exocervix, and many show extensive squamous metaplasia. The stroma of the polyp is usually edematous, with an exudate of lymphocytes, plasma cells, and macrophages. Occasionally it is highly vascular or shows decidual change during pregnancy. If the polyp is ulcerated or infected, neutrophils and other signs of acute inflammation are added. Foci of carcinoma or carcinoma in situ are present in less than 0.5% of endocervical polyps.

Clinical Presentation. Endocervical polyps often cause no symptoms. They may cause irregular or postcoital bleeding. If the polyp

becomes infected, vaginal discharge is common.

Treatment and Prognosis. Endocervical polyps are not neoplastic. Removal by curettage cures.

Microglandular Endocervical Hyperplasia. Microglandular endocervical hyperplasia develops in women taking contraceptive pills containing progestin or during pregnancy. It persists after the pill is withdrawn or after the end of the pregnancy.

The endocervix shows one or more lesions that resemble an endocervical polyp macroscopically. Microscopically, the lesion usually consists of small, closely packed, tubular glands lined by flattened or cuboidal cells. Squamous metaplasia is common. The epithelium is regular and uniform. Less often the epithelial cells grow in a cribriform pattern or in sheets. They have hyperchromatic, irregular nuclei and often have clear cytoplasm.

Microglandular endocervical hyperplasia is not neoplastic. Excision cures.

Condyloma. Condylomata of the cervix uteri are most common in women 20 to 25 years old. They develop in the squamous epithelium of the exocervix and in foci of squamous metaplasia in the endocervix. Frequently they are multiple. Occasionally large numbers of tiny condylomata stud the epithelium of the cervix and vagina.

Lesions. Over 90% of cervical condylomata are flat. They are not apparent macroscopically unless the cervix is painted with acetic acid and examined colposcopically, when they appear as sharply demarcated, white, slightly raised plaques, usually with an irregular surface. The lesions vary from less than 0.1 cm across to more than 3 cm.

Microscopically, the epithelium in a flat condyloma is usually thick and hyperplastic, but maintains its normal pattern of differentiation and shows no cellular atypicality. The surface of the lesion is commonly undulating. Occasionally the epithelium forms small spikes that project from the surface. Mitoses occur only in the basal part of the epithelium and are usually normal, though a few tripolar or diffuse metaphases can occur. Often the granular layer of the epithelium is prominent. Some degrees of hyperkeratosis or parakeratosis is evident. Usually a few cells showing premature keratinization, called dyskeratotic cells, are scattered in the upper part of the epithelium.

Koilocytic cells are present in the upper and middle layers of the epithelium. The name comes from the Greek word meaning hollow or empty. The koilocytes are large, with a peripheral rim of dark cytoplasm that clearly outlines the cells. The nuclei are surrounded by a wide halo of clear cytoplasm that gives the cells an empty look. The nuclei are often pyknotic, show marginal clumping of their chromatin, or are fragmented.

Occasionally a condyloma involves the epithelium of the endocervical glands. The hyperplastic epithelium fills the glands, forming an inverted condyloma, a lesion that seems to project into the tissue rather than standing above it. Occasionally a condyloma accuminatum like that more common on the vulva develops in the cervix.

Some authorities describe an atypical condyloma in which the basal part of the epithelium shows mild disorder and atypicality like those seen in mild epithelial dysplasia. Such lesions are better considered a form of dysplasia.

In 50% of the lesions, electron microscopy shows the crystalline arrays of the human papilloma virus in the nuclei of the koilocytic cells. Immunohistochemistry using an antigen against the virus demonstrates it in the koilocytes in a similar proportion of the lesions. Condylomata contain the high molecular weight keratins found in keratinizing epithelia. Their nuclei are nearly always diploid or polypoid.

Behavior. Most condylomata of the cervix regress spontaneously or are controlled by treatment. In some patients, the lesions recur. In some, especially in those who are untreated, they persist.

In 10% of the patients, some of the cervical condylomata progress to carcinoma in situ or invasive carcinoma. It is not known if the nuclei in the lesions that progress are diploid or polyploid like those in most condylomata or are aneuploid like those in most dysplastic lesions.

Pathogenesis. Condylomata of the cervix uteri are caused by the human papilloma virus. The infection is transmitted by sexual intercourse. The virus in the lesions is fully expressed and infectious. Most condylomata of the cervix are caused by the viruses 6 and 11 that cause condylomata but not carcinoma in situ. Some are caused by the viruses 16 and 18 that also cause carcinoma in situ and invasive carcinoma of the cervix. Probably a few are caused by the viruses 31, 33, and 35 sometimes found in malignant cervical lesions. Sometimes more than one type of papilloma virus is involved.

Treatment and Prognosis. Condylomata on the exocervix are eradicated by cryosurgery or by using a laser beam. Over 90% of the patients are cured. Endocervical lesions require conization, because invasive carcinoma cannot be excluded, though the risk is low. Barrier methods of contraception help reduce the risk of reinfection.

Cervical Intraepithelial Neoplasia. Because dysplasia and carcinoma in situ of the cervical epithelium form a continuity with no clear demarcation between severe dysplasia and carcinoma in situ, many prefer to group cervical dysplasia and carcinoma in situ together, calling them cervical intraepithelial neoplasia, or CIN. Others prefer to maintain the distinction between dysplasia and carcinoma in situ, thinking that dysplasia and carcinoma in situ are different kinds of disease.

Cervical intraepithelial neoplasia can develop at any age, though it is rare before puberty. Most patients with dysplasia are 25 to 30 years old, and most with carcinoma in situ are 30 to 35 years old.

Dysplasia and carcinoma in situ of the cervix are more common in the poorer socioeconomic classes. The incidence of carcinoma in situ between black and white women in the United States differs largely because a greater proportion of black women are in the poorer classes. In the lower socioeconomic classes, the incidence of cervical intraepithelial neoplasia is the same in black and white women.

The incidence of cervical intraepithelial neoplasia is increasing, especially in teenagers and young women, probably because of the change in sexual mores. In the United States, the incidence of carcinoma in situ in girls 15 to 19 years old increased nearly 30 times between 1970 and 1980. In 1981, nearly 2% of sexually active girls 15 to 19 years old had either cervical dysplasia or carcinoma in situ.

Terminology. In dysplasia and carcinoma in situ of the cervix uteri, the squamous epithelium is replaced in part or in whole by atypical cells. In dysplasia, the atypicality is confined to the basal part of the epithelium, with stratification and differentiation evident in its superficial part. In carcinoma in situ, the atypicality extends through the whole thickness of the epithelium.

Those who distinguish between dysplasia and carcinoma in situ divide dysplasia into three stages. In mild dysplasia, the atypicality is confined to the basal third of the epithelium. In moderate dysplasia, the basal

and middle thirds are involved. In severe dysplasia, the atypicality extends into the superficial third, leaving only a narrow zone of stratification and differentiation.

Those who group dysplasia and carcinoma in situ together as cervical intraepithelial neoplasia call mild dysplasia cervical intraepithelial neoplasia 1; moderate dysplasia, cervical intraepithelial neoplasia 2; and group severe dysplasia and carcinoma in situ together as cervical intraepithelial neoplasia 3. Often these terms are abbreviated to CIN 1, CIN 2, and CIN 3.

Lesions. Dysplasia and carcinoma in situ of the exocervix begin in the transformation zone where the glandular mucosa of the endocervix meets the squamous epithelium of the exocervix. The position of the trans-

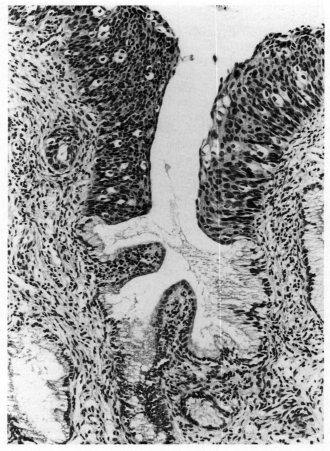

Fig. 41-47. Carcinoma in situ of the cervix uteri extending into the neck of an endocervical gland.

formation zone changes as the patient ages. At puberty, the endocervical mucosa often extends out onto the portio vaginalis, appearing as an erosion. As a woman ages, squamous metaplasia covers the distal part of the endocervical mucosa, spreading in irregular tongues towards the external os of the cervix. After the menopause, the transformation zone is often in the endocervical canal.

In 60% of the patients, dysplasia and carcinoma in situ begin on the anterior lip of the cervix; in 30% on the posterior lip. Only in 10% does the lesion begin in the lateral part of the cervix. The lesion is solitary in 95% of the patients. It may be only a few millimeters across or may extend for several centimeters.

The lesion does not involve the squamous epithelium of the exocervix. The junction between the normal exocervical epithelium and the dysplastic epithelium is sharp and usually oblique. As the lesion grows larger, it extends around the transformation zone and up the endocervix. The abnormal epithelium grows beneath the columnar epithelium of the endocervix and replaces it. Often the endocervical glands are partially or completely filled by the abnormal epithelium.

Macroscopically, a cervix uteri containing a focus of dysplasia or carcinoma in situ usually appears normal when examined with the naked eye. By colposcopy, the lesion may appear as a sharply defined white area when the cervix is cleaned with acetic acid, but often it is apparent only after the cervix is stained with iodine or toluidine blue. Iodine

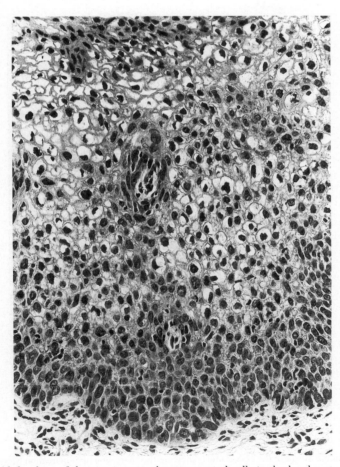

Fig. 41-48. Mild dysplasia of the cervix uteri, showing atypical cells in the basal part of the epithelium.

stains the glycogen present in normal exocervical epithelium, but fails to stain the lesion in 80% of patients with severe dysplasia or carcinoma in situ and in 50% of those with mild or moderate dysplasia. Toluidine blue stains strongly regions in which nuclei are numerous, often showing clearly foci of intraepithelial neoplasia.

At colposcopy, the lesion sometimes shows a mosaic pattern, with irregular polygons outlined in red. Sometimes red dots, called punctuation, are present in it. In carcinoma in situ, abnormal vessels can sometimes be seen beneath the lesion. They show constricted and dilated segments, often with irregular branching.

Microscopically, the atypical cells in cervical dysplasia and carcinoma in situ are arranged in an abnormal fashion. They are often crowded together and appear to overlap. Sometimes they are pleomorphic and arranged in a disorderly manner. Even in the superficial part of the lesion, the atypical cells show no evidence of differentiation.

Most often the atypical cells are small and resemble the basal cells of the epithelium. They have a high nucleocytoplasmic ratio. Their chromatin is coarse and irregular. The nuclei often vary in size and shape. Mitoses are common and sometimes atypical. In moderate and severe dysplasia and in carcinoma in situ, mitoses are commonly present in the middle or superficial part of the epithelium. Dyskeratotic cells are often scattered among the atypical cells.

Less often the atypical cells are larger,

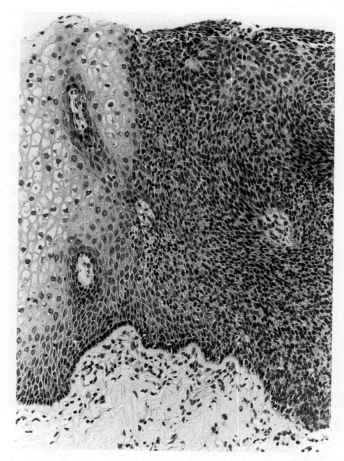

Fig. 41-49. Carcinoma in situ of the cervix uteri, showing the sharp line of demarcation between the normal and the abnormal epithelium.

more like those of the exocervix. They may or may not keratinize. In the keratinizing lesions, intercellular bridges are prominent, nucleoli are large, and often keratin covers the surface of the lesion.

Electron microscopy shows that the atypical cells have less glycogen and fewer filaments than do normal exocervical cells. Desmosomes and other intercellular connections are reduced in number and often ill-formed. Microvilli are present on the surface of the cells. In tissue culture, surface inhibition is impaired.

Immunohistologic stains show that the high molecular weight cytokeratins and involucrum present in normal exocervical epithelium are demonstrable in the atypical cells in 40% of the lesions in mild or moderate dysplasia, but rarely in severe dysplasia or carcinoma in situ. The atypical cells often stain for the epithelial membrane antigen and the carcinoembryonic antigen. In most of the lesions, the atypical cells are aneuploid.

In dysplasia, the cells in the superficial part of the epithelium retain their normal, orderly, stratified pattern. Their nuclei are sometimes larger than normal and slightly hyperchromatic. The demarcation between the atypical cells in the basal part of the epithelium and the differentiated cells in the superficial part is not always clear. Koilocytes are sometimes present in the superficial part of the epithelium, especially in mild and moderate dysplasia.

The blood vessels beneath the lesions are distorted and compressed. The changes are not striking by light microscopy in sections, but are responsible for the polygonal pattern and the punctuation seen at colposcopy.

Behavior. In 50% of untreated patients, mild cervical dysplasia progresses to carcinoma in situ or invasive carcinoma within 10 years. In 10%, it worsens to moderate dysplasia. In 30%, the dysplasia persists. In 10%, it regresses. The more severe the dysplasia, the more likely it is to become carcinoma in situ or invasive carcinoma. The patients in whom the lesion regresses all have mild dysplasia. The patients with mild dysplasia that progress to carcinoma in situ usually do so within three years. Patients with moderate dysplasia that progress to cervical intraepithelial neoplasia 3 usually do so within two years.

In 50% of patients with carcinoma in situ, the lesion progresses to invasive carcinoma, usually after three to 10 years. In 50%, the lesion remains in situ.

In nearly 100% of the lesions that progress and 95% of those that persist, the nuclei in the atypical cells are aneuploid. Over 85% of the lesions that are aneuploid persist or progress, but less than 10% of lesions with diploid or polypoid nuclei.

Diagnosis. The diagnosis of dysplasia and carcinoma in situ of the exocervix depends principally on exfoliative cytologic studies. The lesions produce no symptoms and usually cannot be felt or seen unless a colposcope is used.

In mild dysplasia, the desquamated cells are mainly superficial or intermediate squamous cells, with well-preserved cytoplasm, but with nuclei that are larger than normal and slightly hyperchromatic, like the cells in the superficial part of the dysplastic epithelium. Such cells are called dyskaryotic, from the Greek for wrong and a nut, to emphasize that their nuclei are abnormal.

In moderate dysplasia, the desquamated cells are smaller, round, or ovoid, with a rim of cytoplasm not thicker than the diameter of the nucleus. The nuclei are more hyperchromatic and atypical.

In severe dysplasia or carcinoma in situ, the desquamated cells are usually the small, dark basal cells that make up the lesions. They have atypical nuclei and a narrow rim of cytoplasm. Less often the desquamated cells are larger or are keratinized.

Patients who have abnormal cells in cytologic smears are usually examined by colposcopy, and a history of suspicious regions is needed to establish the diagnosis. If colposcopy is not available, random biopsies are taken. Often an endocervical curettage is performed to ensure that the transformation zone where dysplasia and carcinoma in situ begin is examined.

Pathogenesis. Cervical intraepithelial neoplasia is caused by the human papilloma viruses. By nuclear hybridization, viral deoxyribonucleic acid can be demonstrated in 90% of the lesions. Patients with types 16, 18, 31, 32, and 36 all cause dysplasia and carcinoma in situ. The virus does not usually develop into an infective form. It is often incorporated into the cell's genome.

Treatment and Prognosis. Patients who have repeatedly abnormal cells in their vaginal secretions or who have dysplasia or carcinoma in situ in endocervical curettings but have no lesion by colposcopy are treated by conization. A cone of cervical tissue including the transformation zone is removed and examined microscopically to determine the nature and extent of the lesion. If the lesion is completely removed and abnormal cells disappear from the vaginal secretions, no further treatment is needed. If not, hysterectomy is indicated.

If the lesion is detected at colposcopy and can be entirely visualized, it can be destroyed by cryosurgery or by a laser beam. Nearly 95% of the patients are cured, though a second lesion develops subsequently in 0.1%. If only part of the lesion can be seen, conization is needed. If the lesion is not completely removed, or if abnormal cells persist in the vaginal secretions, hysterectomy is required.

Microinvasive Carcinoma. The term *microinvasive carcinoma of the cervix uteri* is used to describe the earliest form of invasive squamous cell carcinoma detectable in patients with dysplasia or carcinoma in situ of the exocervix. In microinvasive carcinoma, one or more tongues of carcinoma extend down from dysplastic epithelium or from a focus of carcinoma in situ, breaching the basement membrane to invade the underlying connective tissue. There is no agreement as to the definition of microinvasive carcinoma, but a reasonable compromise requires that the invading tongues of carcinoma extend not more than 3 mm beyond the basement membrane and do not invade blood or lymphatic vessels.

Less than 5% of patients with dysplasia or carcinoma in situ have microinvasive carcinoma. Most of the patients are between 40 and 45 years old.

Lesions. Macroscopically, microinvasive carcinoma cannot be differentiated from noninvasive cervical intraepithelial neoplasia with certainty. The presence of abnormal blood vessels beneath the lesion suggests that microinvasion may be present. The diagnosis is made microscopically from a biopsy or conization of the cervix.

The tumor cells in the invading tongues of microinvasive carcinoma are usually larger and look better differentiated than are the cells of the dysplasia or carcinoma in situ in the adjacent epithelium. The invading tongues usually have a ragged, irregular outline, as the carcinoma cells push between the collagen bundles.

Behavior. If not removed, microinvasive carcinomata of the cervix extend more deeply and become invasive squamous cell tumors. The likelihood of metastasis depends on the depth of invasion and the vascular involvement. If the depth of invasion is less than 3 mm and no vessels are involved, less than 0.2% of the patients have metastases in the lymph nodes. If the carcinoma invades vessels but does not penetrate more than 3 mm, 4% of the patients have metastases in the lymph nodes. If it penetrates between 3 and 5 mm, 8% of the patients have metastases.

Treatment and Prognosis. If microinvasive carcinoma penetrates less than 3 mm without vascular invasion, if the lesion is completely removed by conization, and if the lesion is less than 10 mm across, simple hysterectomy cures almost all patients. If it extends more deeply, involves vessels, is more than 10 mm across, or is incompletely removed, the tumor should be considered an invasive squamous cell carcinoma.

Invasive Squamous Cell Carcinoma. It is estimated that in the United States 14,000 women developed invasive squamous cell carcinoma of the cervix uteri in 1986 and 7000 died of it. The incidence is greatest in the poorer socioeconomic groups. The incidence is similar in other developed countries, but is high in countries in which the standard of living is low. Most patients with invasive squamous cell carcinoma of the cervix are between 40 and 60 years old, though the frequency of invasive cervical carcinoma in younger women is increasing.

In North America, Europe, and Australasia, the introduction of cytologic screening to detect carcinoma of the cervix uteri has reduced its incidence greatly. The incidence in the United States fell from 34 per 100,000 in 1947 to 15 per 100,000 in 1970 and continues to fall. In one study, the incidence was 5 per 100,000 in women regularly screened cytologically and 29 per 100,000 in women not screened.

Lesions. Over 95% of invasive squamous cell carcinomata of the cervix begin in the transformation zone. Small tumors are usually confined to this zone. They may be indurated or form a shallow ulcer, but often are slightly raised with a granular surface that bleeds easily. Larger carcinomata invade both the exocervix and the endocervix extensively. Sometimes the carcinoma forms a deep, ragged ulcer; sometimes it forms a large polypoid mass that bulges from the cervix.

Microscopically, squamous cell carcinomata of the cervix form irregular columns of malignant squamous cells that invade down from the surface and are supported by a collagenous stroma. In 5% of the patients, the carcinoma is highly differentiated, with keratinization, epithelial pearls, intercellular bridges, and few mitoses. Occasionally in parts of the tumor there are sheets of pale, cuboidal cells, with sharp cell borders and empty cytoplasm containing glycogen. In 10%, the carcinoma is anaplastic, usually with small, dark, spindle-shaped cells, with only rare foci of keratinization, no intercellular bridges, and many mitoses. Less often, an anaplastic carcinoma is strikingly pleomorphic. In 85% of the patients, the carcinoma is between these extremes, though keratinization is often scant, and the tumor cells tend towards the small, dark, spindle-shaped form.

By electron microscopy, the number of desmosomes and gap junctions between the tumor cells is reduced. Microvilli are present on the surface of the cells. The number of intermediate filaments in the cells is reduced, and often the filaments are clumped together. Commonly the number of mitochondria and ribosomes in the cells is increased. Basement membrane often partially surrounds the columns of invading cells.

In the well-differentiated tumors, the high molecular weight cytokeratins and involucrum found in normal exocervical epithelium are present, but they are not found in the poorly differentiated tumors. Low molecular weight cytokeratins usually persist in the poorly differentiated tumors. Some of the tumors produce the epithelial membrane antigen or

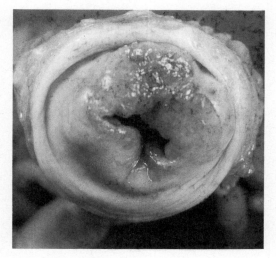

Fig. 41-50. Invasive carcinoma of the cervix uteri, showing the tumor in the upper lip of the cervix.

the carcinoembryonic antigen. The nuclei in the tumor cells are nearly always aneuploid.

Cytologically, the cells desquamated from a squamous cell carcinoma of the cervix uteri are sometimes large and flat, like normal squamous cells, but often they are smaller, rounded, or irregularly shaped. Their cytoplasm is often opaque, instead of finely transparent, as in normal squamous cells. Their nuclei are big, often coarsely hyperchromatic, sometimes irregularly shaped, sometimes with nucleoli. Sometimes the tumor cells have more than one nucleus. Often there are tadpole cells, with an atypical nucleus at one end and a long tail of cytoplasm drawn out behind it. If the carcinoma is made of small, dark spindle cells, the desquamated cells are also small, dark, and spindle-shaped. Often blood and necrotic debris are mixed with the malignant cells, and dyskaryotic cells from an adjacent area of carcinoma in situ or dysplasia may be present. Sometimes the tumor cells are so distorted by necrosis or infection that cytologic diagnosis is difficult.

Behavior. Squamous cell carcinoma of the cervix uteri invades slowly but often extensively. It burrows into the muscle of the cervix and often extends through it into the parauterine tissues and uterine ligaments to reach the bony wall of the pelvis. Not uncommonly, it obstructs one or both ureters. It may invade upwards into the endometrial cavity or downwards into the vagina. Extension into the urinary bladder or the rectum can cause a vesicovaginal or rectovaginal fistula.

When patients come for treatment, 30% of invasive squamous cell carcinomata of the cervix uteri are confined to the cervical muscle. Over 30% have extended beyond the myometrium, but have not reached the pelvic wall or extended beyond the upper two thirds of the vagina. About 30% have reached the pelvic wall or have invaded the lower third of the vagina. Less than 5% have invaded the urinary bladder or the rectum or have extended beyond the pelvis.

The pelvic lymph nodes are involved in 15% of the patients in whom the carcinoma is confined to the myometrium. If it has extended beyond the myometrium but has not reached the pelvic wall or the lower third of the vagina, the lymph nodes are involved in 40% of the patients. If the carcinoma has reached the pelvic wall, the pelvic lymph nodes are involved in 50% of the patients. Late in the disease, the para-aortic lymph nodes in the abdomen are often involved, but the disease does not often spread to the mediastinal lymph nodes or to the lymph nodes in the neck. Occasionally the tumor metastasizes to the external iliac lymph nodes.

Hematogenous metastases usually come late. About 50% of the patients who die of carcinoma of the cervix have distant metas-

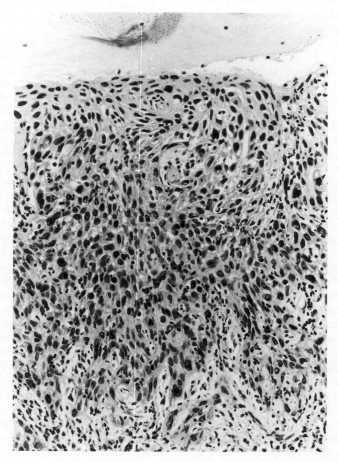

Fig. 41-51. Early invasive carcinoma of the cervix uteri showing the poorly differentiated squamous cells extending into the underlying tissues.

tases, most often in the liver or lungs, though any organ can be involved.

Staging. The International Federation of Gynecologists and Obstetricians has divided carcinoma of the cervix uteri into five stages. In stage 0, the carcinoma is in situ. In stage I, it is confined to the myometrium. In stage II, it has extended into the periuterine tissues, but has not reached the pelvic wall or the lower third of the vagina. In stage III, it has invaded the pelvic wall, the lower third of the vagina, or has obstructed one or both ureters. In stage IV, it has involved the urinary bladder, the rectum, or has spread beyond the pelvis.

Microinvasive carcinomata are staged as Ia1. Tumors that cannot be detected clinically, that penetrate not more than 5 mm, with or without vascular invasion, and are not more than 7 mm across are classed as stage Ia2 and are often called occult carcinomata. Carcinomata that invade more deeply or are more than 7 mm across are considered stage Ib.

Clinical Presentation. Occult squamous cell carcinomata of the cervix usually cause no symptoms. Larger carcinomata cause vaginal bleeding in 99% of the patients, especially after intercourse or douching. Over 10% of the patients complain of discharge or pain radiating to the sacrum.

Pathogenesis. The majority of invasive squamous cell carcinomata of the cervix uteri are caused by the human papilloma virus, types 16, 18, 31, 32, and 36. When the virus is fully expressed and reproduces infective virus, it induces a condyloma. When its replication is imperfect, it can become incorporated into the cell's genome and causes dysplasia, carcinoma in situ, or invasive carcinoma. Viral deoxyribonucleic acid can be demonstrated in 90% of invasive squamous cell carcinomata of the cervix.

Many invasive squamous cell carcinomata begin as dysplasia that progresses to carcinoma in situ, to microinvasive carcinoma, and eventually to invasive carcinoma. The majority of patients with dysplasia are 25 to 30 years old, those with carcinoma in situ are 30 to 35 years old, those with microinvasive carcinoma 40 to 45, and those with invasive carcinoma are 40 to 60 years old, suggesting that the carcinoma progresses in this fashion.

Not all cervical carcinomata follow this sequence. In some, microinvasive carcinoma develops from dysplasia. In some, there is little reason to think that the patient ever had intraepithelial neoplasia.

Many of the factors that increase the risk of developing invasive carcinoma of the cervix probably do so by increasing the risk of infection with the human papilloma virus. The infection is transmitted by sexual intercourse. The earlier intercourse begins, the more frequent it becomes, and the more numerous the sexual partners, the greater the risk of infection with the human papilloma virus. Carcinoma of the cervix is uncommon in nuns and other virgins. It increases 2 or 3 times in women attending venereal disease clinics. It increases 8 times in women whose sexual partner has carcinoma of the penis.

The importance of the herpes simplex virus type 2 in the causation of cervical carcinoma remains uncertain. The virus can transform cells in vitro. It can sometimes be demonstrated in the cells of a carcinoma of the cervix, though it does not become incorporated into the genome of the tumor cells. Some studies have shown that antibody against the virus is found more frequently in women with carcinoma of the cervix than in other women and that women with antibodies against the virus are more likely to develop cervical carcinoma than are other women. Other studies have shown no such association. It has been suggested that infection with the herpesvirus might facilitate infection with the human papilloma virus, or that the virus might initiate the malignant change in the cervix without remaining present in the cells, but neither theory has been proved.

Cervicitis is more common in women infected with the human papilloma virus and may facilitate the infection. Some investigators found that oral contraceptives increase the risk of developing carcinoma of the cervix or accelerate its progression. Others have been unable to confirm the finding. Cigarette smoking increases the risk of developing cervical carcinoma.

The incidence of carcinoma of the cervix is low in Jewish women, in the United States 10% of the incidence in the general population. The circumcision of the male partners does not explain the low incidence, for no correlation between circumcision and the incidence of cervical carcinoma has been found in other racial groups. In India, the incidence of carcinoma of the cervix is the same in Moslems who are circumcised and in Hindus who are not. Genetic factors may be of importance in the Jewish women.

Treatment and Prognosis. Occult invasive squamous cell carcinoma of the cervix is usually treated by radical hysterectomy and pelvic lymphadenectomy. Carcinomata of stage Ib are treated similarly or by intracavitary radiation followed by surgical excision. Over 85% of the patients are alive five years later.

Patients with carcinoma in stage II or III are most often treated by intracavitary and external irradiation. About 70% of those in stage II and 30% of those in stage III live five years. In 30% of the patients, the radiation causes proctitis, necrosis of the vaginal vault, cystitis, obstruction or perforation of the bowel, a vesicovaginal fistula, or major hemorrhage. In 2%, the complications prove fatal.

Patients in stage IV are treated with chemotherapy and sometimes irradiation. Less than 10% live five years.

In nearly 50% of the patients who die of squamous cell carcinoma of the cervix uteri, death is caused by ureteric obstruction, hydronephrosis, pyelonephritis, and renal failure. Less often obstruction or perforation of the bowel, metastases, or hemorrhage causes death.

Verrucous Carcinoma. Verrucous carcinomata of the cervix uteri are uncommon. Rounded projections of well-differentiated squamous cells slowly invade the tissues. Metastases are rare, except in tumors that have been irradiated. Radiation makes the carcinoma more anaplastic and more likely to metastasize. Verrucous carcinomata of the cervix are usually caused by the human papilloma virus 6. Local excision cures, but the tumor is likely to recur if excision is incomplete.

Adenocarcinoma. About 5% of carcinomata of the cervix uteri are adenocarcinomata. Most arise within the endocervical canal, though some begin at the squamocolumnar junction. An adenocarcinoma of the cervix can arise at any age, but most of the patients are over 45 years old.

Lesions. In 50% of the patients with an adenocarcinoma of the endocervix, the carcinoma forms a fungating or polypoid mass protruding from the cervix. Less often, the

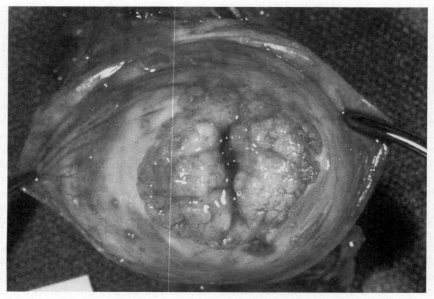

Fig. 41-52. A verrucous carcinoma of the cervix uteri, showing the warty tumor surrounding the cervical os.

carcinoma forms an ulcer or an indurated plaque. In 15% of the patients, the tumor is hidden in the endocervical canal and cannot be detected clinically.

Most often an adenocarcinoma of the cervix forms branching glands that extend down into the myometrium. The glands are usually lined by columnar, mucus-secreting epithelium like that of the endocervix. In some tumors, the epithelium is so highly differentiated that only the invasion shows that the tumor is malignant. More often the tumor cells are moderately differentiated. Occasionally they are anaplastic, forming solid sheets of tumor cells with only occasional acini. The adjacent endocervical epithelium often shows carcinoma in situ. Commonly intraepithelial neoplasia is present in the transformation zone.

Less often the carcinoma resembles a mucinous or serous carcinoma of the endometrium or an endometrioid carcinoma. Foci of squamous metaplasia are sometimes present in the tumor. Psammoma bodies may be present in the stroma. Occasionally the mucus secreted by the tumor cells escapes from the acini to form a colloid carcinoma, or a mucinous carcinoma contains neuroendocrine cells and Paneth cells like those of the bowel. An adenosquamous carcinoma rarely develops in the cervix.

Behavior. Adenocarcinomata of the endocervix behave much as do squamous cell carcinomata of the exocervix, though extension to the pelvic lymph nodes tends to occur earlier.

Treatment and Prognosis. The tumors are treated with radiation or with radiation and hysterectomy. About 50% of the patients survive for five years.

Secondary Tumors. Metastatic tumors of the uterus are rare. The most common is a metastasis of a carcinoma of the ovary to the endometrium. Occasionally a carcinoma implants on the serosa of the uterus.

Vagina

Benign tumors of the vagina are uncommon. They include the fibroepithelial polyp, leiomyoma, fibroma, granular cell tumor, a rare tumor called a rhabdomyoma that has well-differentiated striated muscle fibers in a collagenous stroma, and a mixed tumor that contains islands of well-differentiated squamous epithelium and glands lined by mucus-secreting epithelium in a collagenous stroma. Cysts arising from rests of Gartner's duct and inclusion cysts are more common than the benign tumors.

Secondary carcinoma is the most common malignant tumor in the vagina, but epithelial dysplasia, carcinoma in situ, squamous cell carcinoma, clear cell adenocarcinoma, embryonal rhabdomyosarcoma, leiomyosarcoma, and rarely verrucous carcinoma, basal cell carcinoma, mixed müllerian tumor, alveolar soft part sarcoma, synovial sarcoma, or melanoma can arise in the vagina. Rarely, an endodermal sinus tumor develops in the vagina in a child.

Inclusion Cyst. Inclusion cysts are most common in the posterior vagina near the introitus. They are usually less than 2 cm in diameter and result from the implantation of squamous epithelium into the subepithelial connective tissue, usually during childbirth. The cyst is lined by squamous epithelium and contains the cheesy material resulting from the desquamation of the epithelial cells.

Fibroepithelial Polyp. Fibroepithelial polyps are usually single and less than 1.5 cm across. Macroscopically, they show multiple, finger-like projections. Microscopically, they are covered by intact vaginal epithelium and consist of loose collagenous tissue. In 50% of the patients, large atypical cells are present in the collagenous tissue. Mitoses are few. Excision cures.

Vaginal Intraepithelial Neoplasia. Vaginal intraepithelial neoplasia, or VAIN, constitutes less than 0.5% of the intraepithelial neoplasia of the female reproductive tract. It occurs in 0.3 women per 100,000.

The lesions are often multiple. They are not evident macroscopically. Usually the diagnosis is made when part of the vagina is removed during a hysterectomy for some other disease. In 80% of the patients, the hysterectomy is for intraepithelial neoplasia or invasive carcinoma of the cervix uteri. About 3% of the patients have carcinoma of the vulva. The lesions are similar to those of intraepithelial neoplasia in the cervix.

Squamous Cell Carcinoma. Squamous

cell carcinoma of the vagina makes up 1% of the malignant tumors of the female reproductive tract. In the United States, 1 woman in 100,000 develops a carcinoma of the vagina. Over 75% of the patients are over 50 years old.

Macroscopically and microscopically, a squamous cell carcinoma of the vagina resembles a squamous cell carcinoma of the cervix uteri. The tumors invade locally and metastasize to the lymph nodes in the pelvis and groins, only occasionally more distantly.

Vaginal carcinomata are usually treated by irradiation. If the tumor is confined to the vagina, 90% of the patients will be alive five years later. If it has extended beyond the vagina but has not reached the pelvic wall, 50% live five years. If it has extended further, only 20% of the patients will be alive five years later.

Clear Cell Adenocarcinoma. Clear cell carcinoma of the vagina and cervix uteri is an uncommon tumor that occurs in patients 7 to 30 years old. Fewer than 1000 cases have been reported.

In 50% of the patients, the tumor arises in the upper vagina. In the remainder, it is in the cervix or involves both the cervix and

vagina. Some tumors are small and are found only by microscopy; some are 10 cm across. The larger tumors may be flat, indurated, and ulcerated or may form a polypoid mass. Microscopically, the carcinoma resembles the clear cell carcinomata of the ovaries and endometrium. It may consist of sheets of cells with clear cytoplasm, but more often forms glands or cysts lined by hobnail or flattened cells. Parts of the tumor sometimes have an endometrioid pattern or form glands lined by cuboidal cells with eosinophilic cytoplasm.

A clear cell carcinoma of the vagina or cervix invades locally and metastases by the lymphatic and blood vessels. Metastases in the pelvic lymph nodes are found in 15% of patients with tumors confined to the muscularis of the vagina or cervix, and in 50% of those with tumors that penetrate beyond the wall of the vagina or cervix. Metastases in the supraclavicular lymph nodes or lungs are present in 40% of the patients in whom the tumor recurs.

In 60% of the patients, the patient's mother was given diethylstilbesterol, hexestrol, or dinestrol during pregnancy to reduce the risk of miscarriage, though less than 0.2%

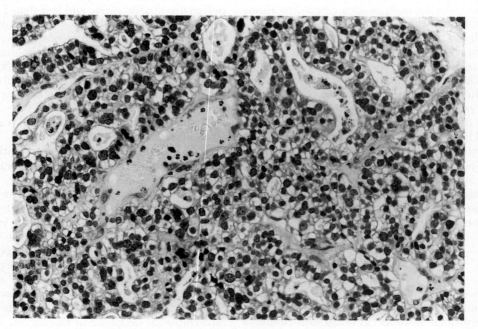

Fig. 41-53. A clear cell adenocarcinoma of the vagina.

of women exposed to these drugs in utero develop a clear cell carcinoma of the cervix or vagina. In another 10% of the patients, the mother was given a drug of unknown nature to reduce the risk of miscarriage. In 30% of the patients, there is no history of exposure to estrogen in utero.

Most of the tumors in patients not exposed to estrogen in utero arise in the cervix, probably from the endocervical glands. In the women exposed to estrogen in utero, the tumor may arise in the cervix or from the adenosis common in the vagina in these people.

Clear cell carcinomata of the vagina and cervix are treated like other cervical or vaginal carcinomata. About 80% of the patients survive five years. If the tumor recurs, it usually does so within three years.

Embryonal Rhabdomyosarcoma. Embryonal rhabdomyosarcoma, also called sarcoma botryoides, is the commonest tumor of the vagina in girls. Over 90% of the patients are under five years old; 70% are less than

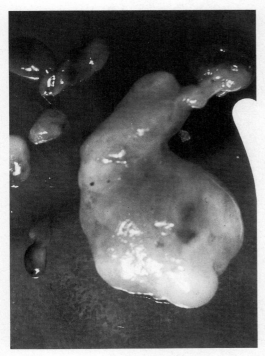

Fig. 41-54. An embryonal rhabdomyosarcoma of the vagina, showing a polypoid mass projecting into the vagina.

two years old. The term *botryoides* is from the Greek for grapes and describes the macroscopic appearance of the tumor.

The sarcoma forms a bulky tumor, with smooth, glistening polypoid masses, which fill the vagina and often protrude through the introitus. The masses look myxomatous, like nasal polyps, and may be red or grayish.

Microscopically, the polypoid masses are covered by intact vaginal epithelium and consist of loose, myxomatous connective tissue. Immediately under the epithelium, the connective tissue becomes much more cellular, with elongated, spindle-shaped cells, which may be atypical. Some of the tumor cells show cross striations, though prolonged search may be necessary before the cross striations are found.

Sarcoma botryoides of the vagina invades extensively and metastasizes to the pelvic lymph nodes. More distant metastases are late in most patients. The prognosis is bad. In spite of surgical excision, irradiation, and chemotherapy, fewer than 50% of the patients live five years.

Secondary Tumors. The vagina is involved in 50% of patients with carcinoma of the cervix, usually by direct extension of the tumor. Less often metastatic deposits of cervical carcinoma result from lymphatic permeation or implantation on the surface of the vagina. Metastases are present in the vagina in 10% of patients with endometrial carcinoma and 20% of those with an endometrial choriocarcinoma. Carcinoma of the ovaries, kidneys, and other organs occasionally metastasize to the vagina. Carcinoma of the vulva can involve the vagina by direct extension.

Vulva

Non-neoplastic cysts of the vulva are common. They include Bartholin's cysts, epidermal cysts like those found in other parts of the skin, mucinous cysts lined by columnar mucus-secreting epithelium formed from obstructed vestibular glands, mesonephric cysts derived from wolffian rests, and cysts lined by mesothelium derived from remnants of the canal of Nuck.

The most frequent benign tumors of the

vulva are condylomata and papillary hidradenomata, but any tumors that occur in the skin can develop in the skin of the vulva, among them the skin tag called an acrochordon, clear cell hidradenoma, syringoma, keratocanthoma, seborrheic keratosis, and the various forms of pigmented nevus. Occasionally an hemangioma, angiokeratoma, hemangiopericytoma, leiomyoma, rhabdomyoma, granular cell tumor, neurofibroma or some other form of benign mesenchymal tumor is found in the vulva.

Intraepithelial neoplasia, Paget's disease, squamous cell carcinoma, verrucous carcinoma, adenocarcinoma, and rarely a basal cell carcinoma can arise in the vulva. Occasionally a leiomyosarcoma, a rhabdomyosarcoma, or some other form of sarcoma develops in the vulva. Malignant melanoma can originate in the vulva. Secondary tumors rarely involve the vulva.

Bartholin's Cyst. Obstruction to the duct of one or both of Bartholin's glands causes a Bartholin's cyst, as the gland becomes dilated by its mucoid secretions. The obstruction sometimes causes pain on coitus when the gland is stimulated to secrete. If necessary, the cyst can be marsupialized.

Condyloma. Each year, over 1,000,000 women in the United States develop condylomata on the vulva, the adjacent skin, the perineum, upper thighs, or around the anus. The incidence is increasing. In 50% of the patients, there are also condylomata on the cervix uteri or in the vagina.

The condylomata of the vulva and adjacent regions are usually warty lesions that project above the surface. They are frequently

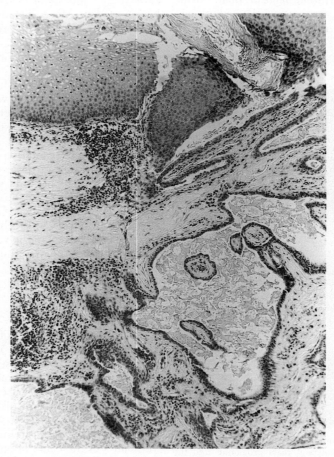

Fig. 41-55. A Bartholin's cyst, showing dilated ducts beneath intact vulvar epithelium.

numerous and vary from the microscopic to several centimeters across. This kind of condyloma is called a condyloma acuminatum, acuminatum from the Latin *acuminatus*, pointed.

Microscopically, a condyloma acuminatum has short, coarse fronds covered by thick squamous epithelium. Often, the epithelium bulges down into the underlying tissue. In most condylomata, the epithelium is orderly and differentiates normally, though mitoses may be present in the basal part of the epithelium. Hyperkeratosis and parakeratosis are usually prominent. In the superficial part of the epithelium, koilocytotic cells with their pyknotic nuclei and empty perinuclear halos are common. The nuclei in the cells are usually diploid or polyploid.

The condylomata of the vulva are a venereal infection caused by the human papilloma viruses. Type 6 is the most commonly isolated, but types 1, 11, 16, and 35 can cause vulvar condylomata.

Condylomata of the vulva sometimes regress. If not, the lesions can be destroyed by applications of podophyllin, electrodessication, cryosurgery, or using a laser beam. Recurrence or reinfection is common. In a few patients, a condyloma acuminatum has progressed to vulvar intraepithelial neoplasia.

Hidradenoma Papilliferum. Hidradenoma papilliferum is a tumor named from the Greek for sweat. With few exceptions, it occurs only on or near the labia majora. Hidradenomata papillifera are not found before puberty and are rare except in white women.

A hidradenoma forms a subcutaneous nodule about the size of a pea, sometimes with red tumor prolapsing through an opening on the skin. Microscopically, the hidradenoma is well circumscribed. It shows some combination of ducts set in fibrous tissue and cysts filled with complex fronds. The ducts and cysts may be lined by a single layer of cuboidal or columnar epithelium, but more often the epithelium has two layers, like the epithelium of the duct of a gland.

Hidradenomata prolifera arise from the apocrine glands present in the labia. With rare exceptions, they are benign and are cured by excision.

Vulvar Intraepithelial Neoplasia. Vulvar intraepithelial neoplasia, called VIN, includes dysplasia, carcinoma in situ, and Paget's disease of the vulva. It is becoming more common in women 20 to 35 years old, though less than 2% of the intraepithelial neoplasias of the reproductive tract involve the vulva. About 50% of the patients have an intraepithelial or invasive neoplasm in some other part of the reproductive tract, most often intraepithelial neoplasia of the cervix uteri.

The lesions are often multiple. They form pink, white, or pigmented plaques or papules that often become confluent. Sometimes the lesions are itchy. Except in the patients with Paget's disease, the lesions are similar to those of intraepithelial neoplasia of the cervix uteri, showing mild, moderate, or severe dysplasia or carcinoma in situ. They show similar atypicality and disorder, though the lesion often has large cells with keratinization and intracellular bridges. Parakeratosis is often prominent on the surface of the lesions. Koilocytes are rarely present. The nuclei are aneuploid.

Vulvar intraepithelial neoplasia lesion regresses in 5% of untreated patients. In many, it persists with little change for 10 or more years. It progresses to invasive carcinoma in 5%. A human papilloma virus can be demonstrated in the lesion in 90% of the patients. Local excision controls the disease.

Paget's Disease. Paget's disease is named after the English surgeon Sir James Paget (1814–1899). It is most frequent in the areola of the nipples but occasionally occurs in the vulva or elsewhere in the milk line. In the vulva, the lesion in the epithelium is similar to that in the breast, with large, pale cells scattered singly or in clumps in the epithelium. The cells stain for neutral and acid mucopolysaccharides and for the carcinoembryonic antigen, but not for dopa. By electron microscopy, they may resemble apocrine cells, eccrine cells, or keratinocytes.

In the breast, an invasive carcinoma nearly always underlies Paget's disease of the nipple. In the vulva, an underlying adenocarcinoma arising from the apocrine or Bartholin's glands is sometimes present, but in 80% of the patients there is no underlying malignancy. It is believed that Paget's disease of the vulva is a type of intraepithelial neoplasia caused by abnormal differentiation of the basal cells of the vulvar epithelium.

Untreated, vulvar Paget's disease slowly becomes more extensive. The lesions are excised locally. Recurrence is not uncommon, perhaps because the lesions are often irregularly shaped or multifocal.

Squamous Cell Carcinoma. About 5% of malignant tumors of the female reproductive tract, less than 1% of all malignant tumors in women, arise in the vulva. In the United States, less than 2 women in 100,000 develop carcinoma of the vulva. The patients are almost all over 50 years old. The older the woman, the greater the risk of developing carcinoma of the vulva.

Lesions. Squamous cell carcinoma of the vulva arises on the labia in 90% of the patients and involves the clitoris in 10%. In 10% of the patients, there is more than one tumor. Occasionally, there are kissing cancers, symmetrically placed carcinomata, one on each side. At first, the carcinoma produces an area of induration without ulceration, but as it enlarges to 2 cm or more across, it usually forms an ulcer with hard, raised edges. Less often, the carcinoma forms a protruding mass.

Microscopically, 90% of squamous cell carcinomata of the vulva are well differentiated, with prominent intercellular bridges and keratinization. Poorly differentiated spindle cell or giant cell carcinomata are uncommon. Occasionally an adenosquamous carcinoma is found.

Behavior. For a long time, perhaps for years, carcinoma of the vulva remains superficial, but if untreated it eventually invades the vagina and other underlying structures. By the time the carcinoma is discovered, 50% of the patients have metastases in the regional lymph nodes in the inguinal region, usually on both sides. Often the carcinoma has spread to the deep inguinal or external iliac nodes. Hematogenous metastases are unusual. A few of the patients develop hypercalcemia.

Staging. The International Federation of Gynecologists and Obstetricians divides carcinoma of the vulva into four clinical stages.

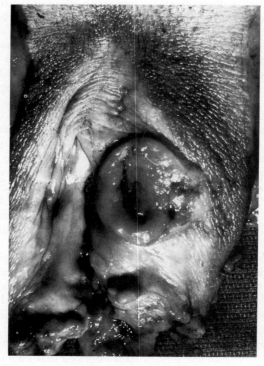

Fig. 41-56. Carcinoma of the vulva.

In stage I, the tumor is less than 2 cm across and there are no suspicious lymph nodes in the groins. In stage II, it is more than 2 cm across, but there are no suspicious lymph nodes in the groins. In stage III, some of the lymph nodes in the groins are suspicious, or the carcinoma has spread beyond the vulva by local invasion. In stage IV, the lymph nodes in the groin contain carcinoma, or there are more distant metastases.

The term *suspicious* is used to describe lymph nodes that suggest involvement by carcinoma, but chronic lymphadenitis cannot be excluded. About 10% of the lymph nodes thought clinically to contain carcinoma prove to be free of tumor, and 20% of those thought to be free of tumor harbor small metastases.

A microinvasive form of squamous cell carcinoma of the vulva called stage Ia is defined as a carcinoma of stage I that does not penetrate more than 1 mm and invades at one site only. It is thought that tumors of stage Ia metastasize rarely. If the carcinoma penetrates 3 mm, 12% of the patients have metastases in the lymph nodes in the groin. If it penetrates 5 mm, 15% have metastases.

Pathogenesis. The relationship of car-cinoma of the vulva to the human papilloma viruses is not clear. The incidence of cervical and vaginal carcinoma is greater in women with a squamous cell carcinoma of the vulva. The incidence of carcinoma of the vulva was increased in textile workers whose clothes became soaked in lubricating oil.

Treatment and Prognosis. If the car-cinoma is microinvasive, local excision may suffice. If it is more advanced, radical re-moval of the carcinoma and dissection of the lymph nodes in both groins is required. If the lymph nodes are free of tumor, 90% of the patients survive five years. If the lymph nodes involved are confined to the groins, 60% live five years. If more distant lymph nodes are involved, 20% survive five years.

Verrucous Carcinoma. Verrucous car-cinomata of the vulva are warty lesions that stand above the skin like large condylomata. Microscopically, large, rounded extensions of the carcinoma invade the underlying tissues. The tumor cells are highly differentiated. The tumor invades slowly, and metastasizes only late in its course. Human papilloma virus 6 can be isolated from most verrucous car-cinomata of the vulva. Less often, another of

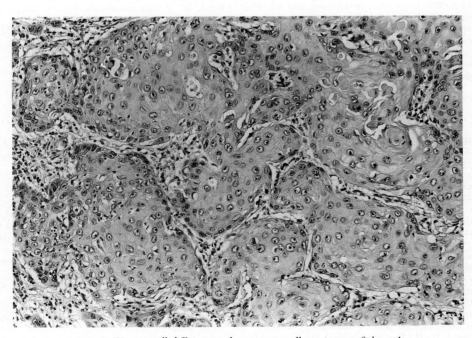

Fig. 41-57. A well-differentiated squamous cell carcinoma of the vulva.

the human papilloma viruses is found. Local excision usually cures. Radiation makes the tumor more aggressive and more dangerous.

Adenocarcinoma. Adenocarcinoma of the vulva is rare. It can arise in a Bartholin's gland, Skene's gland, or from the sweat glands in the labia. Only 50% of the malignant tumors arising in a Bartholin's gland are adenocarcinomata. Most of the rest are squamous cell carcinomata. A few are adenoid cystic tumors, adenosquamous carcinoma, or some other form of carcinoma. After radical excision, 30% of the patients with carcinoma of a Bartholin's gland survive five years.

BIBLIOGRAPHY

General

Blaustein, A.: Interpretation of Endometrial Biopsies, 2nd ed. New York, Raven Press, 1985.

Burghardt, E. (trans. Östör, A. G.): Colposcopy Cervical Pathology. New York, Thieme-Stratton, 1984.

Dallenbach-Hellweg, G. (trans. Dallenbach, F. D.): Histopathology of the Endometrium, 3rd ed. New York, Springer Verlag, 1981.

Fox. H. (Ed.): Haines and Taylor, Obstetrical and Gynaecological Pathology, 3rd ed. Edinburgh, Churchill Livingstone, 1987.

Friedrich, E. G., Jr.: Vulvar Disease, 2nd ed. Philadelphia, W. B. Saunders Co., 1983.

Kurman, R. J. (Ed.): Blausteins's Pathology of the Female Genital Tract, 3rd ed. New York, Springer-Verlag, 1987.

Wilkinson, E. J. (Ed.): Pathology of the Vulva and Vagina. New York, Churchill Livingstone, 1987.

Inflammation

Burnakis, T. G., and Hildebrandt, N. B.: Pelvic inflammatory disease. Rev. Infect. Dis., 8:86, 1986.

Cooper, M. D., and Jeffery, C.: Scanning and transmission electron microscopy of bacterial attachment to mucosal surfaces. Scan. Electron Microsc., (Pt. 3): 1183, 1985.

Corey, L., and Spear, P. G.: Infections with herpes simplex viruses. N. Engl. J. Med., 314:686, 749–757, 1986.

Duff, P.: Pathophysiology and management of postcesarian endomyometritis. Obstet. Gynecol., 67:269, 1986.

Gibbs, R. S., Blanco, J. D., and Bernstein, S.: Role of anaerobic bacteria in endometritis after cesarian section. Rev. Infect. Dis., 7(Suppl. 4):S690, 1985.

Gondos, B., and Riddick, D. H.: Pathology of Infertility. New York, Thieme Medical Publications, 1987.

Handsfield, H. H.: Recent developments in gonorrhea

and pelvic inflammatory disease. J. Med., 14:281, 1983.

Hill, L. V., and Embil, J. A.: Vaginitis. Can. Med. Assoc. J., 134:321, 1986.

Newton, W., and Keith, L. G.: Role of sexual behavior in the development of pelvic inflammatory disease. J. Reprod. Med., 30:82, 1985.

Nilsen, A.: Herpes genitalis. Scand. J. Infect. Dis. (Suppl), 47:51, 1985.

Rapp, F.: The challenge of herpesviruses. Cancer Res., 44:1309, 1984.

Snavely, S. R., and Liu, C.: Clinical spectrum of Herpes simplex virus infections. Clin. Dermatol., 2:8, 1984.

Sobel, J. D.: Epidemiology and pathogenesis of recurrent vulvoaginal candidiasis. Am. J. Obstet. Gynecol., 152:924, 1985.

Swenson, R. M.: Herpes simplex virus genital infections. Clin. Ther., 8:145, 1986.

Wasserheit, J. N., and Holmes, K. K.: Sexually transmitted diseases in women. Emerg. Med. Clin. North Am., 3:47, 1985.

Weström, L., and Mårdh, P.-A.: Current views on the concept of pelvic inflammatory disease. Aust. N.Z. J. Obstet. Gynaecol., 24:98, 1984.

Wildy, P.: Herpes viruses. Br. Med. Bull., 41:339, 1985.

Endometriosis, Adenomyosis, and Endosalpingosis

Bergqvist, A., Ljungberg, O., and Myhre, E.: Human endometrium and endometriotic tissue obtained simultaneously. Int. J. Gynecol. Pathol., 3:155, 1984.

Boyd, M. E.: Endometriosis. Can. J. Surg., 28:471, 1985.

Egger, H., and Weigmann, P.: Clinical and surgical aspects of ovarian endometriotic cysts. Arch. Gynecol., 133:37, 1982.

Other Non-neoplastic Diseases

Coney, P.: Polycystic ovarian disease. Fertil. Steril., 42: 667, 1984.

Ferenczy, A., Gelfand, M. M., and Tzipris, F.: The cytodynamics of endometrial hyperplasia and carcinoma. Ann. Pathol., 3:189, 1983.

Fienberg, R.: Thecosis. Pathol. Annu., 16(Pt. 2):239, 1981.

Fox, H., and Buckley, C. H.: Pathology of female infertility. Rec. Adv. Histopathol., 11:119, 1981.

Fox, H., and Buckley, C. H.: The endometrial hyperplasias and their relationship to endometrial carcinoma. Histopathology, 6:493, 1982.

Futterweit, W.: Polycystic Ovarian Disease. New York, Springer Verlag, 1984.

Hewitt, J.: Lichen sclerosus. J. Reprod. Med., 31:781, 1986.

Hopwood, N. J.: Pathogenesis and management of abnormal puberty. Spec. Top. Endocrinol. Metab., 7: 175, 1985.

Lobo, R. A.: Disturbances of androgen secretion and

metabolism in polycystic ovary syndrome. Clin. Endocrinol. Metab., 15:229, 1986.

Mechanick, J. L., and Futterweit, W.: The aberrant puberty hypothesis of polycystic ovarian disease. Mt. Sinai J. Med., 53:310, 1986.

Molta, L., and Schwartz, U.: Gonadal and adrenal androgen secretion in hirsute females. Clin. Endocrinol. Metab., 15:229, 1986.

Morris, D. V.: Hirsutism. Clin. Obstet. Gynaecol., 12: 649, 1985.

Root, A. W., and Shulman, D. I.: Isosexual precocity: current concepts and recent advances. Fertil. Steril., 45:749, 1986.

Tumors

Andreasson, B., Bock, J. E., Strom, K. V., and Visfeldt, J.: Verrucous carcinoma of the vulvar region. Acta Obstet. Gynaecol. Scand., 62:183, 1983.

Andreasson, B., and Bock, J. E.: Intraepithelial neoplasia in the vulvar region. Gynecol. Oncol., 21:300, 1985.

Aurelian, L.: Herpes simplex virus type 2 and cervical cancer. Clin. Dermatol., 2:90, 1984.

Bell, J., Averette, H., Davis, J., and Toledano, S.: Genital rhabdomyosarcoma. Obstet. Gynecol. Surv., 41:257, 1986.

Berget, A., and Lenstrup, C.: Cervical intraepithelial neoplasia. Obstet. Gynaecol. Surv., 40:545, 1985.

Blaustein, A.: Surface (germinal) epithelium and related ovarian neoplasms. Pathol. Annu., 16(Pt. 1):247, 1981.

Brescia, R. J., Jenson, A. B., Lancaster, W. D., and Kurman, R. J.: The role of human papillomaviruses in the pathogenesis and histologic classification of precancerous lesions of the cervix. Hum. Pathol., 17: 552, 1986.

Buckley, C. H., Butler, E. G., and Fox, H.: Vulvar intraepithelial neoplasia and microinvasive carcinoma of the vulva. J. Clin. Pathol., 37:1201, 1984.

Cangir, A.: Malignant genital tract tumors in children. Curr. Probl. Cancer, 10:301, 1986.

Christopherson, W. M., and Richardson, M.: Uterine mesenchymal tumors. Pathol. Annu., 16(Pt. 1):215, 1981.

Dallenbach-Hellweg, G. (Ed.): Cervical cancer. Curr. Top. Pathol., 70:3, 1981.

Donato, D. M., Sevin, B. U., and Averette, H. E.: Neoplastic pericarditis and gynecologic malignancies. Obstet. Gynecol. Surv., 41:473, 1986.

Dvoretsky, P. M., and Bonfiglio, T. A.: The pathology of vulvar squamous cell carcinoma and verrucous carcinoma. Pathol. Annu., 21(Pt. 2):23, 1986.

Dyall-Smith, D., and Varigos, G.: Human papillomaviruses and cancer. Australas. J. Dermatol., 26:102, 1985.

Fenoglio, C. M., et al.: Herpes simplex virus and cervical neoplasia. Prog. Surg. Pathol., 4:45, 1982.

Ferenczy, A.: Cytodynamics of endometrial hyperplasia and carcinoma. Prog. Surg. Pathol., 4:95, 1982.

Ferenczy, A., Gelfand, M. M., and Tzipris, F.: The cytodynamics of endometrial hyperplasia and carcinoma. Ann. Pathol., 3:189, 1983.

Fox, H.: Endometrial carcinogensis and its relation to oestrogens. Pathol. Res. Pract., 179:13, 1984.

Franceschi, S., La Vecchia, C., and Talamini, R.: Oral contraceptives and cervical neoplasia. Tumori, 72:21, 1986.

Freeman, D. A.: Steroid hormone-producing tumors in man. Endocr. Rev., 7:204, 1986.

Hanjani, P., Petersen, R. O., Lipton, S. E., and Nolte, S. A.: Malignant mixed mesodermal tumors and carcinosarcoma of the ovary, Obstet. Gynecol. Surv., 38: 537, 1983.

Hausen, H. Z.: Herpes simplex virus in human genital cancer. Int. Rev. Exp. Pathol., 25:307, 1983.

Hays, D. M.: Malignant solid tumors of childhood. Curr. Probl. Surg., 23:161, 1986.

Hoffman, M., Roberts, W. S., and Cavanagh, D.: Second pelvic malignancies following radiation therapy for cervical cancer. Obstet. Gynecol. Surv., 40:611, 1985.

Holck, S., and Laursen, H.: Oral contraceptives and cancer. Arch. Geschwulstforsch., 56:155, 1986.

Horwitz, R. I., and Feinstein, A. R.: Estrogens and endometrial cancer. Am. J. Med., 81:503, 1986.

Huggins, G. R., and Zucker, P. K.: Oral contraceptives and neoplasia. Fertil. Steril., 47:733, 1987.

Iversen, O. E., and Laerum, O. D.: Ploidy differences in endometrial and ovarian carcinomas. Anal. Quant. Cytol. Histol., 7:327, 1985.

Johnston, G. A., Klotz, J., and Boutselis, J. G.: Primary invasive carcinoma of the vagina. Surg. Gynecol. Obstet., 156:34, 1983.

Kodama, M., and Kodama, T.: Relation between steroid metabolism of the host and genesis of cancers of the breast, uterine cervix, and endometrium. Adv. Cancer Res., 38:77, 1983.

McCance, D. J.: Human papillomaviruses and cancer. Biochim. Biophys. Acta, 823:195, 1986.

McCaughey, W. T. E.: Papillary peritoneal neoplasms in females. Pathol. Annu., 20(Pt. 2):387, 1985.

McCaughey, W. T. E., Kannerstein, M., and Churg, J.: Tumors and Pseudotumors of the Serous Membranes. Washington, D.C., Armed Forces Institute of Pathology, 1985.

Meisels, A., Morin, C., Casas-Cordero, M., and Rabreau, M.: Human papillomavirus (HPV) veneral infections and gynecologic cancer. Pathol. Annu., 18(Pt. 2):277, 1983.

Morrow, G. P., and Smart, G. E. (Eds.): Gynecological Oncology. Berlin. Springer-Verlag, 1985.

Okagaki, T.: Female genital tumors associated with human papillomavirus infection. Pathol. Annu., 19 (Pt. 2):31, 1984.

Rapp, F.: The challenge of herpesviruses. Cancer Res., 44:1309, 1984.

Roth, L. M.: Application of electron microscopy to diagnosis in gynecologic neoplasms and tumorlike conditions. Ultrastruct. Pathol., 9:131, 1985.

Roth, L. M., and Czernobilsky, B. (Eds.): Tumors and Tumorlike Conditions of the Ovary. New York, Churchill Livingston, 1985.

Schellhammer, P. F., Jordan, G. H., and El-Mahdi, A. M.: Pelvic complications after interstitial and external beam irradiation of urologic and gynecologic malignancy. World J. Surg., 10:259, 1986.

Scully, R. E.: Tumors of the Ovary and Maldeveloped Gonads. Washington, D.C., Armed Forces Institute of Pathology, 1979.

Silverberg, S. G.: Significance of squamous elements in carcinoma of the endometrium. Prog. Surg. Pathol., 4:115, 1982.

Smith, K. T., and Campo, M. S.: Papillomaviruses and their involvement in oncogenesis. Biomed. Pharmacother., 39:405, 1985.

Steeper, T. A., and Mukai, K.: Solid ovarian teratomas. Pathol. Annu., 19(Pt. 1):81, 1984.

Syrjänen, K. J.: Human papillomavirus (HPV) infections of the female genital tract and their associations with intraepithelial neoplasia and squamous. Pathol. Annu., 21(Pt. 1):53, 1986.

Talerman, A.: Germ cell tumours. Ann. Pathol., 5:145, 1985.

Troche, V., and Hernandez, E.: Neoplasia arising in dysgenetic gonads. Obstet. Gynecol. Surv., 41:74, 1986.

Truong, L. D., et al.: Endodermal sinus tumor of the mediastinum. Cancer, 58:730, 1986.

Turner, W. A., Gallup, D. G., Talledo, O. E., and Otken, L. B. Jr.: Neuroendocrine carcinoma of the uterine cervix complicated by pregnancy. Obstet. Gynecol., 67(3 Suppl.):80S, 1986.

Walker, A. N.: Unusual variants of uterine cervical carcinoma. Pathol. Annu., 22(Pt. 1):277, 1987.

White, P. F., Merino, M. J., and Barwick, K. W.: Serous surface papillary carcinoma of the ovary. Pathol. Annu., 20(Pt. 1):403, 1985.

Young, R. H., and Scully, R. H.: Ovarian sex cord-stromal tumors. Int. J. Gynecol. Pathol., 1:101, 1982.

Young, R. H., and Scully, R. H.: Ovarian Sertoli-Leydig cell tumors. A clinicopathological analysis of 207 cases. Am. J. Surg. Pathol., 9:543, 1985.

Zaloudek, C. J., and Norris, H. J.: Mesenchymal tumors of the uterus. Prog. Surg. Pathol., 3:1, 1981.

42

Pregnancy

IT is surprising that so complicated and complex a process as pregnancy so rarely causes difficulty, particularly since most diseases of pregnancy involve two people: the fetus with its membranes and placenta and the mother who harbors and nourishes it. Not only must infection, malformation, immunologic dysfunction, and tumors be considered but also the interaction between the tissues of two different people.

The disorders of pregnancy that affect principally the fetus are abortion, ectopic gestation, and the diseases of the placenta. Toxemia, eclampsia, hyperemesis gravidarum, disseminated intravascular coagulation, pulmonary embolism, and tumors, especially the tumors of the trophoblast, affect principally the mother. Fatty liver of pregnancy is discussed with the diseases of the liver in Chapter 36.

ABORTION

The term *abortion*, from the Latin for a miscarriage, is used to describe the end of a pregnancy before the fetus is independently viable. A spontaneous abortion results from natural causes, without outside interference. An induced abortion is caused by outside interference, for therapeutic or other reasons.

SPONTANEOUS ABORTION. Spontaneous abortion ends 40% of pregnancies, perhaps more, because spontaneous abortion early in pregnancy easily passes unnoticed. Most spontaneous abortions occur in the first three months of the pregnancy.

Lesions. In most spontaneous abortions, the abortion is complete. The fetus dies in utero and is passed per vaginam. The decidua is shed, and normal menstrual cycles resume. No part of the fetus or its placenta remains in the uterus.

In a threatened abortion, partial disruption of the placenta causes vaginal bleeding. The condition may progress to complete or incomplete abortion, but in many women the bleeding is temporary and the pregnancy can be saved.

If fragments of the fetus or placenta remain in the uterus, the abortion is incomplete. Fragments of chorionic villi or fetal parts remain, embedded in the endometrium. Often the retained tissues are necrotic, and the surrounding endometrium is acutely inflamed. Occasionally the remnants become fibrotic or form a placental polyp. The risk of puerperal infection, shock, and disseminated intravascular coagulation is increased.

If the dead fetus is not discharged from the uterus, it may degenerate and disappear or may persist in the uterus with its placenta and membranes. Sometimes the fetus and placenta form a fleshy mass called a carneous mole, from the Latin for flesh and a shapeless mass. Occasionally the fetus becomes mummified or calcified.

Clinical Presentation. The death of the fetus and breakdown of the decidua usually cause vaginal bleeding. The later in the pregnancy the abortion occurs, the more profuse the bleeding is likely to be. Sometimes contractions of the uterus are painful, dilatation of the cervix is evident, or recognizable parts of the fetus or placenta are passed. If the abortion is complete, the bleeding stops and normal menstruation is reestablished. If it is incomplete, irregular bleeding and discharge usually continue. Normal menstruation is not reestablished.

Pathogenesis. Spontaneous abortion is most often caused by an abnormality in the fetus, sometimes by a maternal disorder, and sometimes by a combination of maternal and fetal abnormalities.

Especially in the early weeks of pregnancy, most spontaneous abortions are caused by a chromosomal abnormality in the fetus.

Trisomies are found in 50% of the fetuses that have been examined, triploidy in 20%, and monosomy X in 15%. Tetraploidy, translocations, double trisomy, and mosaicism are less frequent. The earlier in pregnancy the abortion occurs, the more bizarre the chromosomal derangements are likely to be.

Some women who have repeated spontaneous abortions lack an IgG blocking antibody found in the plasma of normal pregnant women. The antibody is thought to facilitate the implantation of the placenta. In other women who suffer spontaneous abortions, the anticoagulant called the circulating lupus anticoagulant is present in the plasma and may interfere with placentation.

Placental abnormalities, infarction, premature separation, faulty placement, syphilis, and placental tumors can cause spontaneous abortion. Premature rupture of the fetal membranes is another cause. The umbilical cord can become knotted or twisted, killing the fetus. Rarely, fatal fetal ischemia results from a hematoma in the umbilical cord or a tumor of the cord.

Maternal rubella, cytomegalic inclusion disease, toxoplasmosis, and other maternal infections can cause a spontaneous abortion. High fever can do so. Maternal heart failure or severe maternal anemia causes fetal hypoxia and abortion. Direct trauma can destroy a fetus. Toxic drugs given to the mother and radiation to the uterus can injure the fetus. Another cause is malformation of the uterus or its distortion by fibroids.

Deficient production of progesterone by the ovaries prevents implantation of the ovum. Failure of the placental trophoblast to secrete proper quantities of gonadotropin, progesterone, and estrogen can stunt fetal growth and bring miscarriage.

Treatment and Prognosis. Complete abortion needs no treatment. Threatened abortion is treated conservatively to preserve the pregnancy. Incomplete abortion requires emptying of the uterus to restore normal menstruation.

INDUCED ABORTION. When an abortion is induced in a hospital before the sixteenth week of conception, the uterine cavity is curetted, often using suction to remove completely the products of conception. If the pregnancy is further advanced, instillation of prostaglandins into the amniotic sac or other techniques are more often used. The uterus is completely emptied. Complications and disability are uncommon.

Criminal abortion can cause major injury. Dangerous substances are sometimes given by mouth or through the vagina. Attempts to pass an instrument or foreign body into the uterus can perforate the uterus or vagina, causing hemorrhage, shock, or peritonitis. A foreign body is sometimes passed by mistake into the urinary bladder. An attempt to inject fluid into the uterus can cause air embolism or allow anisotonic fluid to enter the blood, causing massive hemolysis. Lack of asepsis frequently causes infection. Infection of the fallopian tubes commonly causes salpingitis and sterility.

ECTOPIC PREGNANCY

If a fertilized ovum implants other than in the endometrium, the pregnancy is said to be ectopic. Though the incidence varies in different parts of the world, about 1% of pregnancies are ectopic. Nearly 0.1% of ectopic pregnancies are bilateral. In one pregnancy in 30,000, both an intrauterine pregnancy and an ectopic gestation occur.

In over 95% of ectopic pregnancies, the ovum implants in one of the fallopian tubes. Less often an ovum implants in an ovary, elsewhere in the peritoneal cavity, in the cervix uteri, or in an isolated horn of a malformed uterus. If an ectopic pregnancy initially in a tube ruptures into the peritoneal cavity or into a broad ligament, the fetus may continue to grow in its new position.

TUBAL PREGNANCY. Anything that impedes the movement of the ovum along the tube favors tubal implantation and tubal pregnancy. The trophoblast develops a week or so after ovulation, when the fertilized ovum should be in the uterine cavity and ready to implant there. If the ovum is still in the fallopian tube, it is likely to implant in the tube instead.

Lesion. In 80% of tubal pregnancies, the ovum lodges in the broad, ampullary part of the fallopian tube. In 15%, it embeds in the isthmus of the tube. In 5%, the ectopic pregnancy is in the fimbriated end of a tube. In

55% of the patients, the ectopic gestation is in the right tube.

When an ovum implants in a tube, the trophoblast penetrates into the wall of the tube, exciting a local decidual reaction. The arteries near the site of implantation show intimal thickening, with foam cells in the thickened intima. In 60% of the patients, the tubal epithelium shows a focal proliferation of pale cells with atypical nuclei, similar to the Arias-Stella phenomenon seen in the endometrium in pregnancy.

As the fetus and placenta grow, the tube dilates and its wall grows thinner. If the ectopic gestation is in the ampulla or the fimbriated end of the tube, the tube usually ruptures after 8 weeks. If it is in the isthmus, it ruptures after 12 weeks. The rupture causes intraperitoneal hemorrhage, often massive. The fetus is extruded into the peritoneal cavity and usually disappears. The wall of the tube shows hemorrhage and occasional chorionic villi.

Rarely, the placenta extruded from a ruptured tube implants on the surface of the peritoneum or in the broad ligament, and the fetus continues to grow. Occasionally a peritoneal pregnancy reaches term, but more often hemorrhage separates the placenta from the underlying tissue, and the fetus dies.

In some patients, hemorrhage detaches the placenta from the wall of the tube before the tube ruptures. The fetus and placenta die and are extruded into the lumen of the tube. They may be resorbed and disappear or may pass through the fimbriated end of the tube into the peritoneal cavity and be lost. Rarely, a carneous mole develops in a fallopian tube, or a fetus in a tubal pregnancy is mummified or calcified. A calcified fetus is called a lithopedion, from the Greek words for stone and child. Rarely, the placenta is reimplanted on the surface of the peritoneum, and the fetus continues to grow.

Usually, the uterus grows larger as an ectopic pregnancy advances. Its endometrium nearly always shows decidual changes, like those of a normal pregnancy. If the uterus is curetted while the ectopic fetus is still alive, the decidua re-forms. When the ectopic fetus and its trophoblast die, the decidua is shed within a few days, sometimes as a cast of the uterine cavity, more often in fragments. Normal endometrium re-forms.

In 60% of women with a tubal pregnancy, the endometrium shows foci of atypical hyper-

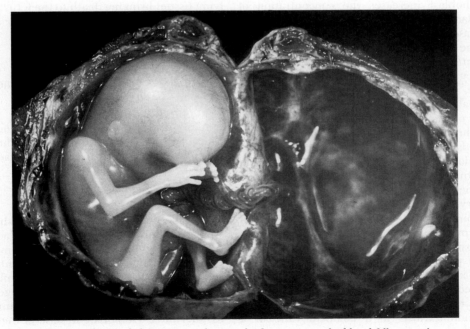

Fig. 42-1. A tubal pregnancy, showing the fetus in a greatly dilated fallopian tube.

plasia, as it often does in a normal, intrauterine pregnancy or in patients with a trophoblastic tumor. This kind of hyperplasia is called the Arias-Stella reaction, after the Peruvian pathologist who described it in 1954. The endometrial glands are irregular, with much papillary infolding. They are lined by tall, columnar cells, with abundant, clear cytoplasm and large, atypical nuclei, often at the luminal margin of the cells. In places, the epithelium is more than one layer thick, and the arrangement of its cells is disorderly. If severe, the hyperplasia can mimic a clear cell carcinoma of the endometrium. In a few patients with an ectopic pregnancy, the endometrium continues to show its normal cyclical progression from the proliferative to the secretory phase.

Clinical Presentation. Some patients with a tubal pregnancy have amenorrhea and other signs of pregnancy. Many have irregular uterine bleeding. In some, the menses continue. Bleeding into the tube often causes attacks of lower abdominal pain. Rupture of the tube causes more massive hemorrhage and more severe pain, sometimes with hypovolemic shock, leukocytosis, and jaundice. If the blood reaches the diaphragm, it causes pain in the shoulder tip. The proliferating trophoblast increases the concentration of human chorionic gonadotropins in the plasma. Ultrasonic examination often reveals a mass in the tube.

Pathogenesis. Most often, a tubal pregnancy is caused by distortion of the fallopian tube, which slows the passage of the ovum and allows it to implant in the tube. In over 50% of the patients, the distortion is caused by chronic salpingitis. Less often, the distortion is caused by a tumor, adhesions, or a previous operation. Occasionally, diverticula of a tube delay the passage of an ovum, as can inefficient tubal contractions or inefficient ciliary action.

Sometimes the corpus luteum develops in one ovary, while the ovum implants in the opposite tube. In this case, the ovum must have passed across the peritoneal cavity to implant in the contralateral tube or must have passed across the uterine cavity, from one tube to the other.

Endometriosis in a fallopian tube or a decidual reaction caused by an intrauterine pregnancy may make a tube more receptive to a developing ovum and a tubal pregnancy more likely. If the ovum is too mature, the risk of implantation in a tube increases. If it is too immature, it may reach the endometrium but fail to implant and later be washed into a tube during menstruation.

Treatment and Prognosis. A tubal pregnancy is treated surgically, by salpingotomy or salpingectomy, to control the bleeding and to remove the conceptus. In the rare ectopic pregnancies that go to term, the child must be delivered surgically, but often the placenta and membranes are left behind, because of the massive hemorrhage that can follow an attempt to remove them.

About 10% of women who suffer a tubal pregnancy develop a second ectopic pregnancy. If the affected tube is preserved, the risk rises to 15%. Most of the distortions of the fallopian tubes that favor development of a tubal pregnancy are incurable and bilateral, explaining why repeated tubal pregnancies are common.

OTHER KINDS OF ECTOPIC PREGNANCY. Other kinds of ectopic pregnancy behave much as do tubal pregnancies. The fetus usually survives for a few weeks. Then hemorrhage separates the placenta from the underlying tissue, bringing death to the fetus. Only rarely has an abdominal pregnancy or a cervical pregnancy gone to term.

DISORDERS OF THE PLACENTA, AMNION, AND UMBILICAL CORD

Many diseases affect the amnion and umbilical cord as well as the placenta. They are considered with the diseases of the placenta.

Placenta

The placenta is often abnormally shaped. In placenta previa, it is abnormally placed in the uterus. In placenta accreta, it invades the myometrium. In abruptio placentae, it separates prematurely. Thrombosis, infarcts, hematomata, and cysts can damage the placenta. Infection can cause chorioamnionitis or villitis. Hemolytic disease of the newborn and diabetes mellitus sometimes injure the placenta. Occasionally a placenta is partially calcified.

MALFORMATION. In 3% of pregnancies, there are two or more separate discs of placental tissue instead of the single plate usually found. Most often, a small disc, called a succenturiate lobe, from the Latin for substitute, is adjacent to the main part of the placenta, but separate from it. The succenturiate lobe is sometimes attached to the larger part of the placenta by a thin isthmus of chorion, sometimes only by the fetal membranes. The umbilical cord usually inserts into the larger disc. The arteries and veins supplying the succenturiate lobe run from the main part of the placenta to the accessory lobe, often in the membranes. Occasionally there is more than one succenturiate lobe.

If the two parts of the placenta are approximately the same size, the placenta is said to be bilobate or bipartite. The umbilical cord usually inserts between the lobes. Rarely, a placenta is multilobate, with three or more equally sized parts.

Placenta extrachorialis is also common. In this condition, the placenta is bigger than its chorionic plate for some or all of its circumference, so that the membranes arise from the surface of the placenta, not from its margins. Two kinds of placenta extrachorialis are distinguished. In placenta marginata, the membranes arise from the edge of the chorionic plate in the usual way. In placenta circumvallata, from the Latin words for around and rampart, the membranes are folded back on themselves and appear to arise a short distance within the chorionic plate. The folded membranes make the edge of the chorionic plate appear thick.

Other malformations of the placenta are uncommon. In a ring placenta, the central part of the placenta is membranous, leaving only an outer rim of villous parenchyma. A fenestrate placenta has holes in which the villi and sometimes the chorionic plate are missing. In placenta membranacea, the placenta is large and thin, with villi covering almost the whole surface of the fetal membranes.

In 70% of placentas, the insertion of the umbilical cord into the placenta is eccentric. In 10%, the cord inserts into the margin of the placenta, an anomaly called a battledore placenta. In 1%, the cord inserts into the membranes, some distance from the placenta,

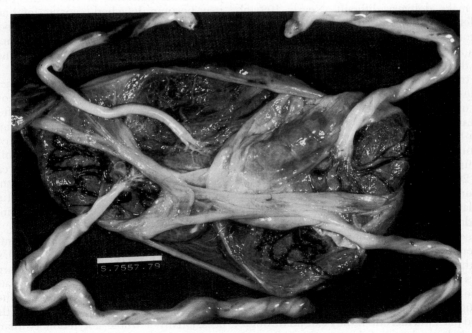

Fig. 42-2. A placenta from a woman with quadruplets, showing the irregularly shaped placenta and the four umbilical cords.

and vessels from the cord ramify across the membranes to reach the placenta. Insertion into the membranes is called velamentous, from the Latin for a veil.

Most malformations of the placenta cause no dysfunction. Occasionally the vessels in the membranes are torn during delivery in patients with a succenturiate lobe, placenta bilobata, or velamentous insertion of the umbilical cord. Placenta extrachorialis increases the risk of premature separation of the placenta. The birth weight of children born to women with a placenta extrachorialis is often low.

PLACENTA PREVIA. In placenta previa, from the Latin for going before, the placenta implants in the lower uterine segment, sometimes partially or completely across the cervical os. Placenta previa occurs in 1 pregnancy in 200.

In 50% of women with placenta previa, the fetus is abnormally placed, most often transversely or obliquely. Sometimes the fetus is poorly oxygenated or nourished. The abnormally placed placenta often becomes separated from the uterine wall after the 30th week of pregnancy, causing painless vaginal bleeding. The abnormal site of the placenta can make delivery difficult. Nearly 10% of the fetuses and 0.1% of their mothers die from hemorrhage. About 10% of the fetuses are born alive and malformed.

If the bleeding is not too severe, conservative treatment can often save the pregnancy. It the fetus is sufficiently mature, early delivery, usually by cesarean section, is indicated.

PLACENTA ACCRETA. In placenta accreta, from the Latin for to fasten to, the placenta is unusually firmly fixed to the wall of the uterus. Estimates of its frequency vary from 1 in 2000 pregnancies to 1 in 70,000.

Normally, the placenta tears free through the large sinuses in the spongy layer of the decidua. In placenta accreta, this basal layer of decidua is missing in all or part of the placenta. The placental villi invade the myometrium, which is separated from the muscle fibers only by fibrin or a little collagenous tissue. If the microvilli extend only part way through the myometrium, the condition is called placenta increta. If they extend through the whole thickness of the myometrium, it is called placenta percreta.

In up to 60% of patients with placenta accreta, the placenta is implanted in the lower uterine segment, or only the part of the placenta in the lower uterine segment is abnormal. In some, the abnormal adherence occurs after a cesarean section. Many of the patients have had several previous deliveries or have some injury or malformation of the uterus.

The fetus usually develops normally, but at delivery the placenta fails to separate. In some of the patients, the abnormal placenta can be removed manually. In many, hysterectomy is necessary.

ABRUPTIO PLACENTAE. Premature separation of the placenta after the twentieth week of gestation is called abruptio placentae, from the Latin for to tear apart. It occurs in 1% of pregnancies. Delivery usually follows rapidly.

Abruptio placentae usually causes vaginal bleeding, sometimes minor but sometimes massive and exsanguinating. Less often, the hemorrhage is concealed, forming a hematoma beneath the central part of the placenta, or is confined to the uterus by the fetal membranes. The separation may affect only a small part of the placenta, or the entire placenta may become detached, causing fetal anoxia. If the bleeding is extensive, the blood infiltrates the myometrium and sometimes extends into the broad ligaments and the retroperitoneum.

In 30% of the patients, abruptio placentae causes few if any symptoms and is discovered only when the placenta is examined after delivery. If the bleeding is severe, the mother may develop hypovolemic shock, and hypoxia can imperil the life of the fetus. Disseminated intravascular coagulation is sometimes caused by the escape of thromboplastin into the circulation. Renal cortical necrosis, renal tubular injury, or infarction of the pituitary gland can follow.

INFARCTION. Infarcts of the placenta are present in 25% of placentas at term. Usually they are multiple and occur at the margin of the placenta. Less often, they are scattered within the placenta. Most infarcts of the placenta are small, 0.5 to 5.0 cm across, though occasionally a whole cotyledon is infarcted. At first the infarcts are wedge-shaped and dark red, but as they age, they become brown, yellow, and at last white. Calcification is common in old infarcts, and sometimes one becomes cystic. Microscopically, the micro-villi in young infarcts are crowded together and are necrotic. Often an infiltrate of neutro-phils is evident. In older lesions, only the ghosts of the villi remain. Fibrosis and repair do not occur. Thrombus may develop at the margin of the infarct, or if the infarct involves the chorionic plate, the overlying fetal vessels may be thrombosed. Unless the infarcts are unusually large, they cause no dysfunction.

Placental infarcts result from a disturbance in the maternal blood supply from the decidua. Occlusion of fetal vessels does not cause in-farction in the placenta. Infarction of the placenta is particularly common in women who have hypertension diabetes, or toxemia of pregnancy. The underlying arterioles in the decidua show changes like those of hyper-tension elsewhere, with medial hyalinization, smudging, and even necrosis. Sometimes large fat-filled cells are prominent in their intima.

THROMBOSIS. Intervillous thrombosis oc-curs in the blood space between the chori-onic villi in from 20 to 50% of placentas. One or more red thrombi develop, usually in the midpart of the placenta. The thrombi are most often 1 to 2 cm in diameter, but may be smaller or much larger. They push the adjacent villi apart. After a few days, the red cells in the thrombus lyse, and the thrombus grows pale, until only a white, laminated mass of fibrin remains. The villi adjacent to the thrombus lose their tropho-blast and atrophy, but no organization of the fibrin occurs. Some think that leakage of fetal blood triggers the thrombosis, even though the thrombus is comprised mainly of the maternal blood that fills the intervillous space. Others think that the thrombus results from injury to the decidua, and the leakage of fetal blood into the thrombus is secondary.

Foci of perivillous fibrin are deposited in 20% of full-term placentas. In the regions involved, large quantities of fibrin separate the villi, which become avascular and atro-phic. The syncytiotrophoblast disappears, but the cytotrophoblast covering the en-trapped villi sometimes proliferates and ex-tends into the fibrin. The cause of perivillous fibrin deposition is unknown. It causes no dysfunction.

Subchorionic fibrin deposits are similar to the perivillous deposits, except that they

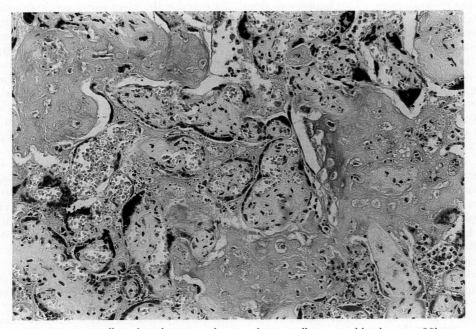

Fig. 42-3. Intervillous thrombosis in a placenta, showing villi separated by deposits of fibrin.

occur against the chorionic plate and contain no villi.

Thrombosis of a fetal artery occurs in 5% of pregnancies. It causes avascularity and hyalinization of the villi affected, usually with prominent syncytiotrophoblastic knots. It causes no dysfunction.

Massive subchorial thrombosis occurs in 0.05% of pregnancies. A thrombus at least 1 cm thick separates the chorionic plate from the placental villi and involves most of the placenta. The lesion is sometimes found in the placenta of a live-born child; sometimes it causes fetal death.

HEMATOMA. A retroplacental hematoma develops between the basal plate of the placenta and the decidua in 5% of pregnancies. It is particularly common in patients with preeclampsia. The part of the placenta overlying the heamtoma is infarcted. If the hematoma is small, it usually does not harm. If it is large, it can cause fetal death or abruptio placentae.

A marginal hematoma occurs where the placenta joins the fetal membranes. It is flattened and often extends into the membranes. Microscopically, the hematoma is usually outside the placenta and causes mild, acute inflammation. Occasionally it is within the intervillous space. The hematoma does not cause the infarction seen with retroplacental hematomata. It causes no dysfunction.

A subamniotic hematoma occurs between the amniotic membrane and the chorionic plate. It causes no dysfunction.

TWIN-TWIN TRANSFUSION SYNDROME. The twin-twin transfusion syndrome develops in 20% of monochorionic twin pregnancies. If the syndrome is severe, one twin is small, pale, and anemic while the other is heavier, edematous, and polycythemic. The organs are larger and heavier in the bigger twin. The heart is hypertrophied in the bigger twin, atrophic in the smaller. In diamniotic twins, the larger twin often has hydramnios, the smaller oligohydramnios. The imbalance between the twins is caused by the diversion of blood from the smaller twin to the larger through anastomoses in the part of the placenta they share.

Both twins are at risk. The mortality may reach 70%. Over 30% of deaths in mono-chorionic twins are caused by the twin-twin transfusion syndrome.

ACARDIA. Acardia develops in 1% of monozygotic twin gestations. One of the twins is severely malformed, with no heart. The other is normal. Blood flow in the acardiac twin is reversed. Blood from the normal twin passes through anastomoses that join the placental arteries of the twins to enter the acardiac twin through the umbilical artery. The blood leaves the acardiac twin through the umbilical vein, and reenters the circulation of the normal twin through anastomoses between the placental veins of the two twins.

FETUS PAPYRACEUS. If one twin dies early in a twin gestation, the dead twin is compressed against the membranes as the other twin grows. It becomes shrunken and flattened, eventually forming an amorphous mass of necrotic tissue. The dead twin is called a fetus papyraceus, from the Latin for paper.

CYST. A cyst is present in 10% of placentas. Usually there is only one, and it is small and easily overlooked. Occassionally a cyst is several centimeters in diameter. Cysts arise in the septa of the placenta and, if large, bulge onto its fetal surface, near the insertion of the umbilical cord. They are linked by flattened cells. They cause no dysfunction.

CHORIOAMNIONITIS. Inflammation of the chorion and amniotic membranes is called chorioamnionitis. Its frequency varies greatly from one part of the world to another. It is most common in the chorion and membranes of infants delivered prematurely. In the United States, almost all spontaneous abortions that occur at 20 weeks of gestation have chorioamnionitis, but less than 10% of pregnancies at term.

Chorioamnioinitis, which is due to infection ascending from the cervix and vagina, begins in the lower part of the uterus. First comes a neutrophilic exudate in the decidua. Acute inflammation extends to the chorionic plate and amniotic membranes. Neutrophils escape into the amniotic fluid, and often the fluid becomes infected. After the twenty-sixth week of gestation, foci of inflammation in the umbilical cord are common, a condition called funisitis from the Latin for cord. Sometimes the skin, eyes, or ears of the fetus are infected, or inhalation of infected amniotic fluid causes fetal pneumonitis or gastroenteritis. Bacteremia in the fetal blood can cause hematogenous infection in the fetus. Macroscopically, the placenta and the membranes usually look normal, but sometimes the chorion and membranes are cloudy or opaque.

The neutrophils come principally from the maternal blood, though if the infection occurs after the twentieth week of gestation fetal neutrophils are also present. The inflammation around the fetal vessels is greatest on the amniotic side of the vessel.

Chorioamnionitis is most common in patients with premature rupture of the membranes, though it is often not clear whether the rupture causes the infection or the infection causes the rupture. In many patients the infection is caused by gram-negative bacteria, most often Escherichia coli, Proteus, Klebsiella, or Pseudomonas. In some, it results from staphylococcal, streptococcal, mycoplasmal, or chlamydial infection. Group B β-hemolytic streptococci sometimes infect the membranes without causing inflammation.

Chorioamnionitis severe enough to cause fever in the mother increases by 50% the perinatal mortality in premature infants. If the mother remains afebrile, chorioamnionitis does not increase perinatal mortality.

VILLITIS. Inflammation of the placental villi is called villitis. In the United States and the United Kingdom, it occurs in 10% of pregnancies.

Villitis is usually multifocal. The chorion and membranes are usually normal. The affected villi can show any of a variety of changes: chronic inflammation, with an exudate of lymphocytes and plasma cells; vasculitis, with a similar exudate; foci of necrosis, with acute or granulomatous inflammation; organizing thrombi in the blood vessels in the villi; an increased number of vessels in the villi; granulation tissue and fibrosis; or only old scarring.

In most patients with villitis, the cause of the inflammation is unknown. In a minority of the patients, it is caused by viral, bacterial, or toxoplasmal infection carried in the maternal blood. Cytomegaloviruses and rubella are the most important viral causes, but herpes simplex, vaccinia, variola, varicella, coxsackievirus B, and hepatitis B can infect the placenta. Treponema pallidum and Listeria monocytogenes are among the more common bacteria causing villitis. Less often, tuberculosis, brucellosis, tularemia, or leprosy involves the villi. Toxoplasmosis is the only protozoal infection likely to cause villitis.

In most patients, villitis is found only after the delivery of a normal child. In a few, especially when it is caused by a known agent, villitis contributes to fetal death.

Cytomegaloviral Villitis. In 10% of the patients, villitis is caused by a cytomegalovirus. The villi affected usually show focal infiltrates of lymphocytes and plasma cells, vasculitis and hemosiderosis, less often necrosis, or scarring and calcification. Viral inclusions are present in endothelial cells, Hofbauer cells, and the trophoblast, but are usually few.

Rubella. At the time of infection, rubella causes multifocal necrotizing villitis and vasculitis. Eosinophilic, intracytoplasmic inclusion bodies are sometimes present in the endothelium, Hofbauer cells, stromal cells, or trophoblast. Foci of chronic inflammation are common in the membranes and umbilical cord. As the infection persists, both necrotic and scarred villi are present. Eventually the placenta becomes small with widespread scarring of the villi.

Syphilis. Syphilitic villitis is now uncommon in most of the world. If it is severe, the placenta is enlarged, pale, and friable. The villi are large, and their vessels show intimal and perivascular fibrosis. A patchy exudate of lymphocytes and plasma cells is present. Treponemata can often be demonstrated in the lesions. The fetus usually shows other signs of syphilitic infection.

Listeriosis. In listeriosis, the villi involved contain abscesses, usually with a neutrophilic exudate and sometimes surrounded by a palisade of macrophages. Occasionally the abscesses are big enough to be visible macroscopically. Nearly always chorioamnionitis and funisitis are also present. Lesions in the fetus are common. Abortion and fetal death are likely.

Toxoplasmosis. In toxoplasmosis, the placenta is usually large and edematous. The villi are swollen, with a patchy exudate of lymphocytes. Occasionally, a villus shows vasculitis or necrosis. The umbilical cord is often involved. The organisms are usually hard to find. The fetus is infected in 50% of the patients if the infection is acquired early in pregnancy, but rarely if the infection is contracted late in pregnancy. If the fetus is severely affected, the lesions of congenital toxoplasmosis become evident soon after birth.

HEMOLYTIC DISEASE OF THE NEWBORN.   In hemolytic disease of the newborn, also called erythroblastosis fetalis, maternal antibodies against the fetal red cells cause severe hemolytic anemia in the fetus. The cause and effects of the disease are discussed in Chapter 49.

If hemolytic disease of the newborn is severe, the placenta is large, bulky, friable, edematous, and pale yellowish white. It may weigh as much as 2 kg. Often the placenta is extrachorial. Commonly the fetal membranes and umbilical cord are also edematous. Usually the umbilical cord and amnion are stained yellow by bile excreted into the amniotic fluid in the fetal urine.

Microscopically, the placental villi are large and edematous. Their blood vessels are prominent, usually at the margin of the villi, and are choked with fetal blood with nucleated red cells. Hofbauer cells are often prominent in the villi. Well-formed cytotrophoblast persists to term, often with many mitoses. Intervillous thrombosis is evident in 50% of the patients.

DIABETES MELLITUS.   In diabetic mothers, the placenta tends to be heavier than normal. The severity of the placental changes varies greatly from one diabetic mother to another. Even if there is severe retinopathy or nephropathy, the placental changes may be slight.

The changes in the placenta are similar to those of hemolytic disease of the newborn. The placental villi are large and edematous, and their vessels are congested, with many nucleated red cells. The trophoblast retains its two layers and often shows mitoses, even at term. The trophoblastic basement membrane is thickened. Intervillous thrombosis is common.

CALCIFICATION.   Foci of calcification in the placenta are common at term. At times the calcification is extensive, but it causes no dysfunction.

Amnion

The quantity of amniotic fluid is sometimes abnormal. Nodules develop on the amnion in amnion nodosum and squamous metaplasia. Occasionally adhesions cross the amnion or bind the fetus to the amnion.

HYDRAMNIOS.   If there is more than 2000 mL of amniotic fluid, the patient is said to have hydramnios. This condition is common in multiple pregnancies, severe hemolytic disease of the newborn, severe diabetes mellitus, and fetal anomalies. The cause is obscure. The fluid is usually normal in composition.

OLIGOHYDRAMNIOS.   If there is too little amniotic fluid, the condition is called oligohydramnios. It is less common, but occurs when there is renal agenesis in the fetus or when there is urinary obstruction in the fetus, suggesting that fetal urine is important in maintaining the quantity of the amniotic fluid.

AMNION NODOSUM.   Amnion nodosum is an unusual condition found when there is serious oligohydramnios. Small yellowish nodules are scattered over the amniotic membrane and can sometimes be picked off it. The nodules consist of vernix, with epidermal cells and hair enmeshed in it. The nodules may lie on top of the epithelium or be covered by it.

SQUAMOUS METAPLASIA.   Small gray or white plaques are often seen on the surface of the amniotic membrane and are called squamous metaplasia. A few show squamous metaplasia microscopically, but most show only focal epithelial hyperplasia.

ADHESIONS.   Adhesions between the amnion and the fetus are uncommon, as are bands running across the amniotic cavity. They sometimes cause fetal abnormalitis, most often deformity or amputation of a limb.

Umbilical Cord

The umbilical cord can be too long, too short, cystic, or have abnormal vessels.

ABNORMAL LENGTH.   The umbilical cord varies from 20 to 120 cm in length, with a mean of 50 cm. If the cord is long, it sometimes spirals or loops around the fetus or becomes knotted, occluding the umbilical vessels and killing the fetus. A short umbilical cord tends to cause abruptio placentae, inversion of the uterus, or hemorrhage into the cord, again imperiling the life of the fetus.

CYSTS. Remnants of the allantoic duct or the omphalomesenteric duct occasionally give rise to epithelium-linked cysts in the cord. More often an excess of Wharton's jelly forms a mucoid cyst without an epithelial lining.

VASCULAR ANOMALIES. In 1% of deliveries, there is only one artery in the umbilical cord. In spontaneous abortions and twins, 3% of umbilical cords have only one artery. In over 30% of the fetuses, other congenital anomalies are present. The birth weight is low. Over 20% of the infants die in the perinatal period. Maternal diabetes mellitus increases the risk of developing the anomaly.

Thrombosis is common in the arteries and veins that ramify across the chorionic plate. The thrombi rarely organize. Rarely, a hematoma develops in the cord. If the hematoma is large, 50% of the infants die in the perinatal period.

PREECLAMPSIA AND ECLAMPSIA

In preeclampsia, sometimes called toxemia of pregnancy, the patients develop hypertension and edema, proteinuria, or both after the twentieth week of gestation. If the condition is more severe, with convulsions or coma, it is called eclampsia, from the Greek for to flash forth. If the patient has only hypertension, edema, or proteinuria, the condition is called gestational hypertension, gestational edema, or gestational proteinuria. Table 42-1 shows a classification of the hypertensive states of pregnancy.

In the United States, toxemia of pregnancy is evident in 7% of pregnancies. In other parts of the world, the incidence varies from 2% of pregnancies in the Far East to 30% in Puerto Rico. Toxemia is more common in the first pregnancy than in subsequent ones, though its frequency rises in mothers over 35 years old. In Scotland, nearly 25% of women developed hypertension during their first pregnancy, but only 8% in subsequent pregnancies. Twins, diabetes mellitus, hy-

TABLE 42-1. HYPERTENSIVE STATES OF PREGNANCY

Gestational disorders
  Gestational edema
  Gestational proteinuria
  Gestational hypertension

Acute disorders
  Preeclampsia
  Eclampsia

Chronic disorders
  Hypertension unrelated to pregnancy

dramnios, and hydatidiform mole increase the risk of toxemia. It is more common in black women than in white. Daughters of women who had eclampsia are at greater risk.

Lesions. Little is known of the lesions in gestational hypertension, gestational edema, gestational proteinuria, or in the milder forms of preeclampsia. The hypertension, edema, or proteinuria are mild, and recovery is usual within 10 days of delivery. If the disorder is more severe, lesions are more prominent in the kidneys, liver, brain, and placenta. Less often the heart, adrenal glands, lungs; or pituitary gland are involved.

The renal lesions of preeclampsia and eclampsia are described in Chapter 27. They affect principally the glomeruli. The endothelium in the glomerular tufts swells. The space between the glomerular endothelium and its basement membrane widens. Fibrin is deposited in the subendothelial space. Lesions of this kind can be found in about 70% of patients with toxemia. Their severity correlates well with the severity of the proteinuria.

The placenta is small in patients with severe preeclampsia and usually contains many large infarcts. In 15% of the patients, a retroplacental hematoma is present. The number of blood vessels in the chorionic villi is reduced. The trophoblast covering the villi is thick with many syncytiotrophoblastic knots. The fetal vessels in the chorionic plate are narrowed or occluded. The invasion of the maternal arteries in the myometrium by the intermediate trophoblast that normally occurs between the sixteenth and twentieth week of gestation is reduced or absent. Acute atherosis develops in the spiral arteries in the decidua and myometrium that are not invaded by trophoblast. Their intima is thickened and contains large, fat-filled macrophages. The media is necrotic. An exudate of lymphocytes and macrophages is present in the adventitia.

Clinical Presentation. Preeclampsia usually begins insidiously after the thirty-second week of gestation. Edema and hypertension come first in most patients, and proteinuria follows. The edema is not usually severe and must be distinguished from the water retention that always occurs during pregnancy. Edema of the eyelids or hands that develops late in pregnancy suggests toxemia. Both systolic and diastolic blood pressure is increased, but the increase is not often great. The proteinuria is usually between 1 and 10 g a day.

If preeclampsia is severe, the blood pressure is likely to exceed 160 mm Hg systolic and 110 mm Hg diastolic. Headache is usual. Often flashes of light, blindness, or other visual disturbances develop. Oliguria, epigastric pain, and vomiting are common. The convulsions and coma of eclampsia may follow.

Pathogenesis. The pathogenesis of preeclampsia is unknown. The plasma volume is probably lower than in a normal pregnancy, suggesting impairment of the retention of sodium and water. The peripheral vascular resistance is higher than in a normal pregnancy, suggesting that an abnormal vasoconstrictor is active. The dysfunction usually subsides promptly after delivery, suggesting that the placenta is at fault.

The placenta normally produces prostaglandins that cause vasodilation and renin. The ischemia caused by the vascular lesions in the decidua and placenta may disturb the balance between renin and the prostaglandins, reducing the absorption of sodium in the renal tubules and causing vasoconstriction.

The lesions in the kidneys and other organs are similar to those in disseminated intravascular coagulation. In most patients with preeclampsia, there is no evidence of abnormal coagulation, but in some, intravascular coagulation may share in the pathogenesis of the lesions.

The liver is involved in 70% of patients with eclampsia, but not in preeclampsia unless it is unusually severe. The liver shows scattered foci of hepatocellular necrosis and periportal or subcapsular hemorrhages. The necrosis and hemorrhage can be extensive.

The brain is affected in 60% of patients dying of eclampsia. Petechiae are frequently present in the cerebral cortex, often with thrombosis of adjacent vessels. Small infarcts a few millimeters across may be scattered throughout the brain. In the cerebral cortex, though rarely elsewhere, the infarcts are sometimes hemorrhagic. There may be more massive hemorrhage into the white matter, the basal ganglia, or the pons.

Occasionally, there are subendocardial hemorrhages in the heart, small hemorrhages in the lungs, or hemorrhages in the adrenal glands. Focal necrosis of the pituitary may occur. Hemolysis is evident in 10% of the patients.

Treatment and Prognosis. In most women with preeclampsia, the hypertension and other signs of the disease regress within two weeks of delivery, though the proteinuria may persist longer. If the blood pressure does not fall to its previous level within six months, the hypertension is probably due to some other cause. Essential hypertension may first become evident during pregnancy, or renal disease may mimic toxemia of pregnancy. Sometimes preeclampsia is superimposed on hypertension of some other type.

Subsequent pregnancies may be normal, but 25% of women who develop preeclampsia in their first pregnancy and 50% of multiparous women who have toxemia develop toxemia again in subsequent pregnancies. Whether toxemia increases the risk of developing hypertension later in life is disputed, but most think that it does so. In one study, 37% of women with toxemia followed for 12 or more years developed hypertension, but only 7% of pregnant women without toxemia.

If toxemia is severe, with convulsions or major neurologic dysfunction, the prognosis is bad, in spite of anticonvulsive and antihypertensive therapy and early emptying of the uterus. Up to 5% of the mothers and 20% of the fetuses die.

OTHER NON-NEOPLASTIC DISEASES

This section considers three unrelated conditions, hyperemesis gravidarum, disseminated intravascular coagulation, and pulmonary embolism.

HYPEREMESIS GRAVIDARUM. Hyperemesis gravidarum takes its name from the Greek words for over much and to vomit. Hyperemesis gravidarum is an accentuation of the nausea and vomiting common in pregnancy severe enough to cause electrolyte imbalance, weight loss, or ketosis. If uncontrolled, it can bring jaundice, hyperpyrexia, albuminuria, vitamin B deficiency, occasionally peripheral neuritis, encephalopathy, and even death. It occurs in 0.3% of pregnancies, usually between the eighth and twelfth weeks.

The excessive vomiting causes dehydration, hemoconcentration, and hypotension. Renal perfusion falls, causing azotemia. The loss of sodium, potassium, and chloride in the vomitus brings hyponatremia, hypokalemia, hypochloremia, and metabolic acidosis.

The cause of hyperemesis gravidarum is unknown. Hormonal, allergic, and psychologic factors have all been suggested. In 1930, the mortality was over 20%. Now, with good maintenance of electrolyte balance and nutrition, both mother and child nearly always survive.

DISSEMINATED INTRAVASCULAR COAGULATION. Disseminated intravascular coagulation is discussed in Chapter 53. It is a serious complication of many of the diseases of pregnancy. Premature separation of the placenta, death of the fetus in utero, amniotic fluid embolism, septic abortion, retained placenta, preeclampsia, and other complications of pregnancy can all cause intravascular coagulation.

PULMONARY EMBOLISM. Fragments of trophoblast can be found in the lungs in 50% of pregnant women. Usually they are small and soon disappear. Rarely, a trophoblastic embolus is large enough to cause pulmonary infarction. Occasionally, fragments of decidua are found in the lungs.

Amniotic fluid emboli are found in the lungs in 1 pregnancy in 25,000, usually after a tumultuous labor. Pulmonary arteries and arterioles are plugged with amniotic fluid or by the squamous cells, hairs, and vernix it contains. Often thrombus develops in or around the emboli. If the patient survives a few hours, a neutrophilic exudate develops in the obstructed vessels. Some patients have intravascular coagulation in other parts of the body.

If amniotic emboli are numerous in the lungs, they cause severe pulmonary edema and hemorrhage. The patients develop the acute respiratory distress syndrome. The dysfunction is probably due principally to the obstruction to the pulmonary blood flow caused by the emboli, but in some patients an anaphylactic response to the antigens in the amniotic fluid increases the dysfunction. If the emboli are widespread, 20% of the patients die within an hour, 80% after a few hours.

TUMORS

With the exception of the hemangiomata, the rare myxomata and myxosarcomata of the umbilical cord, and the tumors of the fetus, all the tumors of pregnancy occur in the placenta. The fetal tumors are described with the neoplasms of the organs affected. The tumors of the placenta are described here.

Hemangiomata are common in the placenta, but almost all the malignant tumors of the placenta arise from the trophoblast. Rarely, a teratoma arises in the placenta or a metastasis involves the placenta.

Four kinds of trophoblastic tumor are distinguished: hydatidiform mole, invasive mole, choriocarcinoma, and the placental site trophoblastic tumor. An exaggerated placental site tumor shows unusually extensive invasion of the endometrium or myometrium by trophoblast that is not neoplastic. The term *gestational trophoblastic disease* includes all four types.

HEMANGIOMA. A hemangioma of the placenta, sometimes called a chorioangioma, is found in 1% of placentas. Similar hemangiomata occur in the umbilical cord. The lesion is often small, but can be over 5 cm across. Sometimes more than one hemangioma is present. Microscopically, the lesion usually has well-differentiated blood vessels separated by loose connective tissue. Less often, poorly differentiated, spindle-shaped endothelial cells are clumped together. Occasionally the connective tissue between the vessels is myxomatous or hyalinized, or the tumor is partially necrotic or calcified.

Hydramnios is common in patients with a large hemangioma in the placenta and often causes premature delivery. Occasionally the fetus has cardiomegaly or congestive failure, perhaps because the hemangioma serves as a shunt.

HYDATIDIFORM MOLE. The hydatidiform mole is the most benign of the tumors of the trophoblast. In the United States, Europe, and Australasia, it occurs in less than 0.1% of pregnancies. The risk of developing a mole is higher in teenagers and in older women. In women over 35 years old, a mole develops in 0.3% of pregnancies; in women over 45 years old, in 3%. The term *hydatidiform* is from the Greek for a drop of water; *mole* is from the Latin for a shapeless mass.

The incidence of hydatidiform moles varies from one part of the world to another. In Mexico, a hydatidiform mole develops in 0.5% of pregnancies; in Paraguay, in 0.02%; in Hong Kong, Taiwan, Indonesia, and the Philippines, in from 1% to 0.5%; in Japan, in 0.2%; and in Nigeria, in 0.3%. The incidence is greatest in the poorer classes.

A previous spontaneous abortion increases the risk of developing a hydatidiform mole. About 1% of women who have had a complete mole develop another in a subsequent pregnancy. The more normal pregnancies a woman has had, the less likely she is to develop a hydatidiform mole.

Two types of hydatidiform mole are distinguished, complete and partial. In a complete mole, almost all the villi are abnormal and a fetus is rarely present. In a partial mole, only some of the villi are involved, and a fetus is often found. Both result from abnormal fertilization of the ovum and have an abnormal complement of chromosomes.

Cytogenetics. In a complete mole, the chromosomes are all derived from the father. Most are 46XX and result from the duplication of a 23X sperm in an ovum that lacks maternal chromosomes. About 10% are 46XY and are caused by the fertilization of an ovum that lacks maternal chromosomes by two sperm, one 23X and one 23Y.

Most partial moles are triploid. In 70%, the chromosomal complement is XXY; in 27%, XXX; and in 3%, XYY. Rarely, the mole is 46XX or is tetraploid. In the triploid moles, two thirds of the chromosomes are paternal. They are caused by the fertilization of a haploid ovum by two haploid sperm, or by the fertilization of a haploid ovum by a diploid sperm.

Lesions. About 70% of hydatidiform moles are complete; 30% are partial. Complete moles usually develop between the eleventh and twenty-fifth weeks of gestation, partial moles between the ninth and thirty-fourth weeks.

Complete Mole. In 70% of patients with a complete mole, the uterus is larger than would be expected. In some, it is small. The cavity of the uterus is filled by grapelike vesicles up to 3 cm in diameter filled with clear fluid and joined by thin, branching stalks. Occasionally a small, macerated fetus is present.

Microscopically, most of the villi in a complete mole are large, round, and edematous. Most are avascular. Often the center of some of the villi is acellular and consists only of a cistern of intercellular substance. Often some of the villi are calcified. In most patients, some or many of the villi are surrounded by a prominent proliferation of cytotrophoblast, intermediate trophoblast, and syncytiotrophoblast. Masses of atypical trophoblast often project into the intervillous blood spaces. In other patients, the trophoblastic proliferation is slight and apparent only in occasional villi. Immunohistochemically, the trophoblast stains strongly for human chorionic gonadotropins but weakly for human placental alkaline phosphatase.

Partial Mole. In a patient with a partial mole, the uterus is often smaller than would be expected. Macroscopically, some of the placental villi are cystic, though smaller than those in a complete mole. Part of the placenta appears normal. Often a fetus is present, but usually shows multiple congenital abnormalities.

Microscopically, some of the chorionic villi are of normal size. They may be fibrotic, but often show little abnormality. Other villi are enlarged and edematous, but not so markedly as in a complete mole. Central cisterns are not usually evident in the edematous villi. Often the margin of the swollen villi is scalloped. Trophoblastic proliferation is less than in a complete mole. Trophoblastic atypicality is rare. The trophoblast stains weakly for human chorionic gonadotropins but strongly for placental alkaline phosphatase.

Behavior. In most patients, a hydatidiform mole remains confined to the uterine cavity and is cured by emptying the uterus. In 15%, the lesion develops into an invasive mole; in 3%, into a choriocarcinoma. About 20% of women with a complete mole develop an invasive lesion, but less than 10% of those with a partial mole.

Clinical Presentation. Vaginal bleeding is commonly the first sign of a hydatidiform mole. It is usually more marked in patients with a complete mole. Occasionally fragments of the mole are passed. The unexpected enlargement of the uterus is evident in most women with a complete mole. The concentration of human chorionic gonadotropins in the plasma and urine is high in patients with a complete mole and usually low or normal in those with a partial mole. Ultrasonography reveals the edematous villi and the absence of a fetus in a complete mole, but is more difficult to interpret with a partial mole.

Complications. Preeclampsia develops in 25% of patients with a complete mole, usually in the first trimester of the pregnancy. It also is common in patients with a partial mole, but tends to begin later in the pregnancy. About 20% of patients with a mole develop hyperemesis gravidarum. Hyperthyroidism of unknown cause develops in 10%. In 20% of the patients, the ovaries are up to 30 cm across and contain multiple follicle cysts with prominent luteinization of the theca interna. In 2%, emboli of trophoblast in the lungs at the time of delivery are sufficiently numerous to cause the acute respiratory distress syndrome.

Treatment and Prognosis. A hydatidiform mole is removed, either surgically or by inducing expulsion medically. If the mole has been completely removed, the level of human chorionic gonadotropin in the plasma falls, usually reaching normal levels within two months. If it remains elevated, the patient probably has an invasive trophoblastic lesion. The complications caused by the mole resolve when it is removed.

INVASIVE MOLE. If a hydatidiform mole invades the myometrium, blood vessels, or extends beyond the uterus, it is called an invasive mole or, less often, a chorioadenoma

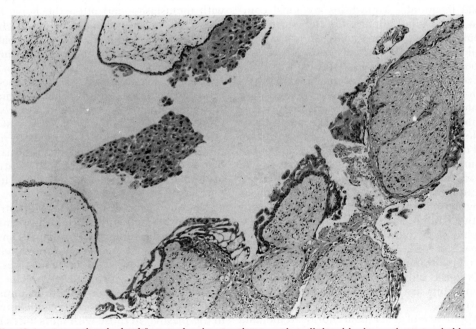

Fig. 42-4. A complete hydatidiform mole, showing the avascular villi lined by hyperplastic trophoblast.

destruens. About 15% of moles are of this type.

Lesions. The invasion of the myometrium is usually evident when a uterus containing an invasive mole is examined macroscopically. The tumor forms a ragged ulcer that extends into the myometrium. The invasion may be superficial or may extend through the whole thickness of the myometrium, sometimes with perforation of the uterus. The vesicles of the mole are often evident in the uterine cavity.

Microscopically, molar villi are present in the myometrium or in extrauterine tissues. The villi are usually less than 0.5 cm across and less edematous than those in an intrauterine hydatidiform mole. Atypical trophoblast is present around the villi. It is sometimes extensive, sometimes sparse.

Metastases are often confined to the blood vessels without invasion of the surrounding tissues. The lesions contain both trophoblast and villi, but frequently the villi are few and difficult to discover.

Behavior. Invasive moles invade locally and sometimes metastasize. The tumor is confined to the uterus in 70% of the patients when the diagnosis is made. In some, the tumor has spread to the vagina, vulva, or broad ligaments. Metastases are most common in the lungs. Before the introduction of chemotherapy, death usually came from the local extension of the disease. Metastases sometimes regress spontaneously.

Treatment and Prognosis. Most patients with persistent trophoblastic disease are treated by chemotherapy, without determining whether the patient has an invasive mole or a choriocarcinoma. Methotrexate and other drugs cause rapid regression of the tumor. Probably almost all patients with an invasive mole are cured.

CHORIOCARCINOMA. A choriocarcinoma is a highly malignant tumor of the trophoblast. In the United States and Europe, a choriocarcinoma develops in 1 pregnancy in 30,000. In parts of Asia, Africa, and South America, it develops in more than 1 pregnancy in 1000. In Nigeria, only carcinoma of the breast and cervix uteri are more common malignancies in women.

About 50% of gestational choriocarcinomata arise from a hydatidiform mole. Some 25% follow a spontaneous abortion. Over 20%

complicate an otherwise normal pregnancy. Less than 5% develop in an ectopic pregnancy. Occasionally a choriocarcinoma develops many years after the last pregnancy.

Lesions. One or more spheroidal, soft, hemorrhagic tumors usually occur in the myometrium of the uterus, often without any communication with the uterine cavity. Occasionally, no tumor can be found in the uterus, even though metastases are present.

Microscopically, a choriocarcinoma consists of sheets of atypical trophoblast. Cytotrophoblast, intermediate trophoblast, and syncytiotrophoblast can all be recognized. The tumor has no stroma. The malignant trophoblast invades the blood vessels in the surrounding tissues, causing hemorrhage into the tumor, which forms large sinusoids lined by ragged masses of trophoblast. Often most of the tumor is necrotic, with viable tissue present only at its margins. No villi are present in the tumor.

Behavior. A choriocarcinoma grows rapidly and metastasizes extensively. The vagina is involved in 20% of the patients. Metastases are often present when the diagnosis is made or appear within a few weeks. The lungs are involved in 90% of the patients with metastases, and often the liver, brain, and kidneys are affected. Before chemotherapy was introduced, 70% of the patients died within five years, most often of hemorrhage or respiratory failure.

Clinical Presentation. Vaginal bleeding is the most common sign of a choriocarcinoma. In some patients, hemoptysis or other symptoms or signs caused by metastases first draw attention to the tumor. Occasionally hyperthyroidism develops. The diagnosis is confirmed by demonstrating a high concentration of human chorionic gonadotropins in the plasma.

Treatment and Prognosis. Methotrexate and other chemotherapeutic drugs cause regression of the tumor and prolonged survival in 80% of patients with a gestational choriocarcinoma without evident metastases, and in 70% of those with metastases. The prognosis is worse in patients with an unusually high level of human chorionic gonadotropins in the plasma, in those with metastases in the brain, and in those developing a tumor after an otherwise normal pregnancy.

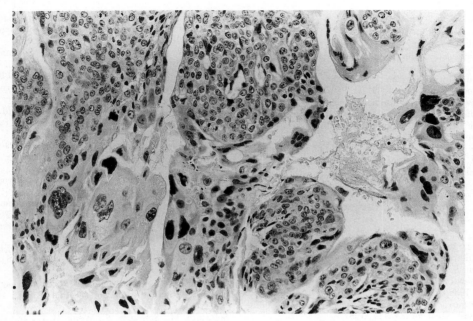

Fig. 42-5. A choriocarcinoma, showing the masses of cytotrophoblast and syncytiotrophoblast that line the blood spaces seen in this tumor.

PLACENTAL SITE TROPHOBLASTIC TUMOR. A placental site trophoblastic tumor is rare. It develops in the reproductive years. The uterus enlarges and macroscopically usually shows a well-defined tumor in the endometrium or myometrium. Occasionally the tumor invades the periuterine structures. It is soft, with little hemorrhage or necrosis.

Microscopically, the tumor consists of intermediate trophoblastic cells growing singly, in cords, or in sheets. Sometimes the trophoblastic cells are spindle-shaped. Vascular invasion is often prominent. The admixture of other types of trophoblastic cell seen in a choriocarcinoma is not present. Villi are not found. The tumor cells stain weakly for human chorionic gonadotropins but strongly for human placental lactogen.

Most placental site trophoblastic tumors are benign, but a few have invaded extensively and metastasized widely. The malignant tumors do not repond as well to chemotherapy as do choriocarcinomata.

EXAGGERATED PLACENTAL SITE. Exaggerated placental site was previously called syncytial endometritis. It describes a pregnancy that is normal except that the trophoblast, mainly intermediate trophoblast, penetrates more deeply into the myometrium than is normal. No treatment is needed.

BIBLIOGRAPHY

General

Fox, H.: Pathology of the Placenta. London, W.B. Saunders, 1978.

Fox, H.: Pathology of the placenta. Clin. Obstet. Gynaecol., *13*:447, 1986.

Gleicher, N.: Pregnancy and autoimmunity, Acta Haematol., *76*:68, 1986.

Kurman, R. J. (Ed.): Blaustein's Pathology of the Female Genital Tract, 3rd ed. New York, Springer-Verlag, 1987.

Lewis, J. E., Coulam, C. B., and Moore, S.B.: Immunologic mechanisms in the maternal-fetal relationship. Mayo Clin. Proc., *61*:655, 1986.

McIntyre, J. A., and Faulk, W. P.: Trophoblast antigens in normal and abnormal human pregnancy. Clin. Obstet. Gynecol., *29*:976, 1986.

Perrin, E. V. D. K. (Ed.): Pathology of the Placenta. New York, Churchill Livingston, 1984.

Redman, C. W.: Immunology of the placenta. Clin. Obstet. Gynecol., *13*:469, 1986.

Toder V., and Beer, A. E. (Eds.): Immunology and Immunopathology of reproduction. Contrib. Gynecol. Obstet., *14*:1, 1985.

Abortion

Beeley, L.: Adverse effects of drugs in the first trimester of pregnancy. Clin. Obstet. Gynaecol., 13:177, 1986.

Eschenbach, D. A.: Acute postpartum infections. Emerg. Med. Clin. North Am., 3:87, 1985.

Gondos, B., and Riddick, D. H.: Pathology of Infertility. New York, Thieme Medical Publications, 1987.

del Junco, D. J.: Association of autoimmune conditions with recurrent intrauterine death. Clin. Obstet. Gynecol., 29:959, 1986.

Lubbe, W. F., and Liggins, G. C.: Lupus anticoagulant and pregnancy. Am. J. Obstet. Gynecol., 153:322, 1986.

Ectopic Pregnancy

Chow, W. H., Daling, J. R., Cates, W. Jr., and Greenberg, R. S.: Epidemiology of ectopic pregnancy, Epidemiol. Rev., 9:70, 1987.

Corson, S. L., and Batzer, F. R.: Ectopic pregnancy. A review of the etiologic factors. J. Reprod. Med., 31:78, 1986.

Decherney, A. H. (Ed.): Ectopic pregnancy. Clin. Obstet. Gynecol., 30:117, 1987.

Edelman, D. A., and Porter, C. W.: The intrauterine device and ectopic pregnancy. Contraception, 36:85, 1987.

Hockberger, R. S.: Ectopic pregnancy. Emerg. Med. Clin. North Am., 5:481, 1987.

Parmley, T. H.: The histopathology of tubual pregnancy. Clin. Obstet. Gynecol., 30:119, 1987.

Patrick, J. D.: Ectopic pregnancy. Ann. Emerg. Med., 11:576, 1982.

Disorders of the Placenta, Amnion, And Umbilical Cord

Altschuler, G.: Placentitis. Contrib. Gynecol. Obstet., 9:113, 1982.

Bosseray, N.: Brucella infection and immunity in placenta. Ann. Inst. Pasteur Microbiol., 138:110, 1987.

Cassell, G. H., Waites, K. B., Gibbs, R. S., and Davis, J. K.: Role of Ureaplasma urealyticum in amnionitis. Pediatr. Infect. Dis., 5 (6 Suppl.):S247, 1986.

Cousins, L.: Pregnancy complications among diabetic women. Obstet. Gynecol. Surv., 42:140, 1987.

Doerr, H. W.: Cytomegalovirus infection in pregnancy. J. Virol. Methods, 17:127, 1987.

Enders, G.: Varicella-zoster infections in pregnancy. Prog. Med. Virol., 29:166, 1984.

Green-Thompson, R. W.: Ante-partum haemorrhage. Clin. Obstet. Gynaecol., 9:479, 1982.

Hayashi, R. H.: Hemorrhagic shock in obstetrics. Clin. Perinatol., 13:755, 1986.

Heifetz, S.A.: Strangulation of the umbilical cord by amniotic bands. Pediatr. Pathol., 2:285, 1984.

Higa, K., Dan, K., and Manabe, H.: Varicella-zoster virus infection during pregnancy. Obstet. Gynecol., 69:214, 1987.

Howell, R. J.: Haemorrhage from the placental site. Clin. Obstet. Gynaecol., 13:633, 1986.

Melchior, J. C., Alegre, A., and Arteche, J. M.: Placenta percreta with bladder involvement. Int. J. Gynaecol. Obstet., 25:417, 1987.

Menser, M. A., Hudson, J. R., Murphy, A. M., and Upfold, L. J.: Epidemiology of congenital rubella. Rev. Infect. Dis., (7 Suppl.) 1:S37, 1985.

Naeye, R. L.: Functionally important disorders of the placenta, umbilical cord, and fetal membranes. Hum. Pathol., 18:680, 1987.

Reece, E. A., and Hobbins, J. C.: Diabetic embryopathy. Obstet. Gynecol. Surv., 41:325, 1986.

Robinson, A., and Henry, G.P.: Prenatal diagnosis by amniocentesis. Annu. Rev. Med., 36:13, 1985.

Sander, C. H.: The surgical pathologist examines the placenta. Pathol. Annu., 20 (Pt. 2):235, 1985.

Sander, C. H., Kinnane, Stevens, N. G., and Echt, R.: Haemorrhagic endovasculitis of the placenta. Placenta, 7: 551, 1986.

Sander, C. H., and Stevens, N. G.: Hemorrhagic endovasculitis of the placenta. Pathol. Annu., 19 (Pt. 1):37, 1984.

Schwartz, M., Schwartz, S., Wenk, R. E., and Cohen, M.: Amniotic fluid and advances in perinatal diagnosis. Clin. Lab. Med., 5:371, 1985.

Stagno, S., and Whitley, R. J.: Herpesvirus infections of pregnancy. N. Engl. J. Med., 313:1270, 1327, 1985.

Preeclampsia and Eclampsia

Alexander, J., Cuellar, R. E., and Van Thiel, D. H.: Toxemia of pregnancy and the liver. Semin. Liver Dis., 7:55, 1987.

Beer, A. E., and Need, J. A.: Immunological aspects of preclampsia/eclampsia. Birth Defects, 21:131, 1985.

Doan-Wiggins, L.: Hypertensive disorders of pregnancy. Emerg. Med. Clin. North Am., 5:495, 1987.

Grünfeld, J. P., and Pertuiset, N.: Acute renal failure in pregnancy. Adv. Exp. Med. Biol., 212:245, 1987.

Hayslett, J. P.: Postpartum renal failure. N. Engl. J. Med., 312:1556, 1985.

Homans, D. C.: Peripartum cardiomyopathy. N. Engl. J. Med., 312:1432, 1985.

Lindheimer, M. D., and Katz, A. I.: Hypertension in pregnancy. N. Engl. J. Med., 313:675, 1985.

Maikranz, P., and Lindheimer, M. D.: Hypertension and pregnancy. Med. Clin. North Am., 71:1031, 1987.

Rubin, P.C.: Hypertension in pregnancy. J. Hypertens., 5: 557, 1987.

Soma, H., Yoshida, K., Mukaida, T., and Tabuchi, Y.: Morphologic changes in the hypertensive placenta. Contrib. Gynecol. Obstet., 9:58, 1983.

Weiner, C. P.: The clinical spectrum of preeclampsia. Am. J. Kidney Dis., 9:312, 1987.

Other-Non-Neoplastic Diseases

Clark, S. L.: Amniotic fluid embolism. Clin. Perinatol., 13:801, 1986.

Dallman, P. R.: Anemia of prematurity. Annu. Rev. Med., 32:143, 1981.

Hoffman, P. C.: Idiopathic thrombocytopenic purpura in pregnancy. Clin. Perinatol., 12:599, 1985.

Lazebnik, N., Jaffa, N., Jaffa, A. J., and Peyser, M. R.: Hemolytic-uremic syndrome in pregnancy. Obstet. Gynecol. Surv., 40:618, 1985.

Pitkin, R. M. (Ed.): Autoimmune disease in pregnancy. Clin. Obstet. Gynecol., 26:519, 1983.

Rutherford, S. E., and Phelan, J. P.: Thrombotic disease in pregnancy. Clin. Perinatol., 13:719, 1986.

Weiner, C. P.: Thrombotic microangiopathies in pregnancy and the postpartum period. Semin. Hematol., 24:119, 1987.

Tumors

Berkowitz, R. S., and Goldstein, D. P. (Eds.): Clinical update on trophoblastic disease. J. Reprod. Med., 32: 621, 1987.

Berkowitz, R. S., et al.: Immunobiology of molar pregnancy and gestational trophoblastic tumor. Cancer Metastasis Rev., 5:109. 1986.

Corson, S. L.: New concepts and questions in gestational trophoblastic disease. J. Reprod. Med., 28:741, 1983.

Elston, C. W.: Gestational tumours of trophoblast. Rec. Adv. Histopathol., 11:149, 1981.

McDonald, T. W., and Ruffolo, E. H.: Modern management of gestational trophoblastic disease. Obstet. Gynecol. Surv., 38:67, 1983.

Ober, W. B.: Pathology of trophoblastic diseases. Hum. Reprod., 2:143, 1987.

Pattillo, R. A., and Hussa, R. O.: Gestational trophoblastic disease and human chorionic gonadotropin measurement. J. Reprod. Med., 32:629, 1987.

Ratnam, S. S., and Ilancheram A.: Disease of the trophoblast. Clin. Obstet. Gynaecol., 9:539, 1982.

Robertson, W. B., et al.: The placental bed biopsy. Am. J. Obstet. Gynecol., 155:401, 1986.

43

Breasts

THE diseases of the breasts are among the commonest of maladies in women, but are less frequent in men. In both women and men, inflammatory lesions, various forms of hyperplasia, and several types of tumor affect the breasts.

INFLAMMATION

Inflammation of the breasts is called mastitis, from the Greek for breast. Acute and chronic mastitis and abscesses can develop in the breasts. Fat necrosis, foreign body reactions, superficial thrombophlebitis, and a galactocele are less common. Occasionally tuberculosis involves a breast, usually by extension from a rib. Syphilis, a fungal infection, or sarcoidosis rarely affects a breast.

ACUTE MASTITIS. Acute mastitis is rare except during the first few weeks of lactation. Bacteria gain entry to a breast through cracks or fissures in the nipple and spread up one or more of the mammary ducts. Staphylococci are the most common invader, though occasionally streptococci or some other organism is involved.

The affected segment of the breast becomes acutely inflamed, red and hot from the congestion, tense and indurated from the edema, painful and tender from the tension in the tissues. Microscopically, there is the usual neutrophilic response of acute inflammation. Sometimes an abscess forms beneath the nipple, in the substance of the breast, or deep to the breast against the pectoral muscles. The regional lymph nodes in the axilla are swollen and tender and show the usual changes of acute lymphadenitis.

Antibiotics and drainage when necessary bring resolution, leaving scarring in the inflamed part of the breast.

MAMMARY DUCT ECTASIA. Ectasia of one or more of the mammary ducts is common in women 40 to 70 years old. At autopsy, 25% of women show dilatation of one or more of the mammary ducts in the subareolar region. The dilated ducts are 3 to 5 mm in diameter, with a thin wall, and are filled with fatty secretions.

Periductal Mastitis. In most women, the ectasia of the ducts causes no symptoms and passes unnoticed. In some, the dilated ducts become inflamed. The inflammation begins beneath the nipple and is usually confined to part of one of the breasts. It slowly spreads into the substance of the breast. The inflammation is sometimes called periductal mastitis, plasma cell mastitis, comedomastitis, or pseudotuberculosis.

The ducts affected are widely dilated and filled with fatty debris. The epithelium lining the ducts is usually thin and inactive. If the inflammation is severe, it is often partially or completely lost. Occasionally foci of squamous metaplasia develop in the epithelium. The walls of the ducts are usually considerably thickened by collagenous tissue. A dense exudate of lymphocytes and macrophages surrounds the ducts and extends into their thickened walls. Sometimes plasma cells are numerous in the exudate. If a duct ruptures, the fatty material escaping from the duct excites a foreign body granulomatous reaction in the surrounding tissue. Occasionally a duct is completely destroyed, and macrophages filled with the fat from the duct accumulate in the core of the lesion. The axillary lymph nodes are enlarged and show chronic lymphadenitis.

Macroscopically, a hard mass that can mimic a carcinoma develops in the breast. The enlarged lymph nodes can be mistaken for metastases. Often the fibrosis in the large ducts beneath the nipple cause retraction of the nipple or dimpling of the overlying skin, as does carcinoma of the breast. The patient may discover the mass, may notice an intermittent brownish or hemorrhagic discharge from the nipple, or may suffer repeated episodes of acute mastitis.

The cause of the inflammation is not known. It may be initiated by leakage of the irritating content of the ectatic ducts into the periductal tissue. Excision cures.

RECURRENT SUBAREOLAR ABSCESS. In young women, recurrent abscesses sometimes develop immediately beneath a nipple. The abscess points or is drained, and healing follows. A few months later, another abscess develops in the same place. The abscesses are caused by squamous metaplasia in one or more of the milk sinuses. Keratin obstructs the sinus, and recurrent infections follow. Excision of the affected sinus or sinuses cures.

FAT NECROSIS. Trauma can disrupt fat cells in a breast, as in any other adipose tissue. Probably minor foci of fat necrosis are common in the breasts, but are too small to attract notice and soon heal. Traumatic fat necrosis sufficiently extensive to be evident clinically is uncommon.

If the lesion is recent, it is often painful, red, and ecchymotic. If it is old, the patient often has a hard mass 2 to 3 cm across, usually close beneath the skin. In some patients, the mass causes retraction of the

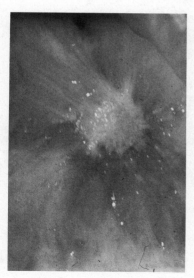

Fig. 43-1. Fat necrosis in a breast, showing a hard, fibrous mass resembling a carcinoma.

nipple and dimpling of the skin. Enlargement of the axillary lymph nodes is unusual.

In an early lesion, neutrophils accumulate among the fat cells in the injured region. Often small pools of neutral fat released from ruptured fat cells are present. Lipophages appear as macrophages begin to take up the fat from the ruptured fat cells.

After a few weeks, the neutrophils disappear and fibrosis becomes the principal feature of the lesion. The fibrosis begins at the periphery of the lesion and gradually extends into its core. Usually there is a moderate exudate mainly of lymphocytes and plasma cells in the fibrous tissue. At first, lipophages are numerous in the core of the lesion, but as it becomes more collagenous the lipophages form small clumps separated by the scar tissue. Occasionally the fat excites a granulomatous reaction, with multinucleated macrophages. Sometimes a focus of fat necrosis becomes cystic, with oily fluid enclosed by a collagenous capsule. Occasionally the lesion calcifies.

The older lesions of fat necrosis in a breast can closely resemble carcinoma, both macroscopically and microscopically. The hard mass with retraction of the nipple is sometimes indistinguishable from a carcinoma. Microscopically, the clumps of lipophages in the lesion can be similar to clumps of tumor cells in a collagenous stroma. Often the lesion must be excised to establish the diagnosis. Excision cures.

FOREIGN BODY REACTION. Various kinds of foreign material have been injected or implanted in the breasts to ameliorate their shape. Such materials often excite a brisk foreign body reaction, with granulomatous inflammation. There is always a risk of infection or excessive scarring.

SUPERFICIAL THROMBOPHLEBITIS. Superficial thrombophlebitis of the breast is uncommon. It is called Mondor's disease, after the French surgeon who described it in 1939. About 25% of the patients are men.

For reasons unknown, one of the subcutaneous veins that drain the chest wall becomes inflamed and thrombosed, usually the vein running from the epigastrium across the lateral aspect of the breast to the axilla. The vein is painful and often tender. The condition subsides after a few weeks as the inflammation subsides and the thrombus organizes.

GALACTOCELE. A galactocele may develop during lactation or a few weeks after it ends. It takes its name from the Greek words for milk and hollow. One or more of the mammary ducts becomes obstructed and dilates to form a thin-walled cyst filled with milky fluid. Often mild acute or chronic inflammation surrounds the cyst. Sometimes the content of the cyst becomes inspissated and cheesy. If the lesion persists, its wall becomes thickened and fibrotic. Rarely, a galactocele becomes infected. Excision cures.

HYPERPLASIA

The most common form of mammary hyperplasia in women is called mammary dysplasia. Less often, the breasts develop prematurely in a girl with precocious puberty, or part of a breast is hyperplastic in a young woman with virginal hyperplasia. Mammary hyperplasia in a man is called gynecomastia.

MAMMARY DYSPLASIA. In mammary dysplasia, the connective tissue of the breasts, the epithelium, or both are hyperplastic. The disease is often called cystic disease of the breasts, fibrocystic disease, cystic hyperplasia, chronic cystic mastitis, less commonly fibro-adenomatosis, or Schimmelbusch's disease after a German surgeon (1860–1895).

Most women have mammary dysplasia, though in many the condition is mild and passes undetected. It is severe enough to be evident clinically in 10% of women. Most of the patients with clinically evident mammary dysplasia are between 35 and 50 years old.

Lesions. Seven kinds of mammary dysplasia are distinguished: intralobular fibrosis, interlobular fibrosis, ductal ectasia, adenosis, sclerosing adenosis, epithelial hyperplasia, and apocrine metaplasia. Each will be described separately, though it is rare that a breast shows only one of these types of reaction. Most lesions show a combination of two or more of these types of response.

Mammary dysplasia is usually patchy, multifocal, and bilateral. It may affect only a

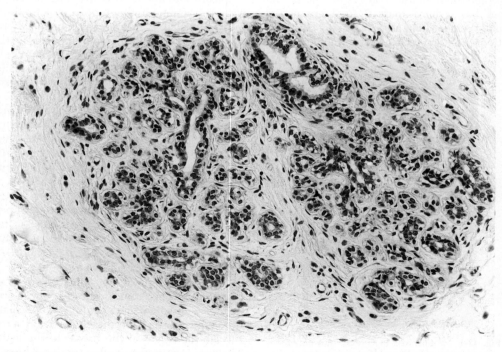

Fig. 43-2. Mammary dysplasia, showing the coarsening of the collagen within a lobule seen in intralobular fibrosis.

few small foci in the breasts or involve most of the parenchyma. Its severity often varies from one part of the breasts to another. Even though much of the parenchyma is involved, only a few of the lesions may be evident clinically. Not uncommonly one dominant lesion seems bigger and different from the disease in other parts of the breasts.

Intralobular Fibrosis. Intralobular fibrosis, sometimes called mazoplasia from the Greek for breast and formation, is one of the commonest forms of mammary dysplasia. Normally, the intralobular stroma has fine collagen and abundant intercellular substance. It is sharply demarcated from the coarser interlobular fibrous tissue, which has thick bundles of collagen, little intercellular substance, and is often partially hyalinized. In intralobular fibrosis, the collagen bundles within the lobules are thickened, and the quantity of intercellular substance is reduced. The intracellular stroma becomes indistinguishable from the interlobular fibrous tissue and merges with it without clear demarcation. Often the quantity of collagenous tissue in the lobules is slightly or moderately increased.

Macroscopically and clinically, intralobular fibrosis is undetectable, though commonly the parts of the breasts involved show also other types of dysplasia.

Interlobular Fibrosis. The quantity of fibrous tissue between the lobules is usually increased in mammary dysplasia. It consists of thick bundles of well-differentiated collagen with little intercellular substance. The fibrosis increases the distance between the lobules and replaces fat. Macroscopically, the parts of the breasts affected show ill-defined bands of firm, white tissue. Clinically, the lesions are often undetectable, though the breasts may feel vaguely granular.

Ductal Ectasia. Slight dilatation of ducts and ductules evident only microscopically is frequent in mammary dysplasia. Usually many of the small and medium-sized ducts are affected. The ectatic ducts have normal ductular epithelium and a normal ductular wall. Less often, a few of the ducts are more markedly dilated, forming cysts up to 5 cm across. In the cysts, the epithelium is usually thin and inactive, and the cyst has a thin collagenous wall.

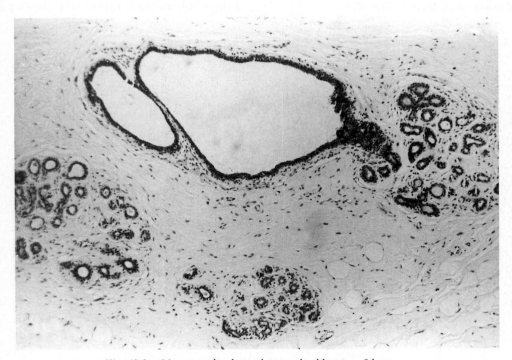

Fig. 43-3.   Mammary dysplasia, showing the dilatation of ducts.

Macroscopically, the cysts bulge from a cut section of the breast and look blue when light is transmitted through their brownish content. The term blue-domed cyst is sometimes used to describe them. Nearly always the affected region shows also interlobular fibrosis. Clinically, the cysts make the affected parts of the breasts feel granular or nodular. Occasionally one cyst is much bigger than the rest and presents as solitary mass.

Adenosis. In adenosis, the mammary lobules are bigger and more numerous than normal. The epithelium in the affected lobules may be normal, but often the epithelial cells become columnar. Sometimes there are several layers of epithelial cells in some of the intralobular ductules, though the epithelial cells show no atypicality and no increase in size, and their arrangement remains orderly. Nearly always, intralobular fibrosis coarsens the intralobular stroma, so that it becomes indistinguishable from the interlobular stroma. Interlobular fibrosis usually joins the affected lobules, without intervening fat.

Macroscopically, the affected parts of the breast are firm, white, and fibrotic. Often the lobules can be seen as pinkish spots. Adenosis cannot be detected clinically.

Sclerosing Adenosis. Sclerosing adenosis usually involves only a few scattered lobules in the breasts. The ductules of the affected lobules proliferate and the lobules are usually considerably enlarged.

In the florid form of sclerosing adenosis, the ductules are closely packed, with little connective tissue between them. They may be larger than normal. Their epithelium is tall and columnar, often filling the ductules, and appears active.

In the sclerotic form of sclerosing adenosis, the ductules in the affected lobule are separated by bands of coarse collagen that merge indistinguishably with the surrounding interlobular stroma. Their epithelium is often cuboidal and looks less active. Often the ductules adopt a swirling pattern.

In both the florid and the sclerotic types of sclerosing adenosis, the margins of the affected lobules are not as well defined as usual. In the sclerotic form, the ductules often fray out into the surrounding fibrous stroma, almost as if they were invading it. Sometimes they extend into fat.

At high power, sclerosing adenosis can look microscopically like carcinoma, though if the whole lesion is considered, the two are

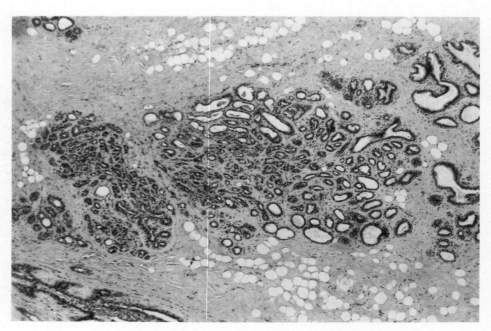

Fig. 43-4.   Mammary dysplasia, showing the enlargement of the lobules seen in adenosis.

usually easily distinguished. Macroscopically, sclerosing adenosis is indistinguishable from adenosis. Sometimes confluent foci of sclerosing adenosis and adenosis joined by interlobular fibrosis form a firm, white mass 2 or 3 cm in diameter. Clinically, such a mass may be impossible to distinguish from carcinoma.

EPITHELIAL HYPERPLASIA. Epithelial hyperplasia can occur in any form of mammary dysplasia. It is most common in slightly ectatic ducts, but can develop in intralobular ductules or cysts.

The affected ducts or ductules are lined by two or more layers of epithelial cells. At times, the lumen of a ductule is filled with epithelial cells. Occasionally small lumina develop in the hyperplastic epithelium. Sometimes the proliferation is principally of the small, dark myoepithelial cells present in the basal part of the ductal and ductular epithelium. The hyperplastic epithelial cells show no atypicality and no enlargement and are arranged in an orderly manner.

Less often, papillary fronds project into a duct or into a cyst. The fronds are usually stumpy, with a fibrous core, and are lined by epithelium that may be mildly hyperplastic.

The epithelial hyperplasia sometimes found in mammary dysplasia cannot be detected macroscopically or clinically. It occurs in association with other forms of mammary dysplasia and is found when these lesions are examined microscopically.

Apocrine Metaplasia. Foci of apocrine metaplasia are common in mammary dysplasia. The normal epithelium of a duct, ductule, or cyst is replaced in whole or in part by tall, well-defined cells with small, pyknotic nuclei and abundant, brightly eosinophilic cytoplasm. Sometimes the apocrine cells bulge into the lumen of the duct or partially fill it. Apocrine metaplasia cannot be detected macroscopically or clinically.

Clinical Presentation. Mammary dysplasia is usually found when a patient finds a cyst or an ill-defined mass in her breast or when a physician finds increased and irregular nodularity in the breasts. Sometimes the induration is sufficient to suggest the possibility of carcinoma. The lesions are painful or tender in a few patients, especially before the menstrual periods. Sometimes a cyst enlarges rapidly before a period and shrinks after it. Discharge from the nipples is uncommon.

Aspiration of a cyst establishes the diag-

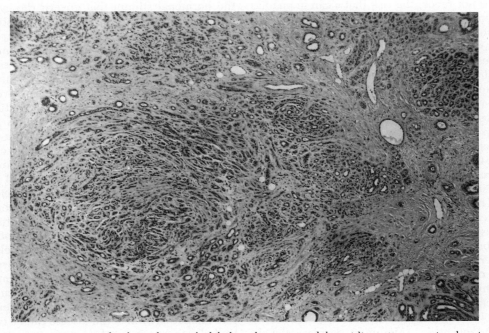

Fig. 43-5. Mammary dysplasia, showing the lobular enlargement and the swirling pattern seen in sclerosing adenosis.

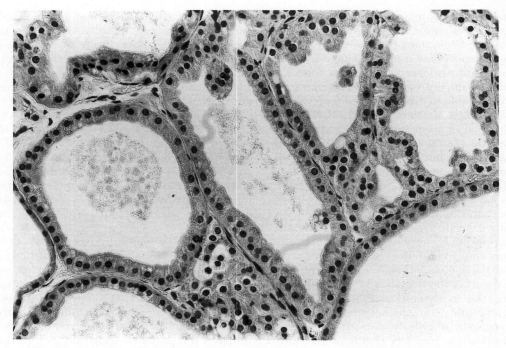

Fig. 43-6. Mammary dysplasia, showing apocrine metaplasia in the epithelium lining dilated ducts.

nosis and often cures the lesion. If the mass disappears completely after aspiration and does not recur, the risk that a carcinoma has been missed is low. If a mass seriously suggests carcinoma, biopsy is needed. Mammography is of considerable help in doubtful cases.

Relation to Carcinoma. Opinions differ as to whether mammary dysplasia increases the risk of developing carcinoma of the breast. Those who doubt that there is any relationship between the two conditions note that carcinoma of the breast and mammary dysplasia are both common. Even if they are unrelated, they are likely often to be both present in the same breast.

Those who consider mammary dysplasia precancerous, agree that sclerosing adenosis does not increase the risk of developing carcinoma. Most think that intralobular fibrosis, interlobular fibrosis, and adenosis increase the risk little if at all, but believe that epithelial hyperplasia and the more severe forms of ductal ectasia increase the risk of developing carcinoma four times.

Pathogenesis. Mammary dysplasia develops during the reproductive years. It is probably due to hormonal imbalance or to failure of the breasts to respond normally to the hormonal stimuli that govern the cyclic changes in the breasts during the menstrual cycle.

Treatment and Prognosis. Mammary dysplasia requires no treatment. The lesions become quiescent or regress after the menopause. Only when a lesion suggests carcinoma is it necessary to establish its nature.

PRECOCIOUS PUBERTY. In precocious puberty, the breasts begin to develop in a girl less than eight years old. In 90% of the children, the cause of the disorder is unknown. Some have a tumor or other disease of the brain or adrenal dysfunction. Precocious pseudopuberty caused by an estrogen-secreting ovarian tumor or, less often, an adrenal tumor, Albright's syndrome, or hypothyroidism causes a similar premature development of the breasts. The breasts are normal in the children with the idiopathic form of the disorder, but may show evidence of hyperestrinism in precocious pseudopuberty. The idiopathic form of the disease can be controlled by giving medroxyprogesterone to suppress the secretion of gonadotropins.

VIRGINAL HYPERPLASIA. Virginal hyperplasia of the breasts, sometimes called adolescent hypertrophy, affects girls at puberty. In the course of a year or so, one or both breasts grow excessively and may come to hang below the umbilicus. Sometimes one breast enlarges more than the other, or one breast remains normal, though the other is enlarged. Occasionally, only part of a breast is affected.

Microscopically, the mammary ducts in the affected breast or breasts usually show little abnormality, though they sometimes show the kind of hyperplasia seen in gynecomastia. The increase in size is due to excessive proliferation of fibrous and fatty tissue.

The hormonal secretion in patients with virginal hyperplasia of the breasts is not abnormal, but the tissue responds excessively to the hormones. The enlargement cannot be reversed. If necessary, the size of the breasts can be reduced surgically.

GYNECOMASTIA. Enlargement of the male breast is called gynecomastia, from the Greek for woman and breast. Four kinds of gynecomastia are distinguished: pubertal, senescent, secondary, and idiopathic.

Pubertal Hyperplasia. Slight enlargement of one or both breasts occurs in 30% of boys between 13 and 17 years old. In 80% of the boys affected the enlargement is bilateral. In most, the enlargement is slight and disappears after six months or more. No treatment is required.

Rarely, the enlargement of one or both breasts is excessive, so that one or both of the boy's breasts come to look like a female breast. Enlargement of this degree is not likely to regress, and mastectomy is required. Microscopy shows elongation and branching of the mammary ducts, sometimes with mild epithelial hyperplasia, but the bulk of the enlargement is due to increase in the fibrous stroma of the breast. The ducts do not form lobules like those of the female breast.

Most of the boys with severe pubertal gynecomastia show no abnormality in hormone production, though some have a slight excess of estrogens or pituitary hormones. In most, probably the reactivity of the breast is a little abnormal, much as in the virginal hyperplasia of girls.

Most boys with pubertal gynecomastia have no abnormality in hormone production, though some show a slight excess of estrogens or gonadotropins. The hyperplasia seems due to abnormal reactivity in the breasts. If the enlargement is great, it is unlikely to regress and mastectomy is needed.

Senescent Hyperplasia. Men over 50 years old occasionally develop enlargement of one and sometimes later the other breast. The hyperplastic tissue forms a disk 2 to 4 cm in diameter beneath the nipple and is often tender. Usually the enlargement regresses after six to nine months.

Microscopically, the appearances are like those of pubertal hyperplasia. There is proliferation of the mammary ducts, but the bulk of the enlargement is due to proliferation of fibrous and fatty tissue. No hormonal imbalance is evident.

Secondary Gynecomastia. Secondary gynecomastia is likely to develop whenever estrogenic activity increases or androgenic activity decreases. The hormonal imbalance may be caused by disease or by drugs.

Atrophy of the testes caused by Klinefelter's syndrome, mumps, other infections, or by trauma reduces the secretion of androgens and can cause gynecomastia. Castration causes gynecomastia. Defective androgen receptors in the hypothalamus and pituitary in testicular feminization and Riefeinstein's syndrome cause gynecomastia by increasing secretion of the luteinizing hormone. The high level of luteinizing hormone in the plasma increases the secretion of both androgen and estrogen by the testes, but reduces the ratio of androgen to estrogen. Increased secretion of gonadotropins in true hermaphroditism, by testicular or pituitary tumors, or by a carcinoma of the lung sometimes causes gynecomastia. Tumors that secrete estrogens can do so. Increased production of androstenedione in congenital adrenal hyperplasia, by adrenocortical tumors, or in hyperthyroidism increases the production of estrogen in the tissues and sometimes causes gynecomastia. Cirrhosis and other severe diseases of the liver impair the capacity of the liver to catabolize androstenedione and so increase the production of estrogen in the peripheral tissues, sometimes enough to cause gynecomastia. Occasionally gynecomastia develops in a patient with tuberculosis or an empyema.

The administration of estrogens to control

carcinoma of the prostate or for other reasons often causes gynecomastia. Adolescents are especially sensitive to estrogens and can develop hyperplasia of the breasts when treated with ointments containing estrogen, or by drinking milk or eating meat from animals given estrogens. Digitalis sometimes causes gynecomastia because of its estrogen-like activity. Alkylating agents reduce the synthesis of androgen in the testes. Spironolactone and cimetidine block the binding of androgen to its receptors. For reasons unknown, tricyclic antidepressant drugs, diazepam, heroin, isoniazid, marijuana, methyldopa, and penicillamine sometimes cause gynecomastia.

The enlargement of the breasts is usually bilateral. It is due mainly to increase in the collagenous and fatty tissue. The ducts proliferate, but acini do not form. The epithelium lining the ducts is often low and inactive, but in some patients it is hyperplastic, irregular, and several layers thick. If the enlargement is troublesome, mastectomy is necessary.

Idiopathic Gynecomastia. Rarely, enlargement of one or both breasts occurs in a young boy without obvious cause. In contrast to other forms of gynecomastia, the proliferating ducts form acini. Microscopically, the enlarged breast or breasts look much like a female breast with mild mammary dysplasia.

CONGENITAL ANOMALIES

Complete absence of one or both breasts is called amastia, from the Greek for without and a breast. More common are polymastia, from the Greek for many and breast, in which there are supernumerary breasts, and polythelia, from the Greek for many and nipple, in which there are supernumerary nipples. Most often the accessory breasts or nipples occur along the milk line, which runs from the axilla to the groin, but they may occur on the thighs, in the midline, or on the back. From 1 to 2% of people have either polymastia or polythelia, with women affected more often than men.

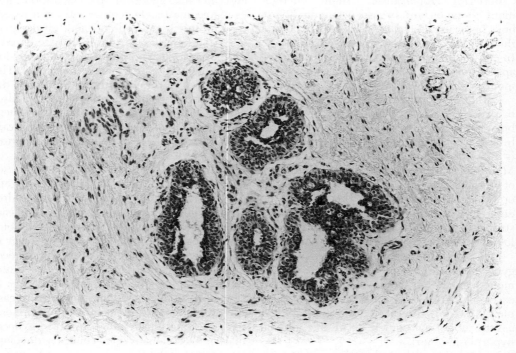

Fig. 43-7. Gynecomastia secondary to the administration of estrogens, showing hyperplasia of the epithelium lining the ducts and a considerable increase in the collagenous tissue around them.

There may be one or more accessory breasts or nipples. Accessory nipples are often small and poorly formed and may be mistaken for moles. Accessory breasts form a mass of normal breast tissue, with or without a nipple. If the anomaly is large enough to cause trouble, it can be removed.

Malformation of the breasts is rare. There may be more than one nipple, in a single areola or each with its own areola. Rarely, the shape of a breast is irregular.

TUMORS

Tumors of the breasts are common in women, rare in men. Fibroadenoma and intraductal papilloma are the most common benign tumors of the breasts, and granular cell tumor sometimes develops in a breast. Rarely an adenoma, with closely packed acini lined by ductal epithelium, is found in a breast. Lipomata and other benign mesenchymal tumors are rare.

Carcinoma is the only common malignant tumor of the breasts. Lobular carcinoma in situ and intraductal carcinoma are forms of carcinoma in situ. Infiltrating ductal carcinoma and infiltrating lobular carcinoma are the most common of the several forms of invasive carcinoma. Paget's disease sometimes involves a nipple. Occasionally a cystosarcoma phylloides develops in a breast. Rarely, an angiosarcoma or some other kind of malignant mesenchymal tumor involves a breast. Secondary tumors of the breasts are uncommon.

FIBROADENOMA. A fibroadenoma, or adenofibroma as some prefer to call it, large enough to be evident clinically develops in 1 woman in 40. Most of the patients are 15 to 35 years old, though some are older. At autopsy, a fibroadenoma can be found in a breast in 10% of women, though more than 80% of these tumors are too small to be detected clinically. In men, fibroadenomata of the breast are unknown.

Lesions. Macroscopically, fibroadenomata detected clinically are usually 2 to 4 cm in diameter. The tumor is within the substance of the breast and is mobile. On palpation, it often slips away beneath the examin-

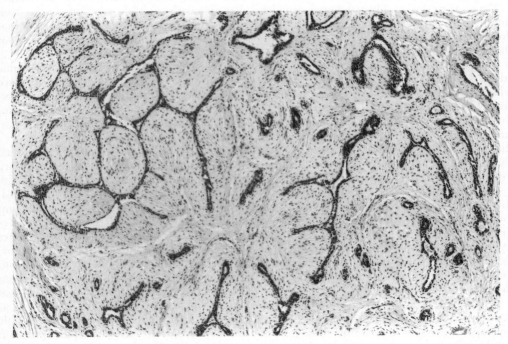

Fig. 43-8. Fibroadenoma of the breast mainly of the intracanalicular type, though a few small round ducts of the pericanalicular type are present.

ing fingers. On cut section, fibroadenomata are usually well defined and form a firm, spheroidal or ovoid mass. The cut surface is white or yellowish and often rather mucoid. The ducts within the tumor often are visible to the naked eye as small cracks or slits in the cut surface of the tumor.

In 15% of patients, fibroadenomata are multiple and may involve both breasts. Rarely, they are numerous and large, so that much of both breasts is replaced by the tumors. Rarely, usually in adolescence, a fibroadenoma grows to be 20 or more cm in diameter.

Microscopically, a fibroadenoma consists of mammary ducts separated by a collagenous stroma. The epithelium lining the ducts is usually two layers thick, as in a normal mammary duct, and shows no sign of activity. Occasionally it is more active, with plump cells, and may be several layers thick. The stroma is usually loose and mucoid, but sometimes is dense, with coarse, hyalinized bundles of collagen. Not uncommonly a fibroadenoma too small to be apparent macroscopically is present in the breast in a patient with mammary dysplasia.

Three varieties of fibroadenoma are distinguished. Most fibroadenomata are predominantly of one or other of these types, though some admixture of the various forms is common. In an intracanalicular fibroadenoma, the stroma compresses the ducts, which are reduced to narrow, anastomosing slits. In a pericanalicular fibroadenoma, the ducts remain cylindrical and are usually small. A sclerotic fibroadenoma is usually of the pericanalicular pattern. Its stroma has thick, coarse bundles of collagen, with little intercellular substance.

Clinical Presentation. A fibroadenoma of the breasts causes no symptoms. Most are found by accident when a young woman is dressing or bathing.

Behavior. A fibroadenoma usually grows slowly for a year or two, then becomes quiescent, and persists with little change for the rest of the patient's life.

Complications. Rarely, a fibroadenoma becomes infarcted. A fibroadenoma does not increase the risk of developing carcinoma of the breast, but carcinoma or lobular carcinoma in situ can develop in a fibroadenoma.

Pathogenesis. Traditionally, a fibroadenoma has been considered to be a mixed tumor, consisting of neoplastic epithelium and neoplastic connective tissue. It seems more likely that the lesion is a form of adenoma, in which the neoplastic epithelium induces an unusually prominent stromal reaction. Some prefer to think that it is a fibroma that excites secondary epithelial proliferation.

Since fibroadenomata occur almost exclusively during the reproductive years, it seems likely that they are caused by hormonal imbalance or an abnormality in the response of the breast to hormones. The nature of the defect or defects is unknown.

Treatment and Prognosis. A fibroadenoma is usually excised. Untreated, the tumor does no harm unless it is unusually large, but excision is desirable to ensure that the lesion is a fibroadenoma, not carcinoma.

INTRADUCTAL PAPILLOMA. Three kinds of intraductal papilloma are distinguished, the solitary intraductal papilloma of large ducts, multiple papillomata of smaller ducts, and the subareolar papilloma. All are uncommon and occur almost exclusively in women. Patients with multiple papillomata are usually 30 to 40 years old; those with a solitary papilloma or a subareolar papilloma are more often 40 to 60 years old.

Lesions. Most intraductal papillomata form fronds with a collagenous core covered by neoplastic epithelium. In some, sheets of epithelium without a fibrous core extend into the duct. The epithelium is usually well differentiated and shows no atypicality.

Solitary Papilloma. A solitary intraductal papilloma usually arises in one of the large ducts beneath the areola. The affected duct is somewhat dilated. The papilloma forms a brown, friable mass, which bulges 2 or 3 mm into the duct and extends along it for 1 to 2 cm or more. Less often, a papilloma is up to 10 cm across, and bulges into a cyst. Such a tumor is sometimes callled a papillary cystadenoma.

Microscopically, a solitary intraductal papilloma consists of fronds of connective tissue covered by ductal epithelium. The fronds are often delicate, but sometimes have a thick fibrous core or are sclerotic. The epithelium covering the fronds usually preserves the normal two layers of the duct and shows little or no evidence of hyperplasia or atypicality. At times the fronds fuse to form glandlike spaces. Sometimes there is apocrine meta-plasia. Sometimes a papilloma becomes scar-red, trapping fragments of epithelium in the scar, in a manner suggestive of carcinoma. Sclerosing adenosis or other evidence of mammary dysplasia is common in adjacent parts of the breast.

Multiple Papillomatosis.   Multiple papil-lomatosis often involves more than one part of the breast affected. In 25% of the patients, the lesions are bilateral.

In the segment or segments of the breasts affected, papillomata fill many of the small ducts and ductules. The papillomata some-times have fronds with a fibrous core covered by neoplastic epithelium. Often the fronds fuse, forming glandlike spaces. In other lesions, fronds consisting only of epithelium project into the ducts, or solid masses of epithelium fill or partially fill the ducts and ductules. Small acini sometimes appear among the epithelial cells filling the ducts. In both types of lesion, the epithelial cells are well differentiated, with no atypicality, are of normal size, and are arranged in an orderly manner. They resemble the cells of normal ductular epithelium or are cuboidal and well defined. Apocrine metaplasia is common in the lesions. Often the adjacent parts of the breasts show mammary dysplasia.

Subareolar Papilloma.   A subareolar pa-pilloma of the nipple develops slowly. Often it has been present for many years by the time the patient seeks advice. The tumor develops in one or more of the milk sinuses in the nipple. At first, it forms a complex papilloma, with fibrous fronds covered by ductular epithelium, which bulges into the milk sinus, filling and distending it. Later, some of the sinuses may become partially or completely filled with sheets of epithelial cells. Often considerable scarring surrounds the affected sinuses, and islands of epithel-ium trapped in the scar tissue look like an invasive carcinoma. The epithelial cells are well-defined and pale. They sometimes show

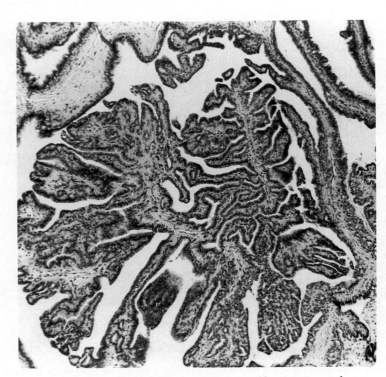

Fig. 43-9.   Intraductal papilloma bulging into a dilated mammary duct.

moderate pleomorphism. Sometimes there is squamous metaplasia or a foreign body reaction around a ruptured duct.

Behavior. Solitary intraductal papillomata are benign, though it is sometimes hard to distinguish between an intraductal papilloma and an papillary carcinoma. Subareolar papillomata are also benign.

Multiple papillomatosis increases the risk of developing carcinoma of the breast. In one series, 40% of the patients developed carcinoma of the breast, though in some patients not until 5 or 10 years after the removal of the papillomata.

Clinical Presentation. Most women with a solitary intraductal papilloma of the breast have an intermittent discharge from the nipple, a few drops of bloody or serous fluid. Less often, a soft mass is palpable. If no mass can be felt, gentle pressure around the areola may cause a drop of fluid to ooze from the nipple.

Women with multiple intraductal papillomatosis usually have a lump in the breast. Discharge from the nipple occurs in 30% of the patients.

A subareolar papilloma first causes intermittent discharge from the nipple. Later, the nipple becomes reddened and inflamed. Eventually, a red, granular tumor 1 or 2 cm across may bulge from the nipple.

Treatment and Prognosis. Local excision of a solitary papilloma or a subareolar papilloma cures. In 50% of patients with multiple papillomatosis treated by local excision, the lesions recur in some other part of the breast or in the other breast within 10 years.

Lobular Carcinoma in Situ. If carcinoma involves the small ducts within the mammary lobules without involvement of large ducts and without evidence of invasion, it is called lobular carcinoma in situ. It is not a common lesion, but is being recognized increasingly frequently. Almost always, the patients are premenopausal.

Lesions. Lobular carcinoma in situ cannot be detected clinically or by macroscopic examination of a breast biopsy. Usually, the carcinoma is found by accident when a biopsy is taken for some other reason, usually for mammary dysplasia.

Microscopically, the affected ducts are

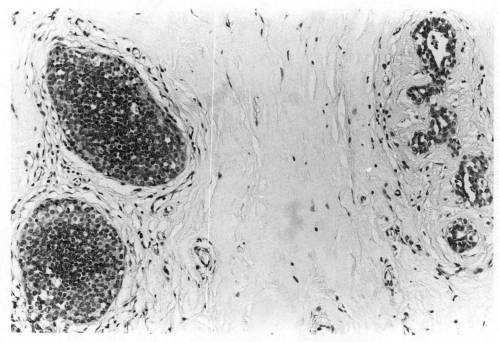

Fig. 43-10.   Lobular carcinoma in situ of the breast. The ducts on the left are filled with carcinoma; on the right a lobule shows mammary dysplasia.

distended and filled with carcinoma cells. The tumor cells are bigger than normal ductular cells and are uniform, with regular spheroidal nuclei and a moderate amount of pale cytoplasm. The cells are arranged in an orderly manner. Mitoses are few or absent. The principal features of the lesion are the large size of the cells and their regularity.

Lobular carcinoma in situ is often multifocal. In 70% of the patients, more than one part of the breast is involved. In 30%, a random biopsy shows lobular carcinoma in situ in the other breast.

Behavior. Lobular carcinoma in situ does not invade and does not metastasize, but increases greatly the risk of developing an infiltrating ductal carcinoma. If a biopsy shows intralobular carcinoma in situ, 25% of the patients will develop an invasive carcinoma in that breast, and 10% will develop an invasive carcinoma in the opposite breast. The invasive tumor may appear soon after the carcinoma in situ is detected or not for 15 or 20 years.

Clinical Presentation. Lobular carcinoma in situ causes no symptoms and cannot be detected clinically. The diagnosis is made only by biopsy.

Treatment and Prognosis. Because lobular carcinoma in situ is so often multifocal and bilateral and increases so greatly the risk of developing an invasive carcinoma, some surgeons treat it by bilateral mastectomy. Others prefer to conserve the breasts, at least in younger women, but to follow the patient closely, so that if an invasive carcinoma develops it can be resected while still small.

Intraductal Carcinoma. Carcinoma in situ of the larger mammary ducts is called intraductal carcinoma. It is a diagnosis always clouded by some doubt. Even if multiple sections are taken through the involved part of the breast, it is never possible to exclude entirely the possibility that somewhere there is a small focus of invasive carcinoma. Extension along the ducts often occurs around an infiltrating ductal carcinoma. If the infiltrating carcinoma is small, it is easily overlooked.

Lesions. Two kinds of intraductal carcinoma of the breast are distinguished, papil-

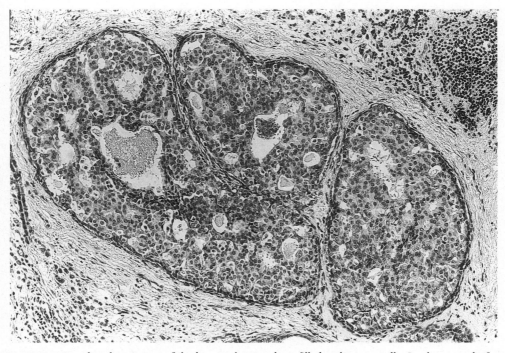

Fig. 43-11. Intraductal carcinoma of the breast, showing ducts filled with tumor cells. In places a cribriform pattern is evident.

lary carcinoma and comedocarcinoma. The distinction between the two types is not sharp, and intermediate forms occur. Tumors that are predominantly intraductal, but show one or more foci of early invasion are sometimes called invasive papillary carcinoma, or invasive comedocarcinoma.

Papillary Carcinoma. About 2% of carcinomata of the breast in women are of the papillary type. They are similar to the multiple intraductal papillomata, and deciding whether such a lesion is benign or malignant is difficult.

A papillary carcinoma of the breast is most common beneath the nipple, where it distends one of the large ducts. Less often, it involves ducts throughout a segment of the breast, or projects into a cyst. The tumor is nearly always large enough to be easily palpable, and at times multiple nodules can be felt in the involved segment of the breast.

Microscopically, the carcinoma sometimes forms fronds with a fine fibrous core. More often, the tumor cells extend into the lumen of the duct without any fibrous framework.

The carcinoma cells are all alike, without the differentiation into two types often evident in benign papillary tumors. The nuclei of the tumor cells are larger than normal and hyperchromatic, though the anaplasia is not usually so marked as to make the diagnosis of carcinoma obvious. Sometimes the carcinoma fills the ducts entirely and forms a cribriform pattern, with multiple glandlike cavities in an otherwise solid mass of tumor cells that distends the duct. Occasionally, a papillary tumor secretes mucus. Often many sections must be taken before deciding whether the degree of atypicality in the tumor cells or the disorder of their arrangement is sufficient to justify a diagnosis of carcinoma, or before a small focus of invasion reveals the nature of the lesion. The cribriform pattern is highly suggestive of carcinoma, even if present only in a small part of the tumor.

Comedocarcinoma. About 5% of the carcinomata of the breast are of the comedo type. The carcinoma involves large ducts, often through much of the breast. The affected ducts are distended by yellowish-

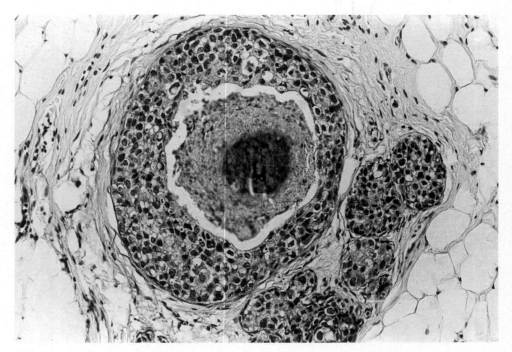

Fig. 43-12.   Comedocarcinoma of the breast, showing a large duct lined by several layers of atypical tumor cells and smaller ducts completely filled with carcinoma.

gray, greasy material, which often can be expressed from the ducts like the core of a comedo in the skin, explaining the name of the carcinoma.

Microscopically, the cells of a comedocarcinoma of the breast are large, pleomorphic, and highly atypical. The affected ducts are dilated and may be filled with carcinoma cells or may show an irregular lining of carcinoma cells several layers thick with necrotic debris in the center of the duct.

Behavior. Papillary carcinomata of the breast grow and extend slowly. If the tumors without evidence of invasion and those with early invasion are considered together, 25% have metastases to the axillary lymph nodes by the time the patient comes to surgery.

Comedocarcinomata of the breast also grow slowly. If the comedocarcinomata without evidence of invasion and those showing early invasion are considered together, 25% of the patients have axillary metastases.

Clinical Presentation. About 50% of patients with a papillary carcinoma have discharge from the nipple. In some, an ill-defined mass or masses are evident, usually beneath the nipple. A comedocarcinoma usually forms a vaguely defined mass.

Treatment and Prognosis. Papillary carcinoma and comedocarcinoma of the breast are usually treated by mastectomy. Over 75% of the patients with a papillary carcinoma are alive 10 years later, and 50% of those who die within 10 years die of causes unrelated to the carcinoma. More than 75% of patients with a comedocarcinoma survive 10 years. The tumors that recur or metastasize presumably do so because a small focus of invasive carcinoma was not detected.

INVASIVE CARCINOMA. In the United States, 25% of malignant tumors in women arise in the breasts. In 1986, 123,000 women in the United States developed carcinoma of the breast and 40,000 died of it. In men, 0.2% of malignant tumors arise in the breasts. In the United States in 1986, 900 men developed carcinoma of the breast and 300 died of it.

In the United States, Canada, the United Kingdom, most of Europe, and in Australasia, from 25 to 30 women in every 100,000 die of the carcinoma of the breast. In Poland, Rumania, Bulgaria, and Greece, 15 to 20 women per 100,000 die of the disease; in Japan and Hong Kong, 5 to 10; in South America, 2 to 15. Women from Japan or Eastern Europe who migrate to the United States tend to show the American incidence of the carcinoma, suggesting that environmental factors are responsible for these differences.

Carcinoma of the breast is rare in women under 25 years old, but after that age the incidence increases as age increases. A woman 80 years old is twice as likely to develop carcinoma of the breast as is a woman 50 years old. In men, the patients are usually over 50 years old.

Lesions. Table 43-1 shows the different kinds of carcinoma in situ and invasive carcinoma of the breast. In women, 90% of the tumors are invasive carcinomata. About 10% are in situ. Paget's disease of the nipple usually complicates an underlying carcinoma.

Infiltrating Ductal Carcinoma. Infiltrating ductal carcinoma is the classic carcinoma of the breast, indeed the classic cancer, known for centuries and well described by the ancient Egyptians. This tumor has given us the words *carcinoma* and *cancer*, from the Greek and Latin for a crab, to describe the claws of carcinoma that invade the surrounding tissues. Over 70% of invasive carcinomata of the breast in women are of this type.

Most infiltrating ductal carcinomata have an abundant, collagenous stroma that makes the tumor stony hard. They are commonly

TABLE 43-1. TYPES OF CARCINOMA OF THE BREAST

In situ
  Papillary carcinoma
  Comedocarcinoma
  Lobular carcinoma in situ

Invasive
  Infiltrating ductal carcinoma
  Infiltrating lobular carcinoma
  Medullary carcinoma
  Colloid carcinoma
  Tubular carcinoma
  Inflammatory carcinoma
  Squamous cell carcinoma
  Carcinoma with metaplastic stroma
  Adenoid cystic carcinoma
  Anaplastic carcinoma

Paget's disease

called scirrhous carcinomata, from the Greek word for hard.

In 52% of the patients, the carcinoma is in the left breast. It is in an upper outer quadrant in 40%, beneath the areola in 30%, in an upper inner quadrant in 15%, in a lower outer quadrant in 8%, in a lower inner quadrant in 5%, over the sternum in 2%, and occasionally in the axillary tail of the gland.

When the patient comes to surgery, 80% of infiltrating ductal carcinomata of the breast are between 1 and 5 cm across. Less than 10% are under 1 cm in diameter.

The carcinoma forms a hard, irregular, often angular mass in the breast. The mass cuts with difficulty, as the knife grates through the dense stroma of the carcinoma. The cut surface is often depressed below the surrounding fat and breast tissue. It is white or yellowish, often with chalky streaks. The carcinoma is well defined. The fibrotic tentacles of carcinoma, which are the claws of the crab, extend a few centimeters into the surrounding fat and pucker it in towards the heart of the cancer.

Microscopically, an infiltrating ductal carcinoma of the breast usually forms long, thin columns of tumor cells, that wind through the dense collagenous stroma they induce and sometimes into the adjacent fat. The tumor cells are sometimes arranged in Indian file, forming columns one cell thick. More frequently the columns of tumor cells are 2, 3, or 4 cells thick and more irregular. Occasionally, the carcinoma forms large clumps of tumor cells or small acini.

Usually, the cells of an infiltrating ductal carcinoma of the breast show little anaplasia. They are larger than normal ductular cells, cuboidal, with spheroidal nuclei and few mitoses. More anaplastic forms and carcinomata with small cells are unusual.

The quantity of stroma varies from one carcinoma to another, but is usually abundant, making up most of the mass. The stroma consists of thick, closely packed bundles of collagen with few fibrocytes. Sometimes the collagen is hyalinized. Condensation of elastic tissue around the remnants of ducts, veins, and to a lesser degree arteries in the tumor is usually prominent and causes the chalky streaks seen macroscopically.

Infiltrating Lobular Carcinoma. About 5% of carcinomata of the breast in women are

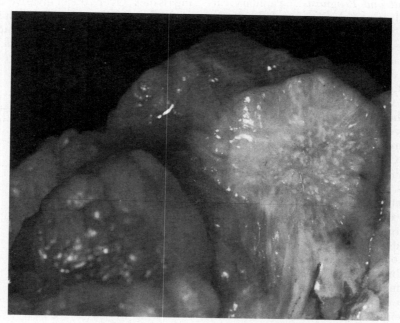

Fig. 43-13. Infiltrating ductal carcinoma of the breast, showing the chalky markings on the cut surface of the tumor.

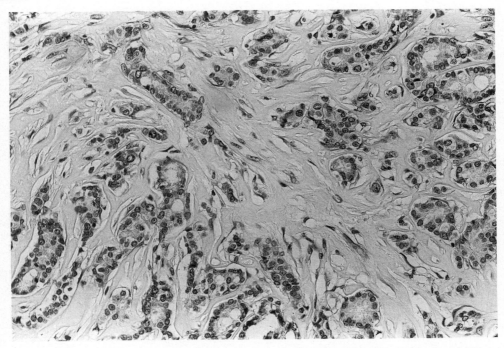

Fig. 43-14. Infiltrating ductal carcinoma of the breast, showing columns of well-differentiated tumor cells, some with acini, separated by a stroma of dense, hyalinized collagen.

of the infiltrating lobular type. Macroscopically, the tumors are indistinguishable from infiltrating ductal carcinomata. They form the same kind of hard, scirrhous mass. Microscopically, infiltrating lobular carcinoma often occurs in association with lobular carcinoma in situ. It forms thin columns of small, regular tumor cells in a dense fibrous stroma. Usually the columns are one cell thick. Sometimes they swirl around small ducts. Sometimes metastases lose their abundant stroma and look like a lymphoma, with masses of small, rounded tumor cells.

Medullary Carcinoma. About 3% of carcinomata of the breast in women are of the medullary type. Most of the patients are about 50 years old. Macroscopically, the tumor is usually 5 to 10 cm across. The overlying skin is sometimes reddened. It is sharply demarcated, soft, grayish-white, usually with extensive necrosis and hemorrhage. Microscopically, the tumor is well demarcated. It consists of sheets of large, pleomorphic cells, with abundant cytoplasm, large vesicular nuclei, and many often bizarre and atypical mitoses. Some of the tumor cells

may be gigantic or multinucleated. Commonly, the central part of the sheets of tumor cells is necrotic. Occasionally, parts of the carcinoma show squamous differentiation. The masses of carcinoma cells are supported by a sparse collagenous stroma, which is usually, but not always, heavily infiltrated by lymphocytes and plasma cells.

Colloid Carcinoma. In 1% of carcinomata of the breast in women mucous secretion is excessive and becomes the most striking feature of the carcinoma. Macroscopically, such carcinomata are usually well demarcated, and on section are soft, slimy, and gelatinous. Microscopically, they may show acini filled with mucus and lined by columnar, mucus-secreting cells, but more often they show small rafts of cuboidal tumor cells floating in a sea of mucus that has escaped into the stroma.

Tubular Carcinoma. Tubular carcinoma of the breast is rare. It consists of small tubules set in a dense stroma of coarse, sometimes hyalinized collagen. The tubules are lined by regular, cuboidal, or flattened cells, often with eosinophilic cytoplasm. The

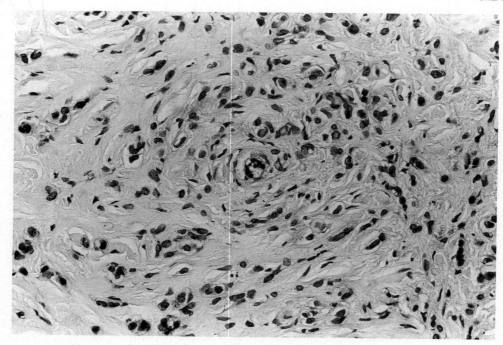

Fig. 43-15. Infiltrating lobular carcinoma of the breast, showing the swirling pattern.

nuclei of the tumor cells are small, regular, and spheroidal.

Inflammatory Carcinoma. Less than 1% of carcinomata of the breast in women is of the inflammatory type. The breast involved becomes firm, edematous, and reddened and is often tender or painful. The edema and reddening often extend rapidly to the surrounding skin or the other breast. The carcinoma is of the infiltrating ductal type. The edema and reddening are caused by massive vascular permeation in the reddened skin and the underlying breast. Lymphatic permeation is especially extensive. There is no inflammatory reaction.

Squamous Cell Carcinoma. Squamous cell carcinoma of the breast is rare. More common are islands of squamous differentiation in a carcinoma, which is predominantly of the infiltrating ductal type.

Carcinoma with Metaplastic Stroma. Rarely, a carcinoma of the breast shows islands of metaplastic cartilage or metaplastic bone in its stroma.

Adenoid Cystic Carcinoma. Rarely, an adenoid cystic carcinoma arises in a breast. The tumor is similar to the adenoid cystic tumors of the salivary glands.

Anaplastic Carcinoma. Rarely, a carcinoma of the breast is anaplastic, with bizarre pleomorphic cells, usually with little stroma.

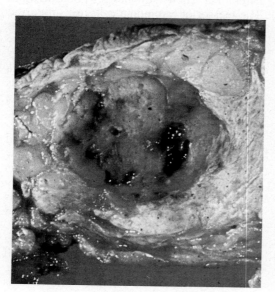

Fig. 43-16. Medullary carcinoma of the breast, showing a large, well-demarcated tumor.

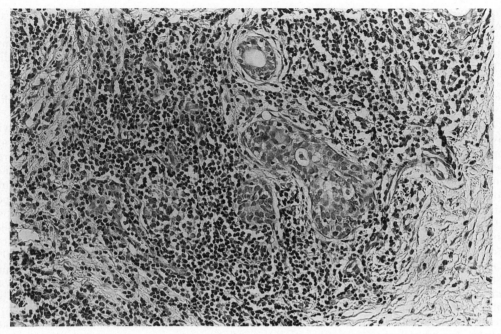

Fig. 43-17. Medullary carcinoma of the breast, showing clumps of large tumor cells and the stoma densely infiltrated with lymphocytes.

Behavior. Most infiltrating intraductal carcinomata of the breast grow slowly. The tumor often takes from 2 to 15 months to double in size. If it is assumed that the growth rate has been constant throughout the life of the tumor, this means that the carcinoma was present for several years before it became evident clinically.

Tentacles of carcinoma cells extend up to 1 cm beyond the apparent margin of an infiltrating ductal carcinoma. They penetrate into fat and extend along lymphatics, ducts, and perineural spaces. As the collagenous stroma of the carcinoma forms around these tentacles, the tumor slowly enlarges. As the collagen matures and contracts, the surrounding tissues are pulled in toward the carcinoma.

Infiltrating ductal carcinomata often grow along lymphatics for a considerable distance. The carcinoma usually remains within the lymphatic vessels, but sometimes escapes into the tissues to establish metastases. Multiple nodules of carcinoma are present in the breast in 15% of the patients. It is often not clear whether they are metastases or multiple primary tumors. Not uncommonly, the lymphatics around the carcinoma are plugged with tumor, causing lymphedema.

Emboli of tumor cells are carried in the lymph to the regional lymph nodes. Infiltrating ductal carcinomata extend to the areola by lymphatic permeation or embolism and then to the lymph nodes in the axilla. Sometimes they extend downward into the lymphatics in the pectoral muscles and then to the axillary or mediastinal lymph nodes. Most of the emboli that reach the lymph nodes die, but in 40% of the patients a few survive and establish metastases. A metastasis in a lymph node usually begins in the peripheral sinus of the node. As it enlarges, it replaces much or all of the lymph node and may invade the surrounding tissue.

Metastases are present in the axillary lymph nodes in 40% of patients with infiltrating ductal carcinoma of the breast by the time the woman comes to surgery. If the carcinoma is in the upper and outer quadrant, more than 50% of the patients have axillary metastases. If it is beneath the nipple, nearly 50% do. If the carcinoma is elsewhere in the breast, between 30 and 40% of the patients have metastases in the axilla.

The larger the carcinoma, the more likely are metastases to the axilla. If the carcinoma is less than 2 cm in diameter, under 25% of the patients have axillary metastases at operation. If the carcinoma is between 5 and 6 cm in diameter, 60% do.

The lymph nodes first involved may be in any part of the axilla. Usually metastases first appear in the lymph nodes in the midpart of the axilla, not in the lymph nodes closest to the primary tumor. As the carcinoma extends, more and more of the nodes in the axilla become involved.

Only microscopic examination can determine with certainty whether an axillary lymph node contains carcinoma. Clinical examination cannot detect the small metastases often present in the axillary nodes, and even if one or more lymph nodes in the axilla of a woman with carcinoma of the breast are large and hard, the enlargement may be due to inflammation rather than to cancer.

Metastases to the mediastinal lymph nodes along the internal mammary artery are also common. They tend to develop later than axillary metastases, usually only after metastases have developed in the axilla. Less than 5% of women with carcinoma of the breast have involvement of the internal mammary nodes without axillary metastases, but 35% of women with axillary metastases have also internal mammary metastases. The more extensive the involvement of the axilla, the more likely are metastases in the internal mammary nodes. Over 50% of patients with axillary metastases who have a carcinoma in the inner half of the breast have metastases in the internal mammary nodes, and nearly 50% of those with a carcinoma in the central part of the breast beneath the areola, but less than 25% of those with a primary tumor in the outer half of the breast.

Late in the disease, the carcinoma extends to other lymph nodes. The supraclavicular lymph nodes are involved in from 10 to 20% of women with metastases in the axillary lymph nodes. The carinal lymph nodes and the nodes at the hilus of the lung may be replaced by carcinoma. The carcinoma often spreads slowly down the chain of para-aortic nodes in the abdomen. Permeation of the peribronchial lymphatics in the lungs is sometimes extensive in patients with carcinoma of the breast. The lymphatics are filled and distended by the carcinoma, which escapes to establish peribronchial metastases. The pleural lymphatics are often also filled and distended by carcinoma.

Hematogenous metastases in patients with an infiltrating ductal carcinoma usually appear soon after the diagnosis is made or are present when the patient is first seen. Occasionally they are long delayed, appearing from 5 to 20 years after the carcinoma has apparently been successfully removed. At autopsy, the lungs contain hematogenous metastases in 70% of patients with an infiltrating ductal carcinoma. The liver is involved in 60%. Metastases are present in the pelvis, spine, femurs, ribs, skull, or humeri in 60%. Usually the bony metastases are osteolytic, but sometimes they are osteoblastic. The skin is involved by metastasis or recurrence in 30% of the patients, most often in the region of the breast. The adrenals, ovaries, or brain, indeed any organ, can be involved.

Some 5% of women with an infiltrating ductal carcinoma in one breast develop a second primary carcinoma in the other. Often the second carcinoma does not appear until many years after the removal of the first.

Infiltrating lobular carcinomata of the breast behave as do infiltrating ductal carcinomata. They invade and metastasize in the same way.

Most medullary carcinomata of the breast are sluggish. Only 30% of the women with a medullary carcinoma have axillary metastases at the time of surgical treatment, even though the tumors are often large. Some suggest that medullary carcinomata grow slowly because the lymphocytes in their stroma mount an immunologic attack on the tumor.

Metastases in the axillary lymph nodes are less common in women with a colloid carcinoma of the breast than in those with an infiltrating ductal tumor. Tubular carcinomata grow slowly, but metastases in the axillary nodes are present in 40% of the patients at tht time of operation. Most adenoid cystic carcinomata remain confined to the breast.

Inflammatory carcinomata grow rapidly and extend widely.

Staging. Carcinoma of the breast is divided clinically into four stages. In stage I, the carcinoma is less than 2 cm across, no metastases are present in the lymph nodes, and no distant metastases are evident. In stage II, the tumor is 2 to 5 cm across. The lymph nodes may contain metastases but are not fixed. No distant metastases are present. In stage III, the carcinoma is over 5 cm in diameter and fixed to the chest wall or the skin, fixed axillary metastases are present, or metastases are present in the supraclavicular lymph nodes. Distant metastases are not detectable. In stage IV, distant metastases are present. Over 60% of carcinomata are in stage I when discovered, 20% in stage II, 10% in stage III and 10% in stage IV.

Clinical Features. Infiltrating ductal carcinomata of the breast produce symptoms only late. In nearly 80% of the patients, the patient discovers a lump or thickening in her breast. About 10% of the patients develop twinges of pain in the region of the carcinoma. Only 2% have a sanguinous or serous dis-

charge from the nipple. Rarely, the skin overlying a carcinoma becomes reddened, or the whole breast becomes shrunken and scarred. Sometimes the patient seeks help only when the carcinoma has ulcerated through the skin in one or more places.

Retraction of the nipple is evident in some patients with carcinoma of the breast. As the collagen in the stroma of the carcinoma matures, thickens, and shortens, it drags on the ducts that pass through the tumor and may distort the nipple, retracting it into the breast, inverting it, or pulling it askew, so that it no longer points in the normal direction.

The carcinoma may become fixed to the skin as it invades the deeper part of the dermis. The carcinoma may pull on the skin, causing a dimple, which often can be made more obvious by raising the arms to lift the breasts, or by pressing the skin over the tumor. The carcinoma often invades the pectoral muscles, becoming fixed to the muscle and no longer able to move over it.

Peau d'orange, or pig skin, develops when widespread obstruction of lymphatics by a

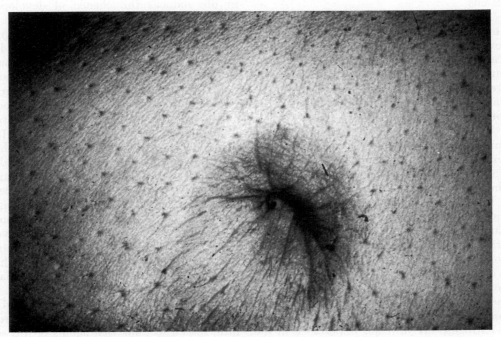

Fig. 43-18. Carcinoma of the breast, showing the retraction of the nipple and peau d'orange.

carcinoma of the breast causes lymphedema in the overlying skin. The skin of the affected part of the breast looks much like the skin of an orange. The ligaments that tether the skin pull it down here and there to give little pits between which the edematous dermis bulges out.

Carcinoma en cuirasse, from the French for the breastplate of a suit of armor, is an unusual form of carcinoma of the breast, usually seen when a carcinoma recurs after mastectomy. In one or more areas, the skin of the chest becomes hard, stiff, and indurated, like stiff leather. Often the affected areas are brown or violaceous. Usually the process begins at the site of the mastectomy, but it may involve much of the skin of the chest. Microscopically, the affected areas show widespread lymphatic permeation, with carcinoma filling the lymphatics in the skin and edema and fibrosis in the dermis.

Mammography is widely used to assist in the diagnosis of carcinoma of the breast. If the tumor is large, the dense carcinoma is seen clearly, in contrast to the more radiolucent fat. Small calcifications are common in carcinomata of the breast, within ducts and in foci of necrosis, but also occur in benign lesions.

Pathogenesis. The pathogenesis of carcinoma of the breast is not clear, and probably several factors interact to cause the tumor. Carcinoma of the breast in rodents has been much studied, but the tumors in the animals are not similar to those in women. The findings in the experimental work should be interpreted with caution.

Genetic factors are of major importance in animals. In some strains of mice, almost all females develop tumors of the breast as they age, but in other strains breast tumors are almost unknown.

In women, the incidence of carcinoma of the breast in the mothers, sisters, and daughters of women with carcinoma of the breast is twice that in women in the general population. How this increased susceptibility is inherited is uncertain, but probably a number of genes are involved. In rare families, the disease is inherited as an autosomal dominant character.

Estrogens are of major importance in the causation of breast tumors in animals. In some strains of mice in which almost all females develop breast tumors, the tumors can be prevented by castrating the animals while they are young. In some strains, breast tumors can be induced in male mice by giving large doses of estrogen.

In women, the importance of estrogens seems equally clear. Any condition that increases the concentration of estrogen in the plasma, increases the ratio of estrogen to progesterone, or increases the time that the breast is exposed to estrogen increases the risk of developing carcinoma of the breast, though the increase in the risk is not great. Carcinoma of the breast is 1.5 times as frequent in women who have never borne children as in women with children. The more children, the less the risk of carcinoma. The earlier the menarche and the later the menopause, the greater the risk of carcinoma. Estrogens favor the development of carcinoma of the endometrium, and the incidence of carcinoma of the breast in women with carcinoma of the endometrium is 1.5 times that in the general population. The types of mammary dysplasia that increase the risk of carcinoma of the breast are probably caused by hormonal imbalance. Oophorectomy early in life reduces the chance of developing carcinoma of the breast.

Radiation increases the risk of developing a carcinoma of the breast in women and in animals. A dose of 0.5 Gy (50 rad) is enough to increase the chance of developing carcinoma of the breast, especially if the radiation is given during adolescence. The incidence of carcinoma of the breast is high in the survivors of the atomic bombs dropped on Japan. It is increased in women with pulmonary tuberculosis who were repeatedly fluoroscoped.

Viruses are an important cause of carcinoma of the breast in mice, but their importance in the causation of human carcinoma is uncertain. Particles like viruses are sometimes present in human milk and occasionally have been found in the cells of an infiltrating ductal carcinoma. Their nature and their role, if any, in the causation of carcinoma of the breast are obscure.

Tumors of the breast can be induced in animals by chemical carcinogens, but there is little reason to think that agents of this sort are important in women. Nor is there any reason to think trauma plays any part in causing carcinoma of the breast.

Treatment and Prognosis. Invasive carcinoma of a breast is treated by excising the carcinoma. Many prefer to do so by a modified radical mastectomy, removing the breast and dissecting the axillary lymph nodes, but leaving the pectoral muscles intact. Others prefer local excision of the carcinoma, especially when it is small and the operation does not cause distortion of the breast. The lymph nodes in the axilla are usually dissected in a separate procedure.

Overall, 80% of patients with an infiltrating ductal carcinoma of the breast of stage I live five years, 65% of those in stage II, 40% of those in stage III, and 10% of patients in stage IV.

The more extensive the carcinoma in the breast and axilla, the more likely local recurrence becomes. In patients with stage II infiltrating ductal carcinoma given no postoperative therapy, the carcinoma will recur locally in 20% of the patients if more than 4 axillary lymph nodes contain carcinoma, in 10% if 1 to 3 nodes are involved, and in less than 5% if no metastases are found in the lymph nodes. If the breast and axilla are irradiated postoperatively or the patient is given postoperative chemotherapy, less than 5% of the tumors recur. The irradiation does not increase the survival rate, but chemotherapy does. It delays or prevents the appearance of distant metastases in many of the patients.

The extent of the disease in the breast and axilla also affects the prognosis. If the lymph nodes are free of carcinoma, 80% of the patients survive 5 years, and nearly 80% live more than 10 years. If 1 to 3 lymph nodes are involved, the 5-year survival is 50%, and the 10-year survival 35%. If 4 or more lymph nodes are involved, 20% of the patients live 5 years and 10% live 10 years. The larger the tumor, the more probable axillary metastases become. If the carcinoma is more than 5.5 cm across, 70% of the patients have axillary metastases. If it is less than 2 cm, 25%.

The better differentiated an infiltrating ductal carcinoma, the better the prognosis. Nearly 50% of women with a well-differentiated tumor, 25% of those with a moderately differentiated tumor, and 20% of those with a poorly differentiated tumor survive 10 years. Some have suggested that hyperplasia of the cells lining the sinuses in the axillary lymph nodes indicates a good prognosis, but later work has failed to confirm the observation.

Most of the less common types of carcinoma of the breast behave much like infiltrating ductal tumors. The prognosis with a medullary carcinoma is better because of its slow course. Most patients who remain tumor free for a few years are cured. The prognosis is also better with a tubular carcinoma. An inflammatory carcinoma grows rapidly. Distant metastases are present at the time of diagnosis in 30% of the patients. On the average, the patients survive 20 months.

If estrogen and progesterone receptors are present in the tumor cells, the prognosis is better. Although the sensitivtiy of the methods used to detect the receptors varies, 80% of infiltrating lobular carcinomata of the breast, 60% of infiltrating ductal carcinomata, and 25% of medullary carcinomata have estrogen receptors, and 50% of infiltrating lobular carcinomata, 40% of infiltrating ductal carcinomata, and 30% of medullary carcinomata have progesterone receptors. The better differentiated the carcinoma, the more likely it is to have estrogen and progesterone receptors. Nearly 90% of well-differentiated carcinomata of the breast have estrogen receptors, but only 40% of poorly differentiated tumors. The carcinomata with receptors tend to have a lower rate of cell division, indicating their less agressive nature. In one group of patients, those with tumors containing estrogen receptors had a median survival of 46 months; those with tumors without receptors a median survival of 21 months. When followed for an average of 18 months, 14% of the patients with tumors containing estrogen receptors suffered recurrence of the carcinoma, but the tumor recurred in 34% of those with tumors without estrogen receptors.

Distant metastases appear sooner or later in 50% of patients with carcinoma of the breast. They can be controlled for a time by hormonal therapy or chemotherapy, though the remission rarely lasts more than one year.

Tamoxifen or other antiestrogens produce a remission in 80% of patients with both estrogen and progesterone receptors in the tumor, 30% of those who have either estrogen or progesterone receptors, and 10% of those with neither. The regression of the tumor is usually evident within eight weeks. If the patient fails to respond to tamoxifen or becomes resistant to it, suppression of adrenal function by aminoglutethimide is sometimes helpful. Sometimes a tumor that does not respond to antiestrogens can be suppressed by giving estrogen. Metastases in the soft tissues are the most likely to respond. Bony metastases are more likely to respond to androgen.

If hormonal therapy fails, or the tumor becomes resistant to it, cytotoxic chemotherapeutic drugs bring partial remission to 80% of patients with carcinoma of the breast, and total remission to 15%.

Paget's Disease. Paget's disease of the nipple is named after the English surgeon Sir James Paget, who described it in 1874. About 3% of women with carcinoma of the breast have Paget's disease. Occasionally it develops in a man. Most of the patients are 40 to 70 years old.

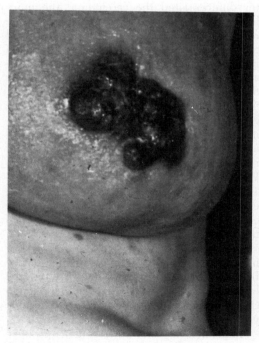

Fig. 43-19. Paget's disease of the nipple, showing replacement of the nipple and areola by the tumor.

Paget's disease of the nipple is almost invariably associated with a carcinoma of the underlying breast. The carcinoma may not be evident when the patient is first seen, but usually becomes obvious within one or two years. In this, Paget's disease of the breast differs from Paget's disease of the vulva, in which there is often no underlying carcinoma.

Lesions. In Paget's disease, the nipple becomes reddened, sometimes smoothed, thickened, or roughened. After months or years, small erosions appear on the nipple. Often they are crusted, bright red, and granular. Serosanguinous fluid oozes from the erosions and may be mistaken for discharge from the nipple. Slowly, as years pass, the erosions extend, to involve much or all of the areola sometimes to involve the skin of the breast.

Microscopically, the affected area shows Paget's cells scattered in the epidermis. The Paget's cells are larger than the epidermal cells, perhaps twice as big, well defined, with pale, empty cytoplasm and spheroidal, vesicular nuclei. They show no prickles but are joined to one another and sometimes to the epidermal cells by desmosomes. Occasionally Paget's cells contain a few granules of melanin, though they do not contain dopa or the other enzymes needed to synthesize melanin. Sometimes they stain with the periodic acid-Schiff reaction or contain small quantities of mucus.

At first, the Paget's cells are few and lie between the epidermal cells, usually in the basal part of the epidermis. Later, they become more numerous and may be scattered in the more superficial part of the epidermis, which often becomes thickened and hyperkeratotic. Still later, the Paget's cells form solid clumps that replace much of the epidermis or form small acini within the epidermis. They may extend into the epidermal appendages, but do not invade the dermis. The dermis beneath the lesion is congested and usually shows a moderate exudate of lymphocytes and plasma cells.

The underlying carcinoma may be of the comedo type, affecting the large ducts leading to the nipple, but often it is of the infiltrating ductal type and lies deep in the breast, without obvious connection to the nipple.

Pathogenesis. Most think that the Paget's

cells are tumor cells from the underlying carcinoma of the breast that have spread up the ducts and are invading the epidermis. Others think that Paget's disease is a form of carcinoma in situ of the epidermis and that the Paget's cells are derived from epidermal cells.

Often the connection between the underlying carcinoma and the erosion of the nipple is far from clear. Random sections from the tissue between the carcinoma and the nipple often fail to show tumor. However, in the few cases that have been studied in detail, a connection between the carcinoma and Paget's disease has always been found, though it may be only a thin column of tumor cells ascending a single duct, between the ductal epithelium and its basement membrane.

Treatment and Prognosis. Paget's disease of the breast is treated like any other carcinoma of the breast. The prognosis depends on the nature and extent of the underlying carcinoma.

Carcinoma of the Male Breast. In men, carcinoma of the breast is rare. Only about 1% of breast carcinomata arise in men. On the average, the patients are 10 years older than are women with carcinoma of the breast. Any of the types of carcinoma of the breast that occur in women can occur in men, though most are intraductal. Usually the patient discovers a mass in his breast, but sometimes discharge from the nipple draws attention to the tumor.

Men with Klinefelter's syndrome have more than 60 times the expected incidence of carcinoma of the breast. Hyperestrinism such as may be caused by damage to the liver by schistosomiasis in Egypt or by starvation has been reported to increase the incidence of carcinoma of the breast in men. Whether the gynecomastia often found in men with carcinoma of the prostate treated with estrogens increases the risk of carcinoma of the breast is debated. Carcinoma does occur in the breasts in these men, but it is usually considered that the tumors are metastatic from the prostate, rather than primary in the breast. In a few men, a genetic predisposition to carcinoma of the breast has been demonstated.

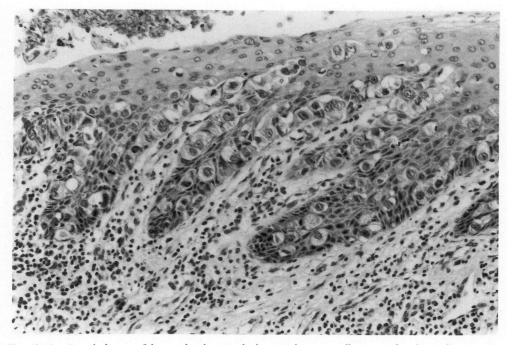

Fig. 43-20.   Paget's disease of the nipple, showing the large, pale tumor cells scattered in the epidermis of the areola.

The prognosis in carcinoma of the breast is bad in men. Probably the small size of the male breast makes it easier for the carcinoma to invade the chest wall or reach the lymph nodes. In 40% of the patients, the carcinoma has extended beyond the limits of resection by the time the man is first seen by a physician.

If the carcinoma appears clinically to be confined to the breast, 50% of the men survive 10 years. If there is clinical evidence of enlargement of the axillary lymph nodes, only 30% survive 10 years. As in women, metastases sometimes appear years after resection of the carcinoma.

CYSTOSARCOMA PHYLLODES. A cystosarcoma phyllodes is a malignant tumor that resembles a fibroadenoma, but has a cellular and atypical stroma between ducts that usually show little atypicality. Some extend the term to include unusually large fibroadenomata of the usual structure, better called giant fibroadenomata. Most women with a cystosarcoma are between 30 and 70 years old.

Lesions. Most cystosarcomata are over 10 cm across when discovered. A few are much larger when the patients seeks advice. A few remain small. The tumor does not become fixed to the underlying tissues and remains freely movable in the breast.

On section, a cystosarcoma phyllodes is sometimes well defined, but often small fingers of tumor extend a short way into the surrounding tissue. The cut surface of the tumor is usually firm and white. Often the lumina of the ducts within it form slits, as in an intracanalicular fibroadenoma. In the bigger tumors, areas of necrosis and hemorrhage are common, and often cystic cavities are present within the tumor. Sometimes the stroma bulges into these cavities, forming the leaflike projections that give the tumor its name, *cysto-*, from the Greek for a cyst and *phyllodes* for leaflike.

Microscopically, a cystosarcoma phyllodes consists of ducts and stroma, like a fibroadenoma. It may show the pericanalicular pattern, the intracanalicular pattern, or both, though most often the ducts are considerably

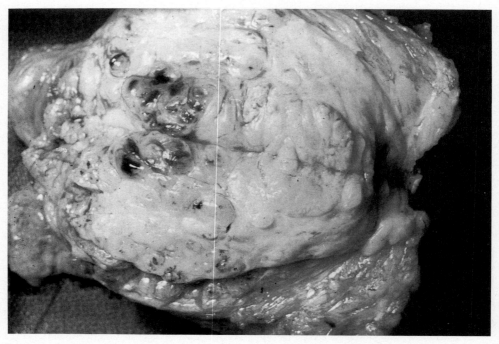

Fig. 43-21. Cystosarcoma phyllodes, which has been cut in half, showing the large tumor replacing much of the breast.

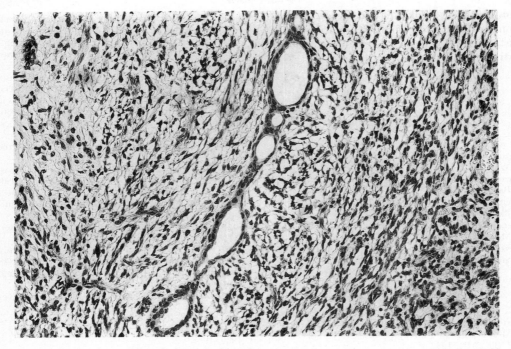

Fig. 43-22. Cystosarcoma phyllodes showing a duct lined by inactive, cuboidal epithelium and surrounded by poorly differentiated, myxoid stroma.

elongated and flattened in the intracanalicular manner. The epithelium lining the ducts may be cuboidal and inactive or may be irregular and several layers thick.

Occasionally, squamous metaplasia is evident in the ducts. Rarely, there is lobular carcinoma in situ or an invasive ductal carcinoma.

The stroma is usually more cellular than is the stroma of a fibroadenoma. The stromal cells are often elongated, like the cells of a well-differentiated fibrosarcoma and grow in a storiform pattern. They may be closely packed, with little collagen, or stellate and separated by myxomatous intercellular substance. Sometimes the stromal cells con-

tain droplets of fat. Occasionally the stromal cells are more anaplastic, with a high mitotic rate. Rarely, foci of bone or cartilage are evident in the stroma.

Behavior. A cystosarcoma phyllodes usually grows rapidly. It invades locally, but metastasizes in less than 10% of the patients. The metastases often consist only of the stromal element of the tumor without its epithelial component.

Treatment and Prognosis. Local excision cures most cystosarcomata. If the excision is too narrow, the tumor recurs. Re-excision is nearly always curative.

SECONDARY TUMORS. Secondary tumors in the breasts are uncommon. Occasionally lymphoma or leukemia involves a breast. Sometimes carcinoma of the prostate metastasizes to a breast in a man treated with estrogens.

BIBLIOGRAPHY

General

Azzopardi, J. G.: Problems in Breast Pathology. London, W. B. Saunders, 1979.

Carter, D.: Interpretation of Breast Biopsies. New York, Raven Press, 1984.

Haagensen, C. D.: Diseases of the Breast, 3rd ed. Philadelphia. W. B. Saunders, 1986.

Hendler, F. J.: Breast diseases and the internist. Am. J. Med. Sci., 293:332, 1987.

Oertel, Y. C.: Fine Needle Aspiration of the Breast. Stoneham MA, Butterworths, 1987.

Hyperplasia

Bartow, S. A., Black, W. C., Waeckerlin, R. W., and Mettler, F. A.: Fibrocystic disease. Pathol. Annu., 17(Pt. 2):93, 1982.

Bussolati, G., et al.: Morphologic and functional aspects of apocrine metaplasia in dysplastic and neoplastic breast tissue, Ann. N. Y. Acad. Sci., 464:262, 1986.

Cook, M. G., and Rohan, T. E.: The patho-epidemiology of benign proliferative epithelial disorders of the female breast. J. Pathol., 146:1, 1985.

Haibach, H., and Rosenholtz, M. J.: Prepubertal gynecomastia with lobules and acini. Am. J. Clin. Pathol., 80:252, 1983.

Mansel, R. E.: Benign breast disease and cancer risk. Ann. N. Y. Acad. Sci., 464:364, 1986.

Mauvais-Jarvis, P., Stiruk-Ware, R., and Kuttenn, F.: Benign breast disease. Breast Cancer, 4:51, 1980.

Thor, A., et al.: ras Gene alterations and enhanced expression of ras p21 expression in a spectrum of benign and malignant human mammary tissues. Lab. Invest., 55:603, 1986.

Wang, D. Y., and Fentiman, I. S.: Epidemiology and endocrinology of benign breast disease. Breast Cancer Res. Treat., 6:5, 1985.

Tumors

Ajaya, D. O. S., Osegbe, D. N., and Ademiluyi, S. A.: Carcinoma of the male breast in West Africans and a review of the world literature. Cancer, 50:1664, 1982.

Bavafa, S., Reyes, C. V., and Choudhury, A. M.: Male breast carcinoma. J. Surg. Oncol., 24:41, 1983.

Beard, D. B., and Haskell, C. M.: Carcinoembryonic antigen in breast cancer. Am. J. Med., 80:241, 1986.

Bogomoletz, W. V.: Elastosis in breast cancer. Pathol. Annu., 21(Pt. 2):347, 1986.

Bulbrook, R. D.: Endocrine aspects of breast and prostatic cancer. Cancer Surv., 5:435, 1986.

Bussolati, G., et al.: Morphologic and functional aspects of apocrine metaplasia in dysplastic and neoplastic breast tissue, Ann. N. Y. Acad. Sci., 464:262, 1986.

Clavel, F., et al.: Breast cancer and oral contraceptives. Contraception, 32:553, 1985.

Coleman, R. E., and Rubens, R. D.: Bone metastases and breast cancer. Cancer Treat. Rev., 12:251, 1985.

Conrad, B., and Kieser, R.: Randomized clinical trials in breast cancer. Arch. Geschwultsforsch., 56:211, 1986.

Cooperman, A. M., and Hermann, R.: Breast cancer. Surg. Clin. North Am., 64:1031, 1984.

DeMay, R. M., and Kay, S.: Granular cell tumor of the breast. Pathol. Annu., 19(Pt. 2):121, 1984.

Elte, J. W., et al.: Osteolytic bone metastases in breast carcinoma. Eur. J. Cancer Clin. Oncol., 22:493, 1986.

Fu, Y. S., et al.: The relationship of breast cancer morphology and estrogen receptor protein status. Prog. Surg. Pathol., 3:65, 1981.

Gambrell, R. D., Jr.: Sex steroids and cancer. Obstet. Gynecol. Clin. North Am., 14:191, 1987.

Grace, W. R. and Cooperman, A. M.: Inflammatory breast cancer. Surg. Clin. North Am., 65:151, 1985.

Holck, S., and Laursen, H.: Oral contraceptives and cancer. Arch. Geschwulstforsch., 56:155, 1986.

Huggins, G. R., and Zucker, P. K.: Oral contraceptives and neoplasia. Fertil. Steril., 47:733, 1987.

Hulka, B. S.: Replacement estrogens and risk of gynecologic and breast cancer. Cancer, 60(8 Suppl.): 1960, 1987.

Jotti, G., Petit, J. Y., and Contesso, G.: Minimal breast cancer. Semin. Oncol., 13:384, 1986.

Kerner, H., and Lichtig, C.: Lobular cancerization: incidence and differential diagnosis with lobular carcinoma in situ of breast. Histopathology, 10:621, 1986.

Kodama, M., and Kodama, T.: Relation between steroid metabolism of the host and genesis of cancers of the breast, uterine cervix, and endometrium. Adv. Cancer Res., 38:77, 1983.

Lagios, M. D., Westdahl. P. R., and Rose, M. R.: The concept and implications of multicentricity in breast carcinoma. Pathol. Annu., 16(Pt. 2):83, 1981.

Lichter, A. S.: Nonmastectomy treatment of breast cancer. Postgrad. Med., 79:93, 1986.

McDivitt, R. W., Stewart, F. W., and Berg, J. W.: Tumors of the Breast. Washington D. C., Armed Forces Institute of Pathology, 1967.

McGuire, W. L.: Prognostic factors in primary breast cancer. Cancer Surv., 5:527, 1986.

Mansel, R. E.: Benign breast disease and cancer risk. Ann. N. Y. Acad. Sci., 464:364, 1986.

Moore, D. H., Moore, D. H., II, and Moore, C. T.: Breast carcinoma etiological factors. Adv. Cancer Res., 40:189, 1983.

Osborne, C. K.: Heterogeneity in hormone receptor status in primary and metastatic breast cancer. Semin. Oncol., 12:317, 1985.

Osborne, C. K., Knight, W. A., III, Yochmowitz, M. G., and McGuire, W. L.: Estrogen receptor and prognosis in breast cancer. Breast Cancer, 4:33, 1981.

Poulsen, H. S.: In vitro tests and hormonal treatment of breast cancer. Prog. Surg. Pathol., 5:37, 1983.

Rosen, P. P.: Clinical implications of preinvasive and small invasive breast carcinomas. Pathol. Annu., 16(Pt. 2):337, 1981.

Sarnelli, R., and Squartini, F.: Multicentricity in breast cancer. Pathol. Annu., 21(Pt. 1):143, 1986.

Schaefer, G., et al.: Breast carcinoma in elderly women. Pathol. Annu., 19(Pt. 1):195, 1984.

Sherry, M. M., et al.: Inflammatory carcinoma of the breast. Am. J. Med., 79:355, 1985.

Shingelton, W. W., and McCarty, K. S., Jr.: Breast carcinoma. Gynecol. Oncol., 26:271, 1987.

Silverman, J. F., et al.: Localized primary (AL) amyloid tumor of the breast. Am. J. Surg. Pathol., 10:539, 1986.

Sledge, G. W., Jr., and McGuire, W. L. Steroid hormone receptors in human breast cancer. Adv. Cancer Res., 38:61, 1983.

Squartini, F., Bistocchi, M., Sarnelli, R., and Basolo, F.: Early pathologic changes in experimental and human breast cancer. Ann. N. Y. Acad. Sci., 464:231, 1986.

Stanford, J. L., Szklo, M., and Brenton, L. A.: Estrogen receptors and breast cancer. Epidemiol. Rev., 8:42, 1986.

Sumpio, B. E., Jennings, T. A., Sullivan, P. D., and Merino, M. J.: Adenoid cystic carcinoma of the breast. Ann. Surg., 205:295, 1987.

Symposium: Estrogen receptor determination with monoclonal antibodies. Cancer Res., 46:4232s, 1986.

Thor, A., et al.: ras Gene alterations and enhanced expression of ras p21 expression in a spectrum of benign and malignant human mammary tissues. Lab. Invest., 55:603, 1986.

Tinkler, M. A., and Wise, L.: The conservative management of breast cancer. Surg. Annu., 19:227, 1987.

Underwood, J. C. E.: Ostrogen receptors in human breast cancer. Diag. Histopathol., 6:1, 1983.

Vorherr, H., Vorherr, U. F., Kutvirt, D. M., and Key, C. R.: Cystosarcoma phyllodes. Arch. Gynecol., 236:173, 1985.

Wellings, S. R.: Development of human breast cancer. Adv. Cancer Res., 31:287, 1980.

Whitehead, M. I., and Fraser, D.: Controversies surrounding the safety of estrogen replacement therapy. Am. J. Obstet. Gynecol., 156:1313, 1987.

Wilkinson, E. J., et al.: Occult axillary lymph node metastases in invasive breast carcinoma. Pathol. Annu., 17(Pt. 2):67, 1982.

Wolff, M., and Reinis, M. S.: Breast cancer in the male. Prog. Surg. Pathol., 3:77, 1981.

44

Pituitary Gland

THE pituitary gland and hypothalamus are closely interrelated. Many of the diseases of the pituitary gland also involve the hypothalamus, and dysfunction of the hypothalamus causes secondary changes in the hypophysis. In addition to non-neoplastic conditions, genital defects, and tumors, other disorders result from overactivity or underactivity of the gland.

NON-NEOPLASTIC DISORDERS

The non-neoplastic conditions that involve the pituitary gland include inflammation, trauma, vascular disorders, and the changes in the gland caused by diseases of other organs.

INFLAMMATION. Inflammation of the pituitary gland is uncommon. Occasionally acute inflammation extends into the gland in meningitis, or an abscess develops in the pituitary gland or hypothalamus in a patient with septicemia.

Sarcoidosis, which occasionally affects the hypothalamus or the pituitary gland, can be extensive enough to cause dysfunction. Rarely, sarcoidosis is confined to the hypothalamus and posterior pituitary, or to the hypothalamus, posterior pituitary, and adrenal glands. Occasionally granulomata with an exudate of neutrophils, lymphocytes, plasma cells, and sometimes eosinophils are found in the hypothalamus and pituitary. Seldom does tuberculosis, a fungal infection, syphilis, or toxoplasmosis involve the hypothalamus or pituitary.

Especially in children, Hand-Schüller-Christian disease may involve the posterior pituitary, its stalk, or sometimes the hypothalamus. The lesions are as in bone, with fat-filled macrophages, sometimes eosinophils,

or lymphocytes and tend to heal by scarring. The mucopolysaccharidoses may involve the anterior pituitary, though they rarely cause dysfunction.

HEMORRHAGE. Hemorrhage from an aneurysm of the circle of Willis or an intracerebral hemorrhage sometimes damages the hypothalamus. A pituitary adenoma or trauma can cause bleeding into the sella turcica. Petechial hemorrhages are prominent in the mammillary bodies in Wernicke's disease.

INFARCTS. Small infarcts or small scars presumably resulting from old infarction are found in the anterior pituitary in 5% of autopsies, but cause no dysfunction. They are particularly common in diabetics, in people with raised intracranial pressure, and in patients maintained on a respirator. They may occur in the newborn. An aneurysm of the circle of Willis sometimes presses on the pituitary stalk, causing focal necrosis. Moderate hypopituitarism becomes evident only when 70% of the anterior pituitary has been destroyed, and severe hypopituitarism develops only when more than 90% of the anterior pituitary has been destroyed.

SHEEHAN'S SYNDROME. Sheehan's syndrome is named after the British pathologist who described it in 1937. In women with massive postpartum hemorrhage, less often in other conditions in which there is severe shock, there is sometimes sudden and almost complete necrosis of the pars distalis of the anterior pituitary, though the pars tuberalis usually survives.

The necrotic pars distalis of the pituitary gland shows coagulative or hemorrhagic necrosis. The stalk and posterior pituitary are spared, though small thrombi are often present in the capillaries of the pituitary stalk in the first few hours after the necrosis and sometimes cause petechial hemorrhages or small foci of necrosis in the stalk. Less often there are similar thrombi in the posterior pituitary.

As months pass, the necrotic pars distalis of the anterior pituitary is converted into a collagenous scar containing only a few, scattered clumps of epithelial cells. The pars tuberalis usually remains normal, though if more than 98% of the pars distalis is destroyed it atrophies.

The posterior pituitary often atrophies as months pass, sometimes shrinking to 10% of its normal volume. It shows subcapsular fibrosis, with the pituicytes packed closely together in the center of the lobe. Sometimes a horizontal band of fibrosis divides the posterior pituitary into two. The proximal part of the lobe remains fairly normal, but the part distal to the septum atrophies almost completely. The stalk of the pituitary usually remains normal.

The atrophy of the posterior pituitary causes secondary shrinkage of the supraoptic and paraventricular nuclei of the hypothalamus. The subventricular nucleus of the hypothalamus is sometimes hypertrophic, probably in response to the low levels of estrogen in the plasma caused by the inability of the anterior pituitary to secrete gonadotropins.

Most think that Sheehan's syndrome is caused by spasm of the arteries that supply the pars distalis of the anterior pituitary. The posterior pituitary and stalk escape because they have a more abundant blood supply. Others think that the necrosis is caused by disseminated intravascular coagulation. The hyperplasia of the pituitary in pregnancy may make it more easily infarcted.

TRAUMA. Surgical division of the pituitary stalk is a common traumatic lesion of the pituitary. Some surgeons divide the stalk to reduce hormonal secretion in patients with carcinoma of the breast or with diabetic retinopathy. Occasionally, a similar injury complicates a fracture of the base of the skull.

The division of the arteries and veins that accompany the stalk causes infarction of from 30 to 90% of the anterior lobe. In the stalk, neurosecretory substances accumulate on either side of the line of resection during the first few weeks, but then disappear. The posterior lobe of the gland atrophies over the course of several months. Its pituicytes persist, but lose their processes and become closely packed. On the hypothalamic side of the line of section, proliferation of the end of the stalk sometimes produces a structure like a little posterior lobe, but there is no

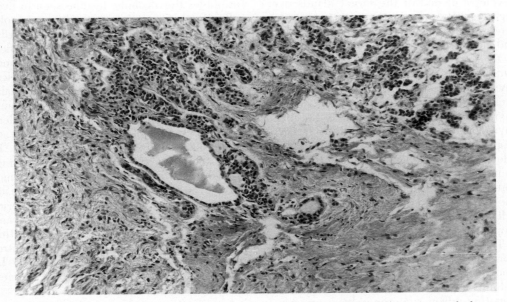

Fig. 44-1. Sheehan's syndrome, showing extensive fibrosis of the anterior lobe of the pituitary in the lower right of the picture, with a little surviving anterior lobe in the upper right and the posterior lobe on the left. (Courtesy of Dr. K. Kovacs)

evidence of neurosecretory secretion after the first few weeks.

In the hypothalamus, the supraoptic and paraventricular nuclei atrophy progressively, until after six months the supraoptic nucleus has only 5 to 10% of its normal complement of neurons. After hypophysectomy, the changes in the upper end of the stalk and in the hypothalamus are similar.

Unless a barrier is interposed to prevent their regeneration, the portal veins rejoin across the line of section, re-establishing a passage by which the release and inhibitory factors of the hypothalamus can reach the surviving anterior pituitary cells.

Tumors, cysts, hydrocephalus, and other space-occupying lesions sometimes compress the hypothalamus or pituitary, causing distortion and atrophy, sometimes with serious dysfunction. Sometimes the pressure causes enlargement of the sella turcica.

SECONDARY CHANGES. The anterior pituitary responds to changes in the secretory activity of the endocrine glands it controls. In general, if the secretion of the target gland is deficient, hyperplasia of the cells in the anterior pituitary produces the tropic hormone for that gland. Occasionally, a tumor of the cells producing the tropic hormone develops. If one of the target glands oversecretes, the cells in the anterior pituitary producing its tropic hormone become small and inactive, but are not reduced in number.

Thyroid Disorders. Severe hypothyroidism, such as occurs in cretins or in severe myxedema, causes hyperplasia and enlargement of the thyrotrophs that produce the thyroid-stimulating hormone. If the hypothyroidism is allowed to continue, a thyrotroph cell adenoma or several small thyrotroph adenomata may develop. Even if there is no tumor, the hyperplasia of the thyrotrophs is sometimes enough to double the weight of the pituitary and cause enlargement of the sella turcica. In thyrotoxicosis, the thyrotrophs are small and shrunken.

The somatotrophs that produce the growth hormone are decreased in severe hypothyroidism. The lack of growth hormone contributes to the dwarfing of cretins. Girls with hypothyroidism sometimes have precocious puberty, suggesting oversecretion of the follicle-stimulating hormone by the pituitary, or girls and women with hypothyroidism may have galactorrhea, suggesting overproduction of prolactin, but changes in the gonadotrophs and prolactin cells have not been identified. Overproduction of the melanocyte-stimulating hormone is rare in hypothyroidism, or diabetes insipidus develops. Administration of appropriate quantities of thyroid hormone reverses all these changes.

Adrenal Disorders. In adrenocortical deficiency, the pituitary may be reduced in size. Both basophils and acidophils seem reduced in number, and large chromophobes become prominent. These large cells result from hypertrophy, hyperplasia, and degranulation of the corticotrophs that secrete the adrenocorticotropic hormone. Administration of glucocorticoids restores the pituitary to normal.

Overactivity of the adrenal cortex or the administration of large doses of adrenocortical steroids causes progressive degranulation of the corticotrophs. Both the nucleus and the cytoplasm of the cells enlarge. One or more large vacuoles may appear in their cytoplasm. Crooke's hyaline, named after the British pathologist who described it in 1935, appears in the cytoplasm of some of the degranulated cells. By light microscopy, Crooke's hyaline resembles the alcoholic hyaline seen in liver cells. By electron microscopy, it consists of a similar tangle of intermediate keratin fibrils.

About 10% of patients with adrenocortical hyperactivity have a corticotroph cell tumor large enough to enlarge the sella turcica. Usually the tumor is an adenoma; occasionally it is a carcinoma. Another 50% of the patients have an adenoma too small to be evident clinically. In 50% of the tumors, the cells are degranulated and stain as chromophobes. In 50%, they retain their basophilic staining. Crooke's hyaline is not evident in the tumor cells, even if it is present in non-neoplastic corticotrophs in other parts of the anterior pituitary. The tumor may be primary and cause the adrenocortical activity by secreting excessive quantities of the adrenocorticotropic hormone or secondary and caused by continued overactivity of the adrenal cortices. cortices.

Sometimes an adenoma in the anterior pituitary of a patient with adrenocortical overactivity becomes evident only after both

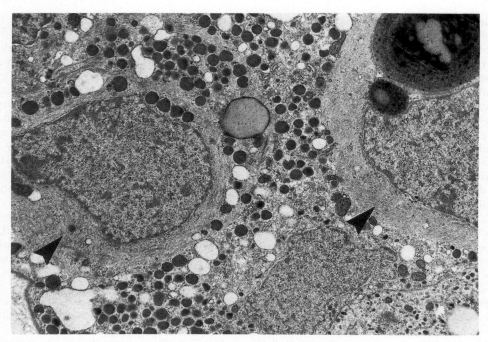

Fig. 44-2. An electron micrograph showing the increase of intermediate filaments (arrow heads) in the cytoplasm of non-neoplastic pituitary cells secreting the adrenocorticotrophic hormone in a woman with Cushing's disease. (Courtesy of Dr. K. Kovacs)

adrenals have been removed. In these people, the adenoma often grows rapidly, compressing or invading neighboring structures and secreting large quantities of the adrenocorticotropic hormone. The combination of bilateral adrenalectomy with the subsequent development of a rapidly growing adenoma of the anterior pituitary is called Nelson's syndrome, after the American physician who described it in 1960.

GONADAL DISORDERS. Castration, the menopause, and other forms of gonadal insufficiency cause increased secretion of the follicle-stimulating hormone. The gonadotrophs become hyperplastic and enlarged. Their ergastoplasm is dilated, so that the cells appear sparsely granulated. Similar changes may be seen in the pituitary of men with Klinefelter's syndrome and in other conditions in which the secretion of the pituitary gonadotropins is increased.

Pregnancy causes enlargement of the pituitary. In some women, the weight of the pituitary doubles. The enlargement is due principally to hyperplasia and enlargement of the prolactin cells. The gonadotrophs become small as the secretion of gonadotropins by the pituitary falls. The changes usually regress after delivery, though in some women after several pregnancies the pituitary remains permanently enlarged.

Little is known of the changes induced in the pituitary by hypersecretion of estrogens or hypersecretion of androgens. In animals, large doses of estrogen cause degranulation of basophils, and hyperplasia, and enlargement of the prolactin cells. In some strains of mouse, prolactin-secreting tumors appear. In rats, administration of testosterone may be followed by hyperplasia of the prolactin cells, perhaps explaining why gynecomastia sometimes accompanies androgen-secreting Leydig cell tumors in men.

CONGENITAL ANOMALIES

Congenital anomalies of the pituitary gland are not uncommon, but usually are small and of no significance.

PHARYNGEAL PITUITARY.   A small clump of anterior pituitary cells called a pharyngeal pituitary is present in the sphenoid bone in the midline in most people. It results from incomplete migration of a few of the anterior pituitary cells from the pharynx during organogenesis. The pharyngeal pituitary is nearly always less than 3 mm in greatest dimension and rarely is of any clinical significance.

EMPTY SELLA.   In the empty sella syndrome, a congenital defect in or absence of the diaphragm of the sella turcica allows the subarachnoid membrane to herniate into the sella turcica, flattening and distorting the pituitary gland. If a pneumoencephalogram is performed, the air in the subarachnoid space extends into the sella turcica, which appears empty. Microscopically, the pituitary gland shows no abnormality, and usually there is no dysfunction.

RATHKE'S CYST.   In 30% of the population, a few clumps of squamous cells, remnants of Rathke's pouch, are present in the stalk of the pituitary, but are of no functional significance. Occasionally, these remnants give rise to an epidermal cyst, sometimes called a cholesteatoma, lined by stratified squamous epithelium and filled with keratin, often with many shimmering cholesterol crystals. The cyst may develop within the pituitary, between the anterior and posterior lobes, but more often lies in the suprasellar region, usually to one side. The cyst may be small, ovoid, or over 5 cm across. If the cyst ruptures, the escaping keratin excites a foreign body reaction in the subarachnoid space. Epilepsy may result. Rarely, a Rathke's cyst contains sebaceous glands and hair follicles in its wall and is filled mainly by greasy sebaceous secretion. Such a cyst is called a dermoid cyst. Occasionally a Rathke's cyst is lined in whole or in part by ciliated, columnar epithelium.

HAMARTOMA.   In 5% of people, one or more small clumps of large cells with dark nuclei and abundant, eosinophilic, granular cytoplasm are present in the posterior lobe or the stalk of the pituitary gland. The granules in the cytoplasm stain strongly with the periodic acid-Schiff reaction. The lesions are rarely more than 1 mm across and rarely cause dysfunction.

Occasionally a hamartoma consisting of neurons and astrocytes is present in the hypothalamus. The lesion can be up to 3 cm across and is sometimes pedunculated, hanging from the tuber cinereum or one of the mamillary bodies.

OTHER ANOMALIES.   In anencephalic mon-

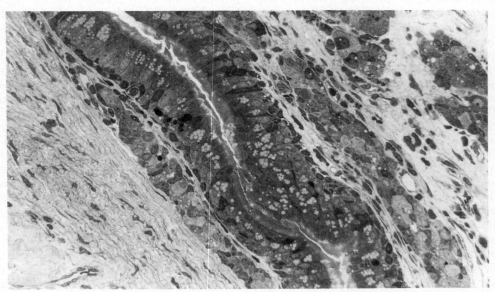

Fig. 44-3.   A Rathke's cyst lined by ciliated, columnar epithelium. The cyst is within the pituitary gland, with the posterior lobe of the pituitary on the left of the picture and the anterior lobe on the right. (Courtesy of Dr. K. Kovacs)

sters, the neurohypophysis often is absent or grossly abnormal. The anterior pituitary is usually present, but is distorted and often misplaced. Dystopia of the pituitary, from the Greek words for wrong and place, is a rare malformation in which the posterior pituitary fails to descend to meet the anterior pituitary in the sella turcica, though it is joined to it by a leash of portal blood vessels. No dysfunction results. Aplasia of the anterior pituitary, in which the anterior pituitary is almost or entirely absent, is rare.

TUMORS

The adenomata that arise in the anterior lobe are the most common tumor of the pituitary. Occasionally a craniopharyngioma arises from remnants of Rathke's pouch, a granular cell tumor or an astrocytoma develops in the posterior lobe of the gland, or a teratoma develops in the region of the pituitary. Rarely, a benign mesenchymal tumor arises in the pituitary, a metastasis develops in the gland, or a meningioma or chordoma arising in a neighboring structure compresses or invades the gland. Carcinoma of the anterior pituitary gland is extremely rare.

ADENOMA. The adenomata of the anterior pituitary are classified according to the secretion they produce (Table 44-1). The different types of cell in the anterior lobe each has its own tumor or tumors. Some of the tumors produce enough of their hormone or hormones to cause dysfunction. Some secrete little or nothing and cause no hormonal imbalance, though they may cause local symptoms.

The classification of pituitary tumors in this way requires immunologic staining to identify the hormone or hormones produced by the tumor cells and electron microscopy. Histologic stains have been devised to identify the different types of cell in the anterior pituitary, but are less reliable than the immunologic methods.

When stained with hematoxylin and eosin, pituitary adenomata can be divided into three groups. In acidophilic adenomata, the cytoplasm of the tumor cells stains pink with eosin. In basophilic adenomata, it stains

TABLE 44-1. TYPES OF PITUITARY ADENOMA

Producing growth hormone
    Growth hormone cell adenoma

Producing prolactin
    Prolactin cell adenoma

Producing growth hormone and prolactin
    Mixed growth hormone cell-prolactin cell adenoma
    Acidophilic stem cell adenoma
    Mammosomatotroph cell adenoma

Producing the adrenocorticotrophic hormone
    Corticotroph adenoma

Producing the thyroid-stimulating hormone
    Thyrotroph adenoma

Producing gonadotropins
    Gonadotroph adenoma

Producing no hormone
    Null cell adenoma
    Oncocytoma

Unclassified adenomata

bluish. In chromophobic adenomata, the cytoplasm shows little staining. The staining depends on the number of secretory granules in the cytoplasm of the tumor cells. Table 44-2 shows the types of pituitary adenoma that are acidophilic or basophilic when the tumor cells contain abundant granules. If the tumor cells contain few secretory granules, all types of adenoma are chromophobic.

Small adenomata that cause no symptoms are found at autopsy in 10% of patients. Most are prolactin cell tumors, null tumors, or oncocytomata. Adenomata that cause symp-

TABLE 44-2. STAINING PROPERTIES OF PITUITARY ADENOMATA

Acidophilic
    Growth cell adenoma
    Prolactin cell adenoma
    Mixed growth cell-prolactin cell adenoma
    Acidophil stem cell adenoma
    Mammosomatotroph adenoma
    Oncocytoma

Basophilic
    Corticotroph adenoma
    Thyrotroph adenoma
    Gonadotroph adenoma

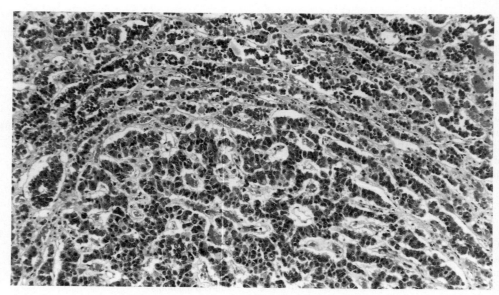

Fig. 44-4. A chromophobe adenoma of the pituitary gland in the lower part of the picture consists of columns of regular cells. The tumor compresses the non-neoplastic part of the anterior lobe seen in the upper part of the picture. (Courtesy of Dr. K. Kovacs)

toms make up less than 5% of symptomatic intracranial tumors. Prolactin cell tumors, growth hormone cell tumors, and corticotroph adenomata are the most common.

Symptomatic adenomata can occur at any age, but most of the patients are 30 to 50 years old. Men and women are affected equally, except that prolactin cell adenomata are especially frequent in women 20 to 40 years old.

Lesion. Adenomata of the pituitary gland range from the microscopic to several centimeters in diameter. The smaller tumors are spheroidal; the larger ones may be lobulated or irregularly shaped. Usually, a thin fibrous capsule surrounds the tumor. Because of its great vascularity, the tumor is usually a dark, reddish brown. It is soft and friable.

By light microscopy, 60% of pituitary adenomata consist of large sheets of regular cells that all look much alike. Usually, the cells are well defined, with homogeneous cytoplasm and regular, spheroidal nuclei. When stained with hematoxylin and eosin, acidophil adenomata have bright red granules in their cytoplasm. Basophil adenomata have bluish granules. Chromophobe adenomata have no cytoplasmic granules. Stroma is

sparse, except for a little collagen around the numerous blood vessels coursing through the tumor. Less often, the tumor has sinusoids, like the sinusoids of the normal anterior pituitary, except that the plates of tumor cells between the sinusoids are several cells thick. Occasionally an adenoma is papillary, with papillary fronds bulging into sinusoidal blood spaces. Sometimes a few of the tumor cells have giant nuclei. Sometimes the tumor cells are mildly pleomorphic. Mitoses are uncommon.

Growth Hormone Cell Adenoma. Two types of growth hormone cell adenoma are distinguished, the densely granulated and the sparsely granulated forms. It is not clear whether these are different forms of the same tumor or different kinds of adenoma. About 10% of pituitary adenomata detected clinically are of the densely granulated type of growth hormone cell adenoma, and 10% are of the sparsely granulated type.

The cells of the densely granulated form of growth hormone cell adenoma are similar to normal somatotrophs. They are round or ovoid, with regular round or ovoid nuclei. They have abundant rough endoplasmic reticulum and a prominent Golgi complex. The cytoplasm contains many spherical secretory granules with an electron dense core and a closely approximated limiting membrane. Most are 350 to 450 nm across. Immunohistochemistry reveals the growth hormone in the tumor cells.

The cells of the sparsely granulated growth hormone cell adenomata are pleomorphic, varying considerably in size and shape. Their nuclei are often crescentic or indented. Multinucleated tumor cells with peripheral nuclei are common. Rough endoplasmic reticulum is abundant, and smooth endoplasmic reticulum may be present. The Golgi apparatus is prominent. Free ribosomes and polysomes are numerous. Mitochondria vary in size and shape and may be numerous. Fibrous bodies consisting of a tangle of microfilaments 10 nm in diameter are often present in the concavity of the crescentic nuclei. Mitochondria and other organelles may be entangled in the fibrous bodies. Some of the tumor cells contain smooth-walled tubules. Centrioles and cilia are common. Spherical secretory granules are present, but are sparse. They have an electron-dense core with a closely applied limiting membrane. Most are 100 to 250 nm in diameter, though some may be larger. The granules can be shown immunologically to contain growth hormone.

Prolactin Cell Adenoma.   Densely granulated and sparsely granulated forms of prolactin cell adenoma are distinguished. Less than 1% of pituitary adenomata detected clinically are of the densely granulated form, but 30% are of the sparsely granulated type.

The cells of the densely granulated form of prolactin cell tumor resemble the normal cells that secrete prolactin. They are oval or oblong, with pleomorphic nuclei. Rough endoplasmic reticulum and Golgi complexes are prominent. The secretory granules have an electron-dense core, separated by an irregular, electron-lucent zone from their limiting membrane. Most are about 600 nm across, with some as much as 1200 nm. Immunologic methods demonstrate prolactin in the tumor cells.

The cells of the sparsely granulated form of prolactin cell adenoma are polyhedral, with large oval, pleomorphic nuclei. Parallel rows and whorls of rough endoplasmic reticulum occupy much of the cytoplasm. The Golgi apparatus is large. The secretory granules are sparse and may be spherical or irregularly shaped. They are electron-dense, with most being 200 to 300 nm across. Abnormal exocytosis with extrusion of secretory granules into the extracellular space in regions distant from capillaries is common. Immunologically, prolactin can be demonstrated in some of the tumor cells.

Mixed Growth Hormone Cell-Prolactin Cell Adenoma.   About 5% of pituitary adenomata consist of a mixture of cells that produce growth hormone and cells that produce prolactin, perhaps reflecting the common origin of these two types of anterior pituitary cell. Microscopically, the tumor cells are similar to those of the pure growth hormone cell and prolactin cell tumors. They may be densely granulated or sparsely granulated. Often there are a few cells like those of the acidophilic stem cell adenoma as well. The different kinds of cell may be jumbled together, or the adenoma may contain little clumps of one type of cell or another. Both growth hormone and prolactin can be demonstrated immunologically in the tumor cells.

Acidophilic Stem Cell Adenoma.   Some 3% of pituitary adenomata consist of acidophilic stem cells. The tumor cells of this type of pituitary adenoma are elongated, with pleomorphic nuclei. The endoplasmic reticulum is often well developed, but the Golgi system is inconspicuous. The mitochondria are usually large, with loss of cristae, and may be numerous. They often contain tubular structures like centrioles. Occasionally a fibrous body like those of the sparsely granulated growth hormone cell tumors is evident. The secretory granules are usually sparse. They are spherical, electron-dense, and 50 to 300 nm across. Abnormal exocytosis, with extrusion of secretory granules in regions distant from capillaries, is common. Immunohistochemical staining shows that the tumor cells contain both growth hormone and prolactin.

Mammosomatotroph Adenoma.   About 1% of adenomata of the pituitary are of the mammosomatotroph type. The cells in the tumor stain strongly for the growth hormone, less strongly for prolactin. By electron microscopy, the cells contain two types of granule.

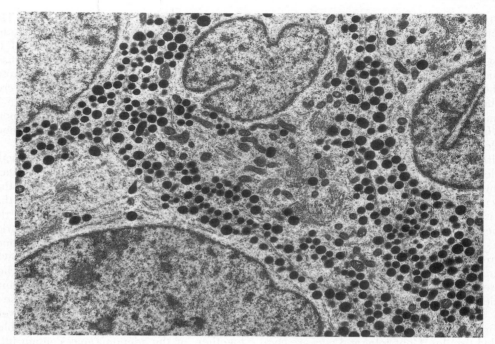

Fig. 44-5. An electron micrograph of a densely granulated growth hormone cell adenoma in a woman with acromegaly, showing the numerous, evenly electron dense secretory granules in the cytoplasm of the tumor cells. (Courtesy of Dr. K. Kovacs)

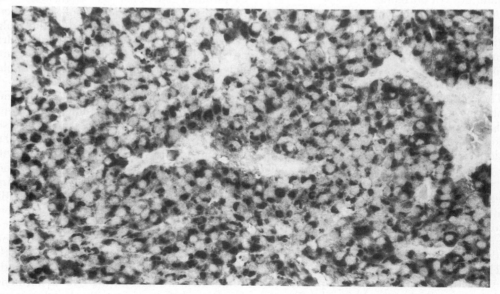

Fig. 44-6. Immunoreactive prolactin in the cytoplasm of the cells of a pituitary adenoma in a woman with galactorrhea and amenorrhea. (Courtesy of Dr. K. Kovacs)

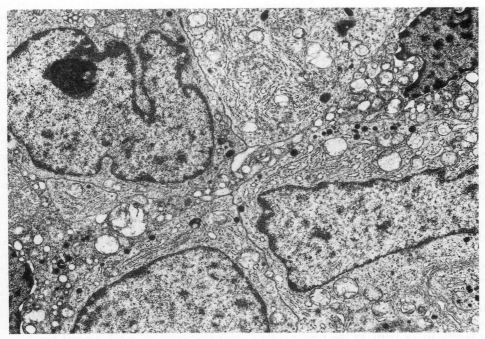

Fig. 44-7. A sparsely granulated, prolactin cell adenoma in the pituitary of a woman with galactorrhea and amenorrhea. Rough endoplasmic reticulum and Golgi apparati are prominent, but secretory granules are few. The arrow head shows misplaced exocytosis. (Courtesy of Dr. K. Kovacs)

Some are 150 to 450 nm across and resemble the granules of the densely granulated growth hormone cell adenomata. Others are irregular or elongated, 350 to 2000 nm across, with a core of varying electron density and a loose limiting membrane. The second type of granule often discharges its content into the intercellular space.

Corticotroph Adenoma. About 15% of pituitary adenomata consist of cells like those producing the adrenocorticotropic hormone. The tumor cells may be densely or sparsely granulated.

In the densely granulated tumors, the cells are ovoid or angular, with spheroidal nuclei and electron-dense cytoplasm. Rough endoplasmic reticulum is abundant, and the Golgi apparatus is prominent. Free ribosomes are numerous. Mitochondria are usually few, though in occasional cells they are numerous. The secretory granules are spherical or irregular and vary in electron density. Most are 250 to 700 nm across. The granules often line up along the cell membrane, but exocytosis is not evident. If the patient has functioning adrenal glands, the tumor cells often have many intermediate filaments in their cytoplasm. The filaments are similar to those that form Crooke's hyaline and may be aggregated into bundles, but do not form larger bodies. Immunohistochemistry demonstrates the adrenocorticotropic hormone, β-lipotropin, and endorphin in the tumors.

In the sparsely granulated corticotroph tumors, secretory granules are few and small, and the cells contain few organelles. The adrenocorticotropic hormone is demonstrable in the granules, but often they are too few for immunologic staining to be evident by light microscopy.

Thyrotroph Adenoma. Less than 1% of pituitary adenomata consist of cells resembling thyrotrophs. The tumor cells are polyhedral, elongated, or irregular, with irregular, indented nuclei. The cytoplasm is usually sparse, occasionally abundant, with well-developed rough endoplasmic reticulum. The Golgi apparatus has 5 or 6 sacculi. Mitochondria are small. Free ribosomes and polysomes are numerous. Microtubules are often common. The few secretory granules have cores of varying electron density, with a prominent halo between the core and the limiting membrane. Most are 100 to 350 nm across. Often the granules line up along the plasma membrane, but exocytosis is not seen. The tumors sometimes fail to stain immunohistochemically for the thyrotropic hormone.

Gonadotroph Adenoma. About 3% of pituitary adenomata are of cells that produce the follicle-stimulating and luteinizing hormones. The tumor cells are small, elongated, or angular, with oval nuclei. Rough endoplasmic reticulum and the Golgi complex are prominent. The tubules of the Golgi apparatus are dilated. Microtubules may be numerous. The secretory granules are spherical, evenly dense, less than 150 nm in diameter, with an electron-lucent halo between their core and the limiting membrane. Exocytosis is not evident. Immunologic stains demonstrate the follicle-stimulating hormone, the luteinizing hormone, or both, in the tumor cells.

Null Cell Adenoma. Nearly 20% of pituitary adenomata are of the null cell type. The tumor cells are small, polyhedral, or irregular, with pleomorphic indented nuclei. Rough endoplasmic reticulum is poorly developed, but the Golgi apparatus is prominent. Microtubules are often abundant. Secretory granules are present in all the tumor cells. They are spherical, less than 250 nm in diameter, with an evenly electron-dense core separated by a halo from their limiting membrane. The secretory granules may line up along the plasma membrane, but exocytosis is not evident. The cells fail to stain by the immunologic methods for anterior pituitary hormones.

Oncocytoma. Over 5% of pituitary adenomata are oncocytomata. The tumor is similar to a null cell adenoma exept that mitochondria are numerous in the cytoplasm of the tumor cells.

Behavior. Nearly 90% of adenomata of the pituitary evident clinically, and almost all those discovered only at autopsy, grow slowly and remain encapsulated or well-defined. The other 10% of the tumors causing symptoms are more aggressive. They slowly invade the adjacent brain or the bones at the base of the skull. Some have grown into the nose.

Metastases are most uncommon. Sometimes the aggressive tumors are called invasive adenomata to emphasize that they do not metastasize.

Complications. Adenomata of the pituitary gland produce symptoms in two ways, by pressing on neighbouring structures and by producing a hormone or hormones.

Compression. If an adenoma of the pituitary is large, it compresses the remainder of the gland against the wall of the sella turcica. The normal part of the gland atrophies. If the adenoma is big enough, it causes hypopituitarism. If the adenoma is removed, the remnant of normal pituitary may regenerate and resume function.

An enlarging adenoma sometimes causes enlargement of the sella turcica. It may erode the anterior or posterior clinoid processes or the tuberculum sellae. It can compress the brain or bulge into a lateral ventricle. Not uncommonly, the tumor compresses or distorts the optic nerves or the optic chiasm, most often causing bitemporal hemianopsia. Sometimes the adenoma pulls on the anterior cerebral arteries, and the tense arteries compress the optic nerves. Paralysis of the third, fourth, or sixth cranial nerves can occur if the tumor is large.

Hormonal Excess. Pituitary adenomata that secrete an excess of the hormone or hormones they produce cause the syndrome associated with that form of endocrine dysfunction. An excess of growth hormone causes acromegaly. In women, an excess of prolactin causes amenorrhea, infertility, and often galactorrhea. In men, it delays puberty and causes hypogonadism. An excess of the adrenocorticotropic hormone causes excessive adrenocortical activity and Cushing's disease. In a person with normal thyroid function, a thyrotroph adenoma causes mild hyperthyroidism. In a person with severe hypothyroidism, it produces little change in thyroid function. In men, a functioning gonadotroph tumor increases the concentration of the follicle-stimulating hormone and sometimes the concentration of the luteinizing hormone in the plasma, but produces few symptoms. In women, the concentration of gonadotropins in the plasma is usually normal, and there are no symptoms.

Clinical Presentation. In 50% of the patients with a pituitary adenoma who develop symptoms, the first manifestation is a disturbance in vision, bitemporal hemianopsia, unilateral blindness, or scotomata caused by pressure on the optic nerves. In 15%, headache is the first symptom, and sooner or later headache develops in 70% of the patients with symptoms. Nearly 15% of the patients have acromegaly, 10% hypopituitarism, 5% amenorrhea, 5% pain other than headache, and 3% Cushing's syndrome. Occasionally the first manifestation is leakage of cerebrospinal fluid from the nose or diabetes insipidus.

Multiple Endocrine Neoplasia. Adenomata of the pituitary develop in multiple endocrine neoplasia type I. The tumor is often a prolactin cell tumor or an adenoma that secretes both prolactin and the growth hormone, though other kinds of adenoma can occur.

Treatment and Prognosis. Pituitary adenomata that cause symptoms are usually removed surgically. If the tumor is functional, the concentration of its hormone in the plasma rapidly falls to normal. The tumor recurs within 10 years in more than 50% of the patients if no postoperative radiation is given. If radiation is added, only 15% of the tumors recur. Radiation alone can control a pituitary adenoma, but the level of hormone in the blood falls only slowly and hypopituitarism develops in 10% of the patients. Small tumors that secrete prolactin can be controlled by the dopamine agonist bromocriptine.

CRANIOPHARYNGIOMA. The tumor arising from remnants of Ratkhe's pouch is called a craniopharyngioma. Its name describes its origin, a rest of pharyngeal epithelium in the cranium. About 5% of intracranial tumors are of this type. Craniopharyngiomata are most common in children. About 50% of them occur in people under 20 years of age. Some occur in young adults and a few in older people.

Lesions. Nearly 95% of craniopharyngiomata arise above the diaphragm of the sella turcica. By the time it is discovered, the tumor often has invaded extensively, eroding the base of the brain, the optic nerves, or other cranial nerves. It can extend into the anterior, middle, or posterior cranial fossa or bulge into the third ventricle. It can destroy the pituitary stalk or penetrate into the sella turcica. Invasion of the bone at the base of the skull is unusual. The tumor is well demarcated, reddish, or gray. Most craniopharyngiomata are cystic, containing multiple smaller or larger cysts.

Microscopically, a craniopharyngioma resembles an ameloblastoma of the jaw. Some call it an ademantinoma. It consists of clumps of epithelial cells separated by a collagenous stroma. The clumps usually have a palisade of tall columnar cells at their periphery with stellate cells in the center. Keratin pearls are often present in some of the clumps. Sometimes part of the tumor consists of sheets of well-differentiated squamous cells. The cysts develop in the clumps of tumor cells. The smaller cysts are lined by columnar cells; the larger cysts, by cuboidal or flattened cells.

The margin of the tumor is usually sharp. It usually compresses the adjacent tissues but does not invade them. Only occasionally does a craniopharyngioma invade the surrounding tissues.

Rupture of one of the cysts releases its content rich in cholesterol into the stroma, exciting a granulomatous reaction. Foci of calcification are evident in 70% of the tumors. Occasionally the stroma of the tumor is ossified. Occasionally a tumor becomes almost completely necrotic, forming a fibrous, calcified mass in which only a few strands of epithelium remain.

Behavior. Craniopharyngiomata invade only to a limited degree and do not metastasize. They have no hormonal activity, but in 30% of the patients cause hypopituitarism by damaging the stalk of the pituitary or compressing the gland. In 15% of the patients, interference with the hypothalamic factors that regulate pituitary function causes hyperprolactinemia. The extension of the tumor often involves the optic nerves and other structures, causing symptoms like those of a pituitary adenoma.

Treatment and Prognosis. Unless the extension of a craniopharyngioma makes complete resection impossible, local excision cures.

GRANULAR CELL TUMOR. Rarely, a granular cell tumor consisting of cells like those of the granular cell hamartomata of the posterior

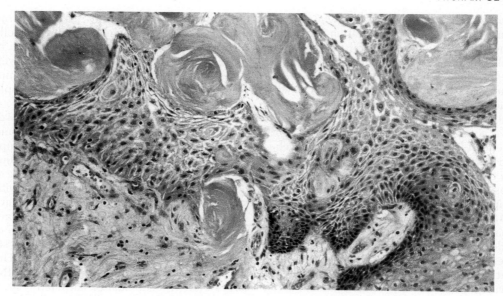

Fig. 44-8. A cranipharyngioma showing keratinizing, stratified squamous epithelium supported by a collagenous stroma. (Courtesy of Dr. K. Kovacs)

pituitary gland arises in the posterior lobe of the pituitary, grows rapidly, and causes symptoms.

ASTROCYTOMA. Rarely, an astrocytoma arises in the posterior lobe of the pituitary, its stalk, or the hypothalamus. The tumor may cause diabetes insipidus or malfunction of the anterior pituitary.

TERATOMA. Occaionally a teratoma arises in the suprasellar region or in the floor of the third ventricle. About 70% of the tumors arise in boys or young men, most of the rest in girls. The tumor is usually malignant and resembles a seminoma. Less often, it consists of a jumble of well-differentiated tissues.

SECONDARY TUMORS. A metastasis is found in the pituitary gland in 3% of patients dying of cancer. Most often it is in the posterior lobe. Carcinoma of the breast is the most common primary site, but carcinoma of the lung, colon, and prostate also spread to the pituitary. Leukemia and malignant melanoma can involve the gland. The metastases are not usually large enough to cause dysfunction.

HYPERPITUITARISM

Hyperpituitarism is caused by oversecretion of one or more of the pituitary hormones.

It can be due to disease of the anterior pituitary, posterior pituitary, or hypothalamus or to secretion of hormones like those of the pituitary by a tumor or other lesion of another organ. The lesion in the pituitary is often an adenoma, but similar dysfunction can be caused by overproduction or underproduction of the hypothalamic hormones that regulate pituitary action.

Excess of the growth hormone causes gigantism or acromegaly. An excess of the adrenocorticotropic hormone causes Cushing's disease. Hyperprolactinemia sometimes causes galactorrhea and amenorrhea. An excess of the thyroid-stimulating hormone can cause hyperthyroidism. Excessive secretion of the gonadotropins usually causes few or no symptoms. Disease of the hypothalamus can cause premature puberty. Inappropriate secretion of the antidiuretic hormone can be caused by disease of the hypothalmus and posterior pituitary but often is due to disease in other organs.

Gigantism. If hypersecretion of growth hormone begins before puberty, the body grows abnormally large. The patient usually has a growth hormone cell adenoma. The child may become a giant as much as 2.7 m high and weighing over 200 kg. At first pituitary giants are strong, but as their adenoma enlarges, hypopituitarism usually follows, bringing muscular weakness and other signs of pituitary insufficiency. Usually, pituitary giants show some degree of acromegaly.

Acromegaly. Acromegaly takes its name from the Greek words for terminal and great and refers to the enlargement of the hands, feet, and jaw characteristic of this disease. It is caused by excessive secretion of the growth hormone in an adult. In the United States, 4 people in 100,000 have the disease. In any one year, fewer than 0.3 people per 100,000 develop acromegaly. Men and women are affected equally. Most patients are 30 to 40 years old when the diagnosis is made, though often it is clear that the disease began insidiously and unrecognized 10 or 20 years earlier.

Lesions. Most tissues in the body enlarge. The hands and feet grow large, soft, and doughy, mainly because of increase in the soft tissues. The lips, ears, and nose grow big and coarse. The skin becomes thick and fleshy, with exaggerated wrinkles, excessive sweating, and sometimes hirsutism. The skin is hyperpigmented in 50% of the patients. Small fibrous polyps called fibromata mollusca develop in 30%.

The bones become thick and coarse. The lower jaw protrudes. The supraorbital ridges become prominent. The bones and cartilages of the chest elongate, increasing the diameter of the thorax. The long bones become massive and may be lengthened or bowed. Osteoarthritis is common. Late in the disease, osteoporosis often develops, sometimes with collapse of vertebrae. Myopathy and peripheral neuritis are common late in the disease.

The internal organs enlarge, sometimes becoming three or more times their normal weight. The tongue is large. The voice deepens as the larynx enlarges. Nodular hyperplasia is common in the endocrine glands. Sometimes adenomata develop in the glands.

Dysfunction. The excess of growth hormone causes insulin resistance in 80% of the patients. About 30% have abnormal glucose tolerance, and 15% develop diabetes mellitus. The metabolic rate is high. Systemic hypertension develops in 25% of the patients. The hypertension is accompanied by retention of sodium and water with low levels of renin and aldosterone. Cardiomegaly and congestive heart failure are common. Hypercalcemia caused by hyperplasia of the parathyroid glands is present in many of the patients. About 20% develop renal stones. Less than 5% have hyperthyroidism.

In normal people, the concentration of growth hormone in the serum is usually less than 2 µg/L (2 ng/mL) 90 minutes after taking 100 g of glucose by mouth, though in some it is as high as 5 µg/L (5 ng/mL). In patients with acromegaly, the concentration is usually greater than 10 µg/L (5 ng/mL), though in some it is between 2 and 10 µg/L.

The concentration of prolactin is increased in 50% of the patients. The increase is sometimes enough to cause amenorrhea, galactorrhea, or reduced libido.

Clinical Presentation. In addition to the deformity produced by the overgrowth of the tissues, enlargement of the sella turcica is evident radiologically in 80% of the patients. Headache is common. Ocular signs develop in 60% of the patients. Paresthesia, muscular weakness, and joint pains are frequent.

Pathogenesis. In 99% of patients with acromegaly, the hypersecretion of growth hormone is caused by an adenoma in the anterior pituitary, usually a growth hormone cell adenoma or a mixed growth hormone cell-prolactin cell adenoma, rarely a mammosomatotroph adenoma or an acidophil stem cell adenoma. In 1%, there is diffuse hyperplasia of the growth hormone cells, suggesting an excess of the growth hormone releasing hormone of the hypothalamus or a deficiency of somatostatin.

Treatment and Prognosis. Removal of the adenoma surgically brings cure in 90% of patients with a localized tumor, but is inadequate when the tumor is extensive or invasive unless postoperative irradiation is given. About 10% of patients with a large tumor develop hypopituitarism. Irradiation can also control the disease, but is more likely to cause hypopituitarism. Bromocriptine lowers the level of growth hormone in the plasma, but alone is unable to control the disease.

CUSHING'S DISEASE. Oversecretion of the adrenocorticotropic hormone by the pituitary causes Cushing's disease, named after the American neurosurgeon who described it in 1932. In 90% of the patients, it is caused by one or more small corticotroph adenomata, less often by a larger adenoma, and rarely by diffuse hyperplasia of the corticotrophs. The excess of the adrenocorticotropic hormone causes oversecretion of cortisol by the adrenal cortices.

Cushing's disease is one form of Cushing's syndrome, a term used to describe the effects of excessive secretion of cortisol. It is similar to Cushing's syndrome caused by secretion of the adrenocorticotropic hormone by a carcinoma of the lung or some other tumor and Cushing's syndrome caused by disease of the adrenal glands. It is discussed further in chapter 46.

HYPERPROLACTINEMIA. Hyperprolactinemia causes amenorrhea, infertility, and galactorrhea in women and reduced libido, impotence, and infertility in men. Rarely, gynecomastia or galactorrhea develops in a man with hyperprolactinemia. Excessive secretion of prolactin is present in over 10% of women with amenorrhea and in 75% of those with both amenorrhea and galactorrhea. In men, hyperprolactinemia is found in 10% of men who are impotent and 5% of those who are infertile.

Lesions. The tissues show little abnormality. If there is amenorrhea, the endometrium is inactive. Gonadal function is depressed.

Dysfunction. The excess of prolactin inhibits the release of the luteinizing hormone releasing factor by the hypothalamus, so reducing the secretion of the gonadotropins by the pituitary. Reduced ovarian activity causes amenorrhea and infertility; reduced testicular activity causes reduced libido, impotence, and infertility. Prolactin stimulates the breasts directly.

Clinical Presentation. In women, hyperprolactinemia is usually discovered early, because of the menstrual disorders, amenorrhea, and galactorrhea it causes. In men, the hypogonadism causes the patient to seek advice in less than 15% of the patients. More often hyperprolactinemia is discovered only when the enlarging tumor in the pituitary causes ocular or other signs.

Pathogenesis. A pituitary adenoma secreting prolactin or growth hormone and prolactin is the most common cause of hyperprolactinemia. In women, 90% of the patients have a small tumor confined to the pituitary. In men, 60% of the patients have a larger tumor that is compressing or invading structures around the pituitary.

Dopamine inhibits the secretion of prolactin. Drugs such as the phenothiazides that block dopamine receptors can cause moderate hyperprolactinemia. Agents such as methyldopa and reserpine that deplete the supply of dopamine can do so. The prolactin release inhibiting factor of the hypothalamus is probably dopamine. Tumors and other conditions that damage the pituitary stalk prevent the flow of the prolactin release inhibiting factor from the hypothalamus to the pituitary and cause hyperprolactinemia.

Hyperprolactinemia develops in 80% of women in renal failure and in 40% of men. Severe hypothyroidism causes a slight increase in the concentration of prolactin in the plasma. Cirrhosis of the liver sometimes increases the secretion of prolactin. Trauma to the chest wall can do so.

Treatment and Prognosis. If the tumor is small and the patient has no important symptoms, a pituitary adenoma causing hyperprolactinemia needs no treatment. If the tumor in the pituitary is small but there are symptoms, the dopamine agonist bromocriptine reduces the secretion of prolactin sufficiently to relieve the symptoms in 90% of premenopausal women. In patients with larger tumors, bromocriptine often causes the tumor to shrink as well as relieving the hormonal symptoms, but surgical removal and postoperative radiation are usually needed. Over 15% of the tumors treated by surgery and irradiation recur.

HYPERTHYROTROPINEMIA. In most patients with hyperthyroidism, the hyperfunction is caused by disease of the thyroid gland, and the pituitary is normal. In a few, it is caused by an excess of thyroid-stimulating hormone. Occasionally, a thyrotroph adenoma of the pituitary secretes enough thyroid-stimulating hormone to cause hyperthyroidism. Occasionally a rising concentration of the thyroid hormone in the plasma fails to suppress the secretion of the thyroid-stimulating hormone by the pituitary, and the continued secretion of the thyroid-stimulating hormone causes hyperthyroidism.

HYPERGONADOTROPINEMIA. Excessive secretion of the gonadotropins by the pituitary or by tumors of other organs rarely causes symptoms. In men and in children, the concentrations of the follicle-stimulating hormone and the luteinizing hormone in the plasma are increased, but in women they are often normal. In a child, hypergonadotropinemia occasionally causes precocious puberty, and in a man it sometimes causes gynecomastia.

Posterior Pituitary and Hypothalamus

Hypersecretion of the antidiuretic hormone is the most common form of hyperpituitarism caused by the hormones of the hypothalamus and posterior pituitary. The dysfunction of the anterior pituitary sometimes caused by disordered secretion of the hypophyseal hormones that regulate its action has already been discussed. Occasionally a tumor or other lesion of the hypothalamus or posterior pituitary causes precocious puberty.

INAPPROPRIATE SECRETION OF THE ANTIDIURETIC HORMONE. Excessive secretion of the antidiuretic hormone, also called vasopressin, causes increased retention of water, loss of sodium in the urine, and intracellular and extracellular hypotonicity. The tissues show no morphologic abnormality.

Clinical Presentation. Patients have increase in weight caused by the retention of water, weakness, lethargy, and mental confusion. The concentration of sodium in the plasma is usually less than 120 mmol/L (120 meq/L), and the concentrations of chloride, creatinine, uric acid, and albumin are low. The osmolality of the plasma is less than 270 mOsmol/kg. The concentration of sodium in the urine usually exceeds 20 mmol/L (20 meq/L).

Pathogenesis. Inappropriate secretion of the antidiuretic hormone is often caused by the synthesis and secretion of the hormone by a tumor. In 80% of the patients it is caused by an oat cell carcinoma of the lung. Less often, the hormone is produced by a carcinoma of the pancreas, a lymphoma, or a thymoma.

In other patients, pulmonary tuberculosis, a lung abscess, pneumonitis, empyema, or obstructive lung disease causes overproduction of the hormone, either because the hormone is synthesized in the lungs, or because reduced blood flow to the left atrium stimulates increased secretion of the hormone by the hypothalamus and posterior pituitary.

Injury to the hypothalamus by trauma, hemorrhage, meningitis, or other disease sometimes causes excessive secretion of the antidiuretic hormone. Inappropriate secretion of the antidiuretic hormone can occur in the Guillain-Barré syndrome, in systemic lupus erythematosus, hypothyroidism, hypoadrenalism, and in acute intermittent porphyria. Drugs such as chlorpropamide, vincristine, cyclophosphamide, carbamazepine, tricyclic antidepressants, clofibrate, anesthetics, and narcotics sometimes stimulate excessive secretion of the hormone.

Treatment and Prognosis. Restriction of the intake of water and replacement of sodium and chloride relieve the symptoms caused by inappropriate secretion of the antidiuretic hormone. Demeclocycline antagonizes the effect of the antidiuretic hormone on the tubules and helps relieve the dysfunction. More permanent relief requires control of the underlying lesion.

PRECOCIOUS PUBERTY. In 10% of girls with precocious puberty, the premature development is caused by a tumor or inflammation of the brain. The gliomata and hamartomata of the hypothalamus are among the lesions that sometimes cause sexual precocity.

HYPOPITUITARISM

In hypopituitarism, one or more of the pituitary hormones is deficient. Usually, the deficiency affects only the anterior pituitary or only the hypothalamus and posterior pituitary. Only if the disease affecting the pituitary gland is unusually extensive are both involved.

Anterior Pituitary

Loss of one or more of the hormones of the anterior pituitary is nearly always caused by destruction of the gland. Usually the secretion of the growth hormone is impaired first, followed by a fall in gonadotropins, and later reduced secretion of the adrenocorticotropic hormone and the thyroid-stimulating hormone. The nature and severity of the symptoms depend on the nature and severity of the deficiency and on the age and sex of the patient.

Compression of the gland by an enlarging adenoma is a common cause of anterior hypopituitarism. Sometimes the gland is compressed by a craniopharyngioma, meningioma, chordoma, or some other tumor of the adjacent tissues or by an aneurysm. Hypophysectomy, division of the pituitary stalk, and irradiation of the pituitary commonly cause anterior pituitary failure. Sheehan's syndrome causes sudden and often almost complete loss of the anterior pituitary hormones. Rarely, tuberculosis or some other infection destroys much of the anterior pituitary, or sarcoidosis involves the gland. Occasionally a congenital defect causes anterior pituitary dysfunction. Occasionally an autoimmune reaction causes pituitary failure.

Growth Hormone Deficiency. In children, growth hormone deficiency sometimes results from a congenital defect, usually inherited as an autosomal recessive character, but sometimes as an X-linked character or an autosomal dominant character. Less often, it is caused by an enlarging tumor, malformation of the tissues around the pituitary fossa, or infarction of the pituitary from trauma at birth. In adults, it is common and can be caused by any of the mechanisms that cause hypopituitarism.

In children, deficiency of growth hormone retards growth. If the deficiency is severe, the child becomes a dwarf. In adults, growth hormone deficiency causes no symptoms and no dysfunction.

A child with a congenital deficiency of growth hormone is normal at birth and remains so for some months. Thereafter, growth is slow. The epiphyses mature slowly. The bone age is less than is appropriate to the child's age. Frontal bossing is common. The child is often plump, with small hands and feet and poorly developed genitalia. The larynx develops poorly. The voice is high pitched. Muscular development is poor. Dentition is late. By the time the child enters school, it is often clear that physical development is retarded. Puberty is usually late. Growth continues longer than normal, but the stature is reduced. Particularly in the first months of life, there may be episodes of hypoglycemia. If the loss of stature is great, the child is called a pituitary dwarf.

Less than 0.1% of children of short stature have growth hormone deficiency. In a few, the tissues fail to respond normally to growth hormone. In most, there is no endocrine abnormality. The child is usually born small and grows slowly. The epiphyses close at the normal age. The person is normal, except for the short stature. If short people without endocrine abnormality intermarry, their children are often of normal stature.

The concentration of growth hormone in the plasma varies considerably in response to metabolic and other factors. To establish that there is a deficiency of the hormone, a provocative test is used. If insulin is given to a fasting person in dose sufficient to reduce the blood sugar to less than 2.2 mmol/L (40 mg/100 mL), the concentration of growth hormone in the serum normally rises to more than 8 µg/L (8 ng/100 mL). In people with deficiency of the hormone, it fails to reach this value, perhaps reaching only 2 µg/L. Exercise, clonidine, and other stimuli can be used in a similar manner to test the ability of the anterior pituitary to produce growth hormone.

In children with a deficiency of growth hormone, hormone given intramuscularly restores normal growth. It is continued until normal adult stature is reached or the epiphyses close. In adults, no treatment is needed. needed.

Progeria. Progeria, from the Greek words for before and old age, is a rare condition of unknown etiology in which a child is born normal, but after a few months or years begins to show all the signs of premature senility. Growth slows. The epiphyses fuse prematurely. The skin becomes wrinkled and atrophic, the head bald. Atherosclerosis and senile dementia advance apace. Death usually comes during childhood from myocardial infarction or cerebral atherosclerosis.

GONADOTROPIN DEFICIENCY. In children, deficiency of the gonadotropins is often congenital. In Kallmann's syndrome, named after the American psychiatrist who described it in 1944, deficiency of the luteinizing hormone releasing hormone of the hypothalamus impairs the release of the gonadotropins and the patients have anosmia, cleft palate, hare lip, or other midline defects. Anorexia nervosa, starvation, and hyperprolactinemia depress the secretion of the luteinizing hormone releasing hormone. An enlarging adenoma of the pituitary and other disorders that damage the anterior pituitary often cause gonadotropin deficiency.

In boys with gonadotropin deficiency, the testes do not develop normally. Because of the lack of androgen, the epiphyses do not close. If the supply of growth hormone is adequate, the limbs continue to grow, so that the arms and legs become abnormally long. Often there is osteoporosis. The penis remains small. The testes are tiny. The prostate is underdeveloped. Pubic hair is fine, axillary hair scant, the beard absent. The larynx is small, and the voice high pitched.

In girls, lack of the gonadotropic hormones causes amenorrhea, and the breasts do not develop. Androgens produced by the adrenal cortex may cause some growth of pubic and axillary hair, or hair in these sites may be absent. The epiphyses may fail to fuse, and the arms and legs become long.

In adults, loss of collagen from the dermis makes the skin fine, with wrinkles at the corners of the mouth. Body hair is reduced or lost. In women, there is amenorrhea. If the deficiency of the gonadotropins is severe, the breasts shrink and the uterus atrophies. In men, the testicles atrophy, with loss of potency and libido.

The concentration of the luteinizing and follicle-stimulating hormones in the plasma is diminished, though because of the episodic secretion of the gonadotropins several samples must be analyzed before it is accepted that the secretion of the gonadotropins is inadequate. In most patients, injection of the luteinizing hormone releasing hormone fails to produce the normal increase in the secretion of the luteinizing hormone. In most, clomiphene citrate, which blocks the hypothalamic suppression of the cells secreting the gonadotropins, fails to produce the normal increase in the concentration of the luteinizing hormone in the serum.

Girls and women with hypogonadotropinemia can be treated with contraceptive pills, which provide a cyclic alternation of estrogens and progesterone to induce menstruation and maintain the development of the breasts. Men and boys are given testosterone in dosage sufficient to maintain the secondary sexual characters. Only if a person who lacks the gonadotropins wishes to become fertile is it necessary to administer human gonadotropins to restore ovarian or testicular function.

Adrenocorticotropic Hormone Deficiency. Deficiency of the adrenocorticotropic hormone is usually associated with deficiency of other of the anterior pituitary hormones. It can develop in childhood as a congenital defect, but usually it is found only when injury to the anterior pituitary is severe.

Lack of the adrenocorticotropic hormone causes adrenocortical deficiency. Stress often brings nausea, vomiting, or collapse. Hypoaldosteronism is usually not present, as the secretion of aldosterone is maintained by the renin system. Pallor of the skin and nipples results from the loss of the melanocyte-stimulating hormones formed together with the adrenocorticotropic hormone. Adrenocortical deficiency is discussed further in Chapter 46.

The deficiency of the adrenocorticotropic hormone can be confirmed by administering a small dose of insulin to induce hypoglycemia, though since people with adrenocortical deficiency are sensitive to insulin, adrenocortical steroids must first be given in sufficient dose to enable the patient to withstand the stress. If the concentration of cortisol in the plasma rises by 150 nmol/L (5 μg/100 mL), or exceeds 500 nmol/L (15 μg/100 mL), secretion of the adrenocorticotropic hormone is adequate. Metyrapone can also be used to test the ability of the anterior pituitary to secrete adequate quantities of the adrenocorticotropic hormone. Metyrapone blocks synthesis of cortisol by the adrenal cortex.

In normal people, the secretion of the adrenocorticotropic hormone by the anterior pituitary increases, stimulating the adrenal cortex to secrete increased quantities of 11β-deoxycortisol and increasing the excretion of 17-hydroxycorticosteroids in the urine. In patients with adrenocorticotropic hormone deficiency, increases in the concentration of 11β-deoxycortisol secretion and in the excretion of 17-hydroxycorticosteroids fail to occur, though it is necessary to confirm that the adrenal cortex can respond normally to the adrenocorticotropic hormone by showing that administration of the adrenocorticotropic hormone restores the normal response.

Deficiency of the adrenocorticotropic hormone is treated by giving hydrocortisone or prednisone. Mineralocorticoids are not needed, as aldosterone secretion continues because of stimulation by the renin system.

Thyroid-Stimulating Hormone Deficiency. Deficiency of the thyroid-stimulating hormone is nearly always associated with deficiency of the growth hormone and gonadotropins, though it can occur as an isolated, congenital defect. The deficiency causes hypothyroidism, though the depression of thyroid function is not usually severe. Other symptoms or signs of hypopituitarism often suggest that the hypothyroidism is due to disease of the pituitary gland rather than of the thyroid gland itself.

In patients with hypothyroidism caused by disease of the thyroid gland, the level of thyroid-stimulating hormone in the serum is high. In people with hypothyroidism caused by disease of the pituitary gland or hypothalamus, the level is low or normal. Most patients with deficiency of the thyroid-stimulating hormone caused by intracranial disease fail to respond to the thyrotropin-releasing hormone, but some do respond normally, and some normal people fail to respond to the hormone. Treatment is as for other forms of hypothyroidism.

Prolactin Deficiency. Deficiency of prolactin causes only a failure to lactate after pregnancy. The diagnosis of hypoprolactinemia can be made by measuring the concentration of prolactin in the serum under basal resting conditions. If necessary, provocative agents such as the thyrotropin-releasing hormone, chlorpromazine, or metoclopramide can be given to determine if the anterior pituitary is still able to respond normally to these stimuli.

Panhypopituitarism. Panhypopituitarism, in which the secretions of the anterior pituitary are almost entirely absent, is often called Simmonds' disease, after the German physician who described it in 1914. The clinical manifestations of panhypopituitarism depend on the severity of the hormone deficiencies. In adults, hypogonadism is usually the predominant feature; in children lack of growth hormone is usually dominant. The patients become weak, easily tired, slothful. They dislike cold. Their skin is pale and finely wrinkled. Axillary and pubic hair is absent. The genitalia are small or ill-developed. Often the patients are overweight, because of hypothyroidism. Sometimes there is diabetes insipidus.

Diagnosis is by demonstration of the multiple deficiencies in the anterior pituitary hormones. Treatment is by replacement of the lost hormones or of the hormones produced in response to them.

Posterior Pituitary and Hypothalamus

Insufficiency of the posterior pituitary and hypothalamus is uncommon. In addition to dysfunction of the anterior pituitary caused by lack of one of the hypothalamic hormones that govern its activity, hypofunction of the posterior pituitary and hypothalamus can cause diabetes insipidus, Frölich's syndrome, the Laurence-Moon-Biedl syndrome, or the diencephalic syndrome. Occasionally a lesion in the hypothalamus causes hypothermia, excessive sleepiness, anorexia, or emotional storms.

DIABETES INSIPIDUS. Deficiency of the antidiuretic hormone causes diabetes insipidus. The renal tubules cannot resorb water normally. The urinary volume is high, causing polyuria. The loss of water causes thirst and polydipsia. Diabetes is from the Greek for syphon, and refers to the increased urinary volume. Insipidus is from the Latin for insipid. The urine tastes insipid, in contrast to the sweet taste of the urine in diabetes mellitus.

Diabetes insipidus can also be caused by disease of the renal tubules that impairs their response to the antidiuretic hormone. The defect in the tubules can be congenital or secondary to severe renal disease. Lithium carbonate, demeclocycline, methoxyfurane, and other drugs depress the tubular response to the hormone.

Diabetes insipidus caused by malfunction of the posterior pituitary or hypothalamus can develop at any age, though most patients are young adults. Men and women are affected equally.

Four kinds of central diabetes insipidus are distinguished. Some patients cannot secrete the antidiuretic hormone, whatever the stimulus. Some respond to dehydration and hypovolemia, but not to increasing osmolality of the plasma. In some the threshold for the release of the hormone is abnormally high, but the patients secrete the hormone if the osmolality of the plasma reaches this level, though the quantity of hormone secreted is often inadequate. In some, normal stimuli bring about the release of the hormone, but the quantity of hormone secreted is inadequate.

In diabetes insipidus caused by disease of the posterior pituitary and hypothalamus, polyuria and polydipsia usually begin suddenly. Most patients pass about 5 L of urine daily, though sometimes the urinary output exceeds 20 L a day. The specific gravity of the urine is less than 1.010, and its osmolality less than 290 mmol/kg (290 mOsm/kg). The ratio of the osmolality of the plasma to the osmolality of the urine is higher than normal. Patients prefer cold drinks and usually drink enough to maintain hydration.

If a patient with diabetes insipidus is deprived of water until the osmolality of the urine becomes constant, perhaps for 12 hours with a loss of 1 kg in weight, and then the antidiuretic hormone is given subcutaneously, the osmolality of the urine will increase by more than 9% if the diabetes insipidus is due to disease of the posterior pituitary or hypothalamus. In normal people, the increase is less than 9%. In people with nephrogenic diabetes mellitus, deprivation of water does little to change the urinary osmolality, and injection of the hormone produces little change in it.

Hypertonic saline can be given intravenously to raise the osmolality of the plasma to determine if there is a threshold at which the secretion of the antidiuretic hormone begins. In most people with diabetes insipidus caused by intracranial disease no threshold can be found, even if the plasma osmolality is raised to over 300 mmol/kg (300 mOsm/kg).

If the intake of fluid becomes inadequate, dehydration develops, with weakness, fever, disorientation, collapse, even death. The osmolality of the plasma rises. The concentration of sodium in the plasma may exceed 175 mmol/L (175 mEq/L).

Compulsive water drinking can closely mimic diabetes insipidus. The patients drink excessive quantities of water and excrete large quantities of hypotonic urine, much as do patients with diabetes insipidus. The ratio of plasma to urinary osmolality remains normal. The patients respond normally to a dehydration test.

In 30% of the patients in whom diabetes insipidus is caused by disease of the posterior pituitary or hypothalamus, a tumor compresses or invades the posterior pituitary or hypothalamus. An adenoma of the anterior pituitary, a craniopharyngioma, pinealoma, leukemia, and metastases can all cause diabetes insipidus in this way. In 20% of the patients, temporary or permanent diabetes insipidus is caused by a surgical proceduse or radiation of the pituitary. In 20%, it results from cerebral trauma. Less often it is caused by histiocytosis X, a vascular lesion, sarcoidosis, or meningitis. In 30% of the patients, no cause for the diabetes insipidus is found, and the condition is called idiopathic. In some kindred, idiopathic diabetes insipidus is inherited as an autosomal dominant character or a sex-linked recessive character. In some of the people with idiopathic diabetes insipidus, there is a reduction of the number of neurons in the supraoptic and paraventricular nuclei, with gliosis.

People with diabetes insipidus caused by an intracranial lesion can be treated with desmopressin or lypressin given intranasally, or by parenteral administration of the hormone. If the patient still has some ability to secrete the antidiuretic hormone, chlorpropamide and clofibrate can increase the release of the hormone from the posterior pituitary and potentiate its action on the renal tubules.

Frölich's Syndrome.   Frölich's syndrome, named after the Austrian neurologist who described it in 1901, or dystrophia adiposogenitalis as it is sometimes called, is an uncommon condition that affects children, boys more often than girls. The gonads fail to develop, and the child becomes obese. Sometimes there is diabetes insipidus, somnolence, mental retardation, or visual disturbances. Most often, Frölich's syndrome is caused by a tumor or some other lesion that damages the hypothalamus, interfering with the production of the gonadotropin-releasing hormone and damaging the eating center, to cause the overeating that leads to the obesity. All fat children with delayed genital development do not have Frölich's syndrome. Most have no hypothalamic lesion.

Laurence-Moon-Biedl Syndrome. The Laurence-Moon-Biedl-syndrome is a rare condition named after a British ophthalmologist (1830–1874), an American ophthalmologist (1844–1914), and a Czech endocrinologist (1869–1933). It is inherited as an autosomal recessive character. The children affected have hypogonadism, obesity, mental retardation, retinitis pigmentosa, polydactyly, syndactyly, and other congenital malformations. The syndrome is believed to be caused by hypothalamic dysfunction, though no lesion has been demonstrated in the hypothalamus.

Diencephalic Syndrome. The diencephalic syndrome occurs in infants and is usually due to destruction of the hypothalamus by an astrocytoma. In spite of eating well, the child becomes extremely emaciated. Nystagmus develops. The children are notably affectionate. The tumor usually brings death within a year. If the child does survive, it may later become obese.

BIBLIOGRAPHY

General

Doniach, I.: Histopathology of the pituitary. Clin. Endocrinol. Metab., *14*:765, 1985.
Ezrin, C., Kovacs, K., and Horvath, E.: Pathology of the adenohypophysis. *In* Endocrine Pathology, 2nd ed. Edited by J. B. M. Bloodworth, Jr. Baltimore, Williams & Wilkins, 1982.
Sheehan, H. L., and Kovacs, K.: Neurohypophysis and hypothalamus. *In* Endocrine Pathology, 2nd ed. Edited by J. B. M. Bloodworth, Jr. Baltimore, Williams & Wilkins, 1982.

Non-Neoplastic Disorders

Asa, S. L., and Kovacs, K.: Functional morphology of the human fetal pituitary. Pathol. Annu., *19* (Pt. 1):275, 1984.
Berger, S. A., Edberg, S. C., and David, G.: Infectious disease in the sella turcica. Rev. Infect. Dis., *8*:747, 1986.

Bhasin, S., and Swerdloff, R. S.: Hypothalamic hypogonadism. Spec. Top. Endocrinol. Metab., 7:237, 1985.
Edwards, O. M., and Clark, J. D. A.: Post-traumatic hypopituitarism. Medicine (Baltimore), 65:281, 1986.
Scheithauer, B.W.: Pathology of the pituitary and sellar region. Pathol. Annu., *20* (Pt. 1):67, 1985.
Veldhuis, J. D., and Hammond, J. M.: Endocrine function after spontaneous infarction of the human pituitary. Endocrinol. Rev., *1*:100, 1980.

Tumors

Becker, L. E., and Halliday, W. C.: Central nervous system tumors of childhood. Perspect. Pediatr. Pathol., 10:86, 1987.
Ciric, I.: Pituitary tumors. Neurol. Clin., *3*:751, 1985.
Gonzalez-Crussi, F.: Extragonadal Teratomas. Washington D. C., Armed Forces Institute of Pathology, 1982.
Howanitz, J. H., and Howanitz, P. J.: Pituitary tumors. Clin. Lab. Med., *4*:643, 1984.
Jordan, R. M., and Kohler, P. O.: Recent advances in the diagnosis and management of pituitary tumors. Adv. Intern. Med., *32*:299, 1987.
Kovacs, K., and Horvath, E.: Tumors of the Pituitary Gland. Washington D. C., Armed Forces Institute of Pathology, 1986.
Lederman, G. S., et al.: Craniopharyngioma in the elderly. Cancer, 60:1077, 1987.
Melmed, S., Braunstein, G. D., Chang, R. J., and Becker, D. P.: Pituitary tumors secreting growth hormone and prolactin. Ann. Intern. Med., *105*:238, 1986.
Roy, S.: Ultrastructure of pituitary adenomas. Prog. Neuropathol., *5*:223, 1983.
Scheithauer, B. W.: Surgical pathology of the pituitary, the adenomas. Pathol. Annu., *19* (Pt. 1):317, (Pt. 2): 269, 1984.
Shalet, S. M.: Pituitary adenomas in children. Acta Endocrinol. (Suppl), *279*:434, 1986.
Snyder, P. J.: Gonadotroph cell adenomas of the pituitary. Endocr. Rev., 6:552, 1985.

Hyperpituitarism

Carpenter, P. C.: Cushing's syndrome. Mayo Clin. Proc., *61*:49, 1986.
Howlett, T. A., Rees, L. H., and Besser, G. M.: Cushing's syndrome. Clin. Endocrinol. Metab., *14*: 911, 1985.
McNicol, A. M.: Cushing's syndrome. Neuropathol. Appl. Neurobiol., *11*:485, 1985.
Magyar, D. M.: Amenorrhea, galactorrhea, and hyperprolactinemia. J. Am. Osteopath. Assoc., *85*:375, 1985.
Melmed, S., Braunstein, G. D., Chang, R. J., and Becker, D. P.: Pituitary tumors secreting growth hormone and prolactin. Ann. Intern. Med., *105*:238, 1986.
Moses, M., and Notman, D. D.: Diabetes insipidus and the syndrome of inappropriate antidiuretic hormone secretion. Adv. Intern. Med., 27: 73, 1982.

Hypopituitarism

Moses, M., and Notman, D. D.: Diabetes insipidus and the syndrome of inappropriate antidiuretic hormone

secretion. Adv. Intern. Med., 27:73, 1982.

Veldhuis, J. D., and Hammond, J. M.: Endocrine function after spontaneous infarction of the human pituitary. Endocrinol. Rev., 1:100, 1980.

45

Pineal Gland

THE pineal gland is small. Its principal diseases are calcification and tumors. Rarely, the gland is absent or malformed. The pineal produces melatonin, but little is known of the properties of melatonin or the consequences of pineal dysfunction.

CALCIFICATION

Calcification of the pineal gland is common. It begins in childhood and is often sufficient to be visible radiologically in adolescents. Small spherules of calcification develop in the stroma of the gland, particularly at its base and in the septa between its lobules. The calcification does not impair the activity of the enzymes that synthesize melatonin.

TUMORS

About 75% of the neoplasms that arise in the pineal gland are germ cell tumors. Most of the rest arise from the tissues of the pineal gland, from the pinealocytes, or the glia that makes up the stroma of the gland. Rarely, an angioma arises in a pineal gland. Some use the term *pinealoma* to include all tumors of the pineal gland. Most restrict it to the tumors that arise from the pinealocytes.

GERM CELL TUMORS. About 80% of the germ cell tumors that arise in the pineal gland are germinomata and resemble a seminoma. Most of the rest are teratomata, though any kind of germ cell tumor can arise in the pineal gland. Precocious puberty develops in 50% of boys with a pineal teratoma. Surgical removal of the tumor is difficult because of its site. About 60% of patients treated by radiation survive more than five years.

PINEALOMA. Two kinds of tumor arise from the pinealocytes. A well-differentiated tumor most common in adults is called a pinealocytoma. A poorly differentiated tumor usually found in children is called a pinealoblastoma.

Lesions. Pinealomata form a soft, gray mass, often with foci of hemorrhage or necrosis. The well-differentiated tumors are well defined and compress the adjacent structures. The poorly differentiated tumors invade the brain.

Microscopically, a pinealocytoma usually consists of small cells that resemble pinealocytes and a proliferation of the astrocytes that make up the stroma of the tumor. The tumor cells that resemble pinealocytes have regular, spheroidal, darkly staining nuclei and eosinophilic cytoplasm. They sometimes grow in clumps separated by a fibrous stroma; sometimes they form rosettes with lumina lined by the tumor cells. Proliferation of the astrocytes forms a lesion like an astrocytoma. Many pinealocytomata show both kinds of differentiation. Some consist predominantly of clumps of pinealocytes or of astrocytoma. Melatonin is present in high concentration in some of the tumors.

A pinealoblastoma consists of masses of large cells with pleomorphic nuclei and many mitoses. Poorly formed rosettes are often present.

Behavior. A pinealocytoma grows slowly and usually produces symptoms only when pressure from the enlarging mass damages some adjacent structure. Injury to the optic nerves causes visual symptoms. Pressure on the third ventricle causes hydrocephalus. Headache is common. Mental deterioration is frequent. Hypogonadism develops in some patients. Precocious puberty develops in 40% of boys with a pinealoma.

A pinealoblastoma grows more rapidly and causes local symptoms earlier. Fragments of tumor carried in the cerebrospinal fluid sometimes implant in distant parts of the subarachnoid space.

Treatment and Prognosis.   A pinealoma is treated surgically. Because of the site of the tumor, complete removal is difficult. Few patients with a pinealoblastoma live more than two years. Most with a pinealocytoma survive for over five years.

BIBLIOGRAPHY

Gonzalez-Crussi, F.: Extragonadal Teratomas. Washington D. C., Armed Forces Institute of Pathology, 1982.

Hoffman, H. J.: Pineal region tumors. Prog. Exp. Tumor Res., *30*:281, 1987.

Moskowitz, M. A., and Wurtman, M. J.: New approaches to the study of the human pineal gland. *In* Endocrine Pathology, 2nd ed. Edited J. M. B. by Bloodworth, Jr. Baltimore, Williams & Wilkins, 1982.

Scheithauer, B. W.: Neuropathology of pineal region tumors. Clin. Neurosurg., *32*:351, 1985.

46

Adrenal Glands

THE diseases of the adrenal glands are divided into infectious conditions, vascular disorders, enzyme deficiencies, primary and secondary forms of hyperplasia and atrophy, congenital defects, and tumors. Since different kinds of adrenal disease cause similar dysfunction, the various kinds of adrenal disease will be discussed first, then the dysfunction they cause.

INFECTION

Infection of the adrenal glands is not common. When it does occur, it affects principally children, especially the newborn.

Infants with generalized listeriosis sometimes show foci of necrosis in the adrenal glands, at first with little inflammation, later with a dense exudate of lymphocytes and macrophages. Listeria monocytogenes can be demonstrated in the lesions.

Tuberculosis used to be the major cause of Addison's disease, but tuberculosis of the adrenal glands has become uncommon in much of world. The tubercle bacilli produce the usual granulomata in the adrenal glands and may form massive caseous abscesses that destroy one or both adrenals. The abscesses are of the usual form seen in tuberculosis, with a caseous core, a sparse granulomatous reaction at the periphery, and often surrounding fibrosis. If the tuberculosis is controlled, the abscesses become stationary and may calcify.

Congenital syphilis can cause interstitial fibrosis in the adrenal glands. Brucellosis or a rickettsial infection occasionally causes focal necorsis. Pyogenic abscesses can develop in septicemia. A terminal infection with a species of candida or aspergillus sometimes occurs in patients with immunologic deficiency or a terminal illness. Histoplas-mosis and toxoplasmosis occasionally involve the adrenal glands.

Cytomegaloviral infection sometimes causes foci of necrosis in the adrenal glands in infants and in adults with immunologic deficiency. The lesions show a core of necrosis surrounded by an exudate of lymphocytes and macrophages. The inclusions of the cytomegalovirus are present in the macrophages and in epithelial cells adjacent to the lesion. Less often, similar necrosis is caused by the herpes simplex virus, usually with extensive necrosis in the liver. Occasionally viral inclusions are found in a gland that shows little or no injury.

ENZYME DEFICIENCY

Deficiency of one of the enzymes needed for the synthesis of the adrenocortical hormones causes serious adrenocortical dysfunction. The deficiencies are divided into two groups, those that cause congenital adrenal hyperplasia and those that have little effect on the size of the adrenal glands. The deficiencies are inherited as an autosomal recessive character. Pseudohypoaldosteronism, a defect of the renal tubules, is also described in this section.

CONGENITAL ADRENAL HYPERPLASIA. Congenital adrenal hyperplasia is caused by deficiency of one of the enzymes needed to synthesize cortisol. It affects one child in 10,000. Nearly 80% of the patients are girls.

Lesions. In congenital adrenal hyperplasia, the adrenal glands are enlarged. In a child, they weigh 10 to 20 g each, instead of the normal 2 to 3 g. In an adult, they weigh 20 to 40 g each. In a normal adult, the adrenal glands together weigh less than 11 g. The enlarged glands are of normal shape. Their surface is convoluted, like the surface of the brain. The glands are brown, rather than the usual yellow.

Microscopically, the enlargement is due to thickening of the adrenal cortex. Almost the whole thickness of the cortex consists of small cells like those of the zona reticularis, with eosinophilic, granular cytoplasm containing fine droplets of lipid. The zona glomerulosa persists against the capsule of the gland, and a thin remnant of the greatly stretched zona fasciculata may be between it and the dominant small granular cells. Lipochrome pigment is often abundant in the cortical cells, especially near the corticomedullary junction.

Pathogenesis. Congenital adrenal hyperplasia is caused by deficiency of one of the enzymes involved in the synthesis of cortisol. Often, the deficiency impairs the production of aldosterone or other of the adrenocortical steroids. Because of the deficiency of cortisol, the secretion of the adrenocorticotropic hormone by the pituitary gland increases. The excess of the adrenocorticotropic hormone causes hyperplasia of the adrenal cortices.

The excess of the adrenocorticotropic hormone causes hyperactivity of those synthetic mechanisms that remain intact in the adrenal cortices. There is overproduction of the precursors of the blocked hormones and the adrenocortical steroids unaffected by the enzyme deficiency.

The effect of the deficiency depends on the function of the enzyme deficient and on the severity of the deficiency. If the enzyme is almost completely lacking, the deficiency of the adrenocortical hormones affected is severe and becomes evident during infancy. If the deficiency of the enzyme is less extreme, the deficiency of the adrenocortical hormones affected is less complete. There may be little or no evidence of adrenocortical dysfunction, or the dysfunction may be recognized only in adult life.

21-Hydroxylase Deficiency. In the majority of the patients with congenital adrenal hyperplasia, 21-hydroxylase is deficient. The abnormal allele is on chromosome 6. Cortisol production is impaired because 17-hydroxyprogesterone cannot be converted adequately into 11-deoxycortisol. Aldosterone production may also be impaired because progesterone cannot be converted adequately into 11-deoxycorticosterone. Since the adrenal androgens do not require 21-hydroxylation, they are produced in excessive quantity as is the precursor of cortisol 17α-hydroxyprogesterone.

Because of the lack of cortisol, the concentration of the adrenocorticotropic hormone in the plasma increases. If aldosterone is lacking, the concentration of renin in the plasma increases. The increased secretion of androgens by the adrenal cortex increases the urinary excretion of 17-ketosteroids. The increased secretion of 17α-hydroxyprogesterone, increases the urinary excretion of pregnanetriol and other of its metabolites.

Virilization caused by an excess of androgens is the major feature of the disorder. In girls, there is masculinization of the external genitalia; cliteromegaly, fusion of the labia to form a pseudoscrotum, and enlargement of the clitoris to form a penis-like organ with the urethra running through it. In boys, it causes sexual precocity and early puberty. Both boys and girls grow rapidly, but the excess of androgens causes premature closure of the epiphyses before growth of the trunk ceases, so that the limbs are short. In women, the excess of androgens brings hirsutism, acne, deepending of the voice, atrophy of the breasts, enlargement of the clitoris, increased muscularity, and a masculine habitus.

In over 50% of infants and children with deficiency of 21-hydroxylase there are episodes of salt loss, with vomiting, dehydration, circulatory collapse, hyponatremia, and hyperkalemia. In some of the patients, the loss of salt is due to aldosterone deficiency, but in others the concentration of aldosterone in the plasma is normal or elevated, and it is thought that the hyponatremia is caused by the excess of the aldosterone antagonists progesterone and 17α-hydroxyprogesterone produced by hyperplastic adrenal cortices.

A diagnosis of 21-hydroxylase deficiency can be confirmed by estimating the concentration of 17-hydroxyprogesterone in the plasma. Normally, an infant 36 hours old has less than 6 nmol/L (1.9 ng/100 mL) of 17-hydroxyprogesterone in the plasma. An infant with 21-hydroxylase deficiency is likely to have more than 200 nmol/L 62 (ng/100 mL). The diagnosis can be made before birth by showing a high concentration of 17-hydroxyprogesterone in the amniotic fluid.

11β-Hydroxylase Deficiency. Deficiency of 11β-hydroxylase is much less common. The conversion of 11-deoxycortisol to cortisol is impaired, causing deficiency of cortisol, and the conversion of 11-deoxycorticosterone to corticosterone is impaired, causing deficiency of aldosterone. Because the production of androgens is not affected, androgens are secreted in excessive quantity by the hyperplastic adrenal glands. Because of the block, the production of 11-deoxycortisol is increased, causing increased excretion of 17-hydroxycorticoids in the urine, and because of the overproduction of androgens by the adrenal the urinary excretion of 17-ketosteroids is increased. Adrenocortical deficiency does not occur, for the weak glucocorticoid 11-deoxycortisol and the weak mineralocorticoid 11-deoxycorticosterone overcome in large part the lack of cortisol and aldosterone.

The deficiency of 11β-hydroxylase causes virilization, much as does deficiency of 21-hydroxylase. In addition, lack of 11β-hydroxylase causes hypertension, though the hypertension may not become evident until some years after virilization is apparent. The hypertension is caused by the accumulation of the mineralocorticoid 11-deoxycorticosterone, much as hypertension is caused in Conn's syndrome. Salt loss does not occur.

The diagnosis of 11β-hydroxylase deficiency is established by measuring the concentration of 11-deoxycortisol in the plasma or the excretion of tetrahydrodeoxycortisol in the urine.

17-Hydroxlase Deficiency. Deficiency of 17-hydroxylase is rare. It causes impairment of the production of cortisol, androgens, and usually of aldosterone. Progesterone, its metabolite pregnanetriol, deoxycorticosterone, and corticosterone accumulate. In boys, the genitalia develop poorly. In girls, the menses fail to begin at puberty, and sexual development is reduced. In both sexes, hypokalemia and hypertension are caused by the accumulation of deoxycorticosterone and corticosterone.

3β-Hydroxysteroid Dehydrogenase Deficiency. Lack of 3β-hydroxysteroid dehydrogenase is a rare defect that impairs the transformation of Δ^5 steroids to Δ^4 steroids in the adrenal glands and the ovaries. The formation of cortisol, aldosterone, androgens, and estrogens is blocked. Instead, pregnenolone and dehydroepiandrosterone are secreted in large quantity. Salt loss is severe, often fatal. Both boys and girls have malformed genitalia, the boys because of the lack of potent androgens, the girls because enough of the weak androgen dehydroepiandrosterone is present to cause partial masculinization.

20,22-Desmolase Deficiency. Deficiency of 20,22-desmolase is rare. It affects the ovaries and testes as well as the adrenal cortices. The synthesis of all adrenocortical steroids is blocked. Loss of salt is severe. Sexual development is imperfect. The affected children rarely survive infancy. The cells of the adrenal cortex become filled with the cholesterol that cannot be utilized to synthesize hormones. Instead of the small cells like the cells of the zona reticularis that are dominant in most forms of congenital adrenal hyperplasia, the cells of the cortex are large and filled with fat.

Treatment. For congenital adrenal hyperplasia, prednisone or some other glucocorticoid is given in dose sufficient to reduce the secretion of the adrenocorticotropic hormone to normal, allowing resolution of the adrenocortical hyperplasia and preventing the overproduction of the unblocked adrenocortical steroids. If the activity of renin in the plasma is increased, showing that there is a deficiency of aldosterone, mineralocorticoids are given as well. If necessary, androgens or estrogens are administered. Malformation of the genitalia is corrected surgically.

NONHYPERPLASTIC DEFICIENCIES. Rarely, deficiency of an adrenocortical enzyme affects only the synthesis of the mineralocorticoids. The production of cortisol is normal. There is no oversecretion of the adrenocorticotropic hormone, and no hyperplasia of the adrenal cortices.

18-Hydroxylase Deficiency. Lack of 18-hydroxylase prevents the conversion of corticosterone to 18-hydroxycorticosterone and aldosterone. Infants with the deficiency have salt loss, dehydration, and fever. The concentration of corticosterone is increased in the plasma, and its metabolite allotetrahydrocorticosterone is present in increased quantity in the urine. The activity of renin in the plasma is increased. Replacement of the missing mineralocorticoid is needed.

18-Hydroxysteroid Dehydrogenase Deficiency. Deficiency of 18-hydroxysteroid dehydrogenase prevents the dehydrogenation of 18-hydroxycorticosterone and the formation of aldosterone. Allotetrahydrocorticosterone, 18-hydroxytetrahydrocorticosterone, and other metabolites of 18-hydroxycorticosterone are excreted in increased quantities in the urine. Salt loss is controlled by giving mineralocorticoids.

PSEUDOHYPOALDOSTERONISM. Pseudohypoaldosteronism is a rare condition that causes salt loss in infancy. Hyponatremia, hyperkalemia, and azotemia are severe. Sometimes there is aminoaciduria or glyosuria. In the plasma the concentration of aldosterone and the activity of renin are increased. The secretion of cortisol and 17-hydroxyprogesterone and the response of the adrenal cortex to the adrenocorticotropic hormone are normal. The administration of mineralocorticoids brings no benefit.

The fault is in the renal tubules and in other tissues whose activity is regulated by aldosterone. The tubules fail to respond to the mineralocorticoids, resulting in salt loss. The salt loss can be controlled by giving the infants a high salt diet. Fortunately, the children grow out of the defect, and after a few years their response to mineralocorticoids becomes normal.

HYPERPLASIA AND ATROPHY

Hyperplasia and atrophy of the adrenal glands usually affect only the cortex. The hyperplasia or atrophy may be primary, caused by disease of the adrenal glands, or secondary, due to excess or lack of the adrenocorticotropic hormone. Hyperplasia of the medulla is uncommon. Atrophy of the medulla occurs only when its blood supply is impaired or there is other serious injury to the gland.

NODULAR ADRENOCORTICAL HYPERPLASIA. In contrast to the congenital adrenal hyperplasia caused by an enzyme deficiency, nodular hyperplasia of the adrenal cortices usually develops in an adult, though it can occur in children. Nodular adrenocortical hyperplasia is uncommon. The patients are usually 40 to 60 years old. About 70% of them are men.

The adrenal glands are enlarged, but preserve their normal shape. They do not show the cerebriform markings of congenital adrenal hyperplasia. The enlargement is due to thickening of the cortex. The medulla is not affected. Usually the cortices are nodular, with multiple nodules from 0.1 to 2.0 cm across.

Microscopically, the hyperplasia is principally of the zona fascicularis. The cortex is thickened by large, pale cells filled with lipid. The nodules consist of similar cells. They compress the adjacent columns of the zona fascicularis, but have no capsule to demarcate them from the zona fascicularis.

Minor degrees of nodular hyperplasia cause no dysfunction. When the condition is more severe, it usually causes hyperaldosteronism but, especially in children, can cause oversecretion of cortisol or other of the adrenocortical hormones.

SECONDARY ADRENOCORTICAL HYPERPLASIA. Secondary hyperplasia of the adrenal cortices is caused by oversecretion of the adrenocorticotropic hormone or the corticotropin releasing hormone. It can be due to disease of the pituitary gland, most often a corticotroph adenoma, or to release of the tropic hormone from an oat cell carcinoma of the lung, some other neuroendocrine tumor, a tumor of the parotid, prostate, kidney, or less frequently some other type of neoplasm.

The adrenal glands usually weigh from 10 to 20 g each. They preserve their normal shape. On section, the cortices are thickened. In 20% of the patients with hyperplasia caused by pituitary dysfunction, they are nodular. The inner part of the cortices is often brown, the outer part bright yellow.

Microscopically, in patients with pituitary dysfunction the inner third of the cortex consists of small, dark cells, like those of the zona reticularis. The rest of the cortex consists mainly of the zona fasciculas, with fat-filled cells, often larger than normal. Collections of fat may lie free between the cells of the zona fascicularis. The zona glomerulosa is sometimes well developed, but often is small, present only here and there around the periphery of the cortex. When nodules are present, they consist of cells like those of the zona fasciculais. At autopsy, the fat of the cortices is usually lost, and the cortices consist almost entirely of small, dark cells extending up to the capsule or appearing to compress the zona glomerulosa.

When a tumor secretes an excess of the tropic hormone, the cortices consist of columns of dark cells, like those of the zona reticularis, but larger than normal. There is little if any zona fasciculata. Instead, clumps of large, pale cells like those of the zona fasciculata are scattered among the columns of dark cells.

Secondary hyperplasia of the adrenal cortices causes oversecretion of cortisol and to a lesser degree of other adrenocortical hormones.

MEDULLARY HYPERPLASIA. Hyperplasia of the medulla of the adrenal glands is uncommon. It sometimes develops in people with multiple endocrine neoplasia type IIa, the condition in which the patients tend to develop hyperplasia or tumors of the parathyroid glands, the medullae of the adrenal glands, and the C cells of the thyroid gland. It sometimes develops without disease of other endocrine glands.

One or both adrenal glands are affected. The gland or glands involved may be of normal size or may weigh as much as 10 g each. Normally, the medulla is confined to the head and body of an adrenal gland, extending into only one of the alae of the body. If medullary tissue is present in the tail of an adrenal gland or in both alae of its body, the medulla is hyperplastic. Morphometry shows that the hyperplastic medulla weighs from 0.8 to 1.6 g, as compared with the normal of under 0.5 g. Often adrenomedullary hyperplasia is nodular, with nodules of medullary tissue up to 1 cm across scattered in the hyperplastic medulla.

Microscopically, the hyperplastic medullary cells are pleomorphic. Some are larger than normal. Some have giant nuclei, and some have several nuclei. Some show mitoses. Some contain hyaline globules in their cytoplasm.

The hyperplastic medulla often secretes inappropriate quantities of catecholamines. The patients develop episodic hypertension and other symptoms like those produced by a pheochromocytoma.

PRIMARY ADRENOCORTICAL ATROPHY. Primary adrenocortical atrophy is uncommon. It may occur at any age. Men and women are affected equally.

The adrenal glands are small, weighing 2 to 5 g each instead of the normal 5 to 6 g. The shape of the glands is preserved. Up to 90% of the cortical cells are lost. The surviving cells are large and eosinophilic, with little fat. They form clumps, separated by the collapsed reticulin framework of the cortices. If the atrophy is not too extreme, foci of adrenocortical hyperplasia are often present in the atrophic cortices or in clumps of adrenocortical cells in the adjacent fat. A moderate exudate of lymphocytes is present in the cortices and may extend into the medulla. Otherwise, the medulla is normal.

In most patients, primary adrenocortical atrophy is probably caused immunologically, much as is Hashimoto's disease of the thyroid gland. Antibodies against the adrenal cortices are present in the plasma in 80% of women with primary adrenocortical atrophy, but in less than 20% of men. As is usual in autoimmune diseases, a similar immunologic attack against other organs is often evident. Some 70% of the patients have antibodies against the thyroid, the parietal cells of the stomach, or the intrinsic factor. Other diseases believed caused by an immunologic derangement are common in people with primary adrenocortical atrophy. Over 15% have insulin-dependent diabetes mellitus. About 10% have Hashimoto's disease of the thyroid; 10% have pernicious anemia; 10% have atrophic gastritis; and 5% have hypoparathyroidism.

If primary adrenocortical atrophy is not severe, it causes little dysfunction. If it is severe, both cortisol and aldosterone are deficient.

Polyglandular Autoimmune Syndromes. In the polyglandular autoimmune syndromes, more than one endocrine organ is damaged by an autoimmune reaction. Type I polyglandular autoimmune syndrome is inherited as an autosomal recessive character. It usually becomes apparent during childhood. The patients have primary adrenocortical atrophy, atrophy of the parathyroid glands, and moniliasis. Sometimes other endocrine glands are also involved. The type II polyglandular autoimmune syndrome usually develops during adult life. The frequency of the HLA antigens B8 and DW3 is increased. Autoimmune injury is evident in two or more organs: Hashimoto's disease, Graves' disease, insulin dependent diabetes mellitus, pernicious anemia, primary hypoparathyrodism, or primary adrenocortical atrophy. Sometimes the patients have vitiligo, alopecia, malabsorption, or myasthenia gravis.

SECONDARY ADRENOCORTICAL ATROPHY. Most often, secondary atrophy of the adrenal cortices is caused by the administration of adrenocortical steroids in dose large enough to reduce the secretion of the adrenocorticotropic hormone. It can follow disease of the pituitary gland, with loss of the adrenocorticotropic hormone. It occurs in wasting diseases, though the mechanism in these patients is unclear.

The adrenal glands are smaller than normal, often weighing about 3 g each, and look thin. Microscopically, their capsules are thick. The cortices consist mainly of a thin zona fasciculata made of small, pale cells. The zona reticularis is thin and may be absent. The medulla is normal.

OTHER NON-NEOPLASTIC DISORDERS

Other non-neoplastic disorders that affect the adrenal cortices are uncommon or of little importance clinically. Among them are the Waterhouse-Friderichsen syndrome, other forms of hemorrhage or necrosis, lipid depletion, tubular change, nodularity, intracytoplasmic inclusions, adrenoleukodystrophy, and amyloidosis.

WATERHOUSE-FRIDERICHSEN SYNDROME. The Waterhouse-Friderichsen syndrome, named after the British physician who described it in 1911 and the Danish pediatrician who discussed it in 1918, is uncommon. Sudden, massive hemorrhage into both adrenal glands is followed by widespread purpura and severe shock. The patients are usually children. Without treatment, death is likely within a few hours.

The adrenal glands are swollen, purple, and hemorrhagic. Sometimes the capsule of a gland ruptures, and blood escapes into the surrounding tissues or into the peritoneal cavity. Microscopically, there is hemorrhagic infarction of the glands, with almost complete destruction of the cortices and medullae. Fibrin thrombi are present in the blood vessels at the margins of the necrosis.

The Waterhouse-Friderichsen syndrome usually complicates meningococcal bacteremia, though bacteremia with other gram-negative bacteria can cause similar adrenal hemorrhage. The infarction and purpura are caused by intravascular coagulation. The collapse is due to sudden loss of the adrenal hormones. Large doses of cortisol are necessary to avert death.

OTHER FORMS OF HEMORRHAGE AND NECROSIS. In adults, trauma, preeclampsia, other forms of disseminated intravascular coagulation, anticoagulant therapy, malignant hypertension, and thrombosis of an adrenal vein can cause hemorrhage into one or both adrenal glands. The hemorrhage is not usually as severe as in the Waterhouse-Friderichsen syndrome, but sometimes causes adrenocortical deficiency. Small foci of necrosis are common in the adrenal cortices in severe septicemia, but are not usually extensive enough to cause dysfunction.

In infants, trauma at birth can cause hemorrhage into an adrenal gland. The hemorrhage is sometimes severe enough to cause a mass in the flank, hypovolemic shock, or adrenocortical deficiency. The fetal cortex of the adrenal glands degenerates soon after birth. Hemorrhage into the degenerating fetal cortex is common, but causes no dysfunction.

LIPID DEPLETION. In patients subjected to prolonged stress, with excessive or long continued oversecretion of adrenocortical steroids, the cells of the zona fasciculata in the adrenal cortices lose much of their fat. Autopsies of patients after a debilitating and fatal illness usually reveal little lipid in the adrenal cortices. In adults, the loss of lipid is usually patchy, with regions devoid of fat alternating with regions in which the zona fasciculata retains much of its lipid. In the regions depleted of lipid, compact, dark cells like those of the zona reticularis extend through the whole thickness of the cortex,

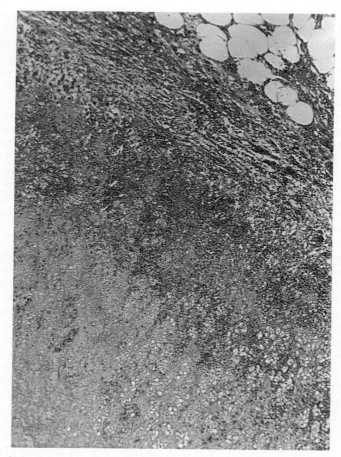

Fig. 46-1. An adrenal gland from a patient with the Waterhouse-Friderichsen syndrome, showing necrosis of the deeper part of the cortex with hemorrhage into its superficial part and into the periadrenal tissues.

from the medulla to the capsule or the inconspicuous zona glomerulosa.

In children with lipid depletion, most of the cortical cells are small and dark, like the cells of the zona reticularis, but scattered among them are large, pale cells filled with lipid, like the cells of the zona fasciculata. Only if the stress has been severe, as in a severe burn, is lipid entirely lost from the cortices.

When fat begins to reappear in the adrenal cortices it accumulates first in the midpart of the zona fasciculata and gradually extends peripherally and centrally until the fat stores of the zona fasciculata are restored, and the small quantities of lipid normally present in the zona reticularis are again evident.

TUBULAR CHANGE. Tubular change in the adrenal cortices is a sign of adrenocortical hyperactivity. In severe trauma, severe burns, severe infections, and other stressful situations, hyaline droplets of protein appear in the cytoplasm of some of the cortical cells. Sometimes a few of the cortical cells become necrotic. The plates of cortical cells in the peripheral part of the zona fasciculata become hollowed to form a central lumen, separated from the adjacent sinusoids by an irregular but usually single layer of cortical epithelium.

NODULARITY. Over 50% of people over 50 years old have multiple nodules in the zona fasciculata of their adrenal cortices. The nodules vary from the microscopic to

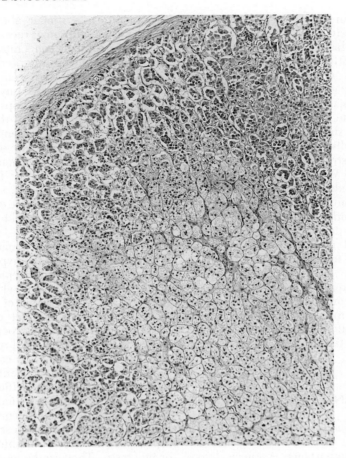

Fig. 46-2. An ill-defined nodule of large, lipid-filled cells in the adrenal cortex of an elderly person with nodular cortical hyperplasia.

0.5 cm in diameter, are spheroidal, and macroscopically look well defined, though microscopically they are not clearly demarcated from the surrounding cortex. The nodules may be within the cortex or may bulge from its surface. Occasionally a nodule lies free in the fat near the adrenal.

The nodules are foci of hyperplasia. The cells in the nodules are arranged much as in the normal cortex, but are often bigger than the cells in the surrounding cortex or contain more lipid. Often the content of enzymes in the cells in a nodule is different from that in the cells of the neighboring cortex.

Probably the nodules are caused by repeated cycles of hyperplasia and regression. The regions that form nodules may react more strongly to the adrenocorticotropic hormone than does the surrounding cortex or may fail to regress when hyperplasia wanes in the surrounding cortex.

INTRACYTOPLASMIC INCLUSIONS. In patients treated with the aldosterone antagonist spironolactone, spheroidal, laminated bodies 2 to 25 μm across appear in the cytoplasm of some of the cells in the zona glomerulosa and zona fasciculata of the adrenal cortices. The spironolactone bodies are eosinophilic and consist in part of phospholipid.

Occasionally, hyaline, eosinophilic spheroids called colloid bodies are found in the cytoplasm of some of the adrenocortical cells. Their nature and significance are unknown.

ADRENOLEUKODYSTROPHY. Adrenoleukodystrophy is a rare condition inherited as a sex-linked recessive character, in which in addition to the changes of leukodystrophy in the brain the patient suffers atrophy of the adrenal cortices. Often the adrenal glands weigh less than 2 g each. The shrunken zona fasciculata is partially replaced by large cells, with pale, hyaline, striated cytoplasm. Electron microscopy shows that the cytoplasm of the abnormal cells contains large quantities of membranous structures.

AMYLOIDOSIS. When amyloidosis affects the adrenal glands, amyloid is usually deposited first in the zona fasciculata, between the sinusoidal endothelium and the cortical epithelium. The deposits may involve much of both adrenal cortices, or the amyloid may be confined to a few foci in one or both adrenal cortices. If amyloidosis is severe, much of the adrenocortical epithelium becomes atrophic or is lost, but the loss is rarely sufficient to cause adrenocortical deficiency. Less often, amyloid is deposited mainly around the blood vessels in the adrenal medulla.

CONGENITAL ANOMALIES

If enzyme deficiencies are excluded, congenital anomalies of the adrenal glands are rarely of clinical importance. Agenesis, hypoplasia, and adrenal rests are the most common malformations. Occasionally two adrenal glands are present on each side.

AGENESIS. The adrenal glands are absent in 10% of children with renal agenesis, in many acephalic monsters, and rarely in infants without other abnormalities. Occasionally, there is enough accessory adrenal tissue in other parts of the body to allow these infants to survive.

HYPOPLASIA. The adrenal glands are small in the anencephalic monsters that have adrenal glands and in infants with other malformations of the pituitary region. In a few kindred, the glands are small in infants without other congenital anomalies.

In the anencephalic monsters, the adrenal glands resemble tiny adult glands macroscopically and microscopically. The fetal cortex normally dominant in the last weeks of pregnancy is absent. In infants without other abnormalities, a similar abnormality is inherited as an autosomal recessive character.

Another form of congenital hypoplasia of the adrenal glands is inherited as an X-linked recessive character and occurs only in boys. The adrenal glands are tiny. The cortices consist of disorderly clumps of large cells that resemble the cells of the fetal cortex. Often giant cells are present. Between the clumps is a loose stroma, sometimes with macrophages containing hemosiderin. Occasionally, remnants of the fetal cortex are present. The medullae are sometimes normal, but sometimes consist of small clumps of medullary cells separated by a collagenous stroma.

Children with the autosomal recessive and X-linked forms of adrenal hypoplasia tend to lose salt and often suffer episodes of hypoglycemia. Both cortisol and aldosterone must be replaced. In all forms of adrenal hypoplasia, the lack of a fetal cortex reduces the production of dehydroepiandrosterone during the later stages of pregnancy and reduces the excretion of estrogen in the mothers' urine. The concentrations of dehydroepiandrosterone and 16α-hydroxypregnenolone in the amniotic fluid are low.

RESTS. Rests of adrenocortical tissue are common. They are often present beneath the capsule of a kidney, in the hilus of an ovary, or in a testis. They can be found in the liver, along the aorta, or in the spermatic cord. Rests of medullary tissue are rare.

TUMORS

Primary tumors of the adrenal cortex or the adrenal medulla are uncommon. Metastatic carcinoma is by far the commonest tumor of the adrenal glands.

Cortical Tumors

An adrenocortical adenoma is the most common tumor of the adrenal cortices. Adrenocortical carcinoma, a hemangioma, or some other mesenchymal tumor of the cortex of an adrenal is uncommon.

ADENOMA. No clear distinction can be drawn between an adrenocortical adenoma

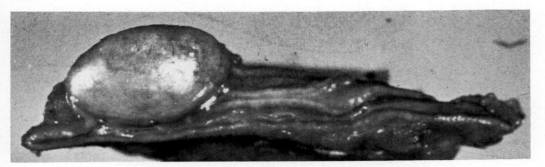

Fig. 46-3. A sharply defined, bright yellow, adrenocortical adenoma.

and the hyperplastic nodules that are common both in hyperplastic adrenal cortices and in adrenal glands otherwise normal. The lesions called adenomata are usually bigger than hyperplastic nodules, often more than 2 cm in diameter. An adenoma is usually solitary; hyperplastic nodules are usually multiple, though occasionally the adrenal glands contain two or three adenomata. The cortex around an adrenocortical adenoma is normal or atrophic; the cortex around hyperplastic nodules is normal or hyperplastic. A lesion big enough to be called an adenoma is found in 2% of autopsies, but many of these lesions are probably hyperplastic, not neoplastic.

Lesions. An adrenocortical adenoma is usually a spheroidal mass, 2 to 5 cm in diameter. Occasionally an adenoma weighs up to 1.5 kg. A thin, collagenous capsule usually demarcates the adenoma from the surrounding cortex. If its cells are like those of the zona fasciculata, the adenoma is usually bright yellow. When it consists mainly of small, dark cells like those of the zona reticularis, it is brown. Occasionally the cells of an adenoma contain so much lipochrome pigment that the tumor is black. If the adenoma is large, there may be foci of hemorrhage, necrosis, or calcification within it.

Microscopically, most adrenocortical adenomata consist mainly of large, fat-filled cells arranged in plates like those of the zona fasciculata. There is usually some admixture of smaller, dark cells, like those of the zona reticularis. Occasionally the dark cells are the predominant component of the tumor. Less often, part of an adenoma resembles the zona glomerulosa. Sometimes, part of an adenoma consists of hybrid cells that contain much fat like the cells of the zona fasciculata, but are smaller, with the higher nucleocytoplasmic ratio characteristic of the zona glomerulosa.

Behavior. Adrenocortical adenomata are benign. They compress the adjacent tissues as they enlarge. Most adenomata grow slowly. Some grow for a time, then cease to enlarge.

In most patients, an adrenocortical adenoma causes no dysfunction. The adenoma is said to be nonfunctional, though it is more probable that it responds to normal stimuli and functions in a normal manner. Nonfunctional adenomata are usually small, though they can weigh over 1 kg. In most, cells like those of the zona fasciculata are predominant, though with some admixture of the other kinds of cell found in adrenocortical adenomata. The adjacent adrenal cortex is normal, except for the compression caused by the tumor.

A few adrenocortical adenomata produce an excess of cortisol. They are usually large, weighing 10 to 70 g or more. They consist mainly of cells like those of the zona fasciculata, though with some admixture of small, dark cells like those of the zona reticularis. Because of the excess of cortisol, the secretion of the adrenocorticotropic hormone is suppressed, and the remainder of the adrenal cortices atrophy.

A few adrenocortical adenomata produce an excess of aldosterone. The tumors sometimes produce cortisol as well as aldosterone, though only aldosterone is produced in ex-

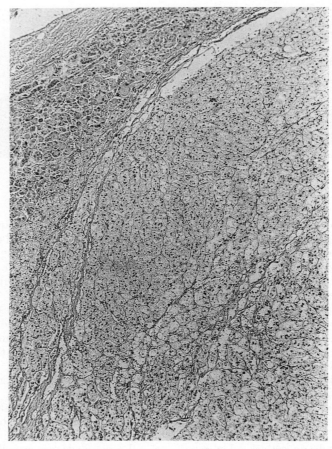

Fig. 46-4.   The ill-defined edge of an adrenocortical adenoma consisting mainly of cells resembling those of the zona fascicularis.

cess. Tumors that secrete aldosterone are usually less than 4 g in weight, though they can weigh as much as 75 g. Microscopically, they consist of a mixture of cells like those of the zona glomerulosa, zona fasciculata, or zona reticularis with hybrid cells intermediate between the cells of the zona fasciculata and the zona glomerulosa. Except for the distortion caused by the tumor, the uninvolved parts of the adrenal cortices are normal.

Less often, an adrenocortical adenoma secretes an excess of androgens or, still less frequently, of androstenedione, which is converted into estrogen in the tissues. These tumors vary from 10 g to over 1 kg in weight. Microscopically, small dark cells like those of the zona reticularis are usually predominant. The uninvolved parts of the adrenal cortices are normal.

Treatment and Prognosis.   Excision of an adrenocortical adenoma cures. If the tumor produces an excess of a hormone, the effects of the hypersecretion gradually wane.

CARCINOMA.   Adrenocortical carcinoma is uncommon. In the United States, fewer than 150 new cases are diagnosed each year. The carcinoma can arise at any age, though most of the patients are adults.

Lesions.   An adrenocortical carcinoma usually weighs over 100 g when discovered. It can weigh as little as 30 g or as much as 4.5 kg. The tumor is usually spheroidal and fairly well demarcated. On section, it is

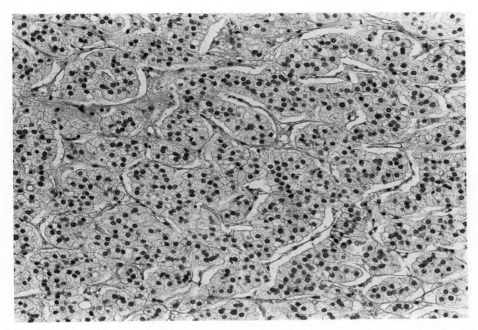

Fig. 46-5. A higher power view of an adrenocortical adenoma, showing well-differentiated cortical cells separated by sinusoids like those of the normal adrenal cortex.

pleomorphic, with yellow, brown, or pink regions intermixed with foci of necrosis, hemorrhage, calcification, of fibrosis.

Microscopically, an adrenocortical carcinoma consists of an admixture of the kinds of cell found in adrenocortical adenomata. Often parts of the tumor are well differentiated, resembling an adrenocortical adenoma, but other parts of the carcinoma are more anaplastic, with large, pleomorphic, bizarre cells, often with several nuclei, and with a high mitotic rate. The tumor cells may form trabeculae, as in an adenoma, or grow in large sheets. In places, they may become spindle-shaped, like the cells of a sarcoma. Invasion of blood vessels or lymphatics is often evident.

If all the tumor is well differentiated, it is hard to distinguish an adrenocortical carcinoma from an adenoma. The larger the tumor, the more likely it is to be malignant. Some think that adrenocortical tumors weighing more than 100 g should be regarded as malignant even if they seem benign on microscopic examination. Sometimes only the presence of metastases shows the tumor is malignant.

Behavior. Adrenocortical carcinomata invade locally, though in most tumors only to a limited degree. Metastases are usually present by the time the diagnosis is made and are often widespread.

Most adrenocortical carcinomata produce an excess of one of the adrenocortical hormones, cortisol, aldosterone, androgen, or of the androstenedione that results in hyperestrinism. The kind of secretion produced by the tumor cannot be predicted from its microscopic appearance, though carcinomata secreting aldosterone usually contain regions resembling the zona glomerulosa or are rich in hybrid cells. Carcinomata producing sex hormones often consist mainly of small, dark cells like those of the zona reticularis.

Treatment and Prognosis. Surgical extirpation of an adrenocortical carcinoma is usually impossible. The drug mitotane (o,p'-DDD) damages the adrenal cortices and induces regression of the carcinoma in 30% of the patients, but its effect is usually only temporary. Few patients live more than two years after the diagnosis is made.

MULTIPLE ENDOCRINE NEOPLASIA. A tumor of the adrenal cortex develops in some

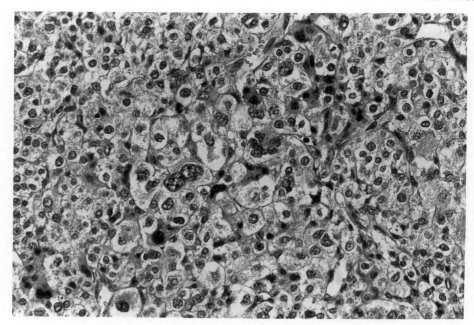

Fig. 46-6. An adrenocortical carcinoma, showing the pleomorphism of the tumor cells, and their resemblance to the cells of a normal adrenal cortex.

patients with multiple endocrine neoplasia type I, in which the patients tend to develop hyperplasia or tumors of the parathyroid glands, the islets of Langerhans, the anterior pituitary gland, and, less often, the adrenal cortices. The adrenal tumors can be functional and are often malignant.

Medullary Tumors

The tumor that arises from the cells of the adrenal medulla is called a pheochromocytoma, from the Greek words for dusky, color, a receptacle or cell, and a tumor, a name given because the cells of the adrenal medulla often stain dusky brown when exposed to chromates. A myelolipoma sometimes arises in an adrenal gland. Rarely, a malignant melanoma or a benign mesenchlymal tumor develops in the adrenal medulla.

PHEOCHROMOCYTOMA. Pheochromocytomata are uncommon. The annual incidence is less than 0.1 per 100,000. The tumor can arise at any age, though most patients are 20 to 60 years old. Men and women are affected equally.

About 10% of pheochromocytomata arise outside the adrenal glands in a chromaffin ganglion. The extra-adrenal tumors are most common in the organ of Zuckerkandl, in the preaortic region in the abdomen, and in the wall of the urinary bladder, but can arise in other parts of the body.

In the adrenal glands, 10% of pheochromocytomata are bilateral. About 5% of the tumors are malignant.

Lesions. Most pheochromocytomata are spheroidal, about 5 cm across, and weigh about 100 g, though the tumor can weigh as little as 1 g or over 3 kg. The small tumors in the adrenal glands have a yellow rim where the adrenal cortex is stretched about them. The larger ones have a collagenous capsule. On section, the tumor is gray or pink, usually with foci of cystic degeneration, hemorrhage, calcification, or fibrosis. Often there is a scar in the center of the tumor.

Microscopically, a pheochromocytoma sometimes consists of columns of cells like those of the normal adrenal medulla. More often, it is made of clumps, columns, or sheets of large, pleomorphic cells, with abundant eosinophilic cytoplasm and reg-

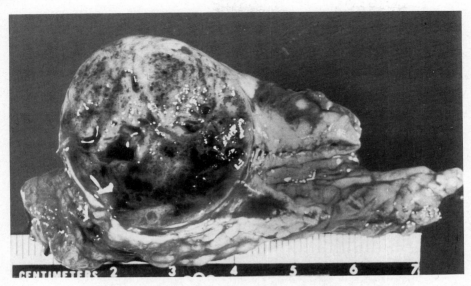

Fig. 46-7.   A pheochromocytoma of an adrenal gland, showing the spheroidal, partially necrotic, partly hemorrhagic tumor.

ular, vesicular nuclei. The clumps are separated by a sparse, richly vascular stroma. Sometimes the center of a clump of tumor cells is necrotic, to give a pseudoglandular pattern. Sometimes part or much of the tumor consists of small spindle cells. Foci of necrosis are common, but mitoses are few. Often secretory droplets that stain brightly with the periodic acid-Schiff stain are present in some of the tumor cells. The droplets may be small or considerably bigger than a nucleus. If the tumor has been fixed in a solution containing chromate, some of the tumor cells usually stain a granular brown. Electron microscopy shows that the tumor cells contain membrane-bound, electron-dense granules containing epinephrine or nor-epinephrine, like those seen in normal adrenal medullary cells.

It is impossible to distinguish microscopically between a benign and a malignant pheochromocytoma. Benign pheochromocytomata can be highly pleomorphic, with many mitoses, can extend through their capsule, and can even invade blood vessels. Malignant pheochromocytomata may show none of these features. Only the development of metastases shows that a pheochromocytoma is malignant.

Behavior. Most pheochromocytomata grow slowly and push aside the adjacent tissues. A few invade, but only to a limited degree. In malignant tumors, metastases develop, most often in the liver or lungs.

Nearly 70% of pheochromocytomata secrete both epinephrine and nor-epinephrine. Most of the rest, including nearly all the pheochromocytomata that arise outside the adrenal glands, secrete only nor-epinephrine. Only rarely does a pheochromocytoma secrete only epinephrine. Occasionally a pheochromocytoma produces increased quantities of dopamine or homovanillic acid. A few tumors that secrete both catecholamines and cortisol have been reported. Rarely, a pheochromocytoma produces erythropoietin.

Clinical Presentation.   In most patients with a pheochromocytoma, the tumor secretes enough norepinephrine and epinephrine to cause symptoms. In a few, the tumor is detected only when an abdominal mass is discovered.

Over 60% of the patients are persistently hypertensive. In some, the blood pressure is only moderately elevated and remains constant, as in essential hypertension. In most, the blood pressure varies from day to day and week to week. Most suffer paroxysms in which the blood pressure rises to as much as 250 mm Hg systolic and 150 mm Hg

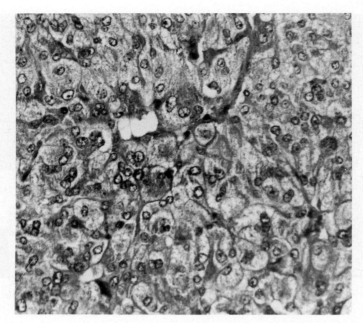

Fig. 46-8. A pheochromocytoma, showing the resemblance of the tumor cells to those of a normal adrenal medulla.

diastolic. The other 40% of the patients are normotensive most of the time, but usually suffer similar paroxysms in which the blood pressure rises greatly.

During a paroxysm, the patient is often apprehensive, with pain or discomfort in the abdomen, a pounding headache, often palpitations, or angina pectoris. In many of the patients, the blood pressure is lower when the patient stands than when supine. The paroxysm may last only a few minutes or persist for several hours. At first a paroxysm may occur only every few weeks or months, but as time passes the paroxysms tend to become more frequent, more severe, and to last longer.

Anything that presses on a pheochromocytoma or displaces it is likely to cause a paroxysm. Exercise may do so. Tight clothing can compress an abdominal pheochromocytoma. Micturition can cause a paroxysm if the tumor is in the urinary bladder. Opiates, histamine, the adrenocorticotropic hormone, and glucagon release catecholamines from a pheochromocytoma and can cause a paroxysm, as can drugs that reduce the neuronal uptake of catecholamines.

Profuse sweating is common in people with a pheochromcytoma. Often the patients lose weight. Often they are anxious. The skin may be pale or flushed. Palpitations, tachycardia, bradycardia, and cardiac arrythmias are common. In 50% of the patients, glucose tolerance is impaired. Reduced plasma volume increases the risk of shock during an operation or after trauma. Rarely, erythropoietin secreted by the tumor causes polycythemia.

Diagnosis. The diagnosis of pheochromocytoma is established by measuring the content of catecholamines or their metabolites in a 24-hour sample of urine. In normal people, the excretion of free catecholamines in the urine is less than 150 µg/day. In most patients with a pheochromocytoma, it is over 250 µg/day. If the urinary excretion of epinephrine is over 50 µg/day, the tumor is probably in an adrenal gland, as only rarely does an extra-adrenal pheochromocytoma secrete significant quantities of epinephrine.

Treatment and Prognosis. In 95% of the patients, a pheochromocytoma can be excised surgically. If the tumor is completely removed, the excretion of catecholamines in the urine falls to normal within a week. The tumor recurs in less than 10% of the patients. Establishment of an α-adrenergic block makes the operation safer, but the induction of anesthesia and handling the tumor are likely to produce sudden and dangerous elevations in the blood pressure and cardiac arrhythmias. In 25% of the patients, hypertension persists because of damage to the kidneys or some other mechanism.

If a pheochromocytoma has metastasized, only about 50% of the patients live five years. All that can be done is to attempt to control the symptoms with adrenergic blocking agents to reduce the production of catecholamines by the tumor.

MYELOLIPOMA. A myelolipoma of the adrenal glands is an uncommon lesion, which usually produces no symptoms and is found only at autopsy. A well-defined, yellow or reddish nodule is present in the medulla of one or both adrenal glands. Usually the nodule is 2 mm to 2 cm in diameter. Rarely, the tumor weighs 500 g or more and causes pain in the loin, dyspnea, or hematuria. In a few instances, a myelolipoma has been associated with virilization, Cushing's syndrome, or the nephrotic syndrome.

Microscopically, a myelolipoma consists mainly of well-differentiated adipose tissue, but scattered through the lesion are small clumps of hematopoietic cells. Usually the myelolipoma pushes the adrenal tissues

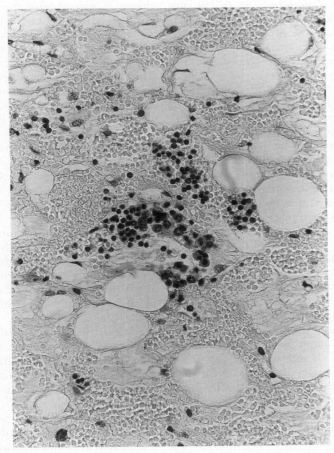

Fig. 46-9.   An island of hematopoietic cells in a predominantly fatty, markedly vascular myelolipoma of an adrenal gland.

aside, but sometimes adrenal cells are intermixed with the adipose and hematopoietic cells.

A myelolipoma is benign. If it is large enough to cause symptoms, excision cures. Some think the lesion is a hamartoma, not a neoplasm.

MULTIPLE ENDOCRINE NEOPLASIA. About 10% of patients with a pheochromocytoma have multiple endocrine neoplasia type II or type IIb, sometimes called type III. People with multiple endocrine neoplasia type II have hyperplasia or a tumor of the C cells of the thyroid gland and perhaps hyperplasia or a tumor of the parathyroid glands as well as hyperplasia or a tumor of the adrenal medulla; people with multiple endocrine neoplasia type IIb have hyperplasia or a tumor of the C cells together with mutliple neuromata, and sometimes café au lait pigmentation of the skin, a habitus like that of Marfan's disease, or other abnormalities, as well as with hyperplasia or a tumor of the adrenal medulla. In both syndromes, the adrenomedullary lesion is usually a pheochromocytoma. More than 50% of the patients have two pheochromocytomata, one in each adrenal gland.

OTHER SYNDROMES. About 5% of patients with a pheochromocytoma have neurofibromatosis; 1% of people with neurofibromatosis have a pheochromocytoma. Rarely, a patient with a pheochromocytoma has the retinal angiomata and cerebellar hemangioblastoma of the von Hippel-Lindau syndrome.

Secondary Tumors

Metastatic tumors are common in the adrenal glands. Emboli of tumors reach the adrenal glands in the blood, or by retrograde extension through the lymphatics, especially when the lymph flow is disturbed by metastases in the lymph nodes in the upper abdomen or lower mediastinum. Nearly always, the metastasis begins in the medulla. Often metastases are bilateral. The metastatic tumor is rarely extensive enough to disturb adrenal function.

Carcinoma of the lung is especially likely to metastasize to the adrenal glands, but carcinoma of the breast, carcinoma of the stomach, and other carcinomata often metastasize to the adrenal glands. Lymphoma and leukemia commonly involve the adrenal glands.

ADRENOCORTICAL HYPERFUNCTION

Oversecretion of cortisol by the adrenal cortices causes Cushing's syndrome. Oversecretion of aldosterone causes Conn's syndrome. Oversecretion of androgens causes adrenal virilization. Rarely, an adrenocortical adenoma secretes an excess of deoxycorticosterone, causing hyporeninism, hypokalemia, and changes like those of Conn's syndrome, though the production of aldosterone is normal or reduced.

CUSHING'S SYNDROME. Cushing's syndrome is named after the American neurosurgeon who described it in 1932. The term is used to describe the lesions and dysfunction caused by hypersecretion of cortisol, whatever the cause of the hypersecretion. The term Cushing's disease is used only when excessive secretion of cortisol is caused by oversecretion of the adrenocorticotropic hormone by the pituitary gland.

If iatrogenic cases are excluded, only 1 patient in every 4000 admitted to a hospital has Cushing's syndrome. About 70% of the patients are women. The syndrome can develop at any age, but is most common in people 20 to 40 years old.

Clinical Presentation. The severity of Cushing's syndrome varies considerably from one patient to another. It may be so slight as to be barely detectable or may evolve rapidly, causing major dysfunction. It may be complicated by the oversecretion of androgens or other steroids, in addition to cortisol.

Almost all patients with Cushing's syndrome are obese. Usually, the obesity affects principally the trunk, contrasting with thin, sticklike arms and legs. Sometimes a prominent pad of fat across the shoulder blades forms a buffalo hump. The face is usually rounded and sometimes seems edematous. The term moon face well describes it.

The increased metabolism of protein caused by the excess of cortisol depletes protein. In children growth is retarded. Adults grow weak. The skeletal muscles become thin and shrunken. The skin and subcutaneous tissue atrophy. The thin skin is easily injured by minor trauma. Often capillaries showing through the thin skin make the moon face red and plethoric. Dependent edema often occurs as fluid leaks from the weakened capillaries. Purple, congested stria develop in the abdomen because the weak subcutaneous tissue tears as it is stretched over the growing obesity. Osteoporosis is often severe, with collapse of the vertebrae, fracture of the ribs or other bones, and loss of lamina dura in the skull. Often there is a mild neutrophilia and sometimes erythremia. The risk of peptic ulcer increases.

Over 80% of the patients are hypertensive, because the excess of glucocorticoids has enough mineralocorticoid activity to retain water and sodium. Over 20% have diabetes mellitus, because the excess of glucocorticoids increases the formation of glucose in the liver and impairs the uptake of glucose by the tissues. Another 30% show impaired glucose tolerance. Up to 50% of the patients have hypercalciuria, because of the wasting of the bones. Nearly 10% suffer urinary stones. Infection, especially of the urinary tract, is common because of the depression of the immunologic system caused by the excess of glucocorticoids, but the excess of cortisol may prevent the usual leukocytosis.

About 20% of the patients with Cushing's syndrome are depressed, and another 20% suffer insomnia, with changes in behavior and mood. Oligomenorrhea, impotence, and infertility are common. Hirsutism develops in 80% of women with hypercortisolemia.

If the secretion of cortisol increases rapidly, as it may do when hypercortisolemia is caused by a malignant tumor, the physical signs of Cushing's syndrome have not time to develop. Instead of obesity, osteoporosis, and striae, the patients become weak, with hypokalemia, sometimes with a sudden onset of diabetes mellitus or systemic hypertension.

Pathogenesis. In the majority of patients, Cushing's syndrome is iatrogenic, caused by the therapeutic administration of adrenocortical steroids. Many of the conditions treated with glucocorticoids respond only when the dose is large enough to cause Cushing's syndrome.

If the patients given large doses of glucocorticoids for a prolonged period are set aside, 80% of the patients with Cushing's syndrome have an adenoma of the anterior pituitary gland. The adenoma secretes excessive quantities of the adrenocorticotropic hormone, causing hyperplasia of the adrenal cortices and oversecretion of cortisol. In 90% of the patients with this form of Cushing's syndrome the pituitary adenoma is small and not easily detected radiologically.

In a few patients, the receptors in the hypothalamus regulating the production of the hypothalamic hormones that govern the production of the adrenocorticotropic hormone by the pituitary may be abnormal, suppressing the production of the adrenocorticotropic hormone only when the concentration of cortisol in the plasma is abnormally high. The pituitary will show diffuse hyperplasia of the corticotropes.

In nearly 20% of the patients with noniatrogenic Cushing's syndrome, the oversecretion of cortisol is caused by disease of one or both adrenal glands. Most of these patients have an adenoma or a carcinoma of one adrenal cortex. About 50% of the tumors are benign; nearly 50% are malignant. Less often, Cushing's syndrome is caused by nodular hyperplasia of the adrenal cortices.

Cushing's syndrome can be caused by a tumor that produces the adrenocorticotropic hormone, the corticotropin releasing hormone, or a substance with similar properties. Most often the tumor is an oat cell carcinoma of the lung, but other types of carcinoma of the lung, carcinomata of other organs, and thymomata sometimes produce an adrenocorticotropic hormone. In most tumors, the quantity of the hormone produced is too small to cause symptoms. Some release large quantities of hormone.

Diagnosis. The concentration of cortisol in the plasma varies so much in normal people that a random measurement of its concentration is of little help in the diagnosis of Cushing's syndrome. In normal people, the concentration of cortisol in the plasma at midnight is less than 50% of the concentration at 0900 hours. In patients with Cushing's syndrome, the concentration is often greater at midnight than at 0900 hours.

The urinary excretion of free cortisol and

of the metabolites of cortisol is increased in most patients with Cushing's syndrome. In normal people, the urinary excretion of free cortisol is less than 400 nmol/day at rest. In patients with Cushing's syndrome, it is usually greater than 1000 nmol/day, sometimes more than 10,000 nmol/day.

In normal people, the potent glucocorticoid dexamethasone suppresses the secretion of the adrenocorticotropic hormone by the pituitary gland and so reduces the secretion of cortisol by the adrenal cortices. If the drug is given in low dose for 2 days, in normal people the concentration of cortisol in the plasma falls to less than 140 nmol/L (5 µg/100 mL), and the excretion of free cortisol in the urine to less than 80 nmol/day (30 µg/day). The excretion of 17-hydroxysteroids in the urine falls to less than 8 nmol/day (3 mg/day). In most patients with noniatrogenic Cushing's syndrome, the concentration of cortisol in the plasma and the excretion of cortisol and its metabolites in the urine remain above these levels. The low dose of dexamethasone does not inhibit the secretion of the adrenocorticotropic hormone by a pituitary adenoma or nonendocrine tumor and does not inhibit the secretion of cortisol by an adrenocortical tumor or nodular adrenocortical hyperplasia.

If a high dose of dexamethasone is given for two days, the secretion of the adrenocorticotropic hormone by a small adenoma of the pituitary is usually suppressed, and the urinary excretion of cortisol and its metabolites falls to less than 50% of their previous level. The excretion of cortisol falls in some patients with nodular adrenocortical hyperplasia, but rarely in patients with Cushing's syndrome caused by a large pituitary adenoma, a nonendocrine tumor, or in patients with an adrenal tumor.

The drug metyrapone inhibits the 11β-hydroxylase that converts 11-deoxycortisol to cortisol. In a normal person, it causes 11-deoxycortisol to accumulate in the plasma, but reduces the production of cortisol. In an attempt to restore normal secretion of cortisol, the production of the adrenocorticotropic hormone by the pituitary gland increases, increasing still more the production of 11-deoxycortisol. Its concentration in the plasma and the excretion of its metab-

olites as 17-hydroxycorticoids in the urine rise to at least twice their basal levels. In 90% of patients with Cushing's syndrome caused by an adenoma of the anterior pituitary gland, the concentration of 11-deoxycortisol in the plasma rises, and the excretion of 17-hydroxycorticoids in the urine increases. In patients with Cushing's syndrome caused by the oversecretion of cortisol by an adrenal tumor, and most of those with Cushing's syndrome caused by a nonendocrine tumor, there is little or no increase in the production of 11-deoxycortisol or of the adrenocorticotropic hormone.

If Cushing's syndrome is caused by an adrenocortical carcinoma, the quantity of cortisol secreted is often greater than in patients with Cushing's syndrome caused by an adenoma of the pituitary gland or an adrenocortical adenoma. Often the synthesis of cortisol by the carcinoma is imperfect, and production of 11-deoxycortisol and other intermediate products of steroid synthesis also is increased. Some carcinomata of the adrenocortical carcinomata produce androgens as well as cortisol, causing virilization in women. Some cause feminization in men, by producing an excess of androstenedione, which is converted into estrogens in the tissues. The production of aldosterone is not increased, but the excess of glucocorticoids produced may have enough mineralocorticoid activity to cause hypokalemia and retention of sodium and water.

When Cushing's syndrome is caused by a nonendocrine tumor, the quantity of the adrenocorticotropic hormone secreted by the tumor is often greater than is usual when the sydrome is caused by overproduction of the adrenocorticotropic hormone by an adenoma of the pituitary. Often the nonendocrine tumor secretes not only intact adrenocorticotropic hormone, but fragments of the hormone, and sometimes β-lipoprotein or other large molecules formed during the synthesis of the adrenocorticotropic hormone.

Pigmentation of the skin in a patient with Cushing's syndrome suggests that the syndrome is due to excessive production of the adrenocorticotropic hormone by a nonendocrine tumor or an adenoma of the pituitary gland. The melanocyte-stimulating hormones are synthesized together with the adrenocorticotropic hormone, but are not produced by the adrenal cortices.

Treatment and Prognosis. The treatment of Cushing's syndrome depends on its cause. If it is due to administration of a glucocorticoid, it may be possible to reduce the dose of the drug. If there is an adenoma of the anterior pituitary gland, it can often be controlled surgically, by the implantation of radioactive isotopes in the pituitary, or by external radiation. If there is an adrenocortical adenoma, it can be removed. If the excessive secretion of cortisol is controlled, the changes of Cushing's syndrome slowly resolve.

If the oversecretion of cortisol cannot be controlled by other means, the drugs metyrapone or aminoglutethimide, which interfere with the synthesis of cortisol, can be tried, or the toxic drug mitotane (o,p'-DDD) can be given to destroy the adrenal cortices.

Bilateral adrenalectomy controls the Cushing's syndrome whatever its cause, but has an operative mortality of 5% in these patients. In 15% of the patients it is followed within 10 years by Nelson's syndrome, a rapidly extending adenoma of the anterior pituitary gland, massive secretion of the adrenocorticotropic hormone, and hyperpigmentation.

CONN'S SYNDROME. Conn's syndrome, named after the American physician who described it in 1956, is caused by oversecretion of aldosterone. The syndrome is uncommon. Its principal feature is hypertension, but only about 1% of patients with hypertension have oversecretion of aldosterone. Nearly 70% of the patients are women. Most are between 30 and 50 years old when the disease is discovered.

Clinical Presentation. The oversecretion of aldosterone causes loss of potassium in the urine and retention of sodium and water. The concentrating power of the renal tubules is reduced, causing polyuria and polydipsia.

In most patients with Conn's syndrome, the retention of sodium and water causes mild hypertension, with an increase principally in the diastolic pressure. Occasionally, malignant hypertension follows. Edema is not usually evident. The loss of potassium usually causes mild hypokalemia, occasionally more severe hypokalemia and hypernatremia. The hypokalemia causes muscular weakness, car-

diac arrhythmias, and sometimes peripheral neuropathy or tetany. If the hypersecretion of aldosterone persists for years, renal failure and azotemia develop.

Pathogenesis. Two types of aldosteronism are disinguished. Primary aldosteronism is caused by disease of the adrenal glands. Secondary aldosteronism results from oversecretion of renin. The adrenal glands are normal, but because of the increased secretion of renin they secrete excessive quantities of aldosterone.

Primary aldosteronism is caused by an adrenocortical adenoma in 70% of the patients. In 30%, it results from nodular hyperplasia of the adrenal cortices. Rarely, it is caused by an adrenocortical carcinoma.

Secondary aldosteronism is most often caused by reduced renal blood flow. Most patients with edema have aldosteronism. Patients with renovascular hypertension and malignant hypertension secrete increased quantities of aldosterone. Less often, secondary aldosteronism is caused by excessive secretion of renin by a tumor of the juxtaglomerular cells or the hyperplasia of the juxtaglomerular apparatus found in Bartter's syndrome.

Diagnosis. In primary aldosteronism, the oversecretion of aldosterone reduces the secretion of renin and the concentration of renin in the plasma. Salt depletion fails to cause a normal increase in the activity of renin in the plasma.

Adrenocortical adenomata secreting aldosterone fail to respond to the expansion of fluid volume caused by salt loading. The administration of 2 L of normal saline solution intravenously in 4 hours suppresses the production of aldosterone in normal people, but fails to do so in people with Conn's syndrome. The adenomata causing Conn's syndrome respond in a normal or excessive way when stimulated by the adrenocorticotropic hormone or an increased intake of potassium.

Treatment and Prognosis. Removal of an adenoma causing Conn's syndrome brings cure in most patients. If this is impossible and when hyperaldosteronism is caused by primary hyperplasia of the adrenal cortices, the oversecretion can usually be controlled by salt restriction and the administration of the aldosterone antagonist spironolactone.

ADRENAL VIRILIZATION. Virilization caused by disease of the adrenal glands is uncommon, but can develop in children with congenital adrenal hyperplasia or in adults with an adrenocortical adenoma or carcinoma. If it is caused by a tumor, there is often Cushing's syndrome as well.

If the oversecretion of androgens begins in childhood, distortion of the external genitalia in girls or precocious puberty in boys is usual. If the oversecretion of androgens begins in adult life, men are little affected, but women develop hirsutism with loss of hair from the scalp, oligomenorrhea or amenorrhea, deepening of the voice, hypertrophy of the clitoris, and often acne. Occasionally an adrenocortical adenoma or carcinoma secretes increased quantities of androstenedione. This is converted into estrogens in the tissues and can cause feminization in men.

Most adrenal lesions casuing virilization secrete large quantities of weak androgens such as dehydroepiandrosterone, in contrast to ovarian lesions causing virilization, which usually secrete testosterone. A high concentration of dehydroepiandrosterone in the plasma or increased excretion of 17-ketosteroids in the urine suggests that virilization results from disease of the adrenal glands.

ADRENOCORTICAL HYPOFUNCTION

Three kinds of adrenocortical hypofunction are distinguished. In primary adrenocortical deficiency, usually called Addison's disease, the dysfunction is caused by disease of the adrenal glands. In secondary deficiency, it is caused by lack of the adrenocorticotropic hormone. In hypoaldosteronism, the secretion of aldosterone is deficient.

ADDISON'S DISEASE. Adrenocortical insufficiency is called Addison's disease, after the British physician who described it in 1855. Addison's disease develops in only 1 person in 100,000. Most of the patients are adult.

Clinical Presentation. Addison's disease usually develops slowly and insidiously. Addison observed "The patient...gradually to fall off in general health; he becomes languid and weak, indisposed to either bodily or mental exertion; the appetite is impaired or entirely lost...the pulse small and feeble... the body wastes...slight pain or uneasiness is from time to time referred to the region of the stomach, and there is occasionally actual vomiting....We discover a most remarkable, and, so far as I know, characteristic discolouration taking place in the skin...a dingy or smoky appearance, or various tints or shades of deep amber or chestnut-brown ....The body wastes...the pulse becomes smaller and weaker...the patient at length gradually sinks and expires."

Languor, fatigue, and asthenia are the principal features, in 90% of patients with Addison's disease. In some patients, the blood sugar is low, and episodes of hypoglycemia are easily induced. Even minor stress causes shock. A few of the patients become irritable and confused, sometimes with delusions, instead of sinking into the languor and exhaustion noted by Addison.

Nearly all the patients show pigmentation of the skin, often like persistent suntan, sometimes bluish, or dirty colored. Areas exposed to the sun and unexposed areas darken equally. Often the pigmentation is accenutated over pressure points such as the elbows, the nipples, or the creases of the hands. Sometimes dark freckles develop. Sometimes there are patches of vitiligo. In more than 80% of the patients, the lips and mucous membranes have patches of brown, bluish, or gray pigmentation. Microscopically, the pigmentation is due to the accumulation of melanin in the epidermal cells and in macrophages in the dermis. Occasionally, patches of hyperkeratosis and acanthosis are associated with the pigmentation.

Hypotension is found in 90% of the patients, sometimes with systolic pressures as low as 80 mm Hg and diastolic pressures of only 50 mm Hg. Sudden movements may cause giddiness or syncope. Gastrointestinal symptoms are present in 90% of patients. Some have only mild anorexia, but some have severe nausea and vomiting, with severe diarrhea. Ill-defined abdominal pain is sometimes severe enough to mimic an abdominal catastrophe. In women, loss of axillary and public hair is common.

Pathogenesis. Addison's disease develops only if more than 90% of the adrenal cortices are destroyed. In over 50% of the patients, the adrenal glands show primary cortical atrophy of the type thought to be caused by an autoimmune reaction. The next most common cause is tuberculosis, with large tuberculous abscesses destroying both adrenal glands. Many of these patients show little evidence of tuberculosis elsewhere, but nearly always a quiescent primary focus can be found in a lung. Less often, the adrenal glands are destroyed by histoplasmosis, coccidioidomycosis, blastomycosis, sarcoidosis, metastatic tumor, leukemia, or amyloidosis. Infants with Addison's disease sometimes have congenital hyperplasia or hypoplasia of the adrenal cortices.

In its early stages, Addison's disease causes little dysfunction. The production of the adrenocortical steroids is reduced, but is still within the normal range. The adrenocortical deficiency can be demonstrated by giving the adrenocorticotropic hormone intravenously for 24 hours. Normally, the concentration of cortisol in the plasma exceeds 1000 nmol/L (40 mg/100 mL), and the urinary excretion of 17-hydroxysteroids exceeds 70 nmol/dl (25 μg/dl). In people with Addision's disease, the response is much less.

The languor, fatigue, and asthenia that are such prominent features of the later stages of Addison's disease in 90% of the patients are due to lack of cortisol. The lack of cortisol also explains the low blood sugar in some patients with Addison's disease and the episodes of hypoglycemia with sweating and weakness. Because the secretion of cortisol cannot be increased, even minor stress causes shock.

Lack of aldosterone with reduced glomerular filtration and acidosis causes hyperkalemia and reduction in the concentrations of sodium, chloride, and bicarbonate in the plasma. The lack of water and sodium causes the hypotension in most patients. In 10% of the patients, there is hypercalcemia. Anemia, a relative lymphocytosis, and eosinophilia are common. Lack of androgen causes the loss of hair in women.

Treatment. Patients with Addison's disease require replacement of the lost gluocorticoids and mineralocorticoids. Usually, cortisol or prednisone is given to replace the lost cortisol, with fludrocortisone to replace the lost aldosterone. If the patient becomes ill or suffers other stress, the dosage must be adjusted accordingly.

SECONDARY ARENOCORTICAL INSUFFICIENCY. Lack of the adrenocorticotropic hormone causes secondary adrenocortical deficiency. Most often, the lack of the adrenocorticotropic hormone is caused by prolonged administration of glucocorticoids. Rarely, it is due to disease of the pituitary gland.

In people treated with large doses of glucocorticoids for a prolonged period, the release of the adrenocorticotropic hormone from the pituitary gland is suppressed, and the adrenal cortices become unresponsive to the hormone. If the glucocorticoids are withdrawn, the patient suffers adrenocortical failure, which persists for days or months before normal pituitary and adrenal function is regained.

Patients with secondary adrenocortical deficiency develop symptoms and signs much like those of Addison's disease. Their skin is not hyperpigmented, because the synthesis of the adrenocorticotropic hormone is suppressed, and with it the production of the melanocyte-stimulating hormones synthesized together with the adrenocorticotropic hormone. Replacement of the lost cortisol is needed, but mineralocorticoids are not required, because stimulation by renin maintains the secretion of aldosterone.

HYPOALDOSTERONISM. Lack of aldosterone with normal secretion of cortisol occurs in patients with a reduced secretion of renin caused by renal disease; in people with a deficiency of the enzyme 18-hydroxysteroid dehydrogenase needed for the synthesis of aldosterone; in patients treated for a long period with heparin; in patients with pretectal disease of the brain; and after removal of a tumor secreting aldosterone.

The patients have hyperkalemia, worsened by salt restriction. Fludrocortisone to replace the aldosterone restores the potassium concentration to normal in some patients. In others, the hyperkalemia is controlled by giving furosamide to increase the excretion of potassium.

BIBLIOGRAPHY

General

Fraser, R.: Disorders of the adrenal cortex: their effects on electrolyte metabolism. Clin. Endocinol. Metab., *13*:413, 1984.

Gould, V. E., and Sommers, S. C.: Adrenal medulla and paraganglia. *In* Endocrine Pathology, 2nd ed. Edited by J. M. B. Bloodworth, Jr. Baltimore, Williams & Wilkins, 1982.

Neville, A. M., and O'Hare, M. J.: The Human Adrenal Cortex. Pathology and Biology—An Integrated Approach. Berlin, Springer-Verlag, 1982.

Neville, A. M., and O'Hare, M. J.: Histopathology of the human adrenal cortex. Clin. Endocrinol. Metab., *14*:791, 1985.

Symington, T.: The adrenal cortex. *In* Endocrine Pathology, 2nd ed. Edited by J. M. B. Bloodworth, Jr. Baltimore, Williams & Wilkins, 1982.

Enzyme Deficiency

Drucker, S., and New, M. I.: Disorders of adrenal steroidogenesis. Pediatr. Clin. North Am., *34*:1055, 1987.

Dunger, D. B., and Grant, D. B.: Endocrine disorders: diabetes mellitus, congenital hypothyroidism, and congenital adrenal hyperplasia. Br. Med. Bull., *42*: 187, 1986.

Hughes, I. A.: Congenital and acquired disorders of the adrenal cortex. Clin. Endocrinol. Metab., *11*:89, 1982.

James, V. H. T., and Few, J. D.: Adrenocorticosteroids: chemistry, synthesis and disturbances in disease. Clin. Endocrinol. Metab., *14*:867, 1985.

McKenna, T. J., Cunningham, S. K., and Loughlin, T.: The adrenal cortex and virilization. Clin. Endocrinol. Metab., *14*:997, 1985.

Miller, W. L., and Levine, L. S.: Molecular and clinical advances in congenital adrenal hyperplasia. J. Pediatr., *111*:1, 1987.

Mininberg, D. T., Levine, L. S., and New, M. I.: Current concepts in Congenital adrenal hyperplasia. Pathol. Annu., *17* (Pt. 1):179, 1982.

New, M. I. (Ed.): Congenital adrenal hyperplasia. Ann. N. Y. Acad. Sci., *458*:1, 1986.

New, M. I.: Molecular genetics and the characterization of steroid 21-hydroxylase deficiency. Endocr. Res., *12*:505, 1986.

New, M. I., et al.: An update of congenital adrenal hyperplasia. Recent Prog. Horm. Res., *37*:105, 1981.

New, M. I., and Speiser, P. W.: Genetics of adrenal steroid 21-hydroxylase deficiency. Endocr. Rev., *7*: 331, 1986.

Savage, M. O.: Congenital adrenal hyperplasia. Clin. Endocrinol. Metab., *14*:893, 1985.

White, P. C., New, M. I., and Dupont, B.: Congenital adrenal hyperplasia. N. Engl. J. Med., *316*:1519, 1580, 1987.

Hyperplasia and Atrophy

Hughes, I. A.: Congenital and acquired disorders of the adrenal cortex. Clin. Endocrinol. Metab., *11*:89, 1982.

Larsen, J. L., Cathey, W. J., and Odell, W. D.: Primary adrenocortical nodular dysplasia. Am. J. Med., *80*: 976, 1986.

Siebermann, R.E.: The pathology of the gonads and adrenal cortex in intersex. Prog. Pediatr. Surg., *16*:149, 1983.

Other Non-Neoplastic Disorders

Moser, H. W., Naidu, S., Kumar, A. J., and Rosenbaum, A. E.: The adrenoleukodystrophies. CRC Crit. Rev. Clin. Neurol., *3*:29, 1987.

Powers, J. M., Moser, H. W., Moser, A. B, and Schaumburg, H. H.: Fetal adrenoleukodystrophy. Hum. Pathol., *13*:1013, 1982.

Tumors

Bravo, E. L., and Gifford, R. W., Jr.: Pheochromocytoma. N. Engl. J. Med., *311*:1298, 1984.

Cance, W. G., and Wells, S. A., Jr.: Multiple endocrine neoplasia Type IIa. Curr. Probl. Surg., *22*(5):1, 1985.

Copeland, P. M.: The incidentally discovered adrenal mass. Ann. Intern. Med., *98*:940, 1983.

Cryer, P. E.: Phaeochromocytoma. Clin. Endocrinol. Metab., *14*:203, 1985.

DeLellis, R. A., et al.: Multiple endocrine neoplasia (MEN) syndromes. Int. Rev. Exp. Pathol., *28*:163, 1986.

Del Gaudio, A., and Solidoro, G.: Myelolipoma of the adrenal gland. Surgery, *99*:293, 1986.

Eckfield, J. H., and Engelman, K.: Diagnosis of pheochromocytoma. Clin. Lab. Med., *4*:703, 1984.

Freeman, D. A.: Steroid hormone-producing tumors in man. Endocr. Rev., *7*:204, 1986.

Gabrilove, J. L., et al.: Virilizing adrenal adenoma. Endocr. Rev., *2*:462, 1981.

Goldfien, A.: Phaeochromocytoma. Clin. Endocrinol. Metab., *10*:607, 1981.

Leshin, M.: Polyglandular autoimmune syndromes. Am. J. Med. Sci., *290*:77, 1985.

Manger, W. M., Gifford, R. W., Jr., and Hoffman, B. B.: Pheochromocytoma. Curr. Prob. Cancer, *9*:1, 1985.

Samaan, N. A., and Hickey, R. C.: Adrenal cortical carcinoma. Semin. Oncol., *14*:292, 1987.

Samaan, N. A., and Hickey, R. C.: Pheochromocytoma. Semin. Oncol., *14*:296, 1987.

Sasano, N., Ojima, M., and Masuda, T.: Endocrinologic pathology of functioning adrenocortical tumors. Pathol. Annu., *15* (Pt. 2):105, 1980.

Sever, P. S., Roberts, J. C., and Snell, M. E.: Phaeochromcytoma. Clin. Endocrinol. Metab., *9*:543, 1980.

Thompson, N. W., and Cheung, P. S. Y.: Diagnosis and treatment of functioning and nonfunctioning adrenocortical neoplasia including incidentalomas. Surg. Clin. North Am., *67*:423, 1987.

Adrenocortical Hyperfunction

Bush. T. L.: The adverse effects of hormonal therapy. Cardiol. Clin., *4*:145, 1986.

Carpenter, P. C.: Cushing's syndrome. Mayo Clin.

Proc., *61*:49, 1986.

Hopwood, N. J.: Pathogenesis and managment of abnormal puberty. Spec. Top. Endocrinol. Metab., 7:175, 1985.

Howanitz, P. J., and Howanitz, J. H.: Hypercortisolism. Clin. Lab. Med., *4*:683, 1984.

Howlett, T. A., Rees, L. H., and Besser, G. M.: Cushing's syndrome. Clin. Endocrinol. Metab., *14*:911, 1985.

McKenna, T. J., Cunningham, S. K., and Loughlin, T.: The adrenal cortex and virilization. Clin. Endocrinol. Metab., *14*:997, 1985.

McNicol, A. M.: Cushing's syndrome. Neuropathol. Appl. Neurobiol., *11*:485, 1985.

Melby, J. C.: Diagnosis and treatment of primary aldosteronism and isolated hypoaldosteronism. Clin. Endocrinol. Metab., *14*:977, 1985.

Molta, L., and Schwartz, U.: Gonadal and adrenal androgen secretion in hirsute females. Clin. Endocrinol. Metab., *15*:229, 1986.

Morris, D. V.: Hirsutism. Clin. Obstet. Gynaecol., *12*: 649, 1985.

Root, A. W., and Shulman. D. I.: Isosexual precocity: current concepts and recent advances. Fertil. Steril., *45*:749, 1986.

Seale, J. P., and Compton, M. R.: Side-effects of corticosteroid agents. Med. J. Aust., *144*:139, 1986.

Adrenocortical Hypofunction

Burke, C. W.: Adrenocortical insufficiency. Clin. Endocrinol. Metab., *14*:947, 1985.

Maclaren, N. K., and Blizzard, R. M.: Adrenal autoimmunity and autoimmune polyglandular syndrome. In The Autoimmune Diseases. Edited by N. R. Rose and I. R. Mackay. Orlando, Academic Press, 1985.

Melby, J. C.: Diagnosis and treatment of primary aldosteronism and isolated hypoaldosteronism. Clin. Endocrinol. Metab., *14*:977, 1985.

Speiser, P. W., Stoner, E., and New, M. I.: Pseudohypoaldosteronism. Adv. Exp. Med. Biol., *196*:173, 1986.

47

Thyroid Gland

THE different forms of thyroidits, the hyperplasia of Graves' disease and nodular goiter, congenital anomalies, and tumors are the principal diseases of the thyroid gland.

THYROIDITIS

Seven types of thyroiditis are distinguished; infectious thyroiditis and six types of chronic thyroiditis, Hashimoto's disease, lymphocytic thyroiditis, chronic nonspecific thyroiditis, granulomatous thyroiditis, and Riedel's struma. The distinction between the different forms of chronic thyroiditis is not sharp. Intermediate forms occur.

INFECTION. Infection of the thyroid gland is uncommon. Acute inflammation in the neck, most often caused by staphylococci, streptococci, or pneumococci, occasionally spreads to the thyroid and causes acute inflammation. Tuberculosis and other granulomatous inflammations are rare in the thyroid. Congenital syphilis can cause diffuse fibrosis, with an exudate of plasma cells and lymphocytes. Viral inclusions are occasionally found in thyroid epithelium. Sarcoidosis, though not an infectious disease, can involve the thyroid.

Infectious thyroiditis rarely causes important dysfunction. The inflammation usually resolves leaving only a little scarring or minor chronic inflammation.

HASHIMOTO'S DISEASE. Hashimoto's disease is named after the Japanese surgeon who described it in 1912. Hashimoto gave the disease the Latin name struma lymphomatosa, a term still often used, *struma* meaning a swelling in the neck, or a goiter, and *lymphomatosa* because lymphocytes are the principal feature of the condition microscopically. The word *goiter* is derived from the Latin for the throat and is used to describe enlargement of the thyroid gland.

Hashimoto's disease affects 60 people in every 100,000. Over 90% of the patients are women, usually between 30 and 50 years old, though the disease can occur in children and older people. The frequency of Hashimoto's disease has increased considerably in the last 30 years, and it seems to be growing still more common.

Lesions. In Hashimoto's disease, the thyroid is moderately enlarged, weighing 100 to 300 g, instead of the usual 25 to 35 g. The enlarged gland is firm, retains its normal shape, and is not attached to the surrounding tissues. When the gland is exposed at surgery, its capsule is intact. On section, the cut surface of the thyroid is hard and white or yellowish, like the surface of a raw potato. Sometimes the cut surface is lobulated.

Microscopically, the thyroid gland is massively infiltrated by a dense exudate of lymphocytes and plasma cells. Often more than 80% of a section from a thryoid with struma lymphomatosa consists of closely packed lymphocytes and plasma cells, with only a few small groups of acini scattered in the exudate. Germinal centers are often present.

Some of the acini are lined by sharply defined, cuboidal epithelial cells with oxyphil cytoplasm that stains brightly with eosin and by dark, spheroidal nuclei. The cells resemble oncocytes and like oncocytes are filled with mitochondria. They are called oxyphil cells or Hürthle cells, after the German histologist born in 1860. Other acini are small and shrunken, with flattened epithelium, and contain only a little inspissated colloid. Occasionally macrophages are present in some of the acini. Electron microscopy shows dense deposits of antigen-antibody complexes in the basement membrane of the acini.

As the years pass, the loss of acini grows

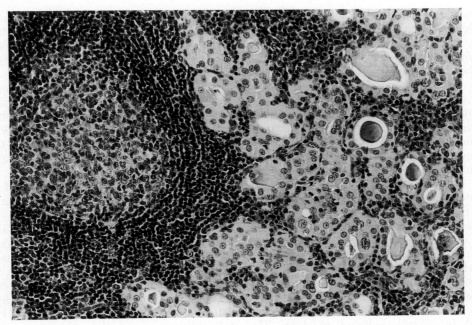

Fig. 47-1. Hashimoto's disease, showing the prominent lymphocytic exudate with a germinal centre and cuboidal Hürthle cells lining the remaining acini.

more severe. The inflammatory exudate persists, the gland slowly becomes increasingly fibrotic.

The relative prominence of the three main features of Hashimoto's disease varies from one patient to another. In most, the exudate of lymphocytes and plasma cells is the most striking feature. Sometimes the Hürthle cells are prominent. Occasionally, there is well-marked fibrosis.

Dysfunction. Early in the course of Hashimoto's disease, most patients are euthyroid. The uptake of iodine by the thyroid is sometimes increased, but the concentrations of thyroxine and triiodothyronine in the plasma are normal.

As the injury to the thyroid becomes greater, the secretion of the thyroid-stimulating hormone increases and for a time maintains homeostasis. Eventually, first the concentration of thyroxine in the plasma and then the concentration of triiodothyronine fall, and hypothyroidism becomes evident.

Clinical Presentation. Hashimoto's disease usually develops slowly. Most often the diagnosis is made when the patient notices that the thyroid gland is englarged, or a goiter is discovered during a routine physical examination. Rarely, the enlargement of the thyroid gland is more rapid, and the gland becomes tender and painful. About 20% of the patients have mild hypothyroidism when first seen, and others become hypothyroid as years pass. In a few patients, hypothyroidism becomes severe.

Occasionally a patient with Hashimoto's disease is hyperthyroid. The hyperthyroidism is sometimes present when the diagnosis is made; sometimes it becomes evident only late in the course of the disease. These patients probably have both Hashimoto's disease and Graves' disease.

Pathogenesis. Hashimoto's disease is caused by an autoimmune reaction against the thyroid. It is sometimes called autoimmune thyroiditis. The injury is probably caused principally by a cell-mediated reaction, though antibodies against the thyroid are present in most patients, usually in high titer.

Over 90% of the patients have antibodies against thyroglobulin in the plasma. Over 80% have antibodies against the microsomes of the epithelial cells that line the acini.

Antinuclear antibodies and antibodies against the receptor for the thyroid-stimulating hormone, thyroxine, triiodothyronine, or another component of colloid are commonly present.

Although immune complexes are present in the basement membrane of the thyroid acini, and in tissue culture, antibodies against the microsomes are cytotoxic, it is unlikely that the antibodies are the major cause of Hashimoto's disease. The antibodies do not damage the metastases of carcinoma of the thyroid. They cross the placenta to reach the fetus, but do not damage the fetal thyroid. The severity of the disease does not correlate with the titer of the antibodies. Similar antibodies are common in people with other kinds of thyroid disease and are present in 5% of normal people, though usually in lower titer than in Hashimoto's disease. Experimentally, antithyroid antibodies injected into monkeys do not cause Hashimoto's disease.

It is more likely that Hashimoto's disease is caused by a cell-mediated reaction. The inflammatory exudate in the lesions is like that seen in other cell-mediated reactions. Electron microscopy shows lymphocytes in intimate contact with damaged epithelial cells. Sometimes the lymphocytes penetrate into the epithelial cells. Lymphocytes from a patient with Hashimoto's disease are activated when cultured with thyroid antigens. In some patients with Hashimoto's disease, a delayed hypersensitivity reaction develops when thyroid antigens are injected into the skin. Experimentally, Hashimoto's disease can be induced by injecting thyroid antigens in Freund's adjuvant in a manner likely to incite a cell-mediated reaction. Lymphocytes from an animal with Hashimoto's disease can transmit the disease to another animal.

The frequent association of Hashimoto's disease with other conditions thought to be caused by an autoimmune reaction—rheumatoid arthritis, Addison's disease, pernicious anemia, Sjögren's syndrome, Graves' disease, and diabetes mellitus—supports the view that Hashimoto's disease is caused by an autoimmune reaction.

Genetic factors are important in the genesis of Hashimoto's disease in some patients. In 50% of the patients, close relatives have antithyroid antibodies in the plasma. In 30%, other members of the family have some form of thyroid disease. Hashimoto's disease sometimes develops in identical twins. The antigen HLA-DR5 is unduly frequent in Caucasians with Hashimoto's disease and HLA-BW35 in Japanese with the disease.

HLA-DR antigens are not normally present on the epithelial cells of the thyroid gland, but are present on the epithelial cells in patients with Hashimoto's disease. When only part of the gland is affected, the HLA-DR antigens appear only in the part of the gland involved.

Some think that the appearance of the HLA-DR antigens is caused by injury to the thyrocytes, perhaps by a viral infection, and that the HLA-DR antigens initiate the autoimmune attack on the thyroid by allowing the immune system to react to antigens normally present on the thyrocytes. Others think that the primary fault is in the suppressor T cells, that the abnormal T cells attack the thyrocytes, and that the expression of the HLA-DR antigens is caused by the autoimmune reaction against the thyroid.

Abnormal iodoproteins are present in the plasma in Hashimoto's disease but are probably the result of the disease, not its cause. In animals, Hashimoto's disease can be induced by altering the antigenicity of thyroglobulin, but there is no evidence that thyroglobulin is abnormal in patients with the disease.

Treatment and Prognosis. Hashimoto's disease is usually treated by giving thyroxine to render the patient euthyroid. The oversecretion of the thyroid-stimulating hormone is suppressed. Particularly in young people, the gland often shrinks, sometimes even to normal. In older patients, the shrinkage is less marked, perhaps because the gland is more fibrotic.

If the gland is large, thyroidectomy may be necessary. The operation takes away the goiter, but increases the severity of the hypothyroidism. Radiation can reduce the size of the goiter, but also increases the severity of the hypothyroidism.

Earlier studies suggest that over 10% of patients with Hashimoto's disease develop carcinoma of the thyroid. More recent investigations have shown little or no increase in the risk of cancer in these people.

PRIMARY ATROPHY. Rarely, the thyroid glands becomes shrunken and fibrotic, weighing 3 to 5 g, instead of its normal 25 to 35 g. Microscopically, there is extensive fibrosis, with a sparse exudate of lymphocytes and plasma cells. Only a few acini remain. They are scattered in the fibrosis and are often lined in part by Hürthle cells. The patient is hypothyroid.

Primary atrophy of the thyroid is probably caused by an immune reaction against the thyroid similar to that in Hashimoto's disease. The patients have in their blood antibodies against the thyroid like those in Hashimoto's disease. The frequency of the HLA-DR3 and HLA-B8 antigens is increased. The difference is that patients with primary atrophy have in the plasma an abnormal immunoglobulin that blocks the action of the thyroid-stimulating hormone. Probably the lack of hormonal stimulation causes the gland to atrophy, while the cell-mediated autoimmune injury causes the fibrosis, inflammation, and the changes in the thyrocytes.

LYMPHOCYTIC THYROIDITIS. Lymphocytic thyroiditis has many names, among them painless thyroiditis, chronic thyroiditis with transient thyrotoxicosis, and hyperthyroiditis. It is often lumped together with Hashimoto's disease. Indeed, some use the term *lymphocytic thyroiditis* to include both Hashimoto's disease and the condition here called lymphocytic thyroiditis. Others consider lymphocytic thyroiditis an early form of Hashimoto's disease.

Lymphocytic thyroiditis is less common than Hashimoto's disease. It usually affects girls and young women, though it does occur in men and in older people. Some 40% of goiters in children are of this type.

The thyroid gland is firm and symetrical, but is enlarged in only 50% of the patients. It is not tender. Microscopically, the thyroid shows an infiltration with lymphocytes and plasma cells like that in Hashimoto's disease. Germinal centers may be present. The epithelium lining the acini remains normal or is slightly hyperplastic. Hürthle cells are few or absent.

Most patients with lymphocytic thyroiditis remain euthyroid. The rest develop hyperthyroidism, usually mild, but sometimes severe. The concentrations of thyroxine and triiodothyronine in the serum rise because the hormones leak from the damaged gland, not because their synthesis is increased. The uptake of radioactive iodine by the thyroid is reduced. The concentration of the thyroid stimulating hormone in the plasma is low. The urinary excretion of iodine is normal.

The etiology and pathogenesis of lymphocytic thyroiditis is unknown. Antithyroid antibodies are present in the plasma in some of the patients, but their titer is low.

Lymphocytic thyroiditis subsides in from 2 to 12 months without treatment. If there has been hyperthyroidism, 40% of the patients become mildly hypothyroid for a few months before returning to euthyroidism. Most of the patients remain well, but 10% suffer one or more recurrences of the thyroiditis. Only supportive treatment is needed.

CHRONIC NONSPECIFIC THYROIDITIS. Chronic nonspecific thyroiditis is common in elderly people, especially in elderly women. It usually causes no symptoms and is found only in at autopsy or when the thyroid gland is removed for some other reason.

Macroscopically, the thyroid gland is usually normal, though occasionally it is a little bigger than normal, or a little shrunken. Microscopically, foci of chronic inflammation are scattered here and there in the parenchyma of the thyroid. In these foci, an exudate predominatly of lymphocytes and plasma cells surrounds or compresses the acini. Germinal centers are sometimes present. Occasionally a few of the acini in the inflamed regions are damaged, and macrophages filled with colloid scavenged from the damaged acini lie among the lymphocytes and plasma cells. Sometimes there is squamous metaplasia of the epithelium in the inflamed foci. A little fibrosis often occurs in the inflamed zones. The parenchyma between the foci of inflammation is normal.

The extent of the inflammation in chronic nonspecific thyroiditis varies from one person to another. A few foci of inflammation of this sort are almost always present in older people. Sometimes the foci of inflammation are more numerous and larger. Occasionally, the inflammation becomes so extensive that the distinction between chronic nonspecific thyroiditis and Hashimoto's disease become obscure.

Most patients with chronic nonspecific thyroiditis are euthyroid. A few have mild

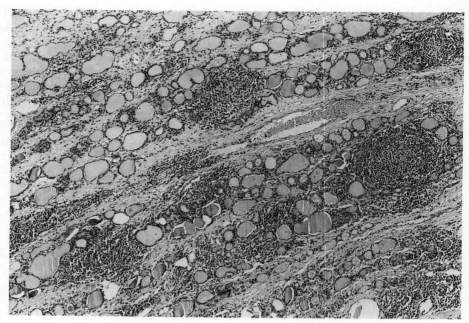

Fig. 47-2. Chronic, nonspecific thyroiditis in an elderly woman, showing a patchy exudate mainly of lymphocytes, a little fibrosis, and some loss of acini.

hypothyroidism. The cause of the inflammation is unknown. Some patients have antithyroid antibodies in the plasma, but they are in low titer. No treatment is needed.

GRANULOMATOUS THYROIDITIS. Granulomatous thyroiditis is often called subacute thyroiditis, or de Quervain's disease, after the Swiss surgeon who described it in 1902. It affects fewer than 10 people in every 100,000. Granulomatous thyroiditis may occur at any age, but most of the patients are about 50 years old. About 80% of the patients are women.

Lesions. In granulomatous thyroiditis, the thyroid is moderately enlarged, perhaps weighing 50 or 60 g, instead of the normal 25 to 35 g. The enlargement may be symmetrical, but often involves principally one side of the thyroid, sometimes only a localized area within one lobe of the thyroid. Sometimes the involved part of the thyroid lightly adheres to the adjacent muscles. On section, the cut surface of the involved part of the thyroid is hard and yellowish white, like the cut surface of a new turnip. At times the lesion mimics a carcinoma.

Microscopically, the involved part of the thyroid shows multiple foci of inflammation, often largely or partly confluent, with an exudate of lymphocytes, plasma cells, macrophages, and neutrophils and usually a good deal of fibrosis. Some of the acini in the inflamed foci are disrupted, with complete or partial loss of their epithelium. The colloid from the disrupted acini is phagocytosed by macrophages, which become filled with colloid and often are multinucleated. Sometimes the multinucleated giant cells around the disrupted acini form granulomata. Less often, there are small abscesses, with an exudate predominantly of neutrophils.

Dysfunction. In the early stages of granulomatous thyroiditis, leakage of thyroid hormones from the damaged acini causes mild hyperthyroidism in 50% of the patients. The concentrations of thyroxine and triiodothyronine in the plasma increase, and the concentration of the thyroid-stimulating hormone falls. The uptake of radioactive iodine is low.

Later in the disease, 25% of the patients become hypothyroid. The stock of hormone in the acini is depleted. The concentrations of thyroxine and triiodothyronine in the plasma fall, and the concentration of the

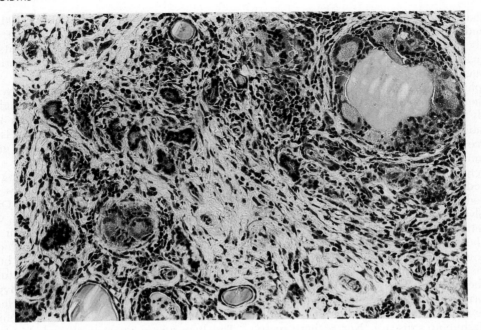

Fig. 47-3. Granulomatous thyroiditis, showing fibrosis, loss of acini, and chronic inflammation with multinucleated giant cells around the colloid in the upper right part of the picture.

thyroid-stimulating hormone rises. The uptake of radioactive iodine remains low.

Clinical Presentation. In granulomatous thyroiditis, pain in the thyroid gland or referred to the lower jaw or ear usually slowly worsens for several weeks, and the gland becomes tender. Less often, the onset is abrupt, with severe pain and tenderness in the gland. In a few patients, the disease is painless, and only the enlargement of the thyroid gland draws attention to the disease.

The pain often begins on one side of the gland and slowly extends to involve much or all of the thyroid. The gland is usually exquisitely tender. Swallowing or turning the head, anything that compresses or distorts the gland, causes pain. Fever, malaise, and sweating are common and sometimes severe. There may be a leukocytosis. The erythrocyte sedimentation rate is high.

Pathogenesis. The cause of granulomatous thyroiditis is uncertain. In many patients it follows an upper respiratory infection, suggesting that it might be initiated by a viral infection. In a few patients, the virus of mumps has been isolated from the gland. The titer of antibody against many viruses increases in the early stages of the disease, but this increase is probably an amnestic reaction. Antibodies against the thyroid gland are in low titer or absent.

Treatment and Prognosis. Prednisone usually brings resolution of granulomatous thyroiditis within a month. The lesions resolve, leaving only minor nonspecific chronic thyroiditis. Thyroid function returns to normal. Untreated, the disease often resolves after several months, but sometimes persists for year or more, with repeated exacerbations and remissions.

RIEDEL'S STRUMA. Riedel's struma, named after the German surgeon who described it in 1896, is rare. Not one thyroidectomy in 2000 shows Reidel's struma. The patients are 30 or more years old. About 60% of them are women. Occasionally a patient with Riedel's struma has also retroperitoneal fibrosis, mediastinal fibrosis, or sclerosing cholangitis.

A stony hard mass develops in the thyroid. The gland becomes firmly fixed to the adjacent muscles and to the trachea, sometimes to the esophagus as well. Often the trachea is compressed.

Microscopically, the thyroid is largely replaced by coarse collagenous tissue, which extends beyond the capsule to bind the gland firmly to the adjacent tissues. Islands of normal acini remain in the scar tissue, and throughout there is a sparse exudate of lymphocytes and plasma cells.

There is usually no dysfunction. Only rarely is hypothyroidism produced.

Patients with Riedel's struma usually seek advice months or years after their goiter first became evident. They are likely to complain of dyspnea, cough, or a feeling of suffocation caused by tracheal compression or dysphagia caused by involvement of the esophagus. Involvement of the recurrent laryngeal nerve sometimes causes paralysis of the vocal cords and hoarseness. The lesion is often difficult to distinguish from carcinoma of the thyroid.

The cause of Riedel's struma is unknown. It does not show any of the immunologic abnormalities of Hashimoto's disease, and there is no reason to think it is the end stage of Hashimoto's disease. Nor is there reason to think that granulomatous thyroiditis sometimes ends as Riedel's struma.

The treatment of Riedel's struma is surgical and is designed to relieve the local symptoms. Once adequate biopsies have been taken to establish the diagnosis, splitting the thyroid isthmus may be all that is needed. Subtotal thyroidectomy is difficult because of the dense fibrosis around the thyroid and does not cure the disease. If hypothyroidism develops, thyroid hormone must be given.

HYPERPLASIA

Three forms of hyperplasia of the follicular epithelium occur in the thyroid gland: Graves' disease, nontoxic goiter, and toxic nodular goiter. Hyperplasia of the C cells is less common.

GRAVES' DISEASE. Graves' disease is named after the Irish physician who described it in 1835. It is also called Parry's disease after an English physician who described it in 1825, Basedow's disease after the German physician von Basedow who described it in 1840, Flajani's disease, after the Italian surgeon who described it in 1802, thyrotoxicosis, exophthalmic goiter, diffuse toxic goiter, or primary hyperthyroidism.

Each year, 20 people in every 100,000 develop Graves' disease. The disease may begin at any age, but most of the patients are 20 to 40 years old. Over 85% of the patients are women.

Lesions. In Graves' disease, the thyroid is moderately and evenly enlarged, weighing 35 to 50 g, rather than its normal 25 to 35 g. On section, the cut surface of the gland is red and meaty and lacks the translucence given by follicles well filled with colloid.

Microscopically, the epithelium lining the follicles is hyperplastic. The follicles are usually small and contain little colloid. Often the periphery of the colloid is scalloped, with a line of vacuoles separating it from the surface of the epithelial cells. This scalloping is an artifact produced during fixation, but is characteristic of Graves' disease. Often stubby papillary projections covered by the hyperplastic epithelium bulge into the follicles to increase the surface area of the epithelium. The hyperplasia involves the whole of the thyroid, but the severity of the hyperplasia often varies from one part of the gland to another.

The epithelial cells are cuboidal or columnar. They have regular, basal nuclei. Mitochondria, Golgi apparati, and other organelles are numerous. The microvilli on the surface of the cells increase in number and length.

The connective tissue between the follicles is vascular and congested, but there is no fibrosis. Sometimes the hyperemia of the gland is so great that a thrill or a bruit is evident over the thyroid. Clumps of lymphocytes and plasma cells, sometimes with germinal centers, are often scattered among the hyperplastic follicles. Occasionally, the inflammation is extensive, suggesting Hashimoto's disease.

Dysfunction. The hyperplastic thyroid in Graves' disease is hyperactive. It synthesizes increased quantities of the thyroid hormones without regard to the needs of the body or the concentration of the thyrotropic hormone in the plasma. The severity of the dysfunction varies from one patient to another and from day to day in the same patient. It may be so mild as to be negligible. Occasionally it becomes extreme.

In most patients with Graves' disease, the uptake of radioactive iodine by the thyroid

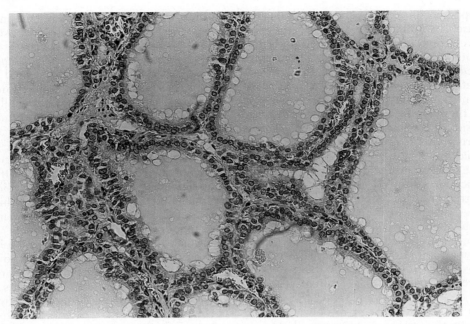

Fig. 47-4.   Graves' disease, showing acini lined by hyperplastic, cuboidal epithelium and the line of vacuoles often seen along the surface of the epithelium in this condition.

increases, sometimes greatly. The turnover of iodine in the gland is more rapid than normal. Production of the thyroxine-binding protein often increases. The concentrations of free and bound thyroxine and triiodothyronine and of other iodinated proteins in the plasma rise. The resin uptake of triiodothyronine increases. The free thyroxine index increases. The degradation of the thyroid hormones increases. The concentration of the thyroid-stimulating hormone in the plasma falls. Administration of the thyrotropin releasing hormone fails to increase the secretion of the thyroid-stimulating hormone. Administration of thyroid hormone fails to reduce the uptake of radioactive iodine to less than 50% of its previous value.

In patients in whom there is little or no evidence of hyperthyroidism, the uptake of radioactive iodine and the concentrations of thyroxine and triiodothyronine in the plasma may be within the normal range. In these people, the diagnosis can be established by demonstrating that the administration of thyroid hormone fails to produce the normal reduction in the uptake of radioactive iodine or that the thyrotropin releasing hormone is

unable to increase the secretion of the thyrotropic hormone.

If adequate quantities of iodine are given to a patient with Graves' disease who has severe hyperthyroidism, the symptoms are greatly ameliorated within a week or 10 days. The patient may become euthyroid. When the iodine is withdrawn, the hyperthyroidism recurs.

The uptake and turnover of iodine by the thyroid is normal or slightly increased in 5% of patients with Graves' disease. The concentration of thyroxine in the plasma is normal, as is the concentration of the thyroxine-binding globulin. Only the concentrations of bound and free triiodothyronine increase. This kind of Graves' disease is called T_3 thyrotoxicosis. Sometimes it precedes the more usual form of Graves' disease. In Chile, more than 10% of patients with Graves' disease have T_3 thyrotoxicosis.

Extrathyroidal Lesions. Graves' disease often affects the eyes and skin as well as lesions in the thyroid gland. The disease of the eyes is called ophthalmopathy; the disease of the skin, dermopathy.

Ophthalmopathy.   Changes in the eyes

are apparent in 70% of patients with Graves' disease. In 10% of the patients, they are severe. Often one eye is affected more than the other. Occasionally only one eye is involved. Often the severity of the ophthalmopathy varies from time to time. In most patients, it develops at the same times as does the hyperthyroidism; in some, it is the first sign of the disease; in others it becomes apparent only long after the onset of hyperthyroidism.

The changes in the eyes are of two types. Retraction of the lids occurs in all forms of hyperthyroidism. Proptosis occurs only in Graves' disease.

Retraction of the lids is caused by the increased secretion of catecholamines caused by hyperthyroidism. The lids are more retracted than is normal and the palpebral fissures are widened. The patient seems to stare or looks pop-eyed. Often the lids lag when the patient looks up or down, allowing a white rim of sclera to appear below or above the iris. Sometimes the retraction is so great that a line of sclera is visible around the iris when the patient looks straight ahead. Sometimes the forehead fails to wrinkle when the patient looks up.

Proptosis is caused by edema of the tissues in the orbit. The eyes are pushed forward and cannot be pressed back into the orbit because of the tense swelling of the orbital tissues. The proptosis can become so severe that the lids can no longer close. In extreme cases, the eyes prolapse completely, and the lids meet behind the globes. Discomfort or pain in the orbits is common.

In patients with proptosis, the conjunctiva, eyelids, and periorbital tissues are often congested and edematous. Lachrymation may be excessive, or the eyes may be dry and gritty. Photophobia is sometimes troublesome. Occasionally the conjunctiva is so swollen that the eyes cannot close. The edematous conjunctiva is easily infected or injured. Ulceration of the corneae can seriously impair vision. Panophthalmitis can destroy the eyes.

The ocular muscles are swollen, sometimes to 10 times their normal diameter. They are edematous, with increased quantities of ground substance between the muscle fibers and an exudate of lymphocytes and plasma cells, sometimes with many neutrophils. If the proptosis is severe, the muscle fibers degenerate. Crescentic deposits of mucopolysaccharide appear beneath their sarcolemma. As the muscle fibers disappear, fat accumulates in the muscles, and they become increasingly fibrotic. As the muscles grow weak, loss of convergence or inability to look up often develops. Sometimes there is diplopia or an external strabismus.

The orbital fat is also edematous, with increased ground substance and an exudate of lymphocytes and plasma cells. If the ophthalmopathy persists, it becomes fibrotic. Occasionally the pressure in the orbits is sufficient to cause papilledema or to damage the optic nerves, causing blindness. The lachrymal glands atrophy and are replaced by loose, edematous collagenous tissue with an exudate of lymphocytes and plasma cells.

Dermopathy.   About 5% of patients with Graves' disease develop dermopathy. In 50% of the patients affected, the dermopathy develops while the patient is still hyperthyroid. In 50%, it develops after the hyperthyroidism has been controlled. Most of the patients affected have severe ophthalmopathy.

Pretibial myxedema is the most common form of dermopathy in Graves' disease. Reddish brown plaques develop over the tibiae and gradually enlarge until they are 10 or 20 cm across and bulge irregularly from the skin. The plaques are firm, with prominent hair follicles and coarse hair. Occasionally the plaques become confluent. Sometimes the plaques are itchy. Usually the severity of the myxedema increases slowly for months or years and then becomes stationary or slowly regresses.

Similar plaques sometimes develop on the dorsum of the feet or the dorsum of the fingers. The process is nearly always bilateral. In thyroid acropachy, from the Greek words for terminal and thick, pretibial myxedema is associated with clubbing of the fingers and osteoarthropathy.

Microscopically, the plaques show an increase in ground substance in the dermis and widely separated collagen fibers. The concentrations of hyaluronic acid and other mucopolysaccharides in the ground substance are greatly increased.

Clinical Presentation.   Graves' disease may begin suddenly, but usually develops gradually and insidiously. In 25% of the patients, the disease follows an emotional disturbance, severe injury, infection, or dieting to lose weight.

As the disease develops, most of the patients show evidence of hyperthyroidism, perhaps slight, often marked. To this is usually added some degree of ophthalmopathy, though hyperthyroidism can develop without eye changes, and eye changes can develop without hyperthyroidism.

Pathogenesis. Graves' disease is caused by an autoimmune reaction against the thyroid. Antibodies react with the receptor for the thyroid-stimulating hormone and other antigens on the surface of the thyrocytes. Some of the antibodies stimulate the thyrocytes, causing hyperplasia. Some block the action of the thyroid-stimulating hormone. Some do not affect the function of the thyrocytes.

The first stimulatory antibody found in the blood of patients with Graves' disease is called the long-acting thyroid stimulator because it causes a long-continued release of iodinated compounds from the thyroid in animals. It or similar stimulatory antibodies are demonstrable in the plasma of almost all patients with Graves' disease and are the principal cause of the hyperplasia.

Antibodies against thyroglobulin or against the microsomes of the thyrocytes are present in 95% of the patients, ususally in higher titer than in patients with a nontoxic goiter or carcinoma of the thyroid, though not in the high titer usual in Hashimoto's disease.

Hashimoto's disease is unduly frequent in the families of patients with Graves' disease, and the incidence of Graves' disease is increased in the families of patients with Hashimoto's disease. Relatives of patients with Graves' disease often have in their blood the antibodies of Hashimoto's disease. Occasionally a patient with Hashimoto's disease develops Graves' disease, or a patient with Graves' disease ends with Hashimoto's disease.

Genetic factors are important in the pathogenesis of Graves' disease in some patients. Abnormal immunoglobulins of Graves' disease are present in the plasma of close relatives in 60% of the patients. The frequency of the antigens HLA-DR3 and HLA-B8 is increased in Caucasians with Graves' disease. HLA-BW36 is unduly common in Japanese; HLA-BW46, in Chinese.

Probably the autoimmune response in Graves' disease is initiated by a mechanism similar to that in Hashimoto's disease. HLA-DR antigens are present on the thyrocytes in patients with Graves' disease, as they are in Hashimoto's disease. Some think they are caused by a viral infection and initiate the autoimmune reaction against the thyroid. Some think that the primary fault is in the suppressor T cells and that the expression of the HLA-DR antigens is caused by the autoimmune reaction.

The pathogenesis of the ophthalmopathy in Graves' disease in unknown. It is not due to the excess of thyroid hormones and is not caused by the thyroid-stimulating hormone. In fish and experimental animals, a factor extracted from the pituitary gland and a fragment of the thyrotropic hormone that no longer has thyrotropic activity have been found able to induce exophthalmos, but there is no evidence that any such factor is involved in Graves' disease.

In the plasma of many patients with exophthalmic Graves' disease is a factor that causes exophthalmos when injected into animals. This exophthalmos-producing substance is not the long-acting thyroid stimulator, is not present in all patients with exophthalmos, and is sometimes present in people who do not have exophthalmos. Its part, if any, in the causation of the proptosis of Graves' disease is unknown.

IgG antibodies that react with orbital tissues have been found in the plasma of patients with exophthalmic Graves' disease. It has been suggested that they might cause the eye changes, by damaging the orbital tissues directly or perhaps in concert with some other factor. Antibodies against thyroglobulin may cross react with the ocular muscles and damage them, though ophthalmopathy does not occur in Hashimoto's disease, in which antibodies against thyroglobulin are commonly in high titer. There is no correlation between the level of the stimulatory antibodies and the occurrence of eye changes.

The cause of the dermopathy found in Graves' disease is unknown.

Treatment and Prognosis. The hyperthyroidism of Graves' disease is treated as are other forms of hyperthyroidism, as is discussed later in the chapter. In up to 50% of the patients, the Graves' disease goes into remission after one or two years, and the treatment can be stopped, leaving the patient euthyroid. Remission is particularly likely if the goiter gets smaller during the treatment, the abnormal immunoglobulins disappear from the plasma, and the administration of thyroid hormone causes a normal reduction in the uptake of radioactive iodine.

Lid retraction usually returns to normal when the hyperthyroidism is controlled. In 80% of patients with proptosis, it becomes stationary. In 10%, it partially regresses. In 10%, it continues to worsen. Progressive proptosis is particularly common in men. If proptosis is severe, adrenocortical steroids can sometimes reduce the swelling. Occasionally an operation or radiation is needed to decompress the orbits. The dermatopathy usually needs no treatment.

NONTOXIC GOITER. Nontoxic goiter and simple goiter are terms used to describe conditions in which the thyroid is large, but there is no hyperthyroidism. Two types of nontoxic goiter are distinguished; endemic goiter in which 10% or more of the population have enlargement of the thyroid and sporadic goiter in which only occasional people are affected.

In many regions in which nontoxic goiter is endemic, most of the population is affected. Usually the thyroid begins to enlarge during childhood in both boys and girls, though the severity of the enlargement varies from one child to another. In men, the enlargement often disappears after puberty or becomes so slight as to pass unnoticed. In women, the enlargement frequently persists or increases. The goiter may become gigantic, half the size of the head. In one goitrous area in Greece, 60% of adolescent boys and girls had a goiter, but by the age of 50 years only 10% of men had an obviously enlarged thyroid, though 50% of women did so.

Sporadic goiter occurs throughout the world. In the United States, from 4 to 8% of people outside the endemic zones have a thyroid large enough to be palpable, though in most of these people the enlargement is not great, About 70% of the people with a big

thyroid are women. Probably the enlargement of the thyroid begins in adolescence. The enlargement may regress after puberty, or the thyroid may continue to enlarge slowly, until it becomes big enough to cause the patient to seek medical advice.

Lesions. In both types of nontoxic goiter, the enlargement of the gland is at first uniform, with all parts of the thyroid affected equally. Usually the enlargement is not great at this stage, though it can be massive.

At the years pass and the gland continues to enlarge, it becomes nodular. Spheroidal nodules from 0.5 to 5.0 cm in diameter bulge from the gland and distort its parenchyma. Usually there are many nodules, and the patient is said to have a multinodular goiter. Occasionally there are only a few, or one nodule is much bigger than the rest. Macroscopically, many of the nodules are gelatinous; some are solid and meaty; some are cystic or hemorrhagic. Some have a fibrous capsule; some merge with the surrounding parenchyma. The parenchyma between the nodules may be fibrotic.

By the time the patient seeks advice, the goiter usually weighs more than 100 g, and especially in endemic regions can weigh 1000 g or more. A normal thyroid gland weighs 25 to 35 g.

Similar nodules sometimes develop in a thyroid gland that is not enlarged. In from 10 to 50% of autopsies, one or more nodules over 1 cm across are present in thyroid glands that are otherwise normal. They are more frequent in women than in men.

When a nontoxic goiter begins to enlarge, its acini are at first small, with little colloid, and are lined by columnar epithelial cells. Papillary projections often bulge into the acini. The gland is hyperemic. The microscopic appearance is similar to that of Graves' disease.

As the years pass, colloid accumulates in the acini. They become larger and are lined by flattened epithelium. Often excessive quantities of colloid distend many of the acini, forming lakes of colloid that are separated only by a thin wall of attenuated epithelium and stroma. The hyperplasia may still be uniform, but often nodules are beginning to appear. Such a goiter is called a colloid goiter.

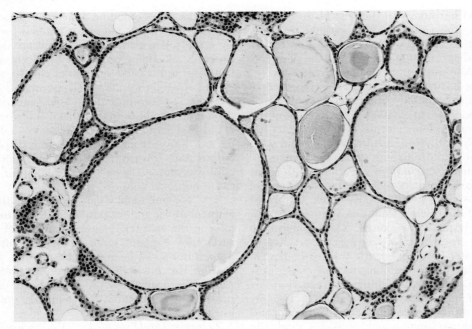

Fig. 47-5. A nodule from a nontoxic, nodular goiter showing acini lined by flattened epithelium and distended with colloid.

The enlarging thyroid undergoes repeated cycles of hyperplasia and involution. When hyperplasia is dominant, the epithelium grows taller, and the acini become smaller. When involution is predominant, the storage of colloid increases, and the epithelium becomes stretched and flattened.

Eventually, the thyroid fails to respond evenly to the stimuli that cause hyperplasia and involution. Some parts of the gland are hyperplastic; in other parts the storage of colloid continues and becomes even more excessive. The foci of hyperplasia and the foci of colloid storage compress the surrounding tissue, and nodules begin to develop. Collagen is laid down between the nodules, demarcating some of them more sharply. The enlarging nodules compress the blood supply within the thyroid, so that the thin walls between the lakes of colloid become atrophic, and cysts form. There may be hemorrhage into some of the nodules. Clumps of cholesterol crystals sometimes lie in the fibrosis between them. Sometimes foci of calcification develop within the gland. The end is a multinodular goiter, with fleshy hyperplastic nodules, gelatinous colloid nodules, cysts, hemorrhages, and fibrosis.

Dysfunction. Most patients with a nontoxic goiter are euthyroid. The uptake of iodine is usually normal unless there is iodine deficiency, where the usual test shows an increased uptake of radioactive iodine. The concentrations of thyroxine and triiodothyronine in the plasma are normal, though the ratio of thyroxine to triiodothyronine may be low because of defective iodination of thyroglobulin. The concentration of the thyroid-stimulating hormone in the plasma is normal.

As years pass, and the goiter becomes nodular, some of the nodules become partially autonomous and fail to respond normally to the stimuli that govern the function of the thyroid. Some take up iodine avidly; some take up little or none. Some produce the appropriate quantity of thyroid hormones; some produce too much or too little.

If one or a few of the nodules have too much of the thyroid hormones, the excess suppresses the secretion of the thyrotropin secreting and the thyroid-stimulating hormones, suppressing the production of the thyroid hormones in the rest of the thyroid gland. For a time, the patient remains euthyroid, though the concentration of the thyroid-stimulating hormone in the plasma is low. Administration of the thyrotropin releasing hormone fails to increase the secretion of the thyroid-stimulating hormone.

Especially in regions in which nontoxic goiter is endemic, some of the patients become hypothyroid. Adults develop mild myxedema. Children show signs of cretinism.

Clinical Presentation. Patients with a nontoxic goiter usually seek assistance because of the unsightly swelling in the neck. Compression of the trachea sometimes causes discomfort, dyspnea, or cough. Occasionally the goiter erodes the cartilages of the trachea. If the goiter is removed, the trachea collapses. Pressure on the esophagus can cause dysphagia. Rarely, stretching of a recurrent laryngeal nerve causes hoarseness. Hemorrhage into a nodule or cyst can cause pain and sudden swelling, which subsides gradually over a week or so. Sometimes the weight of a multinodular goiter causes it to slip beneath the sternum. In such patients, no mass may be apparent in the neck. Instead the patient has the signs and symptoms of a mediastinal tumor.

Pathogenesis. Iodine deficiency is the most common cause of both the endemic and sporadic forms of nontoxic goiter. In all regions in which nontoxic goiter is endemic, the diet is deficient in iodine. In some patients toxic agents called goitrogens are important in the causation of the goiter. In some, an enzyme deficiency causes the enlargement of the thyroid. In many patients with sporadic goiter, the cause of the disease is unknown.

If the intake of iodine is low, its concentration in the plasma and its excretion by the kidneys fall. The thyroid gland is unable to take up enough iodine to maintain normal function and becomes hyperplastic. The hyperplasia may be caused by increased secretion of the thyroid-stimulating hormone caused by a fall in the concentration of the thyroid hormones in the plasma, but more probably iodine deficiency causes the thyroid to respond excessively to a normal concentration of the thyroid-stimulating hormone.

Goitrogens cause nontoxic goiter or enhance the effect of iodine deficiency. In some Himalayan villages, nontoxic goiter is caused by a goitrogen in the drinking water, most probably an agent produced by Esch. coli. Cabbage and related vegetables contain goitrogens related to thiourea. Thiocyanate, perchlorate, paraaminosalicylic acid, and other drugs inhibit the metabolism of the thyroid gland and cause goiter if given for a long period. Fluoride and other halogens displace iodine and contribute to the causation of nontoxic goiter. Even excess of iodine can cause nontoxic goiter.

The enzyme deficiencies that sometimes cause nontoxic goiter in children are discussed later in the chapter. Minor anomalies of this sort may explain some sporadic goiters. Sometimes sporadic goiters are familial, suggesting the possibility of a genetic defect. Antibodies against thyroid antigens are often present in patients with a nontoxic goiter, but their titer is low.

Treatment and Prognosis. Endemic goiter due to iodine deficiency can be prevented, by supplying an adequate quantity of iodine in the diet, usually by adding potassium iodide to table salt. Adding iodine to the diet probably also decreases the incidence of sporadic goiter, but the cause of sporadic goiter is more complex, and other factors are also important.

A nontoxic goiter is managed by giving levothyroxine to suppress the secretion of the thyroid-stimulating hormone. The uptake of radioactive iodine in the first 24 hours should be reduced to less than 5% of the dose. In young people with a goiter that is not yet multinodular, the thyroid usually returns to its normal size within six months, though in most of the patients the administration of levothyroxine must be continued for the rest of the patient's life. If it is stopped, the goiter recurs. In older people with a multinodular goiter, significant shrinkage of the goiter occurs in 30% of the patients. In most of the rest, the growth of the goiter is arrested.

If some of the nodules in a multinodular goiter have become partly autonomous and fail to respond to the normal stimuli governing the thyroid, as shown by the inability of the thyrotropin stimulating hormone to cause a normal increase in the secretion of the thyroid-stimulating hormone, administration of levothyroxine is dangerous. The excessive secretion by the autonomous nodules in the thyroid continues and can cause hyperthyroidism. In such patients, the goiter is best treated as if it were toxic.

A thyroidectomy is indicated only if the goiter is causing compression of the trachea or some other mechanical problem, and when the administration of levothyroxine fails to reduce the size of a large, multinodular goiter. If a partial thyroidectomy is performed, levothyroxine should be given for the rest of the patient's life to prevent the regrowth of the goiter.

TOXIC NODULAR GOITER.   More than 10% of patients who have a multinodular goiter for more than 10 years develop mild hyperthyroidism. Such people are said to have a toxic nodular goiter, or Plummer's disease, named after the American physician who described it in 1928.

Hyperthyroidism caused by a toxic nodular goiter is nearly as frequent as is Graves' disease. It usually occurs in older people, but can develop at any age. About 75% of patients with a toxic nodular goiter are women.

Lesion.   Macroscopically and microscopically, a toxic nodular goiter is indistinguishable from a nontoxic multinodular goiter. The active nodule or nodules are hyperplastic, but so are some of the nodules in nontoxic nodular goiters. Only if a nodule is greatly hyperplastic, with columnar epithelium, papillary infoldings into its acini, and little colloid, is it likely that the nodule is hyperactive.

The normal thyroid parenchyma between the nodules of a toxic nodular goiter is atrophic. The hypersecretion of thyroid hormones by the active nodule or nodules suppresses the secretion of the thyroid-stimulating hormone, causing atrophy of the normal parenchyma.

Dysfunction.   Most patients with a toxic nodular goiter have only mild hyperthyroidism. In 30%, the uptake of radioactive iodine is normal. In the most of the rest, it is slightly increased. A scan of the thyroid after giving radioactive iodine or technetium shows that the active nodules take up the iodine, but the surrounding parenchyma does not. The concentrations of thyroxine and triiodothyronine in the plasma are usually slightly increased. Often the increase in triiodothyro-

nine is greater than the increase in thyroxine. A few patients develop T3 thyrotoxicosis with an increase in triiodothyronine but a decrease in thyroxine. In a few, the increase in thyroxine is greater than the increase in triiodothyronine.

The concentration of the thyroid-stimulating hormone in the plasma is low. Administration of the thyrotropin releasing hormone does not increase the secretion of the thyroid-stimulating hormone. Administration of thyroid hormone to inhibit the secretion of the thyroid-stimulating hormone does not decrease the uptake of iodine by the active nodules or prevent the excessive secretion of the thyroid hormone by the nodules.

Clinical Presentation.   Patients with a toxic nodular goiter usually develop hyperthyroidism so slowly and so mildly that it often goes unnoticed. Cardiac failure, cardiac arrhythmia, muscular wasting, weakness, or emotional lability may be the first sign of the hyperfunction. Sometimes the patient becomes apathetic, rather than hyperactive, as is usual in hyperthyroidism. Ophthalmopathy and dermopathy do not occur. The rare patient with proptosis or lid lag also has Graves' disease.

Pathogenesis.   In a toxic nodular goiter, the autonomy sometimes evident in a few of the nodules in a nontoxic goiter become greater. The quantity of thyroid hormones they secrete increases until the patient becomes hyperthyroid in spite of the inhibition of secretion in the rest of the gland. As time passes, the oversecretion in some nodules may wane, but secretion increases in others, and the hyperthyroidism continues. Often the iodination of thyroglobulin is reduced.

Treatment and Prognosis.   Toxic multinodular goiter is usually treated with radioactive iodine. Care must be taken because of the metabolic instability of elderly people, but the results are usually excellent. Hypothyroidism is unlikely to follow, because the active nodules take up most of the radioactive iodine, sparing the more normal parts of the gland, which are able to resume normal activity.

Jodbasedow Phenomenon (Iodine-induced Hyperthyroidism).   If iodine is added to the diet of a community that has long been deficient, hyperthyroidism develops in some people who have long been euthyroid. Epidemics of hyperthryoidism have been induced in this way.

Similarly, administration of iodine to an elderly person with a nontoxic nodular goiter sometimes causes hyperthyroidism. Even the quantity of iodine in drugs or x-ray contrast media may be sufficient. Presumably, the increased quantity of iodine available allows some of the nodules in the thyroid to secrete increased quantities of the thyroid hormones.

The induction of hyperthyroidism by administering iodine is called the jodbasedow phenomenon, *Jod* being the German for iodine and *basedow* for Basedow's disease. Less often, the administration of iodine causes transient hypothyroidism.

PARAFOLLICULAR CELL HYPERPLASIA. The cells that produce calcitonin are called parafollicular or C cells. In a normal adult thyroid gland, there are usually fewer than 10 parafollicular cells in a high-power field, though in parts of a gland there may be as many as 120. In parafollicular cell hyperplasia, the number of C cells increases, but they remain within the thyroid acini, lying between the thyrocytes and the basement membrane. Often the hyperplastic C cells form clumps, sometimes large enough to fill the lumen of an acinus.

Parafollicular cell hyperplasia is most common in patients with multiple endocrine neoplasia type II or type III. It is nearly always present in patients with these syndromes who have a medullary carcinoma of the thyroid and is frequent in their close relatives. The concentration of calcitonin in the plasma is increased in people with C cell hyperplasia. Secondary C cell hyperplasia can develop in patients with hypercalcemia and in the Zollinger-Ellison syndrome.

OTHER NON-NEOPLASTIC DISEASES

Other non-neoplastic diseases of the thyroid gland are uncommon. Occasionally squamous metaplasia, fatty infiltration, or amyloidosis occurs in the gland.

SQUAMOUS METAPLASIA. Rarely, a small focus of squamous metaplasia is found in the thyroid. The metaplasia is most common in patients with thyroiditis, carcinoma of the thyroid, or multinodular goiter. It is never extensive and causes no dysfunction.

FATTY INFILTRATION. Clumps of adipose cells are sometimes found within the thyroid. In rare cases there is so much fat within the gland that the enlargement is evident clinically.

AMYLOIDOSIS. Amyloidosis can enlarge the thyroid, though it rarely causes dysfunction. Sometimes fatty infiltration is evident in the thyroid gland in a patient with amyloidosis.

CONGENITAL ANOMALIES

The principal congenital anomalies of the thyroid gland are agenesis, malposition, thyroglossal cyst, and enzyme deficiencies that impair the secretion of the thyroid hormones.

AGENESIS. Occasionally the thyroid gland is absent, has only one lobe, or has one lobe with only a vestige of the other. Agenesis, or athyria as it is sometimes called, occurs in 1 live birth in 10,000. It is the most common cause of sporadic cretinism. In most of the infants, there is no evidence of a genetic error. The anomaly is probably caused by injury to the fetus in utero.

MALPOSITION. Malposition of the thyroid gland is uncommon. Part or all of the gland may be abnormally sited anywhere from the base of the tongue to the diaphragm. Carcinoma and other diseases of the thyroid can develop in the abnormally placed part of the gland.

A lingual thyroid is the most common form of malposition. It is found in 1 patient in 4000 coming to surgery for thyroid disease. A mass of otherwise normal thyroid tissue is present in the posterior part of the tongue. In 70% of the patients, there is no other thyroid tissue in the body. In some, thyroid tissue is also present in or near the normal position of the gland.

Less often a nodule of ectopic tissue is present near the hyoid bone or surrounds the bone. Most of these patients have a normally formed gland in the usual place. Often a few thyroid acini are present in the strap muscles near the thyroid. Sometimes small nodules of ectopic thyroid tissue are present in the mediastinum in a person with a normal thyroid in the normal position. Sometimes

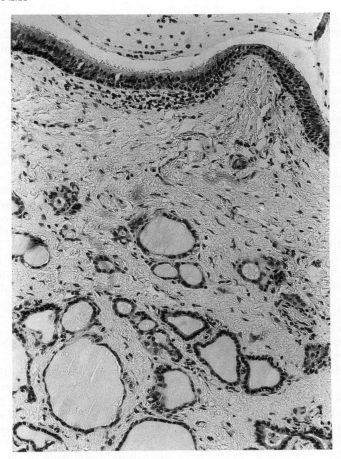

Fig. 47-6. A thyroglossal cyst lined by ciliated epithelium, with thyroid acini in its wall.

the whole thyroid gland is retrosternal, in the anterior mediastinum behind the sternum.

Lateral Aberrant Thyroid. Occasionally a small nodule of apparently normal thyroid is found in a lymph node in the neck. Such a nodule is called a lateral aberrant thyroid. In most patients the nodule is a highly differentiated metastasis of a carcinoma of the thyroid. In a few it is a congenital rest or a metastasis of benign tissue like the metastases thought to cause endometriosis.

THYROGLOSSAL CYST. A thyroglossal cyst is present in 1 person in 3000. The cyst arises from a remnant of the thyroglossal duct and may occur anywhere along the course of the duct, from the foramen cecum in the tongue to the thyroid. Most often it is in the midline just below the hyoid bone.

Thyroglossal cysts are usually discovered in childhood, but sometimes they become evident only in adult life. The cyst is usually 1 to 2 cm in diameter and enlarges slowly. It contains yellowish, mucoid fluid and has a thin, fibrous wall. Microscopically, the cyst may be lined by cuboidal, columnar, or ciliated epithelium. Often there may be considerable squamous metaplasia, with stratified squamous epithelium lining much or all of the cyst. Sometimes the epithelium is eroded, and the cyst is partly or largely lined by granulation tissue.

Occasionally the proximal part of the thyroglossal duct remains patent, and a sinus leads from the cyst to the foramen cecum. Rarely, the cyst ulcerates through the skin. A few thyroid acini are sometimes present in the wall of the cyst. Rarely, a carcinoma of the thyroid develops in a thyroglossal cyst. Excision cures.

ENZYME DEFICIENCIES. Enzyme deficiencies that impair the secretion of the thyroid hormones are uncommon. Most are inherited as an autosomal recessive character. The lack of thyroid hormones causes oversecretion of the thyroid-stimulating hormone, hyperplasia of the thyroid gland, and a goiter. In spite of the hyperplasia, hypothyroidism is usually severe. Unless treated, most children with a deficiency of one of the enzymes needed to synthesize the thyroid hormones become cretins.

In some of the children, the thyroid is unable to concentrate iodine. The salivary glands and gastric mucosa are unable to take up iodine from the blood in the way they do normally. Often the child is mentally retarded.

In other children with an enzyme defect, the thyroid takes up iodine avidly, but cannot attach it to protein. The iodine leaks back into the blood unbound. In most of these children, the enzyme deficient is thyroid peroxidase. The child is usually stunted and mentally retarded and has an enormous, hyperplastic goiter. Less often, the deficiency is less complete. The child remains euthyroid and of normal intelligence, though with a large goiter.

In Pendred's syndrome, name after the English physician who described it in 1896, the children are unable to bind iodine to protein, though the activity of thyroid peroxidase is normal. They are born deaf, because of a defect in the organ of Corti. A child with Pendred's syndrome is euthyroid or mildly hypothyroid and is of normal intelligence. A goiter usually appears only late in childhood.

If iodotyrosine dehalogenase is deficient, the iodine needed for the synthesis of thyroid hormones is not released from the iodotyrosines when thyroglobulin is broken down. The iodotyrosines are lost in the urine. Iodine deficiency develops and causes a nontoxic goiter. Some of the patients are hypothyroid.

In some goitrous cretins, severe hypothyroidism results from deficiency of the iodotyrosyl-coupling enzymes, which join iodotyrosines to form iodothyronines. In some children with a goiter who are euthyroid or hypothyroid, the thyroid fails to form adequate quantities of thyroglobulin and instead makes excessive quantities of iodoalbumin and other iodoproteins.

Rarely, cretinism or hypothyroidism results from a congenital lack of the thyroid-stimulating hormone, from failure of the thyroid gland to respond to the hormone, or from failure of the tissues to respond to the thyroid hormones.

In most children with an enzyme defect that impairs the secretion of the thyroid hormones, thyroid hormone must be given to supply the deficiency. In iodotyrosine dehalogenase deficiency, iodine also is effective. If the deficiency is severe, therapy must be instituted soon after birth if serious impairment of mental and skeletal development is to be avoided.

TUMORS

The primary tumours of the thyroid gland are nearly all epithelial. Most arise from the follicular epithelium; some from the parafollicular cells. The benign tumors are called adenomata; the malignant ones carcinoma. Unless otherwise qualified, the terms *adenoma* and *carcinoma* of the thyroid refer to tumors of the follicular epithelium.

Occasionally a benign teratoma arises in or near the thyroid in an infant and is large enough to compress the trachea or obstruct the esophagus. In adults, a lymphoma sometimes involves the thyroid. Rarely, a benign or malignant mesenchymal tumor arises in the gland.

ADENOMA OF FOLLICULAR EPITHELIUM. It is impossible to draw a clear distinction between an adenoma of the follicular epithelium of the thyroid gland and the nodules of a multinodular goiter. Indeed, the terms *adenoma* and *nodule* are often used vaguely, as if they were interchangeable. Some speak of a multinodular goiter as an adenomatous goiter, as if the nodules were neoplasms. Probably it is best to reserve the term *adenoma* of the thyroid for lesions that arise in a gland that is otherwise uniform, without nodularity.

Adenomata of the thyroid so defined are

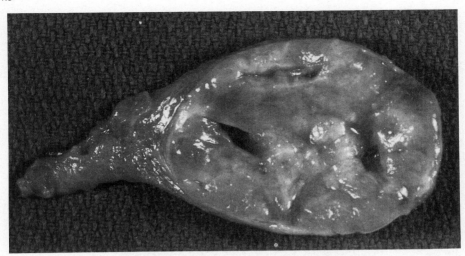

Fig. 47-7. A well-circumscribed adenoma of a thyroid gland, with foci of cystic necrosis in the center of the lesion.

not common. Most occur in people over 30 years old. Over 80% of the patients are women.

Lesions. Adenomata of follicular epithelium of the thyroid are spheroidal, usually 1 to 5 cm in diameter, well defined or encap-

sulated. On section, an adenoma is often reddish brown and translucent if it contains much colloid, but is paler and more homogeneous if it is more cellular. Sometimes an adenoma becomes cystic, a fibrous scar develops in the center of an adenoma, or the

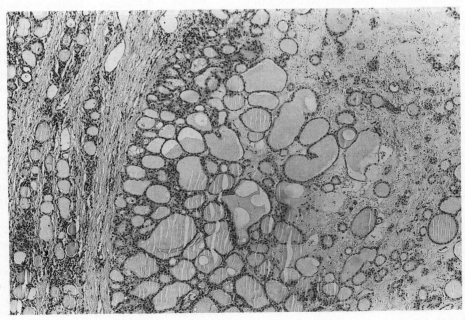

Fig. 47-8. A thyroid adenoma, showing the thin capsule that clearly demarcated the lesion from the adjacent tissue.

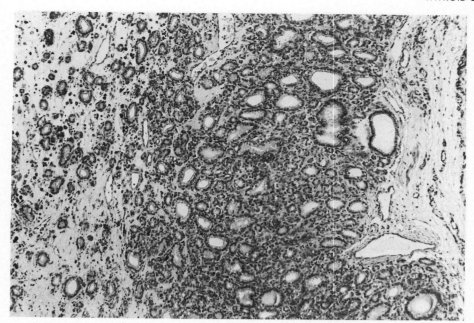

Fig. 47-9. A fetal adenoma of a thyroid gland, showing small acini lined by cuboidal epithelium. On the left the acini are widely separated by an edematous stroma.

lesion is partly calcified. There may be old or recent hemorrhage into a cystic adenoma.

Most adenomata of the thyroid have a thin, collagenous capsule, though it may not be complete. If there is no capsule, the lesion is sharply demarcated from the surrounding parenchyma. Most adenomata grow slowly and compress the surrounding parenchyma.

Microscopically, most adenomata of the thyroid are the same throughout, unless the pattern is altered by necrosis or fibrosis. A number of different kinds of adenoma are distinguished.

Embryonal Adenoma. An embryonal adenoma resembles an embryonal thyroid gland in the early stages of its development. It consists of columns of small, regular epithelial cells, sometimes closely packed, sometimes with abundant, edematous stroma. Follicles are few and small and contain little or no colloid.

Fetal Adenoma. A fetal adenoma resembles the thyroid gland in the later stages of fetal life. It consists of small follicles, often widely scattered in an edematous stroma. The follicles vary in size, but contain little colloid and are lined by low, cuboidal epithe-lium. Central necrosis, with cyst formation or hemorrhage, is common.

Simple Adenoma. Simple adenomata have follicles like those of the normal thyroid. It may be difficult to distinguish such an adenoma from a nodule in a nontoxic goiter.

Colloid Adenoma. Colloid adenomata have large follicles, which vary in size and are distended with colloid. Such an adenoma is often indistinguishable microscopically from a colloid nodule in a multinodular goiter.

Hürthle Cell Adenoma. A Hürthle cell adenoma is uncommon. It consists of large cells with abundant, eosinophilic cytoplasm filled with mitochondria. The tumor cells have spheroidal vesicular or pyknotic nuclei. They are closely packed in cords, with few acini and little stroma.

Papillary Adenoma. Macroscopically, papillary adenomata are often cystic. The cyst has a shaggy wall with innumerable little papillae projecting into it. Microscopically, the peripheral part of the adenoma often consists of follicles like those of a simple adenoma. The central part consists of delicate fronds with a core of fine collagenous tissue covered by low, atrophic-looking epithelium.

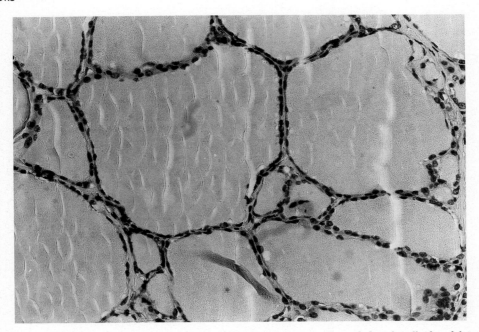

Fig. 47-10. A colloid adenoma of a thyroid gland, showing large acini distended with colloid and lined by flattened epithelium.

Sometimes a few foci of calcification are evident.

Atypical Adenoma.   An atypical adenoma consists of closely packed, somewhat pleomorphic cells often with a few mitoses. The cells form clumps and columns. Follicles are rare. The capsule of the adenoma is intact. Often it is thicker than in other adenomata. The blood vessels or the capsule are not invaded.

Behavior. About 90% of the solitary, encapsulated tumors of the thyroid are benign. They grow slowly and get bigger, but do not invade and do not metastasize. Most are of the fetal type. Some are simple adenomata or colloid adenomata.

The other 10% of encapsulated tumors invade their capsules or invade blood vessels. About 25% of embryonal lesions and 5% of fetal lesions show local invasion of this sort. It is rarely evident in a simple or a colloid lesion. Some call tumors that show only local extension invasive adenomata. Most call them low grade carcinomata. Local excision cures 85% of these lesions, but 15% recur or metastasize.

The Hürthle cell tumors are particularly

dangerous. Some 40% of them show vascular invasion, and 20% recur or metastasize. Many prefer to consider all Hürthle cell tumors low grade carcinomata or use the noncommital term Hürthle cell tumor without indicating whether the lesion is benign or malignant.

A papillary adenoma is hard to distinguish from a papillary carcinoma of the thyroid. If there is any cellular atypicality or any cellular proliferation in the tumor, it must be considered to be malignant. Local excision cures many papillary lesions, but some showing little or no evidence of malignancy metastasize. Because of the difficulty in ensuring that a papillary lesion is benign, some prefer to consider all papillary lesions malignant.

The atypical adenomata are also ominous. Probably these tumors are comparable to the carcinoma in situ of other organs. If there is no invasion, complete excision will almost certainly cure. If an atypical tumor invades the blood vessels or its capsule, it must be considered a carcinoma. In nearly 70% of the patients with an invasive tumor of this sort, the tumor recurs or metastasizes. Nearly 20% of the patients die of their carcinoma.

Dysfunction.   Most adenomata of the thy-

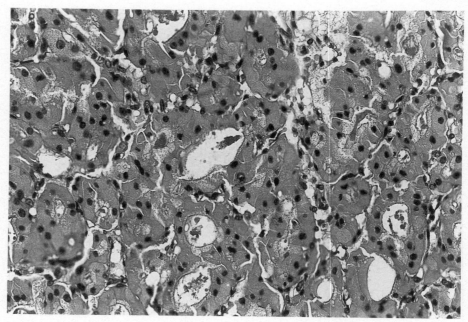

Fig. 47-11. A Hürthle cell tumor of a thyroid gland, showing the large, cuboidal epithelial cells filled with mitochondria.

roid take up iodine and similar substances more avidly than does the surrounding thyroid parenchyma. If radioactive iodine or radioactive technitium is given, the adenoma concentrates the radioactivity more than does the surrounding parenchyma and appears darker than the rest of the parenchyma when the thyroid is scanned. A nodule that appears darker than the surrounding parenchyma is called a warm nodule.

As an adenoma grows larger, its activity tends to increase. It is not fully bound by the factors normally governing the production of the thyroid hormones and produces more of the thyroid hormones than is needed for homeostasis. The patient is euthyroid, but the secretion of the thyroid-stimulating hormone is inhibited, and the activity of the normal part of the parenchyma falls. If radioiodine or radioactive technitium is given, the adenoma concentrates the marker, but the rest of the parenchyma takes up little or none. Only the adenoma appears dark when the thyroid is scanned. Such a nodule is called a hot nodule.

If an adenoma of the thyroid is largely destroyed by hemorrhage or cystic necrosis, it can no longer take up iodine and no longer produces significant quantities of the thyroid hormones. The patient is euthyroid, because the rest of the parenchyma functions normally. The secretion of the thyroid-stimulating hormone is normal. If radioactive iodine or radioactive technitium is given, the normal part of the parenchyma concentrates the marker normally, but the adenoma takes up little or none. A scan will show the parenchyma normally, but the adenoma will appear as a pale zone. Such a nodule is called a cold nodule.

Other adenomata are cold on scanning even though the thyrotrophic hormone binds to the cells of the adenoma and activates adenyl cyclase. A defect in the tumor cells prevents the uptake of the marker.

Toxic Adenoma.   About 10% of adenomata of the thyroid secrete the thyroid hormones in sufficient quantity to cause hyperthyroidism. The tumor is called a toxic adenoma. In a radioactive iodine or technitium scan, the nodule is hot. The oversecretion of the thyroid hormones by the toxic adenoma suppresses the secretion of the thyroid-stimulating hormone and so inhibits the uptake of iodine and technitium by the normal part of the gland.

Both thyroxine and triiodothyronine are secreted in increased quantity, but the ratio between the concentrations of thyroxine and triiodothyronine in the plasma tends to fall. T_3 toxicosis is more common in patients with a toxic adenoma than in other kinds of hyperthyroidism.

Clinical Presentation. A thyroid nodule that to clinical examination appears to be solitary can be found in 1% of the population. Most of these nodules cause no trouble and are never detected by the patient.

In over 90% of these people, the patient has a small multinodular goiter, with only one nodule large enough to be detected clinically. In most of the rest, the lesion is an adenoma. In under 1% of the patients, it is a carcinoma.

It can be difficult to distinguish between these three kinds of thyroid nodule and, in particular, to exclude carcinoma. If a radioiodine or radiotechnitium scan shows that the nodule is hot, or if examination by ultrasound shows it to be cystic, carcinoma is improbable. If the nodule is cold on technitium scan, the risk of carcinoma grows, though fewer than 20% of cold nodules are malignant. The concentration of thyroglobulin in the plasma is often increased in patients with a well-differentiated carcinoma of the thyroid, but it is also often elevated in people with an adenoma of the thyroid, a nontoxic goiter, or Graves' disease. It may be necessary to resort to a needle biopsy or an open, excisional biopsy to exclude carcinoma.

Treatment and Prognosis. Many adenomata of the thyroid gland need no treatment. If the lesion is large, administration of thyroid hormone to suppress the secretion of the thyroid-stimulating hormone often causes the adenoma to shrink. Sometimes surgical excision is needed. A toxic adenoma can be managed by administering radioactive iodine or by excision. When radioactive iodine is given, the adenoma takes up more of the isotope than does the surrounding parenchyma and is more severely injured by the radiation.

ADENOMA OF PARAFOLLICULAR CELLS. The C cells of the thyroid occasionally form a small nodule called an adenoma. Macroscopically, the lesion is encapsulated, solid, and pink or brown. Microscopically, it consists of closely packed clumps and cords of spindle cells or small cuboidal cells. Electron microscopy shows that the cells contain the neurosecretory granules typical of parafollicular cells. Immunohistochemistry shows that they contain calcitonin. The lesion is benign.

CARCINOMA OF FOLLICULAR EPITHELIUM. Less than 1% of malignant tumors arise in the thyroid. Over 95% of them originate from the follicular epithelium. In the United States, each year, 4 people in every 100,000 develop a carcinoma of the thyroid. Over 70% of the patients are women. About 30% of the patients are under 45 years old, 30% are 45 to 65 years old, and 30% are over 65 years old. In other countries the incidence is much the same, though there are differences in the proportion of patients who are women. In Switzerland and Israel, the incidence is two or three times higher.

Carcinoma of the follicular epithelium is divided into five types: papillary carcinoma, follicular carcinoma, anaplastic carcinoma, squamous cell carcinoma, and Hürthle cell carcinoma. Over 60% of thyroid carcinomata are papillary. About 20% of the tumors are follicular and 10% are anaplastic. Squamous cell carcinoma is rare. The Hürthle cell tumors are considered with the adenomata.

Most patients with a papillary carcinoma are 20 to 40 years old. Over 70% of thyroid carcinomata in children are of the papillary type. Patients with a follicular, anaplastic, or squamous carcinoma are usually over 50 years old, and the preponderance of women is less than with the papillary tumors.

Lesions. The different kinds of carcinoma of the thyroid differ macroscopically and microscopically.

Papillary Carcinoma. Papillary carcinomata of the thyroid are often only 1 to 4 mm across. They look like small white scars at the periphery of the thyroid near the capsule. Larger papillary carcinomata sometimes resemble an adenoma, but more often they are hard, grayish-white, and fibrous, without clear demarcation from the surrounding thyroid. Many are 1 to 2 cm across, some 5 cm or more. Sometimes scarring is greatest in the center of the tumor. Sometimes a tumor is calcified. Occasionally, multiple little nodules of papillary carcinoma can be detected in the involved lobe, in addition to the main mass. Rarely, foci of carcinoma are evident to the naked eye in both lobes.

Microscopically, a papillary carcinoma consists of fine, branching fronds, which project into large, glandular spaces. The fronds have a core of delicate collagenous tissue covered with cuboidal epithelium. The tumor cells lining the fronds are fairly regular, with homogeneous, eosinophilic cytoplasm and nuclei with evenly dispersed chromatin. Usually the epithelium is one cell thick, but here and there it may be multilayered. A few Hürthle cells are often scattered among the other tumor cells. In 30% of the carcinomata, a few of the tumor cells have clear cytoplasm. In 45%, small foci of squamous metaplasia are present.

Though the papillary pattern is the main feature of the carcinoma, a papillary carcinoma often forms a few follicles lined by similar epithelium. If a large part of the tumor forms follicles in this way, the tumor is called a mixed papillary and follicular carcinoma.

Laminated, calcified, spheroidal psammoma bodies are present in the stroma in 40% of papillary carcinomata of the thyroid. They are rarely found in other lesions of the thyroid.

Lymphatic permeation can be demonstrated in 80% of papillary carcinomata. Venous invasion is found in 10%.

Some of the papillary carcinomata that are less than 1 cm across consist largely of dense, hyaline scarring, with small islands of papillary carcinoma buried here and there in the scar. The scarring extends irregularly out into the surrounding thyroid and distorts it. Such small carcinomata are sometimes called occult, sclerosing carcinomata.

Multiple deposits of tumor are present in the thyroid in most patients with a papillary carcinoma. The lobe containing the main tumor nearly always contains additional smaller deposits of tumor. The contralateral lobe is affected in over 30% of the patients. Many of the deposits are too small to be visible macroscopically, but they reproduce the papillary structure seen in the main tumor mass. Whether these multiple foci of carcinoma in the thyroid result from lym-

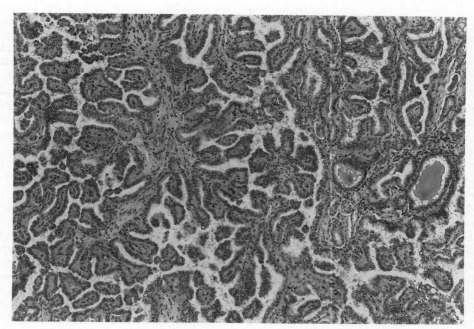

Fig. 47-12.   A papillary carcinoma of a thyroid gland, showing its branching fronds. The fronds have a narrow core of collagenous tissue and are covered by a single layer of cuboidal epithelium.

phatic spread or whether they are multiple primary tumors, is debatable.

Follicular Carcinoma.   About 50% of follicular carcinomata are encapsulated and spheroidal and macroscopically look like an adenoma. The other 50% extend irregularly into the surrounding thyroid. The invasive tumors are from 1 to 10 cm across. They are often hard and sclerotic. They may extend through the capsule of the gland to invade the trachea or the strap muscles. Often there are foci of hemorrhage or necrosis within the tumor.

The encapsulated follicular carcinomata are the tumors some call invasive adenomata. The usually show the embryonal, fetal, or anaplastic pattern of growth, but occasionally resemble a simple or a colloid adenoma. Microscopically, often only invasion of the blood vessels or the capsule distinguishes these tumors from an adenoma. In some, the tumor cells are slightly atypical or slightly pleomorphic.

The invasive follicular carcinomata show microscopically the same follicular patterns seen in the adenomata. At one extreme, the carcinoma may be so well differentiated that it reproduces almost perfectly the structure of the normal thyroid. Sometimes a carcinoma mimics a colloid nodule of a multinodular goiter. Sometimes it is like the hyperplastic thyroid of Graves' disease. Other carcinomata form tiny, closely packed acini or solid columns or tumor cells, with only occasional follicles. Often parts of the carcinoma have a sclerotic stroma, which encloses clumps of follicles lined by cells showing slight atypicality and pleomorphism, perhaps with a few mitoses. A few Hürthle cells may be present, and occasionally there are a few psammoma bodies. Almost always, a follicular carcinoma shows some admixture of papillary carcinoma.

Invasion of blood vessels is usually obvious, and there may be lymphatic invasion. Sometimes there are multiple foci of carcinoma within the thyroid.

Anaplastic Carcinoma.   An anaplastic carcinoma of the thyroid usually forms a hard, irregular mass. It often replaces much of the thyroid, crossing the midline to involve both sides of the neck. Often the carcinoma invades extensively the strap muscles and other structures in the vicinity of the thyroid. On section, the carcinoma may be white and

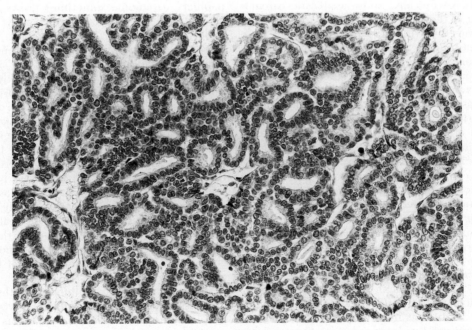

Fig. 47-13.   A follicular carcinoma of a thyroid gland, showing somewhat irregularly shaped acini lined by tall cuboidal epithelium.

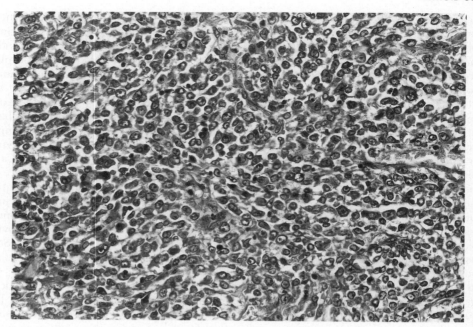

Fig. 47-14. An anaplastic carcinoma of a thyroid gland. The tumor cells are small and round, resembling those of a malignant lymphoma.

fibrous or soft, with extensive necrosis and hemorrhage.

Microscopically, some anaplastic carcinomata of the thyroid form cords or clumps of tumor cells with frequent mitoses but little plemorphism. Sometimes the stroma of these tumors is abundant and hyalinized. In other tumors, the tumor cells resemble lymphocytes and infiltrate the tissue like a lymphoma. Occasionally the tumor cells are large, bizarre, and often multinucleated, like the cells of an adult rhabdomyosarcoma, or the carcinoma consists of spindle cells and resembles a fibrosarcoma. To prove the tumor is a carcinoma it is sometimes necessary to demonstrate by electron microscopy that the tumor cells have desmosomes, microvilli, or other features of epithelial cells or to show immunohistochemically that they contain cytokeratins or other markers for epithelial cells.

Behavior. Papillary carcinoma of the thyroid is an indolent, slow-growing tumor, particularly in children and young adults. It is likely that many papillary carcinomata are present for decades before they are discovered. They grow so slowly that it is a long

time before the primary tumor in the thyroid is big enough to be palpable. In old people, a papillary carcinoma sometimes grows more rapidly and metastasize sooner and more widely.

Metastases come first in the lymph nodes, usually the lymph nodes on the same side of the neck. Sometimes the enlarged lymph nodes are discovered while the primary tumor is still too small to be palpable. If the primary tumor in the thyroid is less than 1.5 cm diameter, 30% of the patients have metastases in the cervical lymph nodes. If the primary is more than 1.5 cm across, 70% of the patients have metastases in the lymph nodes in the neck. More distant metastases are uncommon and usually come only after many years. Less than 5% of the patients develop metastases in the lungs, though spread to the lungs is more common in children. Metastases in bone, liver, or brain are still less frequent.

Rarely, a papillary carcinoma of the thyroid progresses to some more dangerous type, an anaplastic carcinoma or a squamous cell carcinoma.

Follicular carcinomata of the thyroid also

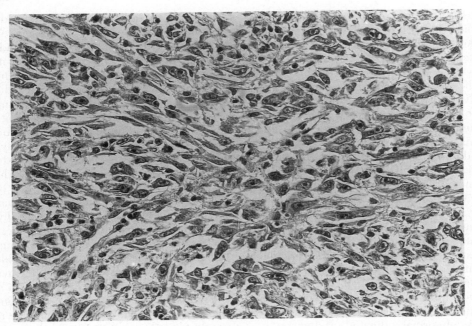

Fig. 47-15. An anaplastic carcinoma of a thyroid gland. The tumor cells are elongated, resembling those of a fibrosarcoma.

grow slowly. Often metastases appear only after the tumor has been present for many years. The encapsulated tumors and the smaller invasive tumors can often be cured by excision.

Metastases develop both in the cervical lymph nodes and by hematogenous extension. Frequently the hematogenous metastases are the more prominent. Like the primary tumor, they often grow slowly and may persist with little change for years. At autopsy, there are metastases in the cervical lymph nodes in the neck or local recurrence of the carcinoma in 90% of the patients, metastases in the lungs in 60%, and metastases in the bones, liver, or brain in 20%.

Anaplastic carcinomata of the thyroid grow rapidly, infiltrate extensively into the tissues of the neck, and metastasize widely to the regional lymph nodes in the neck and then beyond by the blood stream to the lungs, the liver, and bone. Often the rapidly growing carcinoma in the neck, rather than the metastases, brings death.

In some patients with an anaplastic carcinoma of the thyroid, it seems clear that the carcinoma has arisen from an adenoma or a papillary carcinoma. In most, no such progression can be established.

Dysfunction. As they grow less differentiated, most carcinomata of the thyroid lose the ability to concentrate iodine from the plasma, to bind it to protein, and to form the thyroid hormones. Because they cannot take up iodine, most carcinomata fail to show radioactivity when the thyroid is scanned after giving a dose of radioiodine or radiotechnetium and so appear as a cold nodule. Only carcinomata containing well-differentiated follicles are likely to take up iodine in sufficient quantity to appear warm, and even in them the uptake is usually patchy or spotty.

In a few patients, metastases of a follicular carcinoma have maintained the patient in a euthyroid state after the thyroid was completely ablated. In a few, a carcinoma of the thyroid has caused hyperthyroidism. Probably the carcinoma does not produce thyroid hormones efficiently, but the bulk of the carcinoma and its metastases become so large that in spite of its inefficiency the tumor is able to maintain the patient in a euthyroid state or cause hyperthyroidism.

In 10% of carcinomata of the thyroid, the thyroid-stimulating hormone increases the uptake of iodine by the carcinoma and augments its production of thyroid hormones. In some of the more responsive tumors, inhibiting the secretion of the thyrotropic hormone by giving thyroid hormone slows the growth of the carcinoma or causes it to regress.

The concentration of thyroglobulin in the plasma is often increased in patients with a well-differentiated carinoma of the thyroid, as it is in other diseases of the thyroid. If the carcinoma is completely removed, the concentration of thyroglobulin in the plasma returns to normal. If the concentration of thyroglobulin remains elevated or becomes elevated after an interval, there are probably metastases or a recurrence of the carcinoma.

Some carcinomata of the thyroid produce normal thyroglobulin and release normal thyroid hormones into the blood. Some produce an abnormal thyroglobulin. Others release abnormal iodinated products.

About 30% of the patients with carcinoma of the thyroid have antibodies against thyroid antigens in their blood. The titer of the antibodies is usually low, of the order found in patients with a multinodular goiter.

Pathogenesis. Radiation given during infancy to reduce the size of a large thymus is the major cause of carcinoma of the thyroid in children and adolescents. In childhood, even a small dose of radiation increases the risk of developing carcinoma of the thyroid. The greater the dose, the greater the risk. The neck or mediastinum has been irradiated in 80% of children or adolescents with carcinoma of the thyroid. Carcinoma of the thyroid develops in 7% of the children irradiated. The carcinoma usually appears 10 to 20 years after the radiation is given, sometimes later.

Most of the carcinomata in irradiated children and adolescents are papillary, though other kinds of carcinoma occur. The radiation also increases the incidence of adenomata of the thyroid. Adenomata are 10 times as frequent as carcinomata in children irradiated.

In adults, irradiation of the thyroid is less dangerous. Atomic radiation in Japan and the Marshall Islands increased the incidence of nodules and carcinoma of the thyroid in the children irradiated but the increase in the incidence of carcinoma of the thyroid was slight in those who were adult when irradiated and only became evident 30 years after the irradiation. No clear increase in the incidence of carcinoma of the thyroid is evident in patients with Graves' disease who were irradiated between 1930 and 1950, when radiation was often used to treat hyperthyroidism.

In animals, anything that causes long-continued oversecretion of the thyroid-stimulating hormone causes carcinoma of the thyroid. Iodine deficiency, goitrogenic drugs, external radiation, radioactive iodine, or partial thyroidectomy cause sufficient oversecretion of the thyroid-stimulating hormone in animals to cause carcinoma of the thyroid. The thyroid gland in the animals first becomes hyperplastic, then nodular. Adenomata develop and at last carcinomata. There is no clear evidence that prolonged oversecretion of the thyroid-stimulating hormone is carcinogenic in man.

Treatment and Prognosis. Carcinoma of the thyroid is usually treated by unilateral or nearly total thyroidectomy and dissection of the lymph nodes in the neck. Many surgeons prefer an almost total thyroidectomy even when the tumor is localized because of the risk of multiple foci of carcinoma within the thyroid. Postoperatively, the patient is given a diagnostic dose of radioactive iodine. If any unresectable metastases are discovered, or if the primary tumor has not been totally removed, a therapeutic dose of radioactive iodine follows. The patient is maintained on levothyroxine or a similar drug to depress the secretion of the thyroid-stimulating hormone and slow the growth of any remaining tumor. If a slowly growing carcinoma of the thyroid recurs, further therapeutic doses of radioactive iodine or resection of the metastases often allows several years of useful life.

Almost all patients with an occult sclerosing carcinoma can be cured by excising the tumor. With larger papillary carcinomata confined to the thyroid, only 2% of the patients die of their disease. If the carcinoma recurs or has spread beyond the thyroid to the lymph nodes, 15% of the patients die of the carcinoma, though sometimes not for 10 or 20 years. Death is caused by local recurrence in 50% of the patients who die of the carcinoma. The expanding tumor in the neck obstructs the trachea, the esophagus, or the great vessels. Often there is severe and uncontrollable infection around a tracheostomy or in the lungs.

The multiple tumors common in papillary carcinoma of the thyroid do little to worsen the prognosis. In one study in which papillary carcinoma was found in the contralateral lobe in nearly 40% of the patients in whom the contralateral lobe was examined, recurrence on the other side occurred in less than 5% of the patients with papillary carcinoma treated by unilateral lobectomy.

Less than 10% of patients with an encapsulated follicular carcinoma of the thyroid die of their disease. More than 50% of patients with an invasive follicular carcinoma die of the carcinoma within 10 years, usually of metastases. Only 10% of anaplastic carcinomata of the thyroid are resectable. Almost all the patients die within a year, usually from a combination of local recurrence and widespread metastases.

MEDULLARY CARCINOMA. A carcinoma that arises from the parafollicular cells of the thyroid is called a medullary carcinoma. About 5% of carcinomata of the thyroid are of this type. A medullary carcinoma of the thyroid can arise at any age, but most of the patients are over 50 years old. The tumor is more common in men than in women. About 10% of the patients have the multiple endocrine neoplasia syndrome type II or type III.

Lesions. A medullary carcinoma of the thyroid forms a hard, grayish-white mass, usually 2 to 3 cm across, occasionally much bigger or much smaller. Sometimes there are multiple foci of medullary carcinoma within the thyroid. Occasionally the tumor involves both sides of the thyroid.

Microscopically, a medullary carcinoma of the thyroid consists of clumps and cords of tumor cells. The cells may be polyhedral, like the cells of a carcinoid tumor. They may be small and spindle-shaped, like the cells of an oat cell carcinoma of the lung. They may be large and polyhedral. Occasionally, the tumor cells form small acini. Electron microscopy shows that the tumor cells contain neuroendocrine granules 150 to 300 nm in diameter, of the sort seen in parafollicular cells. Immunochemical staining shows that the tumor cells contain calcitonin.

The clumps and cords of tumor cells are usually separated by a prominent, hyaline

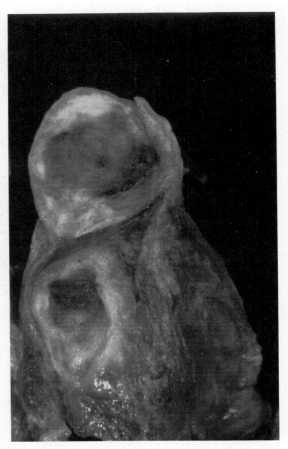

Fig. 47-16. A medullary carcinoma of a thyroid gland. The hard tumor has been bisected and opened like a book.

stroma. In 80% of the tumors, amyloid formed by the polymerization of a precursor of calcitonin is present in the stroma. Often it is abundant. Foci of calcification are commonly present.

In the patients with a multiple endocrine neoplasia syndrome, the carcinoma is often bilateral. C cell hyperplasia is present in the parts of the gland not involved by carcinoma. It usually precedes the development of the carcinoma by several years. C cell hyperplasia is not evident in patients with a medullary carcinoma who do not have a multiple endocrine neoplasia syndrome.

Behavior. Most medullary carcinomata of the thyroid grow slowly. Some enlarge rapidly and spread widely. By the time the tumor is discovered, 70% of the patients have

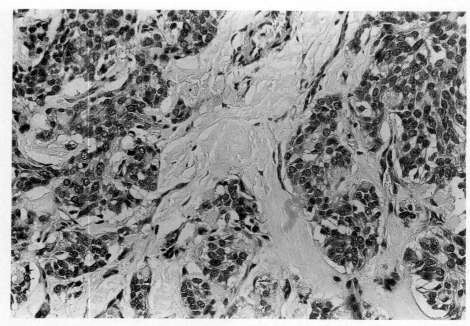

Fig. 47-17.   A medullary carcinoma of a thyroid gland, with polyhedral tumor cells. The structureless material between the tumor cells is amyloid.

metastases in the lymph nodes in the neck. Most distant metastases in the lungs, liver, bones, or other organs often become evident later.

Dysfunction.   Medullary carcinomata of the thyroid produce calcitonin. The tumor may contain as much as 450 µg/g of calcitonin. Normal thyroid contains less than 0.1 µg/g. In 75% of the patients, the concentration of calcitonin in the plasma is increased from 4 to 50 times. If the concentration of calcitonin is normal, the infusion of calcium or pentagastrin often causes excessive secretion of calcitonin. The increased secretion of calcitonin does not usually cause any disturbance in homeostasis. Occasionally there is mild hypocalcemia.

Medullary carcinomata of the thyroid can also secrete other substances, among them the adrenocorticotropic hormone, prolactin, serotonin, the vasoactive intestinal peptide, histamine, and prostaglandins. Diarrhea is present in 30% of the patients and sometimes is the presenting symptom. Sometimes the patients show other features of the carcinoid syndrome. Rarely, the secretion of the ad-

renocorticotropic hormone is sufficient to cause Cushing's syndrome.

Treatment and Prognosis.   A medullary carcinoma of the thyroid is usually treated by bilateral thyroidectomy and dissection of the lymph nodes in the neck. Chemotherapy is of limited value.

If there are no metastases in the regional lymph nodes, the patients have a normal expectation of life, though elevated levels of calcitonin in the blood suggest that there are occult deposits of tumor somewhere in the body in 30% of these people. If the lymph nodes are involved, 50% of the patients die of their carcinoma because of local recurrence or from metastases, usually after 10 to 15 years. If distant metastases become evident, almost all the patients die of the tumor, though often not for more than 10 years. Overall, about 50% of the patients are alive 10 years after the resection of the tumor.

SECONDARY TUMORS.   Metastatic carcinoma is found in the thyroid in 20% of patients dying of carcinoma. Most of these metastases to the thyroid are small and of little importance. Rarely, a metastasis to the thyroid mimics a primary carcinoma of the thyroid.

HYPERTHYROIDISM

Hyperthryoidism, or thyrotoxicosis as it is sometimes called, is caused by the excessive secretion of the thyroid hormones for a prolonged period. Usually, the concentrations of thyroxine and triiodothyronine in the plasma are both increased, with the increase in triiodothyronine being greater than the increase in thyroxine. In patients with T_3 toxicosis, the concentration of thyroxine is normal or depressed, and only triiodothyronine is in excess. In T_4 toxicosis, the concentration of thyroxine is excessive, but the concentration of triiodothyronine in the plasma is normal or low.

The most common cause of hyperthyroidism is the oversecretion of the thyroid hormones in a patient with Graves' disease, a toxic goiter, or a toxic adenoma. Less often it results from the leakage of thyroid hormones from the damaged acini in thyroiditis. Rarely, oversecretion of the thyroid-stimulating hormone, the release of factors that stimulate the thyroid from a trophoblastic tumor, struma ovarii, or metastatic carcinoma of the thyroid causes thyrotoxicosis. Administration of large doses of thyroid hormone induces iatrogenic hyperthyroidism.

Clinical Presentation. The onset of hyperthyroidism is usually insidious, with symptoms developing gradually over months or years. Only in Graves' disease is the onset sometimes abrupt, with severe symptoms developing within several days.

The severity of the dysfunction varies from one patient to another. It may be so mild as to be barely perceptible. It may be so severe as to bring death rapidly unless treated. In any one patient, the severity of the dysfunction often varies from one period to another.

In younger patients, the first symptoms are usually nervousness, palpitations, or fatique. Often there is loss of weight in spite of good appetite, diarrhea, intolerance of heat, and excessive perspiration. The patient is usually restless, fidgets constantly, and is unable to remain still. The patient darts in the door, sits down, jumps up, rushes out, with excessive, jerky rapidity. Emotional lability is common, perhaps irrational bursts of weeping. The patient may be euphoric or may be exhausted by the constant activity. Often there is a fine tremor of the fingers. The tremor of Parkinson's disease is increased. Any tendency towards epilepsy is enhanced, and convulsions become more severe. Reflexes become hyperactive.

Restlessness and irritability are not always evident in old people with a toxic nodular goiter. The patient is often apathetic and dull. Heart failure is often the first sign of the dysfunction.

Dysfunction. The hypersecretion of thyroid hormones causes dysfunction in organs throughout the body. The hyperactivity seen in most patients with hyperthyroidism is due in part to the increased metabolic rate caused by the oversecretion of the thyroid hormones, in part to the increased activity of the catecholamines caused by the hyperthyroidism.

Because of the overactivity of the catecholamines, the patients often seem to stare, with wide palpebral fissures, and rarely blink. The lids may lag when the patient looks up or down. The forehead may fail to wrinkle when the patient looks up. The exopthalmos in some patients with Graves' disease is not seen in other forms of hyperthyroidism.

Changes in the skin are nearly always present and result from the hypermetabolism induced by the hyperthyroidism, with the need to increase the loss of heat, and from the action of the thyroid hormones on the skin. The patients often feel unreasonably hot, and skin in flushed. Sweating is excessive. The skin becomes smooth and silky, without wrinkles. Patchy hyperpigmentation of the skin is common. In a few patients, there are patches of vitiligo. There may be pruritus. The hair becomes fine and straight. Often there is loss of hair, occasionally alopecia areata. The nails, beginning with the fourth fingers, bend upwards away from the nail bed, exposing a ragged, dirty hyponychium. Often there is peripheral edema, in the absence of heart failure. In Graves' disease, pretibial myxedema may be evident.

Weakness of the skeletal muscles is common and sometimes is severe, especially in the extensor muscles. The muscle fibers contract abnormally rapidly, but the duration of the contraction is reduced. The ability of the muscles to take up creatine from the plasma is impaired, causing creatinuria. If the myopathy is severe, the muscles atrophy. The muscle fibers become thin, and fat accumulates between them. Creatinine leaks from the wasted muscles and is lost in the urine. Myasthenia gravis and periodic paralysis are unduly common in thyrotoxicosis.

The excess of thyroid hormones causes increased resorption of bone. The excretion of calcium, phosphorus, and hydroxyproline in the urine increases. A few patients are hypercalcemic, but in most, the concentrations of calcium and phosphorus in the plasma are normal. Increased deposition of new bone sometimes increases the activity of alkaline phosphatase in the plasma. The resorption of bone is not usually severe enough to be evident radiologically, but occasionally causes severe osteoporosis.

The heart rate is increased. The heart sounds are loud. A systolic murmur is usual. Stroke volume and cardiac output are increased, often with elevation of the systolic blood pressure but depression of the diastolic pressure. The peripheral resistance is decreased, with peripheral vasodilation and a shortened circulation time. Extrasystoles are common. Paroxysmal atrial tachycardia or atrial fibrillation occur in 10% of the patients. The patient often complains of palpitations or precordial pain. Congestive heart failure is not uncommon. The effect of digitalis is reduced.

The cardiac hyperactivity results from the excess of the thyroid hormones and from the potentiation of the catecholamines caused by the hyperthyroidism. The foci of necrosis and round cell infiltration sometimes found in the myocardium are caused by the overaction of the catecholamines.

The increased appetite usual in hyperthyroidism results from the hypermetabolic state and serves to reduce the loss of weight that would otherwise occur. Hyperactivity of the intestinal muscle causes diarrhea in 25% of the patients. Sometimes there is abdominal pain. The liver is often palpable. The level of albumin in the plasma may be decreased, and the concentration of globulin increased. There may be hypoprothrombinemia, retention of sulfobromophthalein (Bromsulphalein)

or hypocholesterolemia. Rarely there is jaundice. Biopsy of the liver usually shows little abnormality. Some glycogen may be lost. The mitochondria in the liver cells are swollen, as they are in other cells in hyperthyroidism. In severe hyperthyroidism, there is sometimes necrosis or fibrosis around the terminal hepatic veins.

Mild to moderate hyperplasia of the adrenal cortex is common in hyperthyroidism. The excess of thyroid hormones increases the activity of the enzymes that degrade cortisol in the liver. The concentration of cortisol in the plasma tends to fall, and in consequence the secretion of the adrenocorticotropic hormone increases. Hyperplasia of the adrenal cortex results. The increased turnover of cortisol increases the excretion of 17-hydroxycorticoids in the urine. Hyperthyroidism favors the production of 5-α metabolites of testosterone like androsterone, rather than 5-β metabolites like etiocholanolone.

Menstruation may be normal in women with hyperthyroidism, but often there is oligomenorrhea or amenorrhea. In men, there is occasionally gynecomastia. Fertility is reduced, but libido is sometimes increased.

Mild hypervolemia is common in thyrotoxicosis, with an increase in blood volume of less than 10%. About 30% of the patients have mild normocytic normochromic anemia. Sometimes there is an absolute lymphocytosis. Occasionally the lymph nodes, thymus, and spleen are enlarged.

Oxygen consumption increases in hyperthyroidism, because of the increased metabolic activity caused by the excess of thyroid hormones. The basal metabolic rate increases, though if the hyperthyroidism is mild, the increase may not be great. The utilization of oxygen by the muscles is inefficient, so that muscular work requires 40% more oxygen than in normal people.

Hyperthyroidism increases the absorption of glucose from the gut. If glucose is given by mouth, the concentration of glucose in the plasma rises rapidly to a peak of perhaps 10 mmol/L (200 mg/100 mL) within an hour, but the removal of glucose from the plasma is equally rapid, and its concentration in the blood falls to normal within two hours. There may be glycosuria at the peak of the hyperglycemia. Hyperthyroidism increases the demand for insulin and may aggravate or induce diabetes mellitus.

Both the anabolism and catabolism of protein are increased in hyperthyroidism, with increased excretion of nitrogen. The plasma lipids tend to be in the lower range of normal.

Thyroid Storm. A thyroid storm, or thyroid crisis, is a sudden exacerbation in the severity of hyperthyroidism. It used to occur in the postoperative period in patients who had undergone thyroidectomy while still greatly hyperthyroid, after preparation with iodine, the only drug then available. It has become rare since patients coming to surgery for hyperthyroidism have been prepared with drugs related to thiourea that deplete the stores of hormone in the thyroid. Occasionally a storm is caused by serious infection in a patient with hyperthyroidism.

There is usually a dramatic onset of fever of 41°C or more, with tachycardia, nausea, vomiting, diarrhea, dehydration, often delirium, or coma. Less often, there is apathy, weakness, a little fever, or increase in pulse rate. Any of the manifestations of hyperthyroidism can be exaggerated. Congestive heart failure may worsen rapidly. Cardiac arrhythmia is common. Injury to the liver may bring jaundice. Abdominal pain may be prominent. Many of the patients die, usually of congestive heart failure or hyperpyrexia.

Treatment and Prognosis. Often hyperthyroidism is treated by giving prophylthiouracil or a similar drug to block the synthesis of the thyroid hormones and restore euthyroidism. In many patients, the drug can be withdrawn after one or two years, and the patient will remain euthyroid.

Iodine rapidly suppresses the secretion of the thyroid hormones, though its effect is usually short-lived. It is valuable if hyperthyroidism is severe and a rapid reduction in the secretion of the thyroid hormones is needed. Dexamethasone has a similar effect.

If the antithyroid drugs cannot control the hyperthyroidism, the quantity of thyroid tissue can be reduced by subtotal thyroidectomy or by administering radioactive iodine. Thyroidectomy is usually preferred in people under 40 years old to avoid the risk of carcinoma from irradiation of the thyroid. Radioactive iodine is usually preferred in older people. Especially with radioactive iodine,

hypothyroidism may follow and must be controlled by administering thyroid hormone.

Propranolol or some other adrenergic antagonist reduces the nervousness, tremor, sweating, and other signs of hypercatecholaminism.

HYPOTHYROIDISM

Inadequate secretion of the thyroid hormones for a prolonged period causes hypothyroidism. Severe hypothyroidism in an adult is called myxedema, from the Latin for slime or mucus, or Gull's disease after Sir William Gull, the English physician who described it in 1874. Severe hypothyroidism in a young child is called cretinism, from the Swiss word for Christian. Hypothyroidism in an older child is called juvenile hypothyroidism. Severe hypothyroidism is now rare, and even mild hypothyroidism is unusual.

ADULT HYPOTHYROIDISM. In a adult, hypothyroidism is usually caused by partial destruction of the thyroid by radiation or surgery. It can be caused by thyroiditis, a congenital defect in the enzymes needed for the synthesis of the thyroid hormones, or iodine deficiency. Thiocyanate, para-aminosalicylate, resorcinol, lithium, phenylbutazone, iodides, and other drugs sometimes cause hypothyroidism.

In 5% of the patients, hypothyroidism is due to lack of the thyroid-stimulating hormone caused by disease of the pituitary gland or hypothalamus. Pituitary adenomata, other tumors in the region of the pituitary or hypothalamus, trauma, and Sheehan's syndrome are other causes.

Clinical Presentation. The onset of hypothyroidism is usually slow, taking several years. Only iatrogenic hypothyroidism is likely to develop more rapidly. Often an increasing dislike of cold is one of the first symptoms. Commonly the patient becomes dull, listless, or drowsy. Sometimes constipation, menorrhagia, or gain in weight is the first sign of the disease. Occasionally the slow onset of hypothyroidism passes unnoticed until there is loss of hair, coarsening of the speech, puffiness of the face, or deafness.

Dysfunction. As the lack of thyroid hormones causes a fall in the metabolic rate, the patient becomes increasingly sluggish. All reactions are delayed and depressed. The electroencephalogram is flattened and of low voltage. Numbness and tingling in the limbs are common. Both nerve and conduction deafness are frequent. Nearly 70% of the patients complain of dizziness, vertigo, or tinnitus. Hallucinations, psychosis, and convulsions may develop.

The face becomes swollen, puffy, pale, yellowish, and expressionless. If addressed, the patient smiles and responds only after a delay. The eyelids are particularly swollen. The palpebral fissures are narrowed. The skin is thickened, cold, dry, and rough, often with fine wrinkles or scaliness. The thickened skin does not pit on pressure, but there may be pitting edema around the ankles. The tongue is often large and smooth, sometimes red.

The hair becomes dry and brittle and tends to fall out. The eyebrows may be lost. Shaving and hair cuts are rarely needed. The nails are thick and brittle. The voice becomes deep and coarse, in part from the swelling of the vocal cords, in part from the thickening of the tongue and lips. Speech is slow, deliberate, and often slurred.

The thickening of the skin and other tissues is caused by an increase in ground substance that separates and sometimes splits the collagen bundles. The ground substance is especially rich in hyaluronic acid. The hyaluronic acid and other mucopolysaccharide bind water to add to the swelling of the tissues.

The skeletal muscles may be normal but sometimes are weak and flabby. The duration of the reflexes is increased. The contraction and relaxation of the muscle fibers are slowed. Occasionally, the muscles become hypertrophic. The excretion of creatine in the urine is normal or low. The clearance of creatine from the blood by the muscles is normal or increased.

The capsules of the joints are often thickened. Fluid may be increased in the joint spaces. The formation and resorption of bone are depressed. Occasionally there is hypercalcemia. Parathyroid function is not affected.

The heart beats slowly. It is dilated and hypotonic, and its contractility is reduced. Stroke volume and cardiac output fall, per-haps to half normal. The electrocardiogram may be normal, or its voltage may be low. The peripheral resistance increases. The blood flow to the tissues and the uptake of oxygen by the tissues are reduced. Sometimes there is a pericardial effusion. Some think that myxedema accelerates the development of atherosclerosis.

Rarely, a patient with myxedema has angina pectoris. More often angina pectoris develops as the work of the heart increases when the hypothyroidism is treated. Digitalis does not improve the cardiac dysfunction caused by myxedema, and the patients tolerate it badly. The blood levels of digitalis in patients with myxedema are higher than in normal people given a similar dose.

Anorexia is common in myxedema. The sluggish movements of the intestinal muscle often cause constipation. Gaseous distention may be troublesome. Absorption from the gut is reduced. A glucose tolerance curve rises slowly, to a peak lower than normal, and the return to the baseline is delayed. The activity of the aminotransferases in the plasma may increase. Probably the increase is due to decreased catabolism of the enzymes, not to liver damage. Hypercholesterolemia is common.

Patients with myxedema caused by Hashimoto's disease or primary atrophy of the thyroid often have antibodies against the parietal cells of the gastric mucosa or against the intrinsic factor. About 50% of these people have achlorhydria, and 10% have pernicious anemia.

The level of cortisol in the plasma is usually normal in hypothyroidism. The turnover of cortisol is reduced, as both utilization and production fall. The adrenal cortex reacts slowly and inadequately to stress or to administered adrenocorticotropic hormone. The production of etiocholanolone is increased, and that of androsterone is reduced. The concentration of norepinephrine in the plasma is increased about three times, but the concentration of epinephrine is normal. The urinary excretion of catecholamines is normal, but the response of the body to the catecholamines is reduced.

Menorrhagia is common in premenopausal women with hypothyroidism, though sometimes there is amenorrhea. Libido and fertility are usually decreased. Men with myxedema are often impotent.

Hypovolemia and anemia are frequent. The concentrations of thromboplastins and the antihemophilic globulin in the plasma are often reduced. Capillary fragility is sometimes increased. Several factors combine to cause the anemia. The reduced consumption of oxygen in the tissues increases the oxygen tension in the tissues and inhibits the production of erythropoietin. Often there is malabsorption of vitamin B12 and folic acid. Menorrhagia can cause iron deficiency. The anemia is usually normocytic or macrocytic, but may be hypochromic. The concentration of hemoglobin in the plasma can be as low as 80 g/L (8 g/100 mL).

As oxygen utilization falls in hypothyroidism, the basal metabolic rate falls in severe myxedema to between 50 and 75% of normal. Anabolism and catabolism of protein are both reduced. The nitrogen balance is usually positive.

Iodine uptake is low or absent. The concentration of free and bound thyroxine in the plasma is reduced. The concentration of triiodothyronine in the plasma is reduced, though the reduction is usually less than the reduction in thyroxine. The concentration of the thyroxine-binding globulin may increase. The concentration of the thyroid-stimulating hormone is increased.

Treatment and Prognosis. All signs and symptoms of hypothyroidism in an adult can be reserved by giving thyroid hormone. The concentration of the thyroid-stimulating hormone in the plasma begins to fall within a few hours and reaches normal in one to two weeks. The pulse quickens, the cardiac output increases. Within two or three days, a striking diuresis occurs as the excess of mucopolysaccharides in the ground substance breaks down and the water bound in the tissues escapes, first into the blood to restore the blood volume and then into the urine. The puffiness of the face improves within a few days though it is weeks or months before the coarse skin reverts to normal and the hair regrows. Initiative and activity reappear. Speech improves rapidly.

Occasionally the improvement is too great. Especially in old people, palpitations, angina pectoris, or pains in the muscles occur if treatment is too energetic. Sometimes a patient becomes temporarily psychotic.

CRETINISM. If severe hypothyroidism develops in utero or in infancy, mental and physical development are distorted. The children affected are called cretins. Endemic cretinism used to be common in regions in which iodine was deficient. The occasional cretins found in other parts of the world are said to have sporadic cretinism.

Sporadic Cretinism. In the parts of the world in which endemic cretinism does not occur, hypothyroidism develops in 1 infant in 5000, though it is not always severe. In 70% of infants with sporadic cretinism, the dysfunction is caused by aplasia or hypoplasia of the thyroid. In some it is due to an antithyroid or radioactive drug given during pregnancy. These agents can cross the placenta and severely injure the fetus. Occasionally sporadic cretinism is caused by a deficiency of one of the enzymes needed for the synthesis of the thyroid hormones.

Clinical Presentation. Sporadic cretinism is rarely evident at birth. It becomes manifest only after weeks or months. The expression of the infant becomes heavy, the complexion yellowish, the eyes piglike. Neonatal jaundice is often prolonged, because hypothyroidism delays the maturation of the enzymes needed for the conjugation of bilirubin. Hypothermia is common. The belly is protruberant, often with an umbilical hernia. The skin becomes flabby and coarse. The hair is dry and thick. Constipation is common. Reflexes are slow. Occasionally the heart is enlarged, with congestive heart failure.

As the child ages, the face becomes round, stupid, yellowish, perhaps with a malar flush. The nose is flat and wide, the forehead is narrow, and the lips are thick. Saliva drools from the open mouth, and the big tongue protrudes. The voice is harsh. Respiratory difficulties are common. The pulse is slow. Anemia is usually present. The patient is slow, placid, and stupid.

If the hypothyroidism is severe, the cretin becomes a dwarf, with short, thick neck and with limbs too short in relation to the trunk. The centers of ossification in the limbs fail to develop normally, and the closure of the epiphyses is delayed. When ossification of the epiphyses does occur, it is irregular and patchy, so that in a roentgenogram the bone looks moth-eaten, a change called epiphyseal dysgenesis. The fontanelles are large and slow to close, so that the head grows large. Distortion of the femoral head gives a waddling gait. The appearance of the teeth is delayed. Sexual development occurs late if at all. Often muscular coordination is poor. Sometimes there is spastic diplegia a squint, or the muscles are hypertrophied. The pituitary is enlarged because of the hyperplasia and hypertrophy of the cells that secrete the thyroid-stimulating hormone.

Mental development is impaired. An untreated sporadic cretin may be anything from a helpless idiot to a placid, indolent, but self-sufficient moron.

Hypothyroidism can be diagnosed at birth by estimating the concentrations of thyroxine and thyroid-stimulating hormones in the infant's plasma. In hypothyroidism, the concentration of thyroxine is low, and the concentration of the thyroid-stimulating hormone is high. In some hospitals, all newborn infants are tested, because if an infant is hypothyroid, it is urgent to begin treatment immediately to avoid cretinism.

Treatment and Prognosis. If adequate doses of thyroid hormone are begun within weeks of birth and continued for the rest of the patient's life, normal development and normal intelligence are possible, though they are not always achieved. If treatment is not begun until the child is six months or a year old, some mental retardation, some neurologic deficit, and some distortion of growth are almost inevitable. If treatment is not begun until the child is five or more years old, treatment may only worsen the cretin's disposition, without achieving any improvement of the patient's mental or physical state.

Endemic Cretinism. Iodine deficiency is the major cause of endemic cretinism. In some villages in the Himalayas, Zaire, and the Andes in which there is severe iodine deficiency, more than 10% of the villagers are mentally retarded, though all do not show the other features of cretinism. Less often, goitrogens from plants or bacteria or inbreeding among the villagers cause hypothyroidism. Sometimes, more than one factor is involved.

Clinical Presentation. Two types of ende-

mic cretinism, called myxedematous cretinism and neurologic cretinism, are distinguished. In Zaire, the myxomatous form is predominant; in the Andes the neurologic form is more common; but both types occur in both regions. Some patients show an admixture of the myxomatous and neurologic forms of the disease. Some suffer only some of the abnormalities caused by hypothyroidism. Like sporadic cretinism, endemic cretinism is not evident at birth, but appears months or years later.

Myxomatous cretins have severe mental retardation and severe distortion of growth. They are slow and sluggish and show all the features of severe adult hypothyroidism. They are not deaf or mute. The thyroid is usually of normal size.

The neurologic cretins are also severely retarded mentally, but the retardation of growth is less marked. Most of the. patients are deaf and mute. The deafness appears to be central in origin. Often there is muscular spasticity, squint, or gross muscular incoordination. Flexion deformities are often present. Usually there is a nodular goiter, but sometimes the thyroid is atrophic.

In both forms of endemic cretinism, the diagnosis can be made before severe malformations appear by demonstrating that the concentration of thyroxine in the plasma is low and the concentration of the thyroid-stimulating hormone is high.

Treatment and Prognosis. Endemic cretinism can be prevented. Whether or not iodine deficiency is the only factor involved in its causation, supplementation of the diet with iodine usually prevents the disease. If the disease cannot be prevented, serious malformation can be avoided by giving thyroid hormone to the children born hypothyroid.

JUVENILE HYPOTHYROIDISM. Hashimoto's disease is the most common cause of hypothyroidism in an older child. Less often, the dysfunction is caused by deficiency on one of the enzymes involved in the synthesis of thyroid hormones.

The child shows changes intermediate between those of sporadic creatinism and adult hypothyroidism. Any of the abnormalities of adult hypothyroidism can develop, but they are not often severe. Some degree of mental and physical retardation is usual. Their severity depends on the severity of the hypothyroidism and the age of the child. Puberty is usually delayed, but it may be accelerated. In milder cases, the disease often goes undetected for years.

BIBLIOGRAPHY

General

Barnes, L., and Johnson, J. T.: Clinical and pathological considerations in the evaluation of major head and neck specimens resected for cancer. Pathol. Ann., 21 (Pt. 1): 173, (Pt.2):83, 1986.

Compagno, J.: Diseases of the thyroid. In Surgical Pathology of the Head and Neck. Edited by L. Barnes. New York, Marcel Dekker, 1985.

Livolsi, V. A., and Merino, M. J.: Histopathologic differential diagnosis of the thyroid. Pathol. Annu., 16 (Pt. 2):357–6, 1981.

Sommers, S. C.: Thyroid Gland. In Endocrine Pathology, 2nd ed. Edited by J. M. B. Bloodworth, Jr. Baltimore, Williams & Wilkins, 1982.

Thyroiditis

Bach, J. F.: Antireceptor or antihormone autoimmunity and its relationship to the idiotype network. Adv. Nephrol., 16:251, 1987.

Belfiore, A., et al. Epidemiology of autoallergic human thyroiditis. Monogr. Allergy, 21:215, 1987.

Bigazzi, P. E.: Anti-idiotypic immunity and autoimmunity. Ann. N. Y. Acad. Sci., 475:66, 1986.

Bigazzi, P. E., and Rose, N. R.: Autoimmune thyroid disease. In The Autoimmune Diseases. Edited by N. R. Rose and I. R. Mackay. Orlando, Academic Press, 1985.

Bottazzo, G. F., and Doniach, D.: Autoimmune thyroid disease. Annu. Rev. Med., 37:353, 1986.

Burek, C. L., and Rose, N. R.: Cell-mediated immunity in autoimmune thyroid disease. Hum. Pathol., 17:246, 1986.

Canonica, G. W., Bagnasco, M., and Kong, Y. M.: T-cell mediated mechanisms in autoimmune thyroiditis. Immunol. Res., 5:305, 1986.

Davies, T.F., et al.: Thyroid cell class II antigens: a perspective on the aetiology of autoimmune thyroid disease. Acta Endocrinol. Scand. (Suppl), 281:13, 1987.

Fisher, D. A., Pandian, M. R., and Carlton, E.: Autoimmune thyroid diseases. Pediatr. Clin. North Am., 34:907, 1987.

Hay, I. D.: Thyroiditis: a clinical update. Mayo Clin. Proc., 60:836, 1985.

Kalderon, A. E.: Emerging role of immune complexes in autoimmune thyroiditis. Pathol. Annu., 15 (Pt. 1):23, 1980.

van Ouwerkerk, B. M., et al.: Autoimmunity of thyroid disease. Neth. J. Med., 28:32, 1985.

Piccinini, L. A., Roman, S. H., and Davies, T. F.:

Autoimmune thyroid disease and thyroid cell class II major histocompatibility complex antigens. Clin. Endocrinol., 26:253, 1987.

Straskosch, C. R.: Thyroiditis. Aust. N.Z. J. Med., 16:91, 1986.

Volpé, R.: Autoimmune thyroid disease. Mol. Biol. Med., 3:25, 1986.

Hyperplasia

Bach, J. F.: Antireceptor or antihormone autoimmunity and its relationship to the idiotype network. Adv. Nephrol., 16:251, 1987.

Bigazzi, P. E.: Anti-idiotypic immunity and autoimmunity. Ann. N.Y. Acad. Sci., 475:66, 1986.

Bigazzi, P. E., and Rose, N. R.: Autoimmune thyroid disease. In The Autoimmune Diseases. Edited by N. R. Rose, and I. R. Mackay. Orlando, Academic Press, 1985.

Bottazzo, G. F., and Doniach, D.: Autoimmune thyroid disease. Annu. Rev. Med., 37:353, 1986.

Burek, C. L., and Rose, N. R.: Cell-mediated immunity in autoimmune thyroid disease. Hum. Pathol., 17:246, 1986.

Burman, K. D., and Baker, J. R., Jr.: Immune mechanisms in Graves' disease. Endocr. Rev., 6:183, 1985.

Chopra, I. J., and Solomon, D. H.: Pathogenesis of hyperthyroidism. Annu. Rev. Med., 34:267, 1983.

Davies, T. F., et al., Thyroid cell class II antigens: a perspective on the aetiology of autoimmune thyroid disease. Acta Endocrinol. Scand. [Suppl], 281:13, 1987.

De Lellis, R. A., and Wolfe, H. J.: The pathobiology of the human calcitonin (C)-cell. Pathol. Annu., 16 (Pt. 2):25, 1981.

Fisher, D. A., Pandian, M. R., and Carlton, E.: Autoimmune thyroid diseases. Pediatr. Clin. North Am., 34:907, 1987.

Harrison, L. C.: Antireceptor antibodies. In The Autoimmune Diseases. Edited by N. R. Rose and I. R. Mackay. Orlando, Academic Press, 1985.

Ollis, C. A., Tomlinson, S., and Munro, D. S.: Thyroid stimulating immunoglobulins. Clin. Sci., 69:113, 1985.

van Ouwerkerk, B. M., et al., Autoimmunity of thyroid disease. Neth. J. Med., 28:32, 1985.

Piccinini, L. A., Roman, S. H., and Davies, T. F.: Autoimmune thyroid disease and thyroid cell class II major histocompatibility complex antigens. Clin. Endocrinol., 26:253, 1987.

Rees Smith, B., et al.: Thyrotropin receptor antibodies. Arzneimittelforschung, 35:1943, 1985.

Singh, S. P., Ellyin, F., Singh, S. K., and Yoon, B.: Elephantiasis-like appaearence of the upper and lower extremities in Graves' dermopathy. Am. J. Med. Sci., 290:73, 1985.

Volpé, R.: Autoimmune thyroid disease. Mol. Biol. Med., 3:25, 1986.

Volpé, R., Karlsson, A., Jansson, R., and Dahlberg. P. A.: Evidence that anthithyroid drugs induced remissions in Graves' disease by modulating thyroid cellular activity. Clin. Endocrinol., 25:452, 1986.

Congenital Anomalies

Case. W. G., Ausobsky, J., Smiddy, F. G., and High, A. S.: Primary follicular carcinoma arising in the thyroglossal tract. J. R. Coll. Surg. Edinb., *32*:250, 1987.

Tumors

Bäckdahl, M., et al.: Fine needle biopsy cytology and DNA analysis. Surg. Clin. North Am., *67*:197, 1987.

Bell. R.M.: Thyroid carcinoma. Surg. Clin. North Am., *66*:13, 1986.

Brown, C.L.: The solitary thyroid nodule. Rec. Adv. Histopathol., *11*:203, 1981.

Brunt, L. M., and Wells. S. A., Jr.: Advances in the diagnosis and treatment of medullary thyroid carcinoma. Surg. Clin. North Am., *67*:263, 1987.

Caracangiu, M. L., Zampi, G., and Rosai, J.: Papillary thyroid carcinoma. Pathol. Annu., *20* (Pt. 1):1, 1985.

De Lellis, R. A., and Wolfe, H. J.: The pathobiology of the human calcitonin (C)-cell. Pathol. Annu., *16* (Pt. 2):25, 1981.

DeLellis, R. A., et al.: Multiple endocrine neoplasia (MEN) syndromes. Int. Rev. Exp. Pathol., *28*:163, 1986.

Donnell, C. A., Pollock, W. J., and Sybers, W. A.: Thyroid carcinosarcoma. Arch. Pathol. Lab. Med., *111*:1169, 1987.

Gluck, W. L.: Thyroid and parathyroid cancer. Clin. Geriatr. Med., *3*:729, 1987.

Hamburger, J. I., and Hamburger S. W.: Fine needle biopsy of the thyroid. N. Y. State J. Med., *86*:241, 1986.

Hoffman, E.: Carcinoma of the thyroid. South. Med. J., *80*:741, 1987.

Johannessen, J. V., and Sobrinho-Simoes, M.: Papillary carcinoma of the human thyroid gland. An ultrastructural study. Prog. Surg. Pathol., *3*:111, 1981.

Johannessen, J. V., and Sobrinho-Simoes, M.: Welldifferentiated thyroid tumors. Pathol. Annu., *18* (Pt. 1):255, 1983.

Kahn, N. F., and Perzin, K. H.: Follicular carcinoma of the thyroid. Pathol. Annu., *18* (Pt. 1): 221, 1983.

Kameya, T., Shimosato, Y., Abe, K., and Takeuchi, T.: Morphologic and functional aspects of hormone-producing tumors. Pathol. Annu., *15* (Pt. 1):351, 1980.

Kraemer, B. B.: Frozen section diagnosis and the thyroid. Semin. Diagn. Pathol., *4*:169, 1987.

Mazzaferri, E. L.: Papillary thyroid carcinoma. Semin. Oncol., *14*:315, 1987.

Noguchi, S., and Murakami, N.: The value of lymphnode dissection in patients with differentiated thyroid cancer. Surg. Clin. North Am., *67*:251, 1987.

Oertel, J. E., and Heffess, C. S.: Lymphoma of the thyroid and related disorders. Semin. Oncol., *14*:333, 1987.

Saad, M. F., et al.: Medullary carinoma of the thyroid. Medicine, *63*:319, 1984.

Sheppard, M. C.: Serum thyroglobulin and thyroid cancer. Q. J. Med., *59*:429, 1986.

Sizemore, G. W.: Medullary carcinoma of the thyroid gland. Semin. Oncol., *14*:306, 1987.

Hyperthyroidism

Chopra, I. J., and Solomon, D. H.: Pathogenesis of hyperthyroidism. Annu. Rev. Med., *34*:267, 1983.

Stulberg, B. N., Licata, A. A., Bauer, T. W., and Belhobek, G. H.: Hyperparathryoidism, hyperthyroidism and Cushing's disease. Orthop. Clin. North Am., *15*:697, 1984.

Hypothyroidism

Bastenie, P. A. Bonnyns, M., and Vanhaelst, L.: Natural history of primary myxedema. Am. J. Med., *79*:91, 1985.

Dunger, D. B., and Grant, D. B.: Endocrine disorders: diabetes mellitus, congenital hypothyroidism, and congenital adrenal hyperplasia. Br. Med. Bull., *42*: 187, 1986.

Robuschi, C., et al.: Hypothyroidism in the elderly. Endocr. Rev.,*8*:142, 1987.

48

Parathyroid Glands

HYPERPLASIA and tumors are the major disorders of the parathyroid glands. Inflammation and cysts of the parathyroid glands are uncommon. Congenital anomalies involving the glands rarely cause parathyroid dysfunction.

HYPERPLASIA

Hyperplasia of the parathyroid glands may be primary or secondary. In primary hyperplasia, the cause of the hyperplasia is unknown. There is no abnormality of calcium metabolism other than that which results from the oversecretion of the parathyroid hormone caused by the hyperplasia. Secondary hyperplasia of the parathyroid glands is due to persistent hypocalcemia. The hypocalcemia causes increased secretion of parathyroid hormone. Hyperplasia of the parathyroid glands follows.

PRIMARY HYPERPLASIA. Primary hyperplasia of the parathyroid glands is uncommon. Only 15% of patients with hyperparathyroidism have primary hyperplasia.

Lesions. In primary hyperplasia of the parathyroid glands, all four glands are enlarged. The enlargement is usually greater than in secondary hyperplasia. The four glands weigh together from 150 mg to over 70 g. Their normal weight is 120 to 140 mg. Usually the enlargement affects principally the upper glands, which are often 3 to 30 times as big as the lower glands. Sometimes one of the glands is considerably larger than the other three. The enlarged glands are irregularly shaped and on cross section are often nodular. They are dark brown and soft. Cysts are common within them.

Microscopically, two types of primary hyperplasia of the parathyroid glands are distinguished, chief cell hyperplasia and clear cell hyperplasia. Chief cell hyperplasia is the more common.

Chief Cell Hyperplasia. In primary chief cell hyperplasia, the fat, which normally makes up about 50% of the volume of a parathyroid gland, is reduced or absent. Instead, the glands consist almost entirely of parathyroid cells. At first, the proliferation of the parathyroid cells is uniform throughout the glands. Later, it tends to become nodular. Sometimes the larger nodules compress the adjacent part of the gland. Chief cells are predominant. They are usually of normal size but may be larger than normal. Oxyphil cells are scattered among the chief cells and occasionally form nodules. Often a few clear cells or clumps of clear cells are present. Usually the cells are arranged in sheets and cords, but sometimes they form acini.

Clear Cell Hyperplasia. In primary clear cell hyperplasia, the enlarged glands consist entirely of large, well-defined cells with clear cytoplasm, called water-clear cells (wasserhelle cells—for those who prefer German). The clear cells may be arranged in clumps or cords or may line acini. They vary somewhat in size and have spheroidal, hyperchromatic nuclei. Mitoses are absent.

Dysfunction. Patients with primary hyperplasia of the parathyroid glands have hyperparathyroidism, though it is not usually severe. The parathyroid glands fail to respond to the increasing concentration of ionized calcium in the plasma and secrete inappropriately large quantities of parathyroid hormone.

Multiple Endocrine Neoplasia. Tumors or hyperplasia develop in one or more of the other endocrine glands in 15% of patients with primary hyperplasia of the parathyroid glands. Most have primary chief cell hyperplasia. In multiple endocrine neoplasia type I, the patients have hyperplasia or tumors of

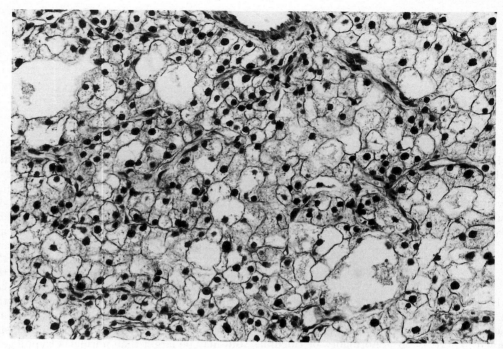

Fig. 48-1. Clear-cell hyperplasia of a parathyroid gland.

the islets of Langerhans, the adrenal cortices, or the pituitary. In multiple endocrine neoplasia type II, they have hyperplasia or tumors of the adrenal medullae or the parafollicular cells of the thyroid.

In some families, primary hyperplasia of the parathyroid glands, usually primary chief cell hyperplasia, is inherited as an autosomal dominant character with incomplete penetrance, but lesions do not develop in other endocrine glands. It may be that these people have an incomplete form of the multiple endocrine neoplasia syndrome.

Treatment and Prognosis. The treatment and prognosis of the various forms of hyperparathyroidism are discussed later in the chapter.

SECONDARY HYPERPLASIA. Secondary hyperplasia of the parathyroid glands develops when increased demand for the parathyroid hormone persists for months or years. Usually, the hyperplasia results from a tendency to hypocalcemia, which causes increased secretion of the parathyroid hormone.

Lesions. Secondary hyperplasia of the parathyroid glands can develop within a week, but the hyperplasia is rarely detected until hypersecretion of the parathyroid hormone has persisted for months or years. All four glands are affected. They may be normal in size or slightly enlarged. Only exceptionally do the four glands weigh together 3 or 4 g, rather than their normal 120 to 140 mg. Often the enlargement is greater in the inferior glands. The hyperplastic glands tend to be cream-colored rather than their normal brown and are often firmer than normal. If the hyperplasia is severe and long continued, the glands become nodular.

Microscopically, secondary hyperplasia of the parathyroid glands cannot be distinguished from primary chief cell hyperplasia. All four glands are affected. The fat normally present within the glands is reduced or lost. The glands consist of a uniform proliferation of parathyroid cells usually arranged in clumps or cords. Occasionally they form acini. Most of the cells are chief cells, but oxyphil cells are scattered among them and occasionally are numerous. Sometimes some of the cells have clear cytoplasm, though they are rarely as large as the cells of primary

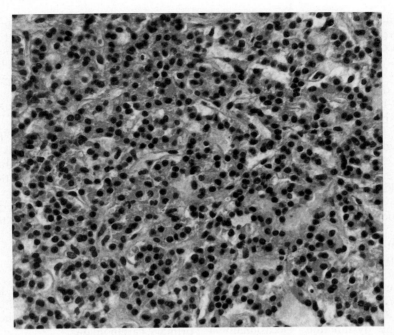

Fig. 48-2. Secondary hyperplasia of a parathyroid gland, showing the loss of fat and a proliferation of chief cells.

clear-cell hyperplasia of the parathyroid glands. If the glands have become nodular, some of the nodules may be comprised entirely of oxyphil cells or clear cells.

Pathogenesis. Chronic renal failure is the commonest cause of secondary hyperplasia of the parathyroid glands. As the glomerular filtration rate falls, the urinary excretion of phosphate becomes inadequate, and the concentration of phosphate in the plasma rises slightly. The hyperphosphatemia causes slight hypocalcemia by increasing the incorporation of calcium into the bones. The hypocalcemia causes increased secretion of the parathyroid hormone, which increases the urinary excretion of phosphate and leaches calcium from the bones into the plasma, restoring homeostasis if the reduction in glomerular filtration is not too great.

The increased concentration of the parathyroid hormone in the plasma also increases the formation of 1,25-dihydroxycholecalciferol in the kidneys. The cholecalciferol increases the absorption of calcium from the gut and augments the resorption of calcium from the bones, tending to restore homeostasis. It also reduces the urinary excretion of

phosphate, which tends to worsen the metabolic disorder.

The increased secretion of the parathyroid hormone in chronic renal failure can maintain homeostasis until the glomerular filtration rate falls to less than 25 mL/min. If the renal failure worsens further, hyperphosphatemia and hypocalcemia cannot be prevented. The bones become resistant to the parathyroid hormone as uremia develops.

Other conditions that demand continuing hypersecretion of the parathyroid hormone to prevent hyperphosphatemia and hypocalcemia cause secondary hyperplasia of the parathyroid glands in similar fashion. Vitamin D deficiency, vitamin D resistance, hyperphosphatemia, intestinal malabsorption, pseudohypoparathyroidism, renal tubular acidosis, and pregnancy, all tend to cause hypocalcemia and hyperplasia of the parathyroid glands. Occasionally hyperplasia of the parathyroid glands occurs in patients with extensive metastases to bone or other tumors for reasons that are not clear.

The concentration of magnesium in the tissue fluid affects the secretion of the parathyroid hormone. If magnesium is deficient, the stimulation of parathyroid function caused by hypocalcemia is inhibited. If magnesium is in excess, parathyroid secretion is stimulated.

Treatment and Prognosis. Secondary hyperplasia of the parathyroid glands is a response to disease elsewhere and usually does not require treatment. If the disease causing the hyperplasia is controlled, the parathyroid glands slowly return to normal.

OTHER NON-NEOPLASTIC DISORDERS

Inflammation of a parathyroid gland is rare. Cysts and congenital anomalies are common, but rarely cause dysfunction.

INFLAMMATION. Infection, infarction, and other inflammatory lesions of the parathyroid glands are rare. Hemorrhage into a parathyroid gland sometimes occurs at childbirth, but as there are four parathyroid glands it does not cause any dysfunction. Occasionally a parathyroid gland in an old person is scarred, perhaps from some long past inflammation, but again there are four parathyroid glands and so no dysfunction.

CYSTS. Microcysts filled with colloid are present in the parathyroid glands in 50% of people. They grow more frequent as age increases. The microcysts cause no dysfunction. Occasionally a parathyroid cyst is big enough to be evident clinically. It may press on the esophagus and cause dysphagia, displace the trachea, or drag on the recurrent laryngeal nerve and cause hoarseness. Large parathyroid cysts are thin-walled, filled with watery fluid, and are lined with flattened epithelium, with only a few remnants of the gland left in the wall of the cyst.

CONGENITAL ANOMALIES. Absence of the parathyroid glands or great reduction in the quantity of parathyroid tissue occurs together with thymic aplasia and other congenital anomalies in the DiGeorge syndrome, described in Chapter 10. Otherwise, aplasia or hypoplasia of the parathyroid glands is rare, though careful dissection may be necessary to find all four of the glands.

Malposition of otherwise normal parathyroid glands is common. Often one or both of the superior glands is embedded in the thyroid. In 10% of people, one or both of the inferior glands lies in the mediastinum, sometimes in the thymus. Sometimes one or more of the glands lies behind the esophagus or in some other part of the neck. The malposition causes no functional disability, but may pose a considerable problem if it is necessary to explore the parathyroid glands surgically.

In 2% of people, accessory parathyroid glands are present in the neck. As many as 12 discrete glands have been described. The accessory glands cause no dysfunction and can be identified only by careful dissection. Rarely, a parathyroid gland is enlarged by a hamartomatous mass of fibroadipose tissue.

TUMORS

Nearly all tumors of the parathyroid glands are primary. Over 99% of them are adenomata. Almost all the rest are primary carcinomata.

ADENOMA. Small adenomata of the parathyroid glands are common. Most produce no local symptoms and are detected only because of some complication of hyperparathyroidism or because the patient is found to be hypercalcemic. More than 80 people in every 100,000 have mild hyperparathyroidism caused by an adenoma.

Lesions. Nearly 75% of the adenomata of the parathyroid glands develop in the inferior glands. About 10% of them lie in the mediastinum, perhaps because of congenital misplacement of the gland, perhaps because the weight of the adenoma pulled the gland down into the mediastinum. The weight of an adenoma in one of the superior glands sometimes drags it down until the gland lies below the inferior gland. Rarely, a patient has more than one parathyroid adenoma.

An adenoma of a parathyroid gland is usually encapsulated, orange or brown, and soft. The tumor may be from 100 mg in weight to over 50 g. Most removed surgically are about 1 cm in diameter. Most are ovoid or lobulated. Often an adenoma contains small cysts filled with clear fluid or shows foci of hemorrhage or fibrosis.

Microscopically, most parathyroid adenomata consist principally of chief cells, arranged in sheets or cords or around acini.

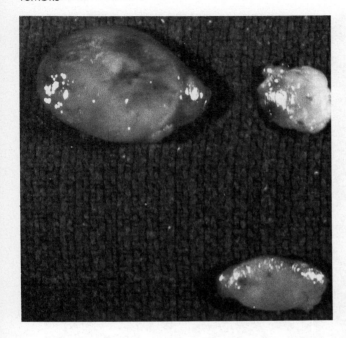

Fig. 48-3. An adenoma of a parathyroid gland. The gland at the upper left is largely replaced by the well demarcated adenoma. The other glands are enlarged by secondary hyperplasia.

Occasionally the acinar pattern is so marked that the adenoma looks like a tumor of the thyroid. In many adenomata, the chief cells are bigger than normal, sometimes twice the normal diameter, that is, 8 times the normal volume. Oxyphil cells and cells with clear cytoplasm are often scattered among the chief cells. Sometimes oxyphil cells or clear cells form clumps within an adenoma. Sometimes the clear cells are large, indistinguishable from the wasserhelle cells of primary clear-cell hyperplasia. Rarely, an adenoma is predominantly of oxyphil cells or clear cells. Occasional cells have large nuclei. Mitoses are rare.

By electron microscopy, the cells of a parathyroid adenoma contain granules like those of normal parathyroid cells. Rough endoplasmic reticulum is abundant, and the Golgi apparatus prominent. The stroma of the adenoma is fine, scant, and vascular. There is no fat in an adenoma. If hyperparathyroidism is severe, calcification of the stroma is common. The gland around the tumor is compressed, but is otherwise normal or shows secondary hyperplasia.

Dysfunction. Most parathyroid adenoma secrete excessive quantities of parathyroid hormone and cause hyperparathyroidism. The oversecretion is not usually great. There is a rough correlation between the size of the adenoma and the severity of the hyperparathyroidism.

Treatment and Prognosis. The treatment and prognosis of an adenoma of a parathyroid gland will be discussed later in the chapter when hyperparathyroidism is considered.

CARCINOMA. Carcinoma of the parathyroid glands is rare. Only about 50 cases have been reported. Almost all the tumors are well differentiated and cause hyperparathyroidism. More anaplastic carcinomata of the parathyroid glands are difficult to distinguish from a carcinoma of the thyroid.

Lesions. Macroscopically, a carcinoma of a parathyroid gland resembles an adenoma or forms a hard, sclerotic mass. Nearly always the carcinoma has extended beyond the parathyroid gland by the time it is discovered. Often it is attached to the esophagus, trachea, or some other neighboring structure.

Microscopically, the carcinoma usually has its cells arranged in a trabecular pattern. The cells are often cylindrical, bigger than the cells of an adenoma. There may be mild atypicality or pleomorphism. Mitoses are

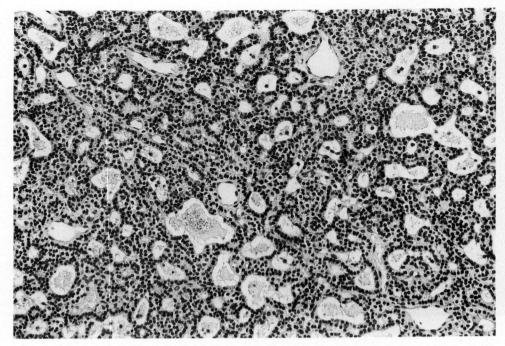

Fig. 48-4.   An adenoma of a parathyroid gland consisting of chief cells. The glandular arrangement sometimes seen in these tumors is evident.

always present and may be numerous. Vascular and lymphatic invasion can often be demonstrated.

Behavior.   A carcinoma of a parathyroid gland usually grows slowly. Most have metastases in the regional lymph nodes by the time the diagnosis is made. More distant metastases are usually late.

Treatment and Prognosis.   Carcinoma of a parathyroid gland is treated surgically. The prognosis is poor. It is usually impossible to remove the carcinoma completely. Recurrence in the neck is usual. Death often comes from uncontrollable hyperparathyroidism.

HYPERPARATHYROIDISM

Hyperparathyroidism is the term used to describe increased secretion of the parathyroid hormone. In primary hyperparathyroidism, the oversecretion results from disease of the parathyroid glands. In secondary hyperparathyroidism, it is caused by disease in some other part of the body. In tertiary hyperparathyroidism, a parathyroid adenoma complicates secondary hyperparathyroidism.

PRIMARY HYPERPARATHYROIDISM.   More than 100 people in every 100,000 secrete excessive quantities of the parathyroid hormone, though in most the excess is slight. Hyperparathyroidism can become evident at any age and becomes increasingly common as age increases. About 70% of the patients are women. Most are over 40 years old.

Nearly 85% of patients with primary hyperparathyroidism have an adenoma in one of the parathyroid glands. Occasionally, more than one gland has an adenoma. About 15% of the patients have primary hyperplasia of the glands, usually chief cell hyperplasia. Less than 1% have carcinoma of a parathyroid gland. In a few patients, a parathormone-like substance secreted by a carcinoma of the lung or some other tumor has caused hyperparathyroidism. In most patients with hypercalcemia caused by a tumor, the hypercalcemia is caused by other mechanisms.

Clinical Presentation.   In 50% of patients

with primary hyperparathyroidism, nephrolithiasis is the first sign of the disease. About 5% of people with renal stones have hyperparathyroidism. In another 30% of the patients, hyperparathyroidism is discovered when the patient is found to be hypercalcemic. Occasionally nausea, fatigue, constipation, weakness, or muscular atrophy is the first sign of the disease.

Dysfunction. In primary hyperparathyroidism, the target organs respond normally to the excess of parathyroid hormone. In the kidneys, the resorption of calcium and the excretion of phosphorus are increased. In the gut, the absorption of calcium is increased, because the parathyroid hormone increases the conversion of 25-hydroxycholecalciferol to 1,25-dihydroxycholecalciferol in the kidneys. In bone, increased quantities of calcium, phosphorus, and matrix are resorbed.

Hypercalcemia is not usually severe. In 30% of the patients, the concentration of calcium in the plasma is below 2.75 mmol/L (11 mg/100 mL). In some, it is in the upper part of the normal range. Many of these people with little increase in the concentration of calcium in the blood plasma have intermittent episodes of more marked hypercalcemia. Repeated estimations of the calcium level may be necessary to detect the elevation. If a patient suspected of hyperparathyroidism has malabsorption, pancreatitis, or some other condition that reduces the concentration of calcium in the plasma, the failure to demonstrate hypercalcemia is of little significance. If the concentration of albumen and other proteins that bind calcium is low in the plasma, the total concentration of calcium in the plasma will be reduced.

The excretion of calcium in the urine is increased in nearly 80% of patients with primary hyperparathyroidism who have good renal function, less often in patients with impaired renal function. The daily loss of calcium in the urine may be as much as twice normal. The resorption of calcium from bone and its absorption from the gut are so great that the increased resorption of calcium by the renal tubules is insufficient to prevent its loss in the urine. The loss of calcium in the urine is less in patients with renal failure because as glomerular filtration falls, the quantity of calcium reaching the tubules becomes less, and so hypercalciuria becomes less likely.

The concentration of phosphate in the plasma is often low, less than 1.1 mmol/L (3.5 mg/100 mL), though in 50% of the patients it is within the normal range. If renal failure or some other condition prevents the excretion of phosphate, its concentration in the plasma is likely to be normal.

The absorption of bicarbonate by the renal tubules is impaired in hyperparathyroidism. Instead, chloride is retained. The concentration of chloride in the plasma is almost always over 100 mmol/L (100 µEq/L). About 30% of the patients have hyperchloremia and mild metabolic acidosis.

The parathyroid hormone activates adenyl cyclase, increasing the production of cyclic adenosine monophosphate in the kidneys and elsewhere. Increased quantities of cyclic adenosine monophosphate escape into the urine, increasing the ratio of cyclic adenosine monophosphate to creatinine in the urine.

In most patients with primary hyperparathyroidism, the concentration of the parathyroid hormone in the plasma is elevated. In some, it is normal, though inappropriate for the level of calcium in the plasma. In a person with normal parathyroid glands, hypercalcemia suppresses the secretion of the parathyroid hormone, and it becomes undetectable in the plasma.

In sarcoidosis, vitamin D toxicity, and other conditions that cause hypercalcemia, administration of prednisone or some other glucocorticoid greatly reduces the hypercalcemia or restores eucalcemia. In primary hyperparathyroidism, the corticosteroids have little or no effect on the hypercalcemia.

The renal stones in primary hyperparathyroidism consist of calcium oxalate, calcium phosphate, or some mixture of the two. Some patients have a history of repeated renal stones, sometimes a history going back many years. Sometimes only one kidney is involved. Urinary obstruction caused by the stones and other complications of nephrolithiasis are common.

Nephrocalcinosis is common in primary hyperparathyroidism. It may be slight, with little affect on function, or may cause progressive renal failure. If the renal damage is severe, relief of the hyperparathyroidism will do little to improve renal function. The scarred, calcified kidneys cannot be repaired. Sometimes the renal damage causes secondary hyperthyroidism, which causes continued hypersecretion of the parathyroid hormone, even if the primary hyperparathyroidism is controlled.

Most patients with primary hyperparathyroidism have only mild changes in the bones. The severe bony disease called osteitis fibrosa cystica, which once was thought characteristic of hyperparathyroidism, is now uncommon.

Radiologically, there may be slight, generalized osteoporosis. Often the bony resorption is seen best radiologically in the terminal phalanges of the fingers, where subperiosteal loss of cortical bone destroys the sharp outline normally found in the terminal phalanges. There may be loss of the lamina densa around the teeth, spotty decalcification of the inner or outer tables of the skull, rarefaction of the distal part of the clavicles, or erosion of the cortex of the symphysis pubis and sacroiliac joints. The bones may become tender or painful or may break easily. In up to 50% of the patients, the resorption of bone is sufficient to cause an increase in the activity of alkaline phosphatase in the plasma and increased excretion of hydroxproline in the urine.

Microscopically, the bones usually show thinning of their trabeculae, with an increase in osteoclasts and osteoclastic activity, and sometimes replacement of the fatty marrow by fibrosis. The more serious bony changes in hyperparathyroidism are described with the diseases of bone in Chapter 59.

Metastatic calcification is common in the soft tissues, though in primary hyperparathyroidism it is not usually severe. There may be foci of calcification in the conjunctivae. Calcification in the corneae can cause hazy bands of opacity concentric with the limbus, an appearance called band keratopathy. There may be calcification of the alveolar walls in the lungs, the mucosa of the stomach, the myocardium, or the arteries. A band of calcification sometimes develops in the articular cartilages.

Mental disturbances are common in hyperparathyroidism. They can range from a minor change in personality or minor mental impairment to major psychosis. If the hypercalcemia becomes high, confusion, stupor, or coma are common.

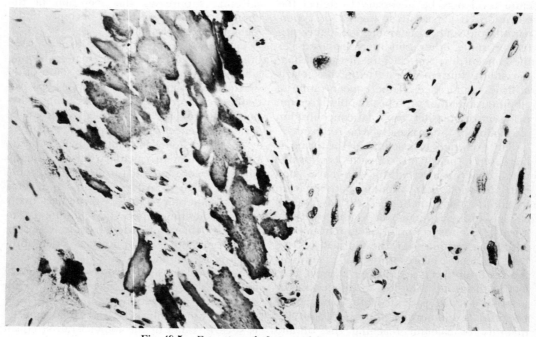

Fig. 48-5. Extensive calcification of the myocardium.

The hypercalcemia can induce muscular weakness and hypotonia, with weak or absent reflexes. Sometimes the weakness and wasting are most prominent in the proximal muscles of the limbs.

A peptic ulcer develops in the duodenum in 15% of patients with hyperparathyroidism. Some of these people have both hyperparathyroidism and the Zollinger-Ellison syndrome, but most of them have no demonstrable abnormality in the islets of Langerhans or their secretions. Acute pancreatitis occurs with increased frequency in people with hyperparathyroidism. Sometimes the pancreatitis renders the patient hypocalcemic, in spite of the hyperparathyroidism. Constipation is common.

The hypercalcemia can interfere with the absorption of sodium in the kidneys, causing polyuria and loss of the power to concentrate the urine. Polydipsia or dehydration can follow.

The concentration of calcium in the plasma bears little relation to the severity of the symptoms in primary hyperparathyroidism. In some people, even a slight increase in the concentration of calcium causes considerable distress. Others have few if any symptoms, even though the concentration of calcium in the plasma is over 3.75 mmol/L (15 mg/100 mL).

Occasionally, the hypercalcemia increases suddenly, perhaps to more than 4.50 mmol/L (18 mg/100 mL). All the symptoms of hyperparathyroidism worsen rapidly. Vomiting, dehydration, azotemia, and stupor often lead to death. Most often a parathyroid crisis of this sort results from hemorrhage into an adenoma or infarction of an adenoma, with sudden release of the hormone stored in the injured cells.

Treatment and Prognosis. In some patients with primary hyperparathyroidism, no treatment is needed. Especially if the patient is old, and there is only mild hypercalcemia, with few if any symptoms, hydration may restore the calcium level to normal. If there are mild symptoms, giving phosphate to raise the concentration of phosphate in the plasma lowers the concentration of calcium and may bring relief, though it increases the risk of metastatic calcification.

If primary hyperparathyroidism is more severe, it is treated surgically. The operation is not easy because the parathyroid glands are small and hard to find. Their position and their number vary from person to person. Usually it is impossible to be sure preoperatively if the patient has an adenoma or primary hyperplasia. If an adenoma is present, it is often impossible to determine its position preoperatively.

If a lesion thought to be an adenoma is found, it is removed. If a quick section confirms that the lesion is an adenoma microscopically, at least one more parathyroid gland is removed. If a quick section shows that it is normal microscopically, some surgeons proceed no further. They assume that the other glands are also normal. Others prefer to take a biopsy of all parathyroid glands to ensure that the patient does not have primary hyperplasia of the parathyroid glands, with a particularly large nodule in one of the glands.

If no adenoma is found, and biopsies of the parathyroid glands show changes that on quick section are consistent with primary hyperplasia, most surgeons remove three of the glands entirely and part of the fourth. Because of the risk of hypoparathyroidism if enough tissue is not left to maintain normal function, some surgeons implant intramuscularly a mince of some of the glandular tissue removed to ensure that the patient will have enough parathyroid tissue to maintain homeostasis.

It is not easy for a pathologist examining a frozen section to decide whether a lesion in a parathyroid gland is an adenoma or primary hyperplasia. The decision is most certain if normal parathyroid tissue can be seen around the adenoma. If the gland is completely replaced by abnormal tissue, it may be impossible to decide whether the lesion is an adenoma or hyperplasia.

If the treatment is successful, the concentration of calcium in the plasma falls to normal within 24 hours of the operation. Mild hypocalcemia may follow and often persists for four or five days before the remaining parathyroid tissue resumes normal function. If too much parathyroid tissue has been taken, more serious hypocalcemia develops and may persist for weeks or months. Hypomagnesemia can also develop postoperatively.

In some patients, hyperparathyroidism recurs after months or years. In primary hyperplasia, the tissue left behind continues to proliferate and eventually can become enough to cause hyperparathyroidism again. In patients with an adenoma, a second adenoma can develop in another of the parathyroid glands. Occasionally damage to the kidneys causes secondary hyperparathyroidism.

SECONDARY HYPERPARATHYROIDISM. In secondary hyperparathyroidism, the parathyroid glands secrete increased quantities of parathyroid hormone to meet an increased demand caused by disease in some other part of the body. Any condition that tends to cause hypocalcemia is likely to cause secondary hyperparathyroidism. Renal disease is its most common cause. The parathyroid glands respond normally, but because of the increased work soon develop secondary hyperplasia.

Clinical Presentation. Patients with secondary hyperparathyroidism have the signs and symptoms of the disease that causes the hyperparathyroidism. Only if the secondary hyperparathyroidism is unusually severe does renal osteodystrophy, calcification of soft tissues, or some other of the complications of hyperparathyroidism become evident.

Dysfunction. Secondary hyperparathyroidism is usually beneficial. In many patients, it restores the concentration of calcium in the tissues to normal and does no harm. Often the concentrations of calcium and phosphorus in the plasma remain normal. The secretion of the parathyroid hormone is increased, but a new equilibrium is established, and homeostasis is maintained.

Only if secondary hyperparathyroidism becomes extreme does it become dangerous. If the glomerular filtration rate falls below 25 mL/min in patients with severe renal disease, the increased secretion of the parathyroid hormone can no longer maintain homeostasis. Hypocalcemia and hyperphosphatemia become evident. The activation of vitamin D in the damaged kidneys is impaired. Acidosis or magnesium deficiency may further disturb the metabolism of calcium and phosphorus.

In adults, renal osteodystrophy follows, with osteoporosis, osteomalacia, osteitis fibrosa, or sometimes osteosclerosis. In children, there may be renal rickets. Sometimes calcification is widespread in the soft tissues, particularly in arteries outside the kidneys. The calcification of the arteries can cause gangrene. Sometimes pruritus is severe because of calcification in the skin. Calcification in the conjunctivae can cause conjunctivitis. Renal stones sometimes develop, though they are less common than in primary hyperparathyroidism.

Treatment and Prognosis. Secondary hyperparathyroidism usually needs no treatment. If the disease that causes the hyperparathyroidism is controlled, parathyroid function reverts to normal. If secondary hyperparathyroidism is severe, restriction of phosphorus in the diet or administration of vitamin D to increase the absorption of calcium may help. If bony disease is severe, partial parathyroidectomy may be necessary, but is likely to lead to hypoparathyroidism.

TERTIARY HYPERPARATHYROIDISM. Tertiary hyperparathyroidism is a complication of secondary hyperparathyroidism. In tertiary hyperparathyroidism, an adenoma develops in one of the glands of a patient with severe secondary hyperparathyroidism, or one or more of the hyperplastic nodules in parathyroid glands with secondary hyperplasia become partially autonomous and secrete excessive quantities of the parathyroid hormone, without regard to the needs of the body.

In tertiary hyperparathyroidism, any of the manifestations of primary hyperparathyroidism can be added to the changes of secondary hyperparathyroidism. Even if the disease that causes the secondary hyperparathyroidism is controlled, the adenoma or autonomous nodules of tertiary hyperparathyroidism continue to secrete excessive quantities of the parathyroid hormones, as in primary hyperparathyroidism, and hyperparathyroidism continues.

HYPOPARATHYROIDISM

If the secretion of the parathyroid hormone is insufficient to meet the body's demands, the patient is said to have hypoparathyroidism. In primary hypoparathyroidism, the deficiency is caused by disease of the parathyroid glands. In pseudohypoparathyroidism, the tissues fail to respond to the hormone. Pseudopseudohypoparathyroidism resembles pseudohypoparathyroidism, but the levels of calcium and phosphorus are normal and the tissues respond normally to the parathyroid hormone.

PRIMARY HYPOPARATHYROIDISM. Most often, primary hypoparathyroidism results from damage to the parathyroid glands caused by a surgical procedure. If too much tissue is removed by partial parathyroidectomy, hypoparathyroidism follows. Damage to the blood supply of the parathyroid glands during exploration of the neck for some other reason can cause hypoparathyroidism. Often the hypoparathyroidism caused by an operation is transient, and after a few days or weeks the parathyroid glands resume normal function. Sometimes it is delayed, becoming evident only weeks or months after the operation.

Idiopathic primary hypoparathyroidism is uncommon. It develops in adults. In some patients, the disease is familial. Some have in addition adrenocortical, thyroid, or ovarian deficiency or pernicious anemia. In these people the damage to the parathyroid glands may be caused immunologically, as in Hashimoto's disease or primary adrenocortical atrophy.

In infants, hypoparathyroidism may be due to the DiGeorge syndrome of thymic aplasia and parathyroid aplasia. It rarely is due to hypoplasia or aplasia of the parathyroid glands alone. More often, hypoparathyroidism in infants is transient and seems due to delayed development of the parathyroid glands. Transient hypoparathyroidism in the child is usual if the mother is hypercalcemic during pregnancy.

Clinical Presentation. If hypoparathyroidism develops quickly, patients have tetany or other signs of neurologic hyperexcitability. If it develops more slowly, changes in the skin or cataracts may first draw attention to the dysfunction of the parathyroid glands.

Dysfunction. The lack of the parathyroid hormone in hypoparathyroidism causes hypocalcemia and hyperphosphatemia. The resorption of calcium by the kidneys is reduced, and phosphate is retained. The resorption of calcium and phosphorus from the bones is reduced. The absorption of calcium from the gut is impaired. The parathyroid hormone is undetectable in the plasma or present in an inappropriately low concentration.

As the concentration of calcium in the tissue fluid falls, the excitability of the nerves increases. If the concentration of calcium becomes low enough, tetany results. Muscle spasm caused by the overactive motor nerves sometimes causes the characteristic main d'accoucheur. There may be spasm of the glottis, abdominal cramps, bronchospasm, or biliary colic. Tapping on a nerve excites muscle spasm in Chvostek's sign. Ischemia induces spasm in Trousseau's sign. Hyperkalemia, excitement, strain, or infection enhances tetany. Hypersensitivity of the sensory nerves causes paresthesia, usually of the hands or feet or around the mouth.

The tendon reflexes are at first increased, but as the hypocalcemia grows profound they disappear. There may be epileptiform seizures. The patient becomes irritable, depressed, confused, and perhaps hallucinatory. Long-continued hypoparathyroidism causes mental retardation in children.

The skin becomes coarse and dry. Eczema and psoriasis are common. The hair becomes thin and scant. The nails are brittle, with transverse grooves, and split easily. In children, the teeth erupt late and are hypoplastic, with defects in the enamel. Cataracts are common in the eyes if the hypoparathyroidism persists for a year or more. Monilial infections of the skin or nails are common in the idiopathic forms. Metastatic calcification may occur in the soft tissues, if the product of the concentrations of calcium and phosphorus in the plasma become high.

Some people are more sensitive to hypocalcemia than are others. Some develop symptoms when the concentration of calcium in the plasma is 2.1 mmol/L (8.5 mg/100 mL); others have no symptoms, though the concentration of calcium is 1.2 mmol/L (5 mg/100 mL). The more rapid the fall in the concentration of ionized calcium in the plasma, the higher the concentration of calcium at which symptoms are likely to appear.

Treatment and Prognosis. The immediate symptoms of tetany can be relieved by giving intravenous calcium. Longer term treatment is more difficult. Parathyroid hormone cannot be given by mouth, and a lifetime of injections is impractible. Sometimes calcium taken by mouth can restore the serum calcium close enough to normal, especially, when the hypoparathyroidism is only temporary. More often both vitamin D and calcium must be given by mouth. A satisfactory level of ionized calcium in the plasma can usually be achieved, but the treatment must be monitored carefully to avoid vitamin D intoxication.

Renal stones sometimes develop in patients with hypoparathyroidism treated with vitamin D and calcium. Without the parathyroid hormone, the kidneys cannot retain calcium normally. Hypercalciuria may be serious, even though the concentration of calcium in the plasma is in the low normal range.

PSEUDOHYPOPARATHYROIDISM.   Pseudohypoparathyroidism is a rare condition in which the kidneys and often other tissues fail to respond normally to the parathyroid hormone. In some patients, the fault is in the receptor that enables the parathyroid hormone to activate adenyl cyclase. In others, a later stage of the response is defective. Pseudohypoparathyroidism is sometimes inherited as an X-linked dominant character or as an autosomal dominant character with variable expressivity. About 70% of the patients are girls.

The disease becomes evident in childhood. The patient is short, thickset, and obese. The face is round; the nose flat. Some of the metacarpals, especially the fourth and fifth, are short because of premature closure of their epiphyses. Some of the metatarsals are affected similarly, though less severely. There may be multiple exostoses. Calcification of the basal ganglia is common. Plaques of calcification or ossification are common in the skin. The teeth appear late. Some patients have cataracts; some have hypertension; some have deficiency of the thyrotropic hormone and hypothyroidism. Mental retardation is common.

Because the renal tubules cannot respond adequately to the parathyroid hormone, calcium is lost in the urine and phosphate is retained. Most patients have hypocalcemia and hyperphosphatemia, though some are at times eucalcemic.

In most patients with pseudohypoparathyroidism, injection of the parathyroid hor-mone brings little or no response in the kidneys. The excretion of calcium and phosphorus in the urine does not change, and there is little or no change in the concentrations of calcium and phosphorus in the plasma. The excretion of cyclic adenosine monophosphate in the urine does not increase. In some patients, the excretion of cyclic adenosine monophosphate in the urine increases normally.

The concentration of the parathyroid hormone in the plasma is usually increased, but may be normal. Because of the continued hypersecretion of the parathyroid hormone, the parathyroid glands often show secondary hyperplasia. Occasionally, the hypersecretion of the parathyroid hormone causes bony changes like those of hyperparathyroidism. Presumably in these patients the receptors for the parathyroid hormone in the bones are relatively intact.

Pseudohypoparathyroidism is treated with calcium and vitamin D as is hypoparathyroidism.

PSEUDOPSEUDOHYPOPARATHYROIDISM.   Pseudopseudohypoparathyroidism is rare. Patients with pseudopseudohypoparathyroidism have the same physical anomalies as do children with pseudohypoparathyroidism, but they have normal levels of calcium and phosphorus in the plasma and respond normally to the parathyroid hormone. Both pseudohypoparathyroidism and pseudopseudohypoparathyroidism have occurred in the same family. Pseudopseudohypoparathyroidism may be an incomplete form of pseudohypoparathyroidism.

BIBLIOGRAPHY

General

Bloodworth, J. M. B., (ed): Endocrine Pathology, 2nd ed. Baltimore, Williams & Wilkins, 1982.
Grimelius, L., Akerström, G., Johansson, H., and Bergström, R.: Anatomy and histopathology of human parathyroid glands. Pathol. Annu., 16 (Pt. 2):1, 1981.
Livolsi, V. A.: Pathology of the parathyroid glands. In Surgical Pathology of the Head and Neck. Edited by L. Barnes. New York, Marcel Dekker, 1985.
Reeve, J., and Zanelli, J. M.: Parathyroid hormone and bone. Clin. Sci., 71:231, 1986.

Hyperplasia

de Bolla, A. R., and Barnes, A. D.: The surgical treatment of parathyroid disease. Surg. Annu., 19:67, 1987.

Cundy, T., et al. Hyperparathyroid bone disease in chronic renal failure. Ulster Med. J., 54 (Suppl.):S334, 1985.

DeLellis, R. A., et al.: Multiple endocrine neoplasia (MEN) syndromes. Int. Rev. Exp. Pathol., 28:163, 1986.

Leshin, M.: Polyglandular autoimmune syndromes. Am. J. Med. Sci., 290:77, 1985.

Tumors

de Bolla, A. R., and Barnes, A. D.: The surgical treatment of parathyroid disease. Surg. Annu., 19:67, 1987.

DeLellis, R. A., et al.: Multiple endocrine neoplasia (MEN) syndromes. Int. Rev. Exp. Pathol., 28:163, 1986.

Fujimoto, Y., and Obara, T.: How to recognize and treat parathyroid carcinoma. Surg. Clin. North Am., 67:343, 1987.

Gluck, W. L.: Thyroid and parathyroid cancer. Clin. Geriatr. Med., 3:729, 1987.

Granberg, P. O., et al.: Parathyroid tumors. Curr. Probl. Cancer, 1, 1985.

Kameya, T., Shimosato, Y., Abe, K., and Takeuchi, T.: Morphologic and functional aspects of hormone-producing tumors. Pathol. Annu., 15 (Pt. 1):351, 1980.

Leshin, M.: Polyglandular autoimmune syndromes. Am. J. Med. Sci., 290:77, 1985.

Hyperparathyroidism

Adler, A. J., and Berlyne, G. M.: Phosphate retention and the genesis of secondary hyperparathyroidism.

Am. J. Nephrol., 6:417, 1986.

Ahrén, B.: Hyperparathyroidism and glucose intolerance. Acta Med. Scand., 220:5, 1986.

Bess, M. A., Edis, A. J., and van Heerden, J. A.: Hyperparathyroidism and pancreatitis. J.A.M.A., 243:246, 1980.

Breslau, N. A.: Update on secondary forms of hyperparathyroidism. Am. J. Med. Sci., 294:120, 1987.

Cundy, T., et al. Hyperparathyroid bone disease in chronic renal failure. Ulster Med. J., 54 (Suppl.):S334, 1985.

Halabé, A., and Sutton R. A. L.: Primary hyperparathyroidism and idiopathic hypercalciuria. Miner. Electrolyte Metab., 13:242, 1987.

Ross, A. J. 3rd, et al.: Primary hyperparathyroidism in infancy. J. Pediatr. Surg., 21:493, 1986.

Sherwood, L. M.: Diagnosis and management of primary hyperparathyroidism. Hospital Prac., 23(3A):9, 1988.

Sitges-Serra, A., and Caralps-Riera, A.: Hyperparathyroidism associated with renal disease. Surg. Clin. North Am., 67:359, 1987.

Sivula, A., and Ronni-Sivula, H.: Natural history of treated primary hyperparathyroidism. Surg. Clin. North Am., 67:329, 1987.

Stulberg, B.N., Licata, A.A., Bauer, T.W., and Belhobek, G.H.: Hyperparathyroidism, hyperthyroidism and Cushing's disease. Orthop. Clin. North Am., 15:697, 1984.

Hypoparathyroidism

Alon, U., and Chan, J. C. M.: Hypocalcemia from deficiency of and resistance to parathyroid hormone. Adv. Pediatr., 32:439, 1985.

Van Dop, C., McNamara, D. J., and Shapiro, J.: Pseudohypoparathyroidism. Annu. Rev. Med., 34:259, 1983.

49

Erythrocytes

THE blood and bone marrow constitute a single organ. Most diseases of the bone marrow are reflected in the blood. Disorders of the blood cause secondary changes in the bone marrow.

Many of the disorders of the blood and bone marrow affect all their elements, the red cells, white cells, platelets, and plasma. Some involve also the lymph nodes, spleen, or thymus. The diseases that affect principally the erythrocytes will be considered first and then the disorders of the different kinds of white cell, faults in coagulation, and the diseases of the spleen and thymus.

The major disorders of the erythrocytes are anemia, in which there is too little hemoglobin in the blood, and polycythemia, in which there are too many red cells in the blood.

ANEMIA

The term *anemia* comes from the Greek words meaning without and blood. If the concentration of hemoglobin in the blood is less than 140 g/L (14 g/100 mL) in a man or 120 g/L (12 g/100 mL) in a woman, or if the hematocrit is less than 0.40 L/L (40%) in a man or 0.37 L/L (37%) in a woman, the person is anemic. So defined, between 2 and 15% of the population is anemic. Most of the people with mild, unrecognized anemia are women.

Table 49-1 shows a classification of the different types of anemia. It is based in part on the morphology of the red cells, in part on the etiology of the anemia, in part on the dysfunction the lack of hemoglobin causes.

Terminology. Erythrocytes that are less than 7 μm in diameter or have a mean cell volume of less than 80 fL are called microcytes. Red cells between 7 and 8.5 μm in diameter with a mean cell volume between 80 and 94 fL are called normocytes. Those with a diameter greater than 8.5 μm or with a mean cell volume of over 94 fL are called macrocytes. Precursors of red cells in the bone marrow that are abnormally large and have abnormally primitive nuclei are called megaloblasts.

If the red cells differ considerably in size, they are said to show anisocytosis, from the Greek for unequal. If they vary greatly in shape, they show poikilocytosis, from the Greek for variegated.

If the mean corpuscular hemoglobin concentration is below 19 mmol/L (31 g/100 mL), the red cells are said to be hypochromic. If the concentration is over 19 mmol/L (31 g/100 mL) they are said to be normochromic.

Dysfunction. In all types of anemia, the ability of the blood to carry oxygen to the tissues is impaired. If the concentration of hemoglobin in the blood is 150 g/L (15 g/100 mL), arterial blood contains about 200 mL/L of oxygen. If the concentration of hemoglobin is 75 g/L (7.5 g/100 mL), it contains only 100 mL/L of oxygen. To combat the tendency to hypoxia, the body adopts a variety of compensatory measures.

In patients with chronic anemia, the concentration of 2,3-diphosphoglyceric acid in the red cells increases. Increased quantities of 2,3-diphosphoglyceric acid are bound to the hemoglobin reducing its affinity for oxygen. At the level of oxygen tension in the capillaries, the decrease in the affinity of hemoglobin for oxygen increases considerably the oxygen supply to the tissues. It may overcome as much as half the deficit. In the lungs, the increase in 2,3-diphosphoglyceric acid impairs the uptake of oxygen by the red cells, but the decrease in uptake is slight.

The heart reacts to anemia by increasing

TABLE 49-1. TYPES OF ANEMIA

Megaloblastic
  Pernicious anemia
    Congenital
    Autoimmune

  Other forms of vitamin B_{12} deficiency
  Folate deficiency
  Deficiency of both folate and vitamin B_{12}
  Impaired deoxyribonucleic acid synthesis
    Drug-induced
    Congenital

  Erythroleukemia

Disorders of iron metabolism
  Iron deficiency anemia
  Anemia of chronic disorders
  Sideroblastic anemia
    Idiopathic
    Hereditary

Hemolytic disorders
  Hereditary
    Hereditary spherocytosis
    Hereditary elliptocytosis
    Acanthocytosis
    Stomatocytosis
    Glucose-6-phosphate dehydrogenase deficiency
    Pyruvate kinase deficiency

  Structural hemoglobinopathy
    Sickle cell disease
    Hemoglobin C disease
    Hemoglobin D disease
    Hemoglobin E disease
    Hemoglobin O Arab disease
    Hemoglobin SC disease
    Hemoglobin SD disease
    Hemoglobin SO Arab disease
    Unstable hemoglobin disease

  Thalassemia
    Carriers of α-thalassemia
    α-Thalassemia minor
    Hemoglobin H disease
    Hemoglobin Bart's disease
    β-Thalassemia major
    β-Thalassemia intermedia
    β-Thalassemia minor
    β-Thalassemia minima
    Hereditary persistence of fetal hemoglobin
    α-Thalassemia
    γβ-Thalassemia
    Thalassemia plus a structural hemoglobinopathy

  Immunohemolytic disorders
    Transfusion reaction
    Hemolytic disease of the newborn
    Warm antibody autoimmunohemolytic anemia
    Cold hemagglutinin disease
    Paroxysmal cold hemoglobinuria
    Drug-induced immunohemolytic anemia

  Fragmentation anemia
  Hemolytic anemia induced by infection

Toxic hemolysis
Burns
Paroxysmal nocturnal hemoglobinuria

Aplastic anemia
  Congenital aplastic anemia
  Acquired aplastic anemia
  Pure red cell aplasia

Other forms of anemia
  Congenital dyserythropoietic anemia
  Leukoerythroblastic anemia
  Acute hemorrhagic anemia
  Anemia of renal disease
  Anemia of hepatic disease
  Anemia in endocrine disease

cardiac output. If the anemia is mild, the increase is achieved largely by increasing the heart rate. People with mild or moderate anemia often have tachycardia at rest or on mild exertion. If the anemia is severe, with a concentration of hemoglobin in the blood of less than 50 g/L (5 g/100 mL), the increased cardiac output is due mainly to an increase in stroke volume.

In chronic anemia, the peripheral resistance to the blood flow is reduced. The blood flow to the muscles and the brain is increased, though the perfusion of the kidneys and the skin is reduced. The diastolic pressure in the lungs falls, but the systolic pressure is maintained. The circulation time is shortened. The arteriovenous oxygen difference is reduced, as the tissues extract a greater proportion of oxygen from the blood.

In old people and in younger people when the concentration of hemoglobin in the blood is less than 50 g/L (5 g/100 mL), the hyperkinetic circulation may overtax the heart, leading to congestive heart failure. Sometimes there is angina pectoris, because the blood can no longer supply enough oxygen to the myocardium.

Dyspnea on exertion is common in people with anemia. During exercise, both oxygen uptake and carbon dioxide production are below normal. Recovery takes longer than normal after exercise, and return to the patient's usual arterial oxygen concentration is delayed.

The poor circulation and hypoxia in the kidneys often bring mild proteinuria. If the anemia is severe, there is occasionally mild fever of less than 38.3°C (101°F).

Clinical Presentation. In all kinds of anemia, the lack of hemoglobin and hypoxia cause weakness, tiredness, and feebleness. Often symptoms of this sort are the first sign of the anemia.

Pallor of the skin may be striking if anemia is severe, but the color of the skin can be misleading. A sun-tanned person with moderate anemia looks better than does a pallid scholar who has a normal concentration of hemoglobin. The severity of the anemia is better estimated by examining the conjunctivae, mucous membranes, or nail beds, where the color of the tissue reflects more accurately the color of the blood.

Headache, roaring or buzzing in the head, giddiness, or spots before the eyes are common in severe anemia. There· is often a bounding pulse, with bruits over the carotid arteries or over the cranium because of the rapid circulation. Sometimes the patient can hear the bruits. Papilledema and retinal hemorrhages sometimes develop if the anemia is unusually severe.

The severity of these changes depends on the severity of the anemia and the speed at which it develops. If the concentration of hemoglobin falls slowly and insidiously over weeks or months, the hematocrit may be under 0.25 L/L (25%) and the concentration of hemoglobin below 80 g/L (8 g/100 mL) before the patient notices anything wrong. If the concentration of hemoglobin falls rapidly, symptoms often become evident when the concentration of hemoglobin in the blood is much higher.

The age of the patient and the state of the heart and lungs are important. Young, healthy people with healthy hearts and lungs compensate much better for anemia than does an old person with reduced cardiac and pulmonary reserves. Anemia rarely brings cardiac failure in children, but often does so in old people.

Megaloblastic Anemia

Pernicious anemia is the commonest of the anemias in which megaloblasts accumulate in the bone marrow, but other forms of vita-min B_{12} deficiency, folate deficiency, deficiency of both vitamin B_{12} and folate, congenital or acquired faults in the synthesis of deoxyribonucleic acid, and erythroleukemia can also cause megaloblastic anemia.

PERNICIOUS ANEMIA. Pernicious anemia is caused by lack of the intrinsic factor in the gastric secretions. The absorption of vitamin B_{12} is impaired, and the vitamin deficiency causes anemia. The term *pernicious anemia* is used only when the deficiency of the intrinsic factor is caused by a congenital defect that prevents formation of the intrinsic factor, or by an autoimmune reaction that destroys the cells that produce the factor. Other kinds of vitamin B_{12} deficiency produce a similar anemia, but are not called pernicious anemia.

Pernicious anemia gained its ominous name because before the introduction of treatment with liver it was almost invariably fatal. Sometimes it is called Addisonian anemia, after the English physician who described it in 1849.

Pernicious anemia is especially common in Scandinavia, England, and Ireland and in the descendants of people from these countries. In Scandinavia, 9 new cases of pernicious anemia are found annually in every 100,000 people, and 1 person in 800 has pernicious anemia. In the south of Europe it is much less common, and in Africa and Asia it is still less frequent. About 60% of the patients are women. The disease does occur in children, but most of the patients are over 30 years old. Pernicious anemia becomes increasingly common as age increases.

Lesions. Pernicious anemia affects not only the bone marrow and the blood. It can cause serious injury to the nervous system, the stomach, and other organs.

Bone Marrow. In pernicious anemia, the bone marrow becomes hyperplastic. If a vertebra is sectioned, the marrow is deep red. If the anemia persists untreated, the red marrow extends peripherally, replacing the fatty marrow of the long bones with soft, gelatinous tissue like red currant jelly.

Microscopically, the quantity of fat in the bone marrow is decreased. If pernicious anemia is severe, the fat is almost all lost and is replaced by proliferating hematopoietic cells.

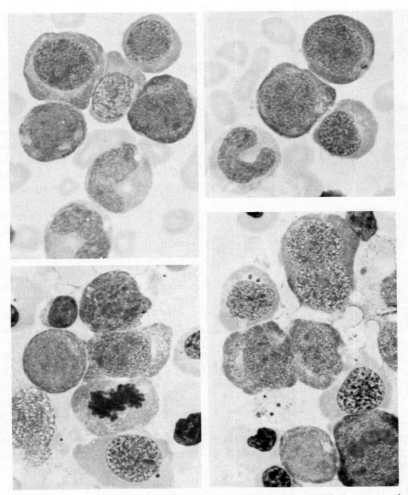

Fig. 49-1.   The bone marrow in pernicious anemia, showing megaloblasts and large metamyelocytes. (From Wintrobe, M. W., et al.: Clinical Hematology. 8th Ed. Philadelphia, Lea & Febiger, 1981.)

The precursors of the red cells in the bone marrow show megaloblastic changes. They proliferate, increasing the proportion of red cells in the bone marrow and replacing the fat. At all stages, they are larger than normal. The maturation of their nuclei is delayed. Instead of the even, dense chromatin of the nuclei of the normoblasts in normal erythropoiesis, the equivalent cells in pernicious anemia have nuclei with fine, delicate, sieve-like chromatin. Even almost completely hemoglobinized red cells that normally have only a pyknotic remnant of a nucleus have larger nuclei, with open granular chromatin.

Mitoses are numerous in the atypical red cells. The proportion of primitive red cells is increased.

Leukopoiesis also increases in the bone marrow, though to a lesser degree. Many of the developing granulocytes look normal. Some are larger than normal and have abnormally larger nuclei that are sometimes irregularly shaped and have irregular chromatin. Some metamyelocytes may be as much as 30 μm in diameter. The large cells are usually hyperdiploid.

The number of megakaryocytes may be reduced, but they usually appear normal.

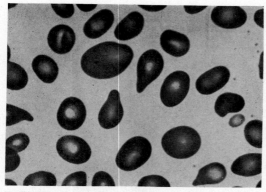

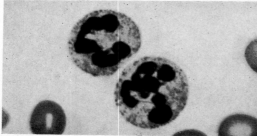

Fig. 49-2. The large, abnormally shaped red cells and hypersegmented neutrophils seen in the blood in pernicious anemia. (From Wintrobe, M. W., et al.: Clinical Hematology. 8th Ed. Philadelphia, Lea & Febiger, 1981.)

Only if pernicious anemia is severe do they show hypersegmentation and other nuclear abnormalities.

The increased production of red and white cells in the bone marrow in pernicious anemia is ineffective. Most of the megaloblasts are destroyed in the bone marrow and never reach the blood. The minority that do reach the blood are defective, and survive only 30 to 70 days instead of the usual 120 days. Many of the granulocytes are destroyed in the bone marrow. If pernicious anemia is severe, there is leukopenia in spite of the hyperplasia of the bone marrow.

Blood. The changes in the blood in pernicious anemia follow from the ineffective erythropoiesis and leukopoiesis in the bone marrow. Anemia and sometimes leukopenia occur.

The concentration of hemoglobin in the blood is usually between 70 and 90 g/L (7 to 9 g/100 mL) when symptoms develop. If pernicious anemia is severe, the concentra-

tion can fall below 20 g/L (2 g/100 mL). The erythrocyte count can fall to less than $1.0 \times 10^{12}/L$ (1,000,000/mm^3).

The circulating red cells are abnormally large. The more severe the anemia, the greater the macrocytosis. If the anemia is slight, the red cells are likely to have mean volume of 95 to 110 fL, as compared with the normal 82 to 92 fL. If it is severe, the mean volume is likely to be between 110 and 130 fL and may be as much as 160 fL.

The concentration of hemoglobin in the circulating red cells is normal unless the disease is complicated by iron deficiency. The cells contain more than the normal quantity of hemoglobin, because they are bigger than normal. Often the mean corpuscular hemoglobin is 33 to 39 pg, as compared with the normal 27 to 31 pg. The bigger the red cells, the more hemoglobin they contain.

The red cells in the blood in pernicious anemia tend to be oval, and their central pallor is often reduced. If the anemia is moderately severe, the increased size of the cells can be appreciated in a blood film, especially by comparison with a normal film. If the anemia is mild, the abnormalities in a blood film are subtle. As the severity of the anemia increases, the red cells show increasing anisocytosis and poikilocytosis. If it is very severe, they vary greatly in size and often assume bizarre shapes. Some of the distorted red cells in the circulation are smaller than normal. Others are much larger than normal.

Instead of the uniform coloration of a normal red cell, some of the red cells in pernicious anemia show blotchy, bluish staining called polychromasia, from the Greek words for many and color. Some of the red cells show dark blue spots called punctate basophilia. Some contain circular or irregularly shaped purple rings, called Cabot's rings, after an American physician (1868–1939). Nucleated red cells sometimes appear in the blood, sometimes with nuclei that show the fine, granular chromatin of the megaloblasts. Some of the red cells may contain a small, pyknotic remnant of a nucleus, called a Howell-Jolly body, after an American physiologist (1860–1945) and a French histologist (1870–1953).

The leukocyte count may be normal in pernicious anemia, but it is usually between 3.0 and 6.0 × 10⁹/L (3000 to 6000/mm³). If the anemia is severe, the count may be as low as 1.0 × 10⁹/L (1000/mm³). The leukopenia is due principally to a lack of neutrophils, caused by the ineffective leukopoiesis in the bone marrow.

Hypersegmentation of the granulocytes in the blood is one of the earliest signs of pernicious anemia, sometimes evident before there is any reduction in the concentration of hemoglobin. Normally, most granulocytes in the blood have nuclei with three lobes or less. Fewer than 25% have four lobes, and a few have five lobes. In pernicious anemia, the proportion of granulocytes with five lobes in their nuclei increases, and some have as many as ten lobes. If any granulocytes in the blood have more than six lobes, if more than 3% have five lobes, or if more than 25% have four lobes, the patient probably has pernicious anemia or one of the other megaloblastic anemias.

The platelet count may be normal in pernicious anemia or may be moderately reduced, perhaps to 100 × 10⁹/L (100,000/mm³). Giant platelets are sometimes found. Sometimes there is evidence of platelet dysfunction, with prolongation of the bleeding time, failure of clot retraction, or purpura.

The transport of iron to the bone marrow increases three or more times in pernicious anemia. Often, the concentration of iron in the plasma is a little increased. Most of the iron carried to the marrow is wasted, making hemoglobin for megaloblasts that die in the marrow. Normally, 80% of the iron delivered to the bone marrow is incorporated into the hemoglobin of circulating red cells. In pernicious anemia, less than 30% of the iron carried to the bone marrow reaches the circulating red cells. The rest leaks back into the plasma and is stored, principally in the liver or the spleen.

Becaused of the increased breakdown of red cells, both in the marrow and in the blood, the production of bile pigments is increased. The concentration of unconjugated bilirubin in the plasma may rise, though the bilirubin level rarely exceeds 35 μmol/L (2 mg/100 mL). The excretion of urobilinogen is increased. If labeled glycine

is given the destruction of megaloblasts in the marrow causes a considerable increase in the early labeled bile pigments.

The destruction of megaloblasts and circulating red cells allows their enzymes to escape into the plasma. The activity of lactic dehydrogenase in the plasma increases to 10 or 20 times normal. The increase is principally in the isoenzymes lactic dehydrogenase 1 and lactic dehydrogenase 2, with the activity of iosenzyme 1 being the greater. The activity of lactic dehydrogenase in the plasma also increases in hemolytic anemias, but the increase is not as large as in pernicious anemia, and in the hemolytic anemias the activity of isoenzyme 2 is greater than that of isoenzyme 1.

The increased destruction of the circulating red cells in pernicious anemia is caused principally by the malformation of red cells, but there is an extracorpuscular hemolytic factor in the blood in pernicious anemia. If normal red cells are transfused into a patient with pernicious anemia, they are destroyed more quickly than is normal.

Nervous System. Before modern therapy was introduced, 95% of patients with pernicious anemia had symptoms of injury to the nervous system, and 30% were disabled by lesions in the spinal cord. With modern treatment, 30% of patients with pernicious anemia have minor neurologic symptoms. Only 5% have evidence of involvement of the spinal cord. The severity of the neurologic injury does not correlate with the severity of the anemia. Rarely, serious neurologic injury occurs in a patient who has no anemia.

The injury to the spinal cord caused by pernicious anemia is called subacute combined degeneration of the spinal cord. In scattered foci, fusiform swellings appear on axons in the white matter of the spinal cord. The myelin around the axons involved breaks down and is taken up by phagocytes. The axons are destroyed. The demyelinization is most severe in the midthoracic part of the cord, usually becoming gradually less above and below this region. The posterior columns are affected first and then the lateral columns. The lesions are always patchy, though they may become confluent. Occasionally the thoracic part of the cord is almost completely demyelinated. Only late in the disease are there sometimes foci of demyelinization elsewhere in the white matter of the spinal cord or in the brain.

Peripheral nerves often show similar patchy demyelination and reduced conduction velocity. Rarely, the optic nerve is affected.

Stomach. In patients with a congenital absence of intrinsic factor the stomach is normal histologically. In patients in whom the disease is caused by an autoimmune reaction, the body of the stomach shows severe gastritis, often gastric atrophy, with thinning of both mucosa and muscularis. Sometimes the body and fundus of the stomach are paper thin, with an abrupt transition to a relatively normal antrum. The volume of gastric secretion is reduced, usually to about 10% of normal. Almost always there is complete achlorhydria. Histamine fails to stimulate either an increase in the volume of gastric juice or the secretion of acid. The secretion of pepsin is reduced. Intrinsic factor is reduced or absent. Only the neuroendocrine cells remain intact in the atrophic mucosa of the body and fundus.

The cells of the gastric epithelium are larger than normal, often about twice the normal size. Their nuclei have fine, clumped chromatin. The nucleocytoplasmic ratio is reduced. Chromosomal abnormalities are unduly frequent.

Tongue. About 50% of patients with pernicious anemia have changes in the tongue. The patient usually has repeated attacks of acute glossitis, most often involving the tip or edges of the tongue, but sometimes affecting the whole dorsum. The affected part of the tongue is painful, swollen, and beefy red. Occasionally the inflammation is more extensive and involves much of the mucosa of the mouth and throat. The glossitis causes loss of the papillae of the tongue. Between the acute attacks, the tongue is smooth, glazed, and red.

Other Organs. Cells throughout the body are enlarged. Their nuclei have fine, clumped chromatin. The nucleocytoplasmic ratio is increased.

The changes once prominent as patients with pernicious anemia neared death are now rarely seen. Severe fatty change was common in the liver, kidneys, and in the dilated, flabby heart. Hemosiderosis of the liver, spleen,

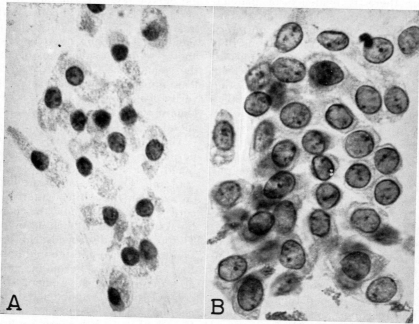

Fig. 49-3. A. Normal gastric epithelial cells. B. The large nuclei and fine chromatin of the nuclei of the gastric epithelium in pernicious anemia. (Courtesy of Dr. Cyrus E. Rubin, from Wintrobe, M. W., et al.: Clinical Hematology. 8th Ed. Philadelphia, Lea & Febiger, 1981.)

kidneys, and other organs became severe as the iron released by the ineffective erythropoiesis accumulated. Congestive heart failure was common. Slight jaundice was usual. Extramedullary hematopoiesis in the liver and the spleen was extensive.

Clinical Presentation. Pernicious anemia develops slowly and insidiously. Often symptoms have been present for a year or more before the patient seeks advice. Weakness, sore tongue, and paresthesia are often the first signs, but diarrhea, some other gastrointestinal upset, congestive heart failure, or mental disturbances may bring the patient to a physician.

As pernicious anemia grows more severe, any of the symptoms and signs of anemia may be present. Pallor is common. If the anemia is severe, the patient's skin is a delicate lemon yellow. Over 20% of the patients with severe pernicious anemia have fever. A poor appetite, diarrhea, abdominal pain, slight enlargement of the liver and spleen, and proteinuria are common.

Subacute combined degeneration can develop rapidly, causing disability within a few weeks, or may worsen slowly, over a year or more. First comes spasticity and ataxia, most severe in the lower limbs, through the upper limbs are sometimes also affected. Often numbness and tingling in the limbs accompany or precede the stiffness. Later comes paraplegia, with anesthesia of the limbs and trunk. Impairment of the memory is common, and sometimes there is confusion, even dementia. Sometimes mild neuropathy suddenly becomes severe, perhaps overnight. More often the symptoms worsen gradually if the anemia is left untreated.

Diagnosis. The diagnosis of pernicious anemia can be confirmed by showing that the concentration of vitamin B_{12} in the plasma is low. Normal people have more than 130 pmol/L (180 pg/mL) of the vitamin in the serum, on the average 330 pmol/L (450 pg/mL). In pernicious anemia, the concentration is usually below 75 pmol/L (100 pg/mL); on the average it is 28 pmol/L (38 pg/mL).

The concentration of folate in the plasma is usually high in patients with pernicious anemia, near or above the upper limit of normal of 34 nmol/L (15 ng/mL). The concentration of folate in the red cells is low, often less than the lower limit of normal of 340 nmol/L (150 ng/mL) because vitamin B_{12} is needed for the transfer of 5-methyltetrahydrofolate from the plasma into the red cells.

The Schilling test, named after the American hematologist who described it in 1953, confirms that there is malabsorption of vitamin B_{12} and that the malabsorption is due to lack of the intrinsic factor. A large dose of nonradioactive vitamin B_{12} is given intramuscularly, and a physiologic dose of radioactive vitamin B_{12} is given by mouth. Normally the radioactive vitamin is absorbed well, but because many of the binding sites for the vitamin have been saturated by the intramuscular dose of the vitamin, more than 10% of the radioactive vitamin is excreted in the urine. In pernicious anemia and other conditions in which there is malabsorption of vitamin B_{12}, less than 1% of the radioactive vitamin appears in the urine. The uptake of the labeled vitamin can also be estimated by measuring its concentration in the plasma or feces, or by whole body counting.

The test is then repeated, giving radioactive vitamin B_{12} bound to intrinsic factor by mouth. If the malabsorption of the vitamin is caused by lack of the intrinsic factor, the excretion of radioactive vitamin in the urine, its concentration in the plasma, and its excretion in the feces are in the normal range. If the malabsorption of the vitamin is caused in some other way, the absorption of the vitamin remains low.

The excretion of methylmalonic acid in the urine is usually increased in pernicious anemia and other forms of vitamin B_{12} deficiency. 5'-Deoxyandenosylcobalamin is needed for the conversion of methylmalonyl coenzyme A to succinyl coenzyme A. If it is deficient, the unused methylmalonyl acid is excreted in the urine. The administration of valine, a precursor of methylmalonic acid, increases the excretion of methylmalonic acid in the urine.

Pathogenesis. Pernicious anemia caused by a congenital lack of the intrinsic factor is rare. The defect is inherited as an autosomal recessive character. The anemia becomes evident early in childhood.

In adults and older children, pernicious anemia is acquired. Patients develop severe atrophic gastritis or gastric atrophy, with severe reduction in gastric secretion or achylia. As the gastritis worsens, the secretion of the intrinsic factor by the parietal cells fails, and pernicious anemia develops.

The gastritis is caused by an autoimmune attack against the intrinsic factor or the parietal cells that produce it. Over 80% of patients with pernicious anemia have in the blood IgG antibodies against the parietal cells, and 60% have IgG antibodies against the intrinsic factor. Some of the antibodies against the intrinsic factor prevent the attachment of vitamin B_{12} to the intrinsic factor and are called blocking antibodies. Others do not affect the attachment of the vitamin to the factor and are called binding antibodies.

There are at least two kinds of binding antibody. Some attach to the intrinsic factor whether or not it has formed a complex with vitamin B_{12}. Others bind to the intrinsic factor more readily when it has formed a complex with vitamin B_{12}.

Antibodies against the intrinsic factor are present in the gastric juice in over 70% of patients with pernicious anemia. Some are IgG; some are IgA.

Whether the antibodies cause the gastritis and deficiency of the intrinsic factor is less certain. A cell-mediated attack against the parietal cells may be more important. In over 90% of patients with pernicious anemia, the intrinsic factor activates the patient's lymphocytes.

Other autoimmune diseases are frequent in patients with pernicious anemia. More than 2% of the patients have Hashimoto's disease, and 2% have Graves' disease. Over 10% of patients with Hashimoto's disease have pernicious anemia, as do 3% of people with Graves' disease. More than 50% of patients with pernicious anemia have antibodies against the thyroid. It may be that Hashimoto's disease, Graves' disease, pernicious anemia, and other such conditions result from an abnormal reactivity of the immunologic system, not from a fault in the organ principally involved.

In some patients with the adult form of pernicious anemia, genetic factors are important. In 10% of the patients, at least one other member of the family has the disease. In such kindred, 20% of the patient's siblings develop pernicious anemia. Antibodies against the parietal cells are demonstrable in 20% of the patient's relatives, and 50% of the relatives have antibodies against thyroid antigens.

The deficiency of vitamin B_{12} that results from the lack of the intrinsic factor impairs the synthesis of deoxyribonucleic acid. Methylcobalamin is required for the reaction that converts homocysteine and N^5-methyltetrahydrofolate to methionine and tetrahydrofolate. If vitamin B_{12} is deficient, N^5-methyltetrahydrofolate accumulates in the cells. The lack of tetrahydrofolate causes a deficiency of the coenzyme N^5N^{10}-methylenetetrahydrofolate needed for the synthesis of thymidylic acid required for the synthesis of deoxyribonucleic acid. Cells throughout the body become abnormal. They grow large, and the maturation of their nuclei is delayed. The chromosomes in the cells usually are normal in number, but often show gaps, breaks, or other abnormalities.

How the deficiency of vitamin B_{12} causes the neuropathy is uncertain. The mechanism is not the same as that which causes anemia. Folate relieves the anemia, presumably by overcoming the block in the formation of N^5N^{10}-methylenetetrahydrofolate, but it does not prevent or ameliorate the neuropathy. Perhaps the neuropathy results from the accumulation of methylmalonic acid caused by the lack of the 5'-deoxyadenosylcobalamin needed to convert methylmalonyl coenzyme A to succinyl coenzyme A, the deficiency in vitamin B_{12} impairs cyanide metabolism.

Treatment and Prognosis. Before treatment with liver was introduced in the 1920s, few patients with pernicious anemia lived for more than three years. Over 80% of the patients enjoyed one or more remissions, but if the anemia was severe enough to cause admission to a hospital, over 50% of the patients died with a month.

Pernicious anemia is now treated by giving cyanocobalamin or hydroxycobalamin by injection for the rest of the patient's life. Once normal stores of vitamin B_{12} have been restored, one injection a month is sufficient to maintain normal hematopoiesis and to prevent neurologic injury. If continued injections are impossible, massive doses of vitamin B_{12} by mouth may be adequate. Porcine intrinsic factor can be given to enhance the absorption of vitamin B_{12}, but antibodies soon develop against the porcine protein and inactivate it.

Folic acid should not be given. It relieves the anemia but does not prevent or arrest the neuropathy. Indeed, the administration of folic acid to patients with vitamin B_{12} deficiency sometimes seems to augment the severity of the neuropathy.

The response to treatment is dramatic. Within 48 hours, the patient feels better. The soreness of the tongue is relieved within a day or two. Within a week its papillae begin to regenerate. Within two weeks, the tongue may be normal.

In the bone marrow, the number of megaloblasts is greatly reduced within 6 to 10 hours. Within 24 to 48 hours, erythropoiesis is normoblastic. Only the giant metamyelocytes persist for a week or so.

In the blood, a reticulocytosis begins within two or three days and reaches a maximum in seven or eight days. The more severe the anemia, the greater the reticulocytosis. More than 50% of the circulating red cells may be reticulocytes at the height of the reaction. The concentration of hemoglobin in the blood begins to rise after a few days, as does the erythrocyte count. The anisocytosis and poikilocytosis gradually lessen. After four to eight weeks, the red cells circulating in the blood are normal. The leukocyte count returns to normal within a week, though there may be at first some excess of primitive granulocytes in the blood. The platelet count becomes normal within a week.

The neurologic damage is arrested by vitamin B_{12}. The lesions heal by gliosis. The symptoms resolve in whole or in part in over 80% of patients with subacute combined degeneration. Often the improvement in the symptoms is slow, but continues for six months or more.

The elevated concentration of iron in the serum falls to normal or below within 48 hours. Serum levels of lactic dehydrogenase become normal in one or two weeks. The serum bilirubin is normal after three or four weeks. The serum urate level may increase in the first week, because of the rapid proliferation of the erythrocytes, but it too is normal within two or three weeks.

Vitamin B_{12} does not reverse the gastritis, though adrenocortical steroids may do so. Between 3 and 5% of patients with pernicious anemia develop carcinoma of the stomach, usually 10 to 15 years after the diagnosis was made.

OTHER FORMS OF VITAMIN B_{12} DEFICIENCY. Other types of vitamin B_{12} deficiency cause anemia with changes in the bone marrow, blood, nervous system, and other organs like those of pernicious anemia, except that in the majority of these disorders the stomach remains normal.

Causes. Table 49-2 lists the causes of vitamin B_{12} deficiency. Most of the conditions listed are uncommon or cause anemia only when they are unusually severe.

Dietary Deficiency. A dietary deficiency of vitamin B_{12} is rare. The vitamin is present in ample quantity in all animal products. Deficiency can develop in extreme vegetarians, but is rarely severe enough to cause anemia. A child born of an extreme vegetarian is likely to become vitamin B_{12}-deficient if breast fed, because the mother's milk contains little or no vitamin B_{12}.

Lack of Intrinsic Factor. Total gastrectomy removes the cells that form the intrinsic factor. Malabsorption of vitamin B_{12} follows, though the stores of vitamin B_{12} in the body are so great that it is 2 to 10 years before anemia becomes evident. Partial gastrectomy

TABLE 49-2. CAUSES OF VITAMIN B_{12} DEFICIENCY

Dietary deficiency

Lack of intrinsic factor
  Pernicious anemia
  Gastrectomy
  Corrosive injury
  Defective intrinsic factor

Competition in the small bowel
  Bacterial overgrowth
  Diphyllobothriasis

Malabsorption
  Crohn's disease
  Surgical resection
  Drug induced
  Secondary
  Congenital

lowers the production of intrinsic factor enough to cause reduced absorption of vitamin B_{12} in 30% of patients, and the malabsorption of the vitamin is severe enough to cause anemia in 20%. Rarely, drinking a corrosive fluid has destroyed the ability of the stomach to produce intrinsic factor. Infrequently, a patient forms an abnormal intrinsic factor, which is unable to promote the absorption of vitamin B_{12}.

Competition. If bacteria or worms grow in the small bowel in sufficient number, they compete for vitamin B_{12} and can fix so much of it that they cause vitamin B_{12} deficiency and anemia. Normally the small bowel is sterile, or nearly so. The gastric acid kills organisms swallowed with food or in the saliva. If there is achlorhydria, the bacteria reach the bowel and grow luxuriantly, sometimes in sufficient numbers to cause vitamin B_{12} deficiency and anemia. Stasis in the small bowel also favors bacterial growth. Diverticula, a blind loop, an anastomosis that allows recirculation of the content of the small bowel, and obstruction by a stricture or adhension can cause stasis and bacterial overgrowth sufficient to cause megaloblastic anemia. Occasionally the tapeworm Diphyllobothrium latum infests the small bowel in such numbers that it causes malabsorption of vitamin B_{12} and anemia.

Malabsorption. Severe Crohn's disease of the terminal ileum, surgical resection of the ileum, and other severe diseases of the ileum prevent the absorption of vitamin B_{12} and can cause anemia. Occasionally paraaminosalicylate, colchicine, neomycin, or ethanol impairs the absorption of vitamin B_{12}, or vitamin B_{12} deficiency develops in a patient with insufficiency of the exocrine pancreas, the Zollinger-Ellison syndrome, or on hemodialysis. Rarely a congenital defect inherited as an autosomal recessive character prevents the absorption of vitamin B_{12}. In a few kindred, the ileal receptors needed for the absorption of the vitamin are defective, or the transcobalamin II needed for its transport in the plasma is absent or defective.

Treatment and Prognosis. Administration of vitamin B_{12} promptly relieves the anemia in all forms of vitamin B_{12} deficiency and prevents or ameliorates injury to the nervous system. If the disorder causing

TABLE 49-3. CAUSES OF FOLATE DEFICIENCY

Dietary deficiency

Malabsorption
  Drug induced
  Congenital
  Surgical resection

Increased demand
  Pregnancy
  Infancy
  Cirrhosis of the liver
  Hyperplasia of the bone marrow

the deficiency cannot be controlled, the vitamin must be continued for the rest of the patient's life.

FOLATE DEFICIENCY. Folate deficiency causes a megaloblastic anemia with changes in the bone marrow and blood like those of pernicious anemia. As in pernicious anemia, cells throughout the body are larger than normal, and the maturation of their nuclei is delayed. Folate deficiency does not cause subacute combined degeneration of the spinal cord or other neurologic injury and is not associated with lesions in the stomach.

Cause. Table 49-3 lists the causes of folate deficiency. The stores of folate in the body are considerable. Even if the intake of folate is low, deficiency does not become apparent for 3 to 6 months.

Dietary Deficiency. Folates are present in many foods and are particularly abundant in green vegetables. They are easily destroyed by boiling. Dietary deficiency is particularly common in the tropics and in countries in which vegetables are thoroughly boiled. Proliferation of bacteria in the small bowel can cause folate deficiency, but more often the organisms produce folate and enhance its absorption.

Malabsorption. Diphenylhydantion primidone, barbiturates, cycloserine, ethanol, and oral contraceptives occasionally cause malabsorption of folate. Occasionally a congenital or acquired deficiency of the glutamyl conjugases necessary to prepare the polyglutamyl folates in the diet for absorption causes folate deficiency. Extensive resection of the ileum can do so.

Increased Demand. Pregnancy increases the demand for folate. From 2 to 50% of pregnant women have folate deficiency, though in most it is not severe enough to cause anemia. Deficiency is most common in the poorer classes, in which the intake of folate in the diet is low.

Infants require 10 times as much folate as adults, relative to their weight, and during the first year of life are largely dependent on the folate in the milk. Overheating can easily reduce the content of folate in the milk by more than 50%. Goat's milk contains little folate, and folate deficiency is common in infants fed on goat's milk.

About 20% of patients with cirrhosis of the liver have megaloblastic anemia caused by folate deficiency, and 50% have less severe deficiency. The deficiency is in part because the diet is poor, in part because ethanol impairs the absorption of folate, in part because the disordered hepatic metabolism increases the demand for folate. Hyperplasia of the bone marrow increases the demand for folate, and can cause folate deficiency if the diet is poor.

Diagnosis. The concentration of folate in the plasma depends on the intake of folate in the diet and can change considerably within a few hours. The concentration of folate in the erythrocytes is a better measure of the body's store. Normally it is over 340 nmol/L (150 ng/mL). In folate deficiency it is below 225 nmol/L (100 ng/mL). In 50% of patients with folate deficiency, the concentration of vitamin B_{12} in the serum is below 130 pmol/L (180 pg/mL) and in 10% it is below 75 pmol/L (100 pg/mL). The concentration of vitamin B_{12} in the serum returns to normal when folate is given.

Formiminoglutamic acid is formed during the conversion of histidine to glutamate. If folate is deficient, the formimino group cannot be transferred to tetrahydrofolate to form glutamate and formiminotetraphydrofolate. Instead, the formiminoglutamic acid, or FIGlu as it is often called, is excreted in the urine. Normal people excrete less than 17 mg of formiminoglutamic acid in the 8 hours after being given 15 g of histidine. People with folate deficiency excrete between 200 and 2000 mg. The excretion of formiminoglutamic acid is also increased in

50% of people with vitamin B_{12} deficiency, though the increase is less than in folate deficiency, rarely exceeding 250 mg in the 8-hour period.

Aminoimidazole carboxamide is an intermediate in purine synthesis that requires folate for its metabolism. It is excreted in excess in the urine in both folate deficiency and in vitamin B_{12} deficiency.

Pathogenesis. Like a deficiency of vitamin B_{12}, folate deficiency impairs the synthesis of deoxyribonucleic acid by causing a lack of N^5N^{10}-methylenetetrahydrofolate and blocking the conversion of deoxyuridylate to thymidylate. The effect on the bone marrow and on nuclear maturation in other tissues is almost the same as that caused by deficiency of vitamin B_{12}.

The cause of the lack of N^5N^{10}-methylemetetrahydrofolate can be demonstrated by growing bone marrow cells in tissue culture. If the lack is caused by vitamin B_{12} deficiency, addition of the vitamin restores the synthesis of deoxyribonucleic acid to normal. If it is caused by folate deficiency, adding vitamin B_{12} is of no effect. Adding folate restores the synthesis of deoxyribonucleic acid to normal in both vitamin B_{12} and folate deficiency.

Treatment and Prognosis. Folate deficiency is treated by giving folate by mouth. The bone marrow and blood show a rapid response like that in pernicious anemia. The blood and other tissues return to normal within two or three months.

Whenever folate deficiency is diagnosed, it is important to exclude vitamin B_{12} deficiency. Large doses of folate cause considerable improvement in the anemia in patients with vitamin B_{12} deficiency, but do not prevent the neurologic injuries.

DEFICIENCY OF BOTH FOLATE AND VITAMIN B_{12}. Tropical sprue and celiac disease often cause deficiency of both folate and vitamin B_{12}. In tropical sprue, folate deficiency is at first the more important, but as years pass, vitamin B_{12} deficiency becomes increasingly prominent. Up to 40% of children with celiac disease have folate deficiency, though iron deficiency is a more common cause of anemia. Vitamin B_{12} deficiency is rare. About 90% of adults with celiac disease have folate deficiency, and in 40% the absorption of vitamin B_{12} is impaired. Anemia is more often due to folate deficiency than to lack of vitamin B_{12}.

The combined deficiency causes a megaloblastic anemia like that in pernicious anemia or folate deficiency. Both folate and vitamin B_{12} must be administered to overcome the dysfunction.

IMPAIRED DEOXYRIBONUCLEIC ACID SYNTHESIS. Drugs that impair the synthesis of deoxyribonucleic acid sometimes cause megaloblastic anemia. Alkylating agents like cyclophosphamide, purine antagonists like 6-mercaptopurine, and pyrimidine antagonists like 5-fluorouracil and cytosine arabinoside cause pancytopenia with megaloblastic changes in the bone marrow and macrocytic anemia. Methotrexate and, less often, other folate antagonists cause megaloblastic anemia by inhibiting dihydrofolate reductase.

A congenital deficiency of one of the enzymes needed for the synthesis of deoxyribonucleic acid is a rare cause of megaloblastic anemia. Some of the patients are mentally deficient or show other abnormalities. Among the defects causing megaloblastic anemia that are inherited as an autosomal recessive character is orotic aciduria, caused by lack of orotidylic decarboxylase, or of both orotidylic decarboxylase and orotidylic pyrophosphorylase; deficiency of N^5-methyltetrahydrofloate transferase; deficiency of formiminotransferase; and lack of dihydrofolate transferase. Lack of hypoxanthine-guanine phosphoribosyl transferase is inherited as an X-linked character.

ERYTHROLEUKEMIA. Megaloblasts sometimes appear in the marrow of patients with the neoplastic proliferation of red and white cells called erythroleukemia, although there is neither deficiency of vitamin B_{12} nor of folate. They are occasionally found in the bone marrow in patients with other forms of acute myeloid leukaemia.

Disorders of Iron Metabolism

Five disorders of iron metabolism impair the formation of hemoglobin and cause anemia. In iron deficiency anemia, the quantity of iron stored in the body is inadequate. In the anemia of chronic disorders, the macrophages fail to release iron into the plasma. In atransferrinemia the plasma lacks the transferrin necessary for the transport of iron to the bone marrow. In congenital hypochromic microcytic anemia with iron overload, the bone marrow fails to take up iron from the plasma. In the sideroblastic anemias, iron accumulates in the precursors of the red cells in the bone marrow.

IRON DEFICIENCY ANEMIA. Iron deficiency is defined as a reduction in the quantity of iron stored in the body. First the quantity of iron stored in the macrophages of the bone marrow, liver, and other organs falls and then the concentration of iron in the plasma.

Iron deficiency is common, especially in women. In Canada, the quantity of iron stored in the body is low in 3% of men, 25% of children, 30% of adolescents, 30% of menstruating women, and 60% of pregnant women. In Finland, it is reduced in 5% of men, 70% of women from 15 to 49 years old, and in 25% of older women. In the United States, 25% of young women attending college have no iron stores, and another 40% have less than the normal quantity of iron.

In most of these people, the iron deficiency is not severe enough to cause anemia. In the United States, less than 1% of men and about 10% of women have iron deficiency anemia. In women, iron deficiency anemia is most common in the reproductive years, especially during pregnancy. In different parts of the United States, from 15 to 50% of pregnant women have iron deficiency anemia. In men, iron deficiency anemia is most common in adolescence.

Lesions. Iron deficiency anemia causes lesions in the bone marrow, the blood, and in other organs. It often causes only minor abnormalities, but can cause severe dysfunction.

Bone Marrow. In iron deficiency anemia, the bone marrow is slightly or moderately hyperplastic, with reduction in the quantity of fat. Erythrocytic precursors are predominant, with some increase in the more primitive forms. Normoblasts are small, with scant, often ragged cytoplasm. The nuclei of the erythrocytic cells mature more rapidly than normal and may be pyknotic in cells containing little hemoglobin. Occasionally, the nuclei of the red cells are distorted. Granulopoiesis and the megakaryocytes are normal.

The iron normally present in the macrophages in the bone marrow is absent or greatly diminished. Normally, about 50% of the normoblasts in the bone marrow contain a few granules of ferritin, which are big enough to be visible by light microscopy when the cells are stained for iron. In iron deficiency anemia, less than 10% of the normoblasts have such granules.

Blood. Iron deficiency anemia often passes unrecognized for months or years. Often the iron deficiency slowly worsens and the anemia slowly becomes more severe.

By the time symptoms develop, the concentration of hemoglobin in the blood is commonly below 80 g/L (8 g/100 mL). The red cells are usually smaller than normal, with a mean volume of between 53 and 93 fL, rather than the normal of from 80 to 94 fL. The mean concentration of hemoglobin in the red cells is low, from 220 to 310 g/L (22 to 31 g/100 mL) in contrast to the normal 320 to 360 g/L (32 to 36 g/100 mL). The red cells contain less hemoglobin than normal, a mean content of from 14 to 29 pg, rather than the normal 27 to 31 pg.

The red cell count and the volume of packed red cells fall less than does the concentration of hemoglobin. The enthrocyte count may be normal, or nearly so and the packed cell volume about 0.30 L/L (30%) even though the concentration of hemoglobin is below 80 g/L (8 g/100 mL).

Because of the lack of hemoglobin, the central pallor of the red cells increased. In severe iron deficiency anemia, there is only a narrow rim of normally stained cytoplasm at the margin of the red cells. Many of the red cells are smaller than normal, but both tiny, hypochromic cells and cells larger than normal are present. Often the big red cells show polychromasia. Poikilocytosis may be prominent, with elongated, pointed or pencil-shaped red cells. Usually a few red cells normally filled with hemoglobin can be found. The fragility of the red cells may be normal in iron deficiency anemia, but often it is decreased, so that little or no hemolysis occurs when the cells are suspended in hypotonic saline solution containing as little salt as 2 g/L (0.2 g/100 mL).

The leukocyte count is normal or slightly lowered. A few hypersegmented granulocytes

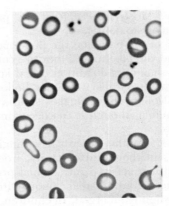

Fig. 49-4. Iron deficiency anemia, showing the increased pallor of the small red cells, some of which are distorted. (From Wintrobe, M. W., et al.: Clinical Hematology. 8th Ed. Philadelphia, Lea & Febiger, 1981.)

are sometimes present, probably because there is mild folate deficiency. If there has been a recent hemorrhage of some volume, there will be a mild leukocytosis. If there is hookworm infestation, there is often eosinophilia.

Often the platelet count is about twice normal, perhaps in response to bleeding rather than because of the iron deficiency.

The concentration of iron in the serum is low in iron deficiency anemia, 2 to 10 μmol/L (10 to 60 μg/100 mL), rather than the normal 10 to 32 μmol/L (60 to 180 μg/100 mL). The saturation of transferrin is always below 0.16 (16%), often about 0.07 (7%), as compared with a normal of 0.20 to 0.45 (20–45%). The total iron-binding capacity is often increased to about 90 μmol/L (500 mg/100 mL), but may be normal or as low as 35 μmol/L (200 mg/100 mL).

The concentration of protoporphyrin in the red cells increases as the concentration of hemoglobin falls. Because of the lack of iron protoprophyrin cannot be converted into heme and accumulates in the erythrocytes.

Other Organs. In 40% of patients with severe iron deficiency anemia, the tongue becomes red and sore, especially when irritated by food or drink. Atrophy of the papillae of the anterior part of the tongue is common, and sometimes the papillae disappear altogether, leaving the tongue smooth and waxy. More than 10% of the patients have angular stomatitis.

In 30% of the patients, the fingernails are brittle and ridged. In 20% they are concave, or spoon-shaped, a condition called koilony-chia, from the Greek words for hollow and a nail. Koilonychnia suggests iron deficiency anemia, though it can occur in other conditions.

About 30% of the patients have tingling or numbness in their limbs. Rarely, iron deficiency causes inceased intracranial pressure and mimics an intracranial tumor. Often the spleen is slightly enlarged. In children, there may be bony changes like those of thalassemia.

About 75% of patients with iron deficiency anemia have gastritis, often mild, superficial gastritis, but sometimes severe atrophic gastritis. About 40% of the patients have hypochlorhydria, and 15% have achlorhydria. In 5%, the intrinsic factor is seriously reduced or absent. Over 30% of patients with iron deficiency anemia have antibodies against the parietal cells.

Ozena is often associated with iron deficiency anemia in southeastern Europe, though not in other parts of the world. In sideropenic dysphagia, discussed in Chapter 33, the patients have iron deficiency anemia, webs in the esophagus, and a high incidence of postcricoid carcinoma. Throughout the body, the activity of enzymes containing iron is reduced, through rarely sufficiently to cause dysfunction.

Clinical Presentation. Iron deficiency anemia develops slowly and insidiously. Lassitude and fatigue are the most common symptoms, though as the anemia worsens any of the symptoms and signs of anemia may occur.

About 50% of patients with severe iron deficiency anemia develop pica, a craving for some unnatural kind of food. The patients have an abnormal appetite for one kind of food, usually something crunchy like ice, celery, or nuts. Hippocrates noted that some of these patients developed a craving to eat earth.

The form of iron deficiency anemia called chlorosis, from the Greek for green, has become rare. It occurred in girls 14 to 17 years old, who developed severe iron de-

ficiency anemia, often with considerable emotional upset, pica, gastrointestinal disturbances, and thrombosis in peripheral veins, especially in the cerebral sinuses. The skin of these girls acquired a distinctive greenish tint. In the 19th century, chlorosis was common. With the dawn of the 20th century, it suddenly disappeared. Girls with severe iron deficiency anemia are pale, but they are no longer green. It has been suggested that chlorosis was caused by the tight lacing of corsets, but the relationship between corsets, iron deficiency, and the green discoloration of the skin is not clear.

Cause. Table 49-4 lists the causes of iron deficiency anemia. Often more than one of these factors combine to cause the anemia.

Blood Loss. Blood loss is the most common cause of iron deficiency anemia. In the United Kingdom, it is the principal cause of the anemia in 80% of people with iron deficiency anemia. The bleeding is not usually dramatic and often passes unnoticed. A

TABLE 49-4. CAUSES OF IRON DEFICIENCY ANEMIA

Blood loss
  Gastrointestinal bleeding
    Aspirin
    Carcinoma
    Diverticulitis
    Diverticulosis
    Hemorrhoids
    Hiatus hernia
    Hookworm infestation
    Peptic ulcer
    Ulcerative colitis

  Other bleeding
    Epistaxis
    Idiopathic pulmonary hemosiderosis
    Paroxysmal nocturnal hemoglobinuria

Inadequate diet

Malabsorption
    Achlorhydria
    Celiac disease
    Gastrectomy
    Pica
    Protein-losing enteropathy
    Vagotomy

Increased demand
    Infancy
    Pregnancy

persistent loss of 3 or 4 mL of blood a day can cause anemia.

Iron deficiency anemia is particularly common in women during the reproductive years because of the loss of iron in the menses. The larger the menstrual flow, the more likely is the loss of iron in the menses to exceed the dietary intake. In Sweden, 70% of women who lost more than 80 mL of blood each menstrual period were anemic, in spite of a dietary intake of about 10 mg of iron a day.

Bleeding from the gastrointestinal tract is a major cause of iron deficiency. The bleeding can be massive, but more often passes unnoticed by the patient. About 15% of people with hiatus hernia bleed enough to become anemic. A peptic ulcer can cause massive bleeding or the continuing loss of a few mL of blood daily. Some 70% of people who take aspirin lose each day a few mL of blood from gastric erosions. In some parts of the world in which hookworm infestation is common, over 30% of the population is anemic. Each worm drinks 0.05 mL of blood a day, and the bowel can contain hundreds of them. Some 5% of people with diverticulosis, 20% of those with diverticulitis, and 80% of those with active ulcerative colitis have iron deficiency anemia. Occult bleeding from a carcinoma of the cecum or some other gastrointestinal tumor can cause iron deficiency. Bleeding from hemorrhoids can do so. Less often, iron deficiency anemia results from overly generous blood donation, paroxysmal nocturnal hemoglobinuria, idiopathic pulmonary hemosiderosis, or repeated bleeding from the nose.

Inadequate Diet. The intake of iron in the diet is rarely so low that it is the major cause of iron deficiency, except in infants. Milk contains little iron, and infants fed only milk may well become iron deficient. More often a diet poor in iron increases the severity of anemia caused by blood loss.

Malabsorption. Malabsorption of iron can cause iron deficiency or increase the severity of iron deficiency produced in other ways. It can be due to disease of the stomach, disease of the small intestine, or to some abnormal substance present in the intestine.

Achlorhydria impairs the absorption of iron. Gastric acid is necessary for the transformation of the ferric iron in the diet to the ferrous form in which it is absorbed. Gastric acid and proteases must split heme from protein before the iron in heme can be absorbed. Gastrectomy and vagotomy tend to cause iron deficiency both by reducing gastric secretion and by increasing the rate of passage through the small bowel where most of the iron is absorbed.

Celiac disease and other forms of malabsorption often cause iron deficiency, especially in children. In infants, protein-losing enteropathy, perhaps due to sensitivity to milk, is often associated with iron deficiency.

Pica is the term used to describe the habitual ingestion of some unusual substance, such as earth, starch, or ice. It sometimes causes iron deficiency if the earth or other matrial ingested contains resins that bind iron and prevent its absorption. In some parts of the world, pica is common especially during pregnancy.

Increased Demand. Pregnancy causes a major increase in the need for iron. The mother loses 700 mg of iron to the fetus and needs another 500 mg to meet her own needs. As most of this demand for iron comes in the third trimester, iron deficiency is common in the later stages of pregnancy. Lactation causes a loss of iron of about the same order as menstruation.

Infancy. Several factors combine to cause the iron deficiency common in infants. The leakage of blood from the fetal to the maternal circulation in utero that occurs in 50% of pregnancies is sometimes enough to cause iron deficiency. If the umbilical cord is clamped early during delivery, much fetal blood is trapped in the placenta, reducing the fetal iron stores. Iron stores are smaller in premature infants than those born at term. Iron stores are low in twins, because they have to share the iron derived from the mother. The rapid growth during the first year of life increases the demand for iron. Milk contains little iron. Gastrointestinal disease and occult bleeding can impair the absorption of iron.

Pathogenesis. Iron deficiency anemia develops when the saturation of transferrin in the plasma falls below 16%. Often it is less than 10%. The total iron-binding capacity is normal or increased.

The iron in the plasma is taken up avidly by the bone marrow. In iron deficiency anemia 50% of a dose of radioactive iron given intravenously disappears from the blood in 20 minutes. Normally, it takes 90 minutes to remove 50% of the radioactivity from the blood. Because of the rapid uptake of iron from the plasma, the daily uptake of iron by the bone marrow is normal or increased. Over 90% of the iron taken up from the plasma is incorporated into hemoglobin. Normally, only 80% is used to manufacture hemoglobin. The quantity of hemoglobin produced is greater than normal.

Anemia develops because many of the red cells produced are defective and are destroyed in the bone marrow. The iron is reincorporated into hemoglobin, but because of the continued destruction of red cells in the bone marrow, the number of red cells delivered to the blood is reduced. The red cells that reach the blood are short-lived, on the average surviving only 70 days instead of the normal 120.

Treatment and Prognosis. Iron cures iron deficiency anemia. Usually ferrous iron is given by mouth and is highly effective, even in those with malabsorption of iron. In therapeutic doses, iron is irritating. About 20% of the patients complain of heartburn, nausea, abdominal cramps, or diarrhea, particularly when too large a dose is given at the outset. Parentrally administered iron is equally effective, but is rarely needed.

Within a week or so, the patient begins to feel better. Reticulocytes begin to increase in the blood after a few days and reach a peak in 5 to 10 days, before falling back to normal. The height of the reticulocytosis depends on the degree of anemia, but often at the peak of the reaction between 5 and 10% of the circulating red cells are reticulocytes. The concentration of hemoglobin in the blood increases more slowly, but regardless of the severity of the anemia, it usually rises half way to normal in three weeks and reaches a normal level in about two months.

Regeneration of the papillae of the tongue begins after two weeks and is usually complete after three months. In a few patients, partial atrophy persists indefinitely. Koilonychia takes up to six months to disappear, as normal nails grow out. In most patients,

the gastritis persists unchanged. If pica was caused by the iron deficiency, it disappears.

ANEMIA OF CHRONIC DISORDERS. Anemia is common in chronic diseases, and can be caused in many ways. To mention only mechanisms already discussed, deficiency of vitamin B_{12} may occur in Crohn's disease; folate deficiency is common in tropical sprue; iron deficiency may complicate a peptic ulcer.

The term *anemia of chronic disorders* is used to describe one of the ways in which chronic diseases cause anemia. It describes a condition in which the concentration of iron in the plasma is low, although there are abundant stores of iron in the liver, bone marrow, and spleen.

Anemia of chronic disorders is common. It is likely to develop in any long continued inflammatory or neoplastic disease, and sometimes occurs without demonstrable cause.

Lesions. The lesions of the anemia of chronic disorders are most severe in the blood. The changes in the bone marrow and other organs are not usually prominent.

Bone Marrow. In the anemia of chronic disorders, from 5 to 20% of normoblasts contain demonstrable deposits of hemosiderin, instead of the normal 30 to 50%. The quantity of iron stored in macrophages in the bone marrow is increased, unless the condition is complicated by iron deficiency. Otherwise, the bone marrow shows little abnormality.

Blood. The anemia of chronic disorders is not severe. The concentration of hemoglobin in the blood is usually between 90 and 110 g/L (9 to 11 g/100 mL). The volume of packed red cells is usually between 30 and 40 L/L (30 to 40%), rarely lower. The concentration of hemoglobin in the red cells is normal or reduced to between 260 and 320 g/L (26 to 32 g/100 mL), rather than the normal 320 to 360 g/L (32 to 36 g/100 mL). The volume of the red cells is usually normal, though if the anemia persists, it is sometimes reduced below the normal mean of 80 to 94 fL, but rarely to a mean of less than 72 fL.

A blood smear shows little abnormality. There may be slight anisocytosis, but poikilocytosis is unusual. The leukocyte count is normal unless affected by the underlying disease.

The concentration of iron in the serum is low, usually between 2 and 10 µmol/L (10 to 60 µg/100 mL). The total iron-binding capacity is low, usually between 35 and 55 µmol/L (200 to 300 µg/100 mL). The saturation of transferrin is less than 16%, often less than 10%. Because of the increased storage of iron, the concentration of ferritin in the plasma is increased.

The concentration of free protoporphyrin increases in the red cells, though only after the anemia is well established. Protoporphyrin is synthesized normally, but cannot be incorporated into hemoglobin because of the lack of iron.

In most patients with the anemia of chronic disorders, the concentration of copper in the serum increases, mainly because of an increase in the concentration of ceruloplasmin. The concentration may be as high as 42 µmol/L (270 µg/100 mL), in contrast to the normal range of from 13 to 23 µmol/L (80 to 150 µg/100 mL). The increased concentration of copper appears before the anemia, and if the infection or tumor is controlled, it disappears before the anemia resolves.

Other Organs.   Increased iron storage is sometimes evident in the liver and spleen in patients with the anemia of chronic disorders.

Clinical Presentation.   The anemia of chronic disorders develops slowly over two or three months and persists as long as the underlying disease continues. The severity of the anemia is roughly proportional to the severity of the underlying disease. It is rarely severe enough to cause serious disability.

Cause.   Table 49-5 lists the causes of the anemia of chronic disorders. Many of these conditions can cause anemia in other ways, and the pathogenesis of the anemia in these patients is often complex.

Pathogenesis.   Three faults combine to cause the anemia of chronic disorders. The life span of the circulating red cells is shortened. The bone marrow fails to respond to the growing hypoxia caused by the anemia. The iron stores fail to release iron normally to transferrin.

The red cells are normal in the anemia of chronic disorders, but are destroyed by an extracorpuscular factor or factors present in the plasma. If red cells from a patient with the anemia of chronic disorders are trans-

TABLE 49-5. CAUSES OF THE ANEMIA OF CHRONIC DISORDERS

Chronic infection
  Infective endocarditis
  Meningitis
  Mycotic infections
  Osteomyelitis
  Pelvic inflammatory disease
  Tuberculosis
  Urinary infections

Collagen disease
  Rheumatic fever
  Rheumatoid arthritis
  Systemic lupus erythematosus

Other forms of chronic inflammation
  Burns
  Myocardial infarction
  Trauma

Tumors
  Carcinoma
  Leukemia
  Lymphoma
  Myeloma

Idiopathic

fused into a normal person, they survive normally. If red cells from a normal person are transfused into a patient with the anemia of chronic disorders, their life is shortened.

The nature of the extracorpuscular factor or factors that shorten the life of the erythrocytes in the anemia of chronic disorders is unknown. Inflammation and tumors might produce a substance that shortens the life of red cells, or the abnormal circulation in the inflamed tissues and in tumors might damage the red cells, shortening their life.

The shortening of the life of the circulating red cells in the anemia of chronic disorders is not great and would be of little note if the marrow responded to the anemia normally. The bone marrow could easily increase the production of red cells enough to compensate for their short life.

In most patients with the anemia of chronic disorders, the marrow fails to increase the production of red cells because the body fails to increase the production of erythropoietin to offset the anemia. Because there is no increase in the production of erythropoietin, there is no stimulus to the marrow to increase production. In most patients, the marrow responds normally if erythropoietin is given.

In some patients with the anemia of chronic disorders, the production of erythropoietin does increase in response to the anemia, but the marrow fails to respond. Whether this failure results from the disordered iron metabolism in these patients or is caused in some other way is not known.

The hypoferremia of the anemia of chronic disorders is caused by failure of the macrophages in the liver, spleen, and bone marrow to release iron to maintain the saturation of transferrin. Possibly a factor released by the phagocytes in the inflammatory lesions prevents the release of iron from the macrophages, or lactoferrin released by the phagocytes binds iron and delivers it back to the macrophages rather than to the bone marrow.

The body responds to the reduced saturation of transferrin much as in iron deficiency. The uptake of iron from the plasma increases, so that a normal or increased quantity of iron reaches the bone marrow. The production of hemoglobin is normal or increased, but the destruction of red cells in the bone marrow prevents the supply of sufficient red cells to the blood.

Treatment and Prognosis. The anemia of chronic disorders can be corrected only by controlling the underlying disease. Iron, vitamin B_{12}, and folate are of no value unless there is also a deficiency of one of these factors.

SIDEROBLASTIC ANEMIA. The sideroblastic anemias are a group of conditions in which iron accumulates in the mitochondria of the precursors of the red cells in the bone marrow. The name comes from the Greek words for iron and for a shoot or sprout. Table 49-6 lists the different forms of sideroblastic anemia. All are uncommon. The idiopathic form is the most frequent.

Idiopathic Refractory Sideroblastic Anemia. Patients with the idiopathic form of sideroblastic anemia are usually over 50 years old, though the disease can develop in younger people. Both men and women are affected.

Lesions. The principal lesions are in the bone marrow and the blood, Other organs show only minor abnormalities.

Bone Marrow. The bone marrow is usually hyperplastic in idiopathic sideroblastic anemia. Often the erythroid cells are as numerous as the myeloid cells. In 80% of the patients, the developing red cells are normoblasts. The other 20% of the patients have folate deficiency and the developing red cells are megaloblasts.

Granules of iron are demonstrable in from 50 to over 90% of the developing red cells. Iron is even present in the early forms of developing red cell, a feature not often seen in other forms of sideroblastic anemia. The iron is stored in the mitochondria as a complex of ferric iron and phosphate. Since the mitochondria are most numerous around the nuclei, the granules of iron form a ring around the nuclei. A nucleated red cell containing iron demonstrable by light microscopy is called a sideroblast. An anucleate

TABLE 49-6. THE SIDEROBLASTIC ANEMIAS

Idiopathic refractory

Hereditary
    Aminolevulinic acid synthetase deficiency
    Coproporphyrinogen oxidase deficiency

Secondary
  To disease
    Blood disease
      Hemolytic anemia
      Leukemia
      Megaloblastic anemia
      Polycythemia vera
    Tumors
      Carcinoma
      Lymphoma
      Multiple myeloma

    Other
      Hyperthyroidism
      Infection
      Myxedema
      Polyarteritis nodosa
      Porphyria
      Rheumatoid arthritis
      Uremia

  To drugs and poisons
    Acetaminophen
    Antineoplastic drugs
    Antituberculous drugs
    Chloramphenicol
    Ethanol
    Lead
    Phenacetin

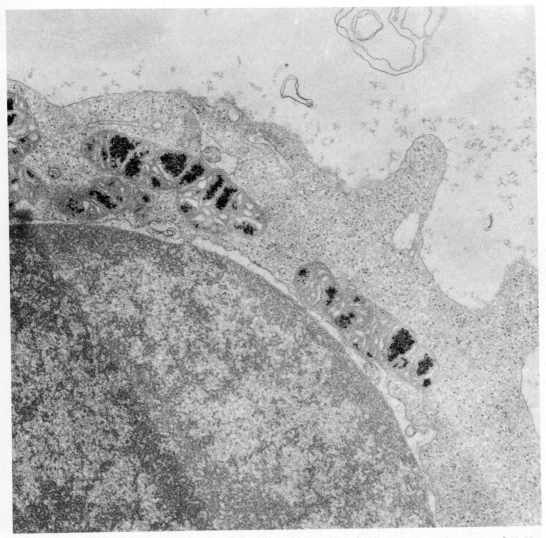

Fig. 49-5. Iron in the mitochondria of a normoblast in a patient with sideroblastic anemia. (Courtesy, of W. N. Jensen from Wintrobe, M. W., et al.: Clinical Hematology. 8th Ed. Philadelphia, Lea & Febiger, 1981.)

red cell containing demonstrable iron is called a siderocyte.

Normally up to 50% of the nucleated red cells in the bone marrow are sideroblasts. They contain a few granules of ferritin free in the cytoplasm or in a vacuole, but iron is not present in the mitochondria. The ferritin is demonstrable by ligh microscopy, but the granules of iron do not form the perinuclear ring seen in sideroblastic anemia.

Blood. In most patients with idiopathic sideroblastic anemia, the concentration of hemoglobin in the blood is between 70 and 100 g/L (7 to 10 g/100 mL). The packed red cell volume is about 0.30 L/L (30%).

The blood shows two populations of red cells. Most are normochromic, but up to 30% of the cells are hypochromic. Because of the predominance of normochromic red cells, the mean corpuscular concentration of hemoglobin is usually normal. The red cells are often the normal size of 80 to 94 fL, but in

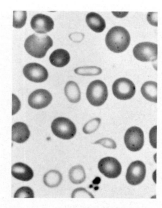

Fig. 49-6. Two populations of red cells seen in the blood in patients with sideroblastic anemia: macrocytic and microcytic. (From Wintrobe, M. W., et al.: Clinical Hematology. 8th Ed. Philadelphia, Lea & Febiger, 1981.)

some patients they are 100 to 120 fL. A few of the circulating red cells may contain granules of hemosiderin.

The leukocyte count is normal or slightly reduced. The activity of alkaline phosphatase in the leukocytes is low in 50% of the patients. The concentration of platelets in the plasma may be normal, low, or increased. In 30% of the patients, the platelet count exceeds 500×10^9/L (500,000/mm^3).

The concentration of protoporphyrin in the red cells increases, sometimes sufficiently to cause photosensitivity. The saturation of transferrin is high, in 30% of the patients over 90%. The total iron-binding capacity is usually normal. The concentration of ferritin in the plasma also is high.

Other Organs.   The amount of iron stored in the macrophages of the liver and spleen increases as the quantity of iron stored in the body grows larger.

Clinical Presentation.   Idiopathic sideroblastic anemia develops slowly. The patient may develop symptoms or signs of mild anemia, or the anemia may be detected during a routine medical examination.

Pathogenesis.   The age at which idiopathic refractory sideroblastic anemia become evident suggests that it is an acquired disorder, not due to a congenital abnormality. The presence of two populations of red cells in the blood is consistent with the theory that an abnormal clone of red cells proliferates in the bone marrow.

About 50% of the patients show chromosomal abnormalities in the bone marrow, most often trisomy 8 or deletion of part of the long arm of chromosome 20. The types of abnormality found are like those in other myeloproliferative diseases. None is consistently present.

The synthesis of hemoglobin in the bone marrow is impaired, probably because of inability to synthesize heme adequately. The aminolevulinic acid synthetase and heme synthetase needed for the synthesis of heme are mitochondrial enzymes and could be inhibited by the iron stored in the mitochondria. The activity of aminolevulinic acid synthetase is usually less than 25% of normal. The activity of other mitochondrial enzymes is reduced.

Because of the impaired synthesis of heme, erythropoiesis is ineffective. The uptake of iron from the plasma is high, and the synthesis of hemoglobin is increased, but many of the developing red cells are destroyed in the bone marrow. The destruction is often sufficient to increase the concentration of bilirubin in the plasma up to 35 µmol/L (2 mg/100 mL) and to increase the excretion of urobilinogen in the urine. The red cells that do reach the blood have a normal life span.

Because the bone marrow cannot utilize iron effectively, iron stores in the body increase. The quantity of iron in the liver and spleen grows, causing the hyperferritinemia and the increased saturation of transferrin.

Treatment and Prognosis.   In 50% of the patients with idiopathic sideroblastic anemia, the anemia is mild and persists with little change for many years. No treatment is required.

If the anemia becomes more severe, large doses of androgens sometimes bring benefit. Pyridoxine is of little value. In some patients, transfusions are the only recourse.

Patients with mild idiopathic sideroblastic anemia live on the average for 15 years. Those who need transfusions survive for a mean of 8 years. Leukemia, usually acute myelomonoblastic leukemia, develops in 7% of the patients, nearly always in people with a normal or low platelet count.

Hereditary Sideroblastic Anemia.   Three types of hereditary sideroblastic anemia have been distinguished. All are rare. In most of the patients, the mitochondrial enzyme δ-aminolevulinic acid synthetase is deficient. This enzyme is needed for the synthesis of the precursor of heme, δ-aminolevulinic acid. The defect is usually inherited as an X-linked recessive character. Nearly all the patients are men, though in some kindreds female heterozygotes show less severe changes. Less often, the deficiency of δ-aminolevulinic acid synthetase is inherited as an autosomal recessive character. Rarely, coproporphyrinogen oxidase, another of the mitochondrial enzymes needed for the synthesis of heme, is deficient.

Lesions. The lesions in the hereditary forms of sideroblastic anemia are similar to those in the idiopathic form of the disease, but are more severe.

Bone Marrow. The bone marrow in people with one of the hereditary forms of sideroblastic anemia shows erythroid hyperplasia. The developing red cells are usually normoblasts, but occasionally are megaloblastic, probably because of folate deficiency. Most of the developing red cells contain granules of iron. The iron forms a ring around the nucleus in up to 50% of the more mature developing red cells. The macrophages in the bone marrow are filled with iron.

Blood. The concentration of hemoglobin in the blood is usually between 60 and 90 g/L (6 to 9 g/100 mL) in the hereditary forms of sideroblastic anemia. Two populatons of red cells are present. In one, the red cells are of normal size, contain a normal quantity of hemoglobin, and appear normal. In the other, the red cells are usually smaller than normal, and the concentration of hemoglobin in their cytoplasm is reduced. This hypochromic, microcytic family of red cells often shows marked anisocytosis and poikilocytosis, with target cells and basophilic stippling. The leukocyte and platelet counts in the blood are usually normal. The saturation of transferrin is light. The concentration of ferritin in the plasma is increased.

The concentration of protoporphyrin in the red cells is low. In a few patients, presumably those with a deficiency of coprophoryrinogen oxidase, coproporphyrin accumulates in the red cells.

Other Organs. The quantity of iron stored in the body is great in the hereditary forms of sideroblastic anemia. The liver and other organs show changes like those in hemochromatosis. Iron is stored in Kupffer cells and hepatocytes, sometimes with fibrosis. Diabetes mellitus develops in 30% of the patients. Occasionally the skin is pigmented. Deposition of iron in the heart can cause cardiac dysfunction.

In 30% of the patients with hereditary sideroblastic anemia, tryptophane metabolism is abnormal. Urinary excretion of xanthurenic acid, kynurenic acid, or both is increased.

Clinical Presentation. In hereditary sideroblastic anemia, the anemia may become evident in childhood, but often it is not detected until the patient is adult, sometimes only in old age. The patient often presents with signs of anemia.

Pathogenesis. The impairment of heme synthesis caused by the enzyme deficiency in the hereditary forms of sideroblastic anemia causes dysfunction similar to that in the idiopathic form of the disease. Erythropoiesis is ineffective, causing the anemia and the increased iron storage.

Treatment and Prognosis. Large doses of pyridoxine restore about 50% of the patients with hereditary sideroblastic anemia nearly to normal. The synthesis of protoporphyrin increases; the concentration of hemoglobin in the blood becomes normal or nearly so; the concentration of iron in the plasma decreases; and tryptophane metabolism returns to normal. Presumably the great excess of pyridoxine compensates for the lack of δ-aminolevulinic acid synthetase in these people. Other patients respond only partially or not at all. The people with deficiency of coprophoryrinogen oxidase are among those who do not respond. In the patients who do not respond to pyridoxine, the increasing load of iron in the tissues can be managed by venesection or by using chelating agents, as in hemochromatosis.

The prognosis should be guarded. Some patients with hereditary sideroblastic anemia do well for years with pyridoxine therapy. In others, the dangers of hemochromatosis, increased risk of infection, or increasing anemia bring death.

Secondary Sideroblastic Anemia. The drugs and diseases listed as causes of secondary sideroblastic anemia rarely cause serious anemia. More often, there are minor sideroblastic changes in the bone marrow, with little or no change in the blood. The changes in the bone marrow, blood, and other organs are similar to those in idiopathic sideroblastic anemia, though they are rarely severe. Folate deficiency is common.

Treatment of secondary sideroblastic anemia is the treatment of its cause. An offending drug should be withdrawn. Any underlying disease should be controlled. Pyridoxine rarely offers any benefit. Some of the patients with multiple myeloma who develop sideroblastic anemia die of leukemia.

Hemolytic Disorders

In the hemolytic disorders, destruction of the circulating red cells is increased, but the bone marrow responds normally and delivers more red cells to the blood in an attempt to maintain the concentration of hemoglobin in the blood. The name comes from the Greek words for blood and loosening or setting free. Conditions such as the megaloblastic anemias and the anemia of chronic disorders in which there is increased destruction of circulating red cells but the bone marrow cannot respond by increasing the number of red cells delivered to the blood are not considered hemolytic disorders.

The bone marrow can increase the production of red cells 6 or 8 times. If the destruction of red cells is not too great, it can compensate for the hemolysis and the concentration of hemoglobin in the blood remains normal. Such a condition is called a compensated hemolytic disorder. If the destruction of circulating red cells is so great that the bone marrow cannot compensate, the patient develops hemolytic anemia.

Table 49-7 lists the different kinds of hemolytic anemia. All shorten the life of the circulating red cells, but the mechanisms involved are different. In the congenital disorders, the defect is in the red cells. In the immunohemolytic disorders, an immune reaction destroys the red cells. In the fragmentation anemias, the red cells are destroyed mechanically. Occasionally infection, drugs, or other conditions cause hemolysis.

TABLE 49-7. HEMOLYTIC DISORDERS

Congenital Anomalies
  Defects in the red cell membrane
    Acanthocytosis
    Hereditary elliptocytosis
    Hereditary spherocytosis
    Stomatocytosis
    Other

  Enzyme deficiencies
    Glucose-6-phosphate dehydrogenase
    Pyruvate kinase
    Other
Structural hemoglobinopathies
    Hemoglobin C disease
    Hemoglobin D disease
    Hemoglobin E disease
    Sickle cell disease
    Unstable hemoglobin disease
    Other

  Thalassemia
    Doubly heterozygous disorders
    Hemoglobin H disease
    Hemoglobin Lepore disease
    Hereditary persistence of fetal hemoglobin
    α-Thalassemia
    β-Thalassemia
    β-Thalassemia
    δβ-Thalassemia

Acquired disorders
  Immunohemolytic disorders
    Cold antibody hemolysis
      Cold agglutinin disorders
      Paroxysmal cold hemoglobinuria
    Hemolytic disease of the newborn
      ABO incompatibility
      Rh incompatibility
    Transfusion reaction
    Warm antibody hemolysis
      Drug-induced
      Idiopathic
      Secondary to other disease

  Fragmentation anemia
    Cardiac anemia
    March hemoglobinuria
    Microangiopathic anemia

  Other hemolytic disorders
    Drug-induced hemolysis
    Hypophosphatemia
    Infectious hemolytic anemia
    Paroxysmal nocturnal hemoglobinuria
    Thermal injury

Two kinds of hemolysis are distinguished. In intravascular hemolysis, the destruction of the red cells occurs in blood vessels throughout the body. The red cells rupture and release hemoglobin and other substances into

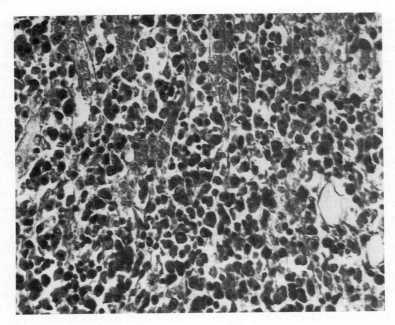

Fig. 49-7. Hyperplastic bone marrow, showing the almost complete absence of fat.

the plasma. In extravascular hemolysis, the red cells are destroyed principally by the macrophages in the spleen and to a lesser degree by the macrophages in the liver and other organs, much as red cells are eventually destroyed in normal people.

The response of the body to hemolysis is similar in all hemolytic disorders. The increased demand for red cells causes hyperplasia of the bone marrow and changes in the blood. The increase in the quantity of hemoglobin and other substances released from the red cells causes changes in the blood and other organs. The response to hemolysis will be discussed first; then the different kinds of hemolytic disorder are considered.

Response to Hemolysis. The hemolytic disorders vary greatly in severity. Some are minor and fully compensated. In others massive destruction of the red cells and severe anemia occur. Some are short-lived and soon pass. Others persist for months, years, or a lifetime. The more severe the hemolysis and the longer it persists, the more severe the lesions in the bone marrow, blood, and other organs.

Bone Marrow. The hemolytic disorders cause erythroid hyperplasia in the bone mar-

row. To meet the increased demand for red cells, the number of erythroid cells in the bone marrow increases. The proportion of fat in the red marrow decreases. If the hyperplasia is severe, the red marrow extends into the long bones, replacing the normal fatty marrow. Normally, from 25 to 40% of the hematopoietic cells in the marrow are erythroid cells. In hemolytic anemia the proportion of erythroid cells increases to from 40 to 70%.

To meet the increased demands of the bone marrow, more iron is carried to the marrow by the blood. Instead of the normal mean of 125 µmol/L/d (0.7 mg/100 mL/d), the marrow takes up from 350 µmol/L/d (2 mg/100 mL/d) to 625 µmol/L/d (3.5 mg/100 mL/d). Because of the increased production of red cells, more iron passes from the marrow to the blood in hemoglobin, 200 µmol/L/d (1.2 mg/100 mL/d) to 350 µmol/L/d (2 mg/100 mL/d) rather than the normal mean of 100 µmol/L/d (0.5 mg/100 mL/d).

Blood. The severity of the anemia varies considerably in the hemolytic disorders, from minimal to most severe. Often the concentration of hemoglobin in the blood is from 70 to 120 g/L (7 to 12 g/100 mL), and the volume of packed red cells is from 25 to 35 L/L (25 to 35%). The life of the circulating red cells is shortened. If hemolysis is severe, the erythrocytes survive for 30 days or less, instead of their normal 120 days.

The hyperactivity of the bone marrow is shown by an increase in the proportion of reticulocytes in the blood. Reticulocytes are red cells that have lost their nucleus, but still retain ribosomes, mitochondria, and a Golgi apparatus. Reticulocytes are 20% larger than normal red cells and irregularly spheroidal, rather than flattened disks. Normally, less than 2.5% of the circulating red cells in men and less than 4% in women are reticulocytes. In the hemolytic anemias, often more than 10% of the red cells are reticulocytes, and at times the proportion reaches 50%. The more active the marrow, the more likely it is to pass immature red cells into the blood, and the greater the reticulocytosis. With them may come a few nucleated red cells, but in the hemolytic anemias less than 1% of the circulating red cells are nucleated.

The red cells in the blood and their precursors in the marrow are often larger than normal. The mean volume of the red cells in the blood is commonly between 100 and 130 fL, instead of the normal 82 to 92 fL. This increase in mean volume occurs in part because of the increased proportion of reticulocytes, which are bigger than other red cells, in part because the mature red cells are bigger. Intense stimulation of the marrow by erythropoietin often results in the production of red cells that are larger than normal. The concentration of hemoglobin in the red cells is usually normal.

Spherocytes appear in the blood in many hemolytic disorders. The name is misleading, for spherocytes are not spherical. They are flattened and have concave surfaces, like other red cells, but are thicker than normal red cells. As the volume of spherocytes is normal, their diameter becomes less as the cell grows thicker. Spherocytosis is caused by damage to the red cell membrane. In some forms of spherocytosis, the damage is due to a congenital defect in the red cells. In some, it is caused by an extracorporeal factor that damages the red cells.

Spherocytes of both types show increased osmotic fragility. If red cells are suspended in a hypotonic solution, they take up water and swell. If the solution is sufficiently hypotonic, they take up so much water that they rupture. Because of their shape, spherocytes can take up less water than normal red cells before rupturing, and so mildly hypotonic solutions that cause little injury to normal red cells cause considerable lysis of spherocytes. If there is only mild spherocytosis, incubating the red cells in the hypotonic solution for 24 hours makes the increased fragility more evident.

The increased breakdown of red cells in the hemolytic disorders increases the production of bilirubin. Often there is mild hyperbilirubinemia. Commonly the concentration of bilirubin in the plasma is between 15 and 50 μmol/L (1 to 3 mg/100mL). It is rarely more than 85 μmol/L (5 mg/100 mL), except in neonates and patients with hepatic dysfunction.

The concentration of bilirubin in the plasma correlates poorly with the severity of the hemolysis. It depends on the efficiency of the liver, as well as on the severity of the hemolysis. In people with good liver function, the level of bilirubin in the plasma may be normal, in spite of hemolysis. In people with poor hepatic function, mild jaundice is the only sign of hemolysis. The marrow can compensate for the increased destruction of the red cells, but the liver cannot excrete the increased load of bilirubin.

The excess of bilirubin in the blood in the hemolytic disorders is not conjugated, and so is not excreted in the urine. An old name for the hemolytic disorders is acholuric jaundice, from the Greek words for without, bile, and urine.

Because of the hyperbilirubinemia, the fecal excretion of urobilinogen is usually increased, but can be normal. Antibiotic therapy reduces the activity of the bacteria in the colon that convert bilirubin to urobilinogen, and in consequence the fecal excretion of urobilinogen remains normal, even though the excretion of bilirubin is increased. The urinary excretion of urobilinogen is often increased in patients with hemolytic disorders, but it too depends on the efficiency of the liver and can be normal, even though there is serious hemolysis.

The endogenous production of carbon

monoxide is a measure of the breakdown of heme. One molecule of carbon monoxide is produced for each molecule of heme degraded to bilirubin. The carbon monoxide forms carboxyhemoglobin. The rate at which carboxyhemoglobin is formed is a measure of the destruction of heme.

The destruction of the circulating red cells allows their lactic dehydrogenase and other enzymes to escape into the plasma. In consequence, the activity of lactic dehydrogenase in the serum increases, sometimes to as much as five times normal. This is less than the increase in lactic dehydrogenase activity of 10 to 20 times caused by the destruction of red cell precursors in the megaloblastic anemias. In contrast to the megaloblastic anemias, the activity of the isoenzyme lactic dehydrogenase 2 is greater than the activity of lactic dehydrogenase 1.

In most hemolytic disorders, the concentration of hemoglobin in the plasma is below its normal upper limit of 0.01 g/L (1 mg/100 mL). Only if there is intravascular hemolysis is it likely to be high. In sickle cell anemia and thalassemia major it may rise to between 0.15 and 0.60 g/L (15 to 60 mg/100 mL). In severe intravascular hemolysis, it may be as much as 10 g/L (1000 mg/100 mL).

The concentration of haptoglobin in the serum is a sensitive measure of intravascular hemolysis. When hemoglobin escapes into the plasma, it binds to haptoglobin. The complex of hemoglobin with haptoglobin is removed from the blood within a few minutes, mainly by the liver. Since hemolysis causes no increase in the synthesis of haptoglobin, the concentration of haptoglobin in the serum soon falls from its normal 1 to 3 g/L to undetectable levels. If the destruction of circulating red cells in twice normal, haptoglobin is undetectable in the serum. The concentration of hemglobin in the plasma often remains in the normal range.

Infections, collagen diseases, cancer, trauma, burns, myocardial infarction, kidney disease, biliary obstruction, and adrenocortical steroids increase the production of haptoglobin, often so greatly that haptoglobin remains present in the plasma, even though there is hemolysis, or reappears in the plasma in a patient in whom it was previously absent. Because haptoglobin is synthesized in the liver, liver disease can reduce its concentration in the plasma.

Once the haptoglobin is exhausted, the dimer of hemoglobin in the plasma is filtered into the urine to cause hemoglobinuria. If there is severe intravascular hemolysis, enough hemoglobin can reach the urine to turn it pink or red, even dark like a cola drink.

Some of the hemoglobin in the urine is taken up by the epithelium of the proximal convoluted tubules, and its iron is stored in the cells as ferritin or hemosiderin. After some days, the tubular epithelial cells are shed, and the hemosiderin they contain can be demonstrated in the urine. Because it is a measure of iron stored in the renal tubular epithelium, hemosiderinuria does not begin until some days after the hemolysis and persists for some time after the hemoylsis has ceased.

Some of the hemoglobin in the plasma is oxidized to methemoglobin. Some heme from the methemoglobin is transferred to albumin or hemopexin. Methemalbumin and hemopexin-heme can be demonstrated in the plasma of patients with hemolysis. Sometimes the concentration of hemopexin in the plasma falls because it is used up by the heme, much as haptoglobin is used up by hemoglobin.

Other Organs.   In the hemolytic anemias, iron accumulates throughout the body, principally in the macrophages of the liver, spleen, and bone marrow. Especially when multiple transfusions are needed, the hemosiderosis can become severe.

The spleen is often enlarged if hemolytic anemia persists for a long time. It is responsible for most of the destruction of the red cells in most forms of hemolytic anemia and because of its increased work becomes hyperplastic. The enlargement is usually moderate, but occasionally becomes great.

Cholelithiasis is common in the congenital hemolytic disorders and may occur if acquired hemolytic disease persists for many years. The continued excretion of excessive quantities of bilirubin in the bile leads to the precipitation of pigment stones in the gallbladder. The stones are uncommon before puberty, but become increasingly common as patients age. In hereditary spherocytosis,

85% of adult patients have pigment stones.

Ulceration of the ankles sometimes occurs in chronic hemolytic anemia, though it is not common. It occurs most often in hereditary spherocytosis and in sickle cell anemia, though it may occur in other hemolytic disorders. The ulcers are bilateral and involve the skin over or above the medial or lateral malleoli. Sometimes the ulcers extend right around the leg. The ulcers are indolent and persist for a long time. If they do heal, they tend to recur. If the hemolysis can be alleviated, the ulcers heal promptly, leaving an indurated, pigmented area in the skin.

If hemolytic anemia is severe in growing children, the hyperplasia of the red marrow may be so great that it distorts the bones. This is particularly likely in thalassemia major, but may occur in sickle cell anemia or, less often, in other congenital hemolytic anemias. The exuberant hyerplasia of the bone marrow can make the diploë of the bones of the skull several times its normal thickness. It can erode and thin the medullary trabeculae in the diploë and greatly thin the inner and outer table of the skull bones. In thalassemia major, the outer table of the bones of the vault of the skull may become invisible to roentgenography, and the trabeculae in the diploë become aligned vertical to the surface of the bone, so that roentgenogram of the skull looks as if the patient's hair were on end. In the tubular bones of the extremities, the marrow cavity is enlarged by the pressure of the red marrow, with thinning of the cortex, and with rarefaction and coarsening of the trabecular pattern in the medulla. The changes are well seen in the metacarpals. As the child grows to adult years, the changes in the long bones regress, but the expansion of the bones of the skull and similar changes in the vertebrae and pelvis persist and may worsen.

Acute Hemolytic Anemia. In most hemolytic disorders, the changes in the bone marrow, blood, and other organs evolve slowly as weeks and months pass. In acute hemolytic anemia, they develop within minutes or hours. An incompatible blood transfusion, an immunologic injury, or some other major attack on the circulating red cells can cause sudden and massive hemolysis. Aching pains develop in the back, abdomen, or limbs. The pain in the abdomen is sometimes severe enough to suggest and abdominal disaster and may be accompanied by muscular rigidity. Often there is malaise, nausea, vomiting, chills, or fever. There may be collapse or shock. Oliguria or anuria is common. Anemia develops rapidly with jaundice. Hemoglobinemia and hemoglobinuria are common. Usually there is a moderate leukocytosis.

Crises. Sudden worsening of the anemia in patients with one of the chronic, congenital forms of hemolytic anemia is called a crisis. Often the crisis is precipitated by a mild infection. Three kinds of crisis are distinguished. Aplastic crises are the most common, but there may be a hemolytic crisis or less often a megaloblastic crisis.

In an aplastic crisis, the production of red cells by the bone marrow is greatly reduced, and reticulocytes disappear from the blood. The concentration of hemoglobin in the blood falls abruptly as hemolysis continues, but the red cells are not replaced. Often mild granulocytopenia and thrombocytopenia occur. After 5 to 15 days, the bone marrow resumes the production of red cells and the crisis passes.

An aplastic crisis is nearly always caused by infection with the parvovirus B19, the agent that causes erythema infectiosum. The virus temporarily depresses the hematopoietic cells in the bone marrow. In normal people, the infection causes mild pancytopenia. In patients with a hemolytic disorder, the depression is more severe. The infection causes immunity, so that a patient with a hemolytic disorder rarely suffers more than one aplastic crisis.

In a hemolytic crisis, the destruction of the circulating red cells suddenly increases. In most patients, the increased hemolysis is caused by increased splenic activity. In some, the spleen enlarges. The bone marrow responds by increasing erythropoiesis. The concentration of reticulocytes in the blood increases. Because of the increased destruction of red cells, the concentration of bilirubin in the plasma increases.

In a megaloblastic crisis, folate deficiency causes a less dramatic increase in the severity of the anemia. The megaloblastic changes caused by folate deficiency are superimposed on the alterations caused by the hemolytic disorder.

HEREDITARY DEFECTS IN THE RED CELL MEMBRANE. In a number of conditions, a hereditary defect in the red cell membrane causes increased hemolysis. In many of these patients, the hemolysis is mild and fully compensated. In some, it is severe. Hereditary spherocytosis and hereditary elliptocytosis are the most common of these disorders.

Hereditary Spherocytosis. Hereditary spherocytosis is the commonest of the congenital hemolytic disorders in people from northern Europe and Great Britain and in their descendants. It is less common in other parts of the world. In the United States, 22 new cases are diagnosed annually in every 100,000 people.

Hereditary spherocytosis is inherited as an autosomal dominant with varying penetrance and expressivity. The abnormal gene is on chromosome 8 or chromosome 12. Occasionally the disease becomes apparent in infancy. More often it is diagnosed during childhood. Occasionally, it is discovered only in old age. Boys and girls are affected equally.

Lesions. In hereditary spherocytosis, some of the red cells are thicker than normal. If the disease is mild, there are only one or two abnormal cells per high power field in a blood smear. If it is severe, there are 20 or 30.

The abnormal red cells are 2.2 to 3.4 μm thick and are 4.0 to 7.2 μm in diameter. Normal red cells are less than 2.0 μm thick and are 7.7 μm in diameter. The volume of the spherocytes is usually between 77 and 87 fL, rather than the normal 82 to 92 fL. Occasionally their volume is as little as 62 fL or is increased up to 125 fL.

The concentration of hemoglobin in the blood is usually between 110 and 140 g/L (11 to 14 g/100 mL) in adults but may be as low as 90 g/L (9 g/100 mL) in adolescents. In some patients, the marrow compensates fully for the hemolysis, and anemia becomes evident only during a crisis. The concentration of hemoglobin in the red cells is high, 340 to 370 g/L (34 to 37 g/100 mL), rather than its normal 320 to 360 g/L (32 to 36 g/100 mL). Usually between 5 and 20% of the circulating red cells are reticulocytes, though the proportion of reticulocytes can be as low as 2% or over 90%.

In a blood smear, the spherocytes of hereditary spherocytosis look smaller than normal red cells. They stain evenly and darkly, without the central pallor of normal red cells. Because of the increased number of reticulocytes, polychromasia is often striking in a blood film.

The thick red cells of hereditary spherocytosis are easily lysed in hypotonic solutions. In severe cases, lysis may be complete in slightly hypotonic solutions that cause little or no lysis of normal red cells. In milder

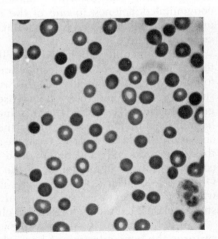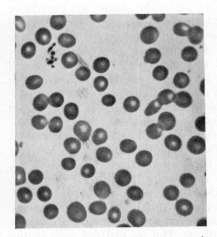

Fig. 49-8.   Blood smears from patients with hereditary spherocytosis, showing darkly staining spherocytes that are smaller than the normal cells with central pallor. (From Wintrobe, M. W., et al.: Clinical Hematology. 8th Ed. Philadelphia, Lea & Febiger, 1981.)

cases of hereditary spherocytosis, in which the proportion of spherocytes in the blood is not great, the increased fragility is less obvious. At times it becomes evident only if the cells are incubated in the hypotonic solution for 24 hours.

If blood from a patient with hereditary spherocytosis is incubated at 37°C, hemolysis occurs sooner and is greater than when blood from normal people is incubated. At a time when less than 5% of normal red cells are destroyed, between 10 and 50% of the red cells from a patient with spherocytosis are lysed. The addition of glucose or adenosine triphosphate to the blood reduces the hemolysis in the blood of the patients with spherocytosis, by providing the adenosine triphosphate the abnormal red cells need to maintain their homeostasis. The spherocytes are more easily damaged by mechanical trauma than are normal red cells.

Clinical Presentation. When hereditary spherocytosis becomes evident in adult life, it is usually mild. The anemia is often too slight to cause disability, except during a crisis. Usually the spleen is mildly or moderately enlarged. Gallstones develop in up to 85% of the patients. Rarely, the ankles ulcerate, or a demyelinating process develops in the spinal cord.

In an infant, hereditary spherocytosis is often more severe, with anemia and jaundice. Occasionally, the hyperplastic marrow causes bony changes.

Pathogenesis. The fault in hereditary spherocytosis is in the membrane of the red cells. The lipid content of the cell membrane is low, and probably spectrin and other proteins that govern the shape of the red cells are abnormal. Increased quantities of sodium enter the abnormal cells and adenosine triphosphate is needed to pump it out again. To maintain the cell's content of adenosine triphosphate, anaerobic glycolysis increases, increasing the cell's requirement for glucose. If sufficient glucose is not available, the cells swell and lyse.

The life of the spherocytes is shortened. They grow increasingly stiff as they circulate and are removed from the blood principally in the spleen. The normal red cells in the blood have a normal life span.

Treatment and Prognosis. Almost in-variably, splenectomy relieves completely the anemia in patients with hereditary spherocytosis, prevents the formation of pigment gallstones, and causes the other manifestations of the disease to heal. After a few weeks, the concentration of hemoglobin in the blood rises to normal. The proportion of reticulocytes falls. The hyperplasia of the bone marrow regresses. The life span of the circulating red cells increases, though usually not quite to normal. Effectively, the disease is cured.

The underlying defect in the red cells persists. There are still spherocytes in the blood after splenectomy, though they may be less numerous. The spherocytes are still fragile and easily destroyed.

Splenectomy increases the risk of infection, especially in young children. For this reason, some prefer to delay splenectomy until adolescence, unless the disease is unusually severe.

Hereditary Elliptocytosis. In hereditary elliptocytosis, or ovalocytosis as it is sometimes called, between 25 and 90% of the red cells in the blood are elliptical or rod-shaped, like the red cells of camels and llamas. The normoblasts in the bone marrow retain their spheroidal shape.

Hereditary elliptocytosis is inherited as an autosomal dominant character. The gene seems to segregate with those of the Rh blood groups. Some 40 people in every 100,000 have the disorder. Sometimes a congenital deficiency in one of the red cell enzymes or an abnormal hemoglobin is associated with the elliptocytosis.

In 90% of people with hereditary elliptocytosis, the defect causes no dysfunction and is found by accident if at all. The oval red cells survive normally and show no increase in fragility. In the other 10%, there is increased hemolysis, but it is usually mild. Increased activity of the bone marrow compensates for the loss of red cells and maintains a normal concentration of hemoglobin in the blood. Only occasionally is there severe anemia, with a reticulocytosis, splenomegaly, gallstones, crises, leg ulcers, or skeletal changes.

If the hemolysis is severe, splenectomy restores the concentration of hemoglobin in the blood to normal and allows the other lesions caused by the anemia to resolve. It

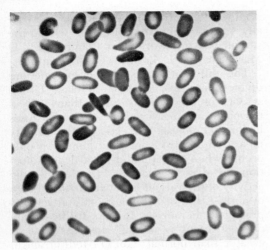

Fig. 49-9. Oval erythrocytes present in the blood in a patient with hereditary elliptocytosis. (From Wintrobe, M. W., et al.: Clinical Hematology. 8th Ed. Philadelphia, Lea & Febiger, 1981.)

does not alter the proportion of elliptocytes in the blood.

Hereditary elliptocytosis is not the only condition in which some of the circulating red cells are oval. Normally, from 1 to 15% of the red cells are elliptical. Oval red cells are common in the megaloblastic anemias and may occur in iron deficiency anemia. They are found in thalassemia, sickle cell anemia, and other congential hemolytic anemias. They may be found when the marrow is replaced by fibrosis or tumor.

Acanthocytosis. In abetalipoproteinemia, many of the red cells in the blood have large, irregular spikes projecting from their surface. These thorn cells are called acanthocytes, from the Greek for thorn and receptacle. Similar cells called spur cells are found in the anemia that accompanies cirrhosis of the liver. Acanthocytes must be distinguished from echinocytes, or burr cells, which occur in many conditions but have shorter, more regular projections.

Acanthocytosis is striking in a blood film, but is of little significance. In most patients with abetalipoproteinemia, the red cells survive normally. A few have episodes of mild hemolysis.

The acanthocytes in abetalipoproteinemia and in liver disease are probably caused by a disturbance in lipid metabolism. In both, the activity of lecithin cholesterol acyltransferase in the serum is reduced. This reduction may play some part in causing the abnormality of the red cell membrane that causes the acanthocytosis.

Stomatocytosis. Stomatocytes are red cells in which the central pallor seen in a blood smear forms a line, rather than the usual circle. The name comes from the Greek for a mouth, as if the line of pallor were a mouth painted on a mask. The stomatocytes are bowl shaped, rather than biconcave like normal red cells.

A few stomatocytes are often present in the blood of alcoholics, and they can appear in other conditions. They are only numerous in a few kindred in which the disorder is inherited as an autosomal dominant character. In some of the kindreds, the concentration of sodium in the abnormal red cells is high and the concentration of potassium is low. In some, the stomatocytes have no Rh antigens. In some, the abnormal red cells show none of these abnormalities.

In many people with hereditary stomatocytosis, there is no anemia, or the anemia is so mild as to be negligible. The concentration of hemoglobin is rarely less than 80 g/L (8 g/100 mL). In most of the patients, the life of the circulating red cells is little shortened, though the osmotic fragility of the red cells is increased. Rarely, the anemia is severe, with a concentration of hemoglobin in the blood of less than 40 g/L (4 g/100 mL). Splenectomy brings no benefit in the patients with severe anemia.

Other. Other hereditary defects in the membranes of the red cells are rare. An excess of phosphatidylcholine in the membranes of the red cells is inherited as an autsomal dominant character in one family with mild anemia. A deficiency of acyltransferase inherited as an autosomal recessive character can cause mild hemolytic anemia. In less than 1 person in 5,000,000 lack of the Rh antigens on the red cells is associated with mild hemolytic anemia. In the McLeod phenotype, lack of the K_x antigen of the Kell blood groups is associated with mild, compensated hemolysis.

In hereditary pyropoikilocytosis, the patients have tiny red cells, with a mean diameter of 2 to 3 μm, and a mean volume of as little as 25 fL. Anisocytosis and poikilocytosis are severe. The little red cells are spherocytes, with increased osmotic fragility. Splenectomy gives some benefit.

ENZYME DEFICIENCY. Reduced activity of one of the enzymes needed for the metabolism of the red cells sometimes causes a hemolytic disorder. Glucose-6-phosphate dehydrogenase deficiency and pyruvate kinase deficiency are the most common of these conditions.

Glucose-6-Phosphate Dehydrogenase Deficiency. Glucose-6-phosphate dehydrogenase deficiency is common. In more than 100,000,000 people the activity of the enzyme in the red cells is less than 25% of normal. In hundreds of millions more, its activity is less drastically reduced. The deficiency is inherited as an X-linked character and is more common in men.

Deficiency of the enzyme is common in Africa, around the Mediterranean, in the Middle East, Southeast Asia, and other regions in which malaria was once common, and in the descendants of people from these regions. It is uncommon in northern Europe and other regions in which malaria was never prevalent, and in people whose ancestors came from these parts of the world. In Africa, the enzyme is deficient in 20% of Bantu men; in northern Europe less than 0.1% of men lack the enzyme. In Sardinia, where malaria was endemic in the lowlands but not in the mountains, glucose-6-phosphate dehydrogenase is deficient in 30% of lowlanders but only 3% of highlanders. In the United States, the activity of the enzyme is normal in most white people, but is less than 25% of normal in 12% of black men and 1% of black women. It is often suggested that the frequency of glucose-6-phosphate dehydrogenase deficiency is high in regions in which malaria was prevalent because the deficiency protects against malaria.

Types of Glucose-6-Phosphate Dehydrogenase. More than 250 variants of glucose-6-phosphate dehydrogenase have been described. The normal form of the enzyme is called G6PD B. The variants common in Africa and the United States are G6PD A and G6PD A−. The variant usual in people from the Mediterranean region is G6PD Mediterranean. The other variants are usually named after the place in which the variant was discovered, for example, G6PD Markham, G6PD Corinth, G6PD Canton.

The different forms of the enzyme are divided into five classes. In class 1, the activity of the variant is less than 10% of normal when measured in vitro and causes lifelong hemolysis. In class 2, the activity measured in vitro is low, but hemolysis only occurs when precipitated by a drug, infection, or diabetic acidosis. In class 3, the activity of the variant is between 10 and 60% of normal, but drugs, infection, and acidosis precipitate hemolysis. In class 4, the activity of the variant is normal. In class 5, it is greater than normal. G6PD Mediterranean is in class 2. G6PD A− is in class 3. G6PD A is in class 4 and causes no disability.

The activity of glucose-6-phosphate dehydrogenase in the red cells falls as the cells age. The half-life of G6PD B is 62 days. The concentration of the enzyme in newly formed red cells is 4 times as great as that in erythrocytes 120 days old. The majority of the abnormal forms of the enzyme are less stable. The half-life of G6PD A− is 13 days, and the half-life of G6PD Mediterranean is several hours.

Lesions. Hemolysis caused by a drug usually begins two to four days after the drug is begun. Hemolysis caused by infection or acidosis begins several days after the onset of the disorder. The concentration of hemoglobin in the blood falls abruptly, often by 30 to 40 g/L (3 to 4 g/100 mL). The hemolysis is intravascular and causes hemogloblinuria. Janundice is common. The bone marrow increases the production of red cells to compensate for the hemolysis, and the proportion of reticulocytes in the blood rises in most patients to about 10% after 7 to 10 days.

In the first few days of the attack, Heinz bodies, named after the German pathologist who described them in 1890, are present in the red cells. The bodies consist of denatured globin, spectrin, and other proteins. They form a mass attached to the cell membrane. The mass distorts the cells and makes them more rigid. The Heinz bodies are removed from the red cells as they pass through the spleen and disappear from the blood in a few days.

In people with G6PD A− in the red cells, an attack induced by a drug lasts about a week. The concentration of hemoglobin in the blood then returns to normal, and the other signs of hemolysis disappear. Hemolysis continues as long as the drug is given, but it is not severe, and the bone marrow is able to compensate.

In people with G6PD Mediterranean in the blood, the initial attack is more severe than in people with G6PD A− and the recovery that comes after a week is less complete. Often the bone marrow is unable to compensate fully and anemia and other signs of hemolysis persist until the drug is withdrawn.

Hemolysis caused by infection or diabetic acidosis is usually mild. Exceptionally, it can be great enough to cause renal failure.

In Italy, Greece, Thailand, and China, infants with glucose-6-phosphate dehydrogenase deficiency often become jaundiced soon after birth. The hyperbilirubinemia is usually transient and not severe, but sometimes an exchange transfusion is necessary to avoid kernicterus. The syndrome does not occur in the United States.

People with an abnormal glucose-6-phosphate dehydrogenase of class 1 become jaundiced and anemic in infancy. The anemia and jaundice persist throughout life.

Glucose-6-phosphate dehydrogenase is also lacking in the white cells and platelets in people with a deficiency of the enzyme. In most of these people the function of the leukocytes is not affected, but in a few the bactericidal activity of the phagocytes is impaired, leading to repeated infections.

Favism. Favism takes its name from the Italian fava, a bean. It is most common in Italy and Greece, but occurs in China and other parts of the world. It does not occur in Africa and is rare in the United States. In favism, hemolytic anemia develops in a person with glucose-6-phosphate deficiency some hours after eating broad beans. The hemolysis is severe and can be fatal. The patient is often a child. The beans alone do not cause the hemolysis, for a person with a similar deficiency eating the same beans may suffer no injury and a person who has recovered from an attack of favism does not always develop hemolysis if similar beans are eaten on another occasion. The nature of the additional factor or factors needed to cause the hemolysis is unknown.

Pathogenesis. The loci governing the structure and synthesis of glucose-6-phosphate dehydrogenase are on the X chromosome. In men, the cells have only one X chromosome. If the allele on that chromosome codes for an abnormal form of the enzyme, the enzyme is abnormal in all the red cells. If the abnormal enzyme is of class 1, hemolytic anemia is inevitable. If it is of class 2 or 3, hemolysis occurs only when precipitated by a drug, infection, or acidosis.

Women have two X chromosomes in their cells. In some cells one of the X chromosomes is active; in some the other. If the allele on one of the X chromosomes is abnormal, but the allele on the other is normal, the enzyme is abnormal in the red cells in which the chromosome bearing the abnormal allele is active, normal in the cells in which the chromosome with the normal allele is active. The woman is a mosaic. Overall, the activity of the enzyme in the red cells is intermediate between the normal and abnormal values. In most heterozygous women, the activity of the enzyme is sufficient to prevent hemolysis. Only if the proportion of abnormal red cells is unusually high, or if both the woman's X chromosomes carry an abnormal allele, is hemolysis likely.

Probably the hemolysis in glucose-6-phosphate dehydrogenase deficiency is caused by increased activity of free radicals in the red cells. Because of their lack of mitochondria, red cells need glucose-6-phosphate dehydrogenase to reduce the nicotinamide adenine dinucleotide phosphate needed for the maintenance of the reduced glutathione required for the detoxification of free radicals.

Table 49-8 lists the drugs that cause hemolysis in people with glucose-6-phosphate deficiency. Probably most do so by increasing the production of free radicals. Some, such as primaquine, tend to cause serious hemolysis. The greater the dose, the greater the risk. Others, such as chloramphenicol or sulfoxone rarely cause hemolysis, even when given in large doses.

People with G6PD Mediterranean in their red cells are more likely to suffer hemolysis than are people with G6PD A− in the ery-

TABLE 49-8. DRUGS CAUSING HEMOLYSIS IN GLUCOSE-6-PHOSPHATE DEHYDROGENASE

Drug	With C6PD A- and G6PD Mediterranean	Only with G6PD Mediterranean
Antimalarials	Chloroquine Pamaquine Pentaquine Primaquine Quinacrine	Quinine
Sulfonamides	Salicylazosulfapyridine Sulfacetamide Sulfamethoxazole Sulfamethoxypyridazine Sulfanilamide Sulfapyridine Sulfisoxazole	
Sulfones	Dapsone Diaminodiphenylsulfone Sulfoxone Thiazosulfone	
Nitrofurans	Furaltadone Furazolidone Nitrofurantoin Nitrofurazone	
Analgesics	Acetanilid Acetophenetidin Acetylsalicylic acid	Aminopyrine Antipyrine
Other	Acetylphenylhydrazine Dimercaprol Isoniazid Methylene blue Nalidixic acid Naphthalene p-Aminosalycilic acid Phenylhydrazine Probeneceid Trinitrotoluene Vitamin K	Chloramphenicol Fava beans Quinidine

throcytes, probably because of the shorter half-life of G6PD Mediterranean, and the hemolysis is more likely to be severe.

Treatment and Prognosis. No treatment is needed in most people with anemia caused by glucose-6-phosphate dehydrogenase deficiency. An offending drug should be withdrawn. If infection or diabetes mellitus is present, it should be controlled. Little can be done for people with an abnormal glucose-6-phosphate dehydrogenase of class 1. Splenectomy is of no benefit.

Pyruvate Kinase Deficiency. Pyruvate kinase deficiency is uncommon. It is found

most often in people from northern Europe, though it can occur in any part of the world. It is inherited as an autosomal recessive character. In homozygotes, the activity of the enzyme is less than 25% of normal. In heterozygotes it is about 50% of normal.

Only the homozygotes develop hemolytic anemia. The severity of the hemolysis varies from one kindred to another. Usually anemia becomes evident during childhood and is moderately severe. In some kindred, the disease brings death in infancy. In some, it is mild and is detected only in adult life.

In most patients, the concentration of

hemoglobin in the blood is between 60 and 120 g/L (6 to 12 g/100 mL). The circulating red cells are often a little bigger than normal and slightly polychromatic. A few nucleated red cells and a few irregularly shaped or elongated erythrocytes are usually present. In children there may be acanthocytes. The osmotic fragility of the red cells is normal, but they lyse more easily than normal on incubation. The defect is corrected by a-denosine triphosphate but not by glucose. Jaundice, gallstones, crises, and splenomegaly are common. Ulceration of the ankles and bony changes are unusual.

Pyruvate kinase is needed by the red cells for the regeneration of adenosine triphosphate from adenosine diphosphate. How the deficiency causes the hemolysis is not clear. There is no correlation between the activity of the enzyme in the red cells and the severity of the hemolysis. Perhaps a deficiency of adenosine triphosphate develops and prevents the red cells from maintaining their membranes.

The increased destruction of the red cells occurs principally in the spleen. Reticulocytes are particularly at risk, being destroyed more actively than are older red cells.

Splenectomy is sometimes beneficial, especially in young children with severe anemia, but it is not as effective as in hereditary spherocytosis. Hemolysis continues after splenectomy, though it is less severe.

Other. Other forms of enzyme deficiency can cause hemolytic anemia. All are uncommon; most are rare. In most of these disorders, the defect is inherited as an autosomal recessive character. Phosphoglycerate kinase deficiency is inherited as an X-linked character.

Deficiency of one of the other enzymes active in the glycolytic pathway in the red cells causes changes like those of pyruvate kinase deficiency. Hexokinase, glucosephosphate isomerase, phosphofructokinase, triosephosphate isomerase, 2,3-diphosphoglyceromutase, phosphoglycerate kinase, enolase, and aldolase have all been found deficient in at least a few patients with hemolytic anemia. The deficiency of some of these glycolytic enzymes affects more than the red cells. In glucosephosphate isomerase

deficiency, the enzyme is also deficient in the leukocytes, though the deficiency does not impair leukocytic function. Phosphofructokinase deficiency also affects the muscles to give type VII glycogen storage disease. Triosephosphate isomerase deficiency affects many tissues, causing severe neurologic disease, repeated infections because of leukocytic dysfunction, and sometimes myocardial dysfunction. Phosphoglycerate kinase deficiency also affects the leukocytes, and some of the patients have been mentally defective.

Hemolytic anemia is caused rarely by a deficiency of one of the enzymes concerned with nucleotide metabolism, pyrimidine 5'-nucleotidase, adenosine triphosphatase, or adenylate kinase. An excess of adenosine deaminase also causes hemolytic anemia. Lactic dehydrogenase may be deficient in the red cells, but does not cause a hemolytic disorder.

Deficiency of the glutathione synthetase, γ-glutamylcysteine synthetase or glutathione reductase involved in the hexose monophosphate path and glutathione metabolism causes anemia like that of glucose-6-phosphate synthetase deficiency. The deficiency of glutathione reductase is sometimes due to an inherited defect; sometimes it is caused by a lack of riboflavin in the diet.

STRUCTURAL   HEMOGLOBINOPATHY.   Two kinds of abnormality occur in the hemoglobin of the red cells. In the structural hemoglobinopathies, one or more of the four polypeptide chains that constitute globin are abnormal. In the thalassemias, one or more of the peptide chains is made in insufficient quantity, though usually all are normal. Some apply the term *hemoglobinopathy* to both forms of malformation. Other reserve it for the structural hemoglobinopathies.

The distinction between the two kinds of abnormality is not absolute. Some patients have both a structural abnormality in one or more of the peptide chains of their hemoglobin and a defect in the rate of production of one or more of the chains. Some forms of structural hemoglobinopathy are best considered with the thalassemias, for their clinical presentation is similar to that of the thalassemias.

Terminology.   When it was first realized

that there was more than one kind of hemoglobin, the different kinds of hemoglobin were designated by letters. Normal adult hemoglobin with its two α chains and two β chains was called hemoglobin A. Fetal hemoglobin with its two α chains and two γ chains was called hemoglobin F. The hemoglobin with two α chains and two δ chains normally present in small quantity in adults was called hemoglobin A_2.

In soon became evident that there were not enough letters in the alphabet to designate all the abnormal hemoglobins in this way. By 1984, 525 structurally abnormal hemoglobins had been reported and more continue to be identified. Instead, the abnormal hemoglobins were given names, usually the name of the place in which the hemoglobin was first identified, for example hemoglobin Vancouver, hemoglobin Christchurch, hemoglobin Zambia, and hemoglobin Wein. In addition, the name of some of the hemoglobins contains a letter, as in hemoglobin G Philadelphia, to show that hemoglobin G Philadelphia has an electrophorectic motility similar to that of the abnormal hemoglobin once called hemoglobin G, or as in hemoglobin M Saskatoon, to indicate that the hemoglobin tends to form methemoglobin. Only the abnormal hemoglobins C, E, H, and S are now designated by letters.

Prevalence. Four abnormal hemoglobins are common: hemoglobin S, hemoglobin C, hemoglobin D Punjab, and hemoglobin E. Each is largely restricted to descendants of people from that part of the world where intermarriage made common the gene that causes the abnormality. Each is found in millions of people.

Hemoglobin S is common in central Africa, from Senegal to Angola in the west and Kenya to Mozambique in the east, and is also frequent in the Malagasy Republic. In parts of eastern Africa, up to 50% of the population have hemoglobin S in their blood. In much of central Africa, from 10 to 20% of the population are affected. In the United States, 8% of black people have hemoglobin S in their blood. In some communities as many as 20% of black people have the abnormal hemoglobin. Hemoglobin S is also frequent in isolated communities in India, Arabia,

and Turkey. It is common in parts of Greece and Italy. In some villages in Greece, 30% of the villagers have hemoglobin S in their blood.

Hemoglobin S is common in regions where malaria used to be common, suggesting that hemoglobin S may protect against malaria. The association between hemoglobin S and falciparum malaria is particularly strong. In parts of Africa, there is an inverse correlation between the frequency of hemoglobin S and the frequency of falciparum malaria.

In northern Ghana, nearly 30% of the people carry the gene for hemoglobin C. It is less common in the south of Ghana, in the neighboring countries, and in Nigeria west of the Niger. In the United States, 3% of black people have the gene for hemoglobin C.

Hemoglobin D Punjab is found in 2% of Sikhs in the Punjab in Gujarat, and in Iran. It is found occasionally in people in other parts of the world.

Hemoglobin E is common in people in the East, from Sri Lanka to southern China, and throughout Southeast Asia to the Philippines. In eastern Thailand, over 50% of the people have hemoglobin E in their red cells. In Burma and Cambodia, over 20% of the people carry the gene. In Vietnam and the south of China it is less common.

Most other abnormal hemogloins are rare, though occasionally one is common in a restricted locality. Hemoglobin J Tongariki is found in 10% of the people living on the island in the Pacific after which it is named. An abnormal hemoglobin of some kind was found in 0.1% of 8000 people from Denmark and Great Britain, but as the method used detected only about a third of the abnormal hemoglobins, the prevalence in these people was probably about 0.5%.

Structure. In most structurally abnormal hemoglobins, the only abnormality is the replacement of a single amino acid in one of the chains that make up the molecule by another amino acid. In hemoglobin J Toronto, aspartic acid is substituted for alanine as the fifth amino acid from the N terminal end of the α chains. The molecule is otherwise normal. The substitution is usually in the α chains or the β chains. Less often it is in the γ chains or the δ chains.

In less than 1% of structurally abnormal hemoglobins there are two substitutions, at different points on the α or the β chains. In the hemoglobin C Harlem, for example, valine is substituted for glutamic acid at the sixth position on the β chains, and asparagine is substituted for aspartic acid at the 73rd position.

In 2% of abnormal hemoglobins, from 1 to 5 amino acids are deleted from adjacent positions in the β chains. In hemoglobin Lyon, for example, lysine and valine are deleted from the 17th and 18th positions of the β chains.

In 1% of structurally abnormal hemoglobins from 5 to 31 amino acids are added to the C terminal end of the α or β chains. Hemoglobin Constant Spring with 31 amino acids added to the α chains is the best known. Occasionally, there are both addition of amino acids to the α or β chains and substitutions within affected chains. In hemoglobin Wayne, five amino acids are added to the α chains, and substitutions alter the last three amino acids of the normal part of the chains. In one abnormal hemoglobin, three additional amino acids are added between the 115th and 118th positions of the α chains.

In 2% of structurally abnormal hemoglobins, the abnormal chains consist of portions of two normal chains fused together. In most the abnormal hemoglobin consists of the N terminal end of a δ chain and the C terminal end of a β chain. The three kinds of hemoglobin Lepore are formed in this way. In hemoglobin Kenya, the abnormal chains have the N terminal end of a γ chain and the C terminal end of a β chain.

In yet other abnormal hemoglobins, the four polypeptide chains making up the molecule are all the same. Hemoglobin Barts has four γ chains, and hemoglobin H has four β chains.

The abnormal hemoglobins are sometimes given descriptive names that indicate the abnormality in their structure. Hemoglobin S can be described as hemoglobin β6(A3) Glu → Val, to show that the abnormality is in the 6th amino acid from the N terminal end of the β chains, the 3rd in the A helix, and consists of the replacement of glutamic acid by valine. The deletion in hemoglobin Freiburg is shown as β23(B5) Val → 0, to show that the abnormality is in the β chain, affects the 23rd amino acid from the N terminal end, the 5th in the B helix, and consists of deletion of a molecule of valine. The deletions in hemoglobin Lyon are shown as β17–18(A14–15) Lys Val missing, to indicate that lysine and valine are missing in the 17th and 18th positions on the β chains. The addition of amino acids is indicated as α + 31C in hemoglobin Constant Spring, which has 31 extra amino acids on the C terminal end of its α chains.

Inheritance. The genes controlling the synthesis of the α chains of hemoglobin and the ζ chains of fetal hemoglobin are in the same region on chromosome 16. The synthesis of the α chains is controlled by four genes, two close together on each chromosome 16. The synthesis of the ζ chains is controlled by two genes, one on each chromosome 16.

The loci for the genes that control the production of the β chains, the two types of γ chain, the γ chains, and the σ chains are grouped together on chromosome 11. There are two genes for each chain, one on each chromosome 11. The two kinds of γ chain differ only in that Gγ has glycine as the 136th amino acid from the N terminal end, while Aγ has alanine.

The genes that regulate the production of the peptide chains of hemoglobin are all codominant. At each locus, the two alleles are expressed equally. Normal people are homozygous and have normal alleles at all loci.

The expression of the genes changes with age. Early in fetal life, hemoglobin Gower II, hemoglobin Gower I, and hemoglobin Portland are predominant, with their ζ and σ chains, together with some α and γ chains. Later in fetal life, hemoglobin F becomes dominant, with α and γ chains. This gradually gives way to the hemoglobin A of adult life, with α and β chains, though some production of γ chains for hemoglobin F continues, and some δ chains are produced for hemoglobin A_2.

If there is one abnormal allele at one locus on one chromosome, an abnormal hemoglobin will be produced. The person is said to be heterozygous for that abnormality. As the normal allele on the other chromosome of the pair affected is also expressed, there will be a mixture of normal and abnormal hemoglobins in the red cells.

In an adult, if the abnormality is in the β chains, about 6% of the hemoglobin is hemoglobin A, with normal α and normal β chains. About 40% is the abnormal hemoglobin, with normal α but abnormal β chains. There is the normal 2 to 3% of hemoglobin A_2, with normal α and δ chains, or a little more, and the normal trace of hemoglobin F with its α and γ chains.

If the abnormality is in the α chains in an adult, over 60% of the hemoglobin is hemoglobin A, with normal α and β chains. There is the usual amount of hemoglobin A_2, with normal α and normal δ chains, and the usual trace of hemoglobin F, with normal α and normal γ chains. About 25% of the hemoglobin is abnormal with abnormal α chains and normal β chains. There are traces of abnormal hemoglobins with abnormal α chains and normal β chains, and with abnormal α chains and normal γ chains. In all, six kinds of hemoglobin are present.

If the same abnormal allele is present on both the chromsomes that control the production of β chains, the person is said to be homozygous for that character. No normal hemoglobin A is produced. In an adult, over 90% of the hemoglobin is abnormal. Hemoglobin A_2 and hemoglobin F remain normal, and both may be present in slightly increased quantity in the red cells. Because of the four genes involved, homozygous production of an abnormal hemoglobin with an α chain abnormality is rare.

If different abnormal alleles are present on the chromosomes that regulate the manufacture of β chains, no normal hemoglobin A is made. The red cells contain a mixture of roughly equal quantities of two abnormal hemoglobins, together with the usual small quantities of hemoglobin A_2 and hemoglobin F. People with this sort of abnormality are called doubly heterozygous. If two abnormal alleles are present, one on a β locus and one on an α locus, the mixture of normal and abnormal hemoglobins is more complex. If there is an abnormal β allele and an abnormal α allele, eight kinds of hemoglobin are present in the red cells; hemoglobin A with normal α and β chains, abnormal hemoglobins with normal α and abnormal β chains, abnormal α and normal β, or abnormal α and abnormal β chains, together with small quantities of normal hemoglobin A_2 with normal α and δ chains, normal hemoglobin F with normal α and γ chains, and traces of abnormal hemoglobins with abnormal α but normal γ and δ chains.

Almost without exception, the substitution of one amino acid for another in the abnormal hemoglobins requires an alteration in only one base in the deoxyribonucleic acid molecule. For example, in hemoglobin New York, glutamic acid is substituted for valine as the 15th amino acid of the G helix of the β chain. If the codon for valine in the deoxyribonucleic acid were cytosine, adenosine, thymidine, the change of adenosine to thymidine would change the codon to cytosine, thymidine, thymidine, which is one of the codons for glutamic acid.

The more complex abnormalities in the hemoglobinopathies probably result from more complex genetic alterations. Cross-over between the chromosomes is often invoked to explain the abnormalities.

Dysfunction. Most structurally abnormal hemoglobins function normally. The substitution of a single amino acid is unlikely to cause dysfunction if the abnormality is on the surface of the folded molecule of hemoglobin.

The few of the modifications of the surface of the folded molecule of hemoglobin that cause dysfunction do so by causing the molecules of hemoglobin to stick together, polymerizing, or crystallizing within the red cells. Hemoglobin S causes sickle cell anemia in this way. The aggregates of hemoglobin distort and stiffen the red cells, bringing about their destruction.

If the abnormality in the hemoglobin is within the folded molecule, serious malfunction is likely. Often the binding of heme is weakened, or heme may fall out of the globin. Water can gain acess to the heme, preventing its function. The whole structure of the folded molecule may be distorted. Often the hemoglobin becomes unstable and tends to precipitate within the red cells. Hemoglobin Köln is the most common example of this sort of hemoglobin.

If tyrosine replaces histidine as the 7th amino acid in the E helix, or the 8th in the F helix, in either the α or the β chains, the iron

in heme forms an ionic bond with the tyrosine. A similar ionic bond can be formed if
glutamic acid replaces valine as the 11th
amino acid of the E helix of the β chain.
Methemoglobin is formed, and the cell
can no longer bind oxygen. Hemoglobin M
Saskatoon is an example of this sort of hemoglobin. Some of the abnormal hemoglobins
that form methemoglobin are also unstable.

About 10% of structurally abnormal hemoglobins bind oxygen more firmly than is
normal, making its release to the tissues
difficult. More than 3% fail to take up oxygen
adequately, impairing oxygenation. Some of
the hemoglobins with abnormal affinity for
oxygen are also unstable. The abnormality in
these hemoglobins is usually in the looser of
the regions in which the α and β chains are
in contact, but sometimes involves the C
terminal end of the β chains. Hemoglobin
British Columbia is an example of a hemoglobin with an increased affinity for oxygen.

Sickle Cell Disease.   Sickle cell anemia is
the term used to describe the disease that
develops in people homozygous for hemoglobin S. Heterozygotes for hemoglobin S
usually develop no disease, though the abnormal hemoglobin is readily detected in
their blood, They are said to have the sickle
cell trait.

Lesions.   In homozygotes, the hemoglobin S in the red cells tends to polymerize
and precipitate, especially when the oxygen
tension is low. The stiff, distorted red cells
are destroyed intravascularly, causing
hemolytic anemia, and clog small blood
vessels, causing ischemia. In most heterozygotes, polymerization of hemoglobin S does
not occur. In some, it can be precipitated by
hypoxia.

Sickle cell disease first becomes evident
when a homozygote is six to nine months
old. Hemoglobin F prevents the polymerization of hemoglobin S. For the first six to nine
months of life, it is present in the red cells
in sufficient quantity to prevent hemolysis.
Only when the proportion of hemoglobin F
in the red cells falls does hemolysis begin. It
continues for the rest of the patient's life. In
most patients, the anemia slowly worsens.
Repeated crises cause sudden but transient
worsening of the patient's condition.

Crises.   The crises that occur in homozygotes are of two kinds, hematologic crises like

those in patients with other forms of hemolytic anemia, and veno-occlusive crises caused
by the occlusion of blood vessels by the
distorted red cells.

Vaso-occlusive crises usually begin in the
first year of life, but in some patients they
are delayed until adolescence or until adult
life. Usually, the crises develop without
apparent cause, but occasionally they are
triggered by a minor infection, chilling, or
travel in an unpressurized aircraft.

In infants, hand and foot crises caused by
obstruction of blood vessels in the hands or
feet often bring swelling, pain, and after
some weeks cortical resorption in the bones
of the hands and feet. The crisis usually
begins suddenly and persists for one or two
weeks. In older children, bone and joint
crises cause obstruction in the sinusoids in
the bone marrow and commonly cause attacks of pain in the long bones. The ischemia
is often severe enough to cause foci of infarction in the long bones or arthritis with
swelling of the knees or elbows. Usually the
attack subsides within a week.

Pulmonary crises result from occlusion of
small blood vessels in the lungs, causing
ischemia and bleeding. There is usually
tachypnea, pain in the chest, leukocytosis,
and roentgenographic evidence of consolida-
tion. Especially in children, bacterial or
mycoplasmal infection often complicates the
injury.

In abdominal crises, ischemia or infarction caused by obstruction of vessels in the
mesentery or gut causes sudden abdominal
pain. The pain usually subsides after a few
days, but may persist much longer.

Obstruction of vessels in the brain causes
hemiplegia in 15% of homozygotes with
sickle cell disease. Convulsions develop in
10% of the patients. Some develop aphasia,
changes in consciousness, or other signs of
cerebral ischemia.

Aplastic crises are usually precipitated by
infection. They are similar to the aplastic
crises that occur in other kinds of hemolytic
anemia. Hemolytic crises caused by increased destruction of the abnormal red cells
in the spleen are particularly likely in people
who have glucose-6-phosphate dehydrogenase deficiency or hereditary spherocytosis
as well as sickle cell anemia. In the United
States, 10% of black men with sickle cell

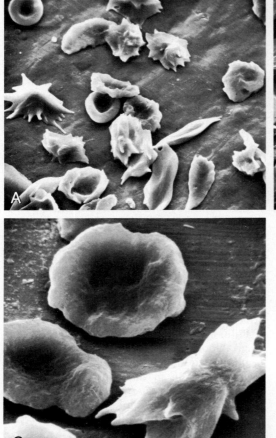
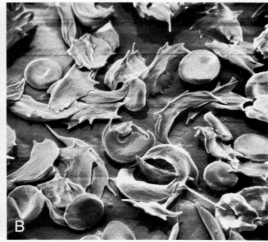

Fig. 49-10. Scanning electron micrographs showing the distortion of red cells containing hemoglobin S caused by hypoxia. (From Wintrobe, M. W., et al.: Clinical Hematology. 8th Ed. Philadelphia, Lea & Febiger, 1981.)

anemia have also glucose-6-phosphate dehydrogenase deficiency, In young children, sequestration of blood in the spleen sometimes causes sudden splenomegaly. The quantity of blood trapped in the spleen is sometimes so great that it causes hypovolemia and shock, even death. Folate deficiency occasionally causes a megaloblastic crisis.

Blood. Between crises, the concentration of hemoglobin in the blood is usually between 60 and 100 g/L (6 to 10 g/100 mL). There is hyperbilirubinemia of from 15 to 35 μmol/L (1 to 2 mg/mL). Because the hemolysis is in part intravascular, the concentration of haptoglobin in the serum is reduced. The osmotic fragility of the red cells is often increased. The erythrocyte sedimentation rate is low.

A blood smear shows little abnormality if the red cells are well oxygenated. If the red cells are deoxygenated by adding a reducing agent, the hemoglobin S precipitates and distorted red cells become numerous. They may be sickle shaped, cigar shaped, or more grossly abnormal, with the prickles and projections sticking out from their surfaces. A reticulocytosis of from 5 to 30% reflects the hyperactivity of the bone marrow caused by the hemolysis. Howell-Jolly bodies or Heinz bodies are sometimes present.

Neutrophilia with a leukocyte of from

8 to 20 × 10^9/L (800 to 20,000/mm^3) is usual. The platelet count averages 450 × 10^9/L (450,000/mm^3), sometimes with megathrombocytes.

Other Organs. The repeated crises and less dramatic episodes of vaso-occlusion slow the growth of the bones during adolescence, though most patients reach normal, adult stature. Many of the patients are tall and thin, with long arms and legs. Foci of necrosis in the medulla of the long bones heal by new bone formation, causing patchy densities visible radiologically. The heads of the femora sometimes collapse, causing Perthes' disease. Damage to the joints caused by foci of bony necrosis can cause arthritis and deformity. The central part of the vertebral plates may be weakened, so that the intervertebral disks bulge into the vertebral bodies.

Because of its increased activity in destroying red cells, the spleen enlarges during infancy. The enlargement persists during childhood, but in adolescence the spleen begins to shrink. Blockage of sinusoids by sickled red cells causes foci of hemorrhage, and blockage of larger blood vessels in the spleen brings infarction. The spleen becomes increasingly fibrotic, with large quantities of iron stored in its macrophages. In an adult homozygous for hemoglobin S, the spleen may be reduced to a scarred remnant less than 30 g in weight.

The anemia causes enlargement of the heart during childhood, with the murmurs and other signs of anemia. Later in life, hemosiderosis sometimes adds to the cardiac dysfunction, especially when many transfusions are given. Some patients develop cardiac failure. Injury to the lungs can cause hypoxia and occasionally pulmonary hypertension.

Renal dysfunction is common in sickle cell anemia. The kidneys are often a little enlarged. Obstruction of small blood vessels by the sickled cells causes small infarcts, foci of interstitial fibrosis, and other signs of ischemia. Acidification of the urine is often impaired. Hematuria is common and can be severe. Some patients develop nul disease, focal glomerulosclerosis, or membranoproliferative glomerulonephritis and the nephrotic syndrome.

The liver enlarges in infancy and remains slightly enlarged throughout life. Its sinusoids are congested. Usually there is hemosiderosis and slight periportal fibrosis. Occasionally cirrhosis develops. Episodes of increased sickling in the liver can cause a sudden, marked, but temporary increase in the concentration of bilirubin in the plasma. Pigment gallstones are common.

Blockage of the vessels in the skin cause persistent ulceration at the ankles in 75% of people with sickle cell anemia in the tropics. Priapism can be troublesome. Occlusion of blood vessels in the eyes can cause ocular injury.

Infection is common in sickle cell anemia, especially in children under five years old. Pneumococcal infections are particularly frequent. The incidence of bacterial meningitis increases 300 times, and in 70% of the children is caused by a pneumococcus. In older patients, infection with gram-negative bacteria is common. The incidence of osteomyelitis is increased, and in 50% of the patients it is caused by a salmonella infection.

When hypoxia causes symptoms in a heterozygote, its most common manifestations are hematuria and infarcts in the spleen.

Pathogenesis. In hemoglobin S, valine is substituted for glutamic acid as the 6th amino acid from the N terminal end of the β-chain. The substitution is on the surface of the folded molecule. When hemoglobin is oxygenated, the substitution causes no dysfunction. Hemoglobin S functions normally.

If the oxygen tension in the blood falls, hemoglobin S releases its oxygen. If the patient is homozygous for hemoglobin S, the deoxygenated molecules of hemoglobin S polymerize, forming stiff rods consisting of six molecules of deoxygenated hemoglobin S twisted together. The rods bond in parallel bundles to form long, rigid, liquid crystals called tactoids. The tactoids stiffen and distort the red cells, often stretching them into the sickle shape that gives the disease its name.

Sickling does not occur immediately. Even if the hemoglobin S in the red cells is completely deoxygenatged, its takes 2 seconds for tactoids to form.

The affinity of deoxygenated hemoglobin S for oxygen is low, but if the oxygen tension in the blood rises, it does take up oxygen. The tactoids dissolve. The distortion of the red cells disppears, and they again become biconcave disks.

As the red cells circulate in a person homozygous for hemoglobin S, they undergo repeated cycles of sickling and unsickling. The unsickling is not always perfect. Spikes caused by the long tactoids pressing against the red cell membrane often break off and are lost in the plasma. Eventually, the red cell are irreversibly damaged and remain sickled, whatever the oxygen tension.

The distortion of the irreversibly sickled cells is not caused by hemoglobin S. Even if the hemoglobin is removed from the cells, they remain sickled. The repeated cycles of sickling injure the spectrin and other structural proteins of the red cells, and it is they that hold the irreversibly sickled cells in their abnormal shape.

In both the reversibly and the irreversibly sickled cells the flux of sodium and potassium across the red cell membrane increases some five times. In the reversibly sickled cells, the osmolality within the red cells remains normal, but in the irreversibly sickled cells the loss of potassium exceeds the gain in sodium. Because of the reduction in osmolality, water is lost from the distorted red cells, increasing the concentration of hemoglobin within them. The concentration of calcium in the red cells is increased in both temporarily and permanently sickled cells.

The life of sickled red cells is 20 to 30 days. About 70% of them are destroyed in the spleen or by macrophages in other organs. The other 30% are destroyed in the blood vessels as bits of red cells break off during unsickling or when the stiff, distorted sickle cells rupture as they are forced through small blood vessels.

The clogging of blood vessels by sickled red cells lowers the oxygen tension in the blood as well as in the tissues supplied by the obstructed vessels. The lowered oxygen tension adds to the sickling, increasing the obstruction and reducing further the oxygen tension.

Even a small reduction in the pH of the blood increases the risk of sickling and shortens the time needed to achieve it. The greater the concentration of hemoglobin S in the red cells, the greater the risk of sickling, and the more rapidly it occurs. The increase in the concentration of hemoglobin that results from the loss of portions of the cytoplasm of the red cells during unsickling is enough to increase the risk of sickling.

The presence of other kinds of hemoglobin in the red cells protects against sickling. Hemoglobin F is the most effective. Even the small quantities of hemoglobin F normally present in the red cells are of some value. Sickle cell anemia does not occur in double heterozygotes with an allele coding for hemoglobin S on one chromosome 11 and an allele that causes persistence of hemoglobin F into adult life on the other, though these people have 70% of hemoglobin S and only 30% of hemoglobin F in their red cells. Hemoglobin A is less effective, but does usually prevent sickling in heterozygotes with 60% of hemoglobin A and 40% of hemoglobin S in their blood.

The high rate of infection in sickle cell anemia is probably caused by malfunction of the spleen. Splenectomy increases the risk of infection, especially pneumococcal infection.

Treatment and Prognosis. No treatment can cure sickle cell anemia. Attempts to prevent the polymerization of hemoglobin S have so far proved unsuccessful. All that can be done is to manage the complications of the disease as they occur.

In Africa, the mortality of sickle cell anemia is high. In Zambia, 50% of children homozoygous for hemoglobin S died before they were three years old. In Zimbabwe, only 10% lived more than 10 years. In Jamaica and in the United States, the prognosis is better. Only 10 to 20% of the patients die in childhood. Some live to old age. In Saudi Arabia and India, the disease is mild and does little to reduce life expectancy. In children, the commonest cause of death is infection. In adults, renal failure is one of the more common causes of death.

Hemoglobin C Disease. Hemoglobin C differs from hemoglobin S in that lysine instead of valine replaces glutamic acid as the 6th amino acid from the N terminal end of the β chain, that is, as the 3rd amino acid of helix A. People homozygous for hemoglobin C have mild, hemolytic anemia. Some have episodes of mild abdominal pain, arthralgia, or hematuria. Heterozygotes suffer no disability.

In some homozygotes, the concentration of hemoglobin in the blood remains normal, but often it is about 100 g/L (10 g/100 mL). The delivery of oxygen to the tissues remains normal, for the low pH of the red cells facilitates the release of oxygen from the hemoglobin.

A blood smear shows that over 90% of the red cells are target cells, with a dark rim and dark center separated by a pale zone. A few are spherocytes. The osmotic fragility of the spherocytes is increased, but the fragility of the target cells is normal. A few of the red cells may show crystals of hemoglobin C if the red cells are allowed to dry or are treated with 3% sodium chloride.

Hemoglobin D Disease. In hemoglobin D Punjab, glutamine replaces glutamic acid as the 121st amino acid from the N terminal end of the β chain, the 4th in the GH segment of the molecule. Heterozygotes with hemoglobin D Punjab have no disability, except perhaps episodes of hematuria. Homozygotes develop a mild or moderate anemia.

Hemoglobin E Disease. In hemoglobin E disease, lysine replaces glutamic acid as the 26th amino acid form the N terminal end of the β chains, the 8th in the B helix. Homozygotes with alleles coding for hemoglobin E on both chromosomes 11 are common in Asia. They have mild hemolytic anemia with

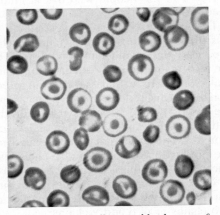

Fig. 49-11. Target cells in a blood smear from a patient with hemoglobin C disease. (From Wintrobe, M. W., et al.: Clinical Hematology. 8th Ed. Philadelphia, Lea & Febiger, 1981.)

many target cells in their blood. Heterozygotes show no dysfunction.

Hemoglobin O Arab Disease. Lysine replaces glutamic acid in the 121st position in the β chain in hemoglobin O Arab. Homozygotes for hemoglobin O Arab have mild hemolytic anemia, with many circulating target cells. The disease has been found in the United States, Jamaica, and the Sudan, as well as in Arabs.

Hemoglobin SC Disease. In parts of Ghana, 25% of the people are doubly heterozygous, with equal quantities of hemoglobin S and hemoglobin C in their blood. Hemoglobin A is absent. Hemoglobin F is present in normal quantity. In the United States and Jamaica, 0.1% of black people have hemoglobin SC disease, as this condition is called.

The patients have mild hemolytic anemia. In 90% of them, the concentration of hemoglobin in the blood is over 100 g/L (10 g/100 mL). A blood smear shows that up to 50% of the red cells are target cells. Crystals of polymerized hemoglobin distort some of the red cells.

In other organs, lesions like those of sickle cell anemia develop. Injury to the eyes and collapse of the femoral heads are more common than in sickle cell disease, and episodes of bone pain are often severe. Fat emboli to the lungs are common during pregnancy. Other complications resemble those of sickle cell disease but are usually mild.

Hemoglobin SD Disease. Most of the hemoglobins that have the electrophoretic mobility of hemoglobin D can be found together with hemoglobin S in double heterozygotes. Most forms of hemoglobin SD disease cause no dysfunction, though people doubly heterozygous for hemoglobin D Pubjab and hemoglobin S develop mild anemia.

Hemoglobin SO Arab Disease. Hemoglobin O Arab reacts readily with hemoglobin S to form polymers. Double heterozygotes with hemoglobin S and hemoglobin O Arab in their blood develop a severe form of sickle cell anemia.

Unstable Hemoglobin Disease. Unstable hemoglobin disease is uncommon. Over 100 unstable hemoglobins are known, but most are rare. Hemoglobin Köln is the most common but is present in fewer than 100 people from 12 families. In hemoglobin Köln, methionine is substituted for valine as the 98th amino acid of the β chain, the 5th of the FG segment.

The unstable hemoglobins tend to precipitate in the red cells. Some, including hemoglobin Köln, lose heme before they precipitate. Others form hemichromes and precipitate, carrying the heme with them. The precipitate appears in the red cells as a Heinz body. The Heinz bodies are removed as the red cells pass through the spleen, leaving a smaller, stiffer red cell, with a short life.

All patients with unstable hemoglobin disease are heterozygotes. Their blood contains both the abnormal hemoglobin and hemoglobin A. Probably the homozygous state is not compatible with life. New mutations occur. In some patients with an unstable hemoglobin, both parents are normal. The gene that codes for an unstable hemoglobin is codominant. If it has been inherited from one of the parents, that parent must have the abnormal hemoglobin in the blood.

Some unstable hemoglobins cause no anemia, though the hemoglobin is unstable when tested in vitro. Most cause only mild hemolysis, with a normal concentration of hemoglobin in the blood, except in hemolytic crises. Only a reticulocytosis of from 5 to 10% shows that the bone marrow is hyperactive to compensate for the hemolysis. Often the diagnosis is made only when a hemolytic crisis draws attention to the disorder. Often the crisis is precipitated by fever or the administration of a sulfonamide.

Some unstable hemoglobins cause moderate anemia, with a concentration of hemoglobin in the blood of from 70 to 120 g/L (7 to 10 g/100 mL). In these patients, the anemia is often first detected in adolescence. In some patients, cholelithiasis, jaundice, or a hemolytic crisis first draws attention to the disorder.

A few unstable hemoglobins cause severe anemia evident in infancy. The concentration of hemoglobin in the blood is less than 70 g/L (7 g/100 mL). Often there is a reticulosis of over 30%. Splenomegaly is usual, though it is uncommon in the milder forms of unstable hemoglobin disease.

The concentration of hemoglobin in the red cells is often low in unstable hemoglobin disease, sometimes as low as 250 g/L (25 g/100 mL), instead of the normal 320 to 360 g/L (32 to 36 g/100 mL). As Heinz bodes form, the unstable hemgolobin is removed in the spleen, leaving only the normal hemoglobin in the red cells. If the anemia is severe, a blood film shows many fragmented red cells and many spherocytes. If it is mild, only the changes usually in hemolytic disorders are evident. Heinz bodies are rarely present in the red cells except in crises and in patients who have undergone splenectomy. In these people, up to 50% of the red cells contain Heinz bodies.

In some patients with an unstable hemoglobin that loses heme, the urine is dark brown or black. Dipyrroles are formed from the heme freed from the hemoglobin and are excreted in the urine.

Splenectomy benefits many patients with moderate or severe unstable hemoglobin disease, though some do not respond. Because of the risk of infection, the spleen should not be removed if the anemia is mild, or the unstable hemoglobin is of a type that does not respond to splenectomy.

Thalassemia. Thalassemia is the name given to a group of disorders in which the rate of synthesis of one or more of the peptide chains of hemoglobin is reduced. The word *thalassemia* is from the Greek for the sea and blood, because the disease was first detected in the people who live around the Mediterranean Sea.

Terminology. The thalassemias are classified according to the chain or chains produced in insufficient quantity. There are two main groups, α-thalassemia and β-thalassemia. In α-thalassemia, the production of α chains is defective. In β-thalassemia, the production of β chains is impaired. In addition, there are a number of less common forms of thalassemia. In δβ-thalassemia, the production of both δ and β chains is reduced. In δβγ-thalassemia, the production of δ, β, and Aγ chains are all inadequate. Rarely, there is inadequate formation only of δ chains or of β and γ chains.

The thalassemias are further subdivided according to the severity of the disease. In α-thalassemia, hemoglobin Bart's disease causes hydrops fetalis and death in infancy. In hemoglobin H disease, the patients have anemia and splenomegaly. In α-thalassemia minor, the patients are usually asymptomatic. Carriers of α-thalassemia suffer no dysfunction. In β-thalassemia, β-thalassemia major is the most severe form, causing sever anemia in infancy and often death in childhood. β-Thalassemia intermedia causes less severe anemia, often with jaundice. β-Thalassemia minor is asymptomatic, with little or no anemia. β-Thalassemia minima causes no dysfunction, though the patient does have an abnormal hemoglobin in the blood.

In some kinds of thalassemia, no α chains are produced. These people are said to have α^D-thalassemia. In other patients, some α chains are produced, though not enough. Such people are said to have $\alpha^\dagger$-thalassemia. In a similar way, β-thalassemia can be divided into α^D thalassemia, in which no β chains are formed, and $\beta^\dagger$-thalassemia, in which their production is insufficient.

Many patients with thalassemia also form a structurally abnormal hemoglobin. Sometimes the chain synthesized in insufficient quantity is the hemgolobin structurally abnormal, as in the hemoglobin Lepore syndromes or with hemgolobin Constant Spring. Other people are double heterozygotes, with one gene coding for a structurally abnormal hemoglobin and another for the underproduction of one of the normal chains. Such diseases are given names like hemoglobin S $\beta-$ thalassemia to indicate the nature of the two defects.

Prevalence. α-Thalassemia is most common in Southeast Asia and the south of China. In Thailand, 225,000 people have one of the forms of α-thalassemia. In parts of the country, up to 10% of the people are affected. It occurs less frequently in India, the Middle East, around the Mediterranean, and in West Africa. In the United States, the synthesis of α chains is impaired in 5% of black people.

β-Thalassemia is common around the Mediterranean. In parts of Sardinia, Italy, and Greece, it affects up to 20% of the population. It is less common in northern and Western Africa, in Middle East, Pakistan, India, Southeast Asia, and southern China.

In Southeast Asia, α-thalassemia is more frequent than is β-thalassemia. In the United States, β-thalassemia is most common in people of Italian or Greek ancestry. About 1% of black people in the United States have β-thalassemia.

Inheritance. Most people with one of the forms of α-thalassemia lack one or more of the four genes controlling the synthesis of α chains. In α-thalassemia 1, both of the loci for α chains are deleted on one or both of the chromosomes 16. In α-thalassemia 2, one of the loci for α chains is missing on one or both of the chromosomes 16.

α-Thalassemia can also be caused if one or more of the loci for α chains is occupied by an allele that reduces the production of α chains. Such people are said to have a nondeletion defect.

The synthesis of hemoglobin Constant Spring or one of the other structurally abnormal hemoglobins with elongation of the α chain also causes α-thalassemia. These hemoglobins are produced only in small quantity, resulting in a lack of α chains.

The synthesis messenger ribonucleic acid is impaired in all forms of α-thalassemia. The greater the number of loci deleted or occupied by inefficient alleles, the more the synthesis of messenger ribonucleic acid is reduced, the smaller the quantity of α-chains produced, and the more severe the disease. If one of the loci for α chains is deleted, the quantity of α chains produced is about 87% of the quantity of β chains. If two of the loci are lost, it falls to 80%. If three are deleted, to 30%. If all four loci for α chains are lost, no α chains are produced.

In β-thalassemia, the genes coding for the β chains seem to be intact. The fault lies in the formation of messenger ribonucleic acid. It is either produced in insufficient quantity or fails to function normally. In patients homozygous for β^+-thalassemia, from 5 to 30% of the normal quantity of messenger ribonucleic acid for β chains is synthesized, with a corresponding reduction in the production of β chains. In some patients homozygous for β^D-thalassemia, no messenger ribonucleic acid for β chains is synthesized. In others, a small quantity of messenger ribonucleic acid is produced, but it fails to function, either because the ribonucleic acid is

defective or because of the lack of some un-
identified cofactor.

In δβ-thalassemia, the gene for β chains is
deleted on one or both of the chromosomes
11, together with part of the gene for δ
chains. In people homozygous for the defect,
neither β nor δ chains are produced.

In γδβ-thalassemia, the genes for β, δ,
and Aγ chains are all deleted. The gene for
Gγ chains remains intact. The hemoglobin
F that is produced contains only Gγ chains.

In the condition called hereditary persistence of fetal hemoglobin, the genes for β
and δ chains are deleted, but the production
of γ chains is increased, almost to equal the
production of α chains. Hemoglobin F continues to be produced in large quantity in
adult life.

In the various kinds of hemoglobin Lepore
disease, part of the gene for β chains and
part of the gene for δ chains are deleted,
together with the segment of the chromosome between them. In homozygotes, β or
δ chains are produced. Instead abnormal
chains are formed, having the structure of
δ chains at their N terminal end and of β
chains at their C terminal end. Three kinds
of hemoglobin Lepore have been distinguished, but in all, the quantity of the abnormal chains produced is low. In homozygotes 5 to 15% of the quantity of α chains
is produced.

In hemoglobin Kenya disease, the genes
for β, δ, and Aγ chains are affected. In
homozygotes, no β, δ, or Aγ chains are
synthesized. The hemoglobin F produced
has only Gγ chains. Instead of the missing
chains, an abnormal chain is produced, having the structure of a γ chain at its N terminal
end and of a β chain at its C terminal end.
The abnormal chain is formed in sufficient
quantity almost to equal the formation of α
chains.

Dysfunction. In the thalassemias, the
failure to produce one or more of the polypeptide chains of hemoglobin has two effects.
Because of the lack of one or more of the
chains, the quantity of hemoglobin formed is
usually reduced. Because the unused chains
precipitate in the red cells and their precursors, the destruction of the red cells is
increased. Usually, the increased hemolysis
is the more serious.

In α-thalassemia, the unused γ chains in
the erythroid cells in the bone marrow in the
fetus and newborn infant polymerize to form
hemoglobin Bart's, with four γ chains. In
older children and in adults, the unused β
chains in the precursors of the red cells in
the bone marrow polymerize to form hemoglobin H, with four β chains.

Both hemoglobin Bart's and hemoglobin H
bind oxygen 10 times more firmly than does
hemoglobin A, releasing little to the tissues.
If the proportion of hemoglobin Bart's or of
hemoglobin H in the blood is high, severe
hypoxia results.

The erythrocytic precursors in the bone
marrow develop normally in α-thalassemia.
They contain hemoglobin Bart's or hemoglobin H, but the abnormal hemgolobin does
not impair their development. Hemoglobin
Bart's and hemoglobin H precipitate only in
the blood. The precipitates make the circulating red cells rigid, causing their early
destruction principally in the spleen.

In β-thalassemia, the unused α-chains
precipitate in the developing red cells in the
bone marrow. If the concentration of free
α-chains is high, the developing red cells are
destroyed. In β-thalassemia major, only from
5 to 30% of the normoblasts reach the blood.
The red cells that do reach the blood contain
smaller concentrations of α-chains, but they
too are soon destroyed, principally in the
spleen and by macrophages in other organs.

In β-thalassemia, the more hemoglobin
F in a circulating red cell, the longer it
survives. Circulating red cells containing
predominantly hemoglobin F have few precipitates of α chains, but in cells containing
mainly hemoglobin A the precipitates are
many and large.

In both α- and β-thalassemia, the precipitates in the red cells damage the cell
membrane. The flux of sodium and potassium across the cell membrane increases,
and potassium is lost from the cells. In
β-thalassemia deoxyribonucleic acid metabolism is depressed in the erythroid cells in
the bone marrow and the formation of heme
is impaired contributing to the ineffective
erythropoiesis prominent in this form of
thalassemia.

Treatment. Patients with thalassemia unable to maintain the concentration of hemo-

globin in the blood above 75 g/L (7.5 g/100 mL) need transfusions to maintain the volume of packed cells above 0.35 L/L (35%). The hyperplasia of the bone marrow is suppressed, and with it many of the signs of the disease.

The transfusions do not increase the hemosiderosis more than does a more sparing use of blood. Indeed, they may reduce the uptake of iron from the bowel. Chelating agents such as deferoxamine can reduce the load of iron in the body, though treatment is expensive.

Splenectomy is needed only if the need for transfusions increases rapidly or if the spleen grows so large that its weight causes discomfort. After splenectomy, the need for transfusions rapidly falls. In hemoglobin H disease, the proportion of red cells containing precipitates of the abnormal hemoglobin increases. In severe β-thalassemia, precipitates of α chains become evident in some of the red cells.

Carriers of α-Thalassemia. Carriers of α-thalassemia have three genes for α chains on chromosomes 16. They are usually heterozygous for α-thalassemia 2. One of their chromosomes 16 has two loci for α chains. The other has one. The carriers have no disease. Their blood and bone marrow are normal. Only in the first few weeks of life can 1 or 2% of hemoglobin Bart's be demonstrated in the blood. Later, neither hemoglobin Bart's nor hemoglobin H is demonstrable. The diagnosis can be made only be mapping the chromosomes 16, or by studying the inheritance of the α-thalassemia 2 defect in the carrier's family.

α-Thalassemia Minor. People with α-thalassemia minor have two genes actively producing α chains on their chromosomes 16. The patient can be homozygous for α-thalassemia 2, with one gene for α chains on each of the chromosomes 16, or heterozygous for α-thalassemia 1, with two genes for α chains on one chromosome 16, none on the other. α-Thalassemia minor also develops in people who have two normal genes for α chains, with the other two loci occupied by nondeletion defects, which produce only a small quantity of α chains, and in people who have two normal genes for α chains, with the other two loci for α chains occupied by the

genes for hemoglobin Constant Spring, which is produced only in small quantity.

People with α-thalassemia minor have no symptoms. The diagnosis is usually made when the blood is examined for some other reason, or when the family of a person with α-thalassemia is investigated.

The concentration of hemoglobin in the blood is normal, or nearly so. A blood smear shows that the red cells are smaller than normal and stain less strongly. There are mild anisocytosis and poikilocytosis. The mean volume of the red cells averages 72 fL, as compared with a normal of from 80 to 95 fL. The mean concentration of hemoglobin in the red cells averages 310 g/L (31 g/100 mL) rather than the normal 320 to 360 g/L (32 to 36 g/100 mL). The mean content of hemoglobin averages 22 pg, against a normal of from 27 to 36 pg.

At birth, the blood contains from 5 to 6% of hemoglobin Bart's. Later in life, no abnormal hemoglobin can be detected. The proportion of hemoglobins A_2 and F in the blood is normal. The diagnosis can be made by mapping the chromosomes 16 or by family studies.

Hemoglobin H Disease. In most patients with hemoglobin H disease, only one gene for α chains is active on the chromosomes 16. The patient may be doubly heterozygous for α-thalassemia 1 and α-thalassemia 2, with deletion of three of the loci for α chains, may be doubly heterozygous for α-thalassemia 1 and for hemgolobin Constant Spring, with deletion of the two loci for α chains on one chromsome 16 and with the allele coding for hemoglobin Constant Spring occupying one of the two loci on the other chromosome 16. Hemoglobin H disease also develops if two of the loci for α chains are lost and the other two are occupied by nondeletion defects, which together produce about as many chains as a normal gene for α chains, or if all four loci are occupied by ineffective nondeletion defects.

People with hemoglobin H disease develop anemia and splenomegaly during infancy and hepatomegaly later. The disease can be mild and easily overlooked but can be severe enough to necessitate blood transfusions. Infection, pregnancy, and oxidant drugs increase the severity of the anemia.

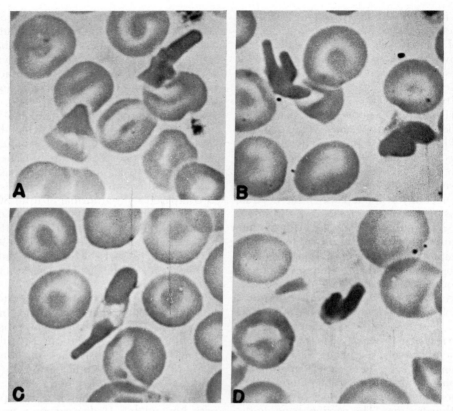

Fig. 49-12.   Hypochromia, anisocytosis, and target cells in the blood of a patient with β-thalassemia major. (By permission of Grune & Stratton, from Diggs, L. W., and Bell, A.: Intraerythrocytic crystals in sickle cell hemoglobin C disease. Blood, 25:218, 1965.)

The concentration of hemoglobin in the blood is usually from 70 to 100 g/L (7 to 10 g/100 mL), with 5 to 10% of reticulocytes. In a blood film, the red cells are small and stain poorly because of their low content of hemoglobin. Target cells are common. Incubation with cresyl blue reveals precipitates of hemoglobin H within the cells. Similar precipitates of hemoglobin H are present in a few of the erythroid cells in the bone marrow.

At birth, from 20 to 40% of the hemoglobin in the blood is hemoglobin Bart's, with four γ chains. In the first few months of life, hemoglobin Bart's disappears almost entirely and is replaced by hemoglobin H, with four β chains, as the synthesis of β chains begins and the synthesis of γ chains falls in the normal way as the infant ages. In adult life, from 5 to 30% of the hemoglobin in the blood of people with hemoglobin H disease is

hemoglobin H. The proportion of hemoglobin A_2 is reduced to about 1.5%, from the normal 2.5%. There may be a trace of hemoglobin Bart's. The rest is hemoglobin A.

Rarely, hemoglobin H appears in the blood of a patient with a myeloproliferative disorder, leukemia, or a refractory sideroblastic anemia. In some of these patients, the abnormal hemoglobin seems to be produced by an abnormal clone of erythrocytes. The production of α chains is deficient in the abnormal clone but normal in the other erythroid cells in the bone marrow. Some of the red cells contain hemoglobin H, some do not.

Hemoglobin Bart's Disease.   Hemoglobin Bart's disease develops when no α chains are produced. It is an important cause of fetal death in Southeast Asia, Greece, and Cyprus. The affected infants are homozygous for α-thalassemia 1. There are no loci for α chains on their chromosomes 16. The disease does not occur in black people with α-thalassemia. The defect in black people with α-thalassemia is α-thalassemia 2, with deletion of one of the loci for α chains from chromosome 16. Even if a black person is homozygous for α-thalassemia 2, two genes remain to produce α chains, and the patient has α-thalassemia minor.

The fetus usually dies in utero, from the 28th to the 40th week of gestation, with hydrops fetalis. If the child is born alive, it dies within a few hours. The child is pale and enormously bloated by edema. The liver and spleen are greatly enlarged by extramedullary hematopoiesis. The placenta is large and friable.

The concentration of hemoglobin in the blood is from 40 to 100 g/L (4 to 10 g/100 mL). A blood smear shows severe anisocytosis and poikilocytosis. The red cells are small, and nucleated red cells are common. The concentration of hemoglobin in the red cells is low.

When death occurs, more than 80% of the hemoglobin in the blood is hemoglobin Bart's. Most of the rest is hemoglobin Portland. There may be a trace of hemoglobin H. Death comes from hypoxia because hemoglobin Bart's cannot oxygenate the tissues. The fetus survives in the early months of pregnancy because the blood contains more of the early fetal hemoglobins Gower I and Portland. Because they have ζ chains, not α chains, they are formed normally in hemoglobin Bart's disease.

β-Thalassemia Major. β-Thalassemia major is sometimes called Cooley's anemia, after the American pediatrician who described it in 1925. It develops when few or no β-chains are produced.

β-Thalassemia major develops in most people who are homozygous for the defect causing $β^D$-thalassemia, who produce no β chains; who are homozygous for $β^+$-thalassemia or doubly heterozygous for $β^D$-thalassemia and $β^+$-thalassemia, who produce too small a quantity of β chains; or are homozygous for hemoglobin Lepore, who produce neither β nor δ chains. Some people with these abnormalities develop only β-thalassemia intermedia. Why some develop the more severe form of the disease while others do not is unknown.

The bone marrow is highly hyperplastic in β-thalassemia major, principally because of an enormous increase in erythropoiesis. In many of the normoblasts, inclusions formed by precipitated α chains are evident. The macrophages in the bone marrow are distended by cellular debris because of the great destruction of red cell precursors in the bone marrow.

The anemia of β-thalassemia major becomes evident when the patient is a few months old. The concentration of hemoglobin in the blood is usually between 25 and 65 g/L (2.5 and 6.5 g/100 mL). The packed cell volume is from 0.11 to 0.24 L/L (11 to 24%). The red cells are small and contain little hemoglobin. The mean cell volume is from 48 to 72 fL, rather than the normal 80 to 95 fL. This mean concentration of hemoglobin in the cells is from 230 to 320 g/L (23 to 32 g/100 mL), not the normal 320 to 360 g/L (32 to 36 g/100 mL). The osmotic fragility of the red cells is decreased. In some patients, the red cells fail to hemolyze even in distilled water.

A blood smear shows severe anisocytosis and poikilocytosis. The red cells vary from 3 to 15 μm in diameter. Most are pale, but a few are normally pigmented. Target cells and basophilic stippling are common. Many of the cells are greatly distorted. The reticulocytosis is between 5 and 15%. More than 10% of the nucleated cells in the blood are red cells. Sometimes nucleated red cells are two or three times more numerous than granulocytes.

The kinds of hemoglobin in the blood differ in the different kinds of β-thalassemia major. In the homozygotes for $β^D$-thalassemia who produce no β chains, there is no hemoglobin A. Over 94% of the hemoglobin is hemoglobin F, with α and γ chains, and almost all the rest is hemoglobin A_2, with α and δ chains. Free α chains are present in the red cells. In the homozygotes for $β^+$-thalassemia and the double heterozygotes for $β^0$-thalassemia and $β^+$-thalassemia, who produce a small quantity of β chains, some hemoglobin A is present, but most of the hemoglobin is hemoglobin F. The proportion of hemoglobin A_2 may be reduced, normal, or increased to as much as 8%. Free α chains may be present. In homozygotes for hemoglobin Lepore, neither β nor δ chains are produced. There is no hemoglobin A and no hemoglobin A_2. Over 75% of the hemoglobin is hemoglobin F, and the rest is hemoglobin Lepore.

In the forms of β-thalassemia major in which both hemoglobin A and hemoglobin F are produced, the proportion of hemoglobin F in the red cells varies from one cell to another. Cells contining a high proportion of hemoglobin F have a normal life span; cells containing mostly hemoglobin A are destroyed in 20 to 30 days.

Ferrokinetic studies show the changes found in other forms of ineffective reythropoiesis. Hyperbilirubinemia and increased excretion of urobilin and urobilinogen in the urine are usual. The urinary excretion of dipyrroles may increase.

If the anemia is not controlled by transfusions, growth is stunted. The head is overly large. The features are distorted by the overgrowth of the facial bones. The abdomen bulges because of hepatosplenomegaly. Puberty is delayed, and sexual development may be imperfect.

Changes in the bones are prominent in β-thalassemia major. The hyperplastic hematopoietic marrow extends far into the long bones. The medulla of the bones is expanded, and the cortex thinned. The skull is greatly thickened, and its inner and outer tables are bearded. Its trabeculae become arranged perpendicular to the surface of the skull, so that an x-ray study of the skull looks like hair on end. The bones of the face are distorted, bulging towards the nose and causing malocclusion. The erosion of the medullae causes mottling in a radiograph of the bones of the hands. Compression fractures may develop in the spine because of the erosion of the vertebrae.

The liver and the spleen are enlarged in childhood because of massive extramedullary hematopoiesis. Later comes increasing hemosiderosis, due in large part to the transfusions needed to control the anemia and to increased absorption of iron from the bowel. In many of the patients, cirrhosis follows.

Pericardial effusions of unknown etiology are common in childhood, but resolve with-

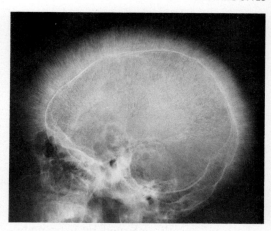

Fig. 49-13. Roentgenogram of the skull of a patient with β-thalassemia major. (From Wintrobe, M. W., et al.: Clinical Hematology. 8th Ed. Philadelphia, Lea & Febiger, 1981.)

out complications. Hemosiderosis causes cardiac dysfunction with arrythymias and congestive heart failure in many of the patients, often before the patient is 20 years old. Most patients with β-thalassemia major die in childhood from infection or from heart failure.

β-Thalassemia Intermedia. Most people who are doubly heterozygous for β°-thalassemia and △ β-thalassemia, for β°-thalassemia and hemoglobin Lepore, β+thalassemia and hemoglobin Lepore, or for δβ-thalassemia and hemoglobin Lepore develop β-thalassemia intermedia. It sometimes occurs in people homozygous for δβ-thalassemia, in a person with one of the genetic disorders that usually cause β-thalassemia major, or in a person with an allele coding for β°-thalassemia on one chromosome 11 and a normal allele on the other. People with both α-thalassemia and β-thalassemia develop a mild anemia like β-thalassemia intermedia.

The changes in the blood and bone marrow are like those of β-thalassemia major, though less severe. The concentration of hemoglobin in the blood is usually maintained at 60 to 90 g/L (6 to 9 g/100 mL) with transfusions. The red cells in the blood are small and hypochromatic, but anisocytosis and poikilocytosis are less severe than in β-thalassemia major. From 3 to 10% of the circulating red cells are reticulocytes. A few nucleated red cells may be present in the blood.

The kinds of hemoglobin found in the blood in β-thalassemia intermedia reflect the genetic defect or defects causing the disease. If neither β chains nor δ chains are produced, there is neither hemoglobin A nor hemoglobin A_2. From 90 to 100% of the hemoglobin in the blood is hemoglobin F. If δ chains are produced, but β chains are not, there is no hemoglobin A. Most of the hemoglobin is hemoglobin F, but there is from 0.3 to 4% of hemoglobin A_2. If some β chains are produced, the ratio of hemoglobin A to hemoglobin F varies considerably from one patient to another. In some, over 60% of the hemoglobin is hemoglobin A, in some, it is less than 20%. The proportion of hemoglobin A_2 varies, but does not exceed 10%. Structurally abnormal hemoglobins are present in the blood only in patients with a gene or genes coding for hemoglobin Lepore and sometimes in people with both α- and β-thalassemia, who may have hemoglobin H in the blood.

Clinically, β-thalassemia intermedia is similar to β-thalassemia major, but less severe. It occurs during childhood, but does not usually affect growth or development. Persistent anemia, splenomegaly, and episodes of jaundice are its principal features. Bony changes are less marked than in β-thalassemia major.

Most patients with β-thalassemia intermedia live into adult life, often for a normal life span. If death is caused by the thalassemia, it is often from myocardial hemosiderosis. The patient do not need many transfusions, but the absorption of iron from the gut is increased 3 to 10 times. By the time the patient is 30 or 40 years old, the iron stores in the body can be massive.

Thalassemia Minor. People heterozygous for β⁰-thalasssemia, β⁺-thalassemia, δβ-thalassemia, or hemoglobin Lepore usually develop β-thalassemia minor. A few of the heterozygotes for β⁰-thalassemia develop β-thalassemia intermedia.

The concentration of hemoglobin in the blood is normal or nearly so in β-thalassemia minor. It is rarely below 120 g/L (12 g/100 mL) in men or 110 g/L (11 g/100 mL) in women. The red cells are smaller than normal, with a mean cell volume averaging 65 fL, rather than the normal 80 to 95 fL. The mean content of hemoglobin in the red cells is low, averaging 20 pg, rather than the normal 27 to 36 pg. Because the red cells are small, the mean concentration of hemoglobin in the red cells is nearly normal, averaging 310 g/L (31 g/100 mL), rather than the normal 320 to 360 g/L (31 to 36 g/100 mL).

Except in heterozygotes for hemoglobin Lepore, about 90% of the hemoglobin in the blood is hemoglobin A. The proportion of hemoglobin A_2 varies from 2.5 to 8%. The rest is hemoglobin F. In heterozygotes for hemoglobin Lepore, up to 15% of the hemoglobin is hemoglobin Lepore, sometimes with as such as 15% of hemoglobin F, but less than 2.5% of hemoglobin A_2.

A blood smear shows small, hypochromatic red cells, with marked anisocytosis and poikilocytosis. Target cells and basophilic stippling are common. Nucleated red cells are not present.

The bone marrow shows only mild hyperplasia. Other organs are affected little, if at all.

β-Thalassemia Minima. In β-thalassemia minima, the gentic defect produces no discernible abnormality. The diagnosis can be established by showing that cultured reticulocytes synthesize fewer β chains than α chains.

Hereditary Persistence of Fetal Hemoglobin. Four kinds of hereditary persistence of fetal hemoglobin are known. In all, there is no synthesis of β or δ chains in homozygotes, but the production of γ chains is increased to compensate for their loss. In the form of the disorder found in black people, both Aγ and Gγ chains are synthesized in about the normal ratio. In Greeks, only Aγ chains are produced. In hemoglobin Kenya disease, the abnormal hemoglobin Kenya replaces the γ chains. In these forms of the disease, the concentration of hemoglobin F is the same in all the red cells. In the heterocellular form of hereditary persistence of fetal hemoglobin, the concentration of hemoglobin F in the red cells varies considerably from one red cell to another.

Hereditary persistence of fetal hemoglobin causes no disability in heterozygotes or in homozygotes. In homozygotes the blood shows changes similar to those of β-thalassemia minor. The concentration of hemoglobin remains normal, or nearly 30.

δ-Thalassemia. Even in homozygotes for δ-thalassemia, the lack of δ chains causes no disability. Hemoglobin A_2 is absent, but there is no defect in the formation of hemoglobin A.

γβ-Thalassemia. The rare γβ-thalassemia causes anemia in childhood, which resolves, leaving the patient with β-thalassemia minor in adult life. The patients have all been heterozygotes. Presumably homozygotes, lacking all γ chains, would die in utero because of the inability to form hemoglobin F.

Thalassemia plus a Structural Hemoglobinopathy. As both thalassemia and some of the structural hemoglobinopathies are common in the same parts of the world, double heterozygotes having both thalassemia and a structural hemoglobinopathy occur.

Double heterozygotes for α-thalassemia and the abnormal α chains of hemoglobin Q or hemoglobin G Philadelphia synthesize no hemoglobin A and develop hemoglobin H disease. A double heterozygote for α-thalassemia and the abnormal α chains of hemoglobin I has 20% of hemoglobin A in the blood and suffers a less severe disease.

The combination of α-thalassemia with one of the structural hemoglobinopathies with abnormal β chains usually does little to modify either the α-thalassemia or the structural hemoglobinopathy. Patients with α-thalassemia have been homozygous or heterozygous for hemoglobin S, hemoglobin C, hemoglobin E, or hemoglobin J Bangkok. Only in a child with α-thalassemia homozygous for hemoglobin S was the sickling ameliorated.

More than 1 black baby in every 2000 in the United States is doubly heterozygous for β-thalassemia and hemoglobin S. Hemoglobin S – β-thalassemia is also common in the Mediterannean countries. The disease is similar to sickle cell anemia, though usually less severe. Hemoglobin S – $β^0$-thalassemia is more severe than hemoglobin S – $β^+$-thalassemia. In hemoglobin S – $β^0$-thalassemia, the blood contains no hemoglobin A. In hemoglobin S – $β^+$-thalassemia, up to 30% of the hemoglobin in the blood is hemoglobin A. The blood and bone marrow show a combination of the features of sickle cell anemia and β-thalassemia.

Hemoglobin S – δβ-thalassemia causes only minor changes in the red cells. People doubly heterozygous for hemoglobin S and hereditary persistence of fetal hemoglobin suffer no disability, because the high concentration of fetal hemoglobin in the red cells prevents sickling. People doubly heterozygous for hemoglobin S and hemoglobin Lepore develop moderately severe sickling disorder.

People doubly heterozygous for hemoglobin C and β-thalassemia remain healthy, though the blood shows changes like those of β-thalassemia minor. People with hemoglobin E-β-thalassemia develop β-thalassemia major. The combination of β-thalassemia with other abnormal hemoglobins produces no disability.

IMMUNOHEMOLYTIC DISORDERS. In the immunohemolytic disorders, an antibody against one of the antigens on the surface of the red cells becomes attached to the red cells and brings about their destruction.

Three kinds of immunohemolytic anemia are distinguished. Preformed antibodies destroy foreign red cells introduced into the circulation in transfusion reactions and in hemolytic disease of the newborn. Antibodies develop against the patient's own red cells in the autoimmunohemolytic anemias. Antibodies that destroy the red cells can be induced by drugs.

Transfusion Reaction. Incompatible blood transfused into a recipient is likely to cause hemolysis. Most often, preformed antibodies in the recipient's plasma attack and destroy any transfused red cells. Less often, transfused antibodies attack the patient's red cells.

Two kinds of hemolytic transfusion reaction occur. Most frequently, the destruction of the red cells is largely intravascular, with release of hemoglobin into the plasma, though some of the transfused cells are destroyed extravascularly by the macrophages of the liver, spleen, and other organs. Less often, the destruction of the red cells is mainly extravascular, with little release of hemoglobin into the plasma.

Lesions. If intravascular hemolysis is predominant in a transfusion reaction, the concentration of hemoglobin in the plasma rises rapidly as the foreign red cells are lysed. Hemoglobinemia and hemoglobinuria persist for a few hours or days. The concentrations of haptoglobin and hemopexin in the plasma fall. The concentration of bilirubin in the plasma rises only if there is also extravascular destruction of red cells by the macrophages of the spleen and liver.

If the destruction of the red cells is predominantly extravascular, hyperbilirubinemia is the principal finding. Little hemoglobin escapes into the plasma. Hemoglobinuria does not occur.

Soon after a transfusion reaction, some of the circulating red cells are coated with antibody. Some are transfused cells that have escaped destruction. Some are the recipient's red cells carrying small quantities of antibody from the donor's blood. The plasma is unlikely to contain the antibodies that caused the reaction. They were fixed to the foreign cells and were destroyed with them.

Clinical Presentation. An intravascular hemolytic transfusion reaction usually begins before the transfusion is finished. The recipient becomes restless and flushed, with tingling in the skin and often pain in the precordial region or the back. The pulse and respiratory rates rise. Nausea and vomiting occur with cyanosis and shock if the reaction is severe. Chills may be followed by a fever over 40°C. Leukopenia is followed by a leukocytosis, usually of from 15 to 20 × 10^9/L (15,000 to 20,000/mm^3). The severity and duration of the reaction varies a good deal, but it usually lasts about 12 hours and then subsides.

Complications. Severe intravascular hemolysis often causes disseminated intravascular coagulation. The concentrations of fibrinogen and of factor VIII in the plasma fall as they are used up by multiple small intravascular thrombi. The concentration of platelets in the blood falls as they are used up. Breakdown products resulting from the lysis of some of the fibrinogen precipitated in the vessels appear in the blood and urine. Even before the transfusion is finished, blood may begin to ooze dangerously from the mucous membranes or from the site of an operation because of the lack of platelets and the depletion of the coagulation factors.

Acute renal failure soucetimes becomes evident about 24 hours after a incompatible transfusion was given. It may be transient or can persist for many days. The severity of the renal injury depends in large part on the quantity of incompatible blood given and the nature of the antibodies against the transfused cells. If a major ABO incompatibility causes intravascular hemolysis, the transfusion of 200 to 500 mL of blood is likely to cause severe tubular injury in the kidneys, sometimes necrosis of the tubular epithelium or bilateral cortical necrosis.

The renal injury is due to ischemia. In part it is caused by disseminated intravascular thrombosis. Small thrombi are common in the renal glomeruli. In part it results from vasomotor nephropathy caused by the deviation of blood away from the renal glomeruli and tubules by vasoactive agents released during the activation of the coagulation system. The hemoglobin excreted by the kidneys probably does little harm.

Extravascular hemolytic transfusion reactions are less dangerous. Malaise and fever are common, but the disseminated intravascular coagulation, renal injury, and shock of massive intravascular hemolysis are rare.

Sometimes a transfusion reaction is delayed for from 2 to 14 days. Probably these recipients do not have antibodies against the transfused red cells circulating in their blood at the time of transfusion, but develop them because of an anamnestic reaction or because the foreign red cells in the blood sensitize the recipient. Delayed hemolytic transfusion reactions can be severe. They are usually caused by antibodies against the JK^a antigen of the Kidd system, the E, c, or D antigens of the Rh system, the Fy^a antigen of the Duffy system, or the K antigen of the Kell system. The hemolysis is predominantly extravascular. Red cells coated with antigen circulate in the blood.

Pathogenesis. Hemolytic transfusion reactions of the intravascular type are caused by complement fixing antibodies. Most often, the reaction is caused by IgM antibodies against the ABH antigens of the transfused red cells. IgG antibodies against these antigens are less important but can cause hemolysis. Occasionally, an intravascular transfusion reaction is caused by complement fixing antibodies against the JK^a antigen of the Kell system, the Le^a antigen of the Lewis system, or the Fy^a antigen of the Duffy system.

IgM antibodies attached to the surface of red cells activate complement efficiently. Every molecular of IgM on the surface of a red cell has the two closely approximated binding sites needed to fix C1q and to initiate the classic pathway for the activation of complement. C3 is split to give C3b, which is bound to the surface of the red cells by the C3b receptors on their surface. C5 is activated, giving C5b, which is also bound to the surface of the red cells, where it fixes C6, C7, C8, and C9.

IgG antibodies activate complement less efficiently. The IgG must be of a type able to activate complement, and the molecules of IgG on the surface of the red cells must be close enough to activate C1q.

The intravascular hemolysis is caused by the complex of C5b with C6, C7, C8, and C9. The complex makes pores in the cell membrane of the red cells, allowing their content to escape into the plasma. The extravascular hemolysis that accompanies intravascular hemolysis is caused by the C3b attached to the surface of the red cells. The C3b binds to the C3b receptors on the phagocytes in the liver, spleen, and other organs, fixing the red cells to the phagocytes. Most of the red cells so attached are phagocytosed and destroyed.

The attachment of red cells to macrophages by C3b is not always followed by phagocytosis. If a red cell remains on the surface of a phagocyte, C3b is split by the C3b inactivator, leaving C3d attached to the red cell. Since C3d does not fix to phagocytes, the cell returns to the circulation. There, it has a normal life span. Red cells carrying C3d are protected against the attachment of more C3b because the C3d occupies its receptors.

Complement activation quickly rids the body of foreign red cells. If a small quantity of red cells is introduced into the blood of a person who has IgM antibodies against the A, B, H antigens of the transfused cells, the

foreign cells are removed from the circulation in less than 2 minutes, principally by attachment to the Kupffer cells in the liver. If a larger quantity of incompatible red cells is transfused, over 80% of their hemoglobin escapes into the plasma as the foreign cells are lysed by C $\overline{566789}$ most of it within 1 minute. A smaller proportion of the red cells becomes attached to phagocytes in the liver, spleen, and other organs. If the volume of incompatible red cells introduced into the circulation is large, their destruction is slower, because there is not enough IgM antibody in the plasma to fill all the receptors on the foreign red cells.

Hemolytic transfusion reactions of the extravascular type are caused by IgG antibodies that do not fix complement. They are most common when red cells carrying the D antigen of the Rh system are transfused into a person who has developed antibodies against the D antigen. The antibodies are mainly IgG1 and IgG2, and so are able to activate complement, but presumably are too far apart to do so. Less often a hemolytic transfusion reaction of the extravascular type is caused by antibodies against other of the Rh antigens or against antigens of the Kidd, Duffy, or Kell systems.

The red cells coated with IgG become attached to phagocytes by the receptors for the Fc portion of IgG1 and IgG2 on the surface of the phagocytes. This method of attachment to the phagocytes is less efficient than is attachment by C3b. The red cells coated with IgG must compete for the receptors on the phagocytes with the IgG in the plasma. Unless the red cells are heavily coated with IgG, few of them will become attached to a phagocyte.

The red cells that are attached to the phagocytes by their receptors for the Fc portion of IgG are phagocytosed and destroyed. The destruction takes place mainly in the spleen, though as the concentration of IgG antibodies against the red cells rises, the proportion of the red cells destroyed by the phagocytes in the liver and elswhere rises.

Because the destruction of the foreign red cells occurs principally in the macrophages of the spleen and liver, little hemoglobin escapes into the plasma. Even if a large quantity of Rh-incompatible blood is given to a person with a high titer of IgG antibodies against the D antigen of the foreign red cells, only about 10% of their hemoglobin escapes into the plasma.

If a small quantity of red cells is introduced into the circulation of a person in whom the concentration of IgG antibodies against the D antigen of the foreign red cells is high, the foreign cells are removed from the circulating blood within a few minutes. If the concentration of antibody against the D antigen is lower, or the quantity of foreign red cells introduced is greater, it takes over an hour to remove half the foreign red cells from the circulating blood.

The antibodies in the transfused plasma rarely do any harm. Even if the donor's blood contains a high concentration of antibodies against the recipient's red cells, they are likely to be so diluted by the recipient's plasma that they cause little damage. Only a high titer of antibody against the major ABO antigens on the recipient's red cells is dangerous.

Treatment and Prognosis. Extravascular hemolytic transfusion reactions are not usually severe enough to need treatment. The incompatible transfusion should be stopped, and the patient allowed to recover.

Severe intravascular hemolytic transfusion reactions are dangerous. The disseminated intravascular coagulation and renal failure are treated as are other forms of these disorders. Shock is treated in the usual way, by giving compatible blood and other fluids. The outcome depends on the severity of the renal injury and of the disseminated intravascular coagulation.

HEMOLYTIC DISEASE OF THE NEWBORN. Many kinds of hemolytic disease occur in the newborn, but the name hemolytic disease of the newborn has become restricted to the disorder caused by the passage of maternal antibodies across the placenta to attack the fetal red cells. Erythroblastosis fetalis is an older name for the condition.

Lesions. Hemolytic disease of the newborn develops in the fetus in utero, though it may not become apparent until after birth. The maternal antibodies attack the fetal red cells, causing hemolysis. If it is not severe,

hemolytic disease of the newborn affects principally the amniotic fluid and blood. If it is severe, the whole body is affected.

Amniotic Fluid. If hemolytic disease of the newborn is severe in utero, a pigment, which is mainly bilirubin, leaks into the amniotic fluid. Instead of its normal straw color, the amniotic fluid becomes bright yellow. The concentration of the pigment can be measured by estimating the optical density of the amniotic fluid or by determining its content of bilirubin. The greater the concentration of pigment, the greater the hemolysis, and the greater the risk to the fetus.

Antibodies against the D antigen escape into the amniotic fluid when an Rh-negative mother bears an Rh-positive child. They do not appear in the amniotic fluid if the child is Rh negative, even if the titer of antibody in the mother's plasma is high. The greater the severity of the hemolytic disease of the newborn, the higher the titer of antibody in the amniotic fluid. If there is hemorrhage from the fetal circulation into the amniotic fluid, the fetal red cells can be typed to determine whether they carry the D antigen.

Blood. If hemolytic disease of the newborn is mild, the concentration of hemoglobin in the blood at birth is within the normal range. If the disease is severe, it can be as low as 30 g/L (3 g/100 mL). In some infants, the concentration of hemoglobin in the blood is normal at birth, but falls rapidly unless treatment is instituted. The concentration of hemoglobin may fall by as much as 30g/L/d (3 g/100 mL/d).

A blood smear shows that great increase in the number of nucleated red cells in the circulation that gave the disease its name of erythroblastosis fetalis. Normally , the concentration of nucleated red cells in the blood of a newborn infant is less than 2×10^9/L (2,000/mm^3). In erythroblastosis fetalis, it is from 10 to 100 $\times$ 10^9/L (10,000 to 100,000/ mm^3). Most of the nucleated red cells are mature, but primitive forms are present. Some of the nonnucleated red cells are normocytic; some are macrocytic. Polychromasia is marked. Up to 60% of the red cells are reticulocytes.

There is often a leukocytosis of more than

30×10^9/L (30,000/mm^3), as compared with the normal 15 to 20 $\times$ 10^9/L (15,000 to 20,000/mm^3) in the newborn. The platelet count is often normal, but is low if the disease is severe.

The concentration of bilirubin in the plasma at birth indicates the severity of hemolytic disease of the newborn. A concentration of over 100 μmol/L (5.5 mg/100 mL) is uncommon and suggests that the disease is severe. If treatment is not begun, the concentration of bilirubin in the plasma rises steadily in the first days after birth, sometimes exceeding 850 μmol/L (50 mg/100 mL). Most of the bilirubin in the plasma is unconjugated, but if the hyperbilirubinemia is allowed to persist, the concentration of conjugated bilirubin also rises.

Many of the red cells in the blood in the first days of life are coated with antibody and react positively with sera against IgG.

Other Organs. Normally, there is little erythropoiesis in the liver or spleen at birth. When hemolytic disease of the newborn is severe, the sinusoids of the liver and spleen are crammed with millions of hematopoietic cells mainly engaged in erythropoiesis. The bone marrow is hyperplastic. Often there is hematopoiesis in the sinusoids of the adrenal glands, in the retroperitoneal tissues, and elsewhere.

If the destruction of fetal red cells is severe, the hyperplasia of the erythropoietic cells in the liver and spleen is so great that it causes hepatomegaly and splenomegaly. The erythopoietic cells in the liver can clog the sinusoids, causing portal hypertension, and compress the hepatocytes, impairing hepatic function. The portal hypertension and hypoalbuminemia cause ascites, hydrothoraces, and eventually severe, generalized edema.

Other changes in the tissue are minor. Iron is often abundant in the macrophages of the liver, spleen, lymph nodes, and elsewhere. Occasionally, bile plugs develop in the liver of jaundiced infants. The islets of Langerhans are bigger than normal.

Clinical Presentation. If hemolytic disease of the newborn is mild, the infant becomes anemic soon after birth. Usually the anemia develops in the first days after birth, but sometimes it is delayed until the child is two to eight weeks old. The concentration of hemoglobin in the blood can fall as low as 50 g/L (5 g/100 mL). There is no jaundice. Recovery comes after six to eight weeks as the red cells coated with antibody are eliminated and replaced by normal red cells.

If the disease is more severe, anemia and jaundice appear during the first 24 hours of life and grow increasingly severe as the concentration of hemoglobin falls rapidly and the concentration of bilirubin in the plasma rises dangerously. If the quantity of unconjugated bilirubin in the plasma exceeds the binding capacity of the circulating albumin, as it is likely to do if the concentration of bilirubin in the plasma exceeds 350 μmol/L (20 mg/100 mL), the unbound bilirubin in the plasma can escape into the basal nuclei of the brain and cause kernicterus.

If hemolytic disease of the newborn is still more severe, the child is usually born prematurely and often is born dead. If the child is live-born, death comes within a few hours in over 80% of the infants. The child is severely edematous, bloated by subcutaneous edema, with massive ascites and large pleural effusions that prevent expansion of the lungs. Anemia is severe. Usually the concentration of hemoglobin in the blood is less than 30 g/L (3 g/100 mL) and rapidly falls still lower. Because bilirubin is cleared from the fetus into the materal blood, the child is pale, not jaundiced. The placenta is large and friable. Such children are said to have hydrops fetalis.

Pathogenesis. Hemolytic disease of the newborn can occur only when the mother has in her plasma IgG antibodies against one of the antigens on the fetal red cells. IgG antibodies can readily cross the placenta and, if present in sufficient quantity in the maternal blood, can injure the fetal red cells. IgM antibodies in the maternal blood are too big to cross the placenta.

In most infants with hemolytic disease of the newborn, the disease is caused by IgG antibodies against the A or B antigens of the ABO system of blood groups. The mother is nearly always group O. Only people of group O develop sufficient IgG antibodies against the A and B antigens to damage the fetal red cells. Other people develop mainly IgM antibodies against these antigens.

The mother is of group O, and the child bears A or B antigens on the fetal red cells in 1 pregnancy in 5, but injury to the fetal red cells caused by antibodies against the A or B antigens is detected in only 1 pregnancy in 150 and is severe enough to cause jaundice in only 1 pregnancy in 750. The hemolytic disease caused by IgG antibodies against the A or B antigens requires exchange transfusion in only 1 pregnancy in 2500.

People of group O are sensitized against the A and B antigens of the ABO system by substances like the A and B antigens in food, and in other ways. Most women of group O have antibodies against the A and B antigens in their blood long before they become pregnant. Pregnancy does little to increase the titer of the antibodies.

Less often, hemolytic disease of the newborn is caused by IgG antibodies against one of the strong Rh antigens. Particular attention has been paid to the disease caused by antibodies against the D antigen of the Rh system, also called Rh_o. It used to be the most common cause of severe hemolytic disease of the newborn.

Hemolytic disease of the newborn caused by antibodies against the D antigen is more dangerous than hemolytic disease caused by antibodies against the A and B antigen. It can be mild but can cause hydrops fetalis. Before the introduction of measures to prevent this form of hemolytic disease of the newborn, 1 child in 200 suffered jaundice or hydrops caused by antibodies against the D antigen.

Hemolytic disease of the newborn caused by antibodies against the D antigen of the Rh system can develop only if the antigen is present on the red cells of the fetus, but not on the red cells of the mother. Only people who do not have the D antigen on their red cells can develop antibodies against it. The antibodies are mainly IgG. They cross the placenta and enter the fetal circulation, but do no harm unless the D antigen is present on the fetal red cells.

People who have the D antigen of the Rh system on their red cells are said to be Rh positive. Those who do not are said to be Rh negative.

A woman who is Rh negative can develop antibodies against the D antigen in two ways. Transfusion of red cells bearing the D antigen into a person who is Rh negative often results in the production of IgG antibodies against the antigen. Leakage of fetal red cells bearing the D antigen into the maternal blod during pregnancy can cause the mother to develop IgG antibodies against the D antigen.

Leakage of fetal blood into the maternal circulation occurs in at least 50% of pregnancies. Usually the quantity of fetal blood escaping into the maternal circulation is small, less than 0.1 mL, though it can be greater, 2 mL or more, especially at the time of delivery. In some pregnancies there may be multiple small leaks of fetal blood into the maternal circulation.

Less than 10% of Rh-negative women who bear an Rh-positive fetus develop antibodies against the D antigen in sufficient titer to be detectable by the usual methods. Another 10% are sensitized against the D antigen, but the sensitization becomes evident only when anti-D antibodies develop rapidly when the woman is again exposed to the D antigen.

In 98% of Rh-negative mothers who develop antibodies against the D antigen because of leakage of Rh-positive fetal blood into the maternal circulation, the antibodies appear only post partum. Presumably the larger quantities of fetal blood that can escape into the maternal circulation at delivery are more efficient in sensitizing the mother than are the small leakages of fetal blood into the maternal circulation during the pregnancy.

An Rh-negative mother with an Rh-positive fetus is three times more likely to develop antibodies against the D antigen if the ABO groups of the mother and fetus are compatible than when they are incompatible. Presumably the fetal red cells leaking into the maternal blood are destroyed by antibodies against incompatible ABO antigens before sensitization to the D antigen can occur. Anti-A antibodies in the maternal circulation destroy A-positive fetal cells more rapidly than anti-B antibodies eliminate fetal cells bearing the B antigen and so offer greater protection against sensitization to the D antigen.

The alleles coding for the D antigen are dominant. Whether the Rh antigens are controlled by three loci on each of the pair of chromosomes involved, as proposed by Fisher, or by one, as proposed by Weiner, an Rh-negative mother has no gene coding for the D antigen. If the fetus is Rh positive, the gene or genes coding for the D antigen must have been inherited from the father. If the father is homozygous, with genes coding for the D antigen on each of the chromosomes involved, the mother is five times as likely to develop antibodies against the D antigen than if the father is heterozygous, with only one gene coding for the D antigen.

The risk of sensitization of an Rh-negative mother by an Rh-positive fetus is greatest when the father is homozygous for the D antigen and the ABO groups of the mother and fetus are compatible. An Rh-negative mother bearing an Rh-positive fetus is 15 times more likely to become sensitized to the D antigen if the father is homozygous for the D antigen, and the ABO groups of the mother and child are compatible, than when the father is heterozygous for the D antigen, and the ABO groups of the mother and child are incompatible.

Occasionally antigens other than A, B, or D cause hemolytic disease of the newborn. The sensitization of the mother against the antigen on the fetal red cells usually is caused by transfusion or by the leakage of fetal blood into the maternal circulation, as in the anti-D form of hemolytic disease of the newborn.

Hemolytic disease of the newborn caused by antibodies against the A or B antigens of the ABO system is as likely in the mother's first pregnancy as in subsequent pregnancies. Most women who are group O develop IgG antibodies against the A and B antigens long before they become pregnant, and pregnancy usually does not increase the titer of the antigen. The first child is at as great a risk as the last.

Unless the mother has been sensitized against the D antigen by transfusion, hemolytic disease caused by antibodies against the D antigen is uncommon in the first pregnancy. Even if an Rh-negative mother bearing an Rh-positive positive fetus becomes sensitized against the D antigen during the first pregnancy, the titer of the antibodies rarely is enough to injure the fetus. It is only when the mother has been sensitized against the D antigen during an earlier pregnancy that an Rh-positive fetus in an Rh-negative mother is at risk. The more often an Rh-negative mother bears an Rh-positive child, the greater the likelihood of sensitization, and the higher the titer of antibody against the D antigen, rendering the risk to a subsequent Rh-positive child great.

The IgG antibodies that attack the fetal red cells do not fix complement. The IgG on coated red cells attaches to the Fc receptors on the surface of the macrophages in the fetal liver and spleen. The fetal red cells are destroyed extravascularly by the phagocytes.

The increased destruction of the fetal red cells releases increased quantities of bilirubin into the fetal plasma. Most of the bilirubin passes across the placenta into the maternal blood and is excreted by the mother. The concentration of bilirubin in the fetal blood increases little if at all. Only if the destruction of the red cells continues after birth does the concentration of bilirubin in the child's plasma rise.

In the newborn, the immature liver is unable to excrete bile efficiently. Even the normal load of bilirubin can overtax it, causing physiologic jaundice. If the production of bilirubin is increased, unconjugated bilirubin accumulates in the plasma and body fluids, bound for the most part to albumin. If the concentration of bilirubin in the plasma exceeds 350 μmol/L (20 mg/mL), there may be not enough albumin to combine with the unconjugated bilirubin, and some of the bilirubin circulates free in the plasma.

The increased destruction of fetal red cells causes the increase in fetal erythropoiesis. The increase is particularly marked in the liver and spleen, though it is evident in the bone marrow and in other organs. The more severe the hemolyses, the greater the increase in erythropoiesis.

Prophylaxis. The sensitization of an Rh-negative mother by an Rh-positive child during pregnancy can be prevented in over 98% of pregnancies by giving the mother an injection of IgG antibody against the D antigen within 72 hours of delivery. Most of the Rh-negative women bearing an Rh-positive child who become sensitized against the D antigen are sensitized post partum. The injection of antibody prevents the sensitization.

In 90% of the Rh-negative mothers with an

Rh-positive child who do become sensitized to the D antigen before delivery, the sensitization can be prevented by giving an injection of antibody against anti-D antibodies at the 28th week of gestation, in addition to the postpartum injection. The injection at the 28th week of gestation does not harm the fetus.

If no prophylactic injection of anti-D antibodies is given, 15% of Rh-negative mothers bearing an Rh-positive child become sensitized at each pregnancy. If a single postpartum injection of antibodies is given, 1.5% become sensitized. If an injection at the 28th week of gestation and one post partum are given, 0.1% are sensitized.

The dose of anti-D antibody given for prophylaxis should be increased if the quantity of fetal blood reaching the maternal circulation is large. It is desirable to give post partum about 20 μg of anti-D IgG for every mL of fetal blood that reaches the maternal circulation.

How the injection of anti-D antibody prevents the sensitization of an Rh-negative mother by Rh-positive fetal blood is uncertain. Only IgG antibody against the D antigen is effective. IgM antibody against the D antigen is of no value. It may be that the injected antibody reacts with the D antigen on the fetal red cells, hiding the antigen, so that it is not recognized by the mother's immunologically competent cells. It could be that the reaction between the D antigen on the fetal cells and the antibody leads to the destruction of the antigen or that the injection of the antibody in some way suppresses the mother's immune mechanisms.

Treatment and Prognosis. In every Rh-negative woman who becomes pregnant, the titer of anti-D antibodies should be determined about the 18th week of gestation, again about the 28th week, and then every one to four weeks until delivery. If sensitization to the D antigen develops, IgM antibodies reactive in saline appear first. They do not harm the fetus, but warn that IgG antibodies reactive in albumin may follow. If the titer of IgG antibodies exceeds 1/16, amniocentesis is indicated to determine if the fetus is in danger.

If the optical density of the amniotic fluid measured at a wavelength of 450 nm is high, the fetal blood is being hemolyzed. In general, the higher the optical density, the greater the risk to the fetus.

If the pregnancy has passed the 34th week of gestation and the ratio of lecithin to sphingomyelin in the amniotic fluid is greater thans 2, showing that the lungs of the fetus are sufficiently mature, labor should be induced without delay. The hemolytic disease is more dangerous than prematurity.

If the pregnancy has not reached this point, packed, Rh-negative red cells can be transfused into the peritoneal cavity of the fetus. The red cells enter the diaphragmatic lymphatics and pass unharmed into the fetal circulation. Anemia is the major cause of fetal injury. The intrauterine transfusions are repeated every two to four weeks to maintain the fetal hemoglobin concentration at about 100 g/L (10 g/100 ML). As soon as it is safe to do so, labor is induced.

An exchange transfusion should be given without delay if an infant with hemolytic disease of the newborn is severely jaundiced or has hydrops fetalis; if the concentration of hemoglobin in the cord blood is less than 120 g/L (12 g/100 mL), or the concentration of hemoglobin in the infant's blood falls below 120 g/L (12 g/100 mL) in the first 24 hours of life; and if the concentration of bilirubin in the cord blood is over 85 μmol/L (5 mg/100 mL), or if the concentration of bilirubin in the infant's blood rises above 350 μmmol/L (20 mg/100 mL).

In an exchange transfusion, 170 mL/kg of the infant's blood is removed and replaced by the same or a slightly smaller volume of Rh-negative blood. About 85% of the fetal red cells coated with antibodies are removed and replaced with healthy red cells. Over 90% of the bilirubin in the plasma is removed, but the unconjugated bilirubin in the extravascular fluid remains and soon flows back into the blood, so that the concentration of bilirubin in the infant's plasma falls by only about 50%. Sometimes albumin is added to the blood transfused into the infant during an exchange transfusion to increase the quantity of albumin available to bind the unconjugated bilirubin in the infant's plasma and reduce the concentration of the unbound, unconjugated bilirubin that causes kernicterus.

Exposure of the infant to blue light reduces the concentration of bilirubin in the plasma by oxidizing bilirubin to biliverdin and then to compounds that are colorless and nontoxic. Some of the bilirubin is converted to photobilirubin, which binds weakly if at all to albumin, but seems to be nontoxic. Blue light alone is not enough to treat serious hemolytic disease of the newborn, but it reduces the number of exchange transfusions needed.

Neither intrauterine nor exchange transfusions are free of risk. An intrauterine transfusion can bring infection, or leakage of amniotic fluid into the mother's blood, causing a coagulopathy, mechanical injury to the fetus or placenta, or premature delivery. Exchange transfusions can cause infection; electrolyte imbalance, heart failure, or clotting defects.

The prognosis for fetuses treated by intrauterine transfusion depends on the severity of the hemolytic disease. If hydrops is present when treatment is begun, less than 20% of the children survive. If there is no hydrops or hydrops is only evident in the fetus at the time of a second intrauterine transfusion, up to 70% of the children survive and grow to normal adults.

Exchange transfusions have greatly altered the prognosis of hemolytic disease of the newborn in infants born alive. More than 99% of the infants survive and grow normally.

Warm Antibody Autoimmunohemolytic Anemia. In warm antibody autoimmunohemolytic anemia, antibodies that react optimally at body temperature form against normal antigens on the surface of the red cells and cause hemolysis. Because it usually develops in children or adults who were previously well, the type of hemolytic disorder is often called an acquired hemolytic anemia.

Two kinds of warm antibody autoimmune hemolytic anemia are distinguished. In some patients, the warm antibody that causes the anemia arises without known cause. Such patients are said to have a primary or idiopathic immunohemolytic anemia. In other patients, the warm antibodies arise in the course of some other disease. Such people are said to have secondary or symptomatic immunohemolytic disease.

The warm antibody hemolytic anemias are not common. In any one year, only 1 person in every 80,000 is likely to develop this sort of anemia.

Lesions. The blood shows changes like those of other kinds of hemolytic anemia. The concentration of hemoglobin is little reduced in many of the patients, but the anemia can be severe, threatening life. Because of the increased destruction of the red cells, many of the red cells are young and bigger than normal. Reticulocytes are usually numerous, but in 25% of the patients they are few or absent. Polychromasia and anisocytosis are marked. Often many microspherocytes are present. Clumps of agglutinated red cells are sometimes evident. The leukocyte count may be normal, low, or increased.

The concentration of bilirubin in the plasma is increased if the anemia is moderately severe, often to 40 to 80 µmol/L (2.5 to 5.0 mg/100/ML). Hemoglobinemia and hemoglobinuria are uncommon, except when the disease is unusually severe.

Clinical Presentation. In most of the patients, warm antibody autoimmunohemolytic anemia is not severe and continues with little change for months or years. Sometimes the patients have cyanotic lips or cheeks, probably caused by the blocking of capillaries by clumps of agglutinated red cells.

Occasionally the anemia develops abruptly and is severe. Especially in children, this fulminant type of autoimmune hemolytic anemia sometimes complicates a viral infection. Sometimes it is of unknown cause. The patients suffer prostration, headache, abdominal pain, vomiting, jaundice, and hemoglobinuria. This type of severe autoimmune anemia is sometimes called Lederer's anemia, after the American pathologist who described it in 1925.

Pathogenesis. The fault in most patients with warm antibody hemolytic anemia is probably in the immune system. In some patients, reduction in the activity of the suppressor T cells has been demonstrated. The depression of suppressor activity permits the formation of antibodies against normal antigens on the surface of the patient's red cells.

There is sometimes a congenital predisposition to develop warm antibody autoimmunohemolytic disease. In some families, several members of the family have developed the disease. Apparently normal members of these families sometimes have antibodies against their red cells circulating in their blood. The HLA antigen B7 is unduly common in people with warm antibody hemolytic anemia.

Secondary warm antibody autoimmune hemolytic disease can complicate a variety of diseases. Some 5% of patients with chronic lymphatic leukemia develop this type of anemia. It occurs in people with lymphoma and other kinds of malignancy. About 5% of people with systemic lupus erythematosus and occasionally people with other collagen diseases develop warm antibody hemolytic anemia. Viral infections can cause it. It may develop in people with immune deficiency caused by defective thymic function.

In most patients with secondary warm antibody autoimmune hemolytic anemia, the fault is in the immune system. In some, other mechanisms are important. The surface of the red cells can be altered by a virus or in some other way, so that a new antigen is produced, which the body mistakes for foreign. In some patients the red cells suffer as innocent bystanders, as in the stibophen type of drug-induced hemolytic anemia.

The increased destruction of the red cells in warm antibody hemolytic anemias is principally extravascular. The red cells coated with antibody are taken up by macrophages in the spleen and other organs. In general, the more antibody on the red cells, the more likely their destruction, though as few as 10 molecules of antibody on a red cell can cause its destruction, and occasionally cells with hundreds of molecules of antibody on their surface survive for a normal span.

Occasionally, clumps of red cells agglutinated by the antibodies form in the circulating blood. The clumps can be large enough to obstruct small blood vessels, causing local ischemia.

The antibodies that cause warm antibody hemolytic anemia are usually IgG, but sometimes they are IgM or IgA. In 40% of the patients, only IgG can be demonstrated on the red cells. In 40%, both IgG and complement are present. In 10% only complement can be demonstrated. IgG3 antibodies are particularly likely to cause hemolysis, for they fix complement more effectively than other forms of IgG, and macrophages have a receptor that binds to the Fc portion of the molecule. IgG1 is less dangerous, though it does activate complement and bind to macrophages. IgG2 and IgG4 do little harm. IgG2 can fix complement weakly, but neither IgG2 nor IgG4 binds to macrophages.

In more than 80% of the patients with warm antibody hemolytic disease, the antibodies bind to some portion of the Rh complex on the red cells. They are not usually specific for the D or other of the Rh antigens important in hemolytic disease of the newborn.

Treatment and Prognosis. Adrenocortical steroids control warm antibody hemolytic anemia in over 70% of the patients. The rate of hemolysis falls sharply within a few days. A low maintenance dose of steroid maintains the remission.

Probably the initial reduction in hemolysis caused by the steroids is due mainly to a reduction of the phagocytosis of the red cells in the spleen and other organs. The reduction in antibody formation caused by the steroids comes later, but is important in the continuing control of the disease. It may be too that the steroids impair the binding of the antibodies to the red cells.

If the adrenocortical steroids fail, splenectomy brings benefit in 50% of the patients, though it also brings the dangers associated with splenectomy. Cyclophosphamide or another cytotoxic drug brings relief in 50% of the patients.

Transfusions must be given with care. The antibodies on the red cells sometimes block their antigens, making it difficult or impossible to type the patient's blood. The antibodies sometimes cause the patient's red cells to agglutinate, making it impossible to carry out the usualy crossmatching. Often, the antibodies in the patient's plasma react with all types of red cell, making it impossible to obtain a match.

Cold Hemagglutinin Disease. Cold hemagglutinin disease is a form of acquired hemolytic anemia caused by antibodies that react with their antigens most efficiently at temperatures below 32°C, usually showing little or no binding to their antigen at 37°C. The antibodies are called cold agglutinins.

Cold hemagglutinin disease is sometimes idiopathic and sometimes secondary to some other disorder. About 30% of patients with acquired autoimmune hemolytic anemia have cold agglutinin disease. Patients with the idiopathic form of the disease are usually over 60 years old though it can occur in younger people. People with secondary cold agglutinin disease are mainly between 30 and 50 years old.

Lesions. The concentration of hemoglobin in the blood is usually normal, or nearly so, in people with secondary cold agglutinin disease. In the idiopathic form of the disease, it rarely falls below 70 g/L (7 g/100 mL). The concentration of bilirubin in the blood is rarely above 50 μmol/L (3 mg/100 mL).

Though the range of temperature at which the cold agglutinins bind to the red cells varies from one patient to another, there is usually no evidence of binding to the red cells if the blood is examined at 37°C. If the examination is repeated at 4°C, the cold agglutinins bind to the red cells and fix complement, causing hemolysis. The complement on the red cells can be demonstrated immunohistochemically, but usually masks the immunoglobulin.

Clinical Presentation. In most patients with cold agglutinin disease, the cold agglutinins in the blood cause no symptoms and no disability. The diagnosis is made by demonstrating the cold agglutinins in the blood.

If there is anemia, it is usually mild, develops slowly, and persists for months or years. In a small proportion of patients with mycoplasmal infections, anemia develops rapidly, but is transient, lasting three or four weeks.

In some patients, the agglutination of the blood in the skin causes acrocyanosis, from the Greek for terminal and dark blue or dusky. The tip of the nose, the ears, and the fingers are most often affected. The skin sometimes becomes white and pallid as the agglutinated red cells obstruct the circulation and sometimes turns dark and purple. The affected parts of the body may be painful. Occasionally gangrene develops. If the condition persists, the affected parts atrophy. Warming the skin rapidly relieves the condition.

Pathogenesis. Cold agglutinin disease is most often secondary to mycoplasmal pneumonia or to lymphoma or some other form of B cell proliferation. It can complicate infectious mononucleosis or, rarely, some other kind of infection.

The antibodies that cause the disease are nearly always IgM, rarely IgG or IgA. When cold agglutinin disease is secondary to mycoplasmal pneumonia, the antibodies are usually directed against the I antigens on the red cells, occasionally against the A, B, or N antigens. When it is secondary to a lymphoproliferative disorder or is idiopathic, the antibodies are usually against the I antigens or the i antigens.

When the disease is secondary to infection, the antibodies are polyclonal. When it complicates a lymphoproliferative disease or is idiopathic, they are monoclonal. Some people with idiopathic cold agglutinin disease develop a lymphoma after months or years, suggesting that the idiopathic form of the disease is due to the proliferation of a clone of abnormal lymphocytes. The anti-I antibodies almost all have κ light chains, while the anti-i antibodies usually have λ light chains. Over 30% of the anti-I antibodies precipitate if the plasma is cooled. The anti-I antibodies do not.

Cold agglutinins do no harm in the interior of the body, where the blood is too warm to allow them to attach to their antigen. They combine with their antigen only in the vessels of the skin and other cool parts of the body, where the temperature of the blood falls to 28°C or less.

The cold agglutinins attached to the red cells fix complement. Some degree of intravascular hemolysis follows, but it is not usually severe. The hemolytic activity of complement falls as the temperature falls. At the temperature in the skin, there is usually little hemolysis before C3b is inactivated by the C3b inhibitor in the plasma, interrupting the hemolytic activity of complement.

The extravascular destruction of red cells by the macrophages in the liver and elsewhere is a more important pathogenic event in most patients. The C3b on the red cells binds to the C3b receptors of the macrophages. Some of the red cells are phagocytosed and destroyed. Others are freed from the macrophages when the C3b inhibitor splits the C3b, leaving the red cells to circulate unharmed, with their C3b receptors blocked by C3d. As the red cells are warmed in the interior of the body, the antibodies are released from the red cells, but the C3d remains.

The cold agglutinins cause the red cells in the skin to clump together. Small vessels in the skin are blocked, causing local ischemia and hypoxia. The agglutinated clumps of red cells are easily damaged by mechanical trauma as they are forced through the blood vessels, adding to their destruction.

Treatment and Prognosis. Most people with cold hemagglutinin disease need no treatment other than to keep warm. If the disease is severe, immunosuppressive drugs or plasmapheresis can be beneficial. Splenectomy and adrenocortical steroids do not help.

Paroxysmal Cold Hemoglobinuria. Paroxysmal cold hemoglobinuria is a rare form of hemolytic anemia caused by cold antibodies. Some, but not all, patients have syphilis.

Patients with paroxysmal cold hemoglobinuria develop acute hemoglobinemia when the body or part of the body is chilled. Often there is pain in the back, legs, or abdomen; malaise with vomiting, diarrhea, and headache; or chills and fever. If the attack is severe, there is hemoglobinuria. If it is mild, there is only hemoglobinemia, perhaps with fever and after a day or so, jaundice.

People with paroxysmal cold hemoglobinuria have in their plasma an IgG antibody called the Donath-Landsteiner antibody after the German immunologist and the Austrian physician who established the pathogenesis of paroxysmal cold hemoglobinuria in 1904. The Donath-Landsteiner antibody is directed against the P antigen on the red cells. It binds to the surface of the red cells most avidly at temperatures below 15°C and fixes complement. At this temperature, complement is inactive. If the blood is warmed, the complement bound to the red cells regains its hemolytic activity, and severe intravascular hemolysis follows.

If the patient has syphilis, control of the syphilis usually brings improvement. If not, avoidance of cold usually prevents hemolysis.

Drug-Induced Immunohemolytic Anemia. In the drug-induced immunohemolytic anemias, the administration of a drug results in the development of warm antibodies that attack and destroy red cells. Three kinds of

TABLE 49-9. DRUGS CAUSING IMMUNOHEMOLYTIC ANEMIA

Hapten type
Cephalothin
Insulin
Penicillins
Streptomycin
Immune complex type
Aminopyrine
p-Aminosalycilic acid
Anhistine
Antaxoline
Chlorpromazine
Dipyrone
Insecticides
Isoniaziad
Phenacetin
Quinine
Quinidine
Rifampin
Stibophen
Sulfonamides
Sulfonylureas
Thiazides
Autoimmune type
Levodopa
Mefenamic acid
α-Methyldopa

drug-induced immune hemolytic anemia are distinguished: the hapten type, the immune complex type, and the autoimmune type. The drugs that cause immune hemolytic anemia are listed in Table 49-9.

Hapten Type. The hapten type of drug-induced immunohemolytic anemia is often called the penicillin type, after the drug that most commonly causes this kind of reaction. The penicillins and cephalosporins mainly cause extravascular hemolysis. Streptomycin causes intravascular hemolysis.

Penicillin-induced immune hemolytic anemia develops only if the dose of penicillin is large, more than 20,000,000 units a day, and usually develops only after the drug has been given for a considerable period or a second course of the drug is given. The concentration of hemoglobin in the blood falls rapidly. Withdrawal of the drug brings a quick end to the hemolysis, though red cells coated with immunoglobulin continue to circulate for weeks, and the direct antiglobulin test remains positive.

The hemolysis is caused by metabolites of penicillin, principally benzylpenicilloyl groups, that serve as a hapten. The benzylpenicilloyl groups are bound to the red cells and other proteins, and IgG antibodies are produced against them. The antibodies react with benzylpenicilloyl groups attached to the red cells. They do not fix complement, but enhance the destruction of the red cells by the macrophages of the spleen and other organs.

Cephalosporins occasionally produce immune hemolytic anemia by a similar mechanism. The antibodies against penicillins and cephalosporins cross-react.

Steroptomycin is bound to the red cells by their M antigens and perhaps by their D antigens. Occasionally IgG antibodies develop against the streptomycin and react with streptomycin bound to the red cells. The antibodies fix complement and cause intravascular hemolysis, sometimes with renal failure.

Immune Complex Type. The immune complex type of drug-induced immunohemolytic anemia is called the stibophen type, after the drug first shown to cause this kind of injury. It is also called the innocent bystander type of drug-induced hemolytic anemia, because the red cells are only secondarily involved.

Only a small dose of the drug is needed to cause the immune complex type of drug-induced hemolytic anemia. The patients develop acute hemoglobinemia and hemoglobinuria. Renal failure develops in 50% of the patients. Injury to the platelets sometimes causes disseminated intravascular coagulation. Withdrawl of the drug stops the hemolysis.

A drug that causes an immune complex type of immunohemolytic anemia acts as a hapten, and IgG, IgM, or both IgG and IgM antibodies form against it. Immune complexes consisting of the drug and antibodies against it circulate in the blood. The complexes become attached to the surface of the red cells by a nonimmunologic mechanism. Complement is activated on the surface of the red cells and cause intravascular hemolysis.

Autoimmune Type. The autoimmune type of hemolytic anemia is the most common of the drug-induced immunohemolytic anemias. It is often called the α-methyldopa type, because autoantibodies frequently develop in patients treated with α-methyldopa. Antinuclear antibodies, rheumatoid factors and antibodies against the gastric mucosa are among the autoantibodies commonly found. The drugs that cause this type of immunohemolytic anemia induce autoantibodies against the Rh complex on the red cells. No antibody is produced against α-methyldopa or the other drugs that cause this kind of immunohemolytic anemia.

Antibodies can be detected on the surface of the red cells in 15% of people taking α-methyldopa, but hemolysis is induced in less than 1% of these patients. The antibodies are IgG and do not fix complement. If hemolysis occurs, it begins only after the drug has been given for weeks or years. The hemolysis is extravascular and results from the destruction of the red cells by macrophages. It begins insidiously and slowly worsens. Usually, it resolves within a few weeks if the drug is withdrawn. If the drug is restarted, it is usually months before hemolysis again becomes evident. If withdrawal of the drug does not bring recovery, adrenocortical steroids usually control the hemolysis.

Probably the drugs that cause the immune complex type of autoimmune hemolytic anemia do so by impairing the activity of the suppressor T cells. The number of circulating T lymphocytes is reduced. The depression of suppressor T-cell function sometimes persists for months after the drug is withdrawn.

A genetic predisposition to this kind of injury may be an important factor. The HLA antigen B7 is unduly common in people with the autoimmune type of drug-induced hemolytic anemia.

FRAGMENTATION ANEMIA. In many conditions, red cells are fragmented by the trauma they suffer in the blood stream. Three kinds of fragmentation anemia are distinguished. In cardiac anemia, the red cells are damaged by lesions in the heart or great vessels. In microangiopathic anemia they are traumatized as they pass through the small vessels. In march hemoglobinuria, they are destroyed by the pounding of the feet on the pavement.

Cardiac Anemia. Any severe lesion of

the heart or great vessels is likely to cause injury to the red cells. Valvular lesions, septal defects, ruptured chordae tendineae, coarctation of the aorta, and other lesions can all do so. Usually the injury is so slight that it passes unnoticed. A few red cells are damaged. Most pass unharmed.

The concentration of hemoglobin in the blood remains normal if the increased destruction of the red cells is fully compensated, but may be less than 50 g/L (5 g/100 mL) if cardiac anemia is severe. Mild hyperbilirubinemia, hemoglobinemia and a reduction in the concentration of haptoglobin in the plasma are sometimes evident. The activity of lactate dehydrogenase in the plasma is increased as the enzyme escapes from the damaged red cells. If cardiac anemia is severe, hemoglobinuria and hemosiderinuria are common.

The blood smear shows many small, distorted red cells called schistocytes, from the Greek word meaning to split. Red cells caught in severe turbulence or directly traumatized by a valve or by being forced through a mesh of fibrin are torn apart. The fragments of the red cells reseal their membranes, forming little, oddly shaped cells that are soon removed by the spleen.

The risk of serious hemolysis is greatest if the cardiac lesion involves the aortic valve. It is especially great if the aortic valve is replaced by a prothesis or a homograft. In most patients with replacement of the aortic valve, there is a measurable reduction in the life of the red cells. In more than 5%, the injury to the red cells is sufficient to cause anemia.

Another cause of cardiac anemia is the repair of a defect within the heart with a polytetrafluorethylene (Teflon) patch. About 5% of these patients develop a significant degree of hemolysis.

The injury to the red cells is due principally to the turbulence caused by the lesion in the heart or vessels. Direct mechanical trauma by a valve or the filtering of red cells through fibrin deposited at the site of the lesion are less important.

The only treatment for cardiac anemia is to repair the lesion causing the fragmentation, usually by replacing a poorly functioning valve or prosthesis.

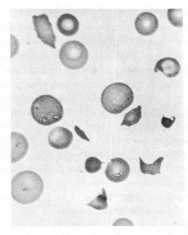

Fig. 49-14. Fragments of damaged red cells in the blood of a patient with microangiopathic anemia. (From Wintrobe, M. W., et al.: Clinical Hematology. 8th Ed. Philadelphia, Lea & Febiger, 1981.)

Microangiopathic Anemia. In microangiopathic anemia, the red cells are damaged by fibrin deposited in small blood vessels. If blood flow continues, the red cells are forced through the mesh formed by the fibrin. Some fold around strands of fibrin like pledgets of sodden dough. Some escape as the eddies in the blood change. Some are torn in half. Some of the fragmented red cells reseal their membrane, forming schistocytes, which circulate for a while, as in cardiac anemia. Other red cells are destroyed altogether, releasing their hemoglobin and enzymes into the plasma.

Microangiopathic anemia is often severe, though it may be only a minor feature of the disease causing the intravascular thrombosis. Hemoglobinemia, mild jaundice, and a leukocytosis are common. Thrombocytopenia often develops because the platelets are used up in the thrombi that cause the anemia.

Anything that causes the deposition of fibrin in the blood vessels but does not prevent blood flow, is likely to cause microangiopathic anemia. The hemolytic uremic syndrome in children causes severe microangiopathic anemia. Thrombotic thrombocytopenic purpura commonly does so. Disseminated intravascular coagulation usually causes less destruction of red cells. Systemic lupus erythematosus, polyarteritis nodosa,

Wegener's granulomatosis, acute glomerulonephritis, eclampsia, and scleroderma occasionally cause microangiopathic anemia. Amyloidosis, fibrin within a hemangioma or metastatic deposits of cancer can do so.

Malignant hypertension sometimes causes microangiopathic anemia. How is not clear. Perhaps there is enough fibrin in the necrotic arterioles to damage the red cells. Perhaps the hypertension forces the red cells close to the endothelium, and red cells are caught on the spurs that project from the endothelial cells near their intercellular junctions.

Microangiopathic anemia is often severe. Hemoglobinemia, mild jaundice, and leukocytosis are common. In many of the patients, there is thrombocytopenia because of the extensive thrombosis. Frequently the microangiopathic anemia is only a minor feature of the disease that causes the intravascular thrombosis.

Microangiopathic hemolytic anemia can be controlled only by treating the condition that causes the intravascular deposition of fibrin. If the mechanical destruction of the red cells is stopped, the anemia resolves.

March Hemoglobinuria. March hemoglobinuria is a rare condition in which strenuous exercise, usually running or marching, so damages the red cells that hemoglobinuria follows and lasts a few hours. The injury to the red cells is mechanical, from the pounding of the feet on the ground. Running on hard ground can cause march hemoglobinuria, but running on soft ground or in well-padded shoes does not. Similar hemoglobinuria has occurred in congo drum players and in a demented man given to slapping his forehead violently. If the exercise is continued, the person often becomes conditioned to it, and the hemolysis ceases.

HEMOLYTIC ANEMIA INDUCED BY INFECTION. This section considers the kinds of hemolytic anemia produced by the few infectious organisms that attack the red cells directly. More frequently, infection precipitates hemolysis indirectly by initiating a crisis in hereditary spherocytosis or some other type of hemolytic anemia, by causing hemolysis in glucose-6-phosphate dehydrogenase deficiency, or by inducing the formation of cold agglutinins.

In malaria, the anemia is partly due to the destruction of red cells by the parasites, partly to reduced marrow activity and immunologic injury. The severe hemolysis in blackwater fever is not due to direct destruction of the red cells by the plasmodia. Its mechanism is uncertain, but an immunologic mechanism may be involved.

Kala-azar causes anemia, which is in part hemolytic, as is the anemia sometimes found in congenital toxoplasmosis. In bartonellosis the bacteria destroy the red cells causing severe hemolytic anemia. Clostridial infections sometimes injure the red cells and cause hemolysis.

TOXIC HEMOLYSIS. A few drugs and poisons damage the red cells directly. More frequently, a drug causes hemolysis indirectly, in a person lacking glucose-6-phosphate dehydrogenase or some other enzyme, or by inducing an immunologic attack on the red cells.

Many of the drugs that damage the red cells in people with glucose-6-phosphate dehydrogenase deficiency do so in normal people if the dose is high enough. Among the drugs more likely to cause hemolysis by attacking the red cells directly are naphthalene, nitrofurantoin, salicylazosulfapyridine, sulfamethoxypyridazine, p-aminosalicylic acid, and sulfoxone. Occasionally phenacetin, phenylsemicarbazide, resorcin, phenylhydrazine, aniline, hydroxylamine, nitrobenzene, phenols, and chlorates do so. All these drugs are oxidants and are thought to cause hemolysis by interfering with the reduction of glutathione in the red cells.

Arsine and copper salts can damage the red cells, though the mechanism is not clear. The accidental entry of distilled water into the blood during a transurethral prostatectomy can cause massive hemolysis by reducing the osmolality of the plasma. Snake and spider venoms sometimes cause dangerous hemolysis.

PHYSICAL INJURY. In severe burns, the heat often damages the red cells, causing hemolytic anemia that continues for one or two days after the injury. Hemolysis occurs if the concentration of phosphate in the plasma falls below 0.03 mmol/L (0.1 mg/100 mL).

PAROXYSMAL NOCTURNAL HEMOGLOBINURIA. Paroxysmal nocturnal hemoglobinuria is sometimes called the Marchiafava-Micheli syndrome, after the Italian pathologist who described it in 1911 and the Italian physician who discussed it in 1931. Paroxysmal nocturnal hemoglobinuria is rare. The disease develops during adult life. It is not congenital or familial. The patients develop hemolytic anemia, usually when they are 30 or 40 years old.

Lesions. The concentration of hemoglobin in the blood is usually less than 60 g/L (6 g/100 mL) in patients with paroxysmal nocturnal hemoglobinuria. Often there are fewer reticulocytes than would be expected in a hemolytic anemia of this severity. Leukopenia and thrombocytopenia are common. The activities of alkaline phosphatase and cholinesterase in the leukocytes are frequently low.

Many of the patients do not have hemoglobinuria, in spite of the name of the disease. Hemosiderinuria is more common. Most of the hemoglobin that reaches the renal tubules is resorbed by the tubular epithelium, and much of its iron is stored in the tubular epithelial cells as hemosiderin. When the tubular epithelial cells are shed, the hemosiderin is carried into the urine with them.

Some of the circulating red cells are abnormally easily lysed by complement. If the patient's red cells are suspended in serum rich in complement, some of them are hemolyzed if the pH is lowered to between 6.5 and 7.0. The reduced pH activates too little complement to lyse normal red cells, but enough to lyse some of the cells in a patient with paroxysmal nocturnal hemoglobinuria. The small quantities of complement activated by diluting citrated or oxalated blood by isotonic sucrose lyses some of the red cells in people with paroxysmal nocturnal hemoglobinuria, but does not harm normal red cells. Acidification of the blood also causes hemolysis in patients with type II dyserythropoietic anemia and in people with many spherocytes in the blood, but dilution with sucrose does not.

The bone marrow shows the hyperplasia of its erythroid elements seen in other kinds of hemolytic anemia. The chromosomal pattern in the hematopoietic cells may be normal, or any of a variety of abnormalities may be found, among them loss of the Y chromosome or trisomy.

Clinical Presentation. The hemolysis begins insidiously in people with paroxysmal nocturnal hemoglobinuria. It may be so slight as to be insignificant or may be severe, disabling, even fatal. Periodic exacerbations in the severity of the hemolysis occur in most patients. They may be initiated by many kinds of stress, but often occur without obvious cause.

About 25% of the patients have hemoglobinuria when first seen by a physician. In some, but not all, of these, the hemolysis is more severe when the patient sleeps, so that hemoglobinuria is only present at night.

Complications. Aplastic anemia is common in patients with paroxysmal nocturnal hemoglobinuria. Usually the aplastic anemia appears first, and the paroxysmal noctural hemoglobinuria is recognized only afterwards, but sometimes the hemoglobinuria comes first.

Thrombosis is frequent in patients with paroxysmal nocturnal hemoglobinuria, particularly in veins. About 50% of the patients who die of the disease have massive intrahepatic thrombosis in the portal veins or cerebral thrombosis. Less widespread cerebral or portal thrombosis causes attacks of headache or abdominal pain. Thrombosis is common in the veins of the legs.

Dysphagia is often caused by powerful contractions of the esophagus. Infections are unduly common, perhaps because a defect in the leukocytes impairs their function.

Pathogenesis. The fault in paroxysmal nocturnal hemoglobinuria is in the red cells. At least three kinds of red cells are produced. Some respond normally to complement. Some are lysed 5 times more easily by complement than are normal red cells. Some are lysed 20 times more easily by complement that are normal red cells.

The patients have in their blood some mixture of these types of red cells. Over 70% of the patients have a mixture of the normal and highly sensitive types, though the proportion of cells highly susceptible to lysis by complement varies greatly from one patient to another. Under 10% have a mixture of the normal and moderately sensitive red cells. Under 10% have all three types of red cell in the blood. Under 5% have a mixture of moderately and highly sensitive red cells. Rarely a patient has only moderately sensitive cells.

The severity of the disease depends on the

proportion of the red cells that are highly sensitive to complement. If less than 20% of the red cells are highly sensitive, the disease is mild or undetectable. If from 20 to 50% of the red cells are highly sensitive, occasional episodes of hemoglobinuria occur. If more than 50% of the cells are highly sensitive, constant hemoglobinuria is usual.

The hemolysis in paroxysmal nocturnal hemoglobinuria is caused by the activation of small quantities of complement. The normal red cells are not harmed, but the highly sensitive red cells are lysed and spill their hemoglobin and enzymes into the plasma. What causes the activation of the complement is unknown. Usually no immunoglobulins are present on the red cells during episodes of hemolysis, and C3 is not detectable on them. The complement may be activated by the alternate pathway.

Scanning electron microscopy shows that the surface of the abnormal red cells is pitted and irregular. Usually acetylcholinesterase is deficient in their cell membrane. The abnormal cells are lysed by hydrogen peroxide more easily than are normal red cells.

Some of the circulating white cells and platelets are abnormally easily lysed by complement in patients with paroxysmal nocturnal hemoglobinuria. The disease sometimes causes leukopenia or thrombocytopenia. The thrombi common in paroxysmal nocturnal hemoglobinuria are probably due in part to lysis of platelets, in part to the thromboplastin released from the lysed red cells. The injury to the leukocytes is in part cause of the increased liability to infection common in the patients.

The increased hemolysis during sleep may be due to the fall in pH that occurs in some organs during sleep. Though the disease is called nocturnal, hemolysis increases if the patient sleeps during the day.

Treatment and Prognosis. No satisfactory treatment is available. Blood transfusions, steroids, androgens, anticoagulants, and bone marrow transplants have been disappointing. Splenectomy is of no benefit.

In a few patients, the disease remits. In many, death comes after 10 years or so, from thrombosis or aplastic anemia. A few patients have developed leukemia.

Aplastic Anemia

Aplastic anemia is caused by hypoplasia of the bone marrow. Usually, all types of hematopoietic cell are deficient. The bone marrow does not contain enough hematopoietic cells to maintain production of the blood cells. The patients have anemia, leukopenia, and thrombocytopenia. Much less often, only the erythroid cells in the bone marrow are affected, a condition called pure red cell hypoplasia.

Three kinds of aplastic anemia are distinguished. The most common is acquired aplastic anemia. Congenital aplastic anemia and pure red cell hypoplasia are rare.

The term *pancytopenia* is often used when red cells, white cells, and platelets are all deficient in the blood. Aplastic anemia often causes pancytopenia, but pancytopenia is more often caused by other diseases that reduce the formation of blood cells or increase their destruction.

CONGENITAL APLASTIC ANEMIA. Congenital aplastic anemia is often called Fanconi's anemia, after the Swiss physician who described it in 1927. Pancytopenia usually becomes evident when the child affected is 5 to 10 years old. The bone marrow is sometimes hyperplastic in the early years of life, but becomes increasingly hypoplastic as the pancytopenia worsens. Chromosomal abnormalities are common in the hematopoietic cells in the bone marrow. The proportion of fetal hemoglobin in the red cells is increased.

Patchy pigmentation of the skin with melanin is common. Often there are congenital anomalies, malformation of the skeleton, dwarfism, microcephaly, an abnormal number of digits, microphthalmia, hypoplasia of the kidneys, or hypoplasia of the spleen. Mental retardation is common. A few of the patients cannot absorb or store folate normally. In a few, the secretions of the exocrine pancreas are deficient.

Fanconi's congenital aplastic anemia is probably caused by a genetic defect inherited as an autosomal recessive character.

Treatment with androgens and adenocortical steroids brings temporary benefit. Most patients die of hemorrhage or infection before they are 20 years old. Some develop leukemia,

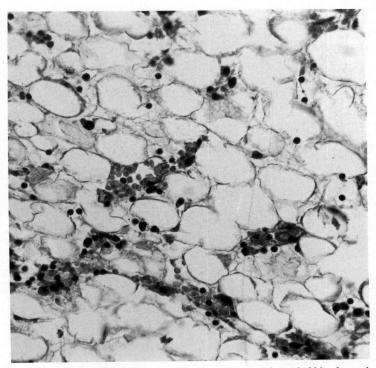

Fig. 49-15. Bone marrow of a patient with aplastic anemia showing fat and distended blood vessels. Few hematopoietic cells remain.

hepatocellular carcinoma, or some other malignant tumor.

ACQUIRED APLASTIC ANEMIA. In any one year, acquired aplastic anemia develops in 1 person in 150,000. In 50% of the patients, the disease is caused by drugs, irradiation, or infection or complicates some other disease. In 50%, its cause is unknown.

Lesions. The severity of the pancytopenia differs from one patient to another. The concentration of hemoglobin in the blood can be as much as 120 g/L (12 g/100 mL) or as little as 30 g/L (3 g/100 mL). The red cells are normal or a little bigger than normal. Reticulocytes are few and nucleated red cells do not occur. If the disease is not severe, lymphocytes are often present in normal concentration, or nearly so, but the concentration of granulocytes is reduced. If it is severe, there are both granulocytopenia and lymphocytopenia. The leukocyte count ranges from 4×10^9/L (4,000/mm^3) to 0.2×10^9/L (200/mm^3). The platelet count can be as

high as 150×10^9/L (150,000/mm^3) or as low as 10×10^9/L (10,000/mm^3).

In the most severe forms of aplastic anemia, no hematopoietic cells are present in the bone marrow. All that remains is fat, with scattered lymphocytes and the macrophages lining the sinusoids. Sometimes the sinusoids are distended and congested.

More often, scattered islands of hematopoietic cells remain in the fatty marrow. Occasionally, these surviving islands of hematopoietic tissue are hyperplastic, though the total number of hematopoietic cells in the bone marrow is greatly decreased.

If the disease is mild or in its early stages, one of the types of hematopoietic cell is often more severely affected than are the others. Sometimes leukopenia or thrombocytopenia precedes more generalized depression of the bone marrow.

Clinical Presentation. Aplastic anemia usually develops insidiously. The nature of the presenting symptoms depends on the

TABLE 49-10. Causes of Aplastic Anemia

DRUGS AND TOXINS	Promazine
Injury Inevitable and Dose Related	Analgesics
Solvents	Acetylsalicylic acid
Benzene	Carbamazepine
Derivatives of benzene	Indomethacin
Trinitrotoluene	Phenylbutazone
Cytotoxic drugs	Antithyroid drugs
Alkylating agents	Methimazole
Busulfan	Potassium perchlorate
Chlorambucil	Propylthiouracil
Cyclophosphamide	Antidiabetic drugs
Melphalan	Chlorpropamide
Antimetabolites	Tolbutamide
Azathioprine	
Cytarabine	Insecticides
6-Mercaptopurine	Chlorophenothane
Methotrexate	Parathion
Thioguanine	Pentachlorophenol
Natural products	Other
Colchicine	Acetazolamide
Vinblastine	Bismuth
Vincristine	Carbon tetrachloride
	Cimetidine
Antibiotics	Dinitrophenol
Daunorubicin	Gold salts
Doxorubicin	Hair dye
	Mercury
Other	Methazolamide
Dichlorovinylcystine	Metolazone
Inorganic arsenic	D-penicillamine
Injury Rare and Not Dose Related	Silver
Antimicrobial agents	Thiocyanate
Amphoteracin B	Tripelennamine
Chloramphenicol	
Organical arsenicals	**RADIATION**
Penicillins	Atomic explosions
Quinacrine	Radioisotopes
Streptomycins	X-rays
Tetracyclines	
Anticonvulsant drugs	**INFECTION**
Ethosuximide	Dengue fever
Mephenytoin	Tuberculosis
Paramethadione	Viral hepatitis
Phenytoin	
Trimethadione	**DISEASE**
Tranquilizers	Diffuse eosinophilic fascitis
Chlordiazepoxide	Simmonds' disease
Chlorpromazine	Systemic lupus erythematosus
Meprobamate	Thyroiditis
Methyprylon	
Pecazine	**UNKNOWN**

nature of the dysfunction in the marrow. If anemia is predominant, weakness, tiredness, pallor, and other signs of anemia are predominant. If thrombocytopenia is severe, bruising is easy. There is often bleeding from the gums or the nose, melena, or menorrhagia. Neutropenia favors infection, ulceration of the throat or gums, and pneumonia.

As the hypoplasia of the marrow grows more severe, all these signs become evident and grow increasingly severe. Anemia deepens. Bleeding becomes more extensive. Cerebral hemorrhage is not uncommon. Infections become uncontrollable.

Pathogenesis. Acquired aplastic anemia is caused by the inability of the stem cells in the bone marrow to proliferate and populate the bone marrow. In most patients, it is not known whether the stem cells are destroyed, or whether their proliferation is prevented by an external factor. In some patients, both mechanisms may be operative. In some, an immunologic mechanism may be involved.

The drugs and other toxic agents that cause aplastic anemia can be divided into two groups. In one group, injury to the marrow is inevitable if the dose of the drug or the toxin is large enough, and the severity of the injury depends on the size of the dose. In the other group, only a small proportion of those exposed to the drug or to the toxin develop hypoplasia of the marrow, and the likelihood of injury is not related to the dose of the drug or toxin.

Benzene is the classic example of an agent that inevitably causes aplastic anemia if the dose is large enough. The size of dose needed varies from one person to another. Some people are very susceptible to injury by benzene. Even a small dose will cause hypoplasia of the marrow. Other people are much more resistant. Benzene and its derivatives are widely used as solvents in industry, and benzene poisoning occurs most often in workers exposed to an excessive concentration of the vapors of these solvents. Benzene is readily absorbed when it is inhaled. Even the fumes from domestic cleaners that contain benzene can be dangerous.

Table 49-10 lists some of the agents that inevitably cause hypoplasia of the marrow if given in large enough doses. Trinitrotoluene and other solvents are dangerous in industry and can cause serious injury to glue-sniffers. Almost all antineoplastic drugs cause depression of the bone marrow, even in therapeutic doses. If the dose is too large, or the patient is unduly sensitive to the drug, hypoplasia of the bone marrow and aplastic anemia results. Too large a dose of the antibiotics daunorubicin and doxorubicin is dangerous. Some people are more susceptible to injury than are others.

Chloramphenicol is a prime example of the agents that cause hypoplasia of the marrow in only a small minority of the people at risk. It has been estimated that of the people given chloramphenicol between 1 in 20,000 and 1 in 60,000 die of aplastic anemia. Why chloramphenicol severely damages the marrow in some people and does no harm in most is uncertain. The dose is not important.

Chloramphenicol affects hematopoiesis in two ways. In 50% of patients given the drug, anemia and reticulocytopenia develop because of impairment of the synthesis of heme and hemoglobin. Sometimes leukopenia and thrombocytopenia also occur. The marrow is normally cellular in these people, but there is vacuolation of the cytoplasm and the nucleus of erythroblasts in the bone marrow and sometimes of the granulocytes. The depression of the marrow is relieved as soon as the drug is withdrawn. The relationship of this transient depression of marrow function to the more serious hypoplasia of the marrow that develops in a small minority of people given chloramphenicol is unknown. Serious hypoplasia of the marrow usually becomes evident only after the course of chloramphenicol has ended.

Some of the other agents that cause hypoplasia of the marrow in only a small minority of the people at risk are listed in Table 49-10. Among the more dangerous of these drugs are the organic arsenical compounds that were once used to treat syphilis; quinacrine used for the prevention of malaria; the anticonvulsants mephenytoin, trimethadione, and paramethadione; the analgesic phenylbutazone; and the gold salts used to treat rheumatic arthritis. With the other agents listed, the risk is low.

Radiation of any kind can destroy the marrow and will cause aplastic anemia if the dose is large enough and enough of the marrow in irradiated.

Occasionally, an infection such as tuberculosis, viral hepatitis, or dengue fever precipitates aplastic anemia. Rarely it complicates pregnancy, Simmonds' disease, or other disorders.

Treatment and Prognosis. If a patient with aplastic anemia is taking any drug that might cause the hypoplasia of the bone marrow, the drug must be withdrawn and never given to the patient again. If the hypoplasia is not severe, it sometimes becomes stable when the drug causing the hypoplasia is withdrawn and no further treatment is needed.

Androgens and adrenocortical steroids sometimes enhance the activity of the bone marrow if the hypoplasia is not too severe. Immunosuppressive drugs bring benefit to 50% of the patients. Bone marrow transplantation is successful in from 50 to 75% of patients with severe acquired aplastic anemia.

If a bone marrow transplant is not performed, acquired aplastic anemia worsens rapidly in many of the patients. The pancytopenia grows more extreme. In 25% of the patients, death comes within a few months, usually from infection or hemorrhage. In some, the disease worsens more slowly. Some of the patients live for years. About 10% recover completely. A few of the patients develop paroxysmal nocturnal hemoglobinuria or leukemia.

PURE RED CELL APLASIA. Pure red cell aplasia is rare. It may be acute or chronic, congenital or acquired.

In acute pure red cell aplasia, erythropoiesis fails suddenly, much as in an aplastic crisis in sickle cell anemia. In some patients the aplasia has followed a minor infection or has complicated viral hepatitis. In some it seems to have been induced by a drug. Salicylates, barbiturates, sulfonamides, anticonvulsants, oral diabetic agents, isoniazid, colchicine, and heparin are among the agents suspected.

A more chronic form of pure red cell aplasia occurs in both children and adults. The anemia is usually severe. The red cells in the blood are normal, or nearly so. Reticulocytes are few or absent. Biopsy of the bone marrow shows a normal population of granulocytes and megakaryocytes, but a marked paucity of erythropoietic cells. An IgG antibody against the nuclei of the erythroblasts has been found in several of these patients.

Over 50% of adults with an acquired, chronic pure red cell aplasia have a thymoma, and 80% of these patients are women. In contrast, 70% of the patients with chronic pure red cell aplasia without thymoma are men.

The congenital form of pure red cell aplasia presents in infancy with severe anemia, with a concentration of hemoglobin as low as 20 g/L (2 g/100 mL). The marrow sometimes shows a lack of erythropoietc cells and sometimes arrest of erythropoiesis at the basophil normoblast stage. Occasionally an abnormality of tryptophane metabolism causes excretion of anthranilic acid in the urine, or bony abnormalities are present.

In most of the children with congenital pure red cell aplasia, the disease persists indefinitely. In 20%, a spontaneous remission occurs after months or years. In 50% of the children, treatment with adrenocortical steroids brings marked improvment. The repeated transfusions necessary may cause serious hemosiderosis.

Other Forms of Anemia

A few other forms of anemia do not fit well into the major groups already discussed.

CONGENITAL DYSERYTHROPOIETIC ANEMIA. The congenital dyserythropoietic anemias are rare disorders, probably genetically determined, in which there is refractory anemia, with bizarre nuclear abnormalities in the erythropoietic cells in the marrow. The severity of the anemia varies considerably. In some patients, it is severe and becomes evident in infancy, with changes like those of thalassemia. In other patients, it is mild and becomes evident only in adults.

The bone marrow is hyperplastic, but the erythropoiesis is ineffective. Most of the red cells produced never reach the blood. As usual with ineffective erythropoiesis, the transport of iron to the marrow is increased, often with hemosiderosis. Because of the destruction of many of the precursors of the red cells in the marrow, hyperbilirubinemia is common. There is no abnormality in the formation of the granulocytes or of the platelets. Three types of congenital dyserythropoietic anemia are distinguished.

Type I. Type I congenital dyserythropoietic anemia is probably inherited as an autosomal recessive character. The erythroid cells in the bone marrow are often binucleated or have multilobed nuclei. Bridges of chromatin join the nuclei of dividing red cells. The nuclear membrane in the precursors of the red cells is sometimes partially deficient.

Some of the erythroid cells in the marrow resemble megaloblasts. The circulating red cells are larger than normal, with a mean cell volume of from 93 to 115 fL, the normal being 80 to 95 fL. Anisocytosis and poikilocytosis are markd, often with polychromasia or Cabot's rings. Splenomegaly is common.

Type II. Type II congenital dyserythropoietic anemia is the commonest of the dyserythropoietic anemias. It is inherited as an autosomal recessive character. The anemia is not usually severe.

Type II congenital dyserythropoietic anemia is called HEMPAS, Hereditary Erythroblastic Multinuclearity associated with a Positive Acidified Serum test. From 10 to 40% of the normoblasts in the bone marrow are binucleate, and the red cells in the blood are easily lysed if the serum in which they are suspended is acidified. The bone marrow does not show the other abnormalities seen in type I or type III congenital dyserythropoietic anemia. The red cells in the blood are of normal size, but show anisocytosis, poikilocytosis, and punctate stippling. Hepatosplenomegaly is common.

The red cells in type II congenital dyserythropoietic anemia have on their surface an abnormal antigen called the HEMPAS antigen. Many normal sera contain IgM antibody against it. The red cells also have on their surface a high concentration of the i antigen usually found only on fetal red cells. Electron microscopy shows that their plasma membrane is in part duplicated.

Type III. Type III congenital dyserythropoietic anemia is inherited as an autosomal dominant character. Up to 30% of the erythroid precursors in the bone marrow are multinucleated. The quantity of deoxyribonucleic acid varies greatly from one normoblast to another.

LEUKOERYTHROBLASTIC ANEMIA. Leukoerythroblastic anemia, or leukoerythroblastosis, is so called because in this condition both nucleated red cells, or erythroblasts, and primitive white cells circulate in the blood. It is caused by partial replacement of the bone marrow by tumor, fibrosis, or some other process. Metastatic carcinoma in bone is the most common cause of leukoerythroblastic anemia. About 10% of patients with multiple myeloma have leukoerythroblastic

anemia. It sometimes develops in people with lymphoma. Patients with myelofibrosis nearly always have leukoerythroblastic anemia. Rarely, it complicates other conditions that injure the bone marrow: Gaucher's disease, Niemann-Pick disease, histiocytosis X, marble bone disease, Paget's disease of bone, tuberculosis, osteomyelitis, amyloidosis, irradiation, or poisoning with bengene or fluorine.

Up to 10% of the nucleated cells in the blood are red cells. Another 3 to 10% are reticulocytes. Anisocytosis and poikilocytosis are often severe. The concentration of hemoglobin in the blood is usually only slightly reduced.

The leukocyte count is increased in 50% of patients with leukoerythroblastic anemia and is decreased in 25%. The increase or decrease is due principally to an increase or decrease in the concentration of neutrophils in the blood. The concentration of eosinophils and basophils is usually increased, even when there is neutropenia. The lymphocyte count is usually normal.

Primitive granulocytes are common in the blood. Between 5 and 10% of the circulating granulocytes are myelocytes. Metamyelocytes are common. An occasional myeloblast is sometimes present. Sometimes hypersegmented neutrophils are evident. The platelet count is increased in some patients with myelofibrosis, but in other forms of leukoerythroblastic anemia the platelet count is usually normal or reduced.

Leukoerythroblastic anemia is sometimes called myelophthisic anemia, from the Greek for marrow and wasting away, but neither the anemia nor the abnormal production of granulocytes is due simply to replacement of the bone marrow. Leukoerythroblastic anemia can develop in patients with carcinoma in whom there is little involvement of the marrow and does not develop in all those in whom involvement of the bone marrow is extensive.

ACUTE HEMORRHAGIC ANEMIA. Acute hemorrhagic anemia is a term used to describe the changes after the sudden loss of a large volume of blood. In a healthy person, the rapid loss of 500 to 1000 mL of blood causes few if any symptoms. Some people faint or become weak, with sweating, nausea, and a temporary fall in blood pressure. If the loss approaches 1500 mL, most people are still comfortable while recumbent, but become dizzy and light-headed because of the fall in blood pressure when they stand. If there is a sudden loss of 2000 mL of blood, most people develop serious symptoms, with confusion or loss of conciousness, shortness of breath, and excessive sweating as the blood pressure, cardiac output, and central venous pressure fall. The pulse becomes thin and thready. The skin is cold and clammy, as blood is shunted from the skin, the muscles, the gut, and the kidneys in an attempt to conserve the blood volume. The patient often becomes thirsty. If the sudden loss of blood is still greater, over 2500 mL, shock and often lactic acid acidosis occur because of hypoxia in the tissues. The danger of death becomes great.

In an acute hemorrhage, whole blood is lost. The blood volume falls sharply, for about three hours. The concentration of hemoglobin in the blood and the volume of packed red cells do not change. After about three hours, fluid begins to enter the blood from the tissue spaces to restore the blood volume. The concentration of hemoglobin in the blood and the volume of packed red cells begin to fall and continue to do so for from 24 to 72 hours, as the blood is increasingly diluted.

Because of the hypoxia, the secretion of erythropoietin increases and causes increased erythropoiesis in the bone marrow. After 24 hours or more, polychromatic red cells and reticulocytes appear in the blood. The reticulocytosis usually reaches a peak about nine days after the hemorrhage, and falls to normal by about the 14th day. The greater the volume of blood lost, the greater the reticulocytosis, though it rarely exceeds 15%.

The leukocyte count usually rises to a peak of from 10 to 20 $\times$ 10^9/L (10,000 to 20,000/mm^3) a few hours after the hemorrhage and falls back to normal within a few days. The leukocytosis is due largely to the mobilization of the neutrophils sequestered in small vessels throughout the body, in what is called the marginal pool. Adrenalin is probably the agent causing this mobilization. The platelet count may fall for a few minutes after the hemorrhage, but then begins to rise, often

to 500 $\times$ 10^9/L (500,000/mm^3), sometimes more. It returns to normal after a few days.

ANEMIA OF RENAL DISEASE. Anemia is almost invariable in severe renal disease. Its severity varies with the concentration of creatinine in the blood. Several factors combine to cause the anemia. Often the damaged kidneys cannot make enough erythropoietin to maintain the production of red cells in the bone marrow. Iron deficiency, folate deficiency, and the anemia of chronic disorders frequently develop. In the hemolytic-uremic syndrome and malignant hypertension, microangiopathic anemia is common.

In many uremic patients, the low concentration of erythropoietin in the blood and increased destruction of the red cells are the principal features of the anemia. The lack of erythropoietin is due in part to the injury to the kidneys, in part to the failure to respond to increased demand that occurs in the anemia of chronic disorders. In some patients, a factor that opposes the action of erythropoietin may be present. The life of the circulating red cells is often 60 days or less, rather than the normal 120 days. The increased destruction is caused by an extracorporeal factor, as in the anemia of chronic disorders.

In patients with severe renal disease, the concentration of hemoglobin in the blood is usually between 50 and 100 g/L (5 and 10 g/100 mL). In most patients the red cells are of the normal size, or a little bigger, and are normally supplied with hemoglobin. Often a few burr cells, with small, regular prickles or a few distorted, triangular or helmet-shaped red cells are present. The reticulocyte aand leukocyte counts are normal or a little increased. The platelet count is normal.

The bone marrow is usually normal, but may be a little hyperplastic or, if the anemia is severe, a little hypoplastic. The iron content of the marrow is usually normal.

Dialysis often brings improvement in the anemia after some months. The production of erythropoietin does not alter, but the marrow does increase the production of red cells. A renal transplant restores the production of erythropoietin, and as the immunosuppressive drugs that depress the marrow are reduced, the concentration of hemoglobin in the blood often returns to normal.

ANEMIA OF HEPATIC DISEASE. The concentration of hemoglobin in the blood is reduced in 75% of patients with advanced cirrhosis of the liver or other severe liver disease. In many of these people, the reduction is caused by an increase in blood volume, and the circulating red cell mass is normal. Only in 40% of the patients with severe liver disease is the circulating red cell mass reduced.

In some of the patients with a reduction in the circulating red cell mass, the anemia is due to iron deficiency, folate deficiency, the depression of the bone marrow caused by ethanol, hypersplenism, or increased hemolysis. In most, it is caused by the disease of the liver.

In such patients, the concentration of hemoglobin in the blood is between 50 and 100 g/L (5 and 10 g/100 mL). In more than 50% of the patients, the red cells are abnormally thin. The diameter of the red cells is increased, but their volume is not. Some of the thin red cells look like target cells. Others are more evenly filled with hemoglobin. If the patient is not drinking alcohol excessively, there is usually a reticulocytosis of 5% or more. If the patient is drinking heavily, there are few if any reticulocytes. If cirrhosis is severe, there are often spur cells, like the acanthocytes of abetalipoproteinemia.

The leukocyte count is often normal, but there may be lymphopenia, neutropenia, or neutrophilia. About 50% of the patients have mild thrombocytopenia. The platelet count is rarely less than 50×10^9/L (50,000/mm^3).

The bone marrow may be mildly hyperplastic, normal, or hypoplastic. In patients with thin red cells, the red cell precursors in the marrow are also thin. Their diameter is increased, though their volume is not. They are sometimes called macronormoblasts. They do not show the nuclear abnormalities found in megaloblasts.

In 70% of patients with severe cirrhosis of the liver, the survival of the circulating red cells is reduced. The maliformation of the spur cells and an extracorporeal factor combine to cause increased destruction of the red cells in the spleen.

The thin red cells and the spur cells are caused by malformation of the red cell membrane. In the thin red cells, the quantity of cholesterol and lecithin in the cell membrane is increased. In the spur cells, the quantity of cholesterol in the membrane is increased, but the quantity of lecithin is normal. The malformation of the red cells is due in part to reduced lecithin-cholesterol acetyltransferase activity in the red cells that develops in severe liver disease, the increase in the ratio of free cholesterol to phospholipid in the plasma, and the retention of bile salts.

ANEMIA IN ENDOCRINE DISEASE. Anemia is common in hypothyrodisim and may occur in hyperthryoidism. It is usual in Addison's disease, Simmonds' disease, and hypogonadism. In some of these people, the anemia is due to iron deficiency or to deficiency of folate or vitamin B_{12}. In some, it is caused by the hormonal disorder.

In hypothyroidism, the anemia caused by the lack of the thyroid hormones is mild, normocytic, and normochromic. It results from reduced production of red cells by the marrow, perhaps because of the lack of thyroid stimulation or because the reduced demand for oxygen in the tissues causes a reduction in the quantity of red cells produced. The anemic blood in hypothyroidism carries enough oxygen to meet the demand in the tissues. Hyperthyroidism usually increases the production of red cells, but occasionally it causes anemia.

In Addison's disease, the mild normocytic normochromic anemia often present can be repaired by replacement therapy. At first, the concentration of hemoglobin falls as the dehydration usually present is corrected, but then the level of hemoglobin climbs to normal.

The mild normocytic normochromic anemia usual in Simmonds' disease probably results from the failure of thyroid, adrenocortical, and gonadal secretions caused by the hypopituitarism. As with hypothyroidism, the reduced need for oxygen in the tissues, rather than the action of the hormones on the erythropoietic cells, may cause the anemia.

Androgens increase the production of erythropoietin, explaining why the concentration of hemoglobin in the blood is higher in men than in women. Estrogens may have a contrary effect. If a man is castrated, the hemoglobin level in the blood falls to the female range.

POLYCYTHEMIA

An excess of red cells in the blood is called polycythemia. The concentration of red cells in the blood, the concentration of hemoglobin, and the volume of packed red cells are all abnormally high.

The term *polycythemia* comes from the Greek words for many, a receptacle and blood. Because the derivation of the word does not show that only the red cells are being considered, some prefer the more accurate term *erythrocytosis*, from the Greek for red, a receptacle, and the general ending used to make nouns.

Two types of polycythemia are distinguished. In both, the concentration of red cells in the blood increases. In true or absolute polycythemia, the total number of circulating red cells is increased. Often the volume of the plasma is also increased, but the increase in the number of red cells is greater than the increase in plasma volume. In relative polycythemia, the number of circulating red cells is normal, but the plasma volume is reduced.

Relative Polycythemia

Two kinds of relative polycythemia occur. Transient polycythemia is caused by temporary dehydration. Gaisböck's syndrome is a form of chronic erythrocytosis.

TRANSIENT POLYCYTHEMIA. Relative polycythemia occurs in any condition in which there is severe dehydration. Persistent vomiting, massive diarrhea, excessive sweating, extensive burns, polyuria, uncontrolled diabetes mellitus, or too vigorous antidiuretic therapy can deplete the body of water, reduce the plasma volume, and cause relative polycythemia. Inadequate intake of water can do so or can augment the dehydration caused by excessive loss of water. The concentration of hemoglobin in the blood is often 180 to 200 g/L (18 to 20 g/100 mL) and

the volume of packed red cells is 0.6 to 0.7 L/L (60 to 70%).

The hemoconcentration caused by the reduction in the volume of plasma also increases the leukocyte count. The leukocyte count often rises more rapidly than does the red cell count, for many of the conditions that cause hemoconcentration also cause leukocytosis.

Correction of the dehydration restores the plasma volume and the concentration of red cells in the blood to normal.

GAISBÖCK'S SYNDROME. Gaisböck's syndrome, also called pseudopolycythemia, benign polycythemia, and stress erythrocytosis, is named after the German physician who described it in 1905. The patients have mild but persistent polycythemia, but no other evidence of disease. The volume of packed red cells is over 0.5 L/L (50%). The circulating red cell volume is normal, but the plasma volume is reduced. The leukocyte count is normal. Most of the patients are men 40 to 50 years old who are tense and strained. Many of them are obese. Some are hypertensive. No treatment is needed. Most of these patients have no disease, though the concentration of red cells in their blood is a little above the usually accepted upper limit of normal.

True Polycythemia

In true or absolute polycythemia, the production of red cells in the bone marrow is increased. Their life span is normal. Three types of true polycythemia are distinguished. Polycythemia vera is of unknown etiology. Secondary true polycythemia is caused by overproduction of erythropoietin. Congenital true polycythemia is caused by a genetic defect.

POLYCYTHEMIA VERA. Polycythemia vera is also called polycythemia rubra vera, from the Latin for red and true, and erythremia from the Greek for red and blood. Each year, less than 1 person in 200,000 develops polycythemia vera. It is more common in Jews than in Caucasians and is uncommon in black people. About 60% of the patients are men. Most are over 40 years old when the disease is diagnosed.

Lesions. Polycythemia affects primarily the bone marrow and the blood, with secondary changes in other organs.

Bone Marrow. The bone marrow is nearly always hyperplastic in polycythemia vera, though occasionally it is of normal cellularity. The quantity of fat in the red marrow is usually reduced. Sometimes the red marrow extends into bones usually filled with yellow marrow. Occasionally the hyperplasia is so great that the sternum and other bones are tender, or there is pain in the limbs.

The erythropoietic cells, granulopoietic cells, and megakaryocytes are all hyperplasic in polycythemia vera. Often the production of red cells is more than doubled, but because of the hyperplasia of the granulopoietic cells and the megakaryocytes the proportion of the cell types remains about normal.

In 10% of untreated patients, the chromosomal pattern is abnormal in the marrow cells. Many different kinds of abnormality are found, with trisomy 9 being the most common. Treatment increases greatly the likelihood that chromosomal abnormalities will be found. In patients who live for many years, the bone marrow eventually becomes fibrotic, and polycythemia vera changes to myelofibrosis.

Blood. Commonly the red count is between 7 and 10 × 10^{12}/L (7,000,000 to 10,000,000/mm^3) and may be as high as 15 × 10^{12}/L (12,000,000/mm^3). The concentration of hemoglobin in the blood rises similarly, often to 180 to 240 g/L (18 to 24 g/100 mL). The volume of packed red cells rises to more than 0.8 L/L (80%). The red cells in the blood are usually normal, and their survival is normal or a little shortened. The reticulocyte count is normal. Only if iron deficiency develops, as it often does, do the red cells become smaller than normal, with less than the normal content of hemoglobin.

The excess of red cells increases the blood volume. Instead of the normal 30 mL/kg body weight, the blood volume is often from 40 to 90 mL/kg. This expansion of the blood volume is caused almost entirely by the excess of red cells. The plasma volume is normal or a little reduced.

The leukocyte count is over 10 × 10^9/L (10,000/mm^3) in over 80% of patients with polycythemia vera. Often it is about 25 × 10^9/L (25,000/mm^3), and it may exceed 50 × 10^9/L (50,000/mm^3). The excess is largely of neutrophils, though eosinophils and basophils may also be increased. A blood smear shows an increase in metamyelocytes and often 1 or 2% of myelocytes. Myeloblasts are not found in the blood. Alkaline phosphatase activity is often greatly increased in the leukocytes.

The platelet count is increased in 70% of the patients, often to 500 to 1000 × 10^9/L (500,000 to 1,000,000/mm^3), sometimes much more. The platelets are sometimes abnormally large or oddly shaped. Coagulation is usually normal, though in some patients with polycythemia vera, platelet factor 3 is deficient, and other abnormalities in the platelets have been described. Continuing intravascular thrombosis may reduce the concentration in the blood of fibrinogen and coagulation factor V.

The excess of red cells increases often the viscosity of the blood two or three times so that the viscid blood is not easily pushed through the capillaries. It may be difficult to draw the thick blood up into a pipette.

Because of the increased activity of the bone marrow, hyperuricemia is evident in 70% of patients with polycythemia vera. About 5% of them develop gout. The increased production and destruction of red cells often increase the concentration of bilirubin in the blood to the upper limit of normal. About 50% of the patients have hypergammaglobulinemia. Often a protein that binds vitamin B$_{12}$ appears in the blood, so that the ability of the plasma to bind vitamin B$_{12}$ is increased. The concentration of erythropoietin in the blood is normal or low.

Other Organs. In polycythemia the skin is strikingly congested. Often the face is a dark brick red or purplish red. The eyes are frequently bloodshot, with prominent, distended blood vessels. Especially in the face, hands, and feet, the blood vessels in the skin are stuffed with semistagnant blood. Because of the increase in blood volume, dermal capillaries normally closed are filled with blood. Because of the increased viscosity of the blood, the circulation in the skin is sluggish. Often so much of the hemoglobin in the red cells is reduced that the skin becomes cyanotic and hypoxemic.

Other tissues are affected similarly. The congestion and slowing of the circulation make ecchymoses common. Sometimes there is bleeding from the gums or epistaxis. Cerebral hemorrhage may bring death.

Thrombosis is common in veins and arteries. Thrombosis in large arteries can cause infarction in the brain, heart, gut, lungs, or legs. Venous thrombosis can injure the brain and oher organs.

The spleen is enlarged in over 70% of the patients. Usually the enlargement is moderate, but occasionally the spleen extends down into the pelvis. Infarcts in the big spleen cause pain or a friction rub as the parietal peritoneum rubs on the inflamed capsule of the spleen. Microscopically, the spleen shows congestion, with sometimes a few small foci of myeloid metaplasia. The liver is moderately enlarged in 40% of the patients, mainly by congestion.

More than 10% of the patients have a peptic ulcer, usually in the duodenum. About 50% have systemic hypertension, thought the hypertension seems coincidental. Control of the polycythemia does not correct the hypertension.

Clinical Presentation. The onset of polycythemia vera is slow and insidious. By the time the patient seeks medical advice, the disease has often been present for many years. Most of the symptoms and signs in polycythemia result from the increase in blood volume or from the slowing of the circulation, caused by the increased viscosity of the blood.

Headache is troublesome in nearly 50% of the patients, and over 40% have episodes of dizziness, both caused by the distention and sluggish circulation in the intracranial blood vessels. Over 30% of the patients have visual disturbances caused by congestion in the retina or by small thromboses and hemorrhages that sometimes develop in the eyes. Pruritus is severe in over 40% of the patients, especially after a hot bath, and may be due to release of histamine from the basophils in the congested blood vessels in the skin. Weakness becomes evident in nearly 50% of the patients. Nearly 30% lose weight. Sweating is troublesome in 30%. Dyspnea on exertion, paresthesias, and pain in the joints develop in about 30% of the patients.

Pathogenesis. Polycythemia vera is caused by an abnormal clone of hematopoietic cells that produces excessive numbers of red cells, granulocytes, and platelets. In tissue culture, the abnormal cells continue to produce red cells in the absence of erythropoietin. Normal marrow cells and marrow cells from a patient with secondary polcythemia rarely do so.

In people heterozygous for the A and B forms of glucose-6-phosphate dehydrogenase, normal hematopoietic cells, like other cells in the body, contain a mixture of the A and B forms of the enzyme. In heterozygotes with polycythemia rubra vera, the hematopoietic cells contain only one form of the enzyme, confirming that the proliferation of hematopoietic cells in polycythemia vera is monoclonal.

People with polycythemia rubra vera respond to a lack of oxygen in the air and to phlebotomy as do normal people. If a person with polycythemia vera ascends to an altitude in which the oxygen tension in the air is low, the concentration of red cells in the blood increases, as it does in a normal person. If the person with polycythemia vera returns to a lower altitude, the red cell count returns to its previous level. If the concentration of red cells in the blood is reduced by phlebotomy in a patient with polycythemia vera, the production of erythropoietin increases and remains high until the red cell count returns to its previous abnormal level.

Most authorities think that polycythmia vera is a neoplasm. They consider that a neoplastic change in a stem cell in the bone marrow gives rise to a clone of hematopoietic cells that proliferate excessively without regard to the needs of the body.

Others think that the hematopoietic cells are normal in polycythemia and that their excessive proliferation is caused by some factor in the plasma or by the excessive sensitivity to erythropoietin of the erythroid cells in the bone marrow.

Polycythemia vera is related closely to myeloid leukemia and other myeloproliferative disorders. In all these disorders, more than one of the types of hematopoietic cell proliferates because of a neoplastic or hyperplastic change in the stem cells in the bone marrow.

Treatment and Prognosis. Untreated, patients with polycythemia vera die within two years of developing symptoms. Most die of thrombosis; a few die of hemorrhage or leukemia. The rest may continue without much change for 10 years or more, but then the polycythemia vera gradually changes to myelofibrosis or less often to acute or chronic myeloid leukemia.

Venesection, to reduce the excess of red cells and reduce the blood volume offers immediate relief. In many patients the remission so obtained persists for months. In some people with polycythemia vera, the removal of 500 or 1000 mL of blood every few months can control the disease.

If venesection proves inadequate, radiation or cytotoxic drugs can be used to reduce the activity of the marrow. Radioactive phosphorus is concentrated in the bones and has proved particularly valuable. In most patients, a remission is achieved and persists for a year or more. Unfortunately, 15% of people treated with radioactive phosphorus develop myeloid leukemia. It is not known whether the radioactive phosphorus causes the leukemia or whether leukemia is one of the natural ends of polycythemia vera, and the increased survival of the people treated with radioactive phosphorus allows time for the leukemia to develop.

With good treatment, about 50% of patients with polycythemia vera are alive and well 10 to 15 years after the onset of symptoms.

SECONDARY TRUE POLYCYTHEMIA. When absolute polycythemia is secondary to some other disease, the increased production of red cells is caused by increased production of erythropoietin. The bone marrow is normal and responds to the increase in erythropoietin in the usual way by increasing erythropoiesis and the output of red cells. Granulopoiesis and the megakaryocytes are not affected.

Lesions. The bone marrow shows hyperplasia of the erythropoietic cells, but not of the granulopoietic cells or of the megakaryocytes. The ratio of the myeloid to the erythroid cells is reduced.

The red cells produced are normal and survive the normal span. The plasma volume remains normal or is slightly reduced. The concentration of red cells in the blood does not usually exceed 8×10^{12}/L (8,000,000/mm^3). The leukocyte count and the platelet count remain normal.

Clinical Presentation. Most patients with secondary polycythemia have no symptoms and no disability. Only if secondary polycythemia grows excessive, do the changes caused by the excess of red cells in polycythemia vera occur.

Pathogenesis. Hypoxia is the most common cause of secondary true polycythemia. Occasionally it is caused by a tumor or by renal disease.

Mountain Sickness. People who ascend quickly to a great altitude often develop a transient illness called acute mountain sickness. Some people can ascend rapidly from sea level to 4000 m without becoming ill. Others develop severe symptoms if they ascend as little as 2000 m.

The symptoms usually begin within a few hours, but may be delayed for some days. The patient feels weak and has a severe headache, often nausea, vomiting, and insomnia. In most people, the symptoms disappear after a few days, as the person become acclimatized to the height. In a few people, acute mountain sickness is more severe, with cerebral or pulmonary edema, and may prove fatal unless the patient is returned to a lower altitude.

The symptoms are believed due to the retention of water caused by oversecretion of the antidiuretic hormone and adrenocortical steroids caused by the hypoxia. Recovery comes as the concentration of 2,3-diphosphoglycerate increases in the red cells, increasing the oxygen supply to the tissues; as the increased secretion of erythropoietin caused by the hypoxia increases the production of red cells; and the excessive secretion of the antidiuretic hormone and the adrenocortical steroids lessens.

People who remain at a considerable altitude develop secondary polycythemia. The severity of the polycythemia varies with the altitude. At 4000 m above sea level, the red cell count is likely to be 7 to 8×10^{12}/L (7,000,000 to 8,000,000/mm^3) and may be higher. The polycythemia usually causes no symptoms. If the person returns to sea level, it soon disappears.

Some people living at high altitude develop chronic mountain sickness, called Monge's disease after the Peruvian physician who described it in 1928, often after many years of succesful adaptation to the height. In these people, the polycythemia becomes more severe than the altitude warrants, and the patient develops many of the features of polycythemia vera. The face is highly congested and turns cyanotic at the least exertion. Often the fingers are clubbed. The tension of carbon dioxide in the blood is abnormally high. Some of the patients have pulmonary emphysema, chronic bronchitis, or some other pulmonary disease that impairs the oxygenation of the blood, augmenting the effect of the high altitude. If the patient descends to a lower altitude, recovery is complete. If the patient reascends, the disease recurs.

Other Causes of Hypoxia. Secondary true polycythemia sometimes complicates pulmonary emphysema, chronic bronchitis, pulmonary arteriovenous shunts, and other diseases of the lungs that cause hypoxia. The red cell count is rarely more than $7 \times 10^{12}/$ L (7,000,000/mm^3). The hypoxia causes increased secretion of erythropoietin, but polycythemia develops in only 50% of the patients. In the others, the bone marrow fails to respond. In some of these patients, infection suppresses the bone marrow. In some, the increased tension of carbon dioxide caused by the pulmonary disease depresses the bone marrow.

Secondary polycythemia can develop in people in whom the respiratory center fails to respond to hypercapnia. These people breathe shallowly in spite of hypercapnia. The oxygen tension in the tissues falls. Polycythemia follows. Some of the patients whose breathing is inadequate are immensely fat and are said to suffer from the pickwickian syndrome, named after the fat boy in Dickens' *Pickwick Papers*. In many of these people, but not all, loss of weight corrects the fault.

Congenital heart disease is a common cause of hypoxia. Any significant right-to-left shunt is likely to cause cyanosis and polycythemia. The red cell count is often 7 to 8 $\times$ $10^{12}/$L (7,000,000 to 8,000,000/mm^3), but may exceed $10 \times 10^{12}/$L (10,000,000/mm^3).

Over 125 structurally abnormal hemoglobins have an increased affinity for oxygen. If one is present in sufficient quantity in the red cells it reduces the supply of oxygen to the tissues. The hypoxia in the tissues stimulates increased secretion of erythropoietin, and polycythemia follows. In most of these patients, the erythropoietin level in the blood is normal when the patient is examined, because the polycythemia has increased the supply of oxygen to the tissues close to normal, and the oversecretion of erythropoietin ceases. If the polycythemia is reduced by bleeding, increased secretion of erythropoietin recurs and continues until the polycythemia is again sufficient to ensure oxygenation of the tissues.

Inappropriate Secretion of Erythropoietin. About 1% of renal cell carcinomata and sometimes a hepatocellular carcinoma, hemangioblastoma of the cerebellum, or leiomyosarcoma of the uterus secretes sufficient erythropoietin to cause polycythemia. Less often, a renal adenoma, renal hemangioma, Wilms' tumor, phenochromocytoma, myxoma of the heart, or a carcinoma of the lung, stomach, prostate, or ovary does so. The increase in the concentration of red cells in the blood is usually slight.

Less often a renal cyst, hydronephrosis, or some other kind of non-neoplastic renal disease causes hypersecretion of erythropoietin. Occasionally nodular hyperplasia of the liver does so.

Treatment and Prognosis. If the cause of the oversecretion of erythropoietin can be controlled, the secondary true polycythemia disappears.

HEREDITARY POLYCYTHEMIA. The abnormal hemoglobins that cause secondary polycythemia cause one form of hereditary polycythemia. In these people, the defect is inherited as an autosomal dominant character. Other forms of hereditary polycythemia are rare. Some are inherited as autosomal dominant, some as autosomal recessive characters. Some kindred are deficient in 2,3-diphosphoglycerate, reducing the delivery of oxygen to the tissues and causing oversecretion of erythropoietin. In a few kindred, the cause of the oversection of erythropoietin is unknown.

METHEMOGLOBINEMIA

Normally, less than 1% of the hemoglobin in the red cells is oxidized to methemoglobin. If this proportion increases, the patient is said to have methemoglobinemia.

Clinical Presentation. If less than 10% of the hemoglobin in the blood is converted to methemoglobin, there are usually no symptoms and no dysfunction. If the proportion of methemoglobin exceeds 15%, the patient becomes cyanosed, but usually has no other disability. Only if the proportion of methemoglobin exceeds 30%, does hypoxia become evident. The methemoglobin both reduces the quantity of hemoglobin available to carry oxygen and impairs the release of oxygen from the remaining hemoglobin. The hypoxia causes dyspnea on exertion, headache, weakness, tachycardia, and dizziness. If the proportion of methemoglobin exceeds 60%, the patient becomes lethargic, with nausea and vomiting, and may become stuporous or unconcious. If it exceeds 70%, death is likely.

Pathogenesis. Methemoglobinemia can be caused by drugs and poisons that prevent the reduction of methemoglobin to hemoglobin. It develops in people deficient in one of the reducing enzymes needed to convert methemoglobin to hemoglobin. It is inevitable in people with a structurally abnormal hemoglobin that irreversibly forms methemoglobin.

Some drugs and chemicals that cause methemoglobinemia are oxidants that act directly on the red cells. Nitrites, chlorates, and quinones produce methemoglobinemia in this way. Other drugs and chemicals cause methemoglobinemia only when they are converted into an active metabolite within the body. The drugs and chemicals that most frequently cause methemoglobinemia are of this type. Among them are phenacetin, sulfonamides, aniline dyes, nitrobenzenes, trinitrotoluene, and nitrates.

Methemoglobinemia caused by phenacetin usually arises in people who have taken the drug for a prolonged period. Antipyrine, acetanilid, and other analgesics cause methemoglobinemia less frequently. Sulfathiazole, sulfapyridine, and sulfamethazole are among the sulfonamides that occasionally cause methemoglobinemia. The sulfones used to treat leprosy sometimes cause methemoglobinemia. Amyl nitrite, ammonium nitrite, benzocaine, bismuth subnitrate, ethyl nitrite, nitroglycerine, quinones, potassium chlorate, resorcin, silver nitrate, and sodium nitrite are among the other drugs that can do so.

In the home, aniline dyes in ink, crayons, shoes, or blankets may cause methemoglobinemia, especially in children who eat or suck these things. Solvents such as nitrobenzene in polishes can do so. Nitrites and nitrates are sometimes used to preserve meat. Sometimes water contains nitrate to cause methemoglobinemia in infants.

In industry, methemoglobinemia can result from nitrobenzene, dinitrobenzene, or trinitrobenzene inhaled or splashed on the skin. Any of the products of aniline can cause it. Welders or silo fillers sometimes inhale enough nitrous oxides to cause methemoglobinemia.

Deficiency of one of the variants of the reduced nicotinamide adenine dinucleotide-dependent methemoglobin reductase can cause methemoglobinemia. Homozygotes usually have about 20% of methemaglobin in the blood, while in heterozygotes the methemoglobinemia is less marked. Some of the patients are mentally deficient.

At least 20 structurally abnormal hemoglobins, called M hemoglobins, form a methemoglobin that cannot be converted to hemoglobin. The proportion of M hemoglobin in the blood is usually about 25%.

Treatment. In many patients with methemoglobinemia, no treatment is needed. If the methemoglobinemia is caused by a drug or chemical, the offending agent should be withdrawn. The normal reducing mechanisms in the red cells will then convert the methemoglobin back to hemoglobin.

In people with methemoglobinemia caused by a deficiency of methemoglobin reductase, and with severe methemoglobinemia caused by a drug or a chemical, the cyanosis and other symptoms can be relieved by giving methylene blue intravenously. The methylene blue increases the conversion of methemoglobin to hemoglobin, reducing the concentration of methemoglobin in the red cells. Ascorbic acid given by mouth acts similarly, though more slowly. Neither methylene blue nor ascorbic acid is of help when methemoglobinemia is caused by an abnormal hemoglobin.

SULFHEMOGLOBINEMIA. The drugs that cause methemoglobinemia sometimes cause sulfhemoglobinemia. Why they produce methemoglobinemia in some people and sulfhemoglobinemia in others is not known. Phenacetin, sulfonamides, and acetanilid are the most likely to do so.

Sulfhemoglobin is unable to carry oxygen. As little as 5 g/L (0.5 g/100 mL) causes cyanosis. There are rarely any other symptoms, even if the concentration of sulfhemoglobin in the blood exceeds 100 g/L (10 g/100 mL).

Withdrawal of the offending drug is the only treatment needed. The cyanosis fades slowly. Sulfhemoglobin cannot be converted to hemoglobin. It persists in the affected red cells until they are destroyed at the end of a normal life span.

BIBLIOGRAPHY

General

Hardisty, R. M., and Weatherall, D. J.: Blood and Its Disorders. 2nd Ed. Oxford, Blackwell, 1982.

Mollison, P. O., Engelfriet, C. P., and Contreras, M.: Blood Transfusion in Clinical Medicine. 8th Ed. Oxford, Blackwell, 1987.

Wickramasinghe, S.N. (Ed.): Blood and Bone Marrow. In Systemic Pathology, 3rd Ed. Edited by Symmers, W. St. C: London, Churchill Livingstone, 1986.

Williams, W. J., Beutler, E., Erslav, A. J., and Lichtman, M. A.: Hematology. 3rd Ed. New York, McGraw-Hill, 1983.

Wintrobe, M. M., et al.: Clinical Hematology. 8th Ed. Philadelphia, Lea & Febiger, 1981.

Wittels, B.: Surgical Pathology of Bone Marrow. Philadelphia, W. B. Saunders, 1985.

Zucker-Franklin, D., Greaves, M. F., Grossi, C. E., and Marmont A. M.: Atlas of Blood Cells. 2nd Ed. Philadelphia, Lea & Febiger, 1988.

Anemia

Anderson, L. J.: Role of parvovirus B19 in human disease. Pediatr. Infect. Dis. J., 6:711, 1987.

Anderson, L. J.: Human parvovirus infections. J. Virol. Methods, 17:175, 1987.

Bagby, G. C. (Ed.): Hematological aspects of systemic disease. Hematol. Oncol. Clin. North Am., 1:167, 1987.

Bank, A.: Genetic disorders of hemoglobin synthesis. Hosp. Pract., 20(9):109, 1985.

Banner, W., Jr., and Tong, T. G.: Iron poisoning. Pediatr. Clin. North Am., 33:393, 1986.

Blacklock, H. A., and Mortimer, P. P.: Aplastic crises and other effects of human parvovirus infection. Clin. Haematol., 13:679, 1984.

Bunn, H. F., and Forget, B. G.: Hemoglobin. Philadelphia, W. B. Saunders, 1985.

Cao, A., Rosatelli, C., and Pirastu, M.: Prenatal diagnosis of inherited hemoglobinopathies. J. Génét. Hum., 34:413, 1986.

Chanarin, I.: Cobalamin-folate interrelations. Blood, 66:479, 1985.

Chanarin, I.: Megaloblastic anaemia, cobalamin and folate. J. Clin. Pathol., 40:978, 1987.

Chanarin, I., et al.: Folate and cobalamin. Clin. Haematol., 14:629, 1985.

Chaplin, H., Jr.: Immune hemolytic anemias. Meth. Hematol., 12:1, 1985.

Chauhan, P. M., Kondlapoodi, P., and Natta, C. L.: Pathology of sickle cell disorders. Pathol. Annu., 18(2):253, 1983.

Dacie, J. V.: The Haemolytic Anaemias. Volume 1. The Hereditary Haemolytic Anaemias, Part 1. 3rd Ed. London, Churchill Livingstone, 1985.

Dallman, P. R.: Anemia of prematurity. Annu. Rev. Med., 32:143, 1981.

Dallman, P. R.: Iron deficiency and the immune response. Am. J. Clin. Nutr., 46:329, 1987.

Doll, D. C., and Weiss, R. B.: Neoplasia and the erythron. J. Clin. Oncol., 3:429, 1985.

Eaton, W. A., and Hofrichter, J.: Hemoglobin S gelation and sickle cell disease. Blood, 70:1245, 1987.

Edelstein, S. J.: The Sickled Cell. Boston, Harvard University Press, 1986.

Escbach, J. W., and Adamson, J. W.: Anemia of end-stage renal disease. Kidney Int., 28:1, 1985.

Fried, W., and Morley, C.: Update on erythropoietin. Int. J. Artif. Organs, 8:79, 1895.

Fucharoen, S., Rowley, P. T., and Paul, N. W. (Eds.): Thalassemia. New York, Alan R. Liss, 1987–1988.

Fucharoen, S., and Winichagoon, P.: Hemoglobinopathies in Southeast Asia. Hemoglobin, 11:65, 1987.

Gardner, P. H.: Refractory anemia in the elderly. Adv. Intern. Med., 32:155, 1987.

Gaston, M. H.: Sickle-cell disease. Semin. Roentgenol., 22:150, 1987.

Habibi, B: Epidemiology of immunohematologic disease. Monogr. Allergy, 21:252, 1987.

Hall, C. (Ed.): The Cobalamins. Edinburgh, Churchill Livingstone, 1983.

Herbert, V.: Megaloblastic anemia. Lab. Invest., 52: 3, 1985.

Honig, G. R., and Adams, J. G., III: Human hemoglobin genetics. Wien, Springer-Verlag, 1985.

Jacobs, A.: Iron Deficiency and Iron Overload. CRC Crit. Rev. Oncol. Hematol., 3:143, 1985.

Kapadia, C. R., and Donaldson, R. M.: Disorders of cobalamin (vitamin B12) absorbtion and transport. Annu Rev. Med., 36:93, 1985.

Kay, M. M.: Senescent cell antigen. Surv. Synth. Pathol. Res., 4:227, 1985.

Lachant, N. A.: Hemoglobin E. Am. J. Hematol., 25:449, 1987.

Lindenbaum, J.: Hematological complications of alcohol

abuse. Semin. Liver Dis., 7:169, 1987.

Linnell, J. C., and Matthews, D. M.: Cobalamin metabolism and its clinical aspects. Clin. Sci., 66:113, 1984.

Marchesi, V. T.: The cytoskeleton system of red blood cells. Hosp. Pract., 20(11):113, 1985.

Marcus, D. L., and Freedman, M. L.: Folic acid deficiency in the elderly, J. Am. Geriat. Soc., 33:552, 1985.

McMillan, R. (Ed.): The immune cytopenias. Edinburgh, Churchill Livingstone, 1983.

Miescher, P. A.: Blood dyscrasia secondary to nonsteroidal anti-inflammatory agents. Med. Toxicol., 1(Suppl 1):57, 1986.

Modell, B., and Berdoukas, V.: The clinical approach to thalassaemia. New York, Grune and Stratton, 1983.

Moses, R. E., Frank, B. B., Leavitt, M., and Miller, R.: The syndrome of type A chronic atrophic gastritis, pernicious anemia and multiple gastric carcinoids. J. Clin. Gastroenterol., 8:61, 1986.

Noguchi, C. T., Rodgers, G. P., Serjeant, C., and Schechter, A. N.: Levels of fetal hemoglobin necessary for the treatment of sickle cell disease. N. Engl. J. Med., 318:96, 1988.

Palek, J., and Coetzer, T.: Clinical expression of alpha spectrin mutants in hereditary elliptocytosis. Blood Cells, 13:237, 1987.

Pearson, T. C., and Messinezy, M.: Polycythaemia and thrombocythaemia in the elderly. Baillière's Clin. Haematol., 1:355, 1987.

Pirofsky, B.: Autoimmune hemolytic anemia. In The Autoimmune Diseases. Edited by Rose, N. R., and Mackay, I. R. Orlando, FL, Academic Press, 1985.

Rappeport, J. M., and Nathan, D. G.: Acquired aplastic anemias. Adv. Intern. Med., 27:547, 1982.

Rifkind, J. M.: Hemoglobin. Adv. Inorg. Biochem., 7:155, 1988.

Rosse, W. F.: Autoimmune hemolytic anemia. Hosp. Pract., 20(8):105, 1985.

Schubert, T. T.: Hepatobiliary system in sickle cell disease. Gastroenterology, 90:2013, 1986.

Sokol, R. J., and Hewitt, S.: Autoimmune hemolysis. CRC Crit. Rev. Oncol. Hematol., 4:125, 1985.

Steinberg, M. H., and Embury, S. H.: Alpha-thalassemia in blacks. Blood, 68:985, 1986.

Stephens, A. D. (Ed.): Haemoglobin. Acta Haematol. (Basel), 78:74, 1987.

Stuart, J.: Erythrocyte rheology. J. Clin. Pathol., 38:965, 1985.

Sullivan, K. M., and Storb, R.: Allogenic bone marrow transplantation. Cancer Invest., 2:27, 1984.

Weatherall, D. J. (Ed.): The Thalassemias. Edinburgh, Churchill Livingstone, 1983.

Weatherall, D. J., and Clegg, J. B.: The Thalassaemia Syndromes. 3rd Ed. Oxford, Blackwell, 1981.

Whittingham, S., and Mackay, I. R.: Pernicious anemia and gastric atrophy. In The Autoimmune Diseases. Edited by Rose, N. R., and Mackay, I. R. Orlando, FL, Academic Press, 1985.

Winter, W. P. (Ed.): Hemoglobin variants in human populations. Boca Raton, FL, CRC Press, 1986.

Worwood, M.: Serum ferritin. Clin. Sci., 70:215, 1986.

Wright, P. E., and Sears. D. A.: Hypogammaglobulinemia and pernicious anemia. South. Med. J., 80:243, 1987.

Young N. S., Leonard, E., and Platanias, L.: Lymphocytes and lymphokines in aplastic anemia. Blood Cells, 13:87, 1987.

Zail, S.: Clinical disorders of the red cell membrane skeleton. CRC Crit. Rev. Oncol. Hematol., 5:397, 1986.

Zoumbos, N., Raefsky, E., and Young, N.: Lymphokines and hematopoiesis. Prog. Hematol., 14:201, 1986.

Zucker, S.: Anemia in cancer. Cancer Invest., 3:249, 1985.

Polycythemia

Berlin, N. I. (Ed.): Polycythemia vera. Semin. Hematol., 23:131, 1986.

Black, V. D.: Neonatal hyperviscosity syndrome. Curr. Probl. Pediatr., 17:73, 1987.

Danish, E. H.: Neonatal polycythemia. Prog. Hematol., 14:55, 1986.

Doll, D. C., and Weiss, R. B.: Neoplasia and the erythron. J. Clin. Oncol., 3:429, 1985.

Peterson, B. A., and Levine, E. G.: Uncommon subtypes of nonlymphocytic leukemia. Semin. Oncol., 14:425, 1987.

Rowley, J. D., and Testa, J. R.: Chromosome abnormalities in malignant hematological diseases. Adv. Cancer Res., 36:103, 1982.

Wiernik, P. H., Canellos, G. P., Kyle, R. A., and Schiffer, C. A.: Neoplastic Diseases of the Blood. 4th Ed. New York, Churchill Livingstone, 1985.

50

Granulocytes

THE diseases of the granulocytes can be divided into four groups, granulocytopenia, in which there are too few granuloytes in the blood; granulocytosis, in which the number of granulocytes in the blood is increased; the conditions in which the function of the granulocytes is abnormal; and the neoplastic and paraneoplastic diseases that involve the granulocytes. Myelofibrosis, a condition in which the bone marrow becomes increasingly fibrotic, will also be discussed in this chapter.

GRANULOCYTOPENIA

A reduction in the concentration of white cells in the blood is called leukopenia. A reduction in the concentration of granulocytes is called granulocytopenia. If only one type of granulocyte is affected, the condition is called neutropenia, eosinopenia, or basophilopenia. The disease that results from a lack of granulocytes is called agranulocytosis. The term -penia comes from the Greek for poverty.

Lesions. Granulocytopenia is not usually severe. In many patients, the leukocyte count is in the normal range, though the proportion of granulocytes is reduced. Only when granulocytopenia is severe does the leukocyte count fall below 2×10^9/L (2000/mm^3). Less than 2% of the circulating white cells are granulocytes. The granulocytes that are present have pyknotic nuclei and vacuolated cytoplasm. Their granules stain poorly.

The bone marrow is sometimes slightly hypocellular in patients with granulocytopenia; sometimes it is hyperplastic. The number of granulocytic precursors in the bone marrow is reduced. If granulocytopenia is severe, no adult granulocytes, metamyelo-cytes, or myelocytes are present. Only a few promyelocytes and myeloblasts remain. The erythroid precursors and the megakaryocytes in the bone marrow are normal. Sometimes the number of lymphocytes and macrophages in the bone marrow increases.

In most patients with granulocytopenia, there is little or no anemia, and the platelet count is normal, or nearly so. The sedimentation rate is often high.

Other organs show no abnormality in granulocytopenia unless the granulocytopenia is severe and a bacterial infection develops. In the absence of neutrophils, the bacteria proliferate exuberantly. The infected region is edematous. Often there is a sparse exudate of lymphocytes and macrophages, but if the granulocytopenia is severe, there are few or no granulocytes. Minor bleeding into the infected region is common. Occasionally there is major hemorrhage.

Clinical Presentation. If granulocytopenia develops suddenly and is severe, the patient has chills, high fever, and prostration. Ulceration of the gums or elsewhere in the oral cavity is common. Less often other mucous membranes are involved. Over 10% of the patients develop infections of the skin. The risk of developing an overwhelming pneumonia or some other major infection is great.

If the granulocytopenia develops more slowly and is less extreme, the major risk is infection. The pathogens that commonly infect the body become more dangerous. Opportunistic invaders that normally can be repelled become able to establish infection. The efficacy of many antibiotics is reduced.

Causes. Table 50-1 lists the causes of granulocytopenia. Most of these agents reduce principally the concentration of neutrophils in the blood.

TABLE 50-1. CAUSES OF GRANULOCYTOPENIA

DRUGS AND TOXINS
  Injury Inevitable and Dose Related
    Cytotoxic drugs
      Alkylating agents
        Busulfan
        Chlorambucil
        Cyclophosphamide
        Melphalan
      Antimetabolites
        Azathioprine
        Cytarabine
        6-Mercaptopurine
        Methotrexate
        Thioguanine
      Natural products
        Colchicine
        Vinblastine
        Vincristine
    Antibiotics
      Daunorubicin
      Doxorubicin

  Injury Rare and Not Dose Related
    Antimicrobial agents
      p-Aminosalicylic acid
      Cephalothin
      Chloramphenicol
      Dapsone
      Isoniazid
      Metronidazole
      Neostibosan
      Nitrofurantoin
      Organic arsenicals
      Pamaquine
      Penicillins
      Primaquine
      Ristocetin
      Streptomycins
      Sulfonamides
      Tetracyclines
      Thiocarbazone
    Anticonvulsant drugs
      Mephenytoin
      Phenytoin
      Trimethadione
    Tranquilizers
      Chlorpromazine
      Diazepam
      Imipramine
      Mepazine
      Meprobamate
      Prochlorperazine
      Promazine
      Thioridazine
    Analgesics
      Acetanalid
      Acetylsalicylic acid
      Aminopyrine
      Carbamazepiue
      Dipyrone
      Indomethacin
      Oxyphenylbutazone
      Phenacetin
      Phenylbutazone
    Antithyroid drugs
      Methimazole
      Propylthiouracil
      Thiouracil
    Antidiabetic drugs
      Carbutamide
      Chlorpropamide
      Tolbutamide
    Antihistamines
      Mepyramine
      Methaphenilene
      Promethazine
      Thenalidine
      Tripelennamine
    Anticoagulants
      Dicumarol
      Phenindione
    Diuretics
      Acetazolamide
      Chlorthalidone
      Chlorothiazides
      Mercurial diuretics
    Other
      Cincophen
      Dinitrophenol
      Gold salts
      D-penicillamine
      Rauwolfia

RADIATION
  Atomic explosions
  Radioisotopes
  X-rays

INFECTION
  Bacterial
    Brucellosis
    Paratyphoid fever
    Typhoid fever
  Rickettsial
    Rickettsialpox
  Viral
    Chickenpox
    Dengue fever
    Hepatitis
    Influenza
    Phlebotomus fever
    Rubella
  Protozoal
    Kala-azar
    Malaria

  Overwhelming infection

DISEASE
  Anaphylactoid shock
  Cachexia
  Cirrhosis of the liver
  Debility

Many of the drugs that cause granulocytopenia also cause aplastic anemia, and most of them cause granulocytopenia more frequently than they induce aplastic anemia. Some inevitably cause granulocytopenia if the dose is large enough. Some cause granulocytopenia in only a small number of patients. The cytotoxic drugs are the most important of the agents that inevitably cause granulocytopenia when given in large dose. Aminopyrine, antithyroid drugs, aspirin, chloramphenicol, chlorpromazine, dipyrone, penicillin, phenylbutazone, promazine and other tranquilizers, and sulfonamides are among the drugs that commonly cause granulocytopenia in a small proportion of patients.

The drugs that inevitably cause granulocytopenia if the dose is large enough usually cause depression of the bone marrow even in therapeutic dosage. If the dose is larger, granulocytopenia becomes more severe. If it is still greater, aplastic anemia is likely to develop.

Some of the drugs that cause granulocytopenia only occasionally cause an abrupt onset of neutropenia. All neutrophils disappear from the blood within six hours or so. Usually the granulocytopenia develops only after the drug has been given repeatedly or for some time. Some people given aminopyrine repeatedly become sensitized to the drug. If even a small dose of aminopyrine is given, severe neutropenia develops within a few hours.

Other drugs that occasionally cause granulocytopenia cause a gradual fall in the concentration of granulocytes, which only becomes evident after the drug has been given for several weeks. Sometimes this fall in the concentration of granulocytes is progressive and becomes increasingly severe if the drug is continued. More often the concentration of granulocytes in the blood becomes stabilized at a low level or returns towards normal, even though the drug is continued. Chlorpromazine acts in this way. Granulocytopenia rarely appears until the drug has been given for at least three weeks.

Some drugs, like the sulfonamides or the antithyroid drugs, sometimes cause an abrupt onset of neutropenia, sometimes a gradual reduction in the concentration of neutrophils in the blood. The frequency with which the drugs that cause granulocytopenia only occasionally cause neutropenia varies from one drug to another. About 1% of people given aminopyrine repeatedly develop granulocytopenia, but in New Zealand only 0.005% of people given phenylbutazone. Between 1 and 10% of people given phenothiazines repeatedly or for a prolonged period develop granulocytopenia. Elderly Caucasian women seem particularly at risk. Less than 1% of people given large doses of sulfonamide develop neutropenia, but up to 4% of people given antithyroid drugs for prolonged periods and as many as 6% of people given anticonvulsant drugs do. Chloramphenicol is more likely to cause aplastic anemia than granulocytopenia.

Radiation causes granulocytopenia if the dose is not large. Large doses of radiation cause aplastic anemia. The infections listed in Table 50-1 commonly cause mild granulocytopenia. Any overwhelming infection is likely to cause severe granulocytopenia.

Aplastic anemia always reduces the production of granulocytes, and pernicious anemia may do so. Rarely, iron deficiency anemia causes granulocytopenia. Cirrhosis of the liver, systemic lupus erythematosus, and Felty's syndrome sometimes cause granulocytopenia. During hemodialysis, neutropenia usually develops during the first 15 minutes, returning to normal in about an hour. Cachexia, debility, endotoxic shock, and anaphylactic shock reduce the concentration of granulocytes in the blood. Hypersplenism usually causes granulocytopenia as well as anemia and thrombocytopenia.

The congenital and idiopathic forms of granulocytopenia are rare. Infantile genetic agranulocytosis, which is inherited as an autosomal recessive character, causes severe neutropenia because of almost complete failure to form neutrophils in the bone marrow. Eosinophils and basophils are formed normally. In other patients, the granulocytes in the marrow fail to develop beyond the myelocytic stage, and the granulocytopenia that results is associated with hypogammaglobulinemia. The defect is sometimes familial, sometimes not. Infants with congenital aleukia have no leukocytes of any kind.

Familial benign chronic neutropenia, which is inherited as an autosomal dominant character, causes a mild granulocytopenia due to impairment of the maturation of the neutrophils beyond the myelocytic stage. The formation of eosinophils is normal. Chronic granulocytopenia of childhood is similar, except that in this condition the neutrophils in the marrow mature normally. Chronic idiopathic neutropenia causes severe neutropenia. The marrow is cellular, but segmented neutrophils are not present. Chronic hypoplastic neutropenia causes severe deficiency of all types of granulocyte and severe hypoplasia of the granulocytic precursors in the marrow.

Cyclic or periodic neutropenia causes episodes of severe neutropenia that recur every three weeks or so and last from three to ten days. During the attack, the precursors of the neutrophils disappear from the marrow. Between attacks, the production of neutrophils seems normal, and the neutrophils in the blood are normal, except that the proportion of segmented neutrophils is often low.

Rarely, an infant is born with neutropenia caused by transplacental passage of a neutropenic factor produced by the mother. Some of the mothers of these infants have been neutropenic; some have not. Rare adults have in their plasma a factor that causes neutropenia.

Pathogenesis. Granulocytopenia can be produced in three ways: by reducing the production of granulocytes by the bone marrow, by increasing the destruction of granulocytes in the tissues, and by increasing the proportion of granulocytes held out of the circulation in the peripheral pool. In a patient with granulocytopenia, any or all of these mechanisms may be operative.

Drugs, infection, cirrhosis of the liver, systemic lupus erythematosus, pernicious anemia, iron deficiency anemia, cachexia, and debility cause granulocytopenia principally by depressing the production of granulocytes in the bone marrow. Many of the drugs interfere with the metabolism of deoxyribonucleic acid, but how the other conditions inhibit the production of granulocytes is unclear.

The destruction of the granulocytes in the tissues is increased in hypersplenism, disseminated lupus erythematosus, pernicious anemia, viral infections, and in Felty's syndrome. In some of the patients with these disorders, immunologic mechanisms or the activation of complement may be involved. Antibodies against the granulocytes have been demonstrated in some patients with granulocytopenia caused by aminopyrine. The increased destruction of the granulocytes is mainly in the spleen.

Increased segregation of the granulocytes in the peripheral pool is the major cause of granulocytopenia in endotoxic shock and anaphylactic shock. The transient neutropenia of hemodialysis is caused by activation of the alternate pathway of complement by the coils of the apparatus, with formation of C5a, and the temporary segregation of granulocytes in the capillaries of the lungs. In many other kinds of chronic granulocytopenia, the proportion of the granulocytes in the blood segregated in the capillaries increases, contributing to the fall in the concentration of granulocytes in the circulating blood.

Treatment and Prognosis. If the agent causing the granulocytopenia can be identified, it must be withdrawn and never used again. Leukocyte transfusions can be given, but the risk of sensitization is great because satisfactory methods for typing leukocytes have yet to be developed. Antibiotics are given as necessary to combat infection.

If the offending drug is stopped or the disease causing granulocytopenia is controlled, recovery usually comes in about a week. Myelocytes and metamyelocytes reappear in the bone marrow, and a day or two later they appear in the blood. Segmented granulocytes follow soon after. Within a few days the concentration of granulocytes rises above normal and then returns to normal. If infection can be held at bay, the patient is cured.

Before the advent of antibiotics, over 80% of patients with severe, acute agranulocytosis died. Antibiotics have improved the prognosis, but severe agranulocytosis is still dangerous. Up to 20% of the patients still die, usually of infection.

GRANULOCYTOSIS

An increase in the concentration of granulocytes in the blood is called granulocytosis. Usually only one type of granulocyte is increased, and the condition is called neutrophilia, eosinophilia, or basophilia.

Lesions. The concentration of the granulocytes in the blood is increased. Usually the circulating granulocytes are normal, though there is often an admixture of more primitive forms than are normally present in the blood. Sometimes the condition causing the granulocytosis produces other changes in the blood, suggesting the cause of the granulocytosis.

Clinical Presentation. Granulocytosis causes no symptoms and no disability. The symptoms and dysfunction associated with granulocytosis are caused by the disorder that induced the granulocytosis.

Causes. Any condition that causes acute inflammation is likely to cause neutrophilia. In adults, the leukocyte count is often 15 to 25×10^9/L (15,000 to 25,000/mm^3). Bacterial infections, burns, surgical procedures, and myocardial infarction are among the conditions that usually cause a neutrophilia. Hemorrhage, strenuous exercise, convulsions, labor, emotional upsets, some kinds of poisoning, and the administration of adrenalin commonly cause neutrophilia. Ketoacidosis, eclampsia, hemolysis, Cushing's syndrome, collagen diseases and malignant tumors sometimes do so.

Two rare diseases cause persistent neutrophilia. In hereditary neutrophilia, the concentration of neutrophils in the blood is high, the liver and spleen are enlarged, and cells like those of Gaucher's disease are present in the spleen. The neutrophils function normally. Occasionally neutrophilia increases the leukocyte count to as much as 40×10^9/L (40,000/mm^3) in a person who is otherwise well. The high leukocyte count persists for months or years.

Eosinophilia is common in allergic disorders and parasitic infections. Pemphigus, dermatitis herpetiformis, and sometimes other types of dermatitis cause eosinophilia. The eosinophilic pneumonias and occasionally a malignant tumor or a collagen disease increase the concentration of eosinophils in the blood. Rarely, a congenital disorder inherited as an autosomal dominant character causes persistent eosinophilia.

Basophilia is uncommon. It sometimes occurs in hypersensitivity reactions and rarely in other conditions.

Pathogenesis. Granulocytosis can be caused by increased production of the type of granulocyte affected or by mobilization of granulocytes held in the peripheral pool. The life span of the granulocytes is rarely much altered.

In most conditions, the increase in the concentration of granulocytes in the blood is caused principally by increased release of granulocytes from the bone marrow. In acute infections, the bone marrow can produce up to 12 times the normal number of granulocytes. Not only does the leukocyte count rise, but the total number of granulocytes in the blood, those circulating and those in the peripheral pool, increases five to six times. The ratio between the circulating granulocytes and those in the peripheral pool varies widely from one patient to another. In infections and other conditions causing neutrophilia, there is often a transient neutropenia, caused by increased segregation of granulocytes in the peripheral pool, before the leukocyte count begins to increase.

In exercise, convulsions, and after the injection of epinephrine, the transient granulocytosis is due mainly to the mobilization of granulocytes from the peripheral pool. There is little or no increase in granulopoiesis.

Treatment and Prognosis. Almost always, granulocytosis is a response to injury and is beneficial. It resolves when the condition causing it is controlled.

ABNORMAL GRANULOCYTES

In several conditions, the granulocytes are abnormal in structure, function, or both. In some of these conditions, the fault is in the granulocytes themselves. In others, the abnormality in the granulocytes is secondary to infection or some other disease.

Primary Defects

The conditions in which the granulocytes themselves are abnormal are all uncommon, often rare. Most are of little importance, but some cause serious disease.

ABNORMAL STRUCTURE BUT NORMAL FUNCTION. In a few conditions, the structure of the granulocytes is abnormal, but their function is normal. The people affected suffer no disability.

Pelger-Huët Anomaly. The Pelger-Huët anomaly is named after the Dutch physicians who described it in 1928 and 1931. The condition is inherited as an autosomal dominant character and occurs in one person in 1000 to 10,000. Normally, over 70% of the neutrophils in the blood have three or more lobes. In heterozygotes with the Pelger-Huët anomaly, over 60% of the neutrophils in the blood have two lobes, and many have only a single round nucleus. Fewer than 10% of the neutrophils have three lobes, and almost none have four or more lobes. In homozygotes, all the neutrophils have a single, spheroidal nucleus. The neutrophils function normally.

Other. A number of other rare malformations of the granulocytes that cause no dysfunction have been described. In the Alder-Reilly anomaly, sometimes inherited as an autosomal recessive character, sometimes found in patients with mucopolysaccharidoses, fragments of mucopolysaccharide in lysosomes appear as granules in the cytoplasm of granulocytes in the marrow and, less often, in the blood. They may also be evident in lymphocytes and monocytes. In the May-Hegglin anomaly inherited as an autosomal dominant character, the granulocytes and monocytes contain aggregates of ribonucleic acid in their cytoplasm, and there is thrombocytopenia with poorly functioning

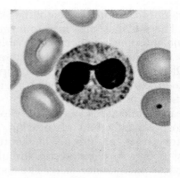

Fig. 50-1. A neutrophil in the blood of a patient with the Pelger-Huët anomaly. (From Wintrobe, M. M., et al.: Clinical Hematology. 8th Ed. Philadelphia, Lea & Febiger, 1981.)

giant platelets. In Jordan's anomaly, the cytoplasm of the granulocytes and of most of the monocytes is vacuolated. Rarely, a family has been found in whom the neutrophils were abnormally large, the neutrophils were hypersegmented, or the eosinophils were hypersegmented.

ABNORMAL STRUCTURE AND ABNORMAL FUNCTION. In the conditions in which the structure and function of the granulocytes are both abnormal, the granules of the granulocytes are malformed. The patients are unusually susceptible to infection, especially staphylococcal infections. The Chédiak-Higashi syndrome is the most studied of these disorders. Rarely, a similar syndrome is produced by a congenital failure to produce the secondary granules of the granulocytes in sufficient quantity.

Chédiak-Higashi Syndrome. The Chédiak-Higashi syndrome, is an uncommon condition named after the French physician who described it in 1952 and the Japanese physician who reported it in 1953. The neutrophils have a few abnormally large lysosomes, formed by fusion of their primary and secondary granules. Similar abnormally large lysosomes are present in eosinophils and sometimes in monocytes and other kinds of cell. Ring-shaped lysosomes, are prominent in monocytes and occasionally can be found in other leukocytes.

The Chédiak-Higashi anomaly is inherited as an autosomal recessive character. The children are born with silvery hair and less than the normal pigmentation of the skin and retina. The melanosomes fuse to form a few large melanosomes, which are unable adequately to darken the hair or to pigment the skin. Often the children have photophobia. The blood contains about half the normal concentration of neutrophils.

Repeated infections develop, especially staphylococcal infections of the skin, upper respiratory tract, or lungs. The neutrophils respond poorly to chemotactic stimuli, but phagocytose bacteria normally. The abnormal lysosomes in the neutrophils fail to fuse with the phagosomes. The bacteria are not exposed to the bactericidal substances in the lysosomes and escape unharmed.

If the child survives the infections, the spleen and lymph nodes enlarge. The neutropenia worsens. Anemia and thrombocytopenia develop. The marrow and the tissues become extensively infiltrated by lymphocytes and histiocytes as what is usually called a lymphoma develops. Often there is peripheral neuropathy because of the cellular infiltration. Hemorrhage is common. Death during childhood almost always is from infection or lymphoma.

The defect in Chédiak-Higashi syndrome is a failure to form normally the microtubules necessary for the movement of the neutrophils in response to chemotaxis and for the movement of the phagosomes and lysosomes in their cytoplasm. If the neutrophils from a patient with Chédiak-Higashi disease are cultured in a medium containing cyclic guanosine monophosphate or cholinergic drugs, which increase the concentration of cyclic guanosine monophosphate in neutrophils, microtubular function is restored to normal, and the lysosomes resume their normal form.

To compound further the inadequacy of the neutrophils in children with the Chédiak-Higashi syndrome, the lysosomes of their neutrophils are deficient in the myeloperoxidase active in killing ingested organisms and in other enzymes. Elastase is almost entirely absent. The concentration of myeloperoxidase is below 50% of normal.

NORMAL STRUCTURE BUT ABNORMAL FUNCTION. In other conditions, the granulocytes are normal structurally but fail to function normally. All are rare, some very rare.

Chronic Granulomatous Disease of Child-hood. In chronic granulomatous disease of childhood, the neutrophils and macrophages are unable to kill catalase-positive organisms. They take up organisms normally. Their phagosomes fuse with the lysosomes normally. Catalase-negative organisms are killed normally, but catalase-positive organisms such as staphylocci, gram-negative bacilli, candida, and aspergilli are not.

Chronic granulomatous disease of childhood is usually inherited as an X-linked character, less often as an autosomal recessive character. The patients are nearly all boys. Boys with the gene causing the X-linked form of the disease on their X chromosome have no normal phagocytes and inevitably develop the disease. Girls heterozygous for the X-linked form of the disease have two populations of phagocytes. One is normal. The other cannot kill catalase-positive microorganisms. Chance determines the size of the two populations. Most of the heterozygous girls have enough phagocytes able to function normally to maintain good health.

In the children affected, infections with staphylococci and gram-negative bacilli begin in childhood. Chronic, suppurative lymphadenitis often causes widespread enlargement of lymph nodes. Eczema is common and often accompanied by stomatitis and rhinitis. Bronchopneumonia, lung abscesses, abscesses in the liver and spleen, enteritis, and anal infections are frequent. Osteomyelitis often develops.

At first the infections cause a normal acute inflammatory reaction. Neutrophils accumulate around the lesions. They phagocytose the bacteria, but cannot kill them. The infection continues. After a week or so, lymphocytes, plasma cells, and macrophages begin to accumulate in the lesions, intermingling with the neutrophils, which persist in their useless endeavor. Often the macrophages become filled with yellow debris, which they cannot digest because their lysosomes are defective. As the lesions grow old, the chronic inflammation becomes predominant. Some of the macrophages become multinucleated, forming giant cells. Often the same organ shows lesions of different ages, some still with many neutrophils, others with chronic, fibrosing inflammation.

The fault in chronic granulomatous disease of childhood is in the mitochondria. The burst of oxidative activity that normally accompanies phagocytosis does not occur. The phagocytes do not form hydrogen peroxide, superoxide, and other active radicals adequately. In most of the patients, the mitochondrial, membrane-bound oxidase needed for the oxidation of reduced nicotinamide adenine dinucleotide phosphate is deficient. In some, another of the enzymes in the oxidative cycle is deficient. Catalase-negative organs like streptococci are killed because they contain the enzymes necessary to overcome the defect in the phagocytes.

Treatment of patients with chronic granulomatous disease is complicated because the bacteria in the phagocytes are protected from many of the antibiotics that would be otherwise effective. Rifampin is sometimes of benefit, because it can kill bacteria within the phagocytes.

The severity of the disease varies. Some of the children progress to death within a few years. In others the defect is less severe, and the patients enjoy long remissions, often lasting several years.

Lazy Leukocyte Syndrome. In the lazy leukocyte syndrome, the neutrophils do not respond to chemotactic stimuli. They do not accumulate at sites of infection. Minor infections that are easily overcome in people with normal neutrophils become more serious.

In some patients with the lazy leukocyte syndrome, the bactericidal power of the phagocytes is normal, but in others it is impaired. In some, the ability of the leukocytes to phagocytose organisms is reduced. In some, the concentration of IgE or IgA in the plasma is increased.

Job's Syndrome. Patients with Job's syndrome develop multiple staphylococcal infections. Their neutrophils do not respond to chemotactic stimuli. The concentration of IgE in their plasma is high. The disorder is described in the Bible in the book of Job.

Myeloperoxidase Deficiency. A few people have no myeloperoxidase in the neutrophils and monocytes. They suffer no ill effects.

Secondary Changes

Secondary changes in the granulocytes circulating in the blood are common in severe infections, burns, and other conditions. The specific granules normally present in the neutrophils become few, or disappear. Instead, toxic granules appear in the cytoplasm of the neutrophils, and sometimes become numerous. Toxic granules are primary lysosomes, that contain peroxidase and acid phosphatase, like other primary lysosomes in neutrophils but do not contain the alkaline phosphatase present in the specific granules of the neutrophils. With the ordinary stains used for blood films, toxic granules stain bluish purple.

Döhle's bodies, named after the German pathologist who lived from 1855 to 1928, may also appear. Döhle's bodies are round or oval, stain bright blue with the usual stains used for blood films, and appear in the peripheral part of the neutrophils. They consist of aggregates of rough endoplasmic reticulum and ribosomes.

The activity of the alkaline phosphatase in the leukocytes is usually moderately increased when leukocytosis is caused by inflammation. It is greatly increased in polycythemia vera and sometimes in myelofibrosis or in idiopathic thrombocytopenia. The increased activity of reduced nicotinamide adenine dinucleotide oxidase in the neutrophils caused by the phagocytosis usual in severe infections can be demonstrated by showing that more than the normal 10% of neutrophils reduce colorless nitroblue tetrazolium to blue-black formazan.

The chemotactic response of the neutrophils is sometimes, though not always, reduced by severe infections or by severe burns. It is sometimes reduced by measles in children. Malnutrition impairs chemotaxis. Hemodialysis, leukemia, and aplastic anemia sometimes reduce the chemotactic response.

MYELOFIBROSIS

Myelofibrosis is an ill-understood disorder in which the bone marrow becomes increasingly fibrotic, and extramedullary hematopoiesis becomes widespread. It is sometimes called agnogenic myeloid metaplasia, or myelosclerosis. *Agnogenic* is from the Greek for unknown and refers to the unknown etiology of the disorder; *myeloid* is from the Greek for marrow. Fibrosis of the bone

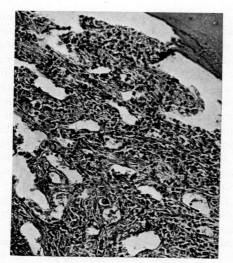

Fig. 50-2. Fibrosis of the bone marrow in a patient with severe myelofibrosis. (From Wintrobe, M. M., et al.: Clinical Hematology. 8th Ed. Philadelphia. Lea & Febiger, 1981.)

marrow occurs in trauma, infections involving bone, and other conditions, but the term *myelofibrosis* is usually reserved for the disorder described in this section.

Myelofibrosis is uncommon. Fewer than 2 people in every 100,000 have the disease. Most patients are Caucasian, middle-aged, or elderly, often 60 or more years old. Men and women are affected equally.

Lesions. The lesions in myelofibrosis affect principally the bone marrow, blood, liver, and spleen. Probably the changes in the bone marrow come first, and the alterations in the other organs follow, but often a biopsy of the bone marrow shows only minor lesions, although the disease is severe in other organs.

Bone Marrow. Early in the disease, the changes in the bone marrow vary from one part of the skeleton to another. In some regions, there is no fibrosis. In others, there is only a slight increase in reticulin fibers. An increase in collagen may be evident only in a few loci. A single biopsy can be misleading. At this stage of the disease, the cellularity of the bone marrow is often normal in most regions. In places, it is sometimes hyperplastic. In other regions, it may be hypoplastic.

As the years pass, the fibrosis of the marrow tends to become more severe. Well-formed collagen replaces much of the bone marrow. The number of hematopoietic cells in the marrow falls. In 50% of the patients, osteosclerosis eventually develops. The cortex and bony trabeculae of the vertebrae and proximal parts of the long bones become thickened. In some patients, osteosclerosis becomes severe, and the remaining marrow is almost entirely replaced by collagenous tissue.

Chromosomal abnormalities are present in the hematopoietic cells of the bone marrow in 40% of the patients. A variety of changes are found. Trisomy 8, trisomy 9, and monosomy 7 are the most common.

Blood. Patients with myelofibrosis are usually anemic, though the anemia is often mild and remains so for many years. Anisocytosis and poikilocytosis are usually marked. Particularly suggestive of myelofibrosis are tear-shaped red cells. Nucleated red cells are often present in considerable numbers.

The leukocyte count is increased in 50% of the patients, to as much as $50 \times 10^9/L$ (50,000/mm³). In 25% of the patients it is reduced, occasionally as low as $2 \times 10^9/L$ (2000/mm³). Often between 10 and 20% of

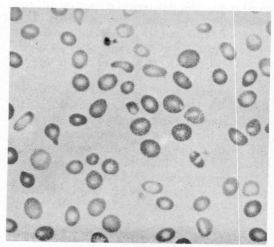

Fig. 50-3. Tear-shaped red cells in the blood of a patient with myelofibrosis. (From Wintrobe, M. M., et al.: Clinical Hematology. 8th Ed. Philadelphia. Lea & Febiger, 1981.)

the granulocytes in the blood are metamyelocytes, myelocytes, or more primitive forms. Eosinophilia and basophilia are usual, even when there is neutropenia. The activity of alkaline phosphatase in the neutrophils is increased in 70% of the patients, normal in most of the rest, but occasionally is low. Lymphocytes circulate in normal numbers.

The platelets are increased, perhaps to $1000 \times 10^9/L$ (1,000,000/mm^3), in 50% of the patients when first seen by a physician. As months and years pass, the platelet count falls, and thrombocytopenia becomes increasingly common. Often large, abnormal platelets appear. Sometimes megakaryocytes or fragments of megakaryocytes appear in the blood. Often an abnormally high proportion of platelets is sequestered in the spleen. In some patients the survival of platelets in the blood is reduced. Often platelet factor 3 is deficient.

Uricacidemia is present in most patients because of the increased turnover of marrow cells and sometimes causes gout or renal stones. Usually the concentration of lactic dehydrogenase in the serum is increased. Often the changes in the bone cause an increase in serum alkaline phosphatase activity. The concentration of vitamin B$_{12}$ in the plasma may be increased because of an increase in transcobalamin I and perhaps of other proteins that carry the vitamin.

Other Organs. As the bone marrow slowly becomes fibrotic, extramedullary hematopoiesis becomes marked in the spleen and liver and may be present in the lymph nodes, adrenal glands, kidneys, retroperitoneal tissues, gut, and the lungs. The spleen is almost invariably enlarged and may reach into the pelvis. The liver is enlarged in 50% of the patients when they are first seen by a physician.

Microscopically, the spleen and liver show clumps of hematopoietic cells in their sinusoids and in the other organs involved. All kinds of hematopoietic cells are present: granulocytic precursors, erythrocytic precursors, and megakaryocytes. The spleen and other organs are otherwise normal. The increase in the size of the spleen is due almost entirely to the accumulation of the marrow cells.

Clinical Presentation. Myelofibrosis de-velops insidiously. In many patients it is probably present for many years before it is recognized. The patient sometimes seeks advice because of the symptoms of anemia or because of discomfort or fullness caused by the large spleen. Occasionally bruising or gout draws attention to the myelofibrosis.

Pathogenesis. At least in some patients, the proliferation of hematopoietic cells in the bone marrow in myelofibrosis is monoclonal, suggesting that the disease is caused by a neoplastic proliferation derived from a primitive cell able to differentiate into granulocytic, erythroid, and megakaryocytic cells. If this is so, myelofibrosis is a neoplastic or quasineoplastic disorder related to myeloid leukemia and the other myeloproliferative disorders.

It is not known why the bone marrow becomes fibrotic. Fibrosis of the bone marrow does sometimes develop in myeloid leukemia, polycythemia vera, and other myeloproliferative disorders. The mechanism in myelofibrosis may be similar.

The extramedullary hematopoiesis in the spleen and other organs in myelofibrosis was originally thought due to the conversion of splenic cells and cells in other organs into hematopoietic cells by metaplasia. This is improbable. It is more likely that the spleen and other organs are colonized by hematopoietic cells carried from the bone marrow by the blood.

The anemia common in myelofibrosis results from the interaction of several factors. In most patients, the production of red cells by the bone marrow and foci of extramedullary hematopoiesis is reduced, though in some it is normal or increased. The destruction of red cells in the spleen is usually increased, so that the life of the circulating red cells is short. In some patients the number of red cells segregated in the spleen is great. As the spleen grows large, the blood volume increases, diluting the red cells and reducing the concentration of hemoglobin in the blood. Folate deficiency is not uncommon. The reduction in the number of granulocytes and platelets common late in the course of myelofibrosis is due in part to reduced production by the bone marrow and the foci of extramedullary hematopoiesis, but usually is due in the main to increased destruction of granulocytes and platelets by the spleen.

Treatment and Prognosis. Patients with myelofibrosis usually live about five years after the diagnosis is made. Some die sooner, and some survive much longer. As the disease slowly worsens, anemia becomes more severe, often neutropenia develops, and thrombocytopenia or platelet dysfunction brings a bleeding tendency. Commonly weight loss is marked. Edema of the lower legs becomes common as the years pass and may be due to the pressure of the large liver and spleen on the inferior vena cava. Sometimes thrombosis of the hepatic or portal veins causes portal hypertension. Infection may become hard to manage, though there seem to be adequate numbers of neutrophils and no immunologic defect.

In the late stages of the disease, it is often hard to distinguish myelofibrosis from chronic myeloid leukemia. The proportion of primitive granulocytes circulating in the blood increases, and myeloblasts become common. The distinction can usually be made by looking for the Philadelphia chromosome. It is present in the granulocytes in 90% of patients with chronic granulocytic leukemia, but is almost never found in myelofibrosis. Fewer than 10% of the patients die with acute leukemia, usually acute myeloid leukemia.

Treatment of myelofibrosis is unsatisfactory. Busulfan can be given if the leukocyte count is high or the spleen is uncomfortably large. Splenectomy may be beneficial if thrombocytopenia or anemia is due in large part to hypersplenism. Otherwise splenectomy serves only to reduce further the functioning hematopoietic tissue. Androgens sometimes stimulate the production of red cells.

TUMORS

In nearly all neoplasms of the granulocytes, all types of granulocytes and usually the monocytes and erythrocytes proliferate. In most of these conditions, the malignant cells circulate in the blood, causing leukemia.

If neoplastic neutrophils are predominant in the blood, the disease is called myeloid leukemia, myelogenous leukemia, or myelo-

cytic leukemia. If neoplastic eosinophils are the most common neoplastic cell in the blood, the disease is called eosinophilic leukemia; if basophils are dominant, it is called basophilic leukemia. In erythroleukemia, both neoplastic erythrocytes and neoplastic granulocytes are numerous in the blood. Rarely, a granulocytic tumor forms a solid mass called a chloroma.

Myeloproliferative Disorders

The neoplastic and quasineoplastic conditions of the hematopoietic cells in the bone marrow are grouped together as the myeloproliferative disorders. Probably all myeloproliferative disorders result from a neoplastic or quasineoplastic change in a primitive bone marrow cell able to differentiate into red cells, granulocytes, and megakaryocytes. Some are clearly neoplastic. In some, it is difficult to decide whether the condition is neoplastic or a response to a stimulus from outside the bone marrow.

Among the myeloproliferative disorders are myeloid leukemia and the other forms of granulocytic leukemia, chloroma, monocytic leukemia, polycythemia vera, the proliferation of megakaryocytes called thrombocythemia, and myelofibrosis. Many of the more benign myeloproliferative disorders tend to progress to a more dangerous form of myeloproliferative disorder.

CHRONIC MYELOID LEUKEMIA. Each year, one person in every 100,000 in the United States dies of chronic myeloid leukemia. About 60% of the patients are men. The disease can occur at any age, but most of the patients are 30 or more years old. The likelihood of developing chronic myeloid leukemia increases as age increases.

Lesions. The neoplastic change in chronic myeloid leukemia occurs in the bone marrow, but its most prominent manifestations are often in the blood, with secondary changes in other organs.

Bone Marrow. In the spine and the flat bones the bone marrow is soft and grayish red. Often the red marrow extends peripherally to replace the proximal part of the yellow marrow.

Microscopically, little fat remains in the

red marrow. Instead, the granulocytic precursors are hyperplastic. Myelocytes are predominant, though the proportion of more primitive white cells in the marrow is increased. Erythropoiesis remains normal, so that the ratio of myeloid to erythroid cells is increased. Often megakaryocytes are prominent. Occasionally, there is some increase in reticulin fibers in the marrow early in the disease. In 50% of the patients, the bone marrow becomes fibrotic late in the disease.

In 95% of the patients with chronic myeloid leukemia, chromosome 22 is abnormal in the neutrophils, eosinophils, basophils, erythrocytic precursors and megakaryocytes. The abnormal chromosome is called the Philadelphia chromosome, because it was first described in Philadelphia in 1960. The Philadelphia chromosome is abnormally small because it has lost part of its long arms by a reciprocal translocation to chromosome 9.

Blood. In over 70% of patients with chronic myeloid leukemia, the leukocyte count is between 100 and $500 \times 10^9/L$ (100,000 and 500,000/mm^3) when the diagnosis is made. It can be as low as $25 \times 10^9/L$ (25,000/mm^3) or can be over $1000 \times 10^9/L$ (1,000,000/mm^3). The leukocytosis is due mainly to an excess of neutrophils, though eosinophils, basophils, and monocytes are usually also increased. The lymphocyte count remains normal.

Most of the granulocytes in the blood are segmented, but more primitive forms are present. Often between 20 and 50% of the granulocytes are metamyelocytes or myelocytes. Usually less than 10% are premyelocytes or myeloblasts, though if the leukocyte count is high, the proportion of blast cells may exceed 20%.

Most patients with chronic myeloid leukemia are mildly anemic when the diagnosis is made. Usually the concentration of hemoglobin in the blood is between 80 and 100 g/L (8 and 10 g/100 mL). The red cells are of normal size and normally supplied with hemoglobin, but there may be some anisocytosis or a slightly increased proportion of reticulocytes.

The platelet count is raised in 50% of the patients when first seen by a physician. Usually the increase is moderate, but at times the concentration of platelets is between 1000 and $3000 \times 10^9/L$ (1,000,000 and 3,000,000/mm^3). Usually the platelets are normal, but occasionally some of them are abnormally large. The platelet count usually falls as the disease progresses.

Alkaline phosphatase activity is low or even absent in the neutrophils in 90% of patients with chronic myeloid leukemia. Uricacidemia is common, because of the increased turnover of marrow cells. Gout may develop, but renal stones are uncommon. The concentration of histamine in the blood is usually increased in chronic myeloid leukemia, probably because of the increased concentration of basophils in the blood. The concentration of vitamin B_{12} in the plasma and vitamin B_{12} binding capacity are increased because of an increased concentration of transcobalamin I and of a third protein that binds the vitamin. The concentration of transcobalamin II, is normal or reduced.

Other Organs. The spleen is nearly always enlarged when the patient is first seen by a physician. Usually the spleen extends beyond the umbilicus, often down into the pelvis. It commonly weighs from 1000 to 4000 g. The spleen is firm and maintains its shape. Infarcts are common. The cut surface of the spleen is homogeneous and brick red. Recent infarcts are a bright yellow, then fade to white, and end as a scar.

Microscopically, the sinusoids in the spleen are distended by innumerable granulopoietic cells. All stages of differentiation are present, from myeloblasts to segmented granulocytes, in much the same proportion as in the marrow. Erythropoietic cells and megakaryocytes are ususally not present. The great increase in the size of the spleen is due almost entirely to the influx of granulocytic precursors.

The liver is enlarged in 50% of the patients at the time of diagnosis. Multiple clumps of granulopoietic cells distend its sinusoids.

Leukemic cells often infiltrate the lymph nodes, kidneys, adrenals, meninges, and other tissues. In most patients with chronic myeloid leukemia, these infiltrates are too small to be of clinical significance at the time the diagnosis is made.

Clinical Presentation. Chronic myeloid leukemia develops insidiously. About 20% of the patients are asymptomatic when the abnormalities in the blood are found during a routine medical examination. Most seek medical advice only when the disease is fully developed, often because of fatigue, fever, loss of weight, or the swelling and discomfort caused by splenomegaly. Splenic infarcts often cause acute abdominal pain as the rough surface of the infarct rubs on the parietal peritoneum. Arthralgia is sometimes severe. A peptic ulcer develops in the stomach or duodenum in 15% of the patients. Bruising, purpura, or bleeding into the retina are less common early signs of the disease. Infiltration of the tissues by the neoplastic cells sometimes causes neurologic signs, priapism, or lesions in the skin.

Pathogenesis. In most patients with chronic myeloid leukemia, the cause of the disease is unknown. The Philadelphia chromosome is not present at birth, but is acquired as chronic myeloid leukemia develops. By the time the disease is diagnosed, the clone derived from the neoplastic precursor carrying the Philadelphia chromosome has almost entirely replaced the normal bone marrow cells. The protooncogene c-abl is translocated from chromosome 9 to the breakpoint cluster region of chromosome 22 and the protooncogene c-sis is present on chromocome 22 near the break point. Activation of these oncogenes could have a part in the pathogenesis of the disease. The translocated c-abl produces a messenger ribonucleic acid and a protein not present in normal cells. In patients with chronic myeloid leukemia who do not have the Philadelphia chromosome, other genetic rearrangements affect the protooncogenes in similar fashion.

Only in a few kindred is the Philadelphia chromosome inherited. In these people, it is present in all the cells of the body, not only in the hematopoietic cells of the bone marrow. The risk of developing chronic myeloid leukemia is high.

Radiation increases the risk of developing chronic myeloid leukemia. In Hiroshima, survivors of the atomic bomb were 20 times more likely to develop leukemia than was the general population. In Nagasaki, the risk of leukemia increased 10 times. The bomb dropped on Hiroshima released more gamma radiation, and the bomb at Nagasaki was richer in neutron radiation. The smaller doses of radiation given therapeutically also increase the risk of developing myeloid leukemia. Irradiation of the spine in ankylosing spondylitis increases the risk of leukemia tenfold if the dose is greater than 2000 rads. Radioactive phosphorus used to treat polycythemia vera increases the risk of myeloid leukemia 10 times.

Treatment and Prognosis. Patients with chronic myeloid leukemia live from a few months to over 20 years from the time of diagnosis. Most survive about three years. For most of this time, the disease can be controlled by busulfan and other cytotoxic drugs. The leukocyte count returns to normal, and primitive cells disappear from the blood. The drug relieves the symptoms but does not eradicate the clone of neoplastic cells carrying the Philadelphia chromosome. Massive doses of chemotherapeutic drugs do not improve the prognosis.

In 85% of the patients, death is caused by a blast crisis. Each year, 25% of patients with chronic myeloid leukemia develop a blast crisis. The crisis often begins abruptly, but sometimes develops gradually, as the leukemia fails to respond to busulfan and other drugs. Occasionally a patient first seeks advice in a blast crisis. If the crisis develops gradually, the leukocyte count rises, and immature cells reappear in the blood. Anemia worsens and the platelet count falls. The patient becomes weak and often feverish. Infiltration of the tissues by leukemic cells increases. The risk of infection and hemorrhage grows greater.

In the blast crisis, more than 20% of the circulating white cells and more than 30% of the hematopoietic cells in the bone marrow are blasts. In 70% of the patients, the blast cells are granulocytes, and the patient develops acute myeloid leukemia. In 30%, the cells are lymphoblasts, and the patient develops acute lymphoid leukemia. Rarely, a patient develops eosinophilic leukemia or erythroleukemia.

The new clone of more malignant cells overgrows the bone marrow. In the patients with acute myeloid leukemia the activity of alkaline phosphatase in the granulocytes is often great. New chromosomal abnormalities appear in the hematopoietic cells in the bone marrow, though the Philadelphia chromosome persists and may be duplicated. The patients with acute lymphoid leukemia usually have terminal deoxynucleotidyl transferase and the common acute lymphoblastic leukemia antigen on the blast cells.

As the crisis worsens, the leukocyte count usually falls. Neutropenia, thrombocytopenia, and anemia grow increasingly severe. The spleen and liver enlarge. The lymph nodes, kidneys, and other organs are often extensively infiltrated by neoplastic cells. The leukemia no longer responds to chemotherapy, though in 20% of the patients vincristine and prednisone bring a short remission. Death usually comes in a few months.

Bone marrow transplantation from a compatible donor after destruction of the bone marrow by chemotherapy and radiation gives long-term survival in 70% of patients treated early in the disease. In a few of these people the disease has recurred. Most are probably cured.

Patients with chronic myeloid leukemia who do not have the Philadelphia chromosome have a poor prognosis. Their disease is often atypical, with features of myelofibrosis. In children one or two years old, this form of chronic myeloid leukemia usually brings death within a year.

ACUTE MYELOID LEUKEMIA. Each year, one person in 100,000 dies of acute myeloid leukemia. About 60% of the patients are men. Acute myeloid leukemia can occur at any age, but most of the patients are 40 or more years old.

Because of the difficulty in disintguishing between acute lymphocytic, acute myeloid, acute monocytic, and acute erythrocytic leukemias, some prefer to group the nonlymphocytic forms together as acute nonlymphocytic leukemia. If acute myeloid leukemia becomes evident in the first weeks of life, it is called congenital leukemia.

Lesions. In acute myeloid leukemia, the bone marrow is replaced by a clone of poorly differentiated malignant cells. Usually, the tumor cells escape into the blood and infiltrate other organs.

The French-American-British (FAB) classification of acute myeloid leukemia divides it into four morphologic types, M1 or undifferentiated leukemia, M2 or differentiated myeloblastic leukemia, M3 or promyelocytic leukemia, and M4 or myelomonocytic leukemia. Monocytic leukemia is classed as M5, erythroleukemia as M6, and megakaryocytic leukemia as M7.

Bone Marrow. Macroscopically, the bone marrow is soft, red, and gelatinous in acute myeloid leukemia. Often red marrow extends into the proximal part of the long bones.

Microscopically, the bone marrow is usually hyperplastic, with little fat remaining. Occasionally it is hypoplastic. Frequently more than 70% of the cells in the marrow are myeloblasts. More differentiated granulocytes are few. Foci of necrosis are sometimes present. Less often the leukemia is less anaplastic, and a greater proportion of more differentiated granulocytes are present among the myeloblasts. Erythropoiesis and megakaryocytes are diminished. Often the red cell precursors are megaloblasts, like those of pernicious anemia.

Chromosomal abnormalities are present in the leukemic cells in 70% of the patients. About 20 structural anomalies occur frequently in acute myeloid leukemia. Trisomy 7 and trisomy 8 are common. A transposition between chromosomes 8 and 21 is found most frequently in acute myeloid leukemia of type M2, transposition between 15 ans 17 is most common in promyelocytic leukemia of type M3, pericentric inversion of chromosome 16 is found principally in myelomonocytic leukemia of type M4 with eosinophilia, and transposition between chromosomes 9 and 11 is found most often in monocytic leukemia of type M5. Other chromosomal abnormalities develop as the leukemia grows more anaplastic. The Philadelphia chromosome is not present.

Blood. In acute myeloid leukemia, the leukocyte count is normal or below normal in 45% of the patients. In 30%, it is less than 5×10^9/L (5000/mm^3). If it is increased, the increase is usually only moderate. Only in 15% of the patients is the leukocyte count over 100×10^9/L (100,000/mm^3).

In 25% of the patients, acute myeloid leukemia is of the M1 or undifferentiated type. From 30 to 90% of the granulocytes in the blood are myeloblasts. Most of the others are segmented, with a few intermediate forms. The myeloblasts have round nu-

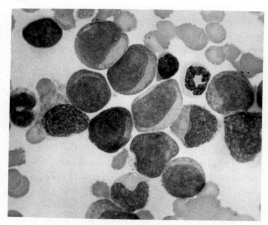

Fig. 50-4. A blood film from a patient with acute myeloblastic leukemia. (Courtesy of Dr. J. H. Crookston)

clei with fine chromatin and prominent nucleoli. Their chromatin contains no granules. They are peroxidase and nonspecific esterase negative.

About 35% of the patients have M2 or differentiated myeloblastic leukemia. The blast cells are like those in type M1, but their cytoplasm contains a few granules that stain for peroxidase but weakly if at all for nonspecific esterase.

In 5% of the patients, more than 50% of the immature granulocytes in the blood have numerous cytoplasmic granules, which stain for peroxidase. Often the granules in the cells are larger than those in normal promyelocytes and are oval rather than round. The nuclei have fine chromatin and prominent nucleoli. These patients have M3 or myelocytic leukemia.

In 35% of the patients the predominant cell in the blood has a folded nucleus with fine, reticular chromatin. The cytoplasm is more abundant than in a myeloblast. Often the cells are irregularly shaped, with pseudopodia. In some of the patients, granules are present in the cytoplasm. Often the cells stain strongly for nonspecific esterase, less strongly for peroxidase. Such people are said to have M4 or myelomonocytic leukemia. Lysozyme is often present in the plasma.

In a few people with acute myeloid leukemia few primitive granulocytes are present in the blood. Such people are said to have

subleukemic leukemia. If no primitive cells can be found in the blood, the person is said to have aleukemic leukemia.

In up to 30% of patients with acute myeloid leukemia, some of the primitive cells in the blood have in their cytoplasm rods or elliptical bodies, which stain red with the usual stains for blood films. These bodies are called Auer rods, after an American physician (1875–1948). They are rare in the blast crises of chronic myeloid leukemia. Up to 50% of patients with acute myeloid leukemia have phi bodies in the cytoplasm of some of the primitive cells in the blood. The phi bodies are shaped like Auer rods, but stain only for catalase or peroxidase.

Immunologic stains are valuable in distinguishing between acute myeloid, acute lymphoid, and acute monocytic leukemia. When ordinary stains are used, the three kinds of malignant cells are similar. The antibodies OKM-1 and Mo-1 react with the leukemic cells in 50% of patients with acute myeloid leukemia; in 80% of the patients these antibodies react with its myeloblastic or myelomonocytic variants. MY-7 reacts with the tumor cells in 80% of patients with myeloid leukemia. MY-3 and MY-4 react with the leukemic cells in 90% of people with the myeloblastic or myelomonocytic types of acute myeloid leukemia. The antibodies cross react with the malignant cells in monocytic leukemia, but not with those of acute lymphoid leukemia. The malignant cells in acute myeloid leukemia do not take the stains for lymphocytes.

The concentration of hemoglobin in the blood is usually between 30 and 80 g/L (3 and 8 g/100 mL) when the patient is first seen by a physician. The red cells may be normocytic and normochromic, or may be larger. Nucleated red cells are sometimes present. Reticulocytes are usually scarce.

Thrombocytopenia is present in 80% of the patients when the diagnosis is made. In 40%, the platelet count is less than $50 \times 10^9/L$ (50,000/mm^3). Large, atypical platelets are sometimes present in the blood.

The activity of alkaline phosphatase in the mature neutrophils is reduced, though there may not be enough of them to make the estimation useful. Uricacidemia is present in 50% of the patients. The urinary excre-

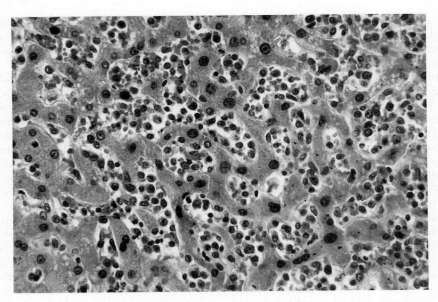

Fig. 50-5. Leukemic cells in the hepatic sinusoids in a patient with myelomocytic leukemia.

tion of uric acid is nearly always increased, though gout is unusual, and renal injury is exceptional, except in patients under treatment with cytotoxic agents. There is often hypergammaglobulinemia.

Other Organs.   The spleen is enlarged in 50% of patients with acute myeloid leukemia at the time the diagnosis is made. It rarely extends more than 5 cm below the costal margin. The enlargement is caused by the accumulation of leukemic cells in the splenic sinusoids. Sometimes leukemic cells can be found in the endothelium-lined spaces in the intima of the trabecular vessels in the spleen, though the invasion of the intima is not as prominent as in acute lymphoid leukemia. Infarcts of the spleen occur in 10% of the patients. The liver is enlarged in 50% of the patients at the time of diagnosis because of the accumulation of leukemic cells in the sinusoids. The lymph nodes are often moderately enlarged, especially in children, sometimes because of infection or infiltration with leukemic cells.

The sternum is tender in 70% of the patients, because of the hyperplasia of the bone marrow. Pain or tenderness in the long bones is common in children with acute lymphoid leukemia, but is found in only 20%

of people with acute myeloid leukemia. Infiltration of the skin with leukemic cells causes diffuse or localized violaceous plaques or reddish-purple nodules in 10% of patients with acute myeloid leukemia. Infiltration of the meninges is less common and usually less extensive than in acute lymphoid leukemia. Often the leukemic cells accumulate in enormous numbers in the kidneys, crowding into the interstitial tissues, often doubling the weight of the kidneys and turning them a uniform yellowish white, often with streaks or blotches of hemorrhage. Renal function is not usually impaired. Sometimes the nephrotic syndrome develops. Leukemic infiltrates sometimes cause ulceration in the stomach or the intestine. Hemorrhages in the fundus of the eyes are present in 15% of the patients. Infiltration of the lungs or other organs can occur.

Infection is common because of the lack of normal neutrophils, especially in the lungs and the skin. Particularly in people with myelomonocytic leukemia, infection of the gums with marked gingival hypertrophy or infection and ulceration in the throat is often striking.

Clinical Presentation.   Weakness and fatigue that develop gradually over several months are often the first sign of acute myeloid leukemia. Over 50% of the patients lose weight. Fever develops in 20%. Bruising or excessive bleeding occurs early in the disease in 10%.

Pathogenesis. In most patients with acute myeloid leukemia, its cause is unknown, or the disease complicates chronic myeloid leukemia. The chromosomal abnormalities are caused by the disease and are not its cause. Only in a minority of the patients is it caused by radiation, benzene poisoning, or occasionally a cytotoxic drug. Its incidence is increased twentyfold in Down syndrome, and it sometimes complicates Fanconi's anemia.

Treatment and Prognosis. Without treatment, most patients with acute myeloid leukemia die within a few weeks or months. Almost none live a year. Spontaneous remissions occur in less than 10% of the patients and are short lived. All features of the disease worsen rapidly. The marrow is increasingly replaced by the tumor. Anemia and thrombocytopenia deepen, and the few functional neutrophils disappear. The concentration of blast cells in the blood may fall, remain much the same, or increase.

In 90% of the patients, death comes from infection, as the neutropenia makes bacterial infection uncontrollable; from hemorrhage caused by the thrombocytopenia; or from some combination of infection and hemorrhage. The hemorrhage is most often subarachnoid or from the gut. Sometimes the leukocyte count becomes so high that the blasts in the blood clog the cerebral vessels and cause intracerebral hemorrhage. Sometimes fungal infections become striking, as the opportunistic fungi prey on the defenseless and dying body.

The cytotoxic drugs—6-mercaptopurine, thioguanine, cytarabine, daunorubicin, vincristine, and others—usually used in combination and together with prednisone, bring remission in more than 50% of the patients. The blast cells may disappear from the blood, and all symptoms disappear. Most remissions last only a few weeks or months. Some last a year or more. Few patients live more than two years. About 10% remain in remission for more than five years, even though treatment has been stopped, and may be cured.

Bone marrow transfusion after destroying the leukemic cells with cytotoxic drugs can cure the leukemia. About 50% of the patients are alive two years after the transplant and may be cured.

The prognosis is best in patients who have a transposition between chromosomes 8 and 21 and is worst in those with abnormalities of chromosome 5. The intensity of the treatment makes little difference in patients with deletion of chromosome 5 or its short limb, but a high dosage of chemotherapeutic drugs improves the survival of patients with a transposition between chromosomes 15 and 17.

EOSINOPHILIC LEUKEMIA. Eosinophilic leukemia is uncommon. Chronic eosinophilic leukemia differs from the usual form of chronic myeloid leukemia only in that eosinophils are the predominant cell in the blood. Acute eosinophilic leukemia is usually a form of promyelocytic leukemia in which most of the neoplastic cells circulating in the blood are eosinophils.

A more highly differentiated form of acute eosinophilic leukemia occurs but is difficult to distinguish from non-neoplastic eosinophilia. The concentration of eosinophils in the blood is high, over $100 \times 10^9/L$ (100,000/mm^3). The eosinophils have segmented nuclei, but are bigger than normal, with few granules. The lungs often show shifting infiltrates, as in Löffler's syndrome. Endomyocardial fibrosis with overlying thrombosis, congestive heart failure, thrombophlebitis with emboli, anemia, neutropenia, and thrombocytopenia sometimes develop. Occasionally blast cells become numerous in the blood in the terminal stage.

BASOPHILIC LEUKEMIA. Chronic basophilic leukemia is like other types of chronic myeloid leukemia, except that basophils are numerous in the blood. Acute basophil leukemia is a promyelocytic leukemia in which most of the circulating leukemic cells are basophils. Both forms of basophil leukemia are rare.

Systemic mastocytosis is also rare. Large numbers of mast cells circulate in the blood. The number of mast cells in the skin and other organs is increased. There is little evidence that the mast cells are neoplastic.

ERYTHROLEUKEMIA AND ERYTHREMIC MYELOSIS. Erythroleukemia and erythremic myelosis are rare conditions in which both neoplastic red cells and neoplastic granulocytes circulate in the blood. In erythroleukemia, sometimes called Di Guglielmo's disease after the Italian physician who described it in 1926, both neoplastic red cells and neoplastic granulocytes are prominent in the blood and bone marrow. In erythremic myelosis, neoplastic red cells predominate.

Chronic erythroleukemia and chronic erythremic myelosis are similar to the usual form of chronic myeloid leukemia. More often erythroleukemia and erythremic myelosis are acute, with neoplastic erythroblasts and myeloblasts in the blood and bone marrow. The cytoplasm of the neoplastic erythroblasts stains strongly with the periodic acid-Schiff reaction. Normal erythroblasts and myeloblasts do not stain.

CHLOROMA. Rarely, localized tumors appear in a patient with acute myeloid leukemia, usually a child or young adult. Occasionally, a local mass appears before other manifestations of leukemia are evident. Most often the tumor is subperiosteal. It is especially common in the orbit, where it may cause exopthalmos.

When sectioned, the tumor turns green for a few minutes, probably because of the myeloperoxidase in the leukemic cells. The green color gives the lesion its name of chloroma, from the Greek for green. Microscopically, the tumor consists of a mass of leukemic cells, like those in the blood.

Myelodysplastic Syndromes

The myelodysplastic syndromes, sometimes called the preleukemic syndromes, are preneoplastic disorders in which an abnormal clone of hematopoietic cells causes changes in the bone marrow and the blood that progress to leukemia. Most patients are over 50 years old and have refractory anemia that does not respond to treatment.

The bone marrow is usually hyperplastic. All types of hematopoietic cell are abnormal. The precursors of the red cells are often multinucleate or have fragmented nuclei. Nucleocytoplasmic asynchrony may be evident. Ringed sideroblasts like those seen in the sideroblastic anemias are often present. The granulocytic precursors usually have few granules. The chromatin in their nuclei is condensed. Hyposegmentation is common. In 50% of the patients, the megakaryocytes are abnormally small or have multiple nuclei.

Most of the patients are anemic. Often some of the red cells in the blood are abnormally shaped, stippled, or nucleated. Reticulocytes are few. In 80% of the patients, about 10% of the hemoglobin in the red cells is hemoglobin F. Many of the patients have granulocytopenia. Commonly the circulating granulocytes are poorly granulated and hyposegmented. Thrombocytopenia is frequent, and often the platelets are abnormal. Some patients have lymphopenia, with a deficiency of helper T cells.

Chromosomal abnormalities are present in the hematopoietic cells in the bone marrow in 50% of patients with a myelodysplastic syndrome. The most common anomalies are monosomy 7, 7q−, trisomy 8, monosomy 5, 5q−, and lack of the Y chromosome.

Several myelodysplastic syndromes have been described. In refractory anemia without ringed sideroblasts, less than 15% of the nucleated cells in the bone marrow are sideroblasts. In refractory anemia with ringed sideroblasts, more than 15% of the nucleated cells are sideroblasts. Patients with refractory anemia with an excess of blasts have up to 20% of blast cells in the bone marrow and up to 5% in the blood. Some patients develop chronic (myelomonocytic leukemia; some have refractory anemia in transition to leukemia.

Leukemia develops in 50% of patients with a myelodysplastic syndrome within a year; in 75%, within 2 years. Most progress to acute myeloid leukemia. In some acute lymphoid leukemia, chronic myeloid leukemia, or myelofibrosis develops. In a few, the condition persists for up to 20 years with little change.

BIBLIOGRAPHY

General

Frisch, B., Lewis, S. M., Burkhardt, R., and Bartl, R.: Biopsy Pathology of Bone and Bone Marrow. London, Chapman and Hall, 1985.

Hardisty, R. M., and Weatherall, D. J.: Blood and Its Disorders. 2nd Ed. Oxford, Blackwell, 1982.

Jandl, J. H.: Blood. Boston, Little, Brown and Co., 1987.

Wickramasinghe, S. N. (ed.): Blood and Bone Marrow. In Systemic Pathology, 3rd Ed. Edited by Symmers, W. St. C: London, Churchill Livingstone, 1986.

Williams, W. J., Beutler, E., Erslav, A. J., and Lichtman, M. A.: Hematology. 3rd Ed. New York, McGraw-Hill, 1983.

Wintrobe, M. M., et al.: Clinical Hematology. 8th Ed. Philadelphia, Lea & Febiger, 1981.

Wittels, B.: Surgical Pathology of Bone Marrow. Philadelphia, W. B. Saunders, 1985.

Zucker-Franklin, D., Greaves, M. F., Grossi, C. E., and Marmont, A. M.: Atlas of Blood Cells. 2nd Ed. Philadelphia, Lea & Febiger, 1988.

Granulocytopenia

Chaplin, S.: Bone marrow depression due to mianserin, phenylbutazone, oxyphenbutazone, and chloramphenicol—Part I. Adverse Drug React. Acute Poisoning Rev., 5:97, 1986.

Lalezari, P.: Autoimmune neutropenia. In The Autoimmune Diseases. Edited by Rose, N. R., and Mackay, I. R. Orlando, FL, Academic Press, 1985.

Lindenbaum, J.: Hematological complications of alcohol abuse. Semin. Liver Dis., 7:169, 1987.

Granulocytosis

Bagby, G. C. (Ed.): Hematological aspects of systemic disease. Hematol. Oncol. Clin. North Am., 1:167, 1987.

Spry, C. J., and Kumaraswami, V.: Tropical eosinophilia. Semin. Hematol., 19:107–115, 1982.

Abnormal Granulocytes

Boxer, G. J., Curnutte, J. T., and Boxer, L. A.: Disorders of polymorphonuclear leukocyte function. Hosp. Pract., 20(3):69, 20(4):129, 1985.

Boxer, L. A., and Morganroth, M. L.: Neutrophil function disorders. Dis. Mon., 32(12):681, 1987.

Cline, M. J. (Ed.): Leucocyte function. Edinburgh, Churchill Livingstone, 1981.

Curnette, J. T.: Phagocytic defects. Hematol. Oncol. Clin. North Am., 2:1, 1988.

Gallin, J. I.: Neutrophil specific granule deficiency. Annu. Rev. Med., 36:263, 1985.

Repo, H.: Defects in phagocytic functions. Ann. Clin. Res., 19:263, 1987.

White, C. J., and Gallin, J. I.: Phagocytic defects. Clin. Immunol. Immunopathol., 40:50, 1986.

Myelofibrosis

Barosi, G., and Polino, G.: Chronic myelofibrosis with myeloid metaplasia. Haematologica, 72:553, 1987.

Tumors

Abbondanzo, S. L., Anagnou, N. P., and Abbondanzo, Sacher, R. A.: Myelodysplastic syndrome with acquired hemoglobin H disease. Am. J. Clin. Pathol., 89:401, 1988.

Aksoy, M. (Ed.): Benzene Carcinogenicity. Boca Raton, FL, CRC Press, 1988.

Alderson, M.: The epidemiology of leukemia. Adv. Cancer Res., 31:2, 1980.

Antin, J. H., and Rosenthal, D. S.: Acute leukemias, myelodysplasia, and lymphomas. Clin. Geriatr. Med., 1:795, 1985.

Austin, H., Delzell, E., and Cole, P.: Benzene and leukemia. Am. J. Epidemiol., 127:419, 1988.

Bagby, G. C., Jr.: The concept of preleukemia. CRC Crit. Rev. Oncol. Hematol., 4:203, 1986.

Beris, P., and Miescher, P. A.: Primary acquired myelodysplastic syndromes. Ergb. Inn. Med. Kinderheit., 56:129, 1988.

Bitter, M. A., et al.: Associations between morphology, karyotype and clinical features in myeloid leukemias. Hum. Pathol., 18:211, 1987.

Bloomfield. C. D.: Chromosomal abnormalities in acute leukemia. Schweiz. Med. Wochenschr., 115:1501, 1985.

Bloomfield, C. D. (Ed.): Acute myeloid leukemia. Semin. Oncol., 14:357, 1987.

Brandt, L.: Environmental factors and leukaemia. Med. Oncol. Tumor Pharmacother., 2:7, 1985.

Brandt, L.: Leukaemia and lymphoma risks derived from solvents. Med. Oncol. Tumor Pharamacother., 4:199, 1987.

Brunning, R. D., and McKenna, R. W.: Immunologic markers for acute leukemia. Monogr. Pathol., 29:124, 1987.

Brusamolino, E., Pagnucco, G., and Bernasconi, C.: Acute leukemia occurring in a primary neoplasia (secondary leukemia). Haematologica, 71:60, 1986.

Butturini, A., and Gale, R. P.: Oncogenes and human leukemias. Int. J. Cell Cloning, 6:2, 1988.

Butturini, A., Sthivelman, E., Canaani, E., and Gale, R. P.: Oncogenes in human leukemias. Acta Haematologica, 78(Suppl 1):2, 1987.

Cacciola, E. (Ed.): Hemato-oncology and hemato-immunology. Acta Haematologica, 78(Suppl 1):1, 1987.

Canellos, G. P., and Griffin, J. D.: Chronic granulocytic leukemia: the heterogeneity of stem cell differentiation within a single disease entity. Semin. Oncol., 12:281, 1985.

Castoldi, G., Cuneo, A., Tomasi, P. and Ferraro, L: Chromosome abnormalities in myelofibrosis. Acta Haematologica, 78(Suppl 1):104, 1987.

Catovsky, D. (Ed.): The Leukemic Cell. Edinburgh, Churchill Livingstone, 1981.

Cazzola, M., and Riccardi, A.: Myelodysplastic syndromes: Biologic and clinical aspects. Haematologica, 71:147, 1986.

Chaganti, R. S. K.: Significance of chromosome change to hematopoietic neoplasms. Blood, 62:515, 1983.

Chaganti, R. S. K.: Cytogenetics of leukemia and lymphoma. Monogr. Pathol., 29:184, 1987.

Champlin, R., Gale, R. P., Foon, K. A., and Golde, D. W.: Chronic leukemias: oncogenes, chromosomes, and advances in therapy. Ann. Intern. Med., *104*:671, 1986.

Chan, J. K. C., Ng, C. S., and Hui, P. K.: A simple guide to the terminology and application of leucocyte monoclonal antibodies. Histopathology, *12*:461, 1988.

Dean, B. J.: Recent findings on the genetic toxicity of benzene, toluene, xylenes and phenols. Mutat. Res., *154*:153, 1985.

Dinsmore, R., and O'Reilly, R. J.: Bone marrow transplantation. Pathobiol. Annu., *12*:213, 1982.

Drexler, H. G.: Classification of acute myelogenous leukemia. Leukemia, *1*:697, 1987.

Drexler, H. G., and Minowada, J.: The use of monclonal antibodies for the identification and classification of acute myeloid leukemias. Leuk. Res., *10*:279, 1986.

Favara, B. E., et al.: The leukemias of childhood. Perspect. Pediatr. Pathol., *9*:75, 1987.

Fong. C.-t., and Brodeur, G. M.: Down's syndrome and leukemia. Cancer Genet. Cytogenet., *28*:55, 1987.

Foon, K. A., and Todd, R. F. III: Immunologic classification of leukemia and lymphoma. Blood, *68*:1, 1986.

Freedman, A. S., and Nadler, L. M.: Cell surface markers in hematologic malignancies. Semin. Oncol., *14*:193, 1987.

Freireich, E. J.: Adult acute leukemia. Hosp. Pract., *21*(6):91, 1986.

Gale, R. P. (Ed.): Acute leukemias. Semin. Hematol., *24*:1, 1987.

Gale, R. P. (Ed.): Chronic myelogenous leukemia. Semin. Hematol., *25*:1, 1988.

Goldman, J. M.: The Philadelphia chromosome from cytogenetics to oncogenes. Br. J. Haematol., *66*:435, 1987.

Greaves, M. F.: Speculations on the cause of childhood acute leukemia. Leukemia, *2*:120, 1988.

Greenberg, P. L.: Biologic nature of the myelodysplastic syndromes. Acta Haematol., *78*(Suppl 1):94, 1987.

Griffin, J. D. (Ed.): Myelodysplastic syndromes. Clin. Haematol., *15*:909, 1986.

Grignani, F.: Chronic myelogenous leukemia. CRC Crit. Rev. Oncol. Hematol., *4*:31, 1985.

Gunz, F. W., and Henderson, E. S. (Eds.): Leukemia. 4th Ed. New York, Grune and Stratton, 1983.

Gössner, W., Gerber, G. B., Hagen, U., and Luz, A. (Eds.): The radiobiology of radium and thorotrast. Mnchen, Urban and Schwarzenberg, 1986.

Hakami, N., and Monzon, C. M.: Acute nonlymphocyte leukemia in children. Clin. Hematol. Oncol. North Am., *1*:567, 1987.

Harris, H.: The genetic analysis of malignancy. J. Cell Biol., Suppl 4:431, 1986.

Heim, S., and Mitelman, F.: Cancer Cytogenetics. New York, Alan R. Liss, 1987.

Hoogstraten, B. (Ed.): Hematologic malignancies. Berlin, Springer-Verlag, 1985.

Infante, P. F., and White, M. C.: Projections of leukemia risk associated with occupational exposure to benzene. Am. J. Indust. Med., *7*:403, 1985.

Ishak, K. G., and Zimmerman, H. J.: Hepatic toxicity of drugs used for hematologic neoplasia. Semin. Liver Dis., *7*:237, 1987.

Jacobs, A.: Myelodysplastic syndromes: pathogenesis, functional abnormalities, and clinical implications. J.

Clin. Pathol., *38*:1201, 1985.

Koeffler, H. P.: Syndromes of acute nonlymphocytic leukemia. Ann. Intern. Med., *107*:748, 1987.

Kolb, H. J.: Allogenic bone marrow transplantation in leukemia. Rec. Res. Cancer Res., *93*:269, 1984.

Konopka, J. B., and Witte, O. N.: Activation of the abl oncogene in murine and human leukemias. Biochim. Biophys. Acta. *823*:1, 1985.

Kurzrock, R., et al.: Expression of c-abl in Philadelphia-positive acute myelogenous leukemia. Blood, *70*:1584, 1987.

Lawler, S. D.: Significance of chromosome abnormalities in leukemia. Semin. Hematol., *19*:257, 1982.

Layton, D. M., and Mufti, G. J.: The myelodysplastic syndromes. Br. Med. J., *295*:227, 1987.

Le Beau, M. M.: Chromosomal fragile sites and cancer-specific rearrangements. Blood, *67*:849, 1986.

Le Beau, M. M., and Rowley, J. D.: Chromosomal abnormalities in leukemia and lymphoma. Adv. Hum. Genet., *15*:1, 1986.

McCoy, E. E., and Epstein, C. J. (Eds.): Oncology and immunology of Down syndrome. Prog. Clin. Biol. Res., *246*:1–2, 1987.

McCulloch, E. A.: Normal stem cells and the clonal hemopathies. Prog. Clin. Biol. Res., *184*:21, 1985.

McCulloch, E. A.: Regulatory mechanisms affecting the blast stem cells of acute myeloblastic leukemia. J. Cell Physiol. [Suppl], *4*:27, 1986.

McDonald, G. B., Shulman H. M., Sullivan, K. M., and Spencer, G. D.: Intestinal and hepatic complications of human bone marrow transplantation. Gastroenterology, *90*:460, 770–784, 1986.

Mes-Masson, A. M., and Witte, O. N.: Role of the abl oncogene in chronic myelogenous leukemia. Adv. Cancer Res., *49*:53, 1987.

Miller, R. W.: Recent advances in the epidemiology of leukemia and lymphoma. Monogr. Pathol., *29*:81, 1987.

Modan, B.: Cancer and leukaemia risks after low-level radiation. Med. Oncol. Tumor Pharmother., *4*:151, 1987.

Mole, R. H.: Leukaemia induction in man by radionuclides and some relevant experimental and human observations. Strahlentherapie Sonderbund, *80*:1, 1986.

Najean, Y.: The iatrogenic leukaemias induced by radio- and/or chemotherapy. Med. Oncol. Tumor Pharmacother., *4*:245, 1987.

Netzel, B., Haas, R. I., and Thierfelder, S.: Allogenic bone marrow transplantation in leukemia. Rec. Res. Cancer Res., *93*:290, 1984.

Nimer, S. D., and Golde, D. W.: The 5q− abnormality. Blood, *70*:1705, 1987.

Oscier, D. G.: Myelodysplastic syndromes. Baillière's Clin. Haematol., *1*:389, 1987.

Papas, T. S., et al.: The cellular ets genes. Cancer Invest., *4*:555, 1986.

Pedersen-Bjergaard, J., and Philip, P.: Chromosome characteristics of therapy-related acute non-lymphocytic leukemia and preleukemia. Leuk. Res., *11*:315, 1987.

Peschle, C. (Ed.): Normal and neoplastic blood cells. Ann. N.Y. Acad. Sci., *511*:1, 1987.

Peterson, B. A., and Levine, E. G.: Uncommon subtypes of nonlymphocytic leukemia. Semin. Oncol.,

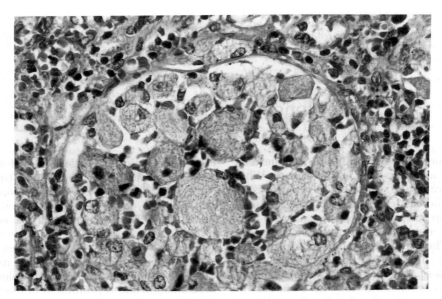

Fig. 51-1. Gaucher cells in the spleen.

tween the normal and that of homozygotes, but do not develop the disease.

Three types of Gaucher's disease are distinguished. The most common and the mildest is the adult type. The juvenile type is of intermediate severity and is the least common. The infantile type is the most severe. In the adult form of the disease, the activity of β-glucocerebrosidase is between 15 and 40% of normal. In the infantile form, it is less than 10% of normal. The adult and juvenile forms of Gaucher's disease can occur in the same kindred, though in different families. In kindred with the juvenile type of the disease, all those affected have the juvenile form.

Adult Type. About 1000 cases of the adult type of Gaucher's disease have been reported. It is particularly common in Ashkanazi Jews, being found in one child in every 2500 born alive. In spite of its name, the adult form of Gaucher's disease can present at any age. Usually it becomes evident in childhood or early adult life. Men and women are affected equally.

Lesions. Macrophages throughout the body become distended with glucosylceramide. The distended macrophages are called Gaucher cells. They have a small eccentric nucleus and abundant, faintly eosinophilic cytoplasm. By light microscopy, the cytoplasm is vaguely striated, resembling crumpled tissue paper or crumpled silk. It stains strongly with the periodic acid-Schiff reaction and for acid phosphatase. The activity of acid phosphatase in the plasma is increased.

Electron microscopy shows that the glucosylceramide accumulates in the lysosomes of the macrophages. It forms tubules 200 to 300 nm in diameter.

The macrophages distended with glucosylceramide accumulate especially in the spleen. In most patients, the spleen is enlarged, sometimes to more than 5000 g. Microscopically, it shows clumps and nodules of Gaucher cells throughout the red pulp. The liver is frequently enlarged by glucosylceramide stored in the Kupffer cells and sometimes in macrophages in the portal triads. Sometimes clumps of Gaucher cells are present in the lungs.

In 70% of the patients, accumulation of glucosylceramide in macrophages in the bone marrow causes swelling or rarefaction of some of the tubular bones. Often the lower end of the femur is swollen and roentgenographically looks like an Erlenmeyer flask, with a thin cortex and a radiolucent core.

Erosion of the bones sometimes causes pathologic fractures, collapse of vertebral bodies, or Legg-Perthe's disease.

In more than 50% of the patients, increased deposition of melanin in the epidermis turns the skin a dirty yellow. The discoloration is particularly marked on the face, hands, and shins. Pigmented pingueculae sometimes develop in the conjunctiva. Gaucher cells distended with glucosylceramide are present in the pingueculae and in the dermis.

Some patients with Gaucher's disease develop hypersplenism, with anemia, thrombocytopenia, or less often granulocytopenia. Epistaxis, bleeding from the gums, and purpura are common in these patients. Occasionally hypersplenism is the principal feature of the disease, with little or no enlargement of the spleen or other organs.

β-Glucosylceramidase is deficient in fibroblasts and other cells as well as in macrophages. The diagnosis of Gaucher's disease can be confirmed by culturing fibrocytes and demonstrating the reduced activity of the enzyme.

Clinical Presentation. The adult form of Gaucher's disease is often discovered accidentally when splenomegaly is found during a routine examination. In some patients, the discomfort caused by the large spleen or pain from splenic infarcts draws attention to the disease. Less often hypersplenism, pain in the bones, a pathologic fracture, or involvement of the lungs is the first sign of the disease.

Treatment and Prognosis. In the adult form of Gaucher's disease, the prognosis is good. Most patients die of some unrelated condition after a normal life span. The deficient enzyme cannot be replaced, but radiation relieves the pain in the bones and splenectomy usually controls hypersplenism.

Juvenile Type. The juvenile type of Gaucher's disease is most common in Sweden. It becomes evident in infancy. Mental retardation and often lesions in the brain stem are added to splenomegaly, hepatomegaly, and lesions in the bones like those in the adult type of the disease. Some of the patients die in infancy. Some survive to adolescence.

Infantile Type. About 15% of patients with Gaucher's disease have the infantile type of the disorder. Severe retardation of growth, strabismus, spasticity, dysphagia, opisthotonos, and other evidence of severe injury to the nervous system appear during the first six months of life. The liver and spleen are usually enlarged, though the bones are rarely involved. Nodules of Gaucher cells in the lungs are common. Cachexia and death come within six months.

The brain of infants with the infantile type of Gaucher's disease shows degeneration and loss of neurons. The cause of the degeneration is not apparent. Glucocerebrosides are rarely found in the neurons, but are sometimes found in macrophages that accumulate around blood vessels in the white matter. In other organs, the lesions are like those of the adult type of Gaucher's disease.

SECONDARY GLUCOCEREBROSIDOSIS. Macrophages like those of Gaucher's disease, with similar accumulations of tubular glucocerebroside in their lysosomes, are sometimes found in the bone marrow or the spleen in patients with chronic myeloid leukemia or thalassemia. In these patients, the activity of β-glucocerebrosidase is normal. Presumably the glucocerebrosides accumulate because the massive destruction of cells caused by the leukemia or thalassemia releases so much glucocerebroside that the macrophages cannot catabolize all of it.

NIEMANN-PICK DISEASE. Niemann-Pick disease is named after the German physicians Niemann, who described it in 1914, and Pick, who described it in 1922. Sphingomyelin accumulates in macrophages throughout the body and sometimes in neurons and other cells. Cholesterol is also present in excess in these cells. Occasionally other kinds of phospholipid are present in abnormal quantity.

Niemann-Pick disease is rare. It is most common in inbred communities, often in Jews. Men and women are affected equally.

Five types of Niemann-Pick disease are distinguished: type A, also called the infantile type; type B, called the visceral type; type C; type D; and type E. All are inherited as an autosomal recessive character.

Infantile Type. In 85% of patients with Niemann-Pick disease, the disease is of the infantile type, also called the classic type or type A. This form of the disease is especially common in Jews from around the Baltic Sea.

The infantile type of Niemann-Pick disease is caused by sphingomyelinase deficiency. The enzyme is deficient in most cells in the body. The diagnosis can be confirmed by showing that its activity in cultured fibrocytes, leukocytes, or hepatocytes is less that 7% of normal.

Sphingomyelin accumulates in macrophages and neurons, and to a lesser degree in hepatocytes, fibrocytes, and other cells. The macrophages are large, with abundant, finely vacuolated cytoplasm. They stain strongly for fat. Similar vacuoles distend the cytoplasm of the neurons. They are present in smaller numbers in the cytoplasm of hepatocytes, fibrocytes, lymphocytes, and monocytes. Electron microscopy shows that the sphingomyelin is in lysosomes. Sometimes it forms laminar arrays; sometimes it is amorphous.

The accumulation of sphingomyelin becomes evident soon after birth and rapidly grows more massive. The neurons involved degenerate and are lost, causing increasing shrinkage and gliosis of the brain. Splenomegaly grows more marked, as the red pulp is largely replaced by macrophages filled with sphingomyelin. Involvement of the Kupffer cells and hepatocytes causes hepatomegaly. Enlargement of the lymph nodes and infiltration of the lungs are common. Fat-filled macrophages in the bone marrow may be so numerous that they cause rarefaction of the bones. In 50% of the infants, a cherry red spot is visible in the eyes near the macula. Almost every organ contains at least a few macrophages filled with sphingomyelin.

The increasing injury to the brain causes mental retardation and increasingly severe neurologic dysfunction. The liver and spleen grow progressively larger. Wasting and infection usually bring death within three years.

Visceral Type. In the visceral type of Niemann-Pick disease, often called type B, the changes in most organs are as in the infantile form of the disease, but there is no evidence of neurologic injury. Sphingomyelinase is deficient, as in type A. Infection or hypersplenism can be troublesome, but patients with this form of Niemann-Pick disease sometimes live many years.

Type C. A third type of Niemann-Pick disease, usually called type C, becomes evident when the child is three or four years old, but then develops much as does the infantile form, to bring death in adolescence. The activity of sphingomyelinase is normal in these children.

Type D. Niemann-Pick disease type D is similar to the type C disease, but is found only in a kindred from Nova Scotia in Canada. As in type C, sphingomyelinase activity is normal.

Type E. Type E Niemann-Pick disease is a mild form found in adults. There are no neurologic manifestations. Sphingomyelin accumulates in the macrophages, but does little or no harm. The activity of sphingomyelinase is normal.

SEA BLUE HISTIOCYTOSIS. Sea blue histiocytosis is a rare condition in which the macrophages throughout the body stain a bright sea blue with the Giemsa stain and similar techniques. Ceroid, sphingolipids, and perhaps other substances accumulate in the lysosomes of the macrophages, presumably because of an enzyme deficiency. In some of the patients, sphingomyelinase is deficient. The lipid in the lysosomes takes the stains for fat, is acid fast, and stains strongly with the periodic acid-Schiff reaction. By electron microscopy, it shows a laminar structure. The condition is probably inherited as an autosomal recessive character.

Sea blue histiocytosis can develop at any age, but most of the patients are under 40 years old when the diagnosis is made. The sea blue macrophages accumulate in the liver and spleen, causing hepatosplenomegaly. They are numerous in the bone marrow. Some 30% of the patients have lesions in the lungs. Rarely, there is involvement of the retina, skin, or brain.

Most patients do well. A few develop hypersplenism. In a few, extension of the disease brings death.

Similar sea blue macrophages are occasionally found in the spleen or bone marrow of patients with idiopathic thrombocytopenic purpura. Electron microscopy shows degenerating platelets and myelin figures in the lysosomes of the macrophages. Sea blue macrophages have also been found in the spleen in patients with chronic myeloid leukemia, polycythemia vera, sickle cell anemia, thalassemia, sarcoidosis, chronic granulomatous disease, other kinds of lipidosis, and other conditions. Presumably in all these conditions the underlying disease has overloaded the macrophages, so that they cannot catabolize the material presented to them. It is possible that some of these patients also have a partial deficiency of one of the enzymes involved.

WOLMAN'S DISEASE. Wolman's disease is a rare condition named after the Israeli pediatrician who described it in 1956. It is probably inherited as an autosomal recessive character. In the infants affected, the lysosomal lipases are deficient. Cholesterol esters and triglycerides accumulate in macrophages and other cells.

Fever, vomiting, diarrhea, malabsorption, and hepatosplenomegaly develop soon after birth. Thrombocytopenia and purpura are common. Death comes within a year.

The liver is large and yellow or orange. Microscopically, it shows fine, lacy vacuolation of the cytoplasm of both Kupffer cells and hepatocytes. Sometimes there is hepatic fibrosis or cirrhosis.

Macrophages filled with fat enlarge the spleen, crowd the lamina propria of the gut, and are numerous in the bone marrow and lymph nodes. The adrenal glands are enlarged and bright yellow. Their cells are filled with fat. Often the zona reticularis is calcified.

CHOLESTEROL ESTER STORAGE DISEASE. Cholesterol ester storage disease is a rare disorder caused by a congenital deficiency of the lysosomal enzymes cholesterol ester dehydrogenase and triglyceride lipase. It is inherited as an autosomal recessive character. Cholesterol esters and triglycerides accumulate in macrophages and other cells.

Lipid in the Kupffer cells and hepatocytes makes the liver large and orange-yellow. Fat-filled macrophages are numerous in the spleen, which may be enlarged. They are abundant in the lamina propria of the gut and in the bone marrow. Droplets of fat are present in the smooth muscle of the intestine. Hyperlipidemia is caused by an increase in the concentration in the plasma of cholesterol esters, phospholipids, and often triglycerides. Both very low density and low density lipoproteins are increased.

The disease becomes evident in infancy, as the liver and spleen enlarge. The children develop normally and have a normal life expectancy.

TANGIER DISEASE. Tangier disease is named after Tangier Island in Virginia, where the first case was discovered. It is inherited as an autosomal recessive character. In homozygotes, cholesterol esters are stored in increasing quantity in macrophages throughout the body. Heterozygotes show similar but milder changes.

The liver, spleen, and lymph nodes enlarge during childhood, as fat-filled macrophages accumulate in them. The tonsils are greatly enlarged and are stippled yellow or orange by the fat-filled cells. Macrophages in the pharyngeal and rectal mucosa often make the mucosa grayish-yellow. In adults, fat-filled macrophages sometimes infiltrate the cornea. Hypersplenism or peripheral neuropathy occasionally develops. Hypercholesterolemia and hypophospholipidemia are common. The concentration of triglycerides in the plasma is normal or increased. High density lipoproteins are greatly reduced.

Tangier disease causes little disability. It might increase the severity of atherosclerosis.

HISTIOCYTOSIS X

Eosinophilic granuloma, Hand-Schüller-Christian disease and Letterer-Siwe disease are grouped together as histiocytosis X, "X" for unknown, because the conditions are of unknown etiology. In all three conditions, the lesions consist of a tumor-like accumulation of macrophages, some of which have the inclusions and markers of the Langerhans' cells of the skin. Some prefer to call histiocytosis X Langerhans' cell histiocytosis.

The nature of the conditions grouped as histiocytosis X is uncertain. Most think that eosinophilic granuloma and Hand-Schüller-Christian disease are nonneoplastic disorders caused by some unknown stimulus. Letterer-Siwe disease progresses more rapidly and may be a neoplasm.

EOSINOPHILIC GRANULOMA. Two forms of eosinophilic granuloma are distinguished. In one, there is a solitary lesion. In the other, multiple lesions are present.

About 60% of patients with histiocytosis X have unifocal eosinophilic granuloma, and 30% of the patients have the multifocal form of the disease. Most of the patients are chil-

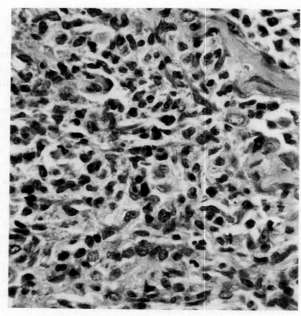

Fig. 51-2. Eosinophilic granuloma of a lung.

dren or young adults. Over 60% of them are men or boys.

Lesions. Eosinophilic granuloma is most frequent in bones. In adults, a rib is the most common site, though any bone can be involved. In children, the skull is the most common site. There is usually only one lesion. In the lungs, many of the patients have more than one lesion, or lesions in the lungs and a lesion in a bone. Rarely, some other organ is involved. The eosinophilic granuloma discussed in this chapter is not related to the forms of eosinophilic gastritis or enteritis sometimes called an eosinophilic granuloma.

When a bone is involved, it is usually swollen. Roentgenographically, the lesion is radiolucent, occasionally with osteosclerosis at its margin. The disease sometimes causes a pathologic fracture or collapse of a vertebra. In the lungs, the lesion forms one or more spheroidal masses that often mimic carcinoma.

Microscopically, the lesion consists largely of an aggregation of macrophages. Many are large and irregularly shaped. Some are multinucleated. Some are small and spindle shaped. Often some of the macrophages contain a few droplets of fat or a few granules of brown pigment. The macrophages are usually packed closely together. Eosinophils are sometimes numerous in the lesions, but often are scant or absent. As the lesions age, they become increasingly fibrotic. In the lungs, the center of the lesion is sometimes cavitated. Often fibrosing interstitital pneumonitis is present around lesions in the lungs.

Electron microscopy shows the rod-shaped or racquet-shaped cytoplasmic inclusions of Langerhans' cells in some of the macrophages. These cells carry the OKT-6 antigen found on thymocytes and Langerhans' cells and stain for the S-100 antigen.

Clinical Presentation. Lesions in bone produce few or no symptoms until the erosion of the bone causes pain or a fracture. In the lungs, eosinophilic grauloma causes cough, dyspnea, and sometimes pain. Spontaneous pneumothorax develops in 10% of the patients.

Treatment and Prognosis. If an eosinophilic granuloma in a bone is still solitary after six months, it is unlikely to become multifocal. Untreated, the lesion often persists for years, but sometimes becomes fibrotic and regresses. Curettage or irradiation usually cures.

In the lungs, the disease becomes stable in many patients. In some, it is progressive and fatal.

HAND-SCHÜLLER-CHRISTIAN DISEASE. Hand-Schüller-Christian disease is named after the American pediatrician who reported a case in 1893, the Austrian neurologist who described it in 1910, and the American physician who discussed it in 1919. It is not clearly demarcated from the multifocal form of eosinophilic granuloma. Usually the term *multifocal eosinophilic granuloma* is preferred when there are multiple lesions in the lungs or bones in an older child or an adult, and the term *Hand-Schüller-Christian disease* is used when the condition develops in a child under five years old.

Lesions. Young children with Hand-Schüller-Christian disease develop multiple lesions in the bones. The skull, mandible, long bones, and pelvis are the most commonly involved. In 30% of the patients, a lesion in an orbital bone causes exophthalmos. Multiple lesions are often present in the lungs. In 50% of the patients, involvement of the liver, spleen, or lymph nodes causes enlargement of one or more of these organs. In 50% of the patients, flat, yellowish-brown macules called xanthoma disseminatum develop in the skin. Involvement of the hypothalamus causes diabetes insipidus in 30% of the patients. Chronic otitis media and mastoiditis are common.

Microscopically, the lesions consist principally of an aggregation of macrophages like that in eosinophilic granuloma. In the young children with numerous lesions, fat is usually abundant in the macrophages. Eosinophils are often present in the lesions, and sometimes there are neutrophils, lymphocytes, or plasma cells. Fibrosis is sometimes extensive in or around the lesions.

Clinical Presentation. Young children with Hand-Schüller-Christian disease often have fever, lesions in the skin, recurrent otitis media or mastoiditis, and repeated upper respiratory infections. In older patients, the symptoms are similar to those of eosinophilic granuloma.

Treatment and Prognosis. In 50% of children with Hand-Schüller-Christian disease, the lesions resolve spontaneously. In the other patients, vinblastine, vincristine, or other cytotoxic drugs usually bring remission and cure. Radiation causes rapid shrinkage of lesions causing symptoms.

LETTERER-SIWE DISEASE. Letterer-Siwe disease was described by the German physicians Letterer in 1924 and Siwe in 1933. It is rare. It develops in infants or occasionally older children.

Aggregates of macrophages develop in organs throughout the body and rapidly grow more numerous and more extensive. Lesions are particularly common in the bones, skin, liver, spleen, and lymph nodes. Microscopically, they consist of macrophages with little admixture of other cells. The nuclei of the macrophages have coarse chromatin and occasional nucleoli. Some of the cells have inclusions of Langerhans' cells in the cytoplasm.

The child loses weight and often is feverish. Scaling papular or ulcerated lesions in the skin are usually extensive. Enlargement of the liver, spleen, and lymph nodes is common. Anemia and thrombocytopenia are frequent.

Chemotherapy controls Letterer-Siwe disease in 70% of the children, but 30% die of the disease. The younger the infant at the onset, the worse the prognosis.

TUMORS

Monocytes give rise to two kinds of tumor. The forms of leukemia in which malignant monocytes circulate in the blood are considered in this chapter. The tumors in which monocytes form a solid mass are discussed with the diseases of the lymphocytes in Chapter 55.

MONOCYTIC LEUKEMIA. Monocytic leukemia is uncommon. It is a form of myeloid leukemia in which malignant monocytes are numerous in the blood, together with malignant granulocytes.

Chronic monocytic leukemia is rare. The term is sometimes used to describe the form of chronic myeloid leukemia in which monocytes are numerous in the blood; sometimes to describe one of the forms of myeloid dysplasia.

Acute monocytic leukemia is type M-5 in the French-American-British classification of acute myeloid leukemia. The malignant monocytes in the blood are usually large, with irregular borders and large, irregular, folded nuclei. The leukocyte count tends to be higher in patients with acute monocytic leukemia than in people with other kinds of acute myeloid leukemia. On the average, the leukocyte count is $40 \times 10^9/L$ $(40,000/mm^3)$ in patients with acute monocytic leukemia, $20 \times 10^9/L$ $(20,000/mm^3)$ in acute myelomonocytic leukemia, less than $15 \times 10^9/L$ $(15,000/mm^3)$ in acute myeloblastic leukemia, and under $10 \times 10^9/L$ $(10,000/mm^3)$ in patients with acute promyelocytic leukemia. Patients with acute monocytic leukemia more often have enlarged lymph nodes, leukemic infiltration of the gums, and lesions in the skin than do people with other types of myeloid leukemia.

BIBLIOGRAPHY

General

Frisch, B., Lewis, S. M., Burkhardt, R., and Bartl, R.: Biopsy Pathology of Bone and Bone Marrow. London, Chapman and Hall, 1985.

Hardisty, R. M., and Weatherall, D. J.: Blood and Its Disorders. 2nd Ed. Oxford, Blackwell, 1982.

Isaacson, P. G., and Wright, D. H.: Histiocytic disorders in lymphoreticular pathology. Rec. Adv. Histopathol., 12:197, 1984.

Jandl, J. H.: Blood. Boston, Little, Brown and Co., 1987.

Wickramasinghe, S. N. (Ed.): Blood and Bone Marrow. In Systemic Pathology, 3rd Ed. Edited by Symmers, W. St.C: London, Churchill Livingstone, 1986.

Williams, W. J., Beutler E., Erslav, A. J., and Lichtman, M. A.: Hematology. 3rd Ed. New York, McGraw-Hill, 1983.

Wintrobe, M. M., et al.: Clinical Hematology. 8th Ed. Philadelphia, Lea & Febiger, 1981.

Wittels, B.: Surgical Pathology of Bone Marrow. Philadelphia, W. B. Saunders, 1985.

Zucker-Franklin, D., Greaves, M. F., Grossi, C. E., and Marmont, A. M.: Atlas of Blood Cells. 2nd Ed. Philadelphia, Lea & Febiger, 1988.

Storage Diseases

Desnick, R. J. (Ed.): Gaucher disease. Prog. Clin. Biol. Res., 95:1, 1982.

Douglas, S. D., and Musson, R. A.: Phagocytic defects—monocytes/macrophages. Clin. Immunol. Immunopathol., 40:62, 1986.

Glew, R. H., Basu, A., LaMarco, K. L., and Prence, E. M.: Mammalian glucocerebrosidase: implications for Gaucher's disease. Lab. Invest., 58:5, 1988.

Repo, H.: Defects in phagocytic functions. Ann. Clin. Res., 19:263, 1987.

White, C. J., and Gallin J. I.: Phagocytic defects. Clin. Immunol. Immunopathol., 40:50, 1986.

Histiocytosis X

Basset, F., Nezelof, C., and Ferrans V. J.: The histiocytoses. Pathol. Annu., 18(2):27, 1983.

Favara, B. E., McCarthy, R. C., and Mierau, G. W.: Histiocytosis X. Hum. Pathol., 14:663, 1983.

Osband, M. E.: Histiocytosis X. Hematol. Oncol. Clin. North Am., 1:737, 1987.

Osband, M. E., and Pochedly, C. (Eds.): Histiocytosis X. Hematol. Oncol. Clin. North Am., 1:1, 1987.

Tumors

Basset, F., Nezelof, C., and Ferrans V. J.: The histiocytoses. Pathol. Annu., 18(2):27, 1983.

Catovsky, D. (Ed.): The Leukemic Cell. Edinburgh, Churchill Livingstone, 1981.

Gunz, F. W., and Henderson, E. S. (Eds.): Leukemia. 4th Ed. New York, Grune and Stratton, 1983.

Hoogstraten, B. (Ed.): Hematologic Malignancies. Berlin, Springer-Verlag, 1985.

Jones, J. F., and Strauss, S. E.: Chronic Epstein-Barr virus infection. Annu. Rev. Med., 38:195, 1987.

Koeffler, H. P.: Syndromes of acute nonlymphocytic leukemia. Ann. Intern. Med., 107:748, 1987.

Peschle, C. (Ed.): Normal and neoplastic blood cells. Ann. N. Y. Acad. Sci., 51:1, 1987.

Peterson, B. A., and Levine, E. G.: Uncommon subtypes of nonlymphocytic leukemia. Semin. Oncol., 14:425, 1987.

Shaw, M. T.: Monocytic leukemias. Hum. Pathol., 11:215, 1980.

Wain, S. L. and Borowitz, M. J.: Practical applications of monoclonal antibodies to the diagnosis and classification of acute leukaemias. Clin. Lab. Haematol., 9:221, 1987.

Wiernik, P. H., Canellos, G. P., Kyle, R. A., and Schiffer, C. A.: Neoplastic Diseases of the Blood. 4th Ed. New York, Churchill Livingstone, 1985.

van der Valk, P., and Meijer, C. J. L. M.: Histiocytic sarcoma. Pathol. Annu., 20(2):1, 1985.

52

Platelets

THE disorders of the megakaryocytes cause disease principally by altering the number or function of the platelets that circulate in the blood. If there are too few platelets in the blood, the patient is said to have thrombocytopenia. If there are too many, the disorder is called thrombocytosis. If the circulating platelets are abnormal, thrombasthenia, thrombopathy, and other terms are used to describe the abnormality.

THROMBOCYTOPENIA

Thrombocytopenia is the commonest cause of abnormal bleeding. If there are not enough platelets to maintain hemostasis, the slightest injury to a small blood vessel is likely to cause hemorrhage.

As shown in Table 52–1, thrombocytopenia is divided into primary and secondary forms. The primary form of the disease is usually called idiopathic thrombocytopenic purpura.

TABLE 52-1.   CAUSES OF THROMBOCYTOPENIA

Primary Thrombocytopenia
   Idiopathic thrombocytopenic purpura

Secondary Thrombocytopenia
   Drug-induced
   Disease of the bone marrow
   Hypersplenism
   Incompatible platelet transfusion
   Massive blood transfusions
   Other immunologic reactions
   Other infections
   Excessive consumption
   Hypothermia
   Defective regulation of thrombopoiesis
   Episodic thrombocytopenia and thrombocytosis
   Congenital thrombocytopenia
   Congenital megakaryocytic hypoplasia
   Hereditary thrombocytopenia

It is the most common form of thrombocytopenia. Drugs, disease of the bone marrow, and hypersplenism are the most frequent causes of secondary thrombocytopenia.

IDIOPATHIC THROMBOCYTOPENIC PURPURA. Idiopathic thrombocytopenic purpura is almost always caused by antiplatelet antibodies or by immune complexes that become attached to the platelets. In children, the disease often follows a viral infection and the abnormal immunologic response is caused by the infection. In adults, the cause of the abnormal antibodies is usually unknown.

The term *idiopathic* was introduced by Galen to describe diseases of unknown cause. It continues to be used to describe this form of thrombocytopenia, though it is no longer entirely appropriate. The term *purpura* describes the small, purple flecks of hemorrhage that are common in all forms of thrombocytopenia. It is derived from the Latin for purple, which in turn was derived from the Greek name of the shellfish from which Tyrian purple was made.

Idiopathic thrombocytopenic purpura is divided into acute and chronic forms, though the distinction between the two is not sharp. Intermediate forms occur. The acute form is most common in children two to six years old, but occasionally develops in an adult. The chronic form can develop at any age, but is most frequent in adults 20 to 40 years old. Over 70% of the patients are women. Onyalai is a form of acute idiopathic thrombocytopenic purpura that occurs in the Bantu, usually in children or young men.

Lesions. The lesions are similar in acute and chronic idiopathic thrombocytopenic purpura. The disease affects principally the blood, though there are changes in the bone marrow and often petechiae or more extensive hemorrhage in other organs.

Bone Marrow. Megakaryocytes are numerous in the bone narrow and often larger than usual. Some have only a single spheroidal nucleus. Some have vacuoles in their cytoplasm. Degenerating megakaryocytes can often be found. Occasionally, there is an admixture of abnormally small megakaryocytes. The other cells in the bone marrow are normal, unless the anemia caused by the bleeding is sufficient to cause hyperplasia of the erythrocytic precursors.

Blood. In the acute form of idiopathic thrombocytopenic purpura, the platelet count is often below 20×10^9/L ($20,000$/mm^3). In the chronic form, it is usually between 30 and 80×10^9/L ($30,000$ and $80,000$/mm^3). Purpura is unusual unless the platelet count is less than 50×10^9/L ($50,000$/mm^3). Often the platelets are bigger than normal, sometimes as much as 10 μm across and bizarrely shaped.

The survival of the platelets in the blood is reduced in most patients with idiopathic thrombocytopenic purpura. The more severe the thrombocytopenia, the shorter their life span. If the platelet count is over 50×10^9/L ($50,000$/mm^3), the life of the circulating platelets is 2 days instead of the usual 9 to 12. If the count is less than 10×10^9/L ($10,000$/mm^3), it is only 1 or 2 hours. The increased destruction of platelets increases the activity of β-glycerol acid phosphatase in the plasma.

In almost all patients with idiopathic thrombocytopenic purpura, immune complexes or IgG antiplatelet antibodies coat the circulating platelets. The concentration of immunoglobulin on the platelets is greater in children with the acute form of idiopathic thrombocytopenic purpura than in adults with the chronic form of the disease. Even when the chronic form of the disease is in remission, IgG is demonstrable on the circulating platelets.

The thrombocytopenia impairs clot retraction, but coagulation is otherwise normal. The bleeding time is prolonged, and the tourniquet test is positive.

Anemia develops only if bleeding is unusually severe. The leukocyte count is normal, unless bleeding is extensive. Some children with the acute form of the disease have eosinophilia or a lymphocytosis.

Other Organs. If the platelet count falls sufficiently in idiopathic thrombocytopenic purpura, purpura is evident in the skin and other organs. More extensive bleeding is unusual in children with acute thrombocytopenia and in adults with chronic thrombocytopenia. Only in adults who develop acute thrombocytopenia is massive hemorrhage likely.

Petechiae appear first in the skin and mucous membranes and often remain confined to them. Purple or red dots less than 0.5 cm across caused by the bleeding are most common in the skin over bony prominences and in areas in which clothing is tight. Occasionally the bleeding into the skin is more extensive, with ecchymoses or hematomata. Minor trauma causes bruising. Minor scratches ooze persistently. Bleeding from the nose is common. Hemorrhagic vesicles sometimes develop in the mouth in children with the acute form of the disease. Less often there is bleeding from the gums, menorrhagia, hematuria, hematemesis, or melena. Petechiae in the meninges are common, and occasionally there is more extensive intracranial hemorrhage. Bleeding into the joints is uncommon.

The spleen is often enlarged in idiopathic thrombocytopenic purpura, weighing 300 or 400 g. Microscopically, it usually shows only congestion. Only if the thrombocytopenia is unusually severe do macrophages filled with cholesterol or ceroid derived from phagocytosed platelets appear in the red pulp.

Clinical Presentation. Acute idiopathic thrombocytopenic purpura usually develops abruptly. In children, it usually arises one to three weeks after a respiratory or some other viral infection. The platelet count falls rapidly. Petechiae may appear, or the child may be noticed to bruise easily and bleed excessively from minor injuries.

In adults with chronic idiopathic thrombocytopenic purpura, the onset is usually insidious. As the platelet count falls, episodes of bleeding last for a few days or weeks, then subside. Between attacks, the platelet count may return to normal, but often remains depressed.

Pathogenesis. In some patients, acute idiopathic thrombocytopenic purpura is caused by immune complexes that bind to the Fc receptors on the platelets and megakaryocytes; in some by antibodies that fix to antigens on the platelets and megakaryocytes. In children, the immune complexes contain viral antigens, and the antibodies are probably antiviral antibodies that cross react with the platelets. The chronic form of the disease is caused by autoantibodies that react with the Ib or IIb-IIIa glycoproteins on the surface of the platelets and megakaryocytes.

The coated platelets are segregated and destroyed in the spleen and, to a lesser degree, in the liver. Estrogens increase the destruction of the platelets in the spleen, perhaps explaining why chronic idiopathic thrombocytopenic purpura is more common in women. The antiplatelet antibodies do not fix complement and do not cause lysis of the platelets. In some patients, the antibody impairs the release of platelet factors from the thrombocytes.

The megakaryocytes respond to the thrombocytopenia by increasing the production of platelets from 2 to 9 times. In patients with chronic idiopathic thrombocytopenic purpura, this is usually sufficient to prevent bleeding except during the episodes in which the destruction of platelets increases.

Cell-mediated immunity may also be involved in the pathogenesis of idiopathic thrombocytopenic purpura. Platelets from patients with the chronic form of the disease can cause transformation of lymphocytes.

The bleeding in idiopathic thrombocytopenic purpura is caused in part by the lack of platelets, in part by damage to the blood vessels. It is greater than is usual in other forms of thrombocytopenia of equal severity. Adrenocortical steroids reduce the bleeding, though they cause little or no increase in the concentration of platelets in the blood. The nature of the injury to the blood vessels is obscure.

Treatment and Prognosis. Over 90% of children with acute idiopathic thrombocytopenic purpura recover completely in from a few days to a few months, usually in four to six weeks. No treatment is needed unless the bleeding is unusually severe, though adrenocortical steroids are often given to reduce the bleeding. Platelet transfusions are of help if bleeding is severe, though they do little to increase the platelet count. Less than 1% of the children die, usually of intracranial hemorrhage. In less than 10% of the children, the disease becomes chronic.

Chronic idiopathic thrombocytopenic purpura in adults usually persists for the rest of the patient's life. It varies in severity, but complete remissions are uncommon.

Adrenocortical steroids benefit up to 90% of the patients, principally by reducing the destruction of the platelets in the spleen. The steroids may also reduce the fragility of the blood vessels, perhaps by reducing the production of prostacyclin by the endothelium and so enhancing the aggregation of platelets.

If the adrenocortical steroids fail to control the bleeding or the dose of steroid needed is too large, splenectomy brings a rapid increase in the platelet count in over 80% of the patients. Within a few days, the count rises dramatically, sometimes to as much as 1000 × 10^9/L (1,000,000/mm^3) The count then slowly falls. In over 50% of the patients, splenectomy restores the platelet count to near normal. In others, it brings considerable amelioration. The antiplatelet antibody is still present in the plasma, and the life of the platelets is lengthened.

If splenectomy brings no lasting benefit, immunosuppressive drugs such as vincristine, cyclophosphamide, or azothioprine can sometimes control chronic idiopathic thrombocytopenia purpura. In some patients, the androgen danazol is beneficial.

If a woman with idiopathic thrombocytopenic purpura becomes pregnant, the chance of spontaneous abortion is doubled and the risk of excessive bleeding at delivery is increased. The antiplatelet antibodies cross the placenta and cause thrombocytopenia and bleeding in the fetus.

SECONDARY THROMBOCYTOPENIA. If the cause of thrombocytopenia is known, the patient is said to have secondary thrombocytopenia. Drugs, disease of the bone marrow, and hypersplenism are its most common causes.

The lesions in the different types of secondary thrombocytopenia are similar to those of idiopathic thrombocytopenic purpura. Often it is only the history that indicates whether the patient has the idiopathic form of the disease or thrombocytopenia caused by a drug.

Drug-Induced. Table 52-2 shows some of

TABLE 52-2. DRUGS AND CHEMICALS CAUSING THROMBOCYTOPENIA

Agents causing reduced thrombopoiesis
  Agents causing aplastic anemia
    (See Table 49-1)

Agents depressing only megakaryocytes
  Chlorothiazides
  Estrogens
  Ethanol
  Tolbutamide

Agents causing immunologic injury
  Anticonvulsants
    Carbamazepine
    Phenytoin
    Valproic acid
  Antidepressants
    Desipramine
  Antidiabetic agents
    Chlorpromamide
  Antihistamines
    Antazoline
    Chlorpheniramine
  Antihypertensive agents
    Methyldopa
  Anti-inflammatory agents
    Gold salts
  Antimicrobials
    Hydroxychloroquinine
    Novobiocin
    Organic arsenicals
    Quinine
    Para-aminosalicylic acid
    Rifampin
    Stibophen
    Sulfonamides
  Diuretics
    Acetazolamide
    Chlorthiazides
  Sedatives
    Apronalide
    Carbromal
    Diazepam
  Other
    Digitoxin
    Lidocaine
    Quinidine

Agents damaging platelets directly
  Ristocetin

Mode of action unknown
  Analgesics
    Acetaminophen
    Aminopyrine
    Codeine
    Meperidine
    Phenacetin
    Salicylates

  Anticonvulsants
    Clonazepam
    Ethotoin
    Paramethadione
    Primidone
    Trimethadione
  Antidiabetic agents
    Carbutamide
    Tolbutamide
  Antihistamines
    Chlorpheniramine
    Promethazine
  Antihypertensive agents
    Diazoxide
    Reserpine
    Spironolactone
  Anti-inflammatory agents
    Oxyphenbutazone
    Phenylbutazone
  Antimicrobials
    Cephalothin
    Chloroquin
    Erythromycin
    Isoniazid
    Lincomycin
    Nitrofurantoin
    Organic arsenicals
    Penicillin
    Pyrazinamide
    Streptomycin
    Sulfonamides
    Tetracyclines
  Antithyroid drugs
    Propyl thiouracil
    Thiourea
  Diuretics
    Chlorthalidone
    Furosemide
    Mercurial diuretics
  Sedatives
    Barbiturates
  Tranquilizers
    Chlorpromazine
    Meprobamate
    Prochlorperazine
  Other
    Bismuth
    Cimetidine
    Copper sulfate
    Dextroamphetamine
    Dinitrophenol
    Disulfiram
    Ergot
    Digitalis
    Digoxin
    Heparin
    Iopanoic acid

TABLE 52-2.   CONT'D

Insecticides
Hair dyes
Heroin
Levodopa
Nitroglycerine
Penicillamine
Potassium iodide
Prednisone
Tetraethylammonium
Toluene diisocyanate
Turpentine

the drugs and other chemicals that can induce thrombocytopenia. A few of these agents cause thrombocytopenia in many of the people exposed to them. Most do so only in a small proportion of the people exposed to the agent.

Some drugs cause thrombocytopenia by depressing the formation of platelets in the bone marrow. Many of these agents also cause aplastic anemia. Other drugs incite an immunologic reaction that leads to increased destruction of the platelets. Ristocetin attacks the platelets directly. Some agents both depress the megakaryocytes and cause increased destruction of the platelets. With many drugs, the mode of action remains obscure.

Cytosine arabinoside and daunorubicin are among the cytotoxic drugs most likely to cause thrombocytopenia by impairing the production of platelets. Busulfan, cyclophosphamide, 6-mercaptopurine and methotrexate are less dangerous. Chlorothiazide and similar diuretics depress the production of platelets in 25% of patients given the drug for a prolonged period, though the thrombocytopenia is not usually severe. The platelet count is usually between 50 and 100 × 10^9/L (50,000 and 100,000/mm^3). Recovery occurs when the drug is withdrawn, but is slow. If chlorothiazide is again administered, thrombocytopenia again develops, though not until the drug has been taken for a long time. Ethanol causes thrombocytopenia if taken in large quantity. It both depresses the formation of platelets and accelerates their destruction. Rarely, estrogens reduce thrombopoiesis. Adrenocortical steroids occasionally increase the severity of thrombocytopenia, but do not cause thrombocytopenia in normal people.

More often, drug-induced thrombocytopenia is caused by an immunologic reaction against the platelets. The risk that antiplatelet antibodies will develop varies from one drug to another. Only 1 person in every 100,000 given quinidine develops thrombocytopenia, but 1 person in every 100 given gold salts does so. Usually the drug or one of its metabolites serves as a hapten. Antibody against the hapten develops and reacts with the drug or its metabolite to form a complex that circulates in the blood. The complex is bound by nonimmunologic means to the platelets and leads to their early destruction in the spleen.

Immunologically mediated, drug-induced thrombocytopenia usually develops suddenly and is severe. If the drug is withdrawn, the platelet count rises promptly. If even a small quantity of the drug is administered subsequently, the platelet count again falls.

Direct chemical injury to the platelets is rare. The antibiotic ristocetin is one of the few agents able to attack the platelets directly.

Probably most of the drugs that cause thrombocytopenia by an unknown mechanism do so by inducing an immunologic reaction. With most of these agents, the risk of thrombocytopenia is low.

In most forms of drug-induced thrombocytopenia, withdrawal of the offending drug restores the platelet count to normal. Only if the platelet count is below 20 × 10^9/L (20,000/mm^3) or the thrombocytopenia persists for an unusually long time after withdrawal of the drug are adrenocortical steroids, platelet transfusion, or plasmapheresis indicated.

Disease of the Bone Marrow.   Any disease that severely injures the bone marrow is likely to cause thrombocytopenia. The replacement of the bone marrow by leukemia, multiple myeloma, metastatic carcinoma, myelofibrosis or osteopetrosis sometimes causes thrombocytopenia. The megaloblastic anemias and paroxysmal nocturnal hemoglobinuria depress thrombopoiesis. The failure of the bone marrow in aplastic anemia is another cause.

Hypersplenism.   Many conditions that cause splenomegaly lead to increased destruction of platelets and other blood cells, a condition called hypersplenism. It is discussed with the diseases of the spleen in Chapter 54.

Incompatible Platelet Transfusion. Transfusion of incompatible platelets results in the destruction of the transfused platelets if the recipient has antibody against them. Less often, transfusion of incompatible platelets causes severe thrombocytopenia, with continuing destruction of the recipient's own platelets, which may persist for months. The platelets of most recipients who suffer this continuing reaction lack the antigen PL^{A1} (Zw^a), and antibody against this antigen is present in their plasma.

Massive Blood Transfusions. Thrombocytopenia is common after mulitple transfusions given for massive hemorrhage. The bleeding depletes the body's store of platelets, and the blood given by transfusion is usually deficient in platelets. The platelet count gradually returns to normal in the course of three to five days.

Other Immunologic Reactions. Antiplatelet antibodies are present in the plasma in 80% of patients with systemic lupus erythematosus. In some of these people, they cause thrombocytopenia and purpura by a mechanism similar to that in idiopathic thrombocytopenic purpura. Less often, antiplatelet antibodies develop in patients with immunohemolytic anemia, leukemia, lymphoma, rheumatoid arthritis or hyperthryoidism. Occasionally an allergic reaction caused by food, inoculation, or an insect bite causes thrombocytopenia, probably because circulating immune complexes become attached to the platelets as in drug-induced immune thrombocytopenia.

Other Infections. In addition to the acute idiopathic thrombocytopenic thrombocytopenia that follows viral infections in children, viruses can cause thrombocytopenia by damaging the megakaryocytes, attacking circulating platelets, or by inducing other immunologic reactions. The virus of measles and other viruses sometimes attack the megakaryocytes, reducing thrombopoiesis. The viruses of rubella and influenza can infect and destroy platelets during the period of viremia. In infectious mononucleosis, cold antibodies against the i antigen on the platelets sometimes cause thrombocytopenia.

Bacterial septicemia can cause thrombocytopenia, especially in children. Malarial parasites can colonize the platelets, destroying them in sufficient number to cause thrombocytopenia.

Excessive Consumption. Excessive consumption of platelets causes thrombocytopenia, in thrombotic thrombocytopenic purpura, disseminated intravascular coagulation, and the hemolytic-uremic syndrome. Occasionally artificial heart valves, other vascular prostheses, or the pump used to maintain extracorporeal circulation during surgery cause thrombocytopenia. In infants, a large cavernous hemangioma sometimes uses so many platelets to repair its leaky endothelium that thrombocytopenia and purpura result.

Hypothermia. Hypothermia of the kind used during surgical procedures causes transient thrombocytopenia. As the temperature falls, the platelets stick to the endothelium of the blood vessels in such numbers that the concentration of platelets in the blood falls. Usually, the platelets return to the circulation when the patient is warmed. Occasionally the process is more severe. Adenosine diphosphate is released from the platelets, platelets clump in the blood, and vessels are occluded by platelet thrombi.

Defective Regulation of Thrombopoiesis. In rare patients, the plasma lacks a substance essential for the production of platelets. Transfusion of normal plasma brings maturation of the inactive megakaryocytes in the bone marrow and normal, though temporary, production of platelets.

Episodic Thrombocytopenia and Thrombocytosis. In a few patients, thrombocytopenia and thrombocytosis alternate at regular intervals. The cause of the alternation is unknown. In tidal platelet dysgenesis, there is hypoplasia of the megakaryocytes in the bone marrow when the platelet count falls and hyperplasia when it rises. In the more common cyclic thrombocytopenia, no hypoplasia of the megakaryocytes occurs when the platelet count falls.

Congenital Thrombocytopenia. Congenital thrombocytopenia is caused by IgG antiplatelet antibodies that cross the placenta from the maternal to the fetal blood. It occurs in chronic idiopathic thrombocytopenic purpura, systemic lupus erythematosus, and occasionally in other conditions. Small hemorrhages of fetal blood into the maternal circulation can sensitize the mother against the fetal platelets. The antibody coats the fetal platelets and increases their destruction in the spleen. The thrombocytopenia in the fetus and newborn child is not often severe. Recovery comes spontaneously as the titer of antiplatelet antibody in the infant's blood falls soon after birth.

Congenital Megakaryocytic Hypoplasia. In congenital megakaryocytic hypoplasia, injury to the fetus in the sixth to eighth week of gestation prevents normal development of the megakaryocytes. The child is born with severe thrombocytopenia and severe bleeding. Megakaryocytes in the marrow are few. Usually other congenital defects are present, such as agenesis of the radius, cardiac defects, or microcephaly. The cause of the injury is usually unknown. In a few cases, tolbutamide is the causative agent. In some, rubella is to blame.

Hereditary Thrombocytopenia. Hereditary thrombocytopenia is rare. Usually the thrombocytopenia is mild, and purpura is not severe. The defect may be inherited as an autosomal dominant character, an X-linked recessive character, or an autosomal recessive character. In other patients, thrombocytopenia is only one manifestation of a more serious genetic abnormality. For example, in the Wiskott-Aldrich syndrome, thrombocytopenia is overshadowed by the deficiency in T and B cells, and in the Chediak-Higashi syndrome the lack of platelets is less important than the functional disorder in the granulocytes.

THROMBOCYTOSIS

Thrombocytosis may be primary or secondary. The primary form of thrombocytosis is usually called thrombocythemia, and the term *thrombocytosis* is used only for the secondary forms.

THROMBOCYTHEMIA. Thrombocythemia, sometimes called essential thrombocytosis, is a myeloproliferative disorder closely related to myelofibrosis, polycythemia vera, and chronic myeloid leukemia. Like the other myeloproliferative disorders, thrombocythe-mia is a quasineoplastic condition. It is rare. Men and women are affected equally.

Lesions. The abnormal megakaryocytes in the bone marrow produce abnormal platelets that circulate in the blood. Lesions develop in the bone marrow, blood, and other organs.

Bone Marrow. The bone marrow shows hyperplasia of the megakaryocytes. They are often bigger than normal and form clumps or sheets. Some megakaryocytes may be malformed or immature. Often there is hyperplasia of the erythropoietic and granulopoietic cells as well. In some patients, the marrow cells have chromosomal abnormalities. In some, virus-like particles are present in the hematopoietic cells.

Blood. In thrombocythemia, the production of platelets increases up to 15 times. The life span of the platelets is usually normal, though in some patients it is shortened. The platelet count is usually over 1000 $\times$ 10^9/L (1,000,000/mm^3), and can exceed 10,000 $\times$ 10^9/L (10,000,000/mm^3). Often the platelets are oddly shaped, with heavy granulation. They are usually larger than normal, but may be small. Fragments of megakaryocytes are sometimes present in the blood.

Hemorrhage is common in thrombocythemia, especially in the gastrointestinal tract. The abnormal platelets in the blood do not aggregate normally to form a hemostatic plug. The bleeding is often extensive. Petechiae are rare.

Thrombosis is less common, but can occur in arteries, veins, or in the microcirculation. It is caused in part by the excess of platelets in the circulation, in part by their malfunction. Thrombi in a limb can cause reddening and swelling of the limb. Thrombi in the skin sometimes cause small areas of gangrene in the fingers or toes. Occlusion of cerebral vessels sometimes causes transient ischemic attacks. Thrombosis of the splenic, mesenteric, or hepatic veins can cause portal hypertension. Pulmonary emboli or thrombi sometimes develop.

Some of the patients are anemic, usually because of iron deficiency resulting from repeated hemorrhages. Other patients show a mild erythrocytosis, with a red count of from 6 to 7 $\times$ 10^{12}/L (6,000,000 to 7,000,000/mm^3). The leukocyte count is usually between

15 and 40 × 10^9/L (15,000 to 40,000/mm^3), with neutrophilia and often slight eosinophilia and basophilia. The proportion of band cells and metamyelocytes in the blood is often increased. There may be a few myelocytes in the circulation.

Because of the cellular proliferation in the bone marrow, the concentration of uric acid in the blood is usually increased. Blood coagulation is usually normal. The bleeding time may be normal or prolonged. Tests of platelet function usually show a deficient release reaction.

Other Organs. Extramedullary hematopoiesis is often present in the spleen, liver, and lymph nodes. Early in the course of the disease, the spleen is enlarged in 80% of the patients. Later it may shrink because of infarcts or thrombosis of the splenic vein.

Clinical Presentation. Patients with thrombocythemia usually have hemorrhage, most often from the gastrointestinal tract or from the nose. Even trivial injuries may cause dangerous hemorrhage. Easy bruising is common. Less often, the first sign is a transient ischemic attack or some other sign of thrombosis.

Treatment and Prognosis. Thrombocythemia usually persists for many years. Long remissions are common. During the remission, the patient is free of all symptoms.

If necessary, the platelet count can be reduced with radioactive phosphorus, busulfan, melphalan, or other cytotoxic drugs. Usually, only a short course of treatment is necessary, and the platelet count then remains at a safe level for many years. Anticoagulants are sometimes helpful, as are drugs like aspirin that inhibit platelet function. In an emergency, thrombocytopheresis reduces the platelet count to a safe level within a few hours.

Splenectomy or atrophy of the spleen are dangerous in thombocythemia. The platelet count is likely to rise to high and uncontrollable levels, sometimes with fatal hemorrhage or thrombosis.

SECONDARY THROMBOCYTOSIS. Secondary thrombocytosis is common. It is usually slight, causes no dysfunction, and is short lived. The platelet count does not often exceed 1000 × 10^9/L (1,000,000/mm^3). Only occasionally is there a tendency to bleed or

an increased risk of thrombosis. Usually, no treatment is needed. Table 52-3 lists the causes of secondary thrombocytosis.

Physiologic. Physiologic thrombocytosis occurs whenever exercise is severe. The increased secretion of epinephrine returns platelets sequestered in the spleen and elsewhere to the circulation. Hypoxia causes thrombocytosis by increasing the production of platelets.

Disease of the Bone Marrow. Anything that increases the activity of the bone marrow is likely to cause thrombocytosis. It often accompanies the erythroid hyperplasia caused by blood loss. It is common in myeloproliferative disorders such as myelofibrosis, polycythemia vera, or chronic myeloid leukemia and in patients recovering from thrombocytopenia. It occasionally develops in iron deficiency anemia, multiple myeloma, and other conditions affecting the bone marrow.

Hyposplenism. Splenectomy usually causes a marked thrombocytosis. The concentration of platelets in the blood begins to rise a few days after the operation and often reaches a peak of 1000 × 10^9/L (1,000,000/mm^3) or more after two or three weeks. Usually the platelet count then slowly falls,

TABLE 52-3.   CAUSES OF SECONDARY THROMBOCYTOSIS

Physiologic
    Exercise
    Hypoxia

Disease of the bone marrow
    Erythroid hyperplasia
    Myeloproliferative disorders
    Post-thrombocytopenia

Hyposplenism
    Splenectomy
    Splenic atrophy

Disease of other organs
    Burns
    Cirrhosis of the liver
    Crohn's disease
    Infection
    Parturition
    Rheumatoid arthritis
    Surgery
    Trauma
    Tumors
    Ulcerative colitis

to return to normal after a few weeks or months. If the splenectomy has been performed to correct anemia, the thrombocytosis persists if the anemia persists and may remain at a high level. The platelet count usually falls to normal if the concentration of hemoglobin in the blood rises to normal. Loss of the spleen caused by disease causes thrombocytosis, though it is usually less severe than after splenectomy.

Disease of Other Organs. Surgical operations, parturition, burns, and other traumatic injuries often cause mild thrombocytosis that usually begins after one to two days and persists for one or two weeks. Carcinoma of the breast, carcinoma of the lung, Hodgkin's disease, and other tumors sometimes increase the concentration of platelets in the blood. Infection occasionally causes thrombocytosis. Ulcerative colitis, Crohn's disease, rheumatoid arthritis, and cirrhosis of the liver sometimes increase the platelet count.

ABNORMAL PLATELETS

In a number of conditions, the platelets fail to function normally. Some of these disorders are inherited; some are acquired. In some, the dysfunction of the platelets is the only abnormality. In others, the dysfunction of the platelets is part of a more complex disorder. Table 52-4 lists conditions in which platelet function is abnormal.

Hereditary Disorders

In a number of genetically determined diseases, the platelets fail to function normally. All are uncommon.

THROMBASTHENIA. Thrombasthenia takes its name from the Greek for a blood clot and weakness or sickliness. In the past, the name has been used loosely, but as now defined thrombasthenia is rare. It is inherited as an autosomal recessive character. Sometimes the condition is called Glanzmann's disease after a Swiss pediatrician (1887–1959).

In thrombasthenia, the platelet count is normal and the platelets look normal. They react with collagen and thrombin normally, but do not bind fibrinogen and fail to

TABLE 52-4.   CAUSES OF PLATELET DYSFUNCTION

Hereditary
　Thrombasthenia
　Bernard-Soulier Syndrome
　Thrombopathic Thrombocytopenia
　Deficient release reaction
　Thrombopathy

Acquired
　Drug induced
　　Antiinflammatory agents
　　　Acetylsalicylic acid
　　　Ibuprofen
　　　Indomethacin
　　　Mefenamic acid
　　　Phenylbutazone
　　　Salycilic acid
　　　Sulfinpyrazone
　　　Sulindac
　　Antidepressant agents
　　　Amitryptyline
　　　Chlorpromazine
　　　Imipramine
　　　Promethazine
　　Antimicrobial agents
　　　Amantadine
　　　Ampicillin
　　　Carbenicillin
　　　Methicillin
　　　Nitrofurantoin
　　　Penicillin
　　Other
　　　Anesthetics
　　　Chloroquine
　　　Clofibrate
　　　Dextrans
　　　Ethanol
　　　Dihydroergotamine
　　　Diphenhydramine
　　　Dipyridamole
　　　Papaverine
　　　Phentolamine
　　　Propanolol
　　　Reserpine
　　　Tolbutamide

　Hematologic disorders
　　Paraproteinemia
　　Myeloproliferative disorders
　　Acute myeloid leukemia

　Other
　　Uremia
　　Fibrinogen degradation products

aggregate when exposed to adenosine diphosphate, thrombin, or epinephrine. They do aggregate when exposed to ristocetin. Clot retraction is impaired. The bleeding time is increased.

The cause of dysfunction in thrombasthenia is in the cell membrane of the platelets. It lacks the glycoprotein IIb-IIIa complex required for fibrinogen binding and for the agglutination mediated by fibrinogen. In some patients, the antigen PL^{A1} (ZW^a) is also deficient.

Homozygotes with thrombasthenia bruise easily and bleed excessively after injury because of the inability of the platelets to initiate hemostasis adequately. Epistaxis, bleeding from the gums, purpura, and other kinds of bleeding are common. Heterozygotes show no abnormality.

No treatment has proved of consistent value.

BERNARD-SOULIER SYNDROME. The Bernard-Soulier syndrome, named after the French physicians who described it in 1948, is inherited as an autosomal recessive character. The patients have giant platelets, some up to 8 μm in diameter, mild thrombocytopenia, and a more severe bleeding tendency than the thrombocytopenia would suggest. The disease is severe in homozygotes and mild in heterozygotes.

In the Bernard-Soulier syndrome, the cell membrane of the platelets lacks the glycoproteins Ib and Is. Because of the deficiency in protein Ib, the platelets cannot bind to the von Willebrand factor and do not adhere normally to the vessel wall. They aggregate normally when exposed to adenosine diphosphate or collagen, but not when exposed to ristocetin. The bleeding time is prolonged. Clot retraction is normal.

THROMBOPATHIC THROMBOCYTOPENIA. Thrombopathic thrombocytopenia is similar to the Bernard-Soulier syndrome but is inherited as an autosomal dominant character.

DEFICIENT RELEASE REACTION. In patients with a deficient release reaction, the platelets are unable to release the adenosine diphosphate and other factors stored in their cytoplasm. If a blood vessel is injured, the platelets react normally to the adenosine diphosphate released from the injured tissue cells and begin to aggregate, but because they are unable to release the adenosine diphosphate in their own cytoplasm, the platelet plug is small, unstable, and soon dissolves.

There are two kinds of hereditary deficient release reaction. In patients with storage pool disease, the quantity of adenosine diphosphate in the platelets is low. In people with a defective release mechanism, the quantity of adenosine diphosphate in the platelets is normal, but they are unable to release it in response to the usual stimuli. In some kindred, the defect is inherited as an autosomal dominant character. In other kindreds, the mode of inheritance is unclear.

The platelets in the blood are normal in number in people with a deficient release reaction and look normal or a little smaller

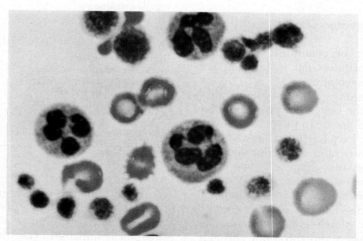

Fig. 52-1. Giant platelets in the blood of a patient with the Bernard-Soulier syndrome. (From Wintrobe, M. M., et al.: Clinical Hematology. 8th Ed. Philadelphia, Lea & Febiger, 1981.)

than usual. Electron microscopy shows a reduction in the number of dark granules that store adenosine diphosphate in the patients with storage pool disease.

Clot retraction is normal. In vitro, a high concentration of adenosine diphosphate causes normal aggregation of the platelets, but a low concentration of adenosine diphosphate causes only partial and temporary aggregation, because the adenosine diphosphate needed to complete the process is not released from the platelets. For the same reason, collagen and epinephrine fail to induce normal aggregation in vitro. The activity of platelet factor 3 may or may not be normal.

Patients with a hereditary deficient release reaction usually show only a mild bleeding tendency, perhaps only easy bruising. The bleeding time is moderately to greatly prolonged and may vary from time to time. No treatment is known.

Some patients with a deficient release reaction have the Chediak-Higashi syndrome or the Wiskott-Aldrich syndrome. The platelets are often abnormally large in people with Marfan's syndrome, the Ehlers-Danlos syndrome, osteogenesis imperfecta, or one of the mucopolysaccharidoses, and in some of these people seem unable to release adenosine diphosphate normally.

People with the Hermansky-Pudlak syndrome, named after the Czechoslovakian physicians who described it in 1959, have albinism and the accumulation of ceroid in macrophages as well as storage pool disease, sometimes with pulmonary fibrosis or inflammatory bowel disease. The Hermansky-Pudlak syndrome is inherited as an autosomal recessive character.

THROMBOPATHY. In people with thrombopathy, the platelets aggregate normally, but little platelet factor 3 is released. The people affected have a mild bleeding tendency. Some consider thrombopathy a variant of the deficient release reaction.

Acquired Disorders

Many drugs and diseases, especially diseases of the hematopoietic system, cause malfunction of the platelets. Usually the dysfunction is mild, but occasionally it is severe enough to cause serious bleedings.

DRUG-INDUCED. Table 52-4 lists some of the many drugs and poisons that can affect the function of the platelets. Usually the dysfunction is too slight to be evident clinically.

Acetylsalicylic acid prevents the release of adenosine diphosphate and other substances from the platelets. Platelets in people taking acetylsalycilic acid adhere normally to the collagen in the intima of the blood vessels, but because the release of adenosine diphosphate from the platelets is reduced, they fail to adhere firmly together. The inhibition caused by a single dose of aspirin persists for the life of the platelets, about a week. Acetylsalicylic acid also inhibits the synthesis of prostaglandins PGE2 and PGFa, the synthesis of thromboxane A2, and to a lesser degree the synthesis of prostacyclin, increasing the hemorrhagic tendency. In most people taking acetylsalicylic acid, the bleeding time is not prolonged beyond the normal limits, but most lose small quantities of blood into the gastrointestinal tract. Some bruise easily. In a few, there is more serious bleeding.

Other nonsteroidal anti-inflammatory agents impair the function of the platelets less than does acetylsalicylic acid, though they too impair the release of adenosine diphosphate and other substances from the platelets and reduce the synthesis of prostaglandins. With most, the injury to the platelets persists for the lifetime of the platelets. Indomethacin and the pyrazoles differ in that the impairment of the function of the platelets is reversible. If the concentration of the drug falls, platelet function returns to normal.

The antimicrobial agents listed in Table 52-4 impair the aggregation of the platelets and reduce the release of adenosine diphosphate and other substances from the platelets. Carbenicillin sometimes causes serious bleeding when given in therapeutic doses, but the other antimicrobial agents listed are unlikely to cause detectable dysfunction in the platelets unless the dose is very high.

Dipyridamole impairs the release of adenosine diphosphate and other substances from the platelets by inhibiting phosphodiesterase in the platelets and so increasing the concentration of cyclic adenosine monophosphate in the platelets. Some of the antidepressents and antihistamines may alter the membranes of the platelets, preventing the release of the content of their granules. Dextrans and similar substances impair the release of adenosine diphosphate from the platelets by coating their surfaces. How the other drugs and toxins listed in Table 52-4 damage the platelets is uncertain.

HEMATOLOGIC. A bleeding tendency sometimes appears in patients with abnormal proteins circulating in the blood, especially in people with macroglobulinemia. In some of these people, the aggregation of the platelets is impaired, or there is reduced release of platelet factor 3. Usually the injury to the platelets is only one of several factors tending to cause bleeding.

In myeloproliferative disorders, the platelets are often irregularly shaped and larger than normal. Often the release of the content of their granules is impaired, or the activity of platelet factor 3 is reduced. The cell membrane of the platelets may be abnormal, with loss of the α-adrenergic receptors or the receptors for thrombin. Ecchymoses, epistaxis, gastrointestinal bleeding, or more serious hemorrhage can follow.

In acute myeloid leukemia and myelodysplasia the platelets are often large, with dilated canaliculi and loss of microtubules. Sometimes giant granules formed by the fusion of normal granules occupy more than 50% of the volume of the platelets. Faults in the aggregation of the platelets and inability to release the content of their granules are common.

OTHER DISEASES. Bleeding can be severe in uremia and is due in large part to the inability of the platelets to release adenosine diphosphate, platelet factor 3, and other substances. The injury to the platelets is caused by a factor circulating in the plasma. The fibrinogen degradation products formed in disseminated intravascular coagulation impair the aggregation of platelets and reduce the release of the content of their granules.

BIBLIOGRAPHY

General

Corrigan, J. J., Jr.: Hemorrhagic and thrombotic diseases in childhood and adolescence. New York, Churchill Livingstone, 1985.

Firkin, B. G.: The Platelet and its Disorders. Lancaster, MTP Press, 1984.

Frisch, B., Lewis, S. M., Burkhardt, R., and Bartl, R.: Biopsy Pathology of Bone and Bone Marrow. London, Chapman and Hall, 1985.

Hardisty, R. M., and Weatherall, D.J.: Blood and Its Disorders. 2nd Ed. Oxford, Blackwell, 1982.

Harker, L. A.: Acquired disorders of platelet function. Ann. N. Y. Acad. Sci., 509:188, 1987.

Ingram, G. I. C., Bronzovic, M., and Slater, N. G. P.: Bleeding Disorders. 2nd Ed. Oxford, Blackwell, 1982.

Jandl, J. H.: Blood. Boston, Little, Brown and Co., 1987.

Levine, R. F., Williams, N., Levin, J., and Evatt, B. L. (Eds.): Megakaryocyte development and function. Prog. Clin. Biol. Res., 215:1, 1986.

Longnecker, G. L. (ed.): The Platelets. New York, Academic Press, 1985.

Weiss, H. J.: Platelets. New York, A. R. Liss, 1982.

Westwick, J., Scully, M. F., MacIntyre, D. E. and Kakkar, V. V. (eds.): Mechanisms of stimulus-response coupling in platelets. Adv. Exp. Med. Biol., 192:1, 1985.

Wickramasinghe, S.N. (ed.): Blood and Bone Marrow. In Systemic Pathology, 3rd Ed. Edited by Symmers, W. St. C. London, Churchill Livingstone, 1986.

Williams, W. J., Beutler, E., Erslav, A. J., and Lichtman, M. A.: Hematology. 3rd Ed. New York, McGraw-Hill, 1983.

Wintrobe, M. M., et al.: Clinical Hematology. 8th Ed. Philadelphia, Lea & Febiger, 1981.

Wittels, B.: Surgical Pathology of Bone Marrow. Philadelphia, W. B. Saunders, 1985.

Zucker-Franklin, D., Greaves, M. F., Grossi, C. E., and Marmont, A. M.: Atlas of Blood Cells. 2nd Ed. Philadelphia, Lea & Febiger, 1988.

Thrombocytopenia

Arthur, C. K., Isbister, J. P., and Aspery, E. M.: The heparin-induced thrombosis-thrombocytopenia syndrome. Pathology, 17:82, 1985.

Aster, R. H.: Idiopathic thrombocytopenic purpura. In The Autoimmune Diseases. Edited by Rose, N. R. and Mackay, I. R. Orlando, Academic Press, 1985.

Bick, R. L.: Hemostasis defects associated with cardiac surgery, prosthetic devices, and other extracorporeal circuits. Semin. Thromb. Hemostas., 11:249, 1985.

Bowie, E. J., and Owen, C. A.: The clinical pathology of intravascular coagulation. Bibl. Haematologica, 49:217, 1983.

Chaplin, S.: Bone marrow depression due to mianserin, phenylbutazone, oxyphenbutazone, and chloramphenicol—Part I. Adverse Drug React. Acute Poisoning Rev., 5:97, 1986.

Colvin, B. T.: Thrombocytopenia. Clin. Haematol., 14:661, 1986.

Edmunds, L. H., Jr.: Thrombotic and bleeding complications of prosthetic heart valves. Ann. Thorac. Surg., 44:430, 1987.

Kagan, R., and Laros, R. K., Jr.: Immune thrombocytopenia. Clin. Obstet. Gynecol., 26:537, 1983.

Kelton, J. G.: Heparin-induced thrombocytopenia. Haemostasis, *16*:173, 1986.

Kelton, J. G., and Murphy, W. G.: Heparin-induced thrombocytopenia and thrombotic thrombocytopenic purpura. Ann. N. Y. Acad. Sci., *509*:205, 1987.

Kitchens, C. S.: The purpuric disorders. Semin. Thromb. Hemostas., *10*:173, 1984.

Lian, E. C.-Y.: Thrombotic thrombocytopenic purpura. Annu. Rev. Med., *39*:203, 1988.

Lindenbaum, J.: Hematological complications of alcohol abuse. Semin. Liver Dis., *7*:169, 1987.

McMillan, R. (ed.): The Immune Cytopenias. Edinburgh, Churchill Livingstone, 1983.

Newland, A. C.: Idiopathic thrombocytopenia and IgG. J. Infect., Suppl 1:41, 1987.

Shende, A.: Idiopathic thrombocytopenic purpura in children, Pediatr. Ann., *14*:609, 1985.

Thomas, H. S., and Bauer, J. H.: Hereditary nephritis, deafness and thrombocytopenia. Mo. Med., *81*:305, 1984.

Vermylen, J., Blockmans, D., Spitz, B., and Deckmyn, H.: Thrombosis and immune disorders. Clin. Haematol., *15*:393, 1986.

Ware, R., and Kinney T. R.: Immunopathology of childhood idiopathic thrombocytopenic purpura. CRC Crit. Rev. Oncol. Hematol., *7*:169, 1987.

Thrombocytosis

Foster, P. N., and Losowsky, M. S.: Hyposplenism. J. R. Coll. Physicians Lond., *21*:188, 1987.

Pearson, T. C., and Messinezy, M.: Polycythaemia and thrombocythaemia in the elderly. Baillière's Clin. Haematol., *1*:355, 1987.

Sills, R. H.: Splenic function. Physiology and splenic hypofunction. CRC Crit. Rev. Oncol. Hematol., *71*:1, 1987.

Abnormal Platelets

Andrassy, K., and Ritz, E.: Uremia as a cause of bleeding. Am. J. Nephrol., *5*:313, 1985.

Balduini, C. L. and Ascari, E.: Acquired autoimmune thrombasthenia. Haematologica, *72*:387, 1987.

Phillips, D. R., Charo, I. F., Parise, L. V., and Fitzgerald, L. A.: The platelet membrane glycoprotein IIb-IIIa complex. Blood, *71*:831, 1988.

Rao, A. K., and Holmsen, H.: Congenital disorders of platelet function. Semin. Hematol., *23*:102, 1986.

Rodgers, G. M., and Shuman, M. A.: Congenital thrombocytic disorders. Am. J. Hematol., *21*:419, 1986.

White, J. G.: Platelet granule disorders. CRC Crit. Rev. Oncol. Hematol., *4*:337, 1986.

53

Disorders of Coagulation

THE disorders of coagulation are divided into hereditary and acquired forms. They are caused by deficiency of one of the coagulation factors, an inhibitor that impairs coagulation, or excessive intravascular coagulation.

HEREDITARY DISORDERS

The hereditary disorders of coagulation include some of the most famous of the diseases that cause excessive bleeding, among them hemophilia, Christmas disease, and von Willebrand's disease.

HEMOPHILIA. Hemophilia is often called hemophilia A, to distinguish it from Christmas disease, commonly called hemophilia B. Hemophilia has been known since ancient times, but only in 1910 was it realized that the excessive bleeding in hemophiliacs was caused by a defect in a plasma protein, now known to be the antihemophilic factor, factor VIII of the coagulation system. The factor VIII that circulates in the plasma in patients with hemophilia is unable to play its part in the coagulation sequence normally, though the other functions of factor VIII are preserved.

About 1 person in 10,000 has hemophilia. It is the most common of the hereditary disorders in which a defect in one of the coagulation factors causes excessive bleeding. In Europe and North America, 80% of people with a hereditary bleeding disorder have hemophilia. It is inherited as an X-linked character.

Lesions. The lesions in hemophilia are caused by hemorrhage. Their severity depends on the coagulant activity of the factor VIII in the plasma.

In severe hemophilia, the coagulant activity of the factor VIII in the plasma is less than 1% of normal. Hemorrhage into the muscles or joints occurs without apparent cause. It is often massive and crippling. Damage to the bones leads to skeletal deformities. Even a minor injury is likely to cause dangerous hemorrhage.

If the coagulant activity is between 1 and 5%, spontaneous bleeding into the joints and muscle is less likely and less massive, but severe bleeding follows even minor injury. Without treatment, the hemorrhage can prove fatal. If the coagulant activity of the factor VIII in the plasma is between 5 and 25% of normal, spontaneous bleeding into joints or muscles is unlikely. There may be enough coagulant activity to control the bleeding from minor injuries. Any major injury or surgical procedure is likely to cause severe hemorrhage. If the coagulant activity is between 25 and 50% of normal, the patient suffers no disability, though bleeding may be unusually profuse during a surgical operation.

The bleeding into the joints results from rupture of small blood vessels in the synovial membrane, no doubt caused by some trivial injury. The knees and other large joints are the most commonly affected. As the cavity of the joint fills with blood, the joint becomes hot, tense, and acutely painful, and inflammation develops in the adjacent tissues. The blood is slowly resorbed in the course of some weeks. The inflammation caused by the hemorrhage subsides. The first time that bleeding occurs, there is usually little permanent injury.

If there are repeated hemorrhages into the same joint, recovery is no longer complete. The synovium of the affected joint becomes thickened and edematous. Villous arborations extend from the synovial membrane into the joint cavity. The synovium becomes brown, as increasing quantities of hemosiderin accumulate from the breakdown of red cells.

Macrophages filled with hemosiderin and chronic inflammatory cells infiltrate the synovium. The cartilage of the joint is eroded and destroyed. Sometimes cystic cavities develop in the bone beneath the cartilage. Because of the pain, the limb is held still, and the inactivity causes the adjacent bone to become osteoporotic. Osteophytes sometimes extend around the joint, restricting its movement. Further bleeding into the joint becomes ever more likely as the villous excrescences from the synovium become large enough to be crushed between the surfaces of the joint. Eventually, the joint may be completely destroyed, with fibrous or bony ankylosis.

Injury to the soft tissues causes hemorrhage into the skin, subcutaneous tissue, or muscles. If the hemorrhage is massive, it causes fever, leukocytosis, and anemia. Compression or spasm of arteries surrounded by hemorrhage can cause ischemic contracture or gangrene distal to the hemorrhage. Compression of nerves sometimes causes peripheral neuritis. If the blood is trapped in a confined space, its high osmolality attracts fluid into the lesion, increasing the pressure on surrounding structures.

Epistaxis, bleeding from the gums, and bleeding from the tongue are common and can endanger life. Hematemesis, melena, and hematuria are frequent. About 5% of the patients have subdural, epidural, subarachnoid, or intracerebral bleeding.

Small cuts do not cause much bleeding in most hemophiliacs. The platelets, with such coagulant activity as the patient's factor VIII retains, are sufficient to control the hemorrhage. Larger injuries sometimes cause massive bleeding immediately after the injury; sometimes slow, persistent oozing continues for weeks.

Delayed bleeding occurs even in mild hemophilia. After an injury, perhaps extraction of a tooth, hemostasis seems normal but after some hours or days, the platelets and the coagulant activity remaining in the patient's factor VIII can no longer control the injury, and hemorrhage, often dangerous hemorrhage, begins.

The partial thromboplastin time is prolonged if the coagulant activity of factor VIII is less than 20% of normal. It can be restored to normal by adding normal plasma containing normal factor VIII. The coagulation time is abnormal only if the coagulant activity is less than 1% of normal. The prothrombin consumption test is normal if the coagulant activity is more than 2% of normal.

Clinical Presentation. Almost all patients with hemophilia are boys or men. If the disease is severe, it becomes apparent soon after birth, often because of bleeding into the scalp caused by injury during delivery. If it is less severe, the bleeding tendency becomes evident only when the child begins to crawl, increasing the risk of trauma to the limbs. If hemophilia is mild, the bleeding tendency may not become obvious until adolescence or adult life.

Pathogenesis. The gene that codes for the part of the factor VIII molecule with coagulant activity is on the long arm of the X chromosome between the locus for color blindness and that for glucose-6-phosphate dehydrogenase. The genes controlling the remainder of the molecule are autosomal. The severity of the defect varies from one kindred to another, though in any one kindred the severity of the disease is the same in all those affected, suggesting that more than one abnormal allele can cause hemophilia.

On the average, girls and women heterozygous for hemophilia have about 50% of the normal coagulant activity of factor VIII. In some of the cells synthesizing factor VIII, the X chromosome with the normal allele is active, and normal factor VIII is produced. In some, the chromosome with the abnormal allele is active, and the factor VIII produced lacks coagulant activity. In individual heterozygotes, the coagulant activity of factor VIII varies widely, from almost normal, to dangerously low. If a girl or woman heterozygous for hemophilia has the misfortune to have the X chromosome bearing the abnormal allele active in most of the cells synthesizing factor VIII, most of her factor VIII lacks coagulant activity. In rare instances the coagulant activity of factor VIII is so low that a heterozygote develops hemophilia. Rarely, a girl is homozygous for an allele causing hemophilia and develops the disease.

New mutations are common in hemophilia. In 30% of the patients, there is no history of the disease in the patient's ancestors. The gene that caused hemophilia in the royal families of Europe probably originated in one of Queen Victoria's parents.

In 90% of patients with hemophilia, antibodies that block the coagulant activity of normal factor VIII fail to react with the abnormal molecules circulating in the hemophiliacs, suggesting that the portion of the molecule of factor VIII responsible for its coagulative activity is either absent or abnormal. In 10% of hemophiliacs, the abnormality in factor VIII is more subtle, and the blocking antibodies react with the abnormal factor VIII present in the patient's plasma.

The bleeding in hemophilia is caused by the inability of the factor VIII to activate the subsequent steps of the coagulation sequence. Hemorrhage occurs whenever damage to a blood vessel is too great to be controlled by a hemostatic plug of platelets and the little coagulant activity that remains.

Treatment and Prognosis. Hemophilia is managed by administering factor VIII to control bleeding. Usually it is sufficient to maintain the coagulant activity of the factor at about 30% of normal for a few days. If there is major bleeding or if an operation is contemplated, the activity of the coagulant activity of factor VIII must be raised to 100% and maintained at that level until healing is complete. Since the half-life of factor VIII given by injection is from 12 to 18 hours, repeated injections are needed.

Some 5% of patients with hemophilia develop antibodies that block the coagulative activity of factor VIII. In such people, plasmapheresis to reduce the quantity of antibody in the blood and large doses of factor VIII or concentrates of factor IX are of value if there is serious bleeding of if an operation is scheduled. Factor VIII prepared from pigs or other animals may be less likely to be inactivated by the antibodies than is the human factor VIII usually given. Because most patients with hemophilia are treated with factor VIII prepared from human blood, the risk that they will develop viral hepatitis or the acquired immune deficiency syndrome is high.

Before the treatment was discovered, severe hemophilia often brought death in childhood and crippled many of those who survived. With care to avoid injury, treatment with factor VIII has improved the prognosis greatly, though the risk of dangerous hemorrhage remains.

CHRISTMAS DISEASE. Christmas disease, also called hemophilia B, is due to deficiency of the plasma thromboplasmic component, factor IX, of the coagulation sequence. The disease is named after the patient in whom hemophilia B was first clearly distinguished from hemophilia A, in 1952. Less than 1 person in every 70,000 has Christmas disease. It is inherited as an X-linked character. New mutations are uncommon.

Lesions and Clinical Presentation. The lesions and clinical presentation in Christmas disease are indistinguishable from those of hemophilia A. Bleeding is severe if the coagulant activity of factor IX is less than 1% of normal. There is little or no bleeding if the activity exceeds 20% of normal.

Pathogenesis. The gene coding for the coagulant activity of factor IX is on the long arm of the X chromosome. More than one genetic abnormality can cause Christmas disease. In most patients, only the portion of the molecule of factor IX responsible for its coagulant activity is defective. In some, no part of the molecule can be detected in the blood. In most patients, the prothrombin time is normal. In others, it is prolonged when the test is performed with bovine brain thromboplastin, though not when other thromboplastins are used.

The coagulant activity of factor IX in girls and women heterozygous for Christmas disease is often less than 25% of normal. Heterozygotes are more likely to bleed abnormally than are heterozygotes for hemophilia A.

Treatment and Prognosis. Christmas disease is treated by giving concentrates of factor IX. Because the concentrates are prepared from human blood, there is a risk of developing viral hepatitis or the acquired immune deficiency syndrome. In most patients, the severity of the disorder remains unchanged throughout the patient's life. In the Leyden variety of Christmas disease, the disorder grows less severe as the patient ages.

VON WILLEBRAND'S DISEASE. von Willebrand's disease is named after the Finnish physician who described it in 1926. In this disease, a defect in factor VIII impairs the adhesion of platelets to the wall of damaged blood vessels. Nearly always, the coagulant activity of factor VIII is also impaired. The incidence of von Willebrand's disease is unclear, for often the disease is mild and passes unrecognized, but probably it occurs in 1 person in 50,000. The milder forms of von Willebrand's disease are inherited as an autosomal dominant character. The severe form seems to be inherited as an autosomal recessive character.

Lesions and Clinical Presentation. The defective adherence of the platelets to the vessel wall in von Willebrand's disease causes easy bruising, epistaxis, bleeding from the gums, gastrointestinal bleeding, hematuria, menorrhagia, and prolonged bleeding from minor injuries. Petechiae are uncommon. The bleeding time is prolonged because of the inability of the platelets to form a hemostatic plug. Bleeding like that in hemophilia occurs in von Willebrand's disease only in the minority of patients in whom the coagulant activity of factor VIII is greatly reduced.

Pathogenesis. The gene governing the synthesis of the von Willebrand factor, the part of factor VIII that facilitates platelet adherence to the vessel wall, is on chromosome 12. Several types of von Willebrand's disease are distinguished.

In type I, the concentration of the von Willebrand factor in the plasma is reduced, but the multimers of the factor that are present are normal, and the ratio of large, intermediate, and small multimers is normal. The binding of platelets to the vessel wall, the coagulant activity of factor VIII, and the aggregation of platelets induced by ristocetin are all impaired. The platelets are normal. They adhere normally to collagen and aggregate normally in vitro. Type I is the most common form of von Willebrand's disease. It is usually mild and is inherited as an autosomal dominant character. The patients are heterozygotes.

In type II, the concentration of the von Willebrand factor in the blood is usually normal, but the proportion of large multimers in the blood is low, and the small multimers are sometimes abnormal. The aggregation of

platelets by ristocetin is impaired, but the coagulant activity of factor VIII is usually normal. In some people with type II disease, the synthesis of the large and intermediate multimers of the factor is impaired. In some, the large multimers are catabolized abnormally rapidly. In some, the large multimers bind inappropriately to circulating platelets and are rapidly cleared from the blood, causing thrombocytopenia and a deficiency of the large multimers. Type II disease is inherited as an autosomal dominant character. The patients are heterozygotes.

The severe form of von Willebrand's disease is sometimes called type III. Little or no von Willebrand factor is present in the plasma. The coagulant activity of factor VIII is greatly depressed. The patients have bleeding like that of hemophilia as well as evidence of platelet dysfunction. This form of the disorder appears to be inherited as an autosomal recessive character, though many of the patients are children of parents both of whom have type I von Willebrand's disease. Probably most patients with severe von Willebrand's disease are double heterozygotes with different genetic abnormalities on their chromosomes 12, or are homozygotes with the same abnormality on each chromosome 12.

Occasionally a patient with a lymphoma or an autoimmune disorder develops antibodies against the von Willebrand factor, a patient with von Willebrand's disease given multiple transfusions develops antibodies against the factor, or a tumor adsorbs the factor. The acquired deficiency of the factor can be severe enough to cause dysfunction.

Treatment and Prognosis. In many patients with von Willebrand's disease, no treatment is needed. If necessary, cryoprecipitate containing both von Willebrand factor and the coagulant activity of factor VIII is given to control the dysfunction.

Patients with type I disease often benefit from 1-desamino-8-D-arginine vasopressin, a drug that raises the concentration of the von Willebrand factor and the activity of factor VIII in the plasma without causing hypertension or fluid retention. The drug is not of help in patients with type II disease.

OTHER HEREDITARY DISORDERS OF CO-AGULATION. In a few patients, one of the other coagulation factors is absent because of an inborn error of metabolism, usually inherited as an autosomal recessive character, occasionally as an autosomal dominant or an X-linked character. Prothrombin, factor V, factor VII, factor X, factor XI, factor XII, and factor XIII have each been found absent in a few kindred. In some of these patients, the deficient factor is replaced by a similar but inactive protein. In some, the quantity of the factor synthesized is reduced.

Most of these deficiencies cause only a mild bleeding tendency, like that of mild hemophilia. Only occasionally is the bleeding severe, with hemarthroses and extensive hemorrhages.

In people with deficiency of factor XII, the Hageman factor, there is little bleeding, Instead the patients are likely to develop thrombosis or emboli.

Rarely, two or more of the coagulation factors are deficient. Deficiency of factors V and VIII or of factors VIII as IX are the most common. In some patients, all the vitamin K-dependent factors are deficient. In rare instances prekallikrein or the high molecular weight kininogen is deficient.

AFIBRINOGENEMIA. Afibrinogenemia is a rare disorder in which the people affected have no fibrinogen. Clotting is impossible. Platelet aggregation cannot occur. The erythrocyte sedimentation rate is usually zero. People with afibrinogenemia bleed excessively after surgery and other forms of trauma, but spontaneous bleeding is uncommon and not often severe. Both afibrinogenemia and a less severe form of the disorder called hypofibrinogenemia are inherited as autosomal recessive characters.

DYSFIBRINOGENEMIA. In dysfibrinogenemia, an abnormal fibrinogen circulates in the plasma. More than 50 kinds of dysfibrinogenemia have been identified since the first was discovered in 1963. All are rare. Some of the abnormal fibrinogens cannot be split by thrombin. Some cannot polymerize normally. Some fail to develop the cross-linkages necessary to stabilize fibrin.

Most forms of dysfibrinogenemia are inherited as an autosomal codominant character. In one kindred, the abnormality is inherited as an X-linked character. The patients are heterozygotes with a mixture of normal and abnormal fibrinogens in the plasma. Many are asymptomatic. Some have a mild bleeding tendency. Some have an increased risk of thrombosis.

ACQUIRED DISORDERS

Vitamin K deficiency, liver disease, inhibitors of coagulation, disseminated intravascular coagulation, fibrinolysis, thrombotic thrombocytopenic purpura, and the hemolytic-uremic syndrome are among the diseases that cause secondary derangement of the coagulation system.

VITAMIN K DEFICIENCY. The liver requires vitamin K for the synthesis of prothrombin and the coagulation factors VII, IX, and X. If adequate quantities of vitamin K are not available to the liver, or if the liver cannot use the vitamin, the concentration of these factors in the plasma falls.

Hemorrhagic Disease of the Newborn. The concentration in the plasma of the coagulation factors dependent on vitamin K is normally low at birth and falls further in the course of the next few days, because of the inability of the newborn liver to synthesize these factors efficiently. If vitamin K is deficient, this fall is accentuated. Serious hemorrhage is likely on the second or third day of life. Melena, large hematomata on the head, purpura, bleeding into the soft tissues, and bleeding from the umbilical stump are common. Parenteral vitamin K brings a dramatic cure, with restoration of the vitamin K-dependent coagulation factors to normal within 24 hours.

Hemorrhagic disease of the newborn, as this form of bleeding is called, used to be common. In most of the world, it has been abolished by the prophylactic administration of vitamin K to all newborn infants.

Prematurity increases the risk of developing hemorrhagic disease of the newborn by reducing the ability of the liver to synthesize coagulation factors. Deficiency of vitamin K in the infant's or the mother's diet makes it more likely. Delay in establishing an intestinal flora able to synthesize the vitamin makes bleeding more likely. Drugs like the coumarins and phenytoin cross the placenta and impair the synthesis of the coagulation factors in the fetal liver.

Vitamin K Deficiency in Adults. In adults, vitamin K is derived from the diet and is synthesized by bacteria in the gut. Only if both are deficient is the intake of vitamin K inadequate. Occasionally a sick person who eats little and is taking antibiotics that reduce the proliferation of bacteria in the gut fails to obtain enough vitamin K. Deficiency of the coagulation factors II, VII, IX, and X can develop rapidly.

Malabsorption caused by celiac disease, sprue, ulcerative colitis, Crohn's disease, resection of the bowel, ascariasis, or other forms of severe diarrhea or steatorrhea can reduce the absorption of vitamin K sufficiently to depress the synthesis of factors II, VII, IX, and X if the injury to the bowel is extensive. Biliary obstruction causes malabsorption of vitamin K and can cause serious deficiency in the coagulation factors related to it. Bile salts are necessary for absorption of the vitamin. If no bile salts reach the bowel and no vitamin K is given parenterally, abnormal bleeding is likely to become evident within two or three weeks.

Drugs such as the coumarins are antagonists of vitamin K and compete with it, reducing the synthesis of the coagulation factors II, VII, IX, and X. Wide-spectrum antibiotics and sulfonamides reduce the synthesis of vitamin K in the bowel. Cholestyramine binds bile salts and prevents the absorption of vitamin K. Mineral oil and other cathartics reduce the absorption of the vitamin if used in excess.

The deficiency in the coagulation factors related to vitamin K rarely causes serious bleeding, except during a surgical procedure or after major trauma. The deficiency is overcome by giving vitamin K parenterally. The activity of the coagulation factors returns to normal within 24 hours.

LIVER DISEASE. Liver disease often causes abnormalities in coagulation, though usually they are not severe enough to cause abnormal bleeding. If the defect is severe, the risk of bleeding from a peptic ulcer, esophageal varices, or some other lesion in the gut increases. Bleeding is likely to be excessive during an operation or after the extraction of a tooth. Occasionally, the nose bleeds, or ecchymoses appear in the skin.

Usually, several factors combine to cause the dysfunction. Malabsorption caused by the lack of bile salts can impair the absorption of vitamin K. The damaged liver may be unable to synthesize adequate quantities of its coagulation factors II, V, VII, IX, X, XI, XII, and XIII. The synthesis of fibrinogen, prekallikrein, the high molecular weight kininogen, plasminogen, antiplasmin, or antithrombin III may be deficient, or the liver may produce an abnormal product, which functions poorly. The abnormal liver may be unable to clear from the blood activated coagulation factors, fibrinolysins, or other substances that interfere with coagulation. Debris escaping from the damaged liver cells can cause intravascular coagulation. Liver disease sometimes causes thrombocytopenia or abnormal platelet function.

INHIBITORS OF COAGULATION. Most inhibitors of coagulation are immunoglobulins. Some are antibodies directed against one of the coagulation factors. Some probably react with phospholipids. Occasionally the abnormal proteins that circulate in the blood in patients with multiple myeloma or some other B cell disorder act as an antithrombin or prevent the polymerization of fibrin.

Antibodies against one of the coagulation factors are most often directed against the coagulant portion of factor VIII. They are present in over 5% of people with hemophilia and sometimes develop in people with rheumatoid arthritis, disseminated lupus erythematosis, ulcerative colitis, or other diseases. Rarely, they appear in elderly people who have no other disease. The antibodies are usually IgG. They activate factor VIII slowly, in a reaction dependent on temperature. Severe bleeding like that in hemophilia can follow. Treatment is difficult. Huge doses of factor VIII bring benefit in some patients. In some, a concentrate of the coagulation factors dependent on vitamin K is of help.

Antibodies against the von Willebrand factor are less common. Antibodies against factor IX develop in 5% of people with Christmas disease. They too are IgG, but inactivate factor IX rapidly. Antibodies against factor V have been found, most often in people given streptomycin. They usually cause no bleeding, and disappear after some time. An inhibitor of factor XIII occurs occasionally, especially in people given isoniazid. Rarely, antibodies have developed against fibrinogen, factor VII, factor XI, or factor XII.

More than 10% of patients with disseminated lupus erythematosus have an anticoagulant in their blood. Less often, a similar anticoagulant develops in a patient with carcinoma, lymphoma, multiple myeloma, macroglobulinemia, myelofibrosis, prostatic hyperplasia, disease of the cardiac valves, or rheumatoid arthritis. The anticoagulant may be IgG or IgM. It acts rapidly. In some patients the anticoagulant reacts with phospholipids. In others it inhibits prothrombinase or is directed against one of the coagulation factors. The anticoagulant persists indefinitely. It rarely causes abnormal bleeding, but it does increase the risk of thrombosis.

DISSEMINATED INTRAVASCULAR COAGULATION. In disseminated intravascular coagulation, fibrin is precipitated within the blood vessels. Sometimes small thrombi are formed. If the process is widespread, the coagulation factors are used up, and their concentration in the blood falls. The concentration of fibrinogen in the plasma often falls greatly. The destruction of platelets may be so great that the patient develops thrombocytopenia.

Most of the fibrin precipitated in the blood vessels is soon lysed. Fibrin degradation products accumulate in the plasma. Often the fibrinolytic activity of the blood is increased.

Disseminated intravascular coagulation is sometimes called a consumption coagulopathy, because of the consumption of the coagulation factors, fibrinogen, and platelets by the widespread thrombosis. Sometimes it is called the defibrination syndrome or the coagulation-fibrinolysis syndrome.

Widespread intravascular coagulation is not common. It can be sudden and devastating or can continue intermittently for months.

Lesions. Changes in the circulating blood occur in all patients with disseminated intravascular coagulation, but the lesions in the blood vessels and other organs vary considerably from one patient to another.

Blood. The platelet count is low in disseminated intravascular coagulation. Often it is between 50 and 100 × 10^9/L (50,000 to 100,000/mm^3), but it can be much lower. Often the fall in the platelet count is the first sign of disseminated intravascular coagulation. The platelets that remain in the circulation often have lost much of the content of their granules and behave like platelets in storage

pool disease. Damage to the platelets sometimes releases 5-hydroxytryptamine and epinephrine into small blood vessels, causing vasoconstriction.

In 50% of the patients, the microthrombi damage the red cells sufficiently to cause schistocytes to appear in the blood. More often, increased activity of lactic acid dehydrogenase or a reduced concentration of haptoglobin in the plasma is evidence of damage to the red cells. Rarely, the injury to the red cells is so extreme that there is hemoglobinemia and hemoglobinuria.

The widespread coagulation in the blood vessels uses up some of the coagulation factors that are consumed during coagulation. In most patients the concentrations of fibrinogen, prothrombin, and factors V, VIII, and XIII fall. The concentration of factor V is especially low. Sometimes the concentrations of factors that are not consumed also fall, especially the concentrations of factors VII, IX, and X. The concentration of prothrombin in the plasma is usually normal. The partial thromboplastin time, prothrombin time, and thrombin time are abnormal.

The concentrations of antithrombin III, α-2 antiplasmin, and fibronectin are sometimes low in severe disseminated intravascular coagulation. Plasminogen is often precipitated together with the fibrin, because of its great avidity for fibrin. The complement system, kallikrein system, and plasmin system are all activated.

The activity of the fibrinolysins in the blood is almost always increased in disseminated intravascular thrombosis. The increased activity is due largely to increased activation of plasmin.

In a few patients, usually people with amniotic fluid embolism, heat stroke, or carcinoma, fibrinogenolysins develop as well as fibrinolysins. The fibrinogenolysins are rarely of much importance clinically.

The degradation products produced by the breakdown of fibrin by fibrinolysins accumulate in the plasma and are powerful antithrombins. They inhibit the polymerization of fibrin and interfere with the function of the platelets.

Other Organs. In many patients with disseminated intravascular coagulation, thrombi in the blood vessels are few and hard to find. The fibrinolysins in the blood lyse the fibrin

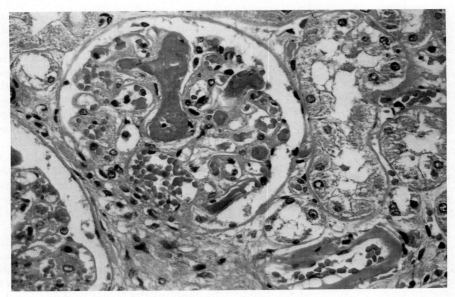

Fig. 53-1.   Thrombi in a renal glomerulus of a patient with disseminated intravascular coagulation.

soon after it is precipitated, and the thrombi that form in small vessels soon disappear.

In some patients, thrombi are found only in the kidneys, for the most part in the glomerular capillaries. They sometimes cause ischemic tubular injury, sometimes tubular necrosis. Occasionally the thrombosis is so extensive that cortical necrosis results.

Only in a minority of the patients are thrombi numerous. They occur in arterioles, capillaries, and venules throughout the body. If the disease is acute, often the liver is the most severely affected. Small vessels in the brain, gut, pancreas, myocardium, lungs, endocrine glands, and skin are commonly involved.

Foci of ischemic change in the gut are common and can develop in patients in whom thrombi are few. Small infarcts sometimes develop in the brain or other organs. Thrombi in the lungs can cause acute alveolar injury. In the pituitary gland, ischemia sometimes results in Sheehan's syndrome. In the adrenal glands, disseminated intravascular thrombosis can cause massive hemorrhage and the Waterhouse-Friderichsen syndrome. In all organs, petechiae and larger hemorrhages are frequent.

Clinical Presentation.   Disseminated intravascular coagulation often develops sud-

denly. Blood begins to ooze from venipuncture sites and around drains. Serious bleeding from surgical wounds or dangerous postpartum bleeding can occur. Purpura and ecchymoses are common in the skin and sometimes become extensive. Some of the ecchymoses may become necrotic, a condition called purpura fulminans. Bleeding from the nose, gums, gut, lungs, or into the urine is frequent. Renal failure, signs of cerebral infarction, or, less often, adrenal or hepatic failure can develop rapidly.

Less often, disseminated intravascular coagulation is less severe and develops more slowly. Repeated epistaxes, repeated hemorrhages into the gut, and persistent ecchymoses in the skin are common signs. Thrombi sometimes develop in unusual sites. Migratory thrombophlebitis can develop in the skin. Dangerous hemorrhage often complicates surgical procedures.

Pathogenesis.   Table 53-1 lists some of the many conditions that can cause disseminated intravascular coagulation. In most of these conditions, disseminated intravascular coagulation is uncommon. In a few, such as thrombotic thrombocytopenic purpura, the hemolytic-uremic syndrome, or eclampsia, widespread intravascular coagulation is an important feature of the disease and is

TABLE 53-1. CAUSES OF DISSEMINATED
INTRAVASCULAR THROMBOSIS

Pregnancy
    Abruptio placentae
    Amniotic fluid embolism
    Eclampsia
    Fetal death in utero
    Septic abortion

Infection
    Bacterial
        Meningococcemia
        Other gram-negative infections
        Septicemia
    Fungal
    Parasitic
    Rickettsial
    Viral

Trauma
    Burns
    Crush injuries
    Fat embolism
    Frostbite
    Gunshot wounds
    Surgery

Tumors
    Carcinoma
    Leukemia

Vascular disease
    Giant hematoma
    Pulmonary emboli
    Shock
    Vasculitis

Hematopoietic disorders
    Hemolytic-uremic syndrome
    Incompatible blood transfusion
    Intravascular hemolysis
    Paroxysmal nocturnal hemoglobinuria
    Thrombotic thrombocytopenic purpura

Other
    Acute alveolar injury
    Acute pancreatitis
    Anaphylaxis
    Diabetic acidosis
    Drugs
    Heat stroke
    Hypoxia
    LeVeen shunt
    Snake bite

responsible for much of the injury it causes.

The entry of thromboplastic substances into the blood is often of major importance in the causation of disseminated intravascular coagulation. In abruptio placentae, thromboplastins from the placenta and blood con-taining activated coagulation factors can enter the maternal blood in large quantity. In amniotic fluid embolism the fluid carries with it large quantities of weak thromboplastins. If a fetus dies in utero, thromboplastins from the fetus slowly leak into the maternal blood. A LeVeen shunt carries thromboplastins from the ascitic fluid into the blood. In severe trauma and following extensive sur-gical procedures, thromboplastins from the injured tissue escape into the blood. Mucus-secreting adenocarcinomata, promyelocyte leukemia cells, and other tumors occasionally release thromboplastic substances into the blood. Some snake venoms are potent throm-boplastins.

Disseminated intravascular coagulation is common in meningococcemia and can occur in other kinds of gram-negative bacteremia and in other kinds of infection. It can be due to injury to the boood vessels caused by the organisms directly, but is more often caused by the endotoxins elaborated by the organ-isms. The endotoxins activate the coagula-tion sequence and cause aggregation of plate-lets. They inhibit fibrinolysins. They damage leukocytes and endothelial cells, releasing thromboplastins into the blood. They acti-vate complement, increasing the tendency to thrombosis. In some patients, they initiate a Shwartzman reaction.

Shock and disseminated intravascular coagulation are often associated, but the relationship between them is complex and is different in different patients. Shock can cause disseminated intravascular coagulation and disseminated intravascular coagulation can cause shock, though not all patients in shock have disseminated intravascular coagu-lation and not all patients with disseminated intravascular coagulation are in shock. Endo-toxemia often causes both shock and dissemi-nated intravascular coagulation. The hypoxia and acidemia caused by shock can join with other factors to cause disseminated intravas-cular coagulation. Acute alveolar injury can cause disseminated intravascular coagulation or be caused by it.

The macrophages, especially the sinusoidal cells in the spleen and the Kupffer cells in the liver, normally remove from the blood most of the substances that initiate intravas-cular coagulation and most of the products that result from it. If disseminated intravascular coagulation is severe, the macrophages become overloaded and can no longer clear the blood of the agents that initiate coagulation or result from it. These substances persist in the blood, perpetuating the disease.

Treatment and Prognosis. Disseminated intravascular thrombosis is best treated by removing its cause, when this is possible. Transfusions to restore blood volume and replace the lost coagulation factors and platelets are important. Often heparin is of value, by interrupting the cycle of thrombosis and fibrinolysis and allowing the concentration of the coagulation factors to return to normal.

The prognosis in disseminated intravascular coagulation is bad. Over 50% of patients with the acute form die, usually of hemorrhage or thrombosis.

FIBRINOGENOLYSIS. The activation of plasmin without thrombosis is less common than disseminated intravascular coagulation. It is usually caused by factors like those that cause disseminated intravascular coagulation or by disease of the liver that prevents the normal clearance of the activators of plasmin from the blood. The concentration of fibrinogen in the plasma is usually normal or a little low because increased production of fibrinogen compensates for the increase in its destruction.

Coagulation is impaired by fibrin degradation products that accumulate in the blood. The clotting time, prothrombin time, and partial thromboplastin time are all abnormal. Clot lysis is increased. Plasmin can attack factor V, factor VIII, and other coagulation factors, adding to the bleeding tendency. The platelet count remains normal.

Treatment with a plasmin inhibitor like episilon aminocaproic acid brings a dramatic cessation of the bleeding caused by fibrinogenolysis. Heparin is sometimes given as well, if there is difficulty in distinguishing between fibrinolysis and disseminated intravascular coagulation.

THROMBOTIC THROMBOCYTOPENIC PURPURA. Thrombotic thrombocytopenic purpura is rare. In the northern United States, its annual incidence is 1 in 1,000,000. The disease can occur at any age, but most of the patients are between 10 and 40 years old. Some 60% of them are girls or women.

Lesions. Patients with thrombotic thrombocytopenic purpura develop multiple small platelet thrombi in arterioles and capillaries throughout the body, most prominently in the heart, brain, kidneys, pancreas, and adrenal glands. Probably it begins with a loose aggregation of platelets in the affected vessels. The platelets then become more tightly bound and surrounded with fibrin. Later, the platelets are gradually lost, and fibrin becomes the principal component of the thrombi. Often some of the thrombi are incorporated into the intima of the affected arterioles.

Often the thrombi form at the bifurcation of vessels. The occluded vessels dilate, forming small aneurysms. The walls of the dilated vessels are greatly thinned.

In the kidneys, though not in other organs, the thrombi often cause a proliferation of endothelial cells. The dilated arterioles become filled with a swirling mass of concentrically arranged, elongated cells. At times the lesions are as large as a glomerulus.

Thrombocytopenia is common in thrombotic thrombocytopenic purpura, because the megakaryocytes cannot compensate for the loss of platelets in the thrombi. Often the platelet count is between 10 and 120 × 10^9/L (10,000 and 120,000/mm^3).

Most patients have microangiopathic anemia. The hemoglobin is rarely above 100 g/L (10 g/100 mL). In 30% of the patients it is less than 50 g/L (5 g/100 mL). Often the intravascular destruction of the red cells causes hyperbilirubinemia. In 50% of the patients, the leukocyte count is increased, sometimes to 20 × 10^9/L (20,000/mm^3). Immature white cells are often present in the blood. In a few patients, there is sufficient breakdown of fibrin in the thrombi to cause fibrin degradation products to accumulate in the blood. Rarely, there is hypofibrinogenemia.

Clinical Presentation. The onset of thrombotic thrombocytopenic purpura is often sudden, with fever and neurologic damage. Over 90% of the patients develop headache, mental changes, hemiparesis, seizures, sensory changes, ataxia, or changes in vision. In some, the neurologic signs and symptoms are intermittent or change suddenly.

Over 90% of the patients develop purpura or ecchymoses in the skin. Often there is bleeding from the nose, gums, gut, or into the urine. Renal dysfunction is evident in

80% of the patients. Over 40% become jaundiced. Occasionally, there is pancreatitis, chest pain, or myalgia.

Pathogenesis. Thrombotic thrombocytopenic purpura is caused by a defect in the systems that normally prevent the formation of platelet thrombi in small blood vessels. The platelets are normal, and there is no fault in the coagulation system.

The thrombi probably develop because the endothelium of the blood vessels fails to synthesize the prostacyclin needed to prevent platelet aggregation and thrombosis, perhaps because a factor normally present in the plasma is deficient. In a few patients, the onset of the disease has followed infection or vaccination. In some, it complicates systemic lupus erythematosus, Sjögren's syndrome, vasculitis, polyarteritis or some other disease that is immunologically mediated. Estrogens may increase the risk of developing thrombotic thrombocytopenic purpura.

Treatment and Prognosis. Antiplatelet drugs, such as acetylsalicylic acid, dipyridamole, cyproheptadine, sulfinpyrazone, or dextran are often of benefit in thrombotic thrombocytopenic purpura, especially when used in combination. Exchange transfusions, plasmapheresis, and plasma infusions give a prolonged remission in some patients. Adrenocortical steroids are of little help, but some patients respond to immunosuppressive agents such as vincristine.

Before the introduction of these forms of therapy, 90% of patients with thrombotic thrombocytopenic purpura died within three months. With modern treatment 70% of the patients now enjoy a prompt and long-lasting remission.

HEMOLYTIC-UREMIC SYNDROME. The hemolytic-uremic syndrome is similar to thrombotic thrombocytopenic purpura, but affects mainly infants, causing acute renal failure. It is discussed with the diseases of the kidneys (Chapter 27).

BIBLIOGRAPHY

General

Bennett, J. S.: Blood coagulation and coagulation tests. Med. Clin. North Am., 68:557, 1984.

Bloom, A. L., and Thomas, D. P.: Haemostasis and Thrombosis. Edinburgh, Churchill Livingstone, 1981.

Colman, R. W., Hirsh, J., Marder, V. J., and Salzman, E. W. (Eds.): Hemostasis and Thrombosis. 2nd Ed. Philadelphia, Lippincott, 1987.

Corrigan, J. J., Jr.: Hemorrhagic and thrombotic diseases in childhood and adolescence. New York, Churchill Livingstone, 1985.

Hardisty, R. M., and Weatherall, D. J.: Blood and its Disorders. 2nd Ed. Oxford, Blackwell, 1982.

Ingram, G. I. C., Bronzovic, M., and Slater, N. G. P.: Bleeding Disorders. 2nd Ed. Oxford, Blackwell, 1982.

Jandl, J. H.: Blood. Boston, Little, Brown and Co., 1987.

Machovich, R.: Blood Vessel Wall and Thrombosis. Boca Raton, CRC Press, 1988.

Thomson, J. M.: Blood Coagulation and Haemostasis. 3rd Ed. Edinburgh, Churchill Livingstone, 1985.

Wickramasinghe, S. N. (Ed.): Blood and Bone Marrow. *In* Systemic Pathology, 3rd Ed. Edited by Symmers, W. St. C. London, Churchill Livingstone, 1986.

Williams, W. J., Beutler, E., Erslav, A. J., and Lichtman, M. A.: Hematology. 3rd Ed. New York, McGraw-Hill, 1983.

Wintrobe, M. M., et al.: Clinical Hematology. 8th Ed. Philadelphia, Lea & Febiger, 1981.

Hereditary Disorders

Bloom, A. L. (Ed.): The Haemophilias. Edinburgh, Churchill Livingstone, 1982.

Coleman, R.: Disorders of thrombin formation. Edinburgh, Churchill Livingstone, 1983.

Furlan, M.: Factor VIII/von Willebrand factor: a multivalent ligand binding to platelets and collagen. Blut, 52:329, 1986.

Holmberg, L., and Nilsson, I. M.: Von Willebrand disease. Clin. Haematol., 14:461, 1985.

Kane, W. H., and Davie, E. W.: Blood coagulation factors V and VIII. Blood, 71:539, 1988.

Larner, A. J.: The molecular pathology of haemophilia. Q. J. Med., 63:473, 1987.

Lillicrap, D. P., White, B. N., Holden, J. J. A., and Giles, A. R.: Carrier detection in the hemophilias. Am. J. Hematol., 26:285, 1987.

McGraw, R. A., et al.: Structure and function of factor IX: defects in haemophilia B. Clin. Haematol., 14:359, 1985.

Meyer, D., et al.: Role of von Willebrand factor in platelet-vessel wall interactions. Ann. N. Y. Acad. Sci., 509:118, 1987.

Moroose, R., and Hoyer, L. W.: Von Willebrand factor and platelet function. Annu. Rev. Med., 37:157, 1986.

Rocha, E., et al., Congenital dysfibrogenemias. Ric. Clin. Lab., 15:205, 1985.

Seligsohn, V., Rimon, A., and Horoszowski, H. (Eds.): Haemophilia. Tunbridge Wells, Castle House Publications, 1981.

Thompson, A. R.: Structure, function, and molecular defects of factor IX. Blood, 67:565, 1986.

Acquired Disorders

Andrassy, K., and Ritz, E.: Uremia as a cause of bleeding. Am. J. Nephrol., 5:313, 1985.

Bick, R. L.: Hemostasis defects associated with cardiac surgery, prosthetic devices, and other extracorporeal circuits. Semin. Thromb. Hemostas., 11:249, 1985.

Brain, M. C., and Neame, P. B.: Thrombotic thrombocytopenic purpura and the hemolytic uremic syndrome. Semin. Thromb. Hemostas. 8:187, 1982.

Byrnes, J. J.: Thrombotic thrombocytopenic purpura. Adv. Intern. Med., 26:131, 1981.

Collen, D., and Lijnen, H. R.: The fibrinolytic system in man. CRC Crit. Rev. Oncol. Hematol., 4:249, 1986.

Editorial: Unravelling HUS. Lancet, 2:1437, 1987.

Edmunds, L. H., Jr.: Thrombotic and bleeding complications of prosthetic heart valves. Ann. Thorac. Surg., 44:430, 1987.

Erickson, L. A., Schleef, R. R., Ny, T., and Loskutoff, D. J.: The fibrinolytic system of the vascular wall. Clin. Haematol., 14:513, 1985.

Francis, C. W., and Marder, V. J.: Concepts of clot lysis. Annu. Rev Med., 37:187, 1986.

Kane, K. K.: Fibrinolysis. Ann. Clin. Lab. Sci., 14:443, 1984.

Kelly, D. A., and Tuddenham, E. G. D.: Haemostatic problems in liver disease. Gut, 27:339, 1986.

Kwaan, H. C. (Ed.): Thrombotic microangiopathy. Semin. Hematol., 24:69, 141–201, 1987.

Levine, M. L.: Risk of haemorrhage associated with long term anticoagulant therapy. Drugs. 30:444, 1986.

Levine, M., and Hirsh, J.: Hemorrhagic complications of long-term anticoagulant therapy for ischemic vascular disease. Stroke, 17:111, 1986.

Marciniak, E.: Antiphospholipid antibody syndrome. J. R. Soc. Med., 80:445, 1987.

McKay, D. G.: Clinical significance of intravascular coagulation. Bibl. Haematologica, 49:63, 1983.

Mergerthaler, H. G., Binsack, T., and Wilmanns, W.: Carcinoma-associated hemolytic-uremic syndrome. Oncology, 45:11, 1988.

Moncada, S. (Ed.): Prostacyclin, thromboxane and leukotrienes. Br. Med. Bull., 39:209, 1983.

Müllertz, S.: Fibrinolysis. Semin. Thromb. Hemostas., 10:1, 1984.

Murgo, A. J.: Thrombotic microangiopathy in the cancer patient including those induced by chemotherapeutic agents. Semin. Hematol., 24:161, 1987.

Mustard, J. F., Kinlough-Rathbone, R. L., and Packham, M. A.: Mechanisms in thrombosis. Agents Actions, 15:9, 1984.

Nield, G.: The haemolytic-uraemic syndrome. Q. J. Med., 63:367, 1987.

O'Grady, J. G., et al.: Coagulopathy of fulminant hepatic failure. Semin. Liver Dis., 6:159, 1986.

Paterson, P. Y., Koh, C. S., and Kwaan, H. C.: Role of the clotting system in the pathogenesis of neuroimmunologic disease. Fed. Proc., 46:91, 1987.

Remuzzi, G.: HUS and TTP. Kidney Int., 32:292, 1987.

Roseman, B.: Disseminated intravascular coagulation. Oral Surg. 59:551, 1985.

Rosenberg, R. D.: The biochemistry and pathophysiology of the prethrombotic state. Annu. Rev. Med., 38:493, 1987.

Schafer, A. I.: Focussing on the clot: normal and pathologic mechanisms. Annu. Rev. Med., 38:211, 1987.

Schwartz, D. B.: Medical diseases in pregnancy. Emerg. Med. Clin. North Am., 5:509, 1987.

Steen, V. M., and Holmsen, H.: Current aspects of human platelet activation and response. Eur. J. Haematol., 38:383, 1987.

Stratta, P.: Hemorrheological approach to thrombotic microangiopathies. Nephron, 40:67, 1985.

Vermylen, J., Blockmans, D., Spitz, B., and Deckmyn, H.: Thrombosis and immune disorders. Clin. Haematol., 15:393, 1986.

Weiner, C. P.: Thrombotic microangiopathies in pregnancy and the postpartum period. Semin. Hematol., 24:119, 1987.

Wu, K. K.: Microvascular thrombosis. Hosp. Pract., 20(5):47, 1985.

54

Spleen

THE diseases of the spleen are divided into those characterized principally by splenomegaly, traumatic injuries, cysts, congenital anomalies, and tumors.

SPLENOMEGALY

Enlargement of the spleen is common. In the United States, from 2 to 6% of people have a speen large enough to be palpable. In from 20 to 40% of these people the cause of the enlargement is obscure. In some tropical areas, over 60% of the population have a palpable spleen.

Table 54-1 lists some of the many causes of splenomegaly. Most of these disorders affect principally other parts of the body, and the involvement of the spleen is only a minor feature of the disease. These conditions are discussed in other parts of the book. Only the diseases in which the enlargement of the spleen is the major feature of the disorder are considered in this chapter.

ACUTE SPLENITIS. Acute splenitis is an unusual condition, found occasionally in severe infections, such as septicemia, massive pneumonia, or bacterial endocarditis. Sometimes the enlargement of the spleen in acute splenitis is called an acute splenic tumor, using the word *tumor* in its Latin sense of a lump.

The spleen is three or four times its normal size, soft, and mushy. On section, its pulp is semiliquid and oozes out over the edge of the organ. Microscopically, the spleen often shows little abnormality, but sometimes the number of neutrophils is increased, or there is hyperplasia of the sinusoidal cells in the pulp.

Infectious mononucleosis and typhoid fever occasionally cause a similar enlargement of the spleen, with a soft semifluid pulp. In these conditions, there is no increase in the number of neutrophils in the pulp. In infectious mononucleosis, atypical lymphocytes can be found in the pulp, In typhoid, clumps of macrophages are present.

CONGESTIVE SPLENOMEGALY. Enlargement of the spleen caused by long-continued congestion is called congestive splenomegaly, or sometimes fibrocongestive splenomegaly. Cirrhosis of the liver is its most common cause. Less often it is due to narrowing or occlusion of the splenic vein or the extrahepatic portal vein, some other kind of intra-

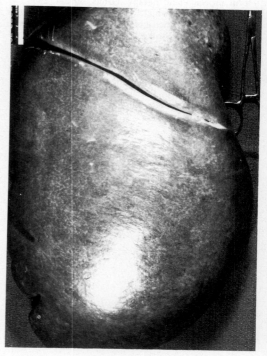

Fig. 54-1. An enlarged spleen in a patient with polycythemia vera. Note the forceps on the upper right of the picture.

1668

Infection
  Acute splenomegaly
    Acute splenitis
    Abscess
    Brucellosis
    Infectious mononucleosis
    Paratyphoid fever
    Typhoid fever
    Typhus

  Chronic splenomegaly
    Echinococcosis
    Histoplasmosis
    Kala-azar
    Malaria
    Schistosomiasis
    Syphilis
    Trypanosomiasis
    Tuberculosis

Hematologic disorders
    Hemolytic anemias
    Hemolytic disease of the newborn
    Leukemias
    Leukoerythroblastic anemia
    Lymphomas
    Megaloblastic anemias
    Multiple myeloma
    Myelofibrosis
    Polycythemia vera
    Structural hemoglobinopathies
    Thalassemias
    Thrombocytopenic purpuras

Congestive splenomegaly
    Cirrhosis of the liver
    Stenosis of the splenic vein
    Stenosis of the portal vein
    Stenosis of the hepatic veins
    Heart failure

Storage diseases
    Gaucher's disease
    Niemann-Pick disease
    Mucopolysaccharidoses

Other
    Amyloidosis
    Berylliosis
    Cysts
    Felty's syndrome
    Graves' disease
    Hamartoma
    Histiocytosis X
    Hyperlipemia
    Metastases
    Sarcoidosis
    Systemic lupus erythematosus
    Tropical splenomegaly

hepatic obstruction to the portal blood flow, or to narrowing of the hepatic veins. Occasionally severe, congestive heart failure causes congestive splenomegaly.

The spleen is moderately enlarged, often 400 to 800 g rather than its normal 150 g, and is firm. Often the capsule of the spleen is thickened by plaques of pearly white fibrosis. When the spleen is sectioned, the cut surface is firm, with prominent trabeculae.

Microscopically, the sinusoids are moderately dilated. The pulp cords are thickened and look stiff and fibrous. There is usually an increase in reticulin fibers in the cords, but little mature collagen is present unless the congestion has persisted for a long time. The white pulp is usually inconspicuous. The trabeculae are thickened. If there are white plaques in the capsule, they are formed of hyaline, acellular fibrosis.

Small hemorrhages into the pulp often cause foci scarring 1 to 2 mm across called Gamna-Gandy nodules or Gandy-Gamna bodies, after an Italian physician born in 1896 and a French physician born in 1872. The coarse collagen bundles in the scar are encrusted with iron and calcium and microscopically resemble bamboo. A few macrophages containing hemosiderin are present among the bundles of collagen.

Congestive splenomegaly usually causes little or no dysfunction. In some patients, hypersplenism develops.

Banti's Syndrome. In 1898, the Italian pathologist Banti described a syndrome in which congestive splenomegaly and anemia preceded the development of liver disease. Few now believe that such a condition exists, but the term *Banti's syndrome* is still sometimes used to describe congestive splenomegaly when its cause is uncertain or to describe the condition in which the patients have both congestive splenomegaly and hypersplenism.

TROPICAL SPLENOMEGALY. Tropical splenomegaly, or the big spleen syndrome, is found in the parts of the tropics in which malaria is prevalent, though it has not been established that the condition is caused by malaria. It occurs in Africa, Arabia, India, China, and New Guinea. The patients are usually young adults.

The spleen is greatly enlarged, often weigh-

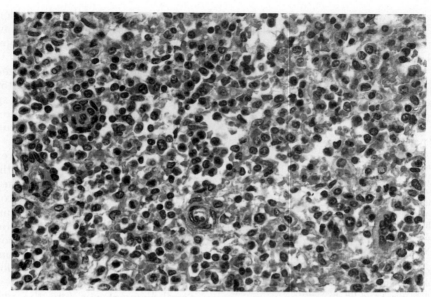

Fig. 54-2.   Acute splenitis in a patient with scarlet fever. Few neutrophils are present in this patient.

ing as much as 5000 g. It is firm, often with infarcts, white plaques on its surface, or Gandy-Gamna nodules. Microscopically, it shows congestion and hyperplasia of the pulp cords.

Many of the patients have hypersplenism, with anemia or pancytopenia. Most have portal hypertension. In some, the splenic veins are narrowed. Occasionally the liver is enlarged and lymphocytes are numerous in the hepatic sinusoids. Usually the concentration of IgM in the plasma is high.

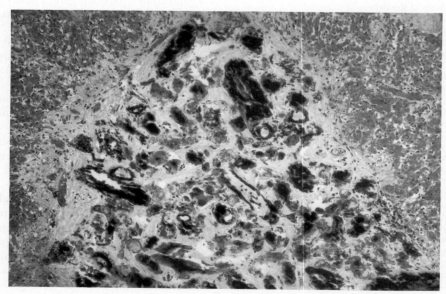

Fig. 54-3.   A Gandy-Gamna nodule in the spleen of a patient with sickle cell anemia showing the encrustation of bundles of collagen with iron and calcium.

Antimalarial therapy usually causes shrinkage of the spleen. The lymphocytes disappear from the liver. Hypersplenism lessens.

PERISPLENITIS. Perisplenitis is common, both when the spleen is enlarged and when it is of normal size. It probably results from episodes of inflammation long in the past. It causes no dysfunction and no symptoms.

The capsule of the spleen is thickened by pearly white fibrosis, usually 3 or 4 mm thick, often almost cartilagenous in consistency. The capsule may be diffusely thickened, or the thickening may form plaques, sometimes smooth, sometimes rough and nodular. Microscopically, the thickening is caused by thick bundles of hyalinized collagen running parallel to the surface of the organ, with few or no fibrocytes evident.

HYPERSPLENISM. The term *hypersplenism* is used to describe the conditions in which the spleen removes blood cells from the blood in such numbers that it causes anemia, leukopenia, thrombocytopenia, or some combination of these conditions. In secondary hypersplenism, the cause of the increased splenic activity is known. In primary hypersplenism, it is not.

Primary hypersplenism can complicate any condition that causes splenomegaly, though in most forms of splenomegaly only a small minority of the patients develop hypersplenism. Secondary hypersplenism is most often due to a defect in the blood cells involved or to an immunologic reaction that leads to their increased destruction.

In both types of hypersplenism, the spleen removes the cells involved from the blood by increasing their segregation in the spleen, by increasing the rate at which they are destroyed, or by some combination of these mechanisms. Up to 40% of the red cells in the blood and as much as 90% of the platelets can be segregated in the spleen. As the blood cell mass falls, the plasma volume increases to maintain the blood volume. The loss of blood cells usually excites hyperplasia of the bone narrow to compensate for the splenic hyperactivity, though in some patients with primary hypersplenism the bone marrow fails to react.

The spleen shows no microscopic abnormality in patients with hypersplenism, except for the lesions caused by the underlying disease. It is not possible to determine whether a patient with splenomegaly has hypersplenism by examining the spleen.

If the underlying condition causing the hypersplenism cannot be controlled, and the loss of blood cells is dangerously large, splenectomy gives relief.

TRAUMA

The spleen, liver, and colon are the abdominal organs most often ruptured by trauma, with the spleen by far the most commonly affected. The trauma may be direct if some object penetrates the abdomen and lacerates the spleen. More often the injury is caused by a sudden blow from some blunt object, such as the seat belt in a motor car or the handlebar of a bicycle. In many patients, the blow causes no apparent injury to the abdominal wall, and the tear in the spleen is the only evidence of injury. Rarely, violent deceleration, as in an aircraft accident, tears the vessels at the hilus of the spleen.

In most patients, the trauma tears the capsule of the spleen, and intra-abdominal hemorrhage follows. The severity of the hemorrhage varies greatly. In some patients, there is only a little bleeding that stops spontaneously. In some, there is massive exsanguinating hemorrhage. In most patients, the blood in the peritoneal cavity causes severe abdominal pain and sometimes pain in the left shoulder from irritation of the diaphragm. Less often, there is nausea or a vague mass in the region of the spleen. The leukocyte count is usually from 15 to 20 × 10^9/L (15,000 to 20,000/mm^3). After some delay, the hematocrit falls as hemodilution develops to restore the blood volume and compensate for the blood loss. Without surgery to remove the spleen and control the bleeding, death is probable.

In 15% of the patients in whom the spleen is injured by blunt trauma, the bleeding is delayed. The injury causes a hematoma within the spleen. For a time, the hematoma is contained by the capsule of the spleen. The patient is often unaware of the injury. Only after a few days, weeks, or months, does the growing pressure within the hematoma rupture the capsule of the spleen. Bleeding into the abdominal cavity begins, just as when the capsule of the spleen is torn at the time of injury. The severity of the delayed hemorrhage varies, but it is no less dangerous than the hemorrhage that follows immediately when the capsule of the spleen is torn at the time of injury.

Some hematomata within the spleen become encapsulated, and as the blood is resorbed form cysts within the spleen. Such cysts are sometimes called pseudocysts, pseudo because they have no epithelial or mesothelial lining.

If fragments of splenic tissue escape into the abdominal cavity when a spleen is ruptured, they often implant on the peritoneum and grow into tiny spleens, like the accessory spleens that develop as a congenital anomaly. If these tiny spleens are numerous, the condition is called splenosis. The implants function like a normal spleen and usually do no harm, though if one is unfortunately placed it can cause obstruction.

HYPOSPLENISM. If splenic function is seriously impaired, abnormalities appear in the blood and the risk of infection increases. Most often hyposplenism is caused by the surgical removal of the spleen, usually after trauma or for hypersplenism, but occasionally it is caused by irradiation, sickle cell disease, or congenital absence of the spleen.

The red cells in the blood of a person who has undergone splenectomy are thinner than normal, often appearing as target cells in a blood smear. Their osmotic fragility is decreased. Nucleated red cells and Howell-Jolly bodies are usually present. Burr cells and Heinz bodies are sometimes evident. The concentration of hemoglobin in the blood may increase or decrease. A leukocytosis of 10 to 15 × 10^9/L (10,000 to 15,000/mm^3) is common, with the increase being principally of neutrophils in the first few weeks after splenectomy but consisting mainly of lymphocytes and monocytes in the months that follow. In 30% of the patients, the platelet count increases to 1500 to 2000 × 10^9/L (1,500,000 to 2,000,000/mm^3) some days or weeks after splenectomy and remains elevated.

Splenectomy increases the risk of fatal infection 200 times. The ability of the body to clear bacteria coated with antibody from the blood is impaired, and the production of antibodies against bacteria is reduced. In 50% of the patients, the infection is pneumococcal. Meningococci, Escherichia coli, Haemophilus influenzae, staphylococci, and streptococci are other organisms commonly found.

CYSTS

Cysts of the spleen are uncommon. They may be a few centimeters in diameter or huge sacs containing as much as 4000 mL. Sometimes there is more than one. The patient is usually an adult.

Some of the cysts are lined in part by stratified squamous epithelium and are derived from an inclusion of epithelium from some neighboring organ or arise by squamous metaplasia of the mesothelium. Other cysts, often in the capsule of the spleen, are lined by mesothelial cells. Often the epithelium or mesothelium lining the cyst is largely lost, and for the most part the cyst is contained only by the fibrous capsule surrounding it. The fluid within the cyst is sometimes clear, especially in mesothelial cysts, but often it contains shimmering crystals of cholesterol or is brown from old hemorrhage.

Cysts contained only by a collagenous wall are more common than those completely or partially lined by epithelium or mesothelium. The wall is sometimes partially calcified. Some cysts of this sort arise from a hematoma. Others are epithelial or mesothelial cysts that have completely lost their lining. Most splenic cysts do no harm and cause no symptoms.

CONGENITAL ANOMALIES

Accessory spleens are the only common congenital anomaly of the spleen. They are usually 2 to 4 cm in diameter, roughly spheroidal, and are most common near the hilus of the spleen. Microscopically, they have sinusoids and white pulp like those of a normal speen.

Accessory spleens are of no significance, except when a splenectomy is performed because of excessive destruction of blood cells in the spleen. If an accessory spleen is left behind, it sometimes enlarges and continues the destruction of the blood cells.

Less often, a circumscribed nodule of splenic tissue called a hamartoma is present within the spleen. The lesion has a collagenous capsule. The splenic tissue in the lesion may be malformed.

TUMORS

Except for the neoplasms of the hematopoietic system, which often involve the spleen, neoplasms of the spleen are uncommon. A hemangioma or a lymphangioma occasionally arises within the spleen. Rarely, a hemangioendothelioma or some other benign or malignant mesenchymal tumor arises in the spleen.

Metastatic carcinoma rarely forms nodules large enough to be recognizable macroscopically in the spleen, though 10% of people with widespread metastatic carcinoma have involvement of the spleen microscopically. Metastases of malignant melanoma or chorionepithelioma sometimes develop in the spleen. spleen.

BIBLIOGRAPHY

General

Baesl, T. J., and Filler, R. M.: Surgical diseases of the spleen. Surg. Clin. North Am., 65:1269, 1985.

Splenomegaly

Cavalli, G., Casali, A. M., and Monari, P.: The microvascular architecture of the spleen in congestive splenomegaly. Pathol. Res. Pract., 174:131, 1982.
Hewlett, D. Jr., and Pitchumoni, C. S.: Tropical splenomegaly syndrome (TSS) and other diseases of the spleen. Baillière's Clin. Gastroenterol., 1:319, 1987.
Nelken, N., Ignatius, J., Skinner, M., and Christensen, N.: Changing clinical spectrum of splenic abscess. Am. J. Surg., 154:27–34, 1987.

Trauma

Bohnsack, J. F., and Brown, E. J.: The role of the spleen in resistance to infection. Annu. Rev. Med., 37:49, 1986.
Di Cataldo, A., et al.: Splenic trauma and overwhelming postsplenectomy infection. Br. J. Surg., 74:343, 1987.
Foster, P. N., and Losowsky, M. S.: Hyposplenism. J. R. Coll. Physicians Lond., 21:188, 1987.
Llende, M., Santiago-Delpin, E. A., and Lavergne, J.: Immunobiological consequences of splenectomy. J. Surg. Res., 40:85, 1986.
Shatney, C. H.: Complications of splenectomy. Acta Anaesthesiol. Belg., 38:333, 1987.
Sills, R. H.: Splenic function. Physiology and splenic hypofunction. CRC Crit. Rev. Oncol. Hematol., 71:1, 1987.
Stoval, T. G., and Ling, F. W.: Splenosis. Obstet. Gynecol. Surv., 43:69, 1988.
Stryker, R. M., and Orton, D. W.: Overwhelming postsplenectomy infection. Ann. Emerg. Med., 17:161, 1988.
Warren, K.S.: The kinetics of hepatosplenic schistosomiasis. Semin. Liver Dis., 4:293, 1984.

Cysts

Brig, K.-F.: Epithelial (true) splenic cysts. Am. J. Surg. Pathol., 12:275, 1988.
Garvin, D. F., and King, F. M.: Cysts and nonlymphomatous tumors of the spleen. Pathol. Annu., 16 (1): 61, 1981.

Tumors

Garvin, D.F., and King, F.M.: Cysts and nonlymphomatous tumors of the spleen. Pathol. Annu., 16(1):61, 1981.
Ng, J. P. et al.: Primary splenic hairy cell leukaemia. Eur. J. Haematol., 39:349, 1987.

55

Lymph Nodes and Lymphocytes

THE diseases of the lymph nodes and lymphocytes are so closely interrelated that they are best considered together. They are divided into the inflammatory conditions called lymphadenitis, conditions in which the lymph nodes are enlarged for other reasons, the immune deficiency diseases, and tumors.

LYMPHADENITIS

Inflammation of the lymph nodes is called lymphadenitis, from the Latin for a water nymph, or by extension clear water, and the Greek for a gland. It is divided into acute, chronic, and granulomatous forms.

ACUTE LYMPHADENITIS. Acute lymphadenitis is common. Almost all kinds of acute inflammation cause acute lymphadenitis in the nodes that receive lymph from the injured tissue. Usually, acute lymphadenitis is mild and transient. Occasionally, it is severe and produces permanent injury.

Lesions. In mild acute lymphadenitis, the affected lymph nodes are two or three times their normal size and may be tender. The swollen glands in the neck caused by a sore throat are a good example.

Microscopically, the affected lymph nodes are congested and edematous, with widely dilated sinusoids. Usually, the follicles are large, with many mitoses and much phagocytosis. Often neutrophils are present in the sinusoids and are scattered in the pulp. If the inflammation persists for a few days, the macrophages in the pulp of the nodes usually proliferate and enlarge. The macrophages often become actively phagocytic, taking up fragments of dying neutrophils and other debris.

If acute lymphadenitis is more severe, the enlargement of the lymph nodes is greater, and they become painful. The edema and neutrophilic exudate in the affected nodes increases. Often the exudate extends through the capsule of the lymph nodes into the adjacent tissues. Foci of necrosis or abscesses sometimes develop within the nodes.

In most patients, acute lymphadenitis subsides, leaving no residual injury. The lymph nodes affected return to normal when the inflammation in the tissue they drain is overcome. If the inflammation does not subside, it slowly merges into chronic lymphadenitis.

Only if acute lymphadenitis is unusually severe, or the same lymph nodes are repeatedly inflamed, is fibrosis likely to follow. The capsule of the lymph nodes becomes thickened, and irregular bands of fibrosis extend into the nodes. Abscesses and the larger foci of necrosis heal by scarring.

Pathogenesis. Usually acute lymphadenitis is caused by chemical irritants carried to the lymph nodes by the lymph from inflamed tissue. Toxins, mediators of inflammation, and other products of inflammation all cause acute lymphadenitis. Less often, a lymph node showing acute lymphadenitis is infected, usually by bacteria or other organisms carried to the node in the lymph from a neighboring site of infection.

The changes in the lymph nodes are much the same in all types of acute lymphadenitis. Only in a few infections such as chancroid or plague does the nature of the lesion suggest its etiology.

CHRONIC LYMPHADENITIS. Chronic lymphadenitis is also common. In the inguinal lymph nodes, it is almost invariable, no doubt due to the frequent minor infections in the tissues these nodes drain. In other lymph nodes, it is less frequent, but still common.

Sometimes chronic lymphadenitis is called reactive hyperplasia of the lymph nodes. If its cause is not apparent, it is often called nonspecific lymphadenitis. Dermatopathic lymphadenitis, lipid lymphadenitis, and vaccinial lymphadenitis are special types of chronic lymphadenitis.

Lesions. Lymph nodes showing chronic lymphadenitis are usually enlarged. They are often firm and easily palpated. They are not tender unless acute lymphadenitis is added to the chronic changes.

Microscopically, the changes in chronic lymphadenitis vary considerably from one person to another. There may be hyperplasia of the follicles; hyperplasia of the paracortical T cells; hyperplasia of the macrophages lining the sinusoids; an infiltrate of macrophages, eosinophils, or neutrophils; edema; or fibrosis. Any or all of these changes or any combination of them may be present. Sometimes one is dominant, sometimes another.

Enlargement of the follicles is common in chronic lymphadenitis. Especially in lymph nodes draining foci of chronic inflammation, it is often the dominant feature of the reaction. The follicles may be several times their normal diameter. Often they are more numerous than normal. Within the follicles, mitoses are numerous. Phagocytosis of nuclear debris and other material by the follicular cells is often striking. A rind of closely packed B cells usually surrounds the enlarged follicles.

Hyperplasia of the T cells in the paracortical region is less often prominent in chronic lymphadenitis. Only in viral infections and occasionally in people with lymphadenitis caused by phenytoin or other drugs is it likely to be the dominant feature. The paracortical region is thickened. Immunoblasts are scattered among the lymphocytes in this region. The immunoblasts are often numberous, and especially in viral infections in children, some of them are often atypical. Sometimes the venules in the paracortical region are prominent.

Hyperplasia of the macrophages lining the sinusoids is common in chronic lymphadenitis, usually in association with follicular hyperplasia. Frequently, the sinusoids are dilated. They often contain scattered macrophages and a few other cells. The macrophages lining the sinusoids are large, with abundant, pale, eosinophilic cytoplasm. Sometimes they show phagocytosis of cells or of cellular debris. Less often, the macrophages lining the sinusoids are hyperplastic. The sinusoids become filled with macrophages with abundant, pale cytoplasm. Especially in the axillary lymph nodes draining a carcinoma of the

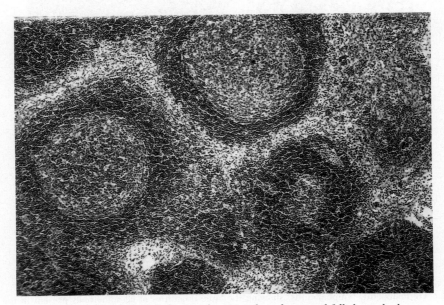

Fig. 55-1. Chronic lymphadenitis, showing enlarged germinal follicles and edema.

breast, this proliferation of the sinusoidal lining cells can be the principal feature of the reaction, a condition called sinus histiocytosis.

Edema is often prominent in lymph nodes showing chronic lymphadenitis. Often the lymphatics leading to the affected lymph nodes are dilated. Occasionally, plasma cells or, less often, macrophages or eosinophils are numerous in the pulp of the lymph nodes. Sometimes a few neutrophils are present. If chronic lymphadenitis persists for weeks or months, the capsules of the involved nodes become thickened, and broad bands of fibrosis extend into the nodes, replacing and distorting them.

If chronic lymphadenitis is severe, an exudate predominantly of lymphocytes but with a few macrophages and occasionally other inflammatory cells often extends through the capsule of the involved lymph nodes into the adjacent fatty tissue.

Chronic lymphadenitis often persists with little change for weeks or years. If its cause is removed, it resolves, at least in part. Only when the lymph nodes have become fibrotic, can they no longer return to normal.

Pathogenesis. Chronic lymphadenitis usually follows repeated attacks of acute lymphadenitis or develops in lymph nodes draining chronically inflamed tissue. It is common in lymph nodes that receive lymph from malignant tumors. Persistent bacterial, viral, and other infections in the tissue drained by the affected lymph nodes commonly cause chronic lymphadenitis, though the nodes themselves are not often infected. Other causes are long continued imunologic stimulation, phenytoin, and other drugs. Often chronic lymphadenitis persists long after the condition that caused it has disappeared.

Dermatopathic Lymphadenitis. Lymph nodes draining skin affected by severe, chronic dermatitis are often enlarged and easily palpable. Because of the unusual changes in the lymph nodes and their association with the dermatitis, this kind of lymphadenopathy is often called dermatopathic lymphadenitis. Occasionally it is called lipomelanotic reticulosis, using reticulosis in an old sense to mean a proliferation of macrophages.

The lymph nodes show chronic lymphadenitis, usually with hyperplasia of the macro-

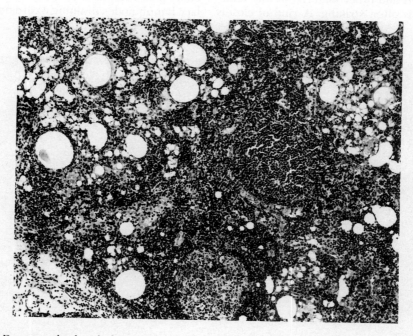

Fig. 55-2. Dermatopathic lymphadenitis, showing the large quantities of fat sometimes present in the lymph nodes in this disorder.

phages lining the sinusoids. The follicles are large and active. Plasma cells, eosinophils, or neutrophils often are numerous in the lymph nodes. Sometimes there are small abscesses or other signs of superimposed acute inflammation. The macrophages contain large quantities of melanin and hemosiderin carried to the lymph nodes in the lymph from the skin. Sometimes the macrophages contain considerable quantities of fat.

Lipid Lymphadenitis. The macrophages lining the sinusoids in the lymph nodes in the porta hepatis and upper part of the abdomen often contain large lipid droplets. At times some of the macrophages become multinucleated to encompass even larger droplets of fat. The fat is probably derived from the chyle that flows through the lymph nodes. Microscopically, the appearance is impressive, but the accumulation of fat is probably temporary and has little affect on the function of the lymph nodes.

The oily solutions used for lymphangiography produce a similar, but more dramatic change in the lymph nodes. The solutions are irritant and first cause acute lymphadenitis, with neutrophils and eosinophils. Within a few days, the oily substances are taken up by the macrophages in the lymph nodes, and the macrophages become filled with fatty droplets. Often there is hyperplasia of the macrophages lining the sinusoids. Sometimes giant cells or granulomata form. As weeks pass, the inflammation subsides, and plasma cells replace the neutrophils and eosinophils. The oil is not metabolized and remains in the macrophages. The lymph nodes become quiescent. Sometimes they become fibrotic.

Vaccinial Lymphadenitis. The lymph nodes draining a site of vaccination often become enlarged. They show chronic lymphadenitis, hyperplasia of the macrophages lining the sinusoids, and often an exudate of eosinophils, neutrophils, and plasma cells. Hyperplasia of the T cells in the paracortical region is often accompanied by a striking proliferation of immunoblasts. Some of the immunoblasts become large and atypical, much as immunoblasts sometimes do in other viral infections.

GRANULOMATOUS LYMPHADENITIS. If granulomata are present in a lymph node, the condition is called granulomatous lymph-

adenitis. Usually the granulomata are superimposed on chronic lymphadenitis.

Table 55-1 shows some of the more common causes of granulomatous lymphadenitis. In some of these conditions, the lesions are characteristic enough to suggest the cause of the granulomata. In some, only a differential diagnosis is possible.

Tuberculosis is still a common cause of granulomatous lymphadenitis. In young lesions, the lymph nodes often contain tuberculous granulomata of the classic type. Their core is a loose aggregation of large, irregular macrophages, often with spaces between them. A little caseous necrosis is often evident in the center of the granuloma. Commonly the granulomata contain large, multinucleated macrophages of the Langhans type.

Tuberculous ganulomata are not always of this classic form. They can resemble the granulomata of sarcoidosis or mimic other kinds of granulomatous lymphadenitis. Tubercle bacilli are usually demonstrable in the granulomata, but failure to find the bacilli does not exclude tuberculosis. If there is reason to suspect that a lymph node contains tuberculous granulomata, a biopsy should be cultured as well as examined histologically.

Older tuberculous lesions in lymph nodes have cores of granular, caseous necrosis surrounded by a collagenous capsule. Often

TABLE 55-1. CAUSES OF GRANULOMATOUS LYMPHADENITIS

Infections
    Tuberculosis
    Histoplasmosis
    Infection with atypical mycobacteria
    Brucellosis
    Cat scratch fever
    Mesenteric adenitis
    Tularemia
    Lymphogranuloma venerum

Sarcoidosis

Other diseases
    Carcinoma
    Crohn's disease

Inert agents
    Beryllium
    Zirconium

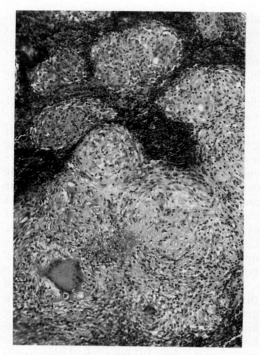

Fig. 55-3. Tuberculous lymphadenitis, showing at the top of the picture granulomata like those of sarcoidosis, in the lower part a larger granuloma with central necrosis.

there is little or no inflammatory reaction where the necrosis meets the capsule. Sometimes there is a palisade of macrophages or a few scattered multinucleated cells, together with lymphocytes at the margin of the necrosis. Tubercle bacilli are rarely demonstrable in old, quiescent lesions.

Histoplasmosis, atypical mycobacteria, and other organisms cause granulomatous lymphadenitis indistinguishable from tuberculous lymphadenitis. Often the organisms can be demonstrated in the lesions, but sometimes they cannot.

In cat scratch fever, mesenteric adenitis, tularemia, and lymphogranuloma venereum, the granulomata in the lymph nodes sometimes resemble the lesions of tuberculosis or sarcoidosis, but more often are larger and irregularly shaped. In most patients, the core of the granuloma is bordered by neutrophils and surrounded by a palisade of macrophages.

Sarcoidosis is a common cause of granulomatous lymphadenitis. In its typical form, the affected lymph nodes are almost replaced by granulomata packed closely together. The granulomata are well defined and compact. They consist of macrophages with abundant, ill-defined, eosinophilic cytoplasm. It is hard to see where one cell ends and the next begins. Some of the macrophages have more than one nucleus, but cells with many nuclei are uncommon. Necrosis is absent or minimal. Less often the granulomata of sarcoidosis are looser, with large, multinucleated macrophages, and resemble the granulomata of tuberculosis. Usually, there is no fibrosis. Only in old lesions do the granulomata become surrounded by a wall of fibrosis, which slowly compresses and replaces the granulomata, until they are reduced to small, spheroidal scars.

The histologic examination of a lymph node alone never permits a certain diagnosis of sarcoidosis. Even if the granulomata are of typical morphology and no organisms can be demonstrated, tuberculosis, histoplasmosis, and other infections cannot be excluded. The granulomata caused by zirconium or beryllium can closely mimic the granulomata of sarcoidosis. To establish a diagnosis of sarcoidosis, the findings in lymph nodes must be interpreted in conjunction with the patient's history and other investigations.

Granulomata are sometimes found in lymph nodes draining a carcinoma, especially a carcinoma of the colon. They are often present in lymph nodes in Crohn's disease. They can be caused by zirconium or beryllium. The collagenous nodules of silicosis can be mistaken for healed granulomata.

HYPERPLASTIC LYMPHADENOPATHY

The hyperplastic lymphadenopathies are benign conditions that cause enlargement of one or more groups of lymph nodes. The disorders often mimic a malignant lymphoma. Anticonvulsant lymphadenitis, sinus histiocytosis, familial hemophagocytic reticulosis, and angiofollicular hyperplasia are conditions of this sort.

ANTICONVULSANT LYMPHADENOPATHY. Anticonvulsant lymphadenopathy develops in a minority of patients given anticonvulsant drugs, most often in people given phenytoin or mephenytoin. One or more groups of lymph nodes become enlarged. The enlargement is painless and suggests lymphoma.

Microscopically, the enlarged lymph nodes show chronic lymphadenitis. The architecture of the lymph nodes is sometimes considerably distorted. Hyperplasia of the T cells in the paracortical region is prominent. Usually immunoblasts are numerous in this region. Some of them are often atypical. Mitoses are common. Hyperplasia of the macrophages lining the sinusoids is often marked. Often there is a diffuse infiltrate of plasma cells, eosinophils, or neutrophils. Foci of necrosis may occur. Sometimes an exudate mainly of lymphocytes extends through the capsules of the lymph nodes into the surrounding tissue. At times, the structure of the lymph node is so distorted that it suggests Hodgkin's disease.

Anticonvulsant lymphadenopathy is benign. It subsides if the drug is withdrawn.

SINUS HISTIOCYTOSIS. Patients with sinus histiocytosis develop massive and painless enlargement of one or more groups of lymph nodes, most often the cervical lymph nodes on one or both sides. With the enlargement come fever, neutrophilia, hypergammaglobulinemia, and a raised erythrocyte sedimentation rate. Most of the patients are black children or young people.

Microscopically, the affected lymph nodes show marked dilatation of their sinusoids, which are filled with macrophages with abundant, pale, eosinophilic cytoplasm. A few of the macrophages are multinucleated, have foamy cytoplasm, or atypical nuclei. The phagocytosis of lymphocytes is often evident in an occasional macrophage, which may contain several lymphocytes in its cytoplasm. Phagocytosis of red cells or other hematopoietic cells is less common. Plasma cells are numerous in the pulp of the lymph nodes. In the later stages of the disease, pericapsular fibrosis is marked.

The cause of sinus histiocytosis is unknown. The enlargement of the lymph nodes persists for months or years with little change, but eventually resolves. No treatment is necessary.

FAMILIAL HEMOPHAGOCYTIC RETICULOSIS. Familial hemophagocytic reticulosis is inherited as an autosomal recessive character.

The disease becomes manifest in infancy, with anorexia, irritability, vomiting, hepatosplenomegaly, and enlargement of one or more groups of lymph nodes. Later come jaundice and thrombocytopenia. There may be hypergammaglobulinemia, immunohemolytic anemia, or other evidence of an immunologic upset. The disorder is benign and resolves as the child grows older.

The lymph nodes show a marked proliferation of macrophages, which fill and dilate the sinusoids. Erythrophagocytosis and the phagocytosis of lymphocytes and other blood cells are prominent. The spleen, liver, and bone marrow show a similar proliferation of macrophages.

ANGIOFOLLICULAR HYPERPLASIA. In angiofollicular hyperplasia, a well-defined mass of lymphoid tissue sometimes several centimeters in diameter is found in the mediastinum or, less often, in some other part of the body. Microscopically, the mass is encapsulated and shows prominent follicles like those in lymph nodes, except that in many of the patients a small blood vessel runs through the center of each follicle. Sometimes the follicular cells swirl around the vessel and look something like a Hassal's corpuscle. Lymphocytes and macrophages fill the space between the follicles. The macrophages may form broad bands, but there are no sinusoids.

In less than 50% of the patients, plasma cells are numerous between the follicles.

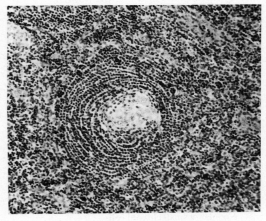

Fig. 55-4. Angiofollicular hyperplasia, showing the swirling pattern common in this condition.

Particularly in these patients, there may be fever, anemia, or hypergammaglobulinemia.

The nature of these masses is obscure, and they have been given many names. Many think they are hamartomata. Some consider they result from infection.

Angiofollicular hyperplasia is benign. The lesion may cause symptoms if it presses on a blood vessel or an airway or may be discovered by accident. Excision cures.

IMMUNE DEFICIENCY DISEASES

The immune deficiency diseases are discussed with the other disorders of the immunologic system in Chapter 10. Many of them are disorders of the lymphocytes and cause major changes in the lymph nodes. If T cells are lacking, the paracortical zone of the lymph nodes is small and atrophic, and the white pulp of the spleen is sparse. If B cells are deficient, follicles disappear from the lymph nodes and spleen, and lymphocytes are few in the medullary cords of the lymph nodes.

TUMORS

Secondary tumors of the lymph nodes are among the commonest of malignant tumors, but interest has centred on the tumors of the lymphocytes, most of which arise in the lymph nodes. Table 55-2 lists the tumors of the lymphocytes and lymph nodes.

TABLE 55-2. TUMORS OF LYMPH NODES
AND LYMPHOCYTES

Lymphoma
  Hodgkin's disease
    Lymphocytic predominance
    Nodular sclerosis
    Mixed cellularity
    Lymphocytic depletion

  Non-Hodgkin's lymphoma
    Well-differentiated lymphocytic lymphoma
      Associated with chronic lymphoid leukemia
      With plasmacytoid differentiation

  Follicle center cell lymphoma
    Nodular of small cleaved cells
    Nodular of mixed small and large follicle center cells
    Nodular of large follicle center cells

Diffuse of small cleaved cells
Diffuse of small and large follicle center cells
Diffuse of large follicle center cells

Immunoblastic lymphoma
  B cell
  T cell
  Undifferentiated

  T-zone lymphoma
  Lennert's lymphoma

Lymphoblastic lymphoma
  Convoluted cell
  Nonconvoluted cell

Adult T cell leukemia/lymphoma

Burkitt's tumour

Cutaneous lymphoma
  Mycosis fungoides
  Sézary syndrome
  Tumors of macrophages
    Histiocytic sarcoma
    Histiocytic medullary reticulosis

Lymphoid Leukemia
  Chronic lymphoid leukemia
    Classic form
    Hairy cell leukemia
    Prolymphocytic leukemia

  Acute lymphoblastic leukemia
    Common
    T cell
    B cell
    Unclassified

Plasma cell tumors
  Plasmacytoma
  Multiple myeloma

Paraproteinemia
  Waldenström's macroglobulinemia
  Heavy chain disease
  Light chain disease
  Benign monoclonal gammopathy
  Cryoglobulinemia

Angioimmunoblastic lymphadenopathy

Secondary tumors

The term *lymphoma* is used to describe the solid tumors arising in the lymph nodes or, less often, in the thymus, spleen, Waldeyer's ring in the pharynx, Peyer's patches in the gut, or lymphoid aggregates in some other organ. The tumors arising from the macrophages in the lymph nodes are grouped together with the tumors of the lymphocytes.

The tumors of lymphocytes in which the principal feature is the presence of malignant cells in the blood and bone marrow are called lymphoid leukemia. Lymphoid leukemia and lymphoma cannot be sharply distinguished. Some tumors of lymphocytes affect principally the lymph nodes. Some involve mainly the blood and bone marrow. Many involve both the lymph nodes and the blood and bone marrow, showing features of lymphoma and lymphoid leukemia.

The tumors of plasma cells are considered separately. Though plasma cells are derived from B cells, and tumors intermediate between lymphoma and multiple myeloma occur, most tumors of plasma cells behave differently from the lymphomata.

The paraproteinemias are a group of conditions in which an abnormal immunoglobulin or part of an immunoglobulin circulates in the blood. They are caused by a proliferation of lymphocytes or plasma cells, most often a tumor of lymphocytes or plasma cells.

The term *lymphoproliferative disorder* is sometimes used to describe the conditions in which there is a neoplastic or quasineoplastic proliferation of lymphocytes or plasma cells.

Lymphoma

Two kinds of lymphoma are distinguished, Hodgkin's disease and non-Hodgkin's lymphoma. Both are subdivided into several subtypes.

HODGKIN'S DISEASE. Hodgkin's disease is named after the British pathologist Hodgkin. In 1832, he described 7 patients with lymphadenopathy and splenomegaly, some of whom had what we now call Hodgkin's disease.

About 40% of patients with lymphoma have Hodgkin's disease. Each year, more than 3 people in every 100,000 develop Hodgkin's disease. About 60% of the patients are men. In the United States, Hodgkin's disease is more common in white people than in black people. Each year, Hodgkin's disease develops in 4 white men but in fewer than 3 black men in every 100,000, and in 3 white women but only 1 black woman.

Except in the underdeveloped countries, Hodgkin's disease is unusual in children. It is most common in young adults, 15 to 35 years old. The risk of developing the disease is less in people 35 to 50 years old, but rises again in people over 50 years old. Elderly Japanese are as likely to develop Hodgkin's disease as are people of other races, but the incidence of the disease in young adults is low in Japan.

The form of Hodgkin's disease called nodular sclerosis differs from the other types of Hodgkin's disease in that it occurs predominantly in young adults and is as common in women as in men.

Classification. As shown in Table 55-3, Hodgkin's disease is divided into the four types defined at a conference held in Rye, New York in 1965. About 20% of the patients have the lymphocyte predominant form of the disease, 35% have nodular sclerosis, 30% have Hodgkin's disease of mixed cellularity, and 15% have the lymphocyte-depleted form of the disease. The distinction between the types is made by light microscopy.

Before the acceptance of the Rye classification, Hodgkin's disease was divided into three types, Hodgkin's paragranuloma, which corresponds more or less to the lymphocytic predominance of the Rye classification; Hodgkin's granuloma, which included nodular sclerosis and Hodgkin's disease of mixed cellularity; and Hodgkin's sarcoma, roughly equivalent to lymphocytic depletion.

Lesions. Hodgkin's disease usually begins with enlargement of a group of lymph nodes. In 40% of the patients, the disease is first evident in the supraclavicular lymph nodes on one side of the neck. In 30%, it appears first in lymph nodes higher on one side of the neck. In 15%, it is first detected in the abdominal lymph nodes; in 10% in the mediastinum; in 4% in some other group of lymph nodes; in 1% in the spleen, the thymus, or some other lymphoid organ.

If the disease is not controlled, it spreads to other groups of lymph nodes, usually by extending from one group of nodes to the

TABLE 55-3. RYE CLASSIFICATION OF
HODGKIN'S DISEASE

Lymphocytic predominance
Nodular sclerosing
Mixed cellularity
Lymphocytic depletion

next. The lymph nodes on the left side of the neck are involved in 70% of the patients, the nodes on the right side of the neck in 60%, and the nodes in the mediastinum in 60%. The abdominal lymph nodes are affected in 30% of the patients, the axillary lymph nodes in 25%, and the inguinal lymph nodes in 15%. The spleen is involved in 10% of the patients. Less often lesions develop in the liver, lungs, skin, bones, or other organs.

Nodular sclerosis differs from the other forms of Hodgkin's disease in that it nearly always arises in the supraclavicular or mediastinal lymph nodes and often remains confined to them.

In an affected group of lymph nodes, all are usually involved, though the degree of involvement often varies from one node to another. In the lymphocyte-predominant form of the disease and in the early stages of its other forms, the lymph nodes remain discrete, clearly separate from one another, but as months pass, the nodes become increasingly matted together in the lymphocyte-depleted form of Hodgkins's disease and to a lesser degree in Hodgkin's disease of mixed cellularity and in nodular sclerosis.

On section, the affected lymph nodes are pale, moist, and homogeneous in the lymphocyte-predominant form of Hodgkin's disease, showing the fish flesh appearance typical of a well-differentiated lymphomata. In nodular sclerosis, the nodularity caused by the scarring within the lymph nodes is often apparent when they are sectioned. In Hodgkin's disease of mixed cellularity and in lymphocytic depletion, necrosis is common. At times, it is extensive, replacing much or all of the involved nodes. Often scarring is evident in and around the lymph nodes in people with disease of mixed cellularity or with lymphocytic depletion. It may be minor and focal or extensive.

Hodgkin's disease in the spleen, the liver, or other organs, often forms spheroidal masses, much like metastatic carcinoma. In other patients, the involvement of these organs is subtle, with tiny deposits of lymphoma only discoverable microscopically.

Microscopically, the different types of Hodgkin's disease can usually be easily distinguished, though lymphocytic predomi-

nance, mixed cellularity, and lymphocytic depletion merge into one another, and intermediate forms occur. Nodular sclerosis is nearly always easily differentiated from the other forms of Hodgkin's disease.

Reed-Sternberg Cells. In all forms of Hodgkin's disease, stress is placed on the presence of Reed-Sternberg cells in the tumor tissue. These cells take their name from the Austrian pathologist Sternberg who described them in 1898 and the American pathologist Dorothy Reed who illustrated them in 1902. Sometimes they are called Reed cells. Reed-Sternberg cells are suggestive of Hodgkin's disease. They always can be found in Hodgkin's disease, though they may be few and hard to find. They are uncommon in other diseases, though similar cells can occur in other forms of lymphoma and other tumors, and can be found in non-neoplastic conditions such as infectious mononucleosis and other viral infections. Some pathologists will not make a diagnosis of Hodgkin's disease unless at least one typical Reed-Sternberg cell is present.

Reed-Sternberg cells are 10 to 40 μm in diameter and roughly spherical. Their margin is well defined, often separated by a little space from the surrounding cells. The cytoplasm is abundant and stains a homogeneous pink with eosin. The cells contain two large nuclei, which fill much of the cell and are set side by side as if one were a mirror image of the other. The chromatin in the nuclei is usually sparse and is concentrated around the nuclear membrane. Each nucleus has a large nucleolus, usually a quarter to a half the diameter of the nucleus, brightly eosinophilic, and structureless. Reed-Sternberg cells are sometimes likened to an owl's head, with the big nuclei as two great eyes, and the nucleoli as two staring pupils.

A typical Reed-Sternberg cell must have two nuclei. Often the lesions of Hodgkin's disease contain cells identical to Reed-Sternberg cells except that they contain only one nucleus with its staring nucleolus or have more than two nuclei. Probably these mononuclear and multinculear cells are closely related to Reed-Sternberg cells, but most authorities do not consider them sufficient to establish a diagnosis of Hodgkin's disease.

Lymphocyte Predominance. The lympho-

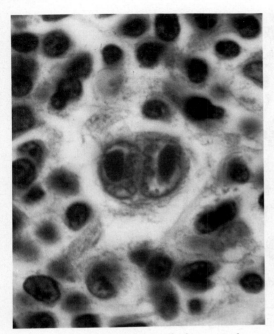

Fig. 55-5. A Reed-Sternberg cell, showing its large size and two prominent nucleoli.

cyte-predominant form of Hodgkin's disease may be nodular or diffuse. In the nodular form of the disease, ill-defined nodules of lymphoma are present in the involved lymph nodes. The nodules often compress or distort the uninvolved parts of the lymph nodes. In the diffuse form of the disorder, the affected lymph nodes are entirely replaced by Hodgkin's tissue. No trace of their sinusoids or follicles remains. All is replaced by the lymphoma.

The lesions consist principally of lymphocytes, which look normal. They are packed closely together and obliterate the structure of the involved lymph nodes. Scattered among the lymphocytes are large, pale macrophages called histiocytes. They may be few or many. Sometimes the macrophages are aggregated into small clumps. Reed-Sternberg cells are few and hard to find. Instead, scattered through the lesion are large cells about the size of a Reed-Sternberg cell, but with a twisted or multilobed nucleus, fine chromatin, and a small nucleolus or nucleoli. Taken in conjunction with the infiltrate of lymphocytes and macrophages, these large cells with twisted nuclei are strongly suggestive of lymphocyte-predominant Hodgkin's disease, though it is desirable to find a few Reed-Sternberg cells to confirm the diagnosis. There are usually no eosinophils, neutrophils, necrosis, or fibrosis in lymphocyte-predominant Hodgkin's disease.

Nodular Sclerosis.   In nodular sclerosis, the involved lymph nodes are usually completely replaced by the lymphoma. At least some of the lymph nodes are divided into nodules by septa of fine, cellular collagen. The collagenous tissue shows no atypicality, nothing to suggest that it is neoplastic. The septa vary in thickness from one patient to another and often from one lymph node to another in the same patient. Sometimes they are so massive that they make up 50% of the volume of the lymph node. Sometimes they are so delicate that they are easily overlooked. In some patients, some lymph nodes have no septa at all.

The nodules between the septa may consist predominantly of a proliferation of lymphocytes and macrophages as in lymphocyte-predominant Hodgkin's disease or may contain a considerable number of eosinophils and neutrophils, sometimes with foci of necrosis, as in Hodgkin's disease of mixed cellularity. Typical Reed-Sternberg cells are few. Instead, there are many large lacunar cells with sharply defined cell borders. Their cytoplasm is pale and seems empty, so that the nucleus floats in space, the lacuna that gives the cells their name. The nuclei have fine, even chromatin and small nucleoli. Often they are divided into several lobes. Lacunar cells are highly suggestive of nodular sclerosis, even if no septa are evident. They are rarely found in other types of Hodgkin's disease or in other kinds of tumor.

Mixed Cellularity.   Hodgkin's disease of mixed cellularity is the classic form of the disease. It replaces the affected lymph nodes entirely, though sometimes the replacement is not complete at the time a biopsy is taken. The lymphomatous tissue shows a mixture of several kinds of apparently normal cells. Usually, lymphocytes are the most numerous, sometimes with an admixture of macrophages, as in the lymphocyte-predominant form of Hodgkin's disease. Eosinophils are commonly abundant and striking, but are not always

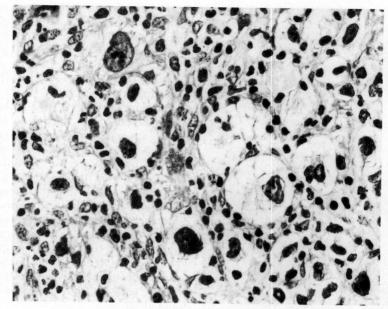

Fig. 55-6.   Lacunar cells in nodular sclerosing Hodgkin's disease.

present. Frequently plasma cells and neutrophils are mixed with the lymphocytes. Reed-Sternberg cells are nearly always numerous, together with mononuclear and multinuclear cells of similar character. Necrosis is common. It may be minor with only small scattered foci of necrosis, or massive, destroying most of the lymph node. Often there is fibrosis, irregularly distributed, but not dividing the lymph node into nodules. The fibrosis is frequently slight and focal but can be extensive, replacing much of the lymph node. Sometimes a few Reed-Sternberg cells or some of the other cells present in the cellular part of the lymphoma persist in the fibrosis.

Lymphocytic Depletion.   There are two forms of lymphocyte-depleted Hodgkin's disease. In one, much of the affected lymph nodes is replaced by fibrosis. In the other, the lymph nodes are replaced by a proliferation of large, highly atypical cells. In some patients, some nodes show the fibrotic form of lymphocyte depletion; others, the cellular form.

In the fibrotic form of lymphocytic depletion, much or all of the affected lymph nodes is replaced by structureless, hyaline fibrosis in which few cells remain. There are few

fibrocytes, only rare lymphocytes or other hematopoietic cells, and few if any Reed-Sternberg cells or other Hodgkin's cells. Usually the fibrosis in diffuse fibrosis shows little birefringence when viewed by polarized light, in contrast to the bright birefringence of the collagen in nodular sclerosis. Fibrosis of this sort is the end of the disease process. Diagnosis might be difficult, if it were not that in most patients islands of mixed cellularity or of some other form of Hodgkin's disease remain to give the diagnosis.

In the cellular form of lymphocyte depletion, the involved lymph nodes are replaced by a proliferation of large, atypical cells, some of which are recognizable as Reed-Sternberg cells. With them may be a few lymphocytes or an occasional neutrophil or eosinophil. Necrosis is often extensive. Often there is some fibrosis. If the fibrotic form of lymphocyte depletion is the death of Hodgkin's disease, its cellular form is the disease's most desperate blaze.

Immunologic Defects.   T-cell function is often defective in Hodgkin's disease. The more extensive the disease, the more likely T-cell dysfunction will be severe. B-cell function and the production of antibodies are

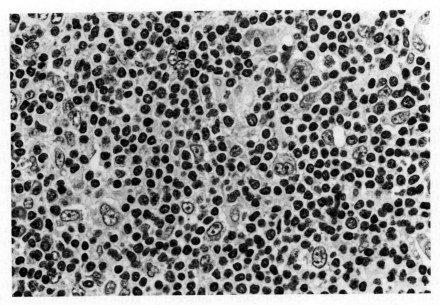

Fig. 55-7. Hodgkin's disease of mixed cellularity, showing a proliferation principally of lymphocytes. A typical Reed-Sternberg cell is present near the center of the picture.

usually normal in people with Hodgkin's disease.

In 40% of the patients, the lymphocyte count in the blood is less than 1.5×10^9/L (1500/mm³). In these people and sometimes in other patients with Hodgkin's disease, the skin often fails to show a delayed hypersensitivity response to antigens to which the patient has probably been exposed in the past. The tuberculin reaction and similar tests become negative. The skin fails to respond to antigens, such as dinitrochlorobenzene, which produce a delayed hypersensitivity reaction in normal people. Mitogens such as phytohemagglutinin fail to activate the patient's lymphocytes. Not all patients with Hodgkin's disease have a great impairment of T-cell function, but if sensitive tests are used, most show some depression of T-cell function.

The T-cell dysfunction is caused by a factor or factors in the plasma. If lymphocytes from a patient with Hodgkin's disease are washed free of plasma, they respond normally to mitogens. A glycoprotein present in the plasma in people with Hodgkin's disease is probably an important cause of the dysfunction. In some patients, antibodies against T-cells or the overproduction of prostaglandin E₂ may play some part. Even if Hodgkin's disease is controlled or cured, the depression of T-cell function usually persists, often for years.

Changes in the Blood. The concentration of hemoglobin in the blood is below 130 g/L (13 g/100 mL) in 25% of patients with early Hodgkin's disease and in over 60% of those with advanced disease. The anemia is usually normochromic and normocytic. Some patients develop an autoimmune hemolytic anemia, but usually only late in the disease.

The leukocyte count is normal in patients in stage I. It is over 10×10^9/L (10,000/mm³) in 20% of patients in stage IIA or IIIA, in 40% of patients in stage IIB or IIIB, and in 60% of patients in stage IV. The increase is usually due to neutrophilia. In some patients, there is also monocytosis. Occasionally, there is eosinophilia. Leukopenia with fewer than 5 $\times 10^9$/L (5000/mm³) circulating leukocytes is present in less than 10% of patients with advanced disease. Reed-Sternberg cells or other large, atypical cells are present in the blood in 10% of patients but are not sufficiently numerous to be easily detected. Only rarely, and late in the disease, do they become numerous.

The erythrocyte sedimentation rate is often elevated and is of value in following the activity of the disease. Often there is hyper-gammaglobulinemia or occasionally hypoalbuminemia. Hyperuricemia occurs only when treatment causes rapid destruction of the Hodgkin's tissue. Disease in the bones or liver is not usually sufficiently extensive to cause hypercalcemia or to increase the activity of alkaline phosphatase in the plasma.

Behavior. In patients with Hodgkin's disease of lymphocytic predominance or mixed cellularity, the disease tends to change for the worse as weeks and months pass. The relatively benign lymphocytic predominance tends to progress to mixed cellularity or lymphocytic depletion, and mixed cellularity tends to progress to lymphocytic depletion. A biopsy of one group of lymph nodes or repeated biopsies show more than one type of Hodgkin's disease in 60% of patients with lymphocytic predominance, mixed cellularity, or lymphocytic depletion.

Nodular sclerosis is different. In 90% of people with this form of Hodgkin's disease, subsequent biopsies continue to show nodular sclerosis.

Staging. The extent of Hodgkin's disease in the body is measured by the criteria developed at a conference in Ann Arbor, Michigan in 1971. Table 55-4 shows a modification of this classification.

TABLE 55-4. STAGING OF HODGKIN'S DISEASE

Stage I	Involvement of a single lymph node region or of a single extralymphatic organ or site.
Stage II	Involvement of two or more lymph node regions on the same side of the diaphragm or the localized involvement of a single extralymphatic organ or site and of one or more lymph node regions on the same side of the diaphragm.
Stage III	Involvement of lymph node regions on both sides of the diaphragm, with or without involvement of an extralymphatic organ or site, the spleen, or both.
Stage IV	Diffuse or disseminated involvement of one or more extralymphatic organs or tissues, with or without involvement of lymph nodes.

Each stage is divided into two groups: A, without general symptoms; and B, with fever, night sweats, or weight loss.

The Ann Arbor system of staging expresses well the gradual extension of Hodgkin's disease from a single group of lymph nodes to adjacent groups and eventually to other organs. In stage I, the disease is confined to a single group of lymph nodes or a single extranodal organ. In stage II, it has involved two or more sites on the same side of the diaphragm. In stage III, lymph nodes or other lymphoid organs on both sides of the diaphragm are involved, but the disease is still confined to the affected lymph nodes or organs. Stage III is divided into stage III_1, in which the disease is confined to the upper part of the abdomen, and stage III_2, in which the lower part of the abdomen is involved. In stage IV, the disease has extended beyond the lymph nodes or other lymphoid tissue in which it originated.

Local extension of the disease into tissues adjacent to involved lymph nodes does not alter the staging. A patient is still classed as stage I if the disease is confined to one group of lymph nodes but has extended into the tissues adjacent to those nodes. The diffuse and disseminated involvement of stage IV means extensive involvement of some organ other than the lymph nodes: the spleen, the thymus, or the lymphoid aggregates of the pharynx and the gut. An exception is made for the liver and the bone marrow. If the liver or bone marrow are involved, however slightly, the disease is classed as stage IV.

Each of the four stages of the Ann Arbor system of staging is divided into two subdivisions, A and B. The patients classed as B have unexplained fever of over 38°C, night sweats, or unexplained loss of more than 10% of the body weight in the six months preceding the diagnosis of Hodgkin's disease. Patients classed as A have no such general symptoms.

In a large group of patients with Hodgkin's disease, 14% were in stage IA when the diagnosis was made, 1% in stage IB, 30% in stage IIA, 12% in stage IIB, 17% in stage IIIA, 15% in stage IIIB, 4% in stage IVA, and 9% in stage IVB. In over 95% of patients in stage I or II, the disease was above the diaphragm. When Hodgkin's disease is detected first in lymph nodes below the diaphragm, it is often already in stage III.

There is a rough correlation between the

type of Hodgkin's disease as judged by the Rye classification and its extent at the time of diagnosis as judged by the Ann Arbor system. The disease is most likely to be localized in people with lymphocytic predominance and most likely to be widespread in people with lymphocytic depletion. About 15% of people with lymphocytic predominance are in stage I at the time of diagnosis, but only 5 to 8% of people with other types of Hodgkin's disease. Less than 5% of people with lymphocytic predominance, less than 15% of people with nodular sclerosis or mixed cellularity, but 25% of people with lymphocytic depletion are in stage IV. From 40 to 50% of the patients are in stage II by the time the diagnosis is made, whatever the type of Hodgkin's disease, and between 20 and 30% are in stage III.

The value of staging Hodgkin's disease depends on the thoroughness of the examination of the patient. In many hospitals, the examination continues to laparotomy, unless it becomes clear earlier that the patient is in stage IV.

When staging a patient with Hodgkin's disease, physical examination should seek especially for enlargement of lymph nodes, splenomegaly, hepatomegaly, and areas of tenderness in bones. X-ray studies evaluate the hilar and mediastinal lymph nodes and demonstrate lesions in the lungs or bones. Computer assisted tomography or sonography detects lesions in the abdomen. Lymphangiography is valuable in detecting involvement of the lymph nodes in the lower abdomen. If it fails to show a lesion, the lower abdominal lymph nodes are probably not involved, but in 20% of patients in whom an abnormality is found it is due to something other than Hodgkin's disease. Bone marrow aspiration is rarely of value, but bone marrow biopsies reveal Hodgkin's disease in 10% of patients. If liver function tests are abnormal, a needle biopsy of the liver may reveal Hodgkin's disease. If a laparotomy is necessary, biopsies of lymph nodes in the porta hepatis or splenic hilus reveal Hodgkin's disease in 20% of patients in whom lymphangiography showed the lymph nodes in the lower abdomen to be free of disease. Removal of an apparently normal spleen shows it to be involved in 20%

of the patients. Biopsies of the liver taken at laparotomy show involvement in 20% of patients with Hodgkin's disease in the abdominal lymph nodes or the spleen.

If lymphangiography and laparatomy are performed routinely, the staging is altered in 50% of the patients. In 30%, unexpected involvement in the abdomen is found. In 20%, the abdomen is found to be free of disease, though earlier investigations had suggested that it was involved.

Clinical Presentation. Most patients with Hodgkin's disease have a painless enlargement of a group of lymph nodes, most often the nodes on one side of the neck. The size of the nodes may fluctuate as weeks pass.

If there is fever, it is usually not more than 38°C, though in more cases it is high and swinging. Recurrent fever, persisting for a week or so and subsiding, only to recur after a few weeks, was once thought typical of Hodgkin's disease but is uncommon. It is called Pel-Ebstein fever after the Dutch physician Pel who described it is 1885 and the German physician Ebstein who reported it in 1887. Fever in a patient with Hodgkin's disease is not necessarily caused by the lymphoma but may be due to infection or some other cause.

Night sweats and weight loss often occur in conjunction with fever. Sometimes pruritus is severe. In less than 20% of the patients, drinking alcohol causes pain, sometimes severe, in some of the lesions. Alcohol rarely causes pain in the lesions of other diseases.

Rarely, a patient with Hodgkin's disease has a cough or other evidence of pulmonary involvement, jaundice from involvement of the liver, or abdominal pain. Compression of the superior vena cava by enlarged lymph nodes or of the spinal cord by deposits of Hodgkin's disease in the spine or meninges can be the first sign of the disease, but like jaundice and pulmonary involvement more often develops late in its course.

Pathogenesis. In the past, many considered that Hodgkin's disease was inflammatory rather than neoplastic. The great accumulation of apparently normal cells in most lesions of Hodgkin's disease was thought to be more suggestive of inflammation than of neoplasia. A variety of infective organisms, from tubercle bacilli to viruses, were suggested as its cause, but none of these claims could be substantiated. Gradually it has become accepted that Hodgkin's disease is a neoplasm, a form of lymphoma.

What is neoplastic in Hodgkin's disease is less clear. The usual view is that the Reed-Sternberg cells are neoplastic, and the lymphocytes, neutrophils, eosinophils, and macrophages that make up the bulk of the lesions are not. If this is true, it is hard to explain how the Reed-Sternberg cells attract so many normal cells and why the normal cells detroy the involved lymph nodes, replacing their normal structure so completely.

The origin of the Reed-Sternberg cells remains uncertain. T cells, B cells, and macrophages have all been proposed. There is little to support the suggestion that Reed-Sternberg cells are altered T cells. Reed-Sternberg cells do not exhibit any of the T-cell markers. Cellular immunity in Hodgkin's disease is not impaired because the T cells are neoplastic, but because a factor or factors in the blood interfere with their activity.

The presence of immunoglobulins in the cytoplasm or on the surface of Reed-Sternberg cells suggested to some investigators Reed-Sternberg cells might be B cells, but the immunoglobulins proved to be polyclonal, with both $\varkappa$ and λ chains. A B cell can produce $\varkappa$ or λ chains, but not both. Presumably the Reed-Sternberg cells take up immunoglobulins, but do not produce them.

Probably the Reed-Sternberg cells are altered macrophages. They contain acid phosphatase and nonspecific esterase, as do macrophages. An antibody has been found that reacts with both Reed-Sternberg cells and the specialized macrophages called the interdigitating reticulum cells found in the parafollicular regions of the lymph nodes, though it is too soon to conclude that the Reed-Sternberg cells are derived from this type of macrophage.

In young adults with Hodgkin's disease, but not in older people, the titer of antibodies to the Epstein-Barr virus is higher than in the general population. Hodgkin's disease is twice as frequent in people who have had infectious mononucleosis as in the general population. It has been suggested that the Epstein-Barr virus or some other virus could be the cause of Hodgkin's disease. Against this suggestion is the failure to find nucleic acid sequences similar to those of the Epstein-Barr virus in the Reed-Sternberg cells, though sequences similar to those of murine leukemia viruses have been found. Both Hodgkin's disease and infectious mononucleosis are more common in young adults of the more affluent classes. It could be that the association between them is only coincidence.

Clusters of patients in the same locality who developed Hodgkin's disease at the same time have been described. It has been suggested that Hodgkin's disease either is infectious and is transmitted from one patient to another or is inherited. Neither suggestion has been established. Coincidence seems the explanation.

Treatment and Prognosis. Without treatment, 50% of patients with Hodgkin's disease die within two years. Less than 10% survive five years. With treatment, most are cured.

Patients with Hodgkin's disease in stage I or II are usually treated by radiotherapy. A dose of 40 Gy (4000 rad) is given to the lymph nodes involved and to adjacent groups of lymph nodes into which the disease may have extended. If the disease is confined to one side of the neck, both sides of the neck, the axillae, and the mediastinum are irradiated. If the disease involves other parts of the body, the extent of the irradiation is adjusted appropriately. Over 80% of patients in stage I and over 70% of those in stage II are free of disease and probably cured five years later. Patients in stage IIA do better than those in stage IIB. Nearly 80% of people in stage IIA but less than 70% of those in stage IIB are free of disease five years after treatment.

Patients in stage IIIA are sometimes treated with radiation, especially if the disease below the diaphragm is confined to the upper abdomen. The neck, axillae, mediastinum, and paraaortic lymph nodes are all irradiated. About 50% of the patients are free of tumor five years after treatment. Others prefer to treat these people with both radiation and chemotherapy, usually with the combination of nitrogen mustard, vincristine, procarbazine, and prednisone called MOPP in addition to the irradiation. About 60% of people in stage IIIA so treated are free of tumor five years later.

Patients with disease in stage IIIB or stage

IV are treated with chemotherapy, usually MOPP. Over 50% of the patients are free of disease five years later, and another 10% enjoy a shorter remission.

Patients with recurrent Hodgkin's disease are treated with radiation or chemotherapy, much as are those treated for the first time. Some prefer to change the drugs used if chemotherapy was given earlier or to add chemotherapy if the patient was treated with radiation alone. The results are inferior to those in patients treated for the first time, but 40% of the patients are free of disease five years later.

The histologic type of Hodgkin's disease affects the prognosis. Over 70% of patients with lymphocytic predominance, 60% of those with nodular sclerosis, 30% of those with mixed cellularity, and 20% of those with lymphocytic depletion are alive five years after diagnosis.

In stages III and IV, the prognosis is better in women than in men. Nearly 60% of women with disease in stages III or IV were free of disease five years later, but only 40% of men. In stages I and II, the prognosis is the same in men and women.

Young adults with Hodgkin's disease do better than do older people. Over 90% of people under 40 years old but only 70% of older people with disease in stage I or stage II are alive five years after the diagnosis. Over 80% of people under 40 years old but only 50% of older people with disease in stages III or IV are alive five years after diagnosis.

Complications. The complications of Hodgkin's disease arise in part from the disease itself, in part from the drugs and radiation used to treat it. Because of the impairment of T-cell function usual in Hodgkin's disease, the patients are prone to infection. Radiation and chemotherapy further impair the efficiency of the immune system. Splenectomy increases the chance of infection, especially in children. The risk of contracting both viral and bacterial infections is increased. Herpes zoster is unduly common. Opportunistic infections with fungi or Pneumocystis carinii sometimes develop.

Radiation and chemotherapy bring their own complications. Both cause nausea and vomiting, injury to the mucosa of the bowel, suppression of the bone marrow, sterility, pneumonitis, or sometimes pulmonary fibrosis. Radiation can cause myelitis. Chemotherapy often causes peripheral neuritis, often with paresthesia.

A second malignant tumor develops within 10 years in 5% of patients treated for Hodgkin's disease, particularly in people given both radiation and chemotherapy. A wide variety of tumors occurs, but most frequently the second malignancy is acute myeloid leukemia or a non-Hodgkin's lymphoma.

NON-HODGKIN'S LYMPHOMA. Most non-Hodgkin's lymphomata are tumors of B cells. Some arise from T cells. A few originate from the macrophages in the lymph nodes. The nature of some is uncertain.

Only the non-Hodgkin's lymphomata that involve lymph nodes and other lymphoid organs or principally the skin are discussed in this chapter. The lymphomata primary to the brain, lungs, gut, and testes are considered with the tumors of those organs.

About 60% of lymphomata are some form of non-Hodgkin's lymphoma. Each year, more than 6 people in every 100,000 develop a non-Hodgkin's lymphoma. About 60% of the patients are men.

In most forms of non-Hodgkin's lymphoma, most of the patients are over 50 years old. The greater the age, the greater the risk of developing a non-Hodgkin's lymphoma. The proportion of male patients increases as age increases.

With the lymphoblastic lymphoma of T cells and Burkitt's lymphoma it is different. Most patients with a lymphoblastic lymphoma of T cells are less than 20 years old, though the disease does occur occasionally in older people. Burkitt's lymphoma is most common in children 3 to 7 years old. It is uncommon in people less than 2 years old or more than 15 years old.

Most forms of non-Hodgkin's lymphoma occur throughout the world. In the United States, non-Hodgkin's lymphoma is more common in white people than in black people. Each year, over 7 white men but only 4.5 black men and 6 white women but only 3 black women in every 100,000 develop a non-Hodgkin's lymphoma.

Burkitt's lymphoma differs from other kinds of non-Hodgkin's lymphoma in that it is common only in central Africa and in New Guinea, though it does occur throughout the world. In Uganda and parts of Nigeria, more than 50% of the malignant tumors of children are Burkitt's lymphoma.

Classification. There is no agreement as to how best to classify the non-Hodgkin's lymphomata. A number of different classifications are in use. Different hospitals use different systems.

For many years, the non-Hodgkin's lymphomata were divided into three main groups: follicular lymphoma, lymphosarcoma, and reticulum cell sarcoma. In a follicular lymphoma, the affected lymph nodes contain nodules of tumor, which by light microscopy look like the follicles of normal lymph nodes. In lymphosarcoma, the involved lymph nodes are completely replaced by a proliferation of cells, which by light microscopy look like lymphocytes. In reticulum cell sarcoma, the lymph nodes are replaced by a proliferation of large, atypical cells.

This old classification is now little used. It has been replaced by newer classifications, most often by the Rappaport classification, the Lukes-Collins classification, the Kiel classification, the Working Formulation, or some modification of one of them.

Rappaport Classification.   One of the most widely used classifications of the non-Hodgkin's lymphomata was introduced in 1956 by the American pathologist Rappaport and revised as the years have passed. Table 55-5 shows one of the modifications of this system now current.

The Rappaport system divides the non-Hodgkin's lymphomata into two groups, nodular tumors, in which the tumor cells form nodules or follicles in the affected lymph nodes, and diffuse tumors, in which the lymphoma replaces the affected lymph nodes completely. Each group is then subdivided according to the appearance of the tumor cells as seen by light microscopy.

The term *histiocytic lymphoma* used in the Rappaport classification is misleading. In most of the histiocytic lymphomata of the Rappaport system, the tumor cells are lymphocytes, usually B cells. Only rarely are the tumor cells derived from a macrophage.

The well-differentiated lymphocytic, poorly differentiated lymphocytic, mixed lym-

TABLE 55-5. RAPPAPORT CLASSIFICATION OF
NON-HODGKIN'S LYMPHOMA

Nodular
  Well-differentiated lymphocytic

  Poorly differentiated lymphocytic

  Mixed lymphocytic and histiocytic

  Histiocytic

Diffuse
  Well-differentiated lymphocytic
    Without plasmacytoid features
    With plasmacytoid features

  Poorly differentiated lymphocytic
    Without plasmacytoid features
    With plasmacytoid features

  Mixed lymphocytic and histiocytic

  Histiocytic
    Without sclerosis
    With sclerosis

  Lymphoblastic
    Convoluted cell
    Nonconvoluted cell

  Burkitt's tumor

  Undifferentiated lymphoma

  Composite lymphoma

  Unclassified

phocytic and histiocytic, and histiocytic lymphomata of the Rappaport system are not sharply distinguished one from another. Rather they show the range of anaplasia seen in the tumors of lymphocytes, from the highly differentiated lymphocytic types, to the most anaplastic of the histiocytic lymphomata. The lymphoblastic tumors and Burkitt's lymphoma have special features, which separate them from the other forms of non-Hodgkin's lymphoma.

Lukes-Collins Classification. In 1974, the American pathologists Lukes and Collins published a new classification of the non-Hodgkin's lymphomata. Table 55-6 shows a modification of this classification.

Lukes and Collins divided the non-Hodgkin's lymphomata into groups by using immunologic markers to determine whether the tumor cells were B cells, T cells, or macrophages. The B-cell and the T-cell tumors were then further subdivided by

TABLE 55-6. LUKES-COLLINS CLASSIFICATION OF
NON-HODGKIN'S LYMPHOMA

B cell
  Small lymphocytic

  Plasmacytoid lymphocytic
  of follicular center cells
    Small cleaved
    Large cleaved
    Small noncleaved
    Large noncleaved

  Immunoblastic sarcoma

T cell
  Small lymphocytic

  Convoluted lymphocytic

  Immunoblastic sarcoma

  Cutaneous
    Mycosis fungoides
    Sézary's syndrome

Histiocytic

U cell

Unclassifiable

their appearance as seen by light microscopy. Lymphomata in which the tumor cells showed no markers were called U cell lymphomata, U for Undefined. Only the rare tumors derived from macrophages were called histiocytic.

Lukes and Collins distinguished four kinds of B-cell tumor. In some, the tumor cells resemble normal lymphocytes. In some, many of the tumor cells resemble lymphocytes, but some show plasmacytoid differentiation. In some, the tumor cells resemble the B cells found in the follicles of normal lymph nodes. In some, the tumor cells are anaplastic and resemble immunoblasts.

Lukes and Collins distinguished four kinds of follicle center cell. They thought that when the B cells in a normal follicle begin to produce immunoglobulin, small cleaved cells present in the follicle grow larger, becoming large cleaved cells, then small noncleaved cells, and finally large noncleaved cells. The large noncleaved cells were thought to leave the follicle, becoming immunoblasts and eventually plasma cells. The tumor cells in the tumors of the follicle center cells can

resemble any of these forms of B cell or form any combination of them.

The T-cell tumors of the Lukes-Collins classification are distinct one from another. Some are well differentiated, some are anaplastic, and some are confined largely to the skin.

Kiel Classification. Yet another classification was developed in Kiel, Germany. Table 55-7 shows a modification of this classification, as it was published in 1981.

The Kiel classification divides the non-Hodgkin's lymphomata into two main groups according to their behavior, tumors of low grade malignancy with a good prognosis and those of high grade malignancy with a poor prognosis. Each group is then subdivided, principally by their appearance when examined by light microscopy, but using immunologic and histochemical markers to determine the nature of the tumor cells when necessary.

TABLE 55-7. KIEL CLASSIFICATION OF
NON-HODGKIN'S LYMPHOMA

Low grade malignancy
  Lymphocytic
    B chronic lymphoid leukemia
    T chronic lymphoid leukemia
    Hairy cell leukemia
    T zone lymphoma
    Cutaneous forms
      Mycosis fungoides
      Sézary's syndrome

  Lymphoplasmacytic immunocytoma
    Plasmacytoid
    Plasmacytic
    Mixed

  Plasmacytic

  Centrocytic

  Centroblastic-centrocytic

High grade malignancy
  Centroblastic

  Immunoblastic
    B cell
    T cell
    Undetermined

  Lymphoblastic
    Burkitt lymphoma
    Convoluted cell
    Unclassified

The well-differentiated forms of B-cell and T-cell lymphoma are called B chronic lymphoid leukemia and T chronic lymphoid leukemia because in these patients leukemia is usually the predominant feature of the disease. The term *lymphoplasmacytic immunocytoma* describes well-differentiated tumors in which many of the cells are lymphocytes, but some resemble plasma cells. In the plasmacytic tumors, most of the tumor cells show plasmacytoid differentiation. The lymphomata that affect principally the skin, and the uncommon hairy cell and T zone tumors are classed with the lesions of low grade malignancy.

The tumors of the follicle center cells are termed centrocytic, centroblastic-centrocytic, or centroblastic lymphoma. The centrocytes are equivalent to the small and large cleaved cells of the Lukes-Collins classification, and the centroblasts to the noncleaved cells. In the better differentiated lesions, the prognosis is good, but in the poorly differentiated follicle center tumors the outlook is poor.

The poorly differentiated B-cell and T-cell tumors are classed as immunoblastic lymphomata, as are poorly differentiated tumors that show neither B- nor T-cell markers. The lymphoblastic, convoluted cell and Burkitt tumors have special features that distinguish them from other lymphomata.

Working Formulation. The introduction of these and other classifications of the non-Hodgkin's lymphomata has caused considerable confusion. Different centers use different systems of classification. The different systems use different criteria to define the different types of lymphoma. Often it is difficult to translate the terms used in one classification into those of another.

To overcome this confusion, a working party was established by the National Cancer Institute of the United States. It considered six widely used classifications of non-Hodgkin's lymphoma and in 1982 proposed a new classification which, it was hoped, could bridge the differences between them. Table 55-8 gives a simplification of the formulation devised by the Institute's working party. Unfortunately, it has not become generally accepted, and the Rappaport, Lukes-Collins, Kiel, and other classifications of the non-Hodgkin's lymphomata continue to be used widely.

The working formulation divides the non-Hodgkin's lymphomata into three groups according to the behavior of the tumor: low grade, intermediate grade, and high grade. Each group is then subdivided by light microscopy. No attempt is made to determine if the tumor cells are B cells, T cells, or macrophages.

TABLE 55-8. WORKING FORMULATION OF NON-HODGKIN'S LYMPHOMA

Low grade
  Small lymphocytic
    Consistent with chronic lymphoid leukemia
    Plasmacytoid

  Follicular, predominantly small cleaved cell
    With diffuse areas
    With sclerosis

  Follicular, mixed small cleaved and large cell
    With diffuse areas
    With sclerosis

Intermediate grade
  Follicular, predominantly large cell
    With diffuse areas
    With sclerosis

  Diffuse, small cleaved cell
    With sclerosis

  Diffuse, mixed small and large cell
    With sclerosis
    With epithelioid cells

  Diffuse, large cell
    Cleaved cell
    Noncleaved cell
    With sclerosis

High grade
  Large cell immunoblastic
    Plasmacytoid
    Clear cell
    Polymorphous
    With epithelioid cells

  Lymphoblastic
    Convoluted cell
    Nonconvoluted cell

  Small noncleaved cell
    Burkitt's lymphoma
    With follicular areas

  Miscellaneous
    Composite
    Mycosis fungoides
    Histiocytic
    Extramedullary plasmacytic
    Unclassifiable

The term *follicular* is used in the working formulation to describe tumors that form nodules in the affected lymph nodes but do not replace them completely. The term *diffuse* describes tumors that replace the lymph nodes entirely. The small cleaved cells are the follicle center cells described by Lukes and Collins.

Comparison Among Classifications. Table 55-9 shows the relationship among the various classifications. It is not exact because the groups defined in different classifications are not always strictly comparable.

Frequency. The frequency of the different kinds of non-Hodgkin's lymphoma is not easy to determine. Different studies have used different criteria, with different findings.

About 80% of people with a non-Hodgkin's lymphoma have a B-cell tumor. About 10% have a T-cell tumor. In 10%, the origin of the tumor cannot be determined. Less than 0.02% have a tumor of macrophages.

Roughly, 5 to 10% of patients with non-Hodgkin's lymphoma have a well-differentiated lymphocytic tumor of the sort usually associated with chronic lymphoid leukemia. In 99% of these patients, the tumor is of B cells. In 1% it is of T cells. Another 5% of people with non-Hodgkin's lymphoma have a well-differentiated tumor in which some of the tumor cells show plasmacytoid differentiation.

From 50 to 70% of non-Hodgkin's lymphomata are of follicle center cells. In 30 to 40% of patients with non-Hodgkin's lymphoma, the tumor forms nodules in the lymph nodes

TABLE 55-9. COMPARISON OF CLASSIFICATIONS

Type of Lymphoma	Rappaport	Lukes-Collins	Kiel	Working Formulation
B Cell Well-differentiated				
	Diffuse well-differentiated lymphocytic without plasmacytoid features	B small lymphocytic	B chronic lymphoid leukemia	Small lymphocytic consistent with chronic lymphoid leukemia
	Diffuse well-differentiated lymphocytic with plasmacytoid features	Plasmacytoid lymphocytic	Immunocytoma, plasmacytoid, or plasmacytic	Small lymphocytic, plasmacytoid
	—	—	Plasmacytic	—
Follicle center	Nodular well-differentiated lymphocytic or Nodular poorly differentiated lymphocytic	Small cleaved cell	centroblastic-centrocytic	Follicular, Predominantly small cleaved cell
	Nodular mixed lymphocytic and histiocytic	Small cleaved cell or Large cleaved cell	centroblastic-centrocytic	Follicular, mixed small cleaved and large cell
	Nodular histiocytic	Large cleaved cell or Noncleaved cell	centroblastic-centrocytic	Follicular, predominantly large cell

TABLE 55-9. CONT'D

Type of Lymphoma	Rappaport	Lukes-Collins	Kiel	Working Formulation
	Diffuse poorly differentiated lymphocytic	Small cleaved cell	Centrocytic	Diffuse, small cleaved cell
	Diffuse mixed lymphocytic and histiocytic	Small cleaved cell or Large cleaved cell or Noncleaved cell	Centroblastic-centrocytic or Immunocytoma, mixed	Diffuse, mixed small and large cell
	Diffuse histiocytic	Large cleaved cell or Noncleaved cell	Centroblastic-centrocytic or Centrocytic or Centroblastic	Diffuse, large cell
Poorly differentiated	Diffuse histiocytic	B-immunoblastic sarcoma	B-cell immunoblastic	Large cell immunoblastic
	Burkitt's tumor	Small noncleaved cell	Burkitt's lymphoma	Small noncleaved cell, Burkitt's lymphoma
T Cell	Diffuse well-differentiated lymphocytic without plasmacytic features	T small lymphocytic	T chronic lymphoid leukemia	Small lymphocytic consistent with lymphoid leukemia
	Diffuse histiocytic	T-immunoblastic sarcoma	T-cell immunoblastic or T zone lymphoma	Large cell immunoblastic
	Lymphoblastic, convoluted cell or nonconvoluted cell	Convoluted lymphocytic	Lymphoblastic, convoluted cell	Lymphoblastic, convoluted cell, or nonconvoluted cell
	—	Mycosis fungoides Sézary syndrome	Mycosis fungoides Sézary syndrome	Mycosis fungoides
Macrophage	Diffuse histiocytic	Histiocytic	—	Histiocytic
Origin Unknown	Diffuse histiocytic	U cell	Lymphoblastic, unclassified	Lymphoblastic, nonconvoluted cell

involved and is predominantly of small cleaved cells. In 20%, it replaces the lymph nodes
entirely and is predominantly of noncleaved
cells.

About 10% of people with non-Hodgkin's
lymphoma have an immunoblastic tumor.
Probably about 3% have a B-cell tumor, 3% a
T-cell tumor, and 3% a tumor that shows
neither B-cell nor T-cell markers. About 5%
of the patients have a T-cell lymphoblastic
lymphoma with convoluted cells.

Lesions. To facilitate description of the
lesions, the non-Hodgkin's lymphomata will
be divided into three main groups: the diffuse, well-differentiated tumors, the tumors
of the cells of the follicle centers, and the
immunoblastic tumors. The lymphoblastic
tumors, Burkitt's tumor, mycosis fungoides,
and Sézary's syndrome will be described
separately.

Macroscopic Findings. In 70% of patients
with non-Hodgkin's lymphoma, one or more
groups of lymph nodes are sufficiently enlarged to be evident clinically at the time the
diagnosis is made. In 30% of the patients, the
cervical or surpraclavicular lymph nodes on
one side are involved, and in 20% the axillary
lymph nodes, though any group of lymph
nodes can be affected. In 5% of patients,
lymph nodes throughout the body are enlarged. In 10%, enlargement of the lymphoid
organs in the throat is apparent, in addition
to the enlargement of one or more groups of
lymph nodes.

In the 30% of patients in whom no
enlargement of lymph nodes is detectable at
the time of diagnosis, the disease begins most
often in the tonsils or elsewhere in the
pharynx, sometimes in the stomach or intestine, in bone, the spleen, or elsewhere. The
lymphoma is usually one of the more anaplastic forms of non-Hodgkin's disease.

In an involved group of lymph nodes, the
degree of enlargement varies from lymph
node to lymph node. In the early stages of
the disease, some lymph nodes may be
affected while others are spared. At times,
the enlarged lymph nodes are 10 cm or more
across.

At first the lymph nodes are discrete,
separate one from another. In the well-differentiated forms of lymphoma they usually remain so. In the more anaplastic types of non-

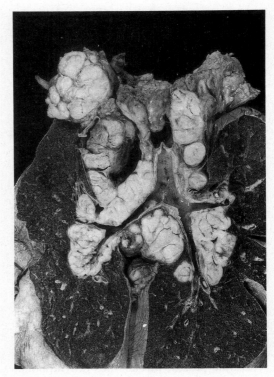

Fig. 55-8. A non-Hodgkin's lymphoma involving the
lymph nodes at the hilus of the lungs and in the
mediastinum.

Hodgkin's lymphoma, the tumor extends out
from the lymph nodes in the later stages of
the disease, infiltrating the connective tissues
and binding the lymph nodes into large,
matted masses.

When a non-Hodgkin's lymphoma involves
an extranodal organ, it may form a discrete
tumor or tumors or may cause diffuse enlargement of the organ. In the tonsils and
stomach, a non-Hodgkin's lymphoma usually
forms a well-defined mass or masses, but in
the spleen numerous small deposits of tumor
in the white pulp often cause enlargement of
the spleen without distorting its shape.

On section, the nodularity of the nodular
or follicular forms of lymphoma is often
apparent. In the diffuse forms, the affected
lymph nodes are usually replaced by uniform,
moist yellowish or grayish tumor, an appearance often likened to fish flesh. The larger
masses in other organs are similar. Only in
the more anaplastic forms of lymphoma is

there sometimes necrosis or hemorrhage in the tumor. Macroscopically, it is usually impossible to decide whether the patient has Hodgkin's disease or one of the forms of non-Hodgkin's lymphoma.

If a non-Hodgkin's lymphoma is not controlled, it spreads to involve more and more lymph nodes. Splenomegaly, hepatomegaly, and lesions of bone are common. The skin, gut, salivary glands, nervous system, lungs, or other organs are less often involved. The lymphoma may form discrete nodules of tumor in the affected organ or organs, or the organ or organs may be enlarged by multiple deposits of tumor too small to be visible macroscopically.

Follicular and Diffuse Forms. In a nodular or follicular non-Hodgkin's lymphoma the involved lymph nodes contain nodules of tumor, often about the size of a normal follicle or a little bigger. The nodules may be in any part of the lymph node and are usually numerous. The part of the lymph node between the nodules may be compressed or distorted, but retains its normal structure.

As time passes, the nodules of lymphoma in the lymph nodes enlarge and often become confluent. Eventually, the affected lymph nodes are completely replaced by lymphoma, as in a diffuse lymphoma, though often some remnant of the nodular pattern remains, at least in some lymph nodes.

In a diffuse non-Hodgkin's lymphoma, the affected lymph nodes are usually completely replaced by the lymphoma, leaving no remnant of the normal structure of the lymph node. Only occasionally is a lymph node partially replaced by a diffuse lymphoma, with part of the lymph node being destroyed by the lymphoma and part retaining its normal structure. Often a diffuse lymphoma extends beyond the capsule of an involved lymph node, flowing out into the surrounding fatty tissue. Late in the disease, this extranodal invasion is sometimes extensive, especially in the more anaplastic lymphomata.

The follicular non-Hodgkin's lymphomata are all B-cell tumors of the follicle center cells. Other kinds of non-Hodgkin's lymphoma are all diffuse. Diffuse follicle center tumors of B cells also occur, sometimes because confluent follicles come to replace the affected lymph nodes completely, sometimes because the lymphoma was diffuse from the start.

Well-Differentiated Lymphocytic Lym-

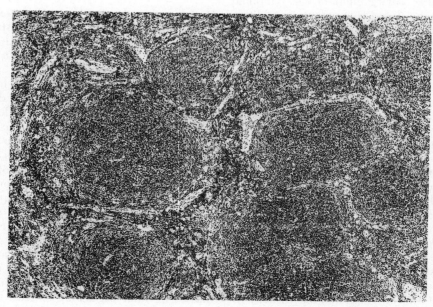

Fig. 55-9. A follicular lymphoma showing the nodules of tumor compressing the uninvolved tissue between them.

phoma. Two kinds of well-differentiated lymphocytic lymphoma are distinguished, the well-differentiated tumors associated with chronic lymphoid leukemia and the tumors that show plasmacytoid differentiation.

In *well-differentiated lymphocytic lymphoma of the kind usually associated with chronic lymphoid leukemia* the affected lymph nodes are completely replaced by a proliferation predominantly of small, well-differentiated lymphocytes showing little or no abnormality. They are the size of the lymphocytes in a normal lymph node or a little larger and have nuclei like those of the lymphocytes in the pulp of a normal lymph node. Mixed with the small lymphocytes are larger lymphocytes, with more abundant cytoplasm, a larger round or ovoid nucleus, finer chromatin, and a prominent nucleolus. The large cells may be few, but in 90% of patients they are grouped together in prominent clumps called proliferation centers. Occasionally, the large cells are the predominant cell in part of a lymph node. The large cells have been called transformed lymphocytes, lymphoblasts, and paraimmunoblasts. Mitoses are few in this kind of lymphoma. When present, they are in the large cells.

It is not possible to determine whether a diffuse, well-differentiated lymphoma of the sort usually associated with chronic lymphoid leukemia is of B cells or T cells without using markers to identify the tumor cells. Postcapillary venules are more prominent in the T-cell tumors, but not sufficiently so to allow a firm diagnosis.

In the B-cell tumors, there is immunoglobulin on the surface of the tumor cells, but not in the cytoplasm. The quantity of immunoglobulin is less than on the surface of normal B cells in the peripheral blood. Because the tumor cells are derived from a single clone, they produce either $\varkappa$ or λ light chains, never both. Most often, they produce both μ and δ heavy chains. The tumor cells usually have receptors for C3d, rarely for C3b. About 60% of the tumor cells form rosettes with mouse red cells. Mixed with the neoplastic B cells are non-neoplastic T cells. The proportion of T cells is rarely more than 10%. The T cells stain with the markers for T cells in the peripheral blood. The tumor cells do not.

In the T-cell tumors, the tumor cells do not carry immunoglobulins and rarely have receptors for complement. They react with the antibodies that identify T cells in the peripheral blood, OKT-1, OKT-3, and anti-Leu-4. Some of them form rosettes with sheep red cells.

In the *well-differentiated lymphocytic lymphomata with plasmacytoid differentiation* the affected lymph nodes are completely replaced by a proliferation predominantly of well-differentiated lymphocytes. Some of the tumor cells resemble normal lymphocytes. Some are larger and show plasmacytoid features. Some are paraimmunoblasts, like those seen in the diffuse, well-differentiated lymphocytic lymphoma usually associated with chronic lymphoid leukemia.

The plasmacytoid cells have more abundant cytoplasm than the small lymphocytes. Rough endoplasmic reticulum develops in their cytoplasm, as it does in plasma cells. Because of the increased content of ribonucleic acids, the cytoplasm becomes amphophilic or basophilic and stains with pyronin. The chromatin in the nucleus of the plasmacytoid cells becomes clumped against the nuclear membrane, as in a plasma cell. In some patients, a few of the tumor cells differentiate into apparently normal plasma cells.

In 50% of the patients, globular aggregations of immunoglobulin are present in the nucleus or cytoplasm of some of the tumor cells. The aggregations can be as large as a nucleus or larger. They stain brightly with the periodic acid-Schiff reaction. Often these aggregates are called Russell bodies, after the Scottish physician who described them in 1890, thinking them an organism that caused cancer.

In almost all patients with a plasmacytoid lymphoma, the tumor cells produce a complete immunoglobulin. In a few, they make only light chains or heavy chains. The immunoglobulin or the chain produced by the tumor cells is present on the surface of the cells. In the tumor cells showing plasmacytoid differentiation, it is also present in the cytoplasm. The tumor cells all produce the same immunoglobulin, the same light chain, the same heavy chain. The immunoglobulin or chain present on the surface of the tumor cells is the same as that in the cytoplasm. More of the tumors produce $\varkappa$ light chains than produce λ light light chains. The commonest of the heavy chains is μ though some plasmacytoid lymphomata produce γ chains or α chains. The tumor cells do not stain with the markers for T cells.

The plasmacytic lymphomata of the Kiel classification are similar, except that the majority of the tumor cells show plasmacytoid features.

Follicle Center Cell Lymphoma. The tumors of the follicle center cells are composed of neoplastic B cells showing one or more of the forms of differentiation seen in the B cells of normal follicles in lymph nodes. The tumor may be nodular or diffuse.

Small cleaved cells are a little bigger than the lymphocytes in the pulp of a normal lymph node. Their cytoplasm is scant and inconspicuous. Their nuclei are irregularly shaped. Some of them show a deep indentation, the cleaving that gives these cells their name. The chromatin of the small cleaved cells is coarse. There are no nucleoli.

Large cleaved cells vary considerably in size, some being two or three times the diameter of a normal, small lymphocyte. They have more cytoplasm than small cleaved cells, though it is still scant. The nuclei are as big as the nuclei of the macrophages in the pulp of a normal lymph node and are irregularly shaped, some showing a deep cleavage. The chromatin is finer than in small cleaved cells. Nucleoli are inconspicuous, if present.

The noncleaved cells are as large as the large cleaved cells or larger. They have more abundant cytoplasm, which becomes increasingly basophilic and pyroninophilic as rough endoplasmic reticulum becomes more abundant in the cells. The nuclei are round or ovoid, smaller than those of the macrophages in the pulp of a normal lymph node in the small noncleaved cells, larger in the large noncleaved cells. The nuclei have fine chromatin, with one or more prominent nucleoli. Often the nucleoli are close to the nuclear membrane.

The tumor cells in follicle center tumors all bear surface immunoglobulin. It is most abundant on the small cleaved cells, less on the large cleaved cells, and still less on the noncleaved follicle center cells. In 50% of the tumors, immunoglobulin is also present within the tumor cells. The tumor cells are derived from a single clone, and the immunoglobulin on and in the tumor cells is the

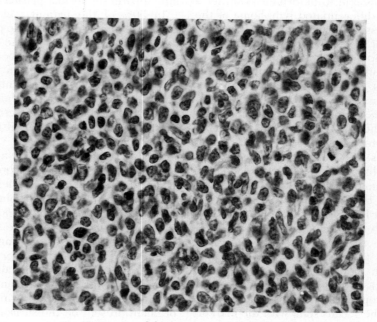

Fig. 55-10. A nodular lymphoma of small cleaved cells.

same in all. In most of the tumors, the tumor cells have receptors for both C3b and C3d, though in the noncleaved cells receptors for C3d usually predominate. In 20% of the tumors, the tumor cells form rosettes with mouse red cells. Non-neoplastic cells are mixed among the tumor cells. Usually from 5 to 20% of the cells in affected lymph nodes are T cells.

The different kinds of follicle center cell lymphoma are not separate diseases. Forms intermediate between the different types are common. The follicle center cell tumors show all patterns of differentiation from the most benign, nodular, small cleaved cell tumor to the most malignant, diffuse, large follicle center cell tumor.

Nodular lymphoma of small cleaved cells is one of the commonest of the non-Hodgkin's lymphomata. The affected lymph nodes usually show nodules of lymphoma compressing and distorting the normal tissue remaining in the lymph nodes but sometimes show more extensive replacement, with only remnants of the follicular pattern remaining. The nodules of tumor consist principally of small cleaved cells. With them are a few small lymphocytes with round nuclei and a few large noncleaved cells, with basophilic, pyroninophilic cytoplasm, fine chromatin, and nucleoli. Mitoses are few.

Nodular lymphoma of mixed small and large follicle center cells is less common. The tumors often have discrete nodules of tumor that distort the lymph nodes, but sometimes show more extensive replacement of the lymph nodes, leaving only remnants of the nodular pattern. The nodules consist of a mixture of small cleaved cells, large cleaved cell, and noncleaved follicle center cells, without a marked predominance of any one type. The larger the proportion of noncleaved cells, the higher the mitotic rate.

In *nodular lymphoma of large follicle center cells* the affected lymph nodes are usually extensively replaced, with the follicular structure of the tumor apparent only occasionally. The tumor cells are mainly large cleaved and noncleaved follicle center cells, though a few small noncleaved cells are often present. Mitoses are often numerous in the noncleaved cells. Especially in the regions in which the lymphoma replaces the lymph node entirely, there is often fibrosis. The scarring, or sclerosis as it is called, begins near the capsule and spreads both into the lymph node and out into the surrounding tissue. It may divide the lymphoma into irregular nodules until eventually part or much or the lymph node is replaced by hyaline scar tissue.

In *diffuse lymphoma of small cleaved cells* the lymphoma replaces the involved lymph nodes completely, with no suggestion of a nodular structure. The tumor consists predominantly of small cleaved cells. With them are often mixed a few large cleaved cells. Mitoses are more numerous than in the follicular tumors predominantly of small cleaved cells. Sometimes sclerosis is evident in the lymph nodes, or reticulin fibers partially surround groups of lymphoma cells.

Some *diffuse lymphomata of mixed small and large follicle center cells* consist of a mixture of small cleaved cells with large cleaved or noncleaved follicle center cells. Some show a mixture of tumor cells that resemble small lymphocytes, larger tumor cells showing plasmacytoid differentiation, and cleaved and noncleaved follicle center cells.

The working formulation also classes as diffuse, small and large cell lymphoma tumors in which the tumor cells vary in size, have irregular but uncleaved nuclei, and bear T-cell markers. These are not tumors of the follicle center cells.

In *diffuse lymphoma of large follicle center cells* the tumor cells are all large cleaved or noncleaved follicle center cells or some mixture of these types of cell. The affected lymph nodes are completely replaced. The large follicle center cells are predominant, but there may be a few small cleaved cells as well. Mitoses are numerous.

Immunoblastic Lymphoma. The lymph nodes involved are replaced completely by large, atypical lymphocytes. In some immunoblastic lymphomata, the tumor cells are B cells. In some, they are T cells. In some, they express neither B-cell nor T-cell markers. Rarely, the tumor cells contain lysozyme and have the markers of macrophages.

In the plasmacytoid form of immunoblastic lymphoma the tumor cells have ample, well-defined cytoplasm. The cytoplasm is ampho-

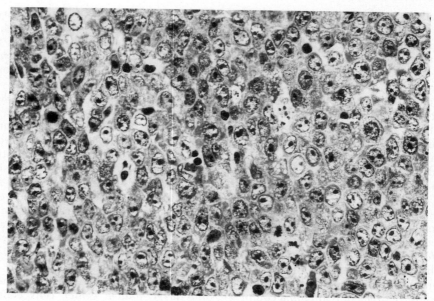

Fig. 55-11. An immunoblastic sarcoma, showing the large, atypical cells with prominent nucleoli that replace the lymph node.

philic or basophilic and stains strongly with pyronin, because of the proliferation of the rough endoplasmic reticulum in the cells. The nuclei of the tumor cells are large, round, or ovoid, with one or more large, centrally placed nucleoli.

In the clear cell type of immunoblastic lymphoma, the tumor cells have abundant, well-defined cytoplasm, which stains weakly and so appears clear by light microscopy. The nuclei of the cells are round or ovoid, with fine chromatin and small, well-defined nucleoli.

In the polymorphous form of immunoblastic lymphoma there is an admixture of small lymphocytes with dark, irregularly shaped nuclei and large cells with clear cytoplasm. Often the large cells are highly pleomorphic, sometimes multinucleated, sometimes resembling Reed-Sternberg cells. The stroma of the tumor is vascular, with small vessels with few branches radiating across the lymph node.

In all types of immunoblastic lymphoma, non-neoplastic macrophages are often mixed among the tumor cells. The macrophages have abundant, pale cytoplasm. Their cytoplasm may be empty or may contain phagocytosed debris. The macrophages may be

scattered singly but sometimes are in small clumps large enough to suggest a granuloma. They may be few or may be numerous. Sometimes there are also clumps of non-neoplastic plasma cells.

The B-cell immunoblastic tumors tend to be of the plasmacytoid type. There is immunoglobulin on the surface of the tumor cells and in over 50% of the patients within the cytoplasm as well. Receptors for C3b, C3d, or both are present in up to 50% of the tumors. The tumor cells may or may not form rosettes with mouse red cells. There is usually some admixture of non-neoplastic T cells.

The T-cell immunoblastic tumors are often of the clear cell type. There is no immunoglobulin on or in the tumor cells. They react with some of the antisera against T cells in the peripheral blood and form rosettes with sheep red cells.

The Kiel classification recognizes a *T-zone lymphoma*, grouped with the immunoblastic tumors in the other classifications. In this form of lymphoma, a proliferation of large, atypical T cells, similar to the cells of the clear cell type of immunoblastic lymphoma, begins in the paracortical region of the affected lymph nodes. Postcapillary venules are numerous and prominent in the affected part of the lymph nodes. For some time, the other parts of the affected lymph nodes remain intact, though perhaps compressed and distorted by the lymphoma. Eventually, the lymphoma replaces the involved lymph nodes completely, becoming an immunoblastic lymphoma.

Also grouped with the immunoblastic lymphomata is a lesion called epithelioid cellular lymphogranulomatosis, or *Lennert's lymphoma*, after the German pathologist who evolved the Kiel classification. In this form of tumor, clumps of large, pale, non-neoplastic macrophages make up much of the tumor. Between them, the neoplastic lymphocytes are for the most part small, with dark, irregularly shaped nuclei. A few large neoplastic lymphocytes like those of the clear cell type of immunoblastic lymphoma are present and sometimes mimic Reed-Sternberg cells. The tumor cells are probably T cells. Occasionally, a Lennert's lymphoma progresses to an immunoblastic lymphoma.

Lymphoblastic Lymphoma.   Two kinds of lymphoblastic lymphoma are recognized. The form with convoluted cells is a T-cell tumor. The form without convoluted cells shows neither B-cell nor T-cell markers.

Convoluted cell lymphoblastic lymphoma usually occurs in patients who are under 20 years of age. Some 80% of the patients have a mass in the mediastinum, usually caused by enlargement of lymph nodes rather than by involvement of the thymus. Lymph nodes elsewhere in the body, and extranodal lymphoid tissues are commonly affected. Over 80% of the patients develop the T-cell form of acute lymphoblastic leukemia at some time during the disease, with neoplastic cells like those in the lymph nodes circulating in the blood. In these people, there is often involvement of the bone marrow, spleen, and liver, as in other forms of acute lymphoblastic leukemia.

Microscopically, the involved lymph nodes are diffusely replaced by a proliferation of uniform tumor cells. The tumor cells are larger than the small lymphocytes predominant in normal lymph nodes, but not as large as large cleaved cells or immunoblasts. The tumor cells have a moderate quantity of ill-defined cytoplasm. Their nuclei have fine,

even chromatin, with small, inconspicuous nucleoli. Usually, most of the nuclei are round, but some have the irregular, indented outline that gives the tumor its name. The cells with convoluted nuclei are not always numerous. In 10% of the patients, all, or almost all, the nuclei are round. Mitoses are frequent. Often non-neoplastic macrophages with abundant, pale cytoplasm are scattered among the tumor cells. Occasionally a few eosinophils are present in the tumor.

The tumor cells usually react with the antibodies against one of the types of T cell found normally only in the thymus. Occasionally, a tumor shows the markers of the T cells in the peripheral blood. The tumor cells often have receptors for C3b or C3d. They show the focal staining for acid phosphatase seen in T cells. In some patients, they form rosettes with sheep red cells.

Nonconvoluted cell lymphoblastic lymphoma is more common in children than in adults. The patients show lymphadenopathy as in other kinds of lymphoma without a predilection for the mediastinum. Microscopically, the changes in the affected lymph nodes are similar to those of convoluted cell lymphoblastic lymphoma, except that the nuclei of the tumor cells are always ovoid or round, never convoluted.

The patients almost all have the common form of acute lymphoblastic leukemia. The tumor cells in the lymph nodes and the blood do not show the markers of either T cells or B cells. Instead, they carry the common acute lymphoblastic leukemia antigen. In a few of the patients, immunoglobulin is present in the cytoplasm of the tumor cells, though not on their surface, suggesting that the tumor cells are perhaps similar to pre-B cells, rather than to the more primitive lymphocytes usual in common acute lymphoblastic leukemia.

Adult T-Cell Leukemia/Lymphoma.   The adult T-cell leukemia/lymphoma is an unusual tumor found principally in southwestern Japan, in the Caribbean, and in the southeastern United States. Only occasional cases are found in other parts of the world.

The patients usually have widespread lymphadenopathy with leukemia. In many, the skin is involved. In some, there is involvement of the leptomeninges. Hypercalcemia is common.

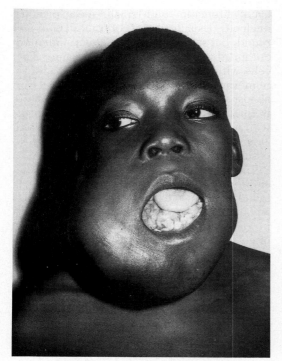

Fig. 55-12. A Burkitt's tumor enlarging and distorting the mandible. (Courtesy of Dr. J. S. Keystone.)

The lymph nodes involved show a proliferation of large, atypical T cells, first evident in the paracortical zone. Later, the lymph nodes are often completely replaced. The blood shows large, pleomorphic T cells with lobate nuclei.

Burkitt's Tumor. Burkitt's tumor is named after the British surgeon who described it in 1961. Most of the patients are children. It is common only in central Africa and New Guinea. The predominant lesion is usually in a jaw or in the abdomen.

In over 70% of young children in Africa with Burkitt's tumor, the lymphoma presents with a massive tumor in the molar or premolar region of the mandible or maxilla. The tumor is often 10 cm or more across, expanding and distorting the face, often displacing an eye or loosening the teeth. Occasionally, the lymphoma is confined to the jaw. More often, it is multifocal, with enlargement of abdominal or retroperitoneal lymph nodes or tumors in the ovaries or gut. The breasts, skin, thyroid gland, salivary glands, bone or brain are occasionally involved. Sometimes there are masses in the liver or spleen. Enlargement of the superficial lymph nodes is unusual.

In older children in Africa and in the occasional patients who develop Burkitt's tumor in the United States, Europe, or other countries, only about 30% of the patients have a lesion in the jaws. More often, the dominant lesion is in the abdomen.

In Burkitt's lymphoma, the involved lymph nodes and other tissues are replaced by closely packed tumor cells. Often the cells are so closely packed that they become polygonal. The tumor cells have a narrow rim of well-defined, amphophilic or basophilic cytoplasm, which is strongly pyroninophilic. Their nuclei are round or ovoid, about the size of the nuclei of normal macrophages. They have coarse, irregular chromatin. Most have several prominent nucleoli. Mitoses are numerous.

In most patients, non-neoplastic macrophages with abundant, pale cytoplasm are scattered among the tumor cells. Often they contain phagocytosed debris of tumor cells. Occasionally an entire tumor cell is engulfed by a macrophage. The pale macrophages scattered among the dark tumor cells give the lesion a starry sky appearance, often striking in Burkitt's lymphoma, but seen also in other kinds of lymphoma and sometimes in toxoplasmosis and other forms of lymphadenitis.

The tumor cells in Burkitt's tumor are B cells. Immunoglobulin is present on the surface of the tumor cells, but not in their cytoplasm. They do not have receptors for complement and do not form rosettes with mouse red cells. Normal T cells are mixed with the tumor cells, but make up less than 10% of the cells present.

Grouped together with the Burkitt's tumor are lymphomata in which the tumor cells are similar to those of Burkitt's lymphoma but more pleomorphic, varying considerably in size and sometimes multinucleated. The nuclei have finer chromatin than in Burkitt's tumor, with less prominent nucleoli.

Cutaneous Lymphoma. Two related types of T-cell lymphoma, mycosis fungoides and Sézary's syndrome, affect principally the skin.

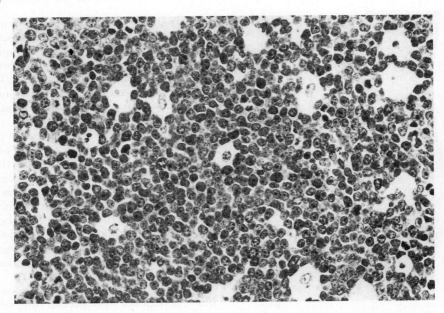

Fig. 55-13.   A Burkitt's tumor, showing pale macrophages scattered among the tumor cells.

Mycosis fungoides affects principally the skin, though late in its course lymph nodes and other internal organs are often involved as well. It is usually a sluggish disease, persisting for many years and changing in character as the years pass. Occasionally, it is rapidly progressive and brings death. Three fairly distinct stages are distinguished, the erythematous stage, the plaque stage, and the tumor stage. Most of the patients are adult.

The name is from the Greek for a mushroom, and the Latin for a fungus. It implies that the disease is a fungal infection, a view that was once popular. It is now agreed that mycosis fungoides is a form of T-cell neoplasm.

In the erythematous stage of mycosis fungoides, the patient usually shows scattered erythematous patches in the skin, irregularly shaped, well defined, scaling, and varying in color from red, to purple, to brown. Itching is often severe. Less often, the erythematous lesions become generalized and cover much of the skin. Because these erythematous lesions are not distinctive, they may be mistaken for eczema, psoriasis, or a number of other conditions.

Microscopically, the skin shows only chronic inflammation with nothing to indicate its cause. Only occasionally do cells like those of the plaque stage of the disease raise a suspicion of mycosis fungoides.

In the plaque stage of mycosis fungoides, the lesions scattered in the skin are irregularly shaped and well defined, but are slightly thickened or indurated. Sometimes the center of a lesion heals, or a whole lesion regresses, leaving the skin thin and atrophic.

Microscopically, the lesions show a prominent cellular infiltrate in the dermis. In the upper dermis, the infiltrate is often diffuse and forms a band a little below the epithelium. In the deeper part of the dermis, the infiltrate forms large, well-demarcated clumps of closely packed cells, often with a blood vessel in the center of the clump. The infiltrate consists mainly of a mixture of lymphocytes, plasma cells, macrophages, and eosinophils, often with a few neutrophils. Scattered among this mixture of normal cells are a moderate number of atypical cells, called mycosis cells. The mycosis cells are about the size of a large lymphocyte, but have hyperchromatic, irregularly shaped nuclei. There may be a few mitoses.

In 50% of the patients with the plaque stage of mycosis fungoides, the infiltrate

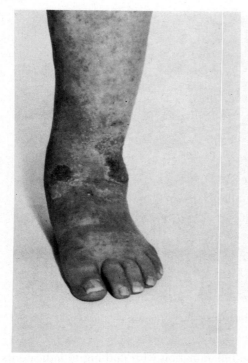

Fig. 55-14. Mycosis fungoides, showing the lesions
in the skin.

extends into the epidermis, forming what are
called Pautrier's microabscesses, named after
the French physician born in 1876. In these
lesions, a few mononuclear cells like those in
the infiltrate in the dermis lie within the
epidermis, usually with a clear space separating them from the epidermal cells.

The epidermis usually shows some acanthosis. Often there is irregular lengthening of
its rete ridges, which extend further than
normal into the dermis.

The lesions of the tumor stage of mycosis
fungoides in the skin form round or irregularly shaped masses, brown or reddish in color,
which bulge above the skin. Some of the
lesions ulcerate.

Microscopically, the lesions show a dense
infiltrate in the dermis which often extends
into the subdermal fat. Usually, the infiltrate
consists of the same mixture of cells as is seen
in the plaque stage, though mycotic cells are
more numerous. Some of them may be
binucleate, and look much like a Reed-
Sternberg cell. Occasionally a lesion consists
almost entirely of mycotic cells.

Early in the course of mycosis fungoides,
the lymph nodes draining the lesions in the
skin often show dermatopathic lymphadenitis. Only late in the course of mycosis fungoides, do the lymph nodes and other internal
organs begin to show foci of cellular infiltrate,
sometimes with a mixture of cells as in the
skin, but often predominantly of mycotic
cells. Only when the tumor stage of mycosis
fungoides is reached, is there likely to be extensive involvement of lymph nodes throughout the body and often of the spleen, liver,
lungs, bowel, or kidneys. The tumor cells
replacing the lymph nodes may resemble the
mycosis cells in the skin or may be more
anaplastic, resembling the cells of a T-cell
immunoblastic lymphoma. The tumor cells
show the markers of T cells, sometimes the
markers of helper T cells.

Mycosis cells are rarely numerous in the
blood of patients with mycosis fungoides, but
an occasional mycosis cell is present in the
blood in more than 20% of the patients.

The *Sézary syndrome*, described by the
French physicians Sézary and Bouvrain in
1938, is a rare form of mycosis fungoides. The
patients show erythema involving much or all
of the skin, with marked hyperkeratosis and
scaling, and intense pruritus.

Microscopically, the skin shows an infiltrate
of lymphocytes, plasma cells, macrophages,
eosinophils, and neutrophils, with many
mycosis cells, or Sézary cells as they are
sometimes called. Pautrier's microabscesses
are often present.

Considerable numbers of Sézary cells circulate in the blood. The leukocyte count is
usually between 10 and 30 × 10^9/L, (10,000
to 30,000/mm^3), sometimes higher, with 5 to
20% of the white cells being Sézary cells.
Some of the tumor cells have round nuclei;
some, deeply convoluted nuclei. The proportion of normal lymphocytes in the blood may
be increased. The lymph nodes are often
enlarged, usually because of dermatopathic
lymphadenitis, but late in the disease sometimes because of infiltration by the neoplastic
T cells.

Tumors of Macrophages. Tumors of
macrophages that resemble lymphoma are
rare. Two types are distinguished, histiocytic
sarcoma and histiocytic medullary reticulosis.

In a *histiocytic sarcoma*, the involved

lymph nodes are diffusely replaced by large tumor cells that have abundant cytoplasm, which is sometimes eosinophilic and opaque, sometimes foamy or vacuolated. Sometimes phagocytosed material is evident in the tumor cells. The nuclei are ovoid or reniform, with a prominent nucleolus or nucleoli. Often some of the tumor cells are multinucleate. Mitoses are common. The cells often contain lysozyme and show some of the markers of macrophages. Electron microscopy usually shows the lysosomes, rough endoplastic reticulum, and the irregular cell borders of macrophages.

The tumor cells contain nospecific esterase and stain for α_1-antitrypsin and lysozyme. They often contain a variety of immunoglobulins, probably because they phagocytose immune complexes.

Histiocytic medullary reticulosis is rare. It usually presents abruptly in older people, with fever, fatigue, weight loss, splenomegaly, and generalized lymphadenopathy. Anemia is severe and for the most part hemolytic. Severe thrombocytopenia is usual. Often there is leukopenia.

The affected lymph nodes are large. The sinusoids are wide and prominent. They are lined and filled by large, neoplastic macrophages, with abundant cytoplasm and large, atypical nuclei. Often the tumor cells contain phagocytosed red cells, occasionally other cells. Some of the tumor cells may be multinucleated. The sinusoids in the spleen show a similar proliferation of malignant macrophages.

Immunologic Defects. Immunologic defects are less common in the non-Hodgkin's lymphomata than in Hodgkin's disease. If an immunologic fault develops, it is usually only late, when the disease is far advanced.

Nearly 40% of patients with a diffuse, well-differentiated lymphoma that shows plasmacytoid differentiation have a monoclonal excess of immunoglobulin in the blood. Usually the abnormal immunoglobulin is IgM, sometimes IgG, but rarely IgA or IgE. Less often a plasmacytoid lymphoma produces an monoclonal excess of a heavy chain or a light chain. Other lymphomata produce an excess of immunoglobulin or one of its chains less frequently.

Changes in the Blood. In most patients with lymphoma, the blood is normal when the diagnosis is made, unless the patient has leukemia or a B-cell tumor producing excessive quantities of an immunoglobulin. As the disease progresses, anemia often develops, occasionally an autoimmune hemolytic anemia. Lymphopenia, neutropenia, and thrombocytopenia are not uncommon. Thrombocytosis is rare. Late in the course, there is often hypoalbuminemia, polyclonal hypergammaglobulinemia or less often hypogammaglobulinemia. A monoclonal excess of a single immunoglobulin or of its light or heavy chain is more probable as the volume of tumor increases. Hyperuricemia and hypercalcemia sometimes develop late in the disease.

Behavior. Non-Hodgkin's lymphoma tends to change for the worse as months pass, and many of the patients develop leukemia.

Progression. Progression to a more serious form of lymphoma is uncommon in patients with the diffuse, well-differentiated lymphoma associated with chronic lymphoid leukemia and in people with a well-differentiated, diffuse, plasmacytoid lymphoma. The tumor changes to an immunoblastic lymphoma in less than 5% of these people, usually only after it has persisted unchanged for years. The well-differentiated forms of lymphoma rarely change to a follicle center cell tumor.

In contrast, progression to the worse is evident in 40% of patients with a tumor of the follicle center cells. The larger, more anaplastic cells tend to become more numerous in the lesions and to replace the smaller cleaved cells. The more benign nodular tumors tend to change to a diffuse lymphoma. A nodular tumor of small cleaved cells can end as a diffuse tumor of large follicle center cells or as an immunoblastic lymphoma.

Progression to the worse also occurs in T-cell tumors. A T-zone lymphoma tends to change to an immunoblastic lymphoma. The more benign form of mycosis fungoides tends to change to plaques or tumors.

Even the poorly differentiated lymphomata tend to become worse if the patient lives long enough. The tumor cells tend to become larger, more anaplastic, and more pleomorphic.

The progression probably is due principally to the instability of the lymphoma cells.

Some of them change to a more active form, which overgrows and replaces the less active tumor cells formerly present. The radiation and drugs used to treat lymphomata are carcinogenic and may favor the emergence of a more dangerous form of the lymphoma or induce a second tumor of a different type.

Leukemia. Almost all patients with a diffuse lymphoma of small, well-differentiated lymphocytes without plasmacytoid differentiation have chronic lymphoid leukemia or develop it. In the diffuse, well-differentiated lymphomata of small lymphocytes with plasmacytoid features, 60% of the patients have more than 4×10^9/L (4000/mm^3) lymphocytes in the blood. Most of the lymphocytes appear normal, but in some patients some of them show plasmacytoid features. Over 80% of patients with a convoluted T-cell lymphoblastic lymphoma have T-cell acute lymphoblastic leukemia. Almost all patients with nonconvoluted lymphoblastic lymphoma have common acute lymphoblastic leukemia.

In other kinds of lymphoma, leukemia is uncommon. Overall, only 20% of children and 10% of adults with non-Hodgkin's lymphoma develop leukemia. A few atypical lymphocytes are often present in the blood, in patients with lymphoma, but they are not sufficiently numerous to justify a diagnosis of leukemia. A patient with lymphoma is said to have leukemia only if there are more than 5 $\times$ 10^9/L (5000/mm^3) lymphocytes in the blood, or if more than 25% of the nucleated cells in the blood are abnormal. The abnormal lymphocytes in the blood of patients with lymphoma are larger than normal, with more abundant cytoplasm and abnormal nuclei. They may resemble the tumor cells seen in the affected lymph nodes. Patients with lymphoma who have considerable numbers of abnormal lymphocytes in the blood are often said to have lymphosarcoma cell leukemia.

A few patients with lymphoma develop an acute or chronic myeloid leukemia. The myeloid leukemia is probably caused by the carcinogenic drugs used to treat the lymphoma. It usually develops 10 or more years after beginning therapy.

Staging. Staging of the sort valuable in Hodgkin's disease is less helpful in non-Hodgkin's lymphoma. At the time of diagnosis, 65% of the patients are in stage IV, as judged by the Ann Arbor system. Only in the forms of lymphoma grouped as diffuse, histiocytic lymphoma in the Rappaport classification are there likely to be more than 30% of patients in stages I or II. Over 80% of patients with a lymphoma of follicle center cells have widespread disease. Patients with a diffuse lymphoma of well-differentiated lymphocytes almost all have chronic lymphoid leukemia. People with a well-differentiated lymphoma with plasmacytoid differentiation usually have widespread disease.

In many patients with non-Hodgkin's lymphoma, physical examination makes it clear that the disease is in stage III or stage IV. In most, a bone marrow biopsy, a liver biopsy, or lymphangiography shows that the disease is in stage III or IV.

Clinical Presentation. Patients with a non-Hodgkin's lymphoma usually have enlargement of one or more groups of lymph nodes. Less than 10% of the patients have fatigue, malaise, weight loss, or night sweats. A few present with abdominal pain, nausea, or vomiting because of involvement of the gastrointestinal tract or abdominal lymph nodes. A few have symptoms caused by involvement of some other extranodal site. Except in children, involvement of the bones is rarely sufficient to cause pain or tenderness in the affected bones. Pruritus is uncommon.

Pathogenesis. Interest in the pathogenesis of the lymphomata has centered on the possibility that they might be caused by a virus. Lymphoid tumors in mice, rats, fowls, cats, hamsters, rabbits, and monkeys are caused by viruses, suggesting that human lymphomata might be caused similarly. This view was strengthened when it was shown that Burkitt's tumor is almost certainly caused by the Epstein-Barr virus and that the adult T-cell leukemia/lymphoma is caused by HTLV-I, the human T cell leukemia virus I, a retrovirus that is a close relative of the human immunodeficiency virus that causes the acquired immune deficiency syndrome. HTLV-I infects helper T cells, altering their function and causing leukemia in some of the people infected.

Chromosomal abnormalities are frequent in patients with well-differentiated lymphocytic lymphoma and chronic lymphoid leukemia. Trisomy 12 and other abnormalities are common in the B-cell form of the disease. Abnormalities of chromosomes 14 are common, especially in Burkitt's tumor. In the more anaplastic lymphomata, chromosomal abnormalities are frequent. In 50% of patients with lymphoblastic lymphoma, the tumor cells are aneuploid. In 10%, they have the Philadelphia chromosome more common in chronic myeloid leukemia.

The activation of oncogenes may be important in some forms of non-Hodgkin's lymphoma, though it is not known whether the altered expression of the oncogenes is the cause of the lymphoma or secondary to a malignant change caused in some other way. In some patients with Burkitt's lymphoma, translocations affect the regulation of the c-myc oncogene. In some with a well-differentiated lymphocytic lymphoma of B cells and chronic lymphoid leukemia, translocation affects the expression of the oncogene bcl-1, and in some with T-cell chronic lymphoid leukemia the oncogene tcl-1 is involved. Abnormal activity of other oncogenes has been detected in well-differentiated lymphocytic lymphomata.

Survivors of atomic radiation show an increase in acute lymphoid leukemia, Hodgkin's and non-Hodgkin's lymphoma, and multiple myeloma, though not in chronic lymphoid leukemia. This increase is much less striking than the increase in myeloid leukemia seen in these people.

Tumors of lymphocytes are common in patients with many of the congenital immune deficiency diseases and in people treated with immunosuppressive drugs. Whether the risk increases because of failure of the immune system or because the drugs are carcinogenic is uncertain. Rheumatoid arthritis and systemic lupus erythematosus increase two or three times the risk of developing a lymphoid tumor. Sideroblastic anemia increases the risk of multiple myeloma. The risk of lymphoma is increased in people with celiac disease.

Treatment and Prognosis. The lymphomata of low malignancy in the Kiel classification and the working formulation usually progress slowly, and for many years cause little or no disability. Some patients need no treatment. In the few patients with a lymphoma of low malignancy, which is stage I or II by the Ann Arbor system, local radiotherapy brings remission that persists for more than 10 years in 75% of the patients, though the disease eventually recurs in some other part of the body. If the disease is more extensive, chemotherapy with a single moderate dose of a single drug such as chlorambucil or cyclophosphamide or with a combination of drugs brings remission that lasts for two to five years in 80% of the patients, though rarely a cure. Even though over 60% of patients with a lymphoma of low malignancy are elderly, over 60% are alive five years after the diagnosis.

The more malignant forms of non-Hodgkin's lymphoma are treated by chemotherapy, using a combination of drugs in high dosage. Local radiation is added if the tumor compresses or obstructs an imporant structure. Radiation of the mediastinum or brain is helpful if the lymphoma involves these structures. Surgical removal of a lymphoma of the gastrointestinal tract is often useful, and occasionally surgical removal of a large mass of tumor is indicated. The chemotherapy brings remission in up to 80% of the patients. In 50% of those treated, the remission persists for several years, and the patient is perhaps cured. Patients who fail to respond to chemotherapy rarely survive more than a year.

Children with a lymphoblastic lymphoma or with Burkitt's tumor usually respond dramatically to chemotherapy. So great is the destruction of tumor cells that the patients often develop hyperkalemia, hypocalcemia, hyperphosphatemia, hyperuricemia, and sometimes renal failure. Irradiation of the brain is necessary because of the frequency of meningeal involvement. With Burkitt's tumor, it is desirable to remove as much of the tumor surgically as is possible. Over 60% of children with lymphoblastic lymphoma are cured. Over 50% of patients with Burkitt's tumor, 90% of those in whom the tumor is confined to a single site, have a prolonged remission and are perhaps cured.

Mycosis fungoides has been treated in many ways. Local application of chemotherapeutic drugs, local irradiation, psoralen to sensitize the lesions to ultraviolet light, and the systemic administration of chemotherapeutic drugs, singly and in combination, have all been used with good effect. The prognosis depends on the stage and extent of the disease. Over 90% of patients with limited plaques survive for more than five years, but those with generalized involvement of the skin, or with tumors, live on the average only three or four years.

The prognosis in patients with a histiocytic sarcoma, histiocytic medullary reticulosis, or adult T-cell leukemia/lymphoma is bad. Whatever the treatment, few patients survive for a year.

Complications. Nearly 50% of patients with lymphoma die of infection, as the body's defenses fail. Bronchopneumonia is a common cause of death. In 20% of the patients, extension of the lymphoma gradually impairs the function of the heart, lungs, liver, or kidneys. There may be involvement of the nervous sytem, compression of the spinal cord, blood vessels, or of lymphatics, or narrowing or perforation of the gut. In 10% of patients with widespread lymphoma, hemorrhage caused mainly by thrombocytopenia contributes importantly to death.

The chemotherapeutic drugs used to treat the lymphomata bring their own complications. Nausea, vomiting, and loss of hair are common and at times very distressing to the patient. Depression of the bone marrow, anemia, neutropenia, and thrombocytopenia is usually transient, but often profound. Rapid destruction of lymphoma cells by chemotherapy can cause hyperuricemia or hyperkalemia. A second malignant neoplasm develops in 5% of the patients who survive for seven or more years. Acute myeloid leukemia is the most common, but other kinds of leukemia and malignant tumors of the gonads and other sites also occur.

Some patients with lymphoma die without obvious cause. The patient gradually becomes weaker, feebler, and more debilitated.

Lymphoid Leukemia

In lymphoid leukemia, the predominant feature of the disease is the presence of malignant lymphocytes in the blood. The bone marrow is always affected, and there is often involvement of lymph nodes and other tissues.

Two principal forms of lymphoid leukemia

are distinguished, chronic lymphoid leukemia, sometimes called chronic lymphatic leukemia, and acute lymphoid leukemia, often called acute lymphoblastic leukemia or occasionally acute lymphatic leukemia. Occasionally a patient develops hairy cell leukemia or prolymphocytic leukemia.

CHRONIC LYMPHOID LEUKEMIA. About 25% of people with leukemia have the chronic lymphoid form of the disease. In the United States, 2 people in every 100,000 die of it. Over 70% of the patients are men. Most are over 60 years old, though the disease can develop in younger people. It is rare in people less than 30 years old. Chronic lymphoid leukemia is uncommon in Japan and China.

Lesions. When the diagnosis is made, most patients with chronic lymphoid leukemia have between 50 and 200 × 10^9/L (50,000 to 200,000/mm³) lymphocytes in the blood. If the disease is untreated, the concentration of lymphocytes in the blood slowly rises as years pass and may come to exceed 1000 × 10^9/L (1,000,000/mm³). In many patients, the concentration of lymphocytes in the blood fluctuates from week to week, sometimes by as much as 50 × 10^9/L (50,000/mm³).

The neoplastic lymphocytes in the blood usually look like normal small lymphocytes. In a few patients, they are a little larger and show plasmacytoid differentiation. Occasionally inclusions, most often of IgM, are evident in the tumor cells.

In 99% of the patients, the tumor cells in the blood are B cells. They have immunoglobulin on their surface and occsionally within their cytoplasm. As the tumor cells are a single clone, the immunoglobulin on or in the tumor cells is the same in all. In less than 1% of the patients, the tumor cells show the markers of the T cells in the peripheral blood.

The malignant lymphocytes are present throughout the bone marrow. By the time the diagnosis is made, usually more than 40% of the cells in the marrow are lymphocytes. In 30% of the patients, the infiltration of the marrow causes pain or tenderness in the sternum.

One or more groups of lymph nodes are enlarged in 90% of the patients at the time of diagnosis. Biopsy usually shows diffuse replacement of the affected lymph nodes by a diffuse, well-differentiated lymphocytic lymphoma. Less often, the tumor cells in the affected lymph nodes show plasmacytoid differentiation.

The spleen is enlarged at the time of diagnosis in 70% of the patients, but rarely extends more than 10 cm below the costal margin. The enlargement is caused by the accumulation of tumor cells in the spleen, principally around the margins of the white pulp.

The liver is enlarged in 50% of the patients, as leukemic cells accumulate principally in the portal tracts. The malignant cells can extend from the blood into other organs, though the involvement is rarely enough to cause dysfunction. They sometimes form masses in the skin or gut.

At the time of diagnosis, 50% of the patients are anemic, 20% are neutropenic, and 40% are thrombocytopenic. The cytopenias are usually mild. Only in 10% of the patients is the packed cell volume less than 0.30 L/L (30%). The platelet count is rarely less than $50 \times 10^9/L$ (50,000/mm³). The anemia is usually normocytic and normochromic, though an occasional patient develops severe autoimmune hemolytic anemia. As the infiltration of the bone marrow grows more extensive, the cytopenias become more severe.

In more than 50% of patients, hypogammaglobulinemia grows increasingly severe as the disease extends. In 5% of the patients, there is a monoclonal excess of an immunoglobulin, usually IgM, or of a light chain.

Clinical Presentation. About 25% of patients with chronic lymphoid leukemia have no symptoms when the diagnosis is made. A high leukocyte count, enlargement of the spleen, or enlargement of lymph nodes is detected during an examination undertaken for some other reason.

About 60% of the patients complain of fatigue, less often of malaise or weight loss. About 20% of the patients seek advice because they discover enlarged lymph nodes. In 30% of the patients, repeated infections lead to the discovery of the leukemia.

Treatment and Prognosis. The course and treatment of chronic lymphoid leukemia are those of the well-differentiated forms of diffuse lymphoma.

Complications. Infection is the major complication of chronic lymphoid leukemia. Nearly 50% of patients die of infection, most often pneumonia. In the late stages of the disease, derangement of the immunologic defenses, and neutropenia are frequent. Herpes zoster is common and can be extensive. Opportunistic fungi or viruses may take advantage of the patient's susceptibility. Damage to the bone marrow caused by the chemotherapy adds to the risk.

Chronic lymphoid leukemia rarely changes to acute leukemia. In the few patients with chronic lymphoid leukemia who have developed acute leukemia, the acute leukemia has been myeloid as often as lymphoid and is probably a second tumor caused by the drugs used in treatment, rather than a progression to the worse in the chronic leukemia. Some have suggested that carcinoma is more common in patients with chronic lympoid leukemia than would be expected, but others have found no excess of carcinoma in their patients.

Most patients with chronic lymphoid leukemia are elderly. Over 30% die of causes unrelated to the leukemia: heart disease, a stroke, carcinoma, or some other of the diseases common in old people.

HAIRY CELL LEUKEMIA. Hairy cell leukemia is a form of chronic lymphoid leukemia. Less than 5% of patients with chronic lymphoid leukemia have this form of the disease. About 80% of the patients are men. Most are middle-aged.

More than 60% of the patients have leukopenia when they seek treatment. The leukocyte count is greater than normal in less than 20%. Nearly 80% of the patients are anemic, and 80% are thrombocytopenic. In 40%, the platelet count is less than $50 \times 10^9/L$ (50,000/mm³).

The hairy cells that give the disease its name are present in the blood in 95% of the patients, but are usually few. In 70% of patients, less than 10% of the leukocytes are hairy cells. In less than 20%, more than 50% of the leukocytes are hairy cells.

As seen in a blood film, the hairy cells are 10 to 20 μm in diameter. They have a nucleus like that of a lymphocyte, but it is often irregularly shaped or reniform. Their cytoplasm may be sparse or more abundant than that of a lymphocyte. Electron microscopy shows that long, irregular cytoplasmic projections extend from the surface of the cells, the hairs that give them their name. The hairs are not always well seen by light microscopy. Complexes of lamellae and ribosomes are present in the cytoplasm of the hairy cells in 50% of the patients.

In 95% of the patients with hairy cell leukemia some of the hairy cells in the blood show granular staining for tartrate resistant acid phosphatase. This enzyme is rarely demonstrable in the circulating tumor cells in other kinds of chronic lymphoid leukemia. It is less useful as a diagnostic aid in the tissues, where the enzyme is widely distributed and other kinds of cell show similar staining. The hairy cells in the blood and tissues stain strongly for nonspecific acid esterase.

In most patients, the hairy cells are B cells. They have immunoglobulin on their surface and sometimes in the cytoplasm. Only one kind of light chain is formed, but there is more than one kind of heavy chain, most often IgM and IgG. Many of the cells have also a receptor for the T-cell growth factor. Less often, the hairy cells are T cells.

The spleen is enlarged in 90% of people with hairy cell leukemia, often greatly, extending below the umbilicus in 50% of the patients. The enlargement is caused by extensive infiltration of the spleen by tumor cells like those in the blood.

One or more groups of lymph nodes are enlarged in 30% of the patients. Microscopically, the involved lymph nodes are infiltrated by tumor cells, first in the B-cell regions and connective tissue septa.

The liver is enlarged in less than 20% of the patients as hairy cells accumulate principally in the sinusoids.

The bone marrow shows widespread replacement by the tumor cells. Usually, there is a considerable increase in reticulin fibers in the marrow, sometimes myelofibrosis. Perhaps because of this, an attempt to aspirate bone marrow is often unsuccessful.

The clinical presentation in hairy cell leukemia is similar to that in the classic form of chronic lymphoid leukemia, often with the

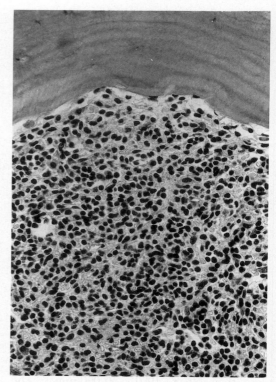

Fig. 55-15.   Hairy cell leukemia, showing infiltration of the bone marrow by the tumor cells.

addition of abdominal discomfort, caused by the weight of the big spleen.

Hairy cell leukemia progresses slowly. Infection, often with an opportunistic organism, is one of its principal dangers. If the cytopenias grow severe, splenectomy usually gives relief. Recombinant α-interferon brings a remission in 90% of the patients. More than 50% of the patients are alive eight years after the diagnosis.

PROLYMPHOCYTIC LEUKEMIA. Prolymphocytic leukemia is a rare variant of chronic lymphoid leukemia. The leukocyte count is usually 100 to 1000 × 10^9/L (100,000 to 10,000,000/mm^3) with the majority of the white cells large, atypical lymphocytes. The cells have abundant, basophilic cytoplasm and round or ovoid nuclei with prominent nucleoli. In most patients, the tumor cells are B cells, though in a few they have been T cells.

The patients usually have marked enlargement of the spleen and liver, caused by infiltration of these organs by the tumor cells. Enlargement of lymph nodes is unusual, but when lymph nodes are involved, they are replaced by a proliferation predominantly of the paraimmunoblasts present in small numbers in the well-differentiated forms of lymphoma.

Symptoms of patients with prolymphocytic leukemia are malaise, weight loss, and often fever. Most are severely anemic, with mild thrombocytopenia.

Prolymphocytic leukemia progresses rapidly. Chemotherapy has proved of little avail. Death is likely within a year.

ACUTE LYMPHOBLASTIC LEUKEMIA. Acute lymphoblastic leukemia is most common in children, though it can develop at any age. In England and Wales, each year 3 boys and 2 girls in every 100,000 under 15 years old develop acute lymphoblastic leukemia. In older people, only 0.6 men and 0.4 women in every 100,000 develop the disease in any one year.

Four kinds of acute lymphoblastic leukemia are distinguished. In T-cell acute lymphoblastic leukemia, the tumor cells bear the markers of T cells, nearly always the markers of one of the forms of T cell found normally only in the thymus. In B-cell acute lymphoblastic leukemia, the tumor cells have the surface immunoglobulin of B cells. In common acute lymphoblastic leukemia, the tumor cells have neither T- nor B-cell markers, but carry what is called the common acute lymphoblastic leukemia antigen. In the unclassified form of actue lymphoblastic leukemia, the tumor cells have none of these markers.

In children, 75% of the patients have common acute lymphoblastic leukemia, 15% have T-cell acute lymphoblastic leukemia, less than 5% have the B-cell acute lymphoblastic leukemia, and the rest have the unclassified form of the disease. In adults, 70% of the patients have the unclassified form of acute lymphoblastic leukemia, 15% have common acute lymphoblastic leukemia, 10% have T-cell leukemia, and 5% have B-cell leukemia.

Lesions. In 50% of patients with acute lymphoblastic leukemia, the leukocyte count is between 10 and 100 × 10^9/L (10,000 and 100,000/mm^3). In 10%, it exceeds 100 × 10^9/L (100,000/mm^3). In 15%, it is between 5 and 10 × 10^9/L (5000 and 10,000/mm^3). In 25%, it is less than 5 × 10^9/L (5000/mm^3). High counts are most common in the T-cell form of the disease.

In most patients, from 30 to 90% of the white cells in the blood are tumor cells. Occasionally, tumor cells are few. Rarely, in people with marked leukopenia, none can be found.

The French-American-British working group distinguish three types of tumor cell in acute lymphoblastic leukemia. Type L1 is the most common in children. Type L2 is the most frequent in adults. Type L3 is seen in people with B-cell acute lymphoblastic leukemia.

In type L1, the tumor cells in the blood are about twice the diameter of a normal lymphocyte. Cytoplasm is scant. The nucleus may be round or ovoid or may be indented, cleft, or folded. The chromatin is sometimes fine, sometimes clumped. Nucleoli are inconspicuous. The appearance of the tumor cells differs from one patient to another, but in a single patient all the tumor cells are alike.

In type L2, the tumor cells in the blood are bigger and vary in size. The cytoplasm is sometimes scant, but more often is abundant and basophilic. The nuclei are irregularly shaped, often indented, cleft, or folded. Chromatin is clumped. One or more prominent nucleoli are present in the cells.

The B cells of type L3 are large. They have abundant, basophilic cytoplasm, which is often vacuolated. The nuclei are round or ovoid, with dense, regular chromatin and one or more prominent nucleoli.

In 80% of patients with acute lymphoid leukemia, the concentration of neutrophils in the blood is reduced, often to less than 1 × 10^9/L (1000/mm^3). If there are enough neutrophils to make the test possible, the activity of alkaline phosphatase in the neutrophils is high, in contrast to the marked reduction in alkaline phosphatase activity usual in acute myeloid leukemia. In 90% of patients, the concentration of platelets in the blood is low, often less than $50 \times 10^9/L$ (50,000/mm^3). Anemia is almost invariable, with the concentration of hemoglobin 80 g/L (8 g/100 mL) or less. In 25% of the patients, myeloblasts or nucleated red cells are present in the blood. Uricacidemia is present in 50% of the patients at the time the diagnosis is made. The concentration of globulins in the blood is usually normal.

At the time of the diagnosis, the spleen is slightly enlarged in 90% of children with acute lymphoblastic leukemia. Tumor cells like those in the blood accumulate in the white pulp. Often they are prominent in endothelium-lined spaces in the intima of arterioles or in the splenic trabeculae. In 70% of the patients, the liver is a little enlarged. The leukemic cells accumulate principally in the portal tracts.

In 70% of patients, one or more groups of lymph nodes are enlarged when the diagnosis is made. In patients with T-cell acute lymphoblastic leukemia, the affected lymph nodes are replaced by a convoluted cell lymphoblastic lymphoma. In patients with common acute lymphoblastic leukemia, the lymph nodes show the nonconvoluted cell form of lymphoblastic lymphoma. In the people with B-cell acute lymphoblastic leukemia, the lymph nodes show Burkitt's tumor or a pleomorphic B-cell tumor.

The bone marrow is extensively replaced by the tumor cells. Up to 80% of the patients have pain or tenderness in the bones or joints. Most have pancytopenia caused by the replacement of the bone marrow by the tumor.

Other organs are often involved, as the tumor cells escape from the blood and infiltrate the tissues. There may be infiltration of the kidneys or lungs. Lesions in the skin and gums are not as striking as in acute myeloid leukemia. Sometimes there is infiltration of the meninges.

Clinical Presentation. Most children with acute lymphoblastic leukemia are listless and seem tired. In 80%, the tumor in the bone marrow causes pain or tenderness in the bones or joints. Fever without evidence of infection or other cause is apparent in 70% of the patients. Nearly 70% of the patients have lost weight. In 60% of the children, a parent discovers a mass. In 50% of the patients,

purpura or other bleeding caused by the thrombocytopenia is prominent.

Treatment and Prognosis. Without treatment, acute lymphoblastic leukemia advances rapidly. Over 90% of the patients die within a year of diagnosis. Unless the disease is controlled, the leukemic cells infiltrate ever more widely into the tissues. Extensive infiltration of the kidneys and of the meninges is common. Cerebral vessels are often plugged by leukemic cells. The ovaries, testes, heart and other organs are frequently involved. Anemia, neutropenia, and thrombocytopenia worsen. Hemorrhage into the brain, meninges, or bowel can bring death. Infection becomes increasingly probable and dangerous. Pneumonia may be uncontrollable.

In over 90% of the children, combination chemotherapy followed by irradiation of the brain brings complete remission, with loss of all signs of the disease, within a few weeks. In 60% of the children, the remission persists for five or more years. Many remain in complete remission years after all treatment has stopped. Probably most of these children are cured.

The prognosis is best in children with common acute lymphoblastic leukemia or the unclassified form of the disease. In adults and in children with the T-cell or B-cell form of acute lymphoblastic leukemia, the outlook is poor. Complete remission can be achieved but does not usually last more than a year. Only 20% of adults survive five years.

Whatever the type of acute lymphoblastic leukemia, the higher the leukocyte count, the worse the prognosis. The prognosis of the T-cell form of the disease is poor in part because the concentration of white cells in the blood is usually high. The outlook is worse in boys than in girls, in part because 80% of children with T-cell acute lymphoblastic leukemia are boys, in part because recurrence in the testes is not uncommon. A mediastinal mass is of ominous significance because it implies that the leukemia is of the T-cell type.

Once remission is achieved, maintenance therapy with 6-mercaptopurine and methotrexate or other drugs is continued, usually for three years or more. About 80% of the patients who remain free from disease for this period continue to be free of disease after the treatment is stopped. The longer the remission, the less the chance of recurrence.

If acute lymphoblastic leukemia recurs during maintenance therapy, the outlook is poor. Further treatment with the drugs that induced the initial remission or with other agents may bring a second remission, but it is likely to be short. Recurrence after treatment has stopped is less dangerous. If other measures fail, bone marrow transplantation has brought prolonged remission and perhaps cure to some patients.

Complications. The principal complications of uncontrolled acute lymphoblastic leukemia are infection due to the profound derangement of the body's defense and bleeding caused mainly by the thrombocytopenia. The power of organisms normally pathogenic is enhanced, and the body can be invaded by any or several of the opportunistic organisms.

The treatment brings its own dangers. The rapid destruction of tumor cells during the initial phase of the therapy can cause hyperuricemia and hyperkalemia sufficient to endanger life unless large quantities of fluid and allopurinol are given to lessen the risk. Nearly 50% of children become feverish during the initial treatment, more often because of the destruction of the tumor than because of infection. The irradiation of the brain brings temporary alopecia. In 60% of the children, it causes temporary somnolence, usually beginning some weeks after the irradiation and persisting for two or three weeks. Rarely, leukoencephalopathy develops, with major injury to the brain. During the maintenance phase of treatment, infection is the main danger because of the immunosuppression caused by the drugs. Measles, varicella, herpes zoster, and infection with a cytomegalovirus can be dangerous. Pneumocystis carinii and other opportunistic organisms can cause serious disease.

Plasma Cell Tumors

The tumors of plasma cells are a form of B-cell tumor but are separated from the lymphomata and lymphoid leukemias because of their different clinical presentation and different behavior. Two kinds of plasma cell tumor are distinguished, a localized lesion called a plasmacytoma and the malignant tumor called multiple myeloma.

PLASMACYTOMA. Plasmacytomata are uncommon. They are found most often in the oral mucosa, the nasal mucosa, or the conjunctiva, but may occur in other parts of the body. The lesion forms a mass a few millimeters across. Microscopically, it consists of closely packed plasma cells, which often look normal. Sometimes they show a little atypicality.

The nature of these little lesions is uncertain. About 70% of them are cured by excision or local radiation. Some think that this sort of plasmacytoma is an inflammatory reaction rather than a neoplasm.

In the other 30% of the patients, the plasmacytoma is only the first sign of multiple myeloma. Other evidence of multiple myeloma may be found when the patient is investigated, but sometimes it is only weeks later that it becomes clear that the patient has multiple myeloma.

MULTIPLE MYELOMA. The malignant tumor of plasma cells is called a multiple myeloma. Myeloma is from the Greek for the bone marrow and indicates the usual site of the lesions. The disease is called multiple because classically multiple areas of bone are affected.

Multiple myeloma occurs in all countries. In the United States, 1 or 2 white people and from 2 to 4 black people in every 100,000 develop multiple myeloma each year. Multiple myeloma is rare in people under 40 years old, but the risk of developing the disease increases steadily as age increases. Some 60% of the patients are men. The incidence of multiple myeloma seems to have doubled in the last 20 years, perhaps because the disease was often overlooked in the past and not because its frequency is increasing.

Lesions. Multiple myeloma affects principally the bone marrow, though lesions can occur in other organs. The excessive production of immunoglobulin by the tumor cells nearly always causes a monoclonal hypergammaglobulinemia.

Bone Marrow. In over 95% of patients, multiple myeloma begins in the bone marrow. Even if the disease at first seems confined to some extraosseous organ, involvement of the bone marrow usually becomes evident later, though sometimes not for months or years.

By the time the diagnosis is made, much or most of the bone marrow is involved. The disease seems localized to one bone in less than 5% of the patients, and in most of these people widespread involvement of the bone marrow later becomes evident. Probably multiple myeloma begins like other tumors by neoplastic transformation of a single cell, but for many years produces no symptoms. Some people have harbored an abnormal clone of plasma cells whose only manifestation was a monoclonal excess of an immunoglobulin in the blood for more than 20 years before multiple myeloma became evident. Only when the disease is widespread do symptoms begin.

The bones normally filled with red marrow — the skull, spine, ribs, and pelvis — are affected first. Later the long bones of the limbs are involved, as the red marrow and malignant plasma cells extend into them.

The malignant plasma cells cause osteoporosis in the bones involved. They secrete an osteoclast stimulating factor and increase the production of prostaglandin E. In 90% of the patients, the rarefaction of the bones is sufficiently advanced to be demonstrable radiologically at the time of diagnosis. First the medullary trabeculae become thin, then the cortex of the bones. In most patients, the rarefaction is at first even and diffuse, involving much of the bones affected. In some, it remains so. In many, foci of more severe rarefaction develop in the bones involved, and appear roentgenologically as sharply defined, round, radiolucent lesions 1 to 2 cm across. In 15% of the patients, a bone or bones become distorted as a mass of tumor cells bulges out from the bone, limited only by a thin rim of cortical bone.

Macroscopically, the bones affected by multiple myeloma usually show diffuse or focal osteoporosis. The normal bone marrow is replaced by soft, gelatinous tumor, often likened to red currant jelly, though it may be gray rather than red. Occasionally, the bones look normal.

Microscopically, malignant plasma cells are present in the parts of the bone marrow involved. They may form clumps or sheets,

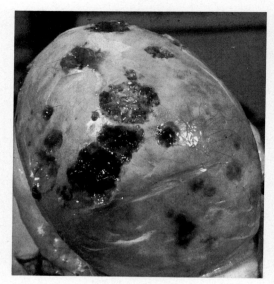

Fig. 55-16.   Multiple myeloma, showing sharply defined lesions in the skull.

which replace the marrow, or may be scattered among the normal hematopoietic cells. Usually, most of the tumor cells are well differentiated. Often tumor cells vary in size. Frequently a few atypical tumor cells are present. Binucleated or, less often, multinucleated plasma cells are sometimes found. Mitoses are unusual. Only occasionally is multiple myeloma more anaplastic, with cells like those of a poorly differentiated B-cell lymphoma.

The spheroidal masses of immunoglobulin called Russell bodies are common in multiple myeloma. They may be found in the tumor cells or free between them. They are often small, but can be bigger than a nucleus. They stain brightly with the periodic acid-Schiff reaction.

The diagnosis of multiple myeloma usually can be established by aspirating a sample of bone marrow, preferably from an area of bony rarefaction, and examining it microscopically. Often, the marrow is hypercellular, with less fat than usual. Usually, from 5 to 30% of the cells in the sample are plasma cells, which show only mild atypicality and pleomorphism, though sometimes the proportion of plasma cells is higher. Sometimes the plasma cells are grouped together in clumps or sheets. If there are not too many myeloma cells, the normal hematopoietic cells persist with little change.

Multiple myeloma is not the only condition in which plasma cells are numerous in the bone marrow. In aplastic anemia, rheumatoid arthritis, lupus erythematosus, cirrhosis of the liver, metastatic carcinoma, and other conditions, 5% or even 10% of the cells in a marrow aspirate may be plasma cells. At times, it is difficult to distinguish between multiple myeloma and a plasmacytosis caused by one of these other conditions. In a secondary plasmacytosis, the plasma cells are normal and are usually scatterred singly in the bone marrow, but in some patients with multiple myeloma the malignant plasma cells look normal and are scattered among the hematopoietic cells. If more than 20% of the cells in a marrow aspirate are plasma cells, if the plasma cells in an aspirate are in clumps or sheets, or if the plasma cells show any pleomorphism, the patient probably has multiple myeloma.

The diagnosis of multiple myeloma can be established by showing that the plasma cells in the bone marrow are a single clone. All have the same immunoglobulin in or on the tumor cells. In the non-neoplastic forms of plasmacytosis of the bone marrow, the plasma cells are polyclonal. Different plasma cells form different immunoglobulins.

Extraosseus Lesions. Extraosseous lesions usually become evident only late in the course of multiple myeloma, if at all. At autopsy, one or more extraosseous organs are infiltrated by malignant plasma cells in 70% of patients, but in most the involvement is too slight to be detected clinically. Only in 25% of the patients is the involvement of the liver sufficient to cause hepatomegaly, and only in 10% is the spleen enlarged. Involvement of the lymph nodes, kidneys, and other organs is usually discovered only by microscopy.

In 50% of patients with multiple myeloma a few atypical plasma cells are present in the blood. Only rarely, usually late in the disease, are they sufficiently numerous to justify a diagnosis of plasma cell leukemia.

Anemia develops in 90% of people with multiple myeloma, though usually only in the late stages of the disease. It is usually normochromic and normocytic, but occasionally deficiency of folate or less often of vitamin B_{12} causes a megaloblastic anemia, or there is a megaloblastic anemia that responds neither to folate nor to vitamin B_{12}. The leukocyte count is usually normal until late in the disease, when it may fall, partly because of replacement of the bone marrow by the tumor, partly because the drugs used to treat the disease depress the bone marrow. The platelet count is usually normal until late in the disease.

In most patients with multiple myeloma, the concentration of the normal immunoglobulins in the blood is low. The excess of abnormal protein produced by the tumor increases greatly the erythrocyte sedimentation rate.

Paraproteinemia. Multiple myeloma is the most common cause of paraproteinemia. In 99% of the patients, an abnormal immunoglobulin or an abnormal light chain can be detected in the plasma. The abnormal protein in the plasma is called an M component, M for myeloma.

In 99% of the patients, the tumor cells all produce the same immunoglobulin. In 50% of the patients, the abnormal immunoglobulin in the plasma is IgG; in 20%, it is IgA; in less than 2%, it is IgD. Rarely, the cells of multiple myeloma produce IgE or IgM. In 60% of the patients, the tumor cells produce both an immunoglobulin and an excess of its light chain. In 20%, only the light chain is detectable in the plasma. In 70% of people with IgG or IgA myeloma, the light chain is ϰ. In 90% of people with IgD myeloma it is λ. If only a light chain is produced, it is ϰ in 55% of patients.

In less than 1% of people with multiple myeloma, the tumor cells produce two kinds of immunoglobulin. Some patients have two clones of malignant plasma cells. One produces one type of immunoglobulin; one, the other. Within each clone, all the tumor cells produce the same immunoglobulin. In other patients, the neoplastic plasma cells produce two kinds of immunoglobulin. Nearly always, they have the same light chain. Nearly 35% of the tumors produce IgG and IgA; 25% produce IgG and IgM; 20% produce two kinds of IgG; less than 10% produce IgM and IgA; and less than 10% produce two kinds of IgM.

In many patients the immunoglobulin and light chains produced by the cells of a multiple myeloma are structurally normal or nearly so. In some patients, the immunoglobulin is able to act as an antibody. In other patients, the immunoglobulin and light chain produced by the tumor are abnormal, usually with deletion of some of the amino acids normally present.

The light chains free in the plasma in 80% of patients with multiple myeloma are small enough to escape into the urine. The light chains in the urine are known as Bence Jones protein, named after the English physician who described in 1848 its curious response when the urine is heated. Unlike the proteins usually present in the urine, which are precipitated irreversibly when the urine is heated, Bence Jones protein in the urine precipitates when the urine is heated to 50 to 60°C, but redissolves when it is heated to 90 to 100°C, only to precipitate again when the urine is cooled.

Clinical Presentation. More than 50% of patients with multiple myeloma seek medical advice because of pain in the bones, usually in the spine or ribs. The pain is usually intermittent, often affecting now one bone, now another, but can be severe. Some patients have a pathologic fracture through a lesion in a bone. Other present with some complication of the disease: renal failure; infection; compression of a nerve root or the spinal cord by a lesion in a vertebra; nausea, vomiting, and dehydration caused by hypercalcemia; some manifestation of amyloidosis; or with bruising, purpura, and epistaxis. Often there is fatigue and vague malaise. In 10% of the patients, the diagnosis is made during investigation of some unrelated condition.

Treatment and Prognosis. Because multiple myeloma advances slowly and can remain aysmptomatic for more than 20 years, treatment is often withheld until symptoms develop. Chemotherapy with melphelan, cyclophosphamide, or some other drug or combination of drugs is the principal method of treatment. Up to 70% of the patients respond, at least in part, as shown by a reduction in the quantity of immunoglobulin or light chain produced by the tumor. Some continue treatment at a lower dose during the remission. Others stop treatment and start again only if there is a relapse. Local radiotherapy is of value to control local lesions, especially the pain caused by lesions in bone.

The prognosis depends on the extent of the tumor. In 25% of the patients, there are no symptoms, there is no evidence of renal failure, and the concentration of hemoglobin in the blood is over 100 g/L (10 g/100mL). Over 75% of these people are alive two years later. In 25%, the disease is sufficient to restrict the patient's mobility, and there is either a hemoglobin concentration of less than 75 g/L (7.5 g/100 mL) or a concentration of urea in the serum of over 10 mmol/L (60 mg/100 mL). Less than 10% of these people are alive two years after diagnosis. Over 50% of the patients in whom the disease is of intermediate severity are alive two years after diagnosis.

Patients with an IgD myeloma and those in whom the tumor produces only λ light chains do badly. These forms of myeloma tend to grow rapidly. Over 50% of the patients die within a year. Patients with IgG myeloma have a somewhat more favorable prognosis than those with other forms of the disease.

Complications. As multiple myeloma extends, rarefaction of the bones increases and becomes more widespread. Pain and distortion of the bones become ever more likely. Pathologic fractures are common. The slightest blow can fracture one of the weakened bones. Collapse of one or more vertebrae sometimes passes unnoticed, but sometimes compresses one or more nerve roots, causing pain in the distribution of the nerve or nerves affected, or compresses the spinal cord, causing paraplegia or quadriplegia. In 5% of the patients, myeloma bulging from a vertebra compresses the spinal cord. Multiple fractures sometimes reduce the stature or cause severe distortion of the thorax.

Hypercalcemia and hypercalciuria are present at the time of diagnosis in 20% of the patients and develop later in many more. The concentration of phosphate and the activity of alkaline phosphatase in the plasma are usually normal. If uncontrolled, the hypercalcemia causes nausea, vomiting, dehydration, hypercalcemic encephalopathy, and death. Rehydration, sometimes with saline solution to increase the excretion of calcium is urgently needed. Prednisone usually brings a prompt fall in the concentration of calcium in the plasma. Furosemide increases its excretion. If other measures fail, mithramycin can often reduce the concentration of calcium in the plasma, probably by inhibiting the resorption of bone.

Nearly 50% of patients with multiple myeloma have renal dysfunction by the time of diagnosis. Many show the tubular injury called myeloma kidney; others have amyloidosis of the glomeruli. About 5% of the patients develop other evidence of amyloidosis, such as cardiac failure or a large tongue.

Petechiae or abnormal bleeding from the nose or gums, in the gut, or into the urine develops in many patients with multiple myeloma as the disease grows extensive. It is due in part to thrombocytopenia caused by the replacement of the bone marrow by the tumor, in part to inactivation of the coagulation factors V, VII, VIII, prothrombin, and fibrinogen by the abnormal protein in the plasma, in part by impairment of platelet function caused by the abnormal protein.

In 5% of the patients, the abnormal immunoglobulin in the blood acts as a cryoglobulin and can cause ischemia of the fingers or any other of the lesions of cryoglobulinemia. In some people, the quantity of abnormal protein produced is sufficient to cause a hyperviscosity syndrome, of the kind that complicates Waldenström's macroglobulinemia.

Hyperuricemia is particularly common when the destruction of the myeloma cells increases sharply as therapy is initiated. It is not as frequent or usually as severe as in chronic myeloid leukemia, acute lymphoid leukemia, polycythemia vera, or myelofibrosis.

Infection becomes increasingly likely and increasingly dangerous in the later stages of multiple myeloma. Pneumococcal pneumonia and infections with one of the gram-negative bacilli are especially common and often bring death.

Peripheral neuropathy like that caused by some lymphomata and carcinomata occurs in 3% of patients with multiple myeloma. Less often, a patient with multiple myeloma develops cerebellar degeneration or one of the other neurologic disorders that sometimes develop in people with malignant tumors.

About 10% of people with multiple myeloma develop a second malignant tumor. Most often, the second tumor is myeloid or monocytic leukemia. Sometimes it is a carcinoma of the breast, gut, or elsewhere. Whether multiple myeloma predisposes to the development of a second malignant tumor or whether the second tumor is caused by the carcinogenic drugs used to treat the disease is uncertain.

People with IgG myeloma tend to have a marked reduction in the production of normal immunoglobulins and are especially liable to infection. They are less likely to develop amyloidosis or hypercalcemia than are people with other types of multiple myeloma. Patients with IgA myeloma are especially likely to develop dangerous hypercalcemia and may develop the hyperviscosity syndrome because of the tendency of IgA to form polymers in the blood. Renal failure, hypercalcemia, and anemia are all common with IgD myeloma.

Paraproteinemia

The paraproteinemias are a group of conditions in which an abnormal immunoglobulin or part of an immunoglobulin circulates in the plasma. Multiple myeloma is the most prominent cause of paraproteinemia, but an abnormal immunoglobulin or one of the chains of an immunoglobulin can appear in the plasma in several of the forms of B-cell lymphoma and in other proliferations of B cells or plasma cells that are less clearly neoplastic.

Table 55-10 lists the causes of paraproteinemia. Multiple myeloma and lymphoma have already been discussed. This section considers the other causes of paraproteinemia.

WALDENSTRÖM'S MACROGLOBULINEMIA. The term *macroglobulinemia* is usually restricted to the disorders in which the plasma has a monoclonal excess of IgM, the macroglobulin that gives the condition its name. Occasionally, the term is used more vaguely to include any condition in which the concentration of IgM in the plasma is increased.

Three kinds of monoclonal macroglobulinemia can be distinguished. Some of the patients have a B-cell lymphoma. Some have

TABLE 55-10. TYPES OF PARAPROTEINEMIA

Multiple myeloma

B-cell lymphoma

Waldenström's macroglobulinemia

Heavy chain disease
  γ Heavy chain disease
  α Heavy chain disease
  μ Heavy chain disease

Light chain disease

Benign monoclonal gammopathy

Cryoglobulinemia

the IgM form of benign monoclonal gammopathy discussed later in this section. In
some, a proliferation of B cells affects principally the bone marrow. Patients with this
form of macroglobulinemia are said to have
Waldenström's macroglobulinemia, named
after the Swedish physician who described
the condition in 1944.

Whether the proliferation of B cells in
Waldenström's macroglobulinemia is neoplastic has been debated. Often the condition
is called a plasma cell dyscrasia, a term used
in medieval Latin to describe a bad mixing of
the humors and now used to imply some fault
or disease.

Patients with Waldenström's macroglobulinemia are usually over 50 years old. About
70% are men. The disease is uncommon.

Lesions. In Waldenström's macroglobulinemia, the bone marrow is highly cellular. The normal hematopoietic cells are
partly or largely replaced by a proliferation of
B cells. The replacement may be diffuse, or
nodules of the abnormal cells may be scattered in the marrow. The abnormal B cells
closely resemble those seen in the plasmacytoid form of diffuse, well-differentiated
lymphoma. Many of the abnormal cells resemble normal lymphocytes. Some are larger,
with more cytoplasm, showing various stages
of plasmacytoid differentiation. Some are
well-developed plasma cells. With them are
mixed a few larger cells, like the paraimmunoblasts of the well-differentiated, diffuse
lymphomata. Russell bodies are often present

in the abnormal cells. Normal mast cells
and basophils are often numerous in the
marrow.

The abnormal cells are a single clone. They
have IgM on their surface and in their
cytoplasm, the same IgM as is present in the
plasma.

As years pass and the disease advances, the
abnormal cells accumulate in the portal triads
in the liver in 40% of the patients in sufficient
number to cause hepatomegaly. In 40%, the
spleen is enlarged because the abnormal cells
accumulate in the white pulp. In 30%, some
lymph nodes are enlarged, because of infiltration by abnormal B cells like those in the
bone marrow. In most patients, the structure
of the lymph nodes is preserved. Diffuse replacement of a lymph node of the sort seen
in a diffuse, well-differentiated lymphoma is
unusual. Less often other organs contain accumulations of the abnormal cells.

For most of the course of Waldenström's
macroglobulinemia, no abnormal cells are
demonstrable in the blood. Only in a few
patients and only when death is near do large
numbers of abnormal B cells like those in the
bone marrow appear in the blood.

The IgM produced by the abnormal B cells
accumulates in the plasma. It gives a sharp
electrophoretic peak, called an M peak, as in
multiple myeloma. In 30% of the patients,
the abnormal cells also produce an excess of
their light chain, which escapes into the
urine as Bence Jones protein. In some
patients, the plasma contains the monomer of
IgM as well as the pentamer. Occasionally μ
heavy chains are free in the plasma, or some
other fragment of the IgM molecule is
present in the blood or urine.

Anemia develops late in the course of
Waldenström's macroglobulinemia, but can
be severe. It is due in part to inadequate
erythropoiesis, in part to hemolysis, in part
to bleeding. The leukocyte count is usually
normal. The platelet count falls late in the
course of the disease in 50% of the patients.

Clinical Presentation. Waldenström's
macroglobulinemia often persists for many
years, causing few if any symptoms. When
symptoms do begin, 50% of the patients complain of weakness and tiredness; 50% have
some form of abnormal bleeding; 20% note
loss of weight; 10% have polyneuropathy or
neurologic symptoms caused by the hyper-

viscosity syndrome; 10% have visual disturbances; less than 5% have signs of cryoglobulinemia.

Treatment and Prognosis. So long as there are no symptoms and no disability, Waldenström's macroglobulinemia needs no treatment. Once symptoms do develop, it is treated by chemotherapy, like a B-cell lymphoma.

Once symptoms develop, some patients die within a few months, as the disease becomes more aggressive. Some enjoy a remission caused by chemotherapy, but most die within two to four years of beginning treatment.

Complications. About 50% of patients with Waldenström's macroglobulinemia eventually develop symptoms caused by the excess of IgM in their blood. The large molecules of IgM increase the viscosity of the blood, making it difficult to maintain blood flow. Often, the retinal veins show alternating dilatation and constriction, like a string of sausages, sometimes with hemorrhages and exudates, sometimes with visual impairment. Changing neurologic signs from headache, dizziness and vertigo to stupor, convulsions, and coma develop. Cerebral hemorrhage sometimes follows. Some patients with the hyperviscosity syndrome become deaf because of injury to the inner ear. Sometimes the cardiac circulation is sufficiently hampered to cause heart failure, or heart failure is caused by the increase in the plasma volume caused by the excess of IgM.

The hyperviscosity syndrome can be controlled temporarily by plasmapheresis, freeing the blood of much of the excess of IgM. The IgM soon accumulates again, making it necessary to repeat the plasmapheresis every week or so.

Abnormal bleeding develops late in the disease in most patients with Waldenström's macroglobulinemia. Often the platelet count is normal, and the bleeding is due principally to the inactivation of clotting factors by the IgM and to the impairment of platelet function caused by the excess of immunoglobulin. Damage to the small vessels caused by the increased viscosity of the plasma adds to the risk. Easy bruising, petechiae, epistaxes, and bleeding from the gums, into the gut, or elsewhere are common.

In 5% of the patients, the IgM acts as a cryoglobulin. Ischemia, necrosis and other signs of cryoglobulinemia develop in the extremities.

Erosion of the bones of the sort common in multiple myeloma is unusual. In spite of the presence of light chains in the urine in 30% of the patients, renal dysfunction is uncommon. Amyloidosis can develop, but is unusual. Deposition of IgM in the wall of the gut can cause malabsorption. About 5% of the patients develop polyneuritis of unknown pathogenesis. In the late stages of Waldenström's macroglobulinemia, infection becomes increasingly probable and increasingly dangerous.

HEAVY CHAIN DISEASES. In the heavy chain diseases, a malignant or premalignant proliferation of B cells produces an excess of one of the heavy chains. Sometimes the conditions are called Franklin's disease, after the American physician who described the first case in 1963. Three kinds of heavy chain disease are distinguished, γ heavy chain disease, α heavy chain disease, and μ heavy chain disease. All are rare. In all, the heavy chains produced are smaller than normal, because of an internal deletion of some of their amino acids.

γ *Heavy Chain Disease.* Patients with γ heavy chain disease are usually over 50 years old, though the disease can develop at any age. The patients have the symptoms and signs of a lymphoma, 85% with widespread lymphadenopathy, 60% with splenomegaly, 55% with hepatomegaly, 25% with involvement of the pharyngeal lymphoid tissues, usually with edema of the uvula.

The involved lymph nodes are replaced by a diffuse, well-differentiated, plasmacytoid lymphoma. The blood shows an excess of the abnormal γ chain. In 50% of the patients, there is more than 20 g/L of the abnormal chain. In 25% of the patients, tumor cells are numerous in the blood. In 25%, anemia is severe; in 50%, neutropenia; in 50%, thrombocytopenia.

The lymphoma usually advances rapidly. Most patients die within a few months, though some have lived for five years or more.

α *Heavy Chain Disease.* α Heavy chain disease is the commonest form of heavy chain disease. It is discussed in Chapter 35 with the other causes of malabsorption.

α Heavy chain disease usually begins in

the small bowel, rarely in the respiratory tract. The patients present with malabsorption, sometimes with enlargement of the abdominal lymph nodes. At first the lamina propria of the small bowel shows a patchy infiltrate of plasma cells and lymphocytes. As months and years pass, the infiltrate extends more deeply into the wall of the intestine. The B cells become more atypical. A few immunoblasts appear in the infiltrate. The abdominal lymph nodes are replaced by a plasmacytoid B-cell lymphoma. Eventually, the lymphoma becomes a B-cell immunoblastic sarcoma, bringing death.

An excess of α heavy chains is demonstrable in the plasma and in the content of the intestine. The heavy chain is usually abnormal, with deletion of over 25% of its amino acids. In the plasma, the α heavy chain does not give a sharp peak of the kind seen in other types of monoclonal gammopathy. The α chains in the plasma are monoclonal, but circulate in varying degrees of polymerization and so give a broad peak or more than one peak.

μ *Heavy Chain Disease.* μ Heavy chain disease is the rarest of the heavy chain diseases. Most of the patients have chronic lymphoid leukemia, a diffuse, well-differentiated, plasmacytoid lymphoma, or a more anaplastic form of B-cell lymphoma. The μ chain produced in excess may be abnormal, with loss of some of its amino acids. In some of the patients, the neoplastic B cells produce a light chain as well as the heavy chain. The light chain appears in the urine, but the heavy chain does not. The course and prognosis are those of the leukemia or lymphoma.

LIGHT CHAIN DISEASE. Some use the term *light chain disease* to include all disorders in which there is excessive production of a light chain or production of an abnormal light chain. Others restrict the term to those disorders in which there is production of an abnormal light chain or of an excess of a light chain without evidence of multiple myeloma.

If an abnormal κ chain is produced, the κ chains may be deposited in the glomeruli and tubules of the kidneys, around the sinusoids in the liver, or in and around blood vessels in other parts of the body. Proteinuria is the usual manifestation, but there may be hepatomegaly or peripheral neuropathy. The deposits are usually small and irregularly distributed. They stain strongly with the periodic acid-Schiff reaction and with the immunofluorescent stain for κ chains. By electron microscopy, they are electron dense and granular and contain arrays of parallel fibrils 11 to 14 nm in diameter. The κ chains can be deposited even though there is no evidence of the abnormal κ chain in the blood or in the urine.

Occasionally, a heavy chain is present in the deposits as well as the κ chains. Rarely, similar lesions have been found in people with an excess of λ chains.

All patients with light chain disease have an abnormal, monoclonal proliferation of plasma cells. Most have multiple myeloma. In some the proliferation is less extensive and less aggressive.

BENIGN MONOCLONAL GAMMOPATHY. In benign monoclonal gammopathy, also called benign monoclonal hypergammaglobulinemia and benign monoclonal paraproteinemia, the patients have in the plasma a monoclonal excess of an immunoglobulin, though they show no evidence of multiple myeloma, lymphoma, or any other kind of proliferation of plasma cells or of B cells. Benign monoclonal gammopathy is common. As age increases, it grows more common. A monoclonal excess of an immunoglobulin can be detected in the plasma of 1% of people over 25 years old and in 3% of people over 70 years old.

The abnormal immunoglobulin in the blood is IgG in 85% of the patients and IgA or IgM in most of the rest. Free light chains are rarely found. The quantity of the abnormal protein in the plasma is rarely more than 30 g/L (3 g/100 mL), in contrast to the large quantities of abnormal immunoglobulin often present in the plasma of people with multiple myeloma.

The bone marrow is normal in 30% of the patients. In the rest, it shows a slight increase in the number of plasma cells, rarely to more than 10% of the marrow cells. The plasma cells appear normal.

The abnormal immunoglobulin persists in the blood with no change in nature or concentration for years, sometimes for the rest of the patient's life. Less than 5% of the patients eventually develop multiple myeloma or some form of B-cell lymphoma.

Presumably, the patients have somewhere in the body a clone of abnormal plasma cells, which produce the abnormal immunoglobulin. It is not known why the abnormal clone develops nor why it so rarely progresses to a more dangerous form of B-cell proliferation. Many of the patients have chronic infections, carcinoma or some other malignant tumor, one of the collagen diseases, liver disease, or some other serious illness. Whether these conditions initiate the proliferation of the abnormal clone of plasma cells or whether benign monoclonal gammopathy is discovered in these patients only because they are more likely to have an electrophoretic analysis of their plasma is uncertain.

CRYOGLOBULINEMIA. Cryoglobulins are proteins that circulate in the plasma, precipitate when the plasma is cooled, and redissolve when the plasma is rewarmed. Most cryoglobulins are immunoglobulins, though occasionally fibrinogen or some other plasma protein can be precipitated by cold in this way. Three kinds of cryoglobulinemia are distinguished.

Types. In 30% of the patients, the cryoglobulin is a monoclonal excess of an immunoglobulin. The immunoglobulin is IgG in 50% of the patients, IgM in 40%, IgA in 10%. Rarely, a light chain acts as a cryoglobulin.

In 20% of the patients, the cryoglobulin is an immune complex in which a monoclonal proliferation of an immunoglobulin acts as an antibody against one or more of the normal, polyclonal immunoglobulins present in the plasma. In 90% of these people, the monoclonal immunoglobulin is IgM, and it binds polyclonal IgG to form the complexes. In 5%, monoclonal IgM binds both polyclonal IgG and polyclonal IgA. In 5%, monoclonal IgG binds polyclonal IgG.

In 50% of the patients, the cryoglobulin is an immune complex in which a polyclonal immunoglobulin acts as an antibody against one or more of the other polyclonal immunoglobulins present in the plasma. In 90% of these people, polyclonal IgM binds polyclonal IgG to form the complexes. In 10%, polyclonal IgM binds both polyclonal IgG and polyclonal IgA. Occasionally, polyclonal IgA binds polyclonal IgG.

Lesions. Patients in whom a monoclonal immunoglobulin acts alone as a cryoglobulin usually have multiple myeloma if the immunoglobulin is IgG or IgA and Waldenström's macroglobulinemia if it is IgM. Occasionally a patient has a B-cell lymphoma. Sometimes the origin of the abnormal immunoglobulin is not apparent. Such people are said to have essential monoclonal cryoglobulinemia.

About 50% of the people in whom a monoclonal immunoglobulin acts as an antibody binding one or more of the normal polyclonal immunoglobulins in the plasma have multiple myeloma, lymphoma, macroglobulinemia, or some other form of B-cell proliferation. Some have hepatitis, a collagen disease, or some other illness. In some, said to have essential mixed cryoglobulinemia, the cause of the cryoglobulinemia is not apparent.

About 50% of the people in whom the cryoglobulin is a complex of two or more polyclonal immunoglobulins have some form of collagen disease. In others, the cryoglobulinemia seems secondary to viral, bacterial, fungal, or parasitic infection. In some, it is secondary to cirrhosis of the liver or hepatitis. Occasionally this form of cryoglobulinemia is familial. When it has no obvious cause, the patients are also said to have essential mixed cryoglobulinemia.

Clinical Presentation. About 50% of people in whom a single monoclonal immunoglobulin acts as a cryoglobulin have no symptoms and suffer no disability. When symptoms do develop, they are usually caused by the precipitation of the cryoglobulin in the dermal blood vessels when the skin is cooled. Raynaud's phenomenon develops in 40% of the patients. About 40% suffer necrosis of the tip of the nose, the tips of the fingers or toes, or the ears. In 15% the extremities easily become cyanotic when cooled. In 15%, purpura develops in the skin. Less than 10% suffer a chronic ulcer above the malleoli at the ankle. About 25% of the patients develop renal lesions of the sort described in Chapter 27. The glomerular capillaries are clogged with cryoglobulin, or a type I membranoproliferative glomerulonephritis caused by subendothelial deposits of cryoglobulin develops. Peripheral neuritis develops in 15% of the patients. There may be bleeding from the nose, lungs, or gut. Rarely, there is thrombosis of a major artery.

Patients with one of the forms of mixed cryoglobulinemia, in which the cryoglobulin is an immune complex, all develop purpura in the skin at some time during the disease. Biopsy shows the bleeding to be due to vasculitis caused by the precipitation of the cryoglobulin in small vessels in the dermis. In many of the patients, IgM, IgG, and complement can be demonstrated in the lesions. Raynaud's phenomenon is evident in 25% of the patients. Arthralgia and stiffening develop in the hands, knees, or ankles when the limbs are exposed to cold in over 60% of the patients. Over 30% develop ulcers above the malleoli at the ankles. Hepatomegaly is evident in 70% of the patients, though apart from increased activity of alkaline phosphatase in the plasma there is usually little hepatic dysfunction except in people in whom the cryoglobulinemia is caused by liver disease. The spleen is enlarged in 60% of the patients. Over 50% develop renal disease, azotemia, edema, or hypertension. Microscopically, the kidneys usually show a type I membranoproliferative glomerulonephritis, with deposits of cyroglobulin subendothelially and in the mesangia. Less often, there is a membranous glomerulonephritis, or the glomerular capillaries become clogged with cryoglobulin. Vasculitis is often present in small vessels in the kidneys and may be evident in other organs.

Treatment. The major factor in the treatment of cryoglobulinemia is to keep the skin warm. If the temperature of the blood does not fall, cryoglobulins do not precipitate. Treatment of the disease causing the production of the abnormal immunoglobulin ameliorates the condition. Especially when a single monoclonal immunoglobulin acts as a cryoglobulin, plasmapheresis to reduce the quantity of cryoglobulin in the plasma is helpful.

Other Lymphoproliferative Disorders

Other lymphoproliferative disorders of neoplastic or preneoplastic character are discussed with the diseases of the organ they principally affect, microgliomatosis with the diseases of the brain, lymphogranulomatosis with the diseases of the lungs, reticulum cell sarcoma of bone with the diseases of bone, and so on. Only angioimmunoblastic lymphadenopathy will be discussed here.

ANGIOIMMUNOBLASTIC LYMPHADENOPATHY. Angioimmunoblastic lymphadenopathy is an

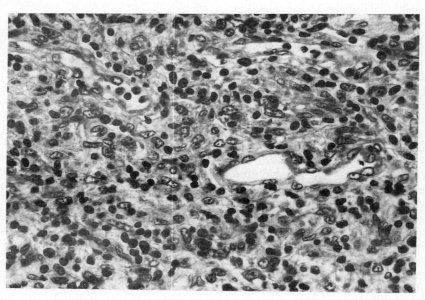

Fig. 55-17. Angioimmunoblastic lymphadenopathy, showing the proliferation of vessels and the immunoblasts lying among the smaller lymphocytes and plasma cells.

uncommon condition found most often in people 40 to 60 years old. It causes widespread enlargement of the lymph nodes, enlargement of the liver and spleen, often fever and malaise, and loss of weight. Most patients have polyclonal hypergammaglobulinemia. Often there is lymphopenia. Some develop hemolytic anemia. Some have an erythematous, maculopapular rash in the skin.

The structure of the involved lymph nodes is distorted. Branching postcapillary venules with thick endothelium and thick basement membranes are numerous and prominent. Throughout the lymph node, clumps of immunoblasts are mixed with plasma cells and lymphocytes. Some of the immunoblasts are multinucleated. Macrophages are sometimes scattered throughout the lymph node or sometimes form clumps. Eosinophils are present in 30% of the patients. A homogeneous, eosinophilic material that stains with the periodic acid-Schiff reaction is present between the cells. Sometimes it is so extensive that the lymph node looks hypocellular. Electron microscopy shows that the homogeneous material consists of debris from dead cells. A similar proliferation of abnormal cells is present in the bone marrow in 70% of the patients.

The cellular proliferation in angioimmunoblastic lymphadenopathy is predominantly of B cells. It is a polyclonal proliferation, not a monoclonal proliferation of the sort seen in B-cell lymphomata.

The prognosis is bad. Less than 50% of the patients live for 18 months, though some do survive several years. Death usually comes from infection. In 10% of the patients, the condition progresses to an immunoblastic sarcoma.

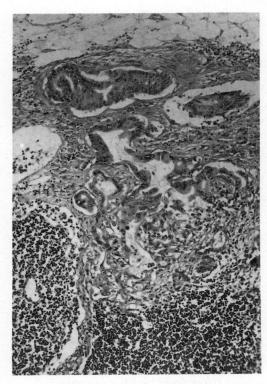

Fig. 55-18. Metastatic adenocarcinoma extending into a lymph node from its peripheral sinus.

nodes in the lymph. Most begin in a peripheral sinus. The lymphatics enter the convexity of the lymph node and discharge their lymph into the peripheral sinus. Once established, the metastasis grows and commonly replaces much or all the lymph node. It may penetrate the capsule of the node and invade the surrounding tissues. It can give rise to further emboli that are carried in the lymph or blood to more distant sites.

Secondary Tumors

Secondary tumors of the lymph nodes are more common than are primary tumors. Most carcinomata, malignant melanoma, and tumors of the ovaries and testes commonly spread to the lymph nodes. Neuroblastomata often involve the lymph nodes, and sometimes a sarcoma does so.

Almost all metastases in lymph nodes are caused by emboli of tumor cells carried to the

BIBLIOGRAPHY

General

Bagby, G. C. (Ed.): Hematological aspects of systemic disease. Hematol. Oncol. Clin. North Am., 1:167, 1987.
Frisch, B., Lewis. S. M., Burkhardt, R., and Bartl, R.: Biopsy Pathology of Bone and Bone Marrow. London, Chapman and Hall, 1985.
Hardisty, R. M., and Weatherall, D. J.: Blood and its Disorders. 2nd Ed. Oxford, Blackwell, 1982.

Jandl, J. H.: Blood. Boston, Little, Brown and Co., 1987.

Robb-Smith, A. H. T., and Taylor, C. R.: Lymph Node Biopsy. New York, Oxford University Press, 1981.

Stansfeld, A. G. (Ed.): Lymph Node Biopsy Interpretation. Edinburgh, Churchill Livingstone, 1985.

Wickramasinghe, S. N. (Ed.): Blood and Bone Marrow. In Systemic Pathology, 3rd Ed. Edited by W. St. C Symmers. London, Churchill Livingstone, 1986.

Williams, W. J., Beutler, E., Erslav, A. J., and Lichtman, M. A.: Hematology. 3rd Ed. New York, McGraw-Hill, 1983.

Wintrobe, M. M., et al.: Clinical Hematology. 8th Ed. Philadelphia, Lea & Febiger, 1981.

Wittels, B.: Surgical Pathology of Bone Marrow. Philadelphia, W. B. Saunders, 1985.

Wright, D. M., and Isaacson, P. G.: Biopsy Pathology of the Lymphoreticular System. London, Chapman and Hall, 1983.

Zucker-Franklin, D., Greaves, M. F., Grossi, C. E., and Marmont, A. M.: Atlas of Blood Cells. 2nd Ed. Philadelphia, Lea & Febiger, 1988.

Lymphadenitis

Strickler, J. G., Warnke, R. A., and Weiss, L. M.: Necrosis in lymph nodes. Pathol. Annu., 22(2):253, 1987.

Hyperplastic Lymphadenopathy

Baden, E., Caverivière, P., and Carbonnel, S.: Sinus histiocytosis with massive lymphadenopathy (Destombes-Rosai-Dorfman syndrome) occurring in a single submandibular node. Oral Surg., 64:320, 1987.

Basset, F., Nezelof, C., and Ferrans V. J.: The histiocytoses. Pathol. Annu., 18(2):27, 1983.

Headington, J. T., Roth, M. S., and Schnitzer, B.: Regressing atypical histiocytosis. Semin. Diagn. Pathol., 4:28, 1987.

Isaacson. P. G., and Wright, D. H.: Histiocytic disorders in lymphoreticular pathology. Rec. Adv. Histopathol., 12:197, 1984.

Levine, A. M., Gill, P. S., and Rasheed, S.: Human retrovirus-associated lymphoproliferative disorders in homosexual men. Prog. Allergy, 37:244, 1986.

List, A. F., Greco, F. A., and Volger, L. B.: Lymphoproliferative diseases in immunocompromized hosts: the role of the Epstein-Barr virus. J. Clin. Oncol., 5:1673, 1987.

Tumors

Aghai, E.: Hodgkin's disease. Leuk. Res., 10:1267, 1986.

Alderson, M.: The epidemiology of leukemia. Adv. Cancer Res., 31:2, 1980.

American Cancer Society Symposium: Staging in Hodgkin's disease. Cancer Res., 31:1707, 1971.

Antin, J. H., and Rosenthal, D. S.: Acute leukemias, myelodysplasia, and lymphomas. Clin. Geriatr. Med., 1:795, 1985.

Azevedo, S. J., and Yunis, A. A.: Angioimmunoblastic lymphadenopathy. Am. J. Hematol., 20:301, 1985.

Bacsky, P.: Hodgkin's disease. The Sternberg-Reed cell. Blut, 55:413, 1987.

Batsakis, J. G., and Manning, J. T.: Soft tissue tumors. Otolaryngol. Clin. North Am., 19:659, 1986.

Berard, C. W., Dorfman, R. F., and Kaufman, N. (Eds.): Malignant lymphoma. Monogr. Pathol., 29:1, 1987.

Bonn, J. M., and Garcia, J. H.: Primary malignant non-Hodgkin's lymphoma of the central nervous sytem. Pathol. Annu., 22(1):353, 1987.

Brandt, L.: Environmental factors and leukaemia. Med. Oncol. Tumor Pharmacother., 2:7, 1985.

Brandt, L.: Leukaemia and lymphoma risks derived from solvents. Med. Oncol. Tumor Pharmacother., 4:199, 1987.

Brunning, R. D., and McKenna, R. W.: Immunologic markers for acute leukemia. Monogr. Pathol., 29:124, 1987.

Brusamolino, E., Pagnucco, G., and Bernasconi, C.: Acute leukemia occurring in a primary neoplasia (secondary leukemia). Haematologica, 71:60, 1986.

Burke, J. S.: Histological criteria for distinguishing between benign and malignant extranodal lymphoid exudates. Semin. Diagn. Pathol., 2:152, 1985.

Burke, J. S.: Malignant lymphomas of the skin. Semin. Diagn. Pathol., 2:169, 1985.

Butturini, A., Sthivelman, E., Canaani, E., and Gale, R. P.: Oncogenes in human leukemias. Acta Haematologica, 78(Suppl 1):2, 1987.

Butturini, A., and Gale, R. P.: Oncogenes and human leukemias. Int. J. Cell Cloning, 6:2, 1988.

Cacciola, E. (Ed.): Hemato-oncology and hemato-immunology. Acta Haematol., 78(Suppl 1):1, 1987.

Carvalli, G., et al.: Chronic lymphocytic leukemia (B cell) in the course of polycythemia vera. Tumori, 73:639, 1987.

Catovsky, D. (Ed.): The Leukemic Cell. Edinburgh, Churchill Livingstone, 1981.

Catovsky, D., Linch, D. C., and Beverley, P. C. L.: T cell disorders in haematological diseases. Clin. Haematol., 11:661, 1982.

Chaganti, R. S. K.: Significance of chromosome change to hematopoietic neoplasms. Blood, 62:515, 1983.

Chaganti, R. S.: Cytogenetics of leukemia and lymphoma. Monogr. Pathol., 29:184, 1987.

Champlin, R., Gale, R. P., Foon, K. A., and Golde, D. W.: Chronic leukemias: oncogenes, chromosomes, and advances in therapy. Ann. Intern. Med., 104:671, 1986.

Chan, J. K. C., Ng, C. S., and Hui, P. K.: A simple guide to the terminology and application of leucocyte monoclonal antibodies. Histopathology, 12:461, 1988.

Chan, W. C., and Winton, E. F., and Waldmannm T. A.: Lymphocytosis of large granular lymphocytes. Arch. Intern. Med., 146:1201, 1986.

Chan, W. C., and Zaatari, G.: Lymph node interdigitating reticulum cell sarcoma. Am. J. Clin. Pathol., 85:739, 1986.

Clendenning, W. E.: Perpectives on cutaneous T cell lymphoma. Clin. Exp. Dermatol., 11:109. 1986.

Cohen, H. J.: Monoclonal gammopathies and aging. Hosp. Pract., 23(3A):75, 1988.

Colby, T. V., and Carrington, C. B.: Lymphoreticular tumors and infiltrates of the lung. Pathol. Annu., 18(1):27, 1983.

Cooper, B. T., and Read, A. E.: Small intestinal lymphoma. World J. Surg., 9:930, 1985.

Cooper, B. T., and Read, A. E.: Coeliac disease and lymphoma. Q. J. Med., 63:269, 1987.

Corley, R. B., Dexter, C. M., and Ovnic, M.: Inducible lymphokines of T cell tumors. CRC. Crit. Rev. Immunol., 6:71, 1986.

Cossman, J.: T-cell neoplasms and Hodgkin's disease. Monogr. Pathol., 29:104, 1987.

Cossman, J., et al.: Molecular genetics and the diagnosis of lymphoma. Arch. Pathol. Lab. Med., 112:117, 1988.

Croce, C. M.: Chromosomal translocations, oncogenes, and B-cell tumors. Hosp. Pract., 20(1):41, 1985.

Croce, C. M., and Nowell, P. C.: Molecular genetics of human B cell neoplasia. Adv. Immunol., 38:245, 1986.

Dabbs, D. J., Morel-Maroger Striker, L., Mignon, F., and Striker, G.: Glomerular lesions in lymphomas and leukemias. Am. J. Med., 80:63, 1986.

Dalla-Favera, R., et al.: Mechanism of activation and biological role of the c-myc oncogene in B-cell lymphomagenesis. Ann. N. Y. Acad. Sci., 511:207, 1987.

DeVita, V. T.: Non-Hodgkin's lymphomas. Hosp. Pract., 21(9):103, 1986.

De Vita, V. T., Jr., et al.: The lymphomas: biologic implications of therapy and therapeutic implications of the new biology. Monogr. Pathol., 29:249, 1987.

Doll, D. C., and Weiss, R. B.: Malignant lymphoma of the testis. Am. J. Med., 8:515, 1986.

Drexler, H. G., Amlot, P. L., and Minowada, J.: Hodgkin's disease—derived cell lines—conflicting clues for the origin of Hodgkin's disease. Leukemia, 1:629, 1987.

Edelson, R. L.: Cutaneous T cell lymphoma. J. Dermatol., 14:397, 1987.

Ernberg, I.: The role of Epstein-Barr virus in lymphomas of homosexual males. Prog. Allergy, 37:301, 1986.

Farhangi, M. (Ed.): Plasma cell myeloma and the myeloma proteins. Semin. Oncol., 13:259, 1986.

Favara, B. E., et al.: The leukemias of childhood. Perspect. Pediatr. Pathol., 9:75, 1987.

Fong, C.-t., and Brodeur, G. M.: Downs's syndrome and leukemia. Cancer Genet. Cytogenet., 28:55, 1987.

Foon, K. A., and Todd, R. F. III: Immunologic classification of leukemia and lymphoma. Blood, 68:1, 1986.

Freedman, A. S., and Nadler, L. M.: Cell surface markers in hematologic malignancies. Semin. Oncol., 14:193, 1987.

Freireich, E. J.: Adult acute leukemia. Hosp. Pract., 21(6):91, 1986.

Gale, R. P. (Ed.): Acute leukemias. Semin. Hematol., 24:1, 1987.

Gale, R. P. (Ed.): Chronic lymphocytic leukemia. Semin. Hematol., 24:209, 1987.

Galton, D. A., and Brito-Babapulle, F.: The management of myelomatosis. Eur. J. Haematol., 39:385, 1987.

Godal, T., and Funderund, S.: Human B-cell neoplasia in relation to normal B-cell differentiation and maturation processes. Adv. Cancer Res., 36:211, 1982.

Golomb, H. M.: Hairy cell leukemia. Adv. Intern. Med., 29:245, 1984.

Greaves, M. F.: Speculations on the cause of chilhood acute leukemia. Leukemia, 2:120, 1988.

Gregson, N. A., and Liebowitz, S.: IgM paraproteinaemia, polyneuropathy and myelin-associated glycoprotein (MAG). Neuropathol. Appl. Neurobiol., 11:329, 1985.

Gunz, F. W., and Henderson, E. S. (Eds.): Leukemia. 4th Ed. New York, Grune and Stratton, 1983.

Gutensohn, N., and Cole, P.: Epidemiology of Hodgkin's disease. Semin. Oncol., 7:92, 1980.

Hamblin, T. J.: Chronic lymphatic leukaemia. Baillière's Clin. Haematol., 1:449, 1987.

Hansen, O. P., and Galton, D. A. G.: Classification and prognostic variables in myelomatosis. Scand. J. Haematol., 35:10, 1985.

Harris, H.: The genetic analysis of malignancy. J. Cell Biol., Suppl 4:431, 1986.

Harris, N. L.: Lymphoma 1987. An interim approach to diagnosis and classification. Pathol. Annu., 22(2):1, 1987.

Heim, S., and Mitelman, F.: Cancer Cytogenetics. New York, Alan R. Liss, 1987.

Hoogstraten, B. (Ed.): Hematologic malignancies. Berlin, Springer-Verlag, 1985.

Hoppe, R. T.: The non-Hodgkin's lymphomas: pathology, staging, treatment. Curr. Probl. Cancer, 11:363, 1987.

Howard, D. R.: Hodgkin's disease: pathology and pathogenesis. CRC Crit. Rev. Clin. Lab. Sci., 14:109, 1981.

Isaacson, P. G., and Wright, D. H.: Histiocytic disorders in lymphoreticular pathology. Rec. Adv. Histopathol., 12:197, 1984.

Ishak, K. G., and Zimmerman, H. J.: Hepatic toxicity of drugs used for hematologic neoplasia. Semin. Liver Dis., 7:237, 1987.

Jaffe, E. S.: Relationship of classification to biologic behavior of non-Hodgkin's lymphomas. Semin. Oncol., 13(4 Suppl 5):3, 1986.

Jaffe, E. S.: Malignant lymphomas: pathology of hepatic involvement. Semin. Liver Dis., 7:257, 1987.

Jaffe, E. S., et al.: The pathologic spectrum of adult T-cell leukemia/lymphoma in the United States. Am. J. Surg. Pathol., 8:263, 1984.

Jansen, J.: Hairy cell leukemia. CRC Crit. Rev. Oncol. Hematol., 7:183, 1987.

Jones, D. B.: The histogenesis of the Reed-Sternberg cell and its mononuclear counterparts. J. Pathol., 151:191, 1987.

Jones, J. F., and Straus, S. E.: Chronic Epstein-Barr virus infection. Annu. Rev. Med., 38:195, 1987.

Kamps, W. A., and Humphrey, G. B.: Heterogenicity of childhood acute lymphoblastic leukemia. Semin. Oncol., 12:268, 1985.

Kaplan, H. S.: Hodgkin's Disease. 2nd Ed. Cambridge, Harvard University Press, 1980.

Kebler, R., Kithier, K., and McDonald, F. D., and Cadnapaphornchai, P.: Rapidly progressive glomerulonephritis and monoclonal gammopathy. Am. J. Med., 78:133, 1985.

Kelly, J. J., Jr.: Peripheral neuropathies associated with monoclonal proteins. Muscle Nerve, 8:138, 1985.

Klein, G.: Chromosomal translocations in B-cell derived tumors. Prog. Clin. Biol. Res., 246:75, 1987.

Knowles, D. M., II: The human T-cell leukemias: cytomorphologic, immunophenotypic, and genotypic characteristics. Hum. Pathol., 17:14, 1986.

Konopka, J. B., and Witte, O. N.: Activation of the abl oncogene in murine and human leukemias. Biochim. Biophys. Acta, 823:1, 1985.

Korsmeyer, S. J.: Antigenic receptor genes as molecular markers of lymphoid neoplasms. J. Clin. Invest., 79:1291, 1987.

Korsmeyer, S. J.: B-lymphoid neoplasms: immunoglobulin genes as molecular determinants of clonality, lineage, differentiation and translocation. Adv. Intern. Med., 33:1, 1988.

Kosmo, M. A., and Gale, R. P.: Plamsa cell leukemia. Semin. Hematol., 24:202, 1987.

Krikorian, J. G., Portlock, C. S., and Mauch, P. M.: Hodgkin's disease presenting below the diaphragm. J. Clin. Oncol., 4:1551, 1986.

Kyle, R. A.: Diagnosis and management of multiple myeloma and related disorders. Prog. Hematol., 14:257, 1986.

Kyle, R. A.: Monoclonal gammopathy and multiple myeloma in the elderly. Baillière's Clin. Haematol., 1:533, 1987.

Langman, A. W., and Kaplan, M. J.: Hodgkin's disease and tonsilectomy. Otolaryngol. Clin. North Am., 20:399, 1987.

Lawler, S. D.: Significance of chromosome abnormalities in leukemia. Semin. Hematol., 19:257, 1982.

Le Beau, M. M.: Chromosomal fragile sites and cancer-specific rearrangements. Blood, 67:849, 1986.

Le Beau, M. M., and Rowley, J. D.: Chromosomal abnormalities in leukemia and lymphoma. Adv. Hum. Genet., 15:1, 1986.

Lee, F. D.: Hodgkin's disease. Histopathology, 11:1211, 1987.

Lembersky, B. C., and Golomb, H. M.: Hairy cell leukemia. Cancer Metastasis Rev., 6:283, 1987.

Lennert, K.: Malignant Lymphomas. Berlin, Springer-Verlag, 1978.

Lennert, K.: Histopathology of Non-Hodgkin's Lymphoma. Berlin, Springer-Verlag, 1981.

Lenoir, G. M., O'Connor, G. T., and Olweny, C. L. M. (Eds.): Burkitt's lymphoma. Lyon, I. A. R. C. Sci. Publ. 60, 1985.

Levine, A. M.: Non-Hodgkin's lymphoma and other malignancies in the acquired immune deficiency syndrome. Semin. Oncol., 14(2 Suppl 3):34–9, 1987.

Levine, A. M., Gill, P. S., and Rasheed, S.: Human retrovirus-associated lymphoproliferative disorders in homosexual men. Prog. Allergy, 37:244, 1986.

List, A. F., Greco, F. A., and Volger, L. B.: Lymphoproliferative diseases in immunocompromized hosts: the role of the Epstein-Barr virus. J. Clin. Oncol., 5:1673, 1987.

Lukes, R. J., and Collins, R. D.: Immunologic charac-

terization of human malignant lymphomas. Cancer, 34:1488, 1974.

Luzzatto, L., and Foroni, L.: DNA rearrangements of cell lineage specific genes in lymphoproliferative disorders. Prog. Hematol., 14:303, 1986.

McCoy, E. E., and Epstein, C. J. (Eds.): Oncology and immunology of Down syndrome. Prog. Clin. Biol. Res., 246:1, 1987.

McCulloch, E. A.: Normal stem cells and the clonal hemopathies. Prog. Clin. Biol. Res., 184:21, 1985.

McElwain, T. J., and Lister, T. A. (Eds.): The lymphomas. Baillière's Clin. Haematol., 1:1, 1987.

Magrath, I. T.: Malignant non-Hodgkin's lymphoma in children. Clin. Hematol. Oncol. North Am., 1:577, 1987.

Matis, L. A., Young, R. C., and Longo, D. L.: Nodular lymphomas. CRC Crit. Rev. Oncol. Hematol., 5:171, 1986.

Meier, C.: Polyneuropathy in paraproteinemia. J. Neurol., 232:204, 1985.

Mellstedt, H., Holm, G., and Björkholm, M.: Multiple myeloma, Waldenström's macroglobulinemia, and benign monoclonal gammopathy. Adv. Cancer Res., 41:257, 1984.

Miedema, F., and Melief, C. J.: Immunobiology of the expanded T cells in T cell leukemia and T-gamma lymphocytosis. Leuk. Res., 10:469, 1986.

Miller, D. R.: Clinical and biological features of childhood acute lymphoblastic leukemia. Clin. Pediatr., 26:623, 1987.

Miller, R. W.: Recent advances in the epidemiology of leukemia and lymphoma. Monogr. Pathol., 29:81, 1987.

Modan, B.: Cancer and leukaemia risks after low-level radiation. Med. Oncol. Tumor Pharmother., 4:151, 1987.

Mole, R. H.: Leukaemia induction in man by radionuclides and some relevant experimental and human observations. Strahlentherapie Sonderbund, 80:1, 1986.

Montserrat, E., and Rozman, C.: Bone marrow biopsy in chronic lymphocytic leukemia. Blood Cells, 12:315, 1987.

Mueller, N.: Epidemiologic studies assessing the role of the Epstein-Barr virus in Hodgkin's disease. Yale J. Biol. Med., 60:321, 1987.

Murphy, G. F.: Cutaneous T cell lymphoma. Adv. Pathol., 1:131, 1988.

Najean, Y.: The iatrogenic leukaemias induced by radio- and/or chemotherapy. Med. Oncol. Tumor Pharmacother., 4:245, 1987.

Nathwani, B. N.: Classifying non-Hodgkin's lymphomas. Monogr. Pathol., 29:18, 1987.

Netzel, B., Haas, R. I., amd Thierfelder, S.: Allogenic bone marrow transplantation in leukemia. Rec. Res. Cancer Res., 93:290, 1984.

Ng, J. P., et al.: Primary splenic hairy cell leukaemia. Eur. J. Haematol., 39:349, 1987.

Norton, A. J., and Isaacson, P. G.: The diagnosis of malignant lymphoma using monoclonal antibodies reactive in routinely fixed wax embedded tissue. J. Pathol., 151:183, 1987.

Notter, D. T., Grossman, P. L., Rosenberg, S. A., and Remington, J. S.: Infection in patients with Hodgkin's disease. Rev. Infect. Dis., 2:761, 1980.

O'Brien, C., Lampert, I. A., and Catovsky, D.: The histopathology of adult T-cell lymphoma/leukemia in blacks from the Caribbean. Histopathology, 7:349, 1983.

O'Connor, N. T.: Genotypic analysis of lymph node biopsies. J. Pathol., 151:185, 1987.

Ochs, H. D., and Wedgwood, R. J.: IgG subclass deficiencies. Annu. Rev. Med., 38:325, 1987.

Oertel, J. E., and Heffess, C. S.: Lymphoma of the thyroid and related disorders. Semin. Oncol., 14:333, 1987.

Osserman, E. F., Merlini, G., and Butler, V. P., Jr.: Multiple myeloma and related plasma cell dyscrasias. J. Am. Med. Assoc., 258:2930, 1987.

Pandolfi, F.: T-CLL and allied diseases: new insights into classification and pathogenesis. Diagn. Immunol., 4:61, 1986.

Papas, T. S., et al.: The cellular ets genes. Cancer Invest., 4:555, 1986.

Patterson, S. D.: Immunologic techniques in the evaluation of lymphoma. Ultrastruct. Pathol., 9:195, 1985.

Pick, A. I. (Ed.): Plasma cell dyscrasias. Acta Haematol., 68:167, 1982.

Piette, W. W.: Myeloma, paraproteinemias, and the skin. Med. Clin. North Am., 70:155, 1986.

Plesner, T., Wilken, M., and Avnstr M. S.: The contribution of immunologic methods to the classification of leukemias and malignant lymphomas. Clin. Lab. Med., 2:579, 1982.

Purtilo, D. T.: Immunopathology of infectious mononucleosis and other complications of Epstein-Barr virus infections. Pathol. Annu., 15(1):253, 1980.

Purtilo, D. T., et al.: Epstein-Barr virus as an etiological agent in the pathogenesis of lymphoproliferative and aproliferative disorders in immune deficient patients. Int. Rev. Exp. Pathol., 27:113, 1985.

Ramsay, A. D., et al.: T-cell lymphomas in adults. J. Pathol., 152:63, 1987.

Rappaport, H.: Tumors of the Hemopoietic System. Washington D. C., Armed Forces Institute of Pathology, 1966.

Raskind, W. H., and Fialkow, P. J.: The use of cell markers in the study of human hematopoietic neoplasia. Adv. Cancer Res., 49:127, 1987.

Ratner, L., et al.: Mechanism of leukemogenesis by human T-cell leukemia virus types I and II. Cancer Detect. Prev., 10:411, 1987.

Reynolds, C. W.: Large granular lymphocyte lymphoproliferative diseases: natural cytotoxic tumors in man and experimental animals. CRC Crit. Rev. Oncol. Hematol., 2:185, 1985.

Richards, M. A.: Lymphoma of the colon and rectum. Postgrad. Med. J., 62:615, 1986.

Rimm, I. J., et al.: Brain tumors after cranial irradiation for childhood acute lymphoblastic leukemia. Cancer, 59:1506, 1987.

Rosenberg, S. A., and Kaplan, H. S. (Eds.): Malignant Lymphomas. New York, Academic Press, 1982.

Rowland, K. M., Jr., and Murthy, A.: Hodgkin's disease: long term effects of therapy. Med. Pediatr. Oncol. 14:88, 1986.

Rowley, J. D.: Biological implications of consistent chromosome rearrangements in leukemia and lymphoma. Cancer Res., 44:3159, 1984.

Rowley, J. D., and Testa J. R.: Chromosome abnormalities in malignant hematological diseases. Adv. Cancer Res., 36:103, 1982.

Sandberg, A. A.: Application of cytogenetics in neoplastic diseases. CRC Crit. Rev. Clin. Lab. Sci., 22:219, 1985.

Sandberg, A. A., et al.: Chromosomes and the causation of human cancer and leukemia. Cancer Genet. Cytogenet., 7:95, 1982.

Sandler, D. P., and Collman, G. W.: Cytogenetic and environmental factors in the etiology of the acute leukemias in adults. Am. J. Epidemiol., 126:1017, 1987.

Savitz, D. A., and Calle, E. E.: Leukemia and occupational exposure to electromagnetic fields. J. Occup. Med., 29:47, 1987.

Schaadt, M., et al.: The cell of origin in Hodgkin's disease. Int. Rev. Exp. pathol., 27:185, 1985.

Sharma, S., Mehta, S. R., and Ford, R. J.: Growth factor, viruses and oncogenes in human lymphoid neoplasia. Lymphokine Res., 6:245, 1987.

Shaw, G. M., Broder, S., Essex, M., and Gallo, R. C.: Human T cell leukemia virus. Adv. Intern. Med., 30:1, 1985.

Sherr, C. J., and Look, A. T.: Cytogenetics of leukemia and lymphoma. Monogr. Pathol., 29:225, 1987.

Showe, L. C., and Croce, C. M.: The role of chromosome translocations in B- and T-cell neoplasia. Annu. Rev. Immunol., 5:253, 1987.

Silva, F. G., Pirani, C. L., Mesa-Tejada, R., and Williams, G. S.: The kidney in plasma cell dyscrasias. Prog. Surg. Pathol., 5:131, 1983.

Slater, D. N.: Lymphoproliferative conditions of the skin. Rec. Adv. Histopathol., 12:83, 1984.

Slater, D. N.: Recent developments in cutaneous lymphoproliferative disorders. J. Pathol., 153:5, 1987.

Solomon, A. R.: Retroviruses and lymphoproliferative disease. Dermatol. Clin., 3:615, 1985.

Spencer, J., and Isaacson, P. G.: Immunology of gastric lymphoma. Baillière's Clin. Haematol., 1:605, 1987.

Steinherz, P. G.: Acute lymphoblastic leukemia of childhood. Hematol. Oncol. Clin. North Am., 1:549, 1987.

Sterry, W.: Mycosis fungoides. Curr. Top. Pathol., 74:167, 1985.

Suchi, T., et al.: Histopathology and immunohistochemistry of peripheral T cell lymphomas. J. Clin. Pathol., 40:995, 1987.

Sugden, B.: Epstein-Barr virus: a human pathogen inducing lymphoproliferation in vivo and in vitro. Rev. Infect. Dis., 4:1048, 1982.

Sullivan, M. P.: Hodgkin's disease in children. Hematol. Oncol. Clin. North Am., 1:603, 1987.

Sutcliffe, S. B. (Ed.): Immunology of the Lymphomas. Boca Raton, CRC Press, 1985.

Sweetenham, J. W., and Williams, C. J.: Malignant lymphoma in the elderly. Baillière's Clin. Haematol., 1:493–511, 1987.

The Non-Hodgkin's Lymphoma Pathologic Classification Project: National Cancer Institute sponsored study of classifications of non-Hodgkin's lymphomas. Cancer, 49:2112, 1982.

Thiel, E.: Cell surface markers in leukemia. CRC Crit.

Rev. Oncol. Hematol., 2:209, 1985.

Thomas, E. D.: Bone marrow transplantation in hematologic malignancies. Hosp. Pract., 22(2):77, 1987.

Toback, A. C., and Edelson, R. L.: Pathogenesis of cutaneous T-cell lymphoma. Dermatol. Clin., 3:605, 1985.

Tsiftsoglou, A. S., and Robinson, F. H.: Differentiation of leukemic cell lines. Int. J. Cell Cloning, 3:349, 1985.

Tubiana, M., et al.: Non-Hodgkin's lymphoma. Cancer Surv., 4:377, 1985.

van der Valk, P., and Meijer, C. J. L. M.: Histiocytic sarcoma Pathol. Annu., 20(2):1, 1985.

Volkman, D. J., Popovic, M., Gallo, R. C., and Fauci, A. S.: Human T cell leukemia/lymphoma virus-infected antigen specific T cell clones. J. Immunol., 134:4237, 1985.

Wain, S. L., and Borowitz, M. J.: Practical applications of monoclonal antibodies to the diagnosis and classification of acute leukaemias. Clin. Lab. Haematol., 9:221, 1987.

Warnke, R. A., and Link, M. P.: The identification and significance of cell markers in leukemia and lymphoma. Annu. Rev. Med., 34:117, 1983.

Watanabe, S., Shimosato, Y., and Shimoyama, M.: Lymphoma and leukemia of T-lymphocytes. Pathol. Annu., 16(2):155, 1981.

Weiss, L. M., Crabtree, G. S., Rouse, R. V., and Warnike, R. A.: Morphologic and immunologic characterization of 50 peripheral T cell lymphomas. Am. J. Pathol., 118:316, 1985.

Wiernik, P. H., Canellos, G. P., Kyle, R. A., and Schiffer, C. A.: Neoplastic Diseases of the Blood. 4th Ed. New York, Churchill Livingstone, 1985.

Williams, S. F., and Golomb, H. M.: Perspective on staging approaches in the malignant lymphomas. Surg. Gynecol. Obstet., 163:193, 1986.

Wright, D. H.: T-cell lymphomas. Histopathology, 10:321, 1986.

Yunis, Y. Y.: Genes and chromosomes in human cancer. Prog. Med. Virol., 32:58, 1985.

Zola, H.: Differentiation and maturation of human B lymphocytes. Pathology, 17:365, 1985.

56

Thymus

THE diseases of the thymus are divided into hyperplasia, immunologic deficiency disorders, congenital anomalies, and tumors.

HYPERPLASIA

Both enlargement of the thymus and its failure to involute are called hyperplasia. Failure to involute occurs in children and is called juvenile hyperplasia. Hyperplasia in an adult is usually associated with an increase in the number of germinal follicles in the thymus and is called follicular hyperplasia.

Juvenile Hyperplasia

The thymus increases in size until a child has reached the age of 15 years or so and then begins to atrophy, so that in the adult the gland is largely replaced by fat, often with only a few vestiges of thymic tissue remaining. At all ages, the size of the normal thymus varies greatly from one person to another. In a child 7 years old, the normal thymus may weigh from 13 to 48 g, and in an adult 60 years old from 2 to 27 g. Infection and other forms of stress sometimes cause sudden reduction in the size of the thymus, with destruction of many of its lymphocytes and phagocytosis of the fragments by macrophages.

Until recently, the great variation in the size of the normal thymus was not realized. Particularly in children, a large thymus was thought to be abnormal and the child was said to have juvenile hyperplasia of the thymus. In many of these children, the thymus was irradiated to reduce its size. The radiation reduced the size of the thymus, but in 7% of the children who were irradiated carcinoma of the thyroid appeared 10 to 20 years later. There seems no doubt that the radiation caused the carcinoma.

Status Thymolymphaticus. The decision to irradiate a big thymus in a child was often inspired by fear of what was called status thymolymphaticus, a mythical disorder, now known to have no basis in reality. At the time, it was believed that children with a big thymus and large lymph nodes were likely to die suddenly for no obvious reason of what we now call the sudden infant death syndrome. The big thymus had nothing to do with the death of these children, but the legacy of carcinoma of the thyroid is a somber memorial to this mistaken hypothesis and the unnecessary irradiation that resulted from it.

FOLLICULAR HYPERPLASIA. The considerable variation in the size of the normal thymus makes it hard to decide when the gland is hyperplastic, in the sense of containing an increased number of cells. Even a considerable increase in the size of a thymus would probably leave it within the normal range.

Instead, attention has fixed on the number of germinal follicles in the cortex of the gland. In a normal adult, germinal follicles are usually few or absent. If they are numerous, the patient is said to have follicular hyperplasia of the thymus, though in most patients with follicular hyperplasia the gland is of normal size or only slightly enlarged.

Many patients with follicular hyperplasia have the disease of muscle called myasthenia gravis. About 80% of people with myasthenia gravis have follicular hyperplasia of the thymus. Less often follicular hyperplasia of the thymus develops in a patient with hyperthyroidism, acromegaly, Addison's disease, gonadal hypofunction, systemic lupus erythematosus, scleroderma, rheumatoid arthri-

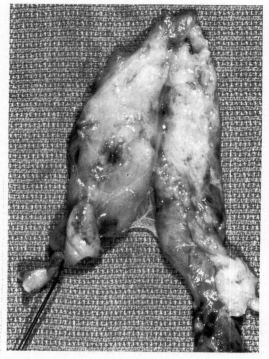

Fig. 56-1. Thymic hyperplasia in an adult with myasthenia gravis.

tis, cirrhosis of the liver, or some other hepatic disorder or is found in a person without other disease.

IMMUNOLOGIC DEFICIENCY DISEASES

The immunologic deficiency diseases are discussed in Chapter 10. In most forms of T-cell deficiency, the number of lymphocytes in the thymus is reduced. Sometimes nothing remains of the thymus except clumps of spindle-shaped epithelial cells. In the Di-George syndrome, it is sometimes completely absent. Only in the Wiskott-Aldrich syndrome is the thymus likely to be normal or only slightly reduced in size.

CONGENITAL ANOMALIES

Congenital anomalies of the thymus are rarely of clinical importance. Sometimes a parathyroid gland is included in the thymus. Sometimes the thymus or, more often, accessory fragments of thymic tissue fail to descend completely and remain in the neck. In 20% of people, tiny fragments of thymic tissue can be found in relation to the parathyroid or thyroid glands.

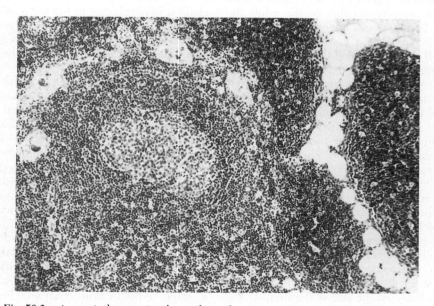

Fig. 56-2. A germinal center in a hyperplastic thymus in a patient with myasthenia gravis.

Thymic Cysts

Small epithelial cysts are present in the thymus in 3% of people over 50 years old. The cysts are usually multiple and may be as much as 5 mm in diameter. They probably result from cystic degeneration of Hassall's corpuscles.

Larger thymic cysts are rare. They occur along the line of descent of the thymus and probably result from the persistence of a segment of the thymopharyngeal duct. In children, they are most frequent in the neck; in adults, in the mediastinum. The cyst may be unilocular or multilocular. It contains clear or murky fluid. It is lined by cuboidal, columnar, or stratified squamous epithelium supported by a fibrous wall, or by some combination of these types of epithelium. Its thymic nature is shown by the presence of thymic tissue somewhere around its periphery.

TUMORS

The tumor that arises from the thymus is called a thymoma and consists of thymic epithelium, usually together with a considerable number of lymphocytes. The thymus can be involved by lymphoma. At times a germ cell tumor, carcinoid tumor, or thymolipoma arises in relation to the thymus.

THYMOMA. Thymomata are uncommon, though they are the most common tumor of the anterior superior mediastinum. Most of the patients are adult. The risk of developing a thymoma increases with age.

Thymomata consist of a mixture of thymic epithelium and lymphocytes. Whether both the epithelium and the lymphocytes are neoplastic is uncertain. Perhaps the best view is that the epithelium is neoplastic and that the lymphocytes are attracted to it, but are not themselves neoplastic.

Lesions. Most thymomata arise in the anterior superior mediastinum. A few arise in the neck or extend into it. A few involve the posterior mediastinum. The tumor usually arises in the midline, is bosselated and roughly spheroidal. Most thymomata are 5 to 10 cm across when discovered. A few are smaller. Some have weighed as much as 5000

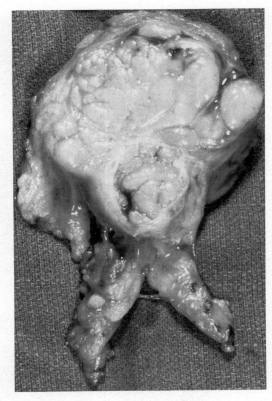

Fig. 56-3. A thymoma replacing and expanding the upper part of the thymus gland.

g. A few form a plaque applied to the chest wall.

The majority of thymomata are encapsulated. They have a firm, collagenous capsule that is often partially calcified or ossified. A few breach the capsule and invade the surrounding tissue.

On section, most thymomata are soft, pink, yellowish, or gray and homogeneous macroscopically and resemble a lymphoma. Some are clearly lobulated. Cysts are evident in 50% of the tumors. Occasionally the cysts are large and numerous, almost replacing the tumor. Foci, hemorrhage, or necrosis is unusual.

Microscopically, thymomata have a thick, collagenous capsule from which broad, collagenous septa extend into the tumor, dividing it into sharply defined clumps of highly cellular tissue. In the clumps, both epithelial cells and lymphocytes are nearly always evi-

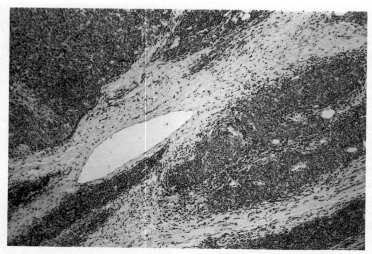

Fig. 56-4. A thymoma showing the broad bands of collagenous tissue that separate the clumps of tumor cells.

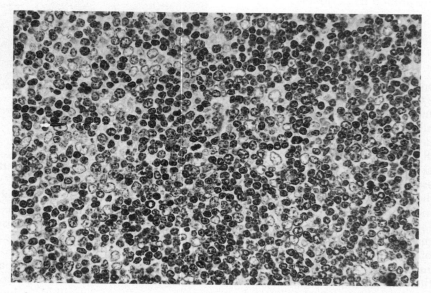

Fig. 56-5. A thymoma showing the mixture of large, pale epithelial cells and the small, dark lymphocytes usual in the cellular part of these tumors.

dent. There is often a good deal of variation from one part of a tumor to another. In 20% of the tumors, epithelial cells are predominant in the cellular clumps. In 40%, both epithelial cells and lymphocytes are abundant in the clumps. In 40%, lymphocytes are predominant. In the predominantly epithelial tumors, lymphocytes may be few or even absent. In the tumors in which lymphocytes are predominant, there is always a meshwork of epithelial cells in the cellular clumps, with the lymphocytes crowded into its interstices.

The epithelial cells are sometimes elongated and look like plump fibrocytes; sometimes they are large and irregularly shaped, resembling macrophages. They usually have spheroidal or ovoid nuclei with fine chromatin and a small nucleolus. Occasionally some of the nuclei are large and hyperchromatic. Electron microscopy shows that the epithelial cells have numerous desmosomes and prominent tonofibrils.

In 80% of thymomata, the large epithelial cells are the more common. They lie singly or form small clumps, joined by their long, thin processes. Often some of the cells have clear cytoplasm. In many thymomata, some of them are squamoid or show frank squamous metaplasia. Rarely, they are anaplastic and pleomorphic.

If the elongated, spindle-shaped epithelial cells are predominant in a tumor or part of a tumor, they often form swirling bundles. Sometimes the spindle-shaped cells surround clumps of large epithelial cells intermixed with lymphocytes.

The lymphocytes in a thymoma are much like the lymphocytes in a normal thymus. Most are T cells and bear the markers of the forms of T cell found normally in the thymus. Some of the lymphocytes are larger than normal and show evidence of activation. Mitoses are often evident. Occasionally, large, pale macrophages filled with debris are scattered among the lymphocytes.

In 60% of thymomata, perivascular spaces are prominent around capillaries and venules. The spaces are bordered by the basement membrane of the blood vessel on their inner side and by the basement membrane of a palisade of epithelial cells on their outer side. They may be empty, but are often filled with lymphocytes, red cells, or macrophages. Eventually, some of the spaces are filled with hyalinized collagen.

In 30% of thymomata, foamy macrophages are present in the perivascular spaces or elsewhere in the tumor. In 20%, Hassall's corpuscles develop. In 20%, rosettes consisting of a ring of epithelial cells surrounding a core of eosinophilic, fibrillar material are present in parts of the tumor. In 10%, germinal centers are present within the tumor. Occasionally a few plasma cells or eosinophils are scattered in the cellular part of the tumor or in its collagenous septa.

In 20% of thymomata, glandular spaces or slit-like lumina lined by cuboidal epithelial cells with microvilli on their surfaces are present in the cellular part of the tumor or in its collagenous septa. In 20%, microcysts formed when a cell or clump of cells become necrotic develop in the cellular part of the tumor. Occasionally part of a thymoma consists of large, irregular spaces lined by flattened epithelial cells.

Clinical Presentation. In 50% of the patients, a thymoma produces no symptoms and is found by accident when a roentgenogram is taken or becomes evident only at autopsy. In 20% of the patients, local symptoms such as cough, dyspnea, or chest pain draw attention to the tumor. In 30% of the patients, myasthenia gravis or some other condition associated with thymomata draws attention to the tumor.

Treatment and Prognosis. At least 75% of thymomata are well encapsulated and benign. Excision cures. In the other 25%, the tumor invades the mediastinal tissues, sometimes extending to the pleura or pericardium. Excision usually cures, if it is possible. If not, irradiation shrinks the tumor and may cure.

Thymomata rarely metastasize. When they do, there is often only a single metastasis in a lung. Widespread metastases are most uncommon. Microscopically, the thymomata that metastasize are similar to the more common benign or locally invasive tumors.

Complications. More than 30% of patients with a thymoma develop myasthenia gravis, red cell aplasia, hypogammaglobulinemia, or, less often, a collagen disease, myocarditis, or leukemia.

Myasthenia Gravis. Though figures differ considerably from one series to another, 20 to 30% of patients with a thymoma develop myasthenia gravis, and 10% of patients with myasthenia gravis have a thymoma. The myasthenia gravis associated with a thymoma may not develop until several years after the appearance of the tumor; sometimes it does not begin until months or years after the removal of the tumor. The thymoma usually weighs 150 g or less and may be benign or malignant.

Microscopically, the epithelial cells in the tumor are nearly always predominantly of the macrophage-like type, though rarely a thymoma predominantly of spindle-shaped epithelial cells is associated with myasthenia gravis. The proportion of lymphocytes in the tumor bears no relation to the likelihood of myasthenia gravis. Hassall's corpuscles and germinal centers are more common in thymomata associated with myasthenia gravis than in those that are not. Rosettes and glandular spaces are rarely found in the thymomata associated with myasthenia gravis. Germinal centers are present in normal thymus outside the tumor in over 50% of the patients with myasthenia gravis, but rarely in patients without myasthenia gravis.

In 25% of the patients with a thymoma and myasthenia gravis, removal of the tumor causes amelioration of the myasthenia gravis, though it may be months or years before the benefit is evident.

Red Cell Aplasia.   About 5% of patients with a thymoma develop red cell aplasia. About 50% of patients with red cell aplasia have a thymoma. In 30% of the people affected, granulocytopoiesis or thrombocytopoiesis is also depressed. Sometimes red cell aplasia develops months or years after the appearance of a thymoma, sometimes only after it has been removed. About 10% of patients with a thymoma and red cell aplasia have also myasthenia gravis.

The thymoma may be benign or malignant. Usually its epithelial cells are predominantly of the spindle-cell type. Removal of the tumor sometimes ameliorates the aplasia.

Hypogammaglobulinemia.   About 10% of patients with a thymoma have hypogammaglobulinemia, with deficiency particularly of IgG and IgA. These people have also a defect in cell-mediated immunity, as shown by delay in rejecting allografts in the skin. Some 30% of patients with hypogammablobulinemia have also red cell aplasia. Some have myasthenia gravis or all three disorders. The hypogammaglobulinemia leads to repeated infections. Thymectomy does not improve the hypogammaglobulinemia.

LYMPHOMA.   Most lymphomata that involve the mediastinum affect the mediastinal lymph nodes rather than the thymus, but any kind of lymphoma can occur in the thymus. Of the non-Hodgkin's lymphomata, the poorly differentiated types are the most common in the thymus. In children, T-cell, convoluted cell lymphoblastic lymphoma frequently involves the thymus.

Any kind of Hodgkin's disease can occur in the thymus, but the nodular sclerosing form of the disease is the most common. In the past, this form of Hodgkin's disease was often mistaken for a thymoma.

GERM CELL TUMORS.   Germ cell tumors of the mediastinum are rare, but any of the kinds of germ cell tumor found in the testes or ovaries can occur in the mediastinum. Seminoma, or germinoma as it is called in the mediastinum, is the most common. The germ cell tumors are not tumors of the thymus but may involve it or arise within it.

Grossly and microscopically the germ cell tumors of the mediastinum are like the germ cell tumors of the gonads and behave like them.   Well-differentiated teratomata are benign and often cystic like a dermoid cyst of an ovary. In 90% of the patients, a germinoma can be cured by surgical excision followed by radiation. The prognosis is bad in patients with an anaplastic germ cell tumor, such as an embryonal cell carcinoma or a choriocarcinoma.

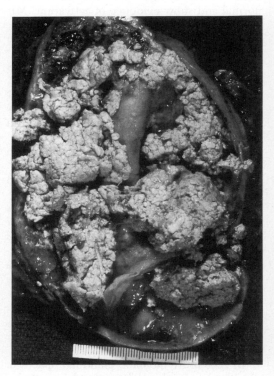

Fig. 56-6.   A well-differentiated benign, cystic teratoma of the mediastinum.

CARCINOID TUMOR. Rarely, a carcinoid tumor grossly and microscopically like a carcinoid tumor of a lung arises in the thymus. Some of these tumors are well encapsulated and are cured by excision. Some are locally invasive. A few give rise to distant metastases. Some of the patients develop Cushing's syndrome. Some also have adenomata in one or more of the endocrine organs.

The origin of the carcinoid tumors of the thymus is obscure. They could arise from a teratoma, like the carcinoid tumors of the ovary, or by aberrant differentiation of the epithelial cells of the thymus.

THYMOLIPOMA. The thymolipoma is a rare, benign tumor in which both the fatty tissue within the thymus and the thymic tissue proliferate. By the time it is discovered, the tumor usually weighs over 500 g, often over 2 kg, sometimes as much as 16 kg. The tumor is usually lobulated and looks like a lipoma, with a smooth, yellow surface. Because it consists mainly of fat, a thymolipoma is radiolucent. Microscopically, it consists of normal looking adipose tissue in which there are streaks of normal looking thymic tissue. Germinal centers are not found. No patient with a thymolipoma has had myasthenia gravis, though one had aplastic anemia. Excision cures.

BIBLIOGRAPHY

General

Arya, S., Gilbert, E. F., Hong, R., and Bloodworth, J. M. B., Jr.: The thymus. *In* Endocrine Pathology. 2nd Ed. Edited by J. M. B. Bloodworth, Jr. Baltimore, Williams & Wilkins, 1982.

von Gaudecker, B.: The development of the human thymus microenvironment. Curr. Top. Pathol., 75:1, 1986.

Janossy, G., et al.: Cellular differentiation of lymphoid subpopulations and their microenvironments in the human thymus. Curr. Top. Pathol., 75:89, 1986.

Müller-Hermelink, H. K. (Ed.): The human thymus. Curr. Top. Pathol., 75:1, 1986.

Steinmann, G. G.: Changes in the human thymus during ageing. Curr. Top. Pathol., 75:43, 1986.

Hyperplasia

Judd, R. L.: Massive thymic hyperplasia with myoid cell differentiation. Hum. Pathol., 18:1180, 1987.

Wekerle, H., and Müller-Hermelink, H. K.: The thymus in myasthenia gravis. Curr. Top. Pathol., 75:179, 1986.

Immunologic Deficiency Diseases

Dourov, N.: Thymic atropy and immune deficiency in malnutrition. Curr. Top. Pathol., 75:127, 1986.

Lindner, J.: The thymus gland in secondary immunodeficiency. Arch. Pathol. Lab. Med., 11:1118, 1987.

Neselof, C.: Pathology of the thymus in immunodeficiency states. Curr. Top. Pathol., 75:151, 1986.

Tumors

Baud, M., Stamenkovic, I., and Kapanci, Y.: Malignant thymomas. Prog. Surg. Pathol., 3:129, 1981.

Mullen, B., and Richardson, J. D.: Primary anterior mediastinal tumors in children and adults. Ann. Thorac. Surg., 42:338, 1986.

Müller-Hermelink, H. K., Marino, M., and Palestro, G.: Pathology of thymic epithelial tumors. Curr. Top. Pathol., 75:207, 1986.

Osborne, B., Mackay, B., and Battifora, H.: Thymoma. Pathol. Annu., 20(2):289, 1985.

Rosai, J.: The pathology of thymic neoplasia. Monogr. Pathol., 29:161, 1987.

57

Nervous System

THe diseases of the nervous system include both the disorders that affect the brain, spinal cord, or meninges and those that involve the peripheral nerves and their ganglia. They include infections, vascular disorders, trauma, metabolic derangements, demyelinating diseases, neuronal diseases, epilepsy, syringomyelia, peripheral neuropathy, congenital anomalies, and tumors.

INFECTION

Infection of the central nervous system and the meninges that cover it is common and at times devastating. Bacteria, fungi, viruses, prions, and parasites can all infect the central nervous system. Infection of the peripheral nerves is less common.

Four kinds of infection of the central nervous system are distinguished. Epidural infections, also called extradural infections, occur between the bone encasing the central nervous system and the dura mater. Subdural infections occur in the subdural space between the dura mater and the arachnoid mater. Leptomeningitis, more often called meningitis, involves the subarachnoid space between the arachnoid mater and the pia mater. Infection of the brain is called encephalitis, and infection of the cord myelitis. Occasionally epidural and subdural infections are grouped together and called pachymeningitis.

Bacterial Infections

Bacterial infections of the central nervous system most often result from hematogenous infection, in which organisms from the blood escape to infect the meninges, brain, or spinal cord. Less often infection spreads directly from the nasal sinuses, middle ear, osteomyelitis of a vertebra, or some other infection in a tissue adjacent to the central nervous system. Trauma greatly favors local infection by breaching the bony case and tough dura mater that protect the central nervous system.

Leptomeningitis is the most common bacterial infection of the central nervous system. It is five times as common as are brain abscesses, and brain abscesses are five times more common than subdural infections. Epidural abscesses are less frequent.

EPIDURAL INFECTIONS. Bacterial epidural abscesses are uncommon within the skull, except in relation to the frontal and mastoid sinuses, though occasionally an epidural abscess complicates osteomyelitis of one of the skull bones. In the skull, the outer layer of the dura mater is firmly bound to the periosteum of the skull bones, leaving no potential space in which infection can become established. When an epidural abscess does occur within the skull, it is usually small and flattened between the tense dura and the underlying bone. Pneumococci, staphylococci, and streptococci are the organisms most often involved.

In the spinal canal, the dura mater is separated from the periosteum of the vertebrae by loose tissue in which infection can more easily become established and can spread along the spine. Most often, the infection is secondary to osteomyelitis of a vertebra. Usually the organism is a staphylococcus, though other organisms such as S. typhi are sometimes found. Occasionally, an epidural infection in the spine is secondary to infection in the pleura or in the retroperitoneum.

Some epidural infections in the spine become widespread. Some are limited by adhesions and fibrosis and remain localized. A localized epidural abscess can compress the spinal cord or obstruct the subarachnoid space, causing xanthochromia in the inferior part of the spinal canal as the concentration of protein in the cerebrospinal fluid inferior to the obstruction rises to high levels.

Drainage of an epidural abscess offers good hope of cure, for the strong underlying dura protects the leptomeninges and the brain or cord.

SUBDURAL INFECTIONS. Subdural infections are more common within the cranium than in the spine. Most are secondary to infection in a neighboring structure, usually infection of a nasal or mastoid sinus, osteomyelitis in a skull bone, or a brain abscess. The infection sometimes reaches the subdural space by penetrating the dura mater or pia mater, sometimes extends along a vein that passes through the dura, often causing thrombosis of the vein. The infection is likely to spread widely in the loose subdural space, becoming bilateral in 25% of the patients. Often the subdural space contains 100 to 200 mL of pus. If the infection is widespread and not localized into abscesses, it is called a subdural empyema. Aerobic or anaerobic streptococci, staphylococci, and gram-negative bacilli are the organisms most often involved. Often more than one bacterium is active. There may or may not be also an epidural abscess.

The dura mater is at first acutely inflamed, with an exudate predominantly of neutrophils, but the arachnoid mater shows little response. Granulation tissue extends from the dura mater into the exudate and organizes it. Sometimes the granulation tissue isolates one or more abscesses in the subdural space as it matures, often at sites distant from the origin of the infection. Veins and sinuses in the dura mater commonly thrombose, adding to the injury. The cerebrospinal fluid contains neutrophils and lymphocytes, the leukocyte count in the fluid being from 50 to 1000 × 10^6/L (50 to 1000/mm^3). The concentration of protein rises to between 0.75 and 3.00 g/L (75 to 300 mg/100 mL). The concentrations of chloride and sugar remain normal. Bacteria are not present in the cerebrospinal fluid.

The patient complains of headache, fever, nausea, and vomiting. After a few days, pressure on the brain causes localizing signs such as seizures, hemiplegia, or aphasia. Papilledema or other evidence of increased intracranial pressure is evident in 50% of the patients. Stupor or coma often develops rapidly.

Without treatment, most patients with a subdural empyema or abscess die within one or two weeks. Early drainage of the subdural space and antibiotic therapy reduce the mortality to less than 20%. Some of those who survive have seizures, hemiplegia, or other signs of local injury to the brain. In the meninges, only thickening of the dura mater remains to show the site of the infection.

LEPTOMENINGITIS. Each year, between 5 and 10 people in every 100,000 develop bacterial leptomeningitis. About 70% of the patients are less than five years old, though meningitis can develop at any age.

Most often leptomeningitis is caused by hematogenous infection, though only a tiny proportion of people with bacteremia develop meningitis. The bacteria reach the cerebrospinal fluid from blood vessels in the pia mater or through the choroid plexus. Less frequently, leptomeningitis is caused by direct extension of an infection from a nasal or mastoid sinus, by an injury that carries bacteria into the meninges, or by a brain abscess. Sometimes infection is introduced by a shunt inserted for hydrocephalus.

In infants, Esch. coli, other gram-negative bacilli, group B streptococci, and pneumococci are common causes of leptomeningitis. In children, Hemophilus influenzae causes the infection in 50% of the patients, meningococci in 30%, and pneumococci in 5%. In adults, pneumococci are responsible in 40% of the patients, and meningococci in 25%. Gram-negative bacilli cause the infection in 20% of people over 50 years old who develop meningitis.

Staphylococci and gram-negative bacilli are common when meningitis is caused by trauma. Pneumococcal meningitis complicates otitis media in 25% of patients with this form of meningitis, pneumonia in 25%, and a head injury in 15%. Shunts are most often infected by staphylococci. Listeria monocytogenes is an increasingly common cause of meningitis in the debilitated and the immunodeficient. Occasionally clostridia, brucellae, gonococci, salmonellae, shigellae, or other bacteria cause meningitis.

Lesions. Leptomeningitis begins with

congestion, edema, and an exudate of neutrophils in the meninges in the region infected. The bacteria soon reach the cerebrospinal fluid, where they multiply rapidly and are carried throughout the subarachnoid space. Often the bacteria are so numerous that they make the cerebrospinal fluid opalescent. Within a few days, neutrophils escape into the cerebrospinal fluid in enormous numbers. Bacteria are usually present in the neutrophils and between them. As the concentration of neutrophils in the cerebrospinal fluid increases, the subarachnoid space becomes filled with yellowish pus.

As meningitis grows more severe, the subarachnoid space becomes increasingly distended, and the leptomeninges increasingly inflamed. Pus fills the sulci of the cerebrum and then as the exudate increases, covers the gyri as well. Flakes of pus float in the cerebrospinal fluid in the ventricles, and exudate may coat their surfaces. In the spinal canal, exudate is usually greatest posteriorly and in the thoracic region. The subdural space is little involved in adults, but in 15% of children with leptomeningitis the quantity of fluid in the subdural space increases. The underlying brain is slightly congested and edematous.

In meningococcal meningitis, the exudate is usually at the base of the brain, where it distends the basal cisterns. If the infection is mild, meningococcal meningitis is often confined to this region. Hematogenous pneumococcal meningitis is usually most marked over the convexities of the cerebral hemispheres. When meningitis results from extension of infection from a neighboring site, the inflammation is usually most severe around the site of infection.

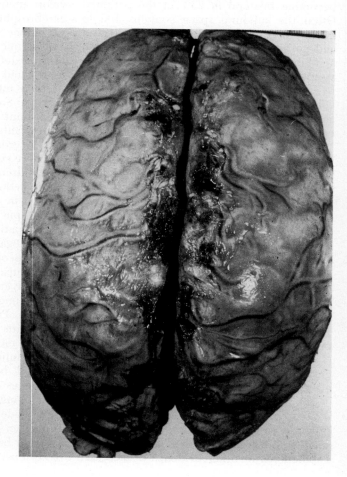

Fig. 57-1. Pyogenic leptomeningitis, showing a thick blanket of exudate filling the subarachnoid space and obscuring the underlying gyri. (Courtesy of Dr. J. H. N. Deck)

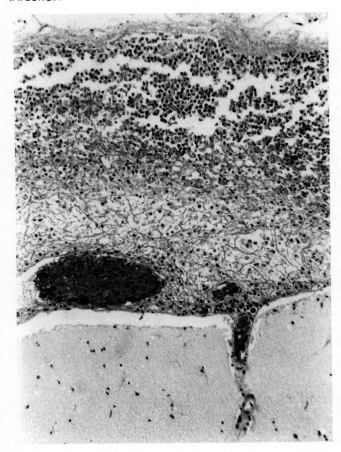

Fig. 57-2. Pyogenic leptomeningitis, showing a fibrinous, neutrophilic exudate distending the subarachnoid space, but little reaction in the underlying brain. (Courtesy of Dr. J. H. N. Deck)

The pressure of the cerebrospinal fluid rises to 500 to 1000 mm of cerebrospinal fluid. The leukocyte count in the fluid is usually between 5000 and 10,000 × 10^6/L (5000 to 10,000/mm^3), but can be as great as 100,000 × 10^6/L (100,000/mm^3). At first neutrophils are predominant, but as days pass increasing numbers of lymphocytes and macrophages appear. The concentration of protein in the cerebrospinal fluid increases to 0.5 to 5.0 g/L (50 to 500 mg/100 mL). The bacteria and neutrophils utilize glucose, and the concentration of glucose in the cerebrospinal fluid falls to less than 2.5 mmol/L (45 mg/100 mL), often to less than 0.5 mmol/L (10 mg/100 mL). The concentration of chloride in the fluid is commonly between 110 and 115 mmol/L (110 to 115 mEq/L).

Clinical Presentation. In 25% of patients with bacterial leptomeningitis, a fulminating illness develops within 24 hours. In 50%, the meningitis slowly worsens for up to a week, usually in association with a respiratory infection. In 20%, the meningitis begins two or three weeks after the onset of a respiratory infection.

The patients have fever, nausea, and headache. Usually the neck is stiff because the patients resist any movement that stretches the inflamed meninges. Kernig's sign is positive. Often that patient is confused, sometimes comatose. Seizures and transient paralyses sometimes occur. Papilledema is unusual, in spite of the increased intracranial pressure.

Treatment and Prognosis. Bacterial leptomeningitis is treated with antibiotics. Without treatment, the disease is almost invariably fatal. With energetic treatment, more than 85% of the patients survive. Pneumococcal meningitis and infections with gram-negative bacilli are the most dangerous. Up to 50% of patients infected with a gram-negative bacilli die. About 10% of children with meningitis caused by Hemophilus influenzae die. Meningococcal meningitis is less dangerous, unless the patient develops adrenal hemorrhage or some other complication.

In most patients who recover, the exudate in the meninges is resorbed. All returns to normal, except for minor, patchy thickening of the leptomeninges and sometimes foci of minor, superficial gliosis on the surface of the brain or spinal cord.

Complications. The longer that lepto-meningitis continues and the more severe it is, the more likely complications become. Damage to a cranial nerve causes temporary paralysis in 15% of the patients. Permanent deafness develops in 10% of children with meningitis, most often in those with a pneumococcal or meningococcal infection.

Thrombosis of blood vessels in the pia mater sometimes causes small infarcts in the superficial part of the brain. Especially in children with a poorly treated infection with H. influenzae, the lesions are sometimes extensive enough to cause mental retardation or epilepsy. Extension of infection into the Virchow-Robin spaces sometimes causes a cerebral abscess or abscesses. The exudate at the base of the brain or collagenous adhesions that develop in the subarachnoid space as the inflammation subsides occasionally obstruct the flow of the cerebrospinal fluid and cause hydrocephalus. Occasionally adhesions isolate a locule of fluid that compresses the brain or spinal cord, causing paraplegia, vertigo, or other symptoms. Sometimes exudate or adhesions prevent the return of cerebrospinal fluid from the spine to the cranium, increasing the concentration of protein in the spinal fluid to more than 10 g/L (1000 mg/100 mL) and causing xanthochromia, as a yellow discoloration of the cerebrospinal fluid is called.

BRAIN ABSCESS. In 40% of patients with a brain abscess, infection spreads directly to the brain from an adjacent focus of infection, most often from a nasal or mastoid sinus or the middle ear. In 15%, the bacteria reach the brain in the blood, usually from the lungs. In 15% of the patients, the abscess is caused by trauma, and in 15%, the origin of the infection cannot be identified.

Streptococci are the most common cause of a brain abscess. Less often, species of Bacterioides, enteric bacilli, staphylococci, or other organisms cause an abscess or abscesses in the brain. Aerobic or anaerobic organisms may be involved. Sometimes there is a mixed infection.

Traumatic abscesses are nearly always caused by staphylococci. Infections with an enteric bacillus most often complicate otitis media or mastoiditis. Abscesses caused by anaerobic streptococci are usually secondary to infection in a lung. Patients with cyanotic congenital heart disease or a left to right shunt in the lungs are particularly likely to develop a brain abscess.

Lesions. Brain abscesses are most common in the cerebral hemispheres, especially in the frontal and parietal lobes. They are less frequent in the cerebellum and basal ganglia and are uncommon in the brain stem.

Abscesses that result from extension of infection from an adjacent structure or from trauma develop in the part of the brain adjacent to the site of infection and are usually solitary. Abscesses caused by hematogenous infection usually begin at the junction of the gray and white matter in a cerebral hemisphere and are often multiple. Abscesses of unknown origin are most often solitary and are most frequent in the parietal region.

A brain abscess may be unilocular and roughly spherical or may be multilocular. A chain of abscesses is sometimes joined by narrow sinuses or bands of acutely inflamed brain tissue. As a brain abscess enlarges, it erodes the white matter, but the gray matter over the abscess is usually spared, even when the abscess is caused by extension of infection from an adjacent site.

A brain abscess begins as a focus of acute inflammation, with congestion, edema, an increasing exudate of neutrophils, and usually many petechial hemorrhages. As the bacteria proliferate and the inflammation grows more intense, the core of the lesion becomes necrotic and begins to liquefy. At first the wall of the abscess is ill defined, and the pus in the core of the lesion merges with inflamed brain tissue that shows edema, congestion and a massive exudate of neutrophils. The

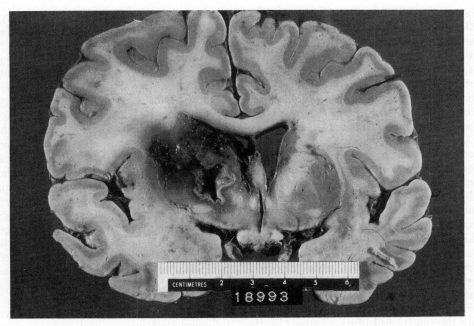

Fig. 57-3. A brain abscess, showing the cavity in the left basal ganglia and the reaction in the surrounding brain. (Courtesy of Dr. J. H. N. Deck)

meninges overlying the abscess show first acute and later chronic inflammation.

After about a week, astrocytes a short distance from the abscess cavity become swollen and begin to form a wall of gliosis to encapsulate the abscess. Often macrophages filled with debris lie between the astrocytes. They are derived from the microglia and from monocytes that escape from the blood. The neutrophilic exudate persists near the cavity of the abscess, but more peripherally lymphocytes and plasma cells become numerous and form cuffs around the blood vessels. After two or three weeks, granulation tissue begins to line the abscess cavity. The granulation tissue is derived principally from the collagenous tissue surrounding the blood vessels. Its extent varies considerably from one abscess to another. It may or may not extend completely around the cavity. Usually the granulation tissue is greatest on the cortical side of the abscess and may be confined to this part of its perimeter. If the abscess becomes quiescent, the granulation tissue matures to form a capsule of collagenous tissue, often a few millimeters thick, that merges with the surrounding gliosis. Often

part of an abscess is bordered only by gliosis. The surrounding inflammation lessens, though edema and an exudate of lymphocytes and plasma cells persist for a long time.

The pressure of the cerebrospinal fluid is likely to be between 200 and 300 mm of water. The leukocyte count in the cerebrospinal fluid is usually less than 100×10^6/L (100/mm³) with lymphocytes predominating, though some neutrophils are present. The concentrations of glucose and chloride are usually normal. The concentration of protein in the cerebrospinal fluid is often about 1 g/L (100 mg/100 mL).

Clinical Presentation. A brain abscess may present as an infection, with fever, malaise, and headache; as a tumor, with the signs of a space-occupying lesion; or with some combination of these symptoms and signs. The onset of symptoms is sometimes sudden, sometimes slow and gradual. The course may be precipitous, with death within a week, or may be slow, like the evolution of a tumor. The signs and symptoms depend upon the size and position of the abscess or abscesses and the severity of the surrounding edema. Hemiplegia is the most common finding. Seizures occur in 30% of the patients. Papilledema is evident in 25%.

An abscess in the frontal lobe tends to cause drowsiness and intellectual impairment, sometimes seizures or mutism. In the parietal lobe it is more likely to cause loss of position sense, homonymous hemianopia, and other visual abnormalities, dysphagia, and sensory or motor signs. In the temporal lobe, an abscess may cause inability to name objects, to read, or understand speech or homonymous hemianopia and other eye signs. Sometimes the signs of meningitis develop, usually because of rupture of the abscess into a ventricle.

Treatment and Prognosis. If a brain abscess is detected before it has cavitated, antibiotic therapy often brings resolution, leaving only a small focus of gliosis. If the abscess is larger, continues to grow, or causes major dysfunction, surgical drainage or excision is necessary. About 90% of the patients recover, though the gliosis and fibrosis caused by the abscess or by surgical excision cause epilepsy or other neurologic dysfunction in many of them.

TUBERCULOSIS. Tuberculosis of the central nervous system occurs in young children in those parts of the world where tuberculosis is common and resistance is low, but in most of the world it is found only occasionally, for the most part in adults. In children, the infection of the nervous system is often secondary to miliary dissemination of the disease, but in adults it usually complicates pulmonary tuberculosis, without other evidence of dissemination beyond the lungs and their lymph nodes. Often the pulmonary disease seems quiescent at the time tuberculosis of the central nervous system is diagnosed.

Tuberculosis can involve the nervous system in three ways. Tuberculous meningitis is the most common. Less often one or more tuberculous abscesses develop within the brain. Sometimes tuberculous osteomyelitis of the spine compresses the spinal cord or its nerves.

In most patients the infection is hematogenous. The tubercle bacilli establish a focus of infection in the brain, meninges, or choroid plexus and the infection spreads to the leptomeninges from this focus, or forms an abscess within the brain. In a few patients, tuber-culous infection of the central nervous system results from extension from a neighboring tuberculous osteomyelitis.

Tuberculous Meningitis. In tuberculous meningitis, the exudate is greatest at the base of the brain, where the cisterns and subarachnoid space are distended with a gelatinous, grayish-green exudate. The exudate often extends up the cerebral hemispheres in their sulci. Often white tubercles a few millimeters across can be seen along blood vessels at the margin of the exudate or on the inner side of the overlying dura mater.

Microscopically, the exudate in the subarachnoid space consists of lymphocytes, plasma cells, and macrophages, together with much fibrin. The leptomeninges show a similar exudate, usually without well-formed tubercles, except along the blood vessels at the margin of the exudate or on the dura mater.

The meningeal arteries are often severely inflamed, sometimes with intimal thickening, sometimes with thrombosis. The arteritis sometimes causes superficial infarcts in the underlying brain, and the necrotic tissue may become secondarily infected by the tubercle bacilli. Involvement of the perforating vessels can cause infarcts in the basal ganglia. Sometimes the nerves at the base of the brain are trapped and compressed by the inflammation.

Changes in the cerebrospinal fluid develop slowly in tuberculous meningitis and may be absent early in the disease. The pressure of the cerebrospinal fluid rises as the disease worsens, often to over 300 mm of water. The leukocyte count in the cerebrospinal fluid is usually between 50 and 200 $\times$ 10^6/L (50 to 200/mm^3), but can be higher. Lymphocytes are predominant, with small numbers of macrophages. Only early in the disease are neutrophils numerous. The concentration of protein in the cerebrospinal fluid rises slowly to as much as 2 g/L (200 mg/100 mL). The concentration of glucose is commonly less than 1 mmol/L (20 mg/100 mL). Late in the disease the concentration of chloride often falls to less than 110 mmol/L (100 mEq/100 mL). Tubercle bacilli can be found in a smear of the cerebrospinal fluid in 25% of the patients and can be cultured from it in 75%.

Tuberculous meningitis begins like other bacterial leptomeningitides, though symptoms often evolve slowly. Energetic treatment with antituberculous drugs and adrenocortical steroids brings resolution in over 75% of the patients, though 25% are left with serious injury to the nervous system, causing paralysis, blindness, deafness, cranial palsies, or hydrocephalus.

Tuberculoma. A tuberculous abscess in the brain is called a tuberculoma. When tuberculosis was rife, tuberculomata of the brain were common, especially in children, and were found most often in the cerebellum. Now tuberculous abscesses of the brain are rare in most of the world, though when one does occur it is frequently in the cerebellum.

Tuberculous abscesses in the brain are often multiple. They may be several centimeters across. The abscess has a core of caseous necrosis surrounded by a collagenous capsule. A zone of gliosis surrounds the capsule. Granulomata are sometimes present at the margin of the necrosis, but often the capsule shows only chronic inflammation with an exudate of lymphocytes, plasma cells, and macrophages.

A tuberculous abscess in the brain enlarges slowly. It causes signs and symptoms like those of a tumor.

SYPHILIS. Neurosyphilis has become rare, though minor and asymptomatic syphilitic infections of the central nervous system are still common if treatment is inadequate or delayed. The lesions are described in Chapter 16.

Fungal Infections

The mycotic diseases are described in Chapter 19. Several of them can affect the meninges or the brain. Most often, the fungus reaches the central nervous system in the blood, though occasionally a mycotic infection of the nervous system originates from a neighboring focus of infection.

Cryptococcosis is the most common mycotic meningitis. The fungus reaches the meninges in the blood, usually from the lungs, and multiples in the cerebrospinal fluid. The subarachnoid space is distended by an immense host of organisms, many with their thick mucoid capsules. With them are mixed lymphocytes and occasionally a few neutro-

phils, but often the cellular response is sparse, both in the cerebrospinal fluid and in the leptomeninges. The concentrations of sugar and chloride in the cerebrospinal fluid both fall greatly, and there is usually some increase in protein. Characteristic of cryptococcosis are cysts, a few millimeters across, in the superficial part of the cortex, caused by innumerable cryptococci crowded into Virchow-Robin spaces, with little reaction round about.

Less often an acute leptomeningitis, a granulomatous leptomeningitis like tuberculous meningitis, or some combination of acute and chronic meningitis occurs in North American blastomycosis, coccidioidomycosis, or histoplasmosis. These fungi may cause granulomata or abscesses in the brain, as may actinomycosis.

If the patient's resistance is reduced by disease or immunosuppressive therapy, the likelihood of fungal infections increases, and a number of opportunistic fungi become able to infect the brain or its meninges. Candida albicans, Aspergillus fumigatus, or less often one of the fungi that cause mucormycosis or the fungus-like bacterium Nocardia asteroides becomes able to cause an abscess or abscesses in the brain. They produce first a hemorrhagic infarct, which later develops into an abscess with acute inflammation or less frequently granulomatous inflammation round about. Less often an opportunistic fungus causes leptomeningitis, nearly always an acute meningitis, like that caused by the pyogenic bacteria. The mycelia or yeast forms of the organism are usually abundant in the exudate.

Viral Infections

Many of the viral infections discussed in Chapter 18 involve the central nervous system. Some cause severe injury, resulting in death; some cause only a minor and transient meningitis. Most cause immediate injury to the nervous system, which follows infection with little delay, but in the slow virus infections the injury is delayed. Except in herpes zoster, the peripheral nervous system is usually less strikingly affected.

Most viral infections of the central nervous system begin by causing a meningoencephalomyelitis, involving both the brain and the spinal cord, as well as the meninges. The lesions are similar in most viral infections of the central nervous system, though the distribution of the lesions within the brain and spinal cord and the severity of the different features of the reaction differ considerably from one kind of viral infection to another.

ASEPTIC MENINGITIS. Aseptic meningitis, or benign lymphocytic meningitis as it is sometimes called, is the commonest viral infection of the central nervous system. In most patients, the disease is mild. The few patients in whom anything is known of the lesions in the central nervous system have an exudate of lymphocytes, plasma cells, and macrophages in the leptomeninges. A few have also mild encephalitis of the kind seen in viral infections. The cerebrospinal fluid shows an increase in cells, at first neutrophils but soon predominantly lymphocytes, and a slight increase in protein, but no other abnormality.

The patient has fever, malaise, headache, stiffness of the neck, and other signs of meningeal irritation. Complete recovery comes within a few days or a week or two. Only occasionally is the disease more severe, with fever of up to 40°C and confusion or coma. Even so, recovery is almost universal.

Polioviruses, echoviruses, coxsackieviruses, the viruses of herpes simplex and encephalomyocarditis, and some of the arboviruses can all cause aseptic meningitis. More than half the patients with mumps have aseptic meningitis, though it is usually asymptomatic. Only occasionally is mumps meningitis severe, with greatly increased cerebrospinal pressure and pleocytosis in the cerebrospinal fluid, and persists for several weeks. Rarely, mumps meningitis results in deafness. Aseptic meningitis can also be caused by the chlamydiae that cause psittacosis.

VIRAL ENCEPHALITIS. The term *encephalitis* comes from the Greek for the brain and so means inflammation of the brain, though the term is often used loosely to include the inflammation of both the brain and the spinal cord found in many kinds of viral infection of the central nervous system. More accurately, inflammation of the spinal cord is called myelitis, from the Greek for the marrow, or inner part. Sometimes the term *encephalo-*

myelitis is used to indicate inflammation of both the brain and the spinal cord.

The different kinds of viral encephalitis are described in Chapter 18, where different syndromes that result from different kinds of viral infection and the special features of the lesions caused by the different kinds of virus are described. Among the more important of the viral encephalitides are the infections with Herpesvirus hominis types 1 and 2, Herpesvirus simiae and the cytomegaloviruses; the infections caused by the arboviruses, equine encephalitis of the eastern, western, and Venezuelan types, St. Louis encephalitis, California encephalitis, Japanese encephalitis, Murray Valley encephalitis, Russian spring-summer encephalitis, Central European tick-borne encephalitis, louping ill, Powassan encephilitis, and other kinds of tick-borne or mosquito-borne arbovirus infection; poliomyelitis; the encephalitides caused by the coxsackieviruses and the echoviruses; rabies; and encephalitis lethargica.

The slow virus infections, subacute sclerosing panencephalitis and progressive multifocal leukoencephalopathy, differ from the usual forms of viral encephalitis, as do the diseases caused by prions, Creutzfeld-Jacob disease, and kuru. They are described in Chapter 18.

Lesion. The lesions found in the different kinds of viral encephalitis are described in Chapter 18. Only a general account of the changes seen in acute viral encephalitis is given here.

If a patient dies of an acute viral infection of the nervous system, the brain, spinal cord, and meninges sometimes look normal macroscopically. In other patients, the brain is a little edematous, slightly swollen, and a little softer than normal. Sometimes foci of necrosis, which may be hemorrhagic, are scattered in the affected part of the brain or spinal cord. So much tissue may be lost that the spinal cord or affected part of the brain is shrunken.

Microscopically, inflammatory cells accumulate around the blood vessels, a process called perivascular cuffing. The cuffing is greatest in the part of the brain or spinal cord most severely affected, but is often evident to a lesser degree through much of the brain and spinal cord. Early in a viral infection, neutrophils are the predominant cells around

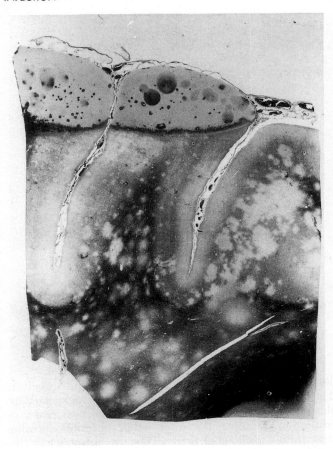

Fig. 57-4. Progressive multifocal leukoencephalopathy. A section stained for myelin shows the multiple pale areas of demyelination caused by this infection. (Courtesy of Dr. J. H. N. Deck)

the vessels, but by the time the diagnosis is made, the cells in the perivascular cuffs are lymphocytes, plasma cells, and macrophages, with plasma cells becoming more numerous after the first week or so. The cells in the perivascular cuffs are in the Virchow-Robin spaces. Only a single layer of inflammatory cells surrounds small blood vessels, but around larger vessels the cuffs are usually several cells thick. Usually the inflammatory cells are confined to the Virchow-Robin spaces and do not extend into the surrounding tissue.

Necrosis of neurons is usually evident. Most of the damaged neurons show first chromatolysis. The damaged cells swell. Their nuclei move to the periphery of the cell. Their cytoplasm becomes vacuolated. The neurons disintegrate and die. Less often a damaged neuron becomes hyalinized or pyknotic.

Foci of edema often loosen the structure of the brain. Sometimes the edema causes well-defined foci of rarefaction, in which all cells disappear, and only a few scattered fibrils remain, strung like a cobweb across a tiny cyst. Sometimes foci of necrosis are more extensive, like infarcts, often just below the pia mater. The gray matter is the most severely injured, but foci of necrosis can extend from the gray matter into the white matter, or injury to the gray matter may result in foci of demyelination of the white matter.

An inflammatory reaction is most severe around the foci of necrosis or injury, but often is evident throughout the brain and spinal cord. The microglial cells and some of the monocytes that escape from the blood enlarge and often become rod shaped, with elongated, twisted, or folded nuclei. Frequently microglial cells and altered mono-

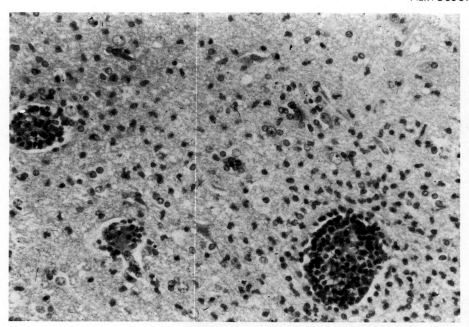

Fig. 57-5.   Perivascular cuffing around blood vessels in a patient with viral encephalitis. (Courtesy of Dr. J. H. N. Deck)

cytes accumulate in clumps called glial nodules. The cells often surround a dying neuron, a process called neuronophagia, an eating up of the neuron. If a glial nodule is in the white matter or unrelated to a neuron, the cluster of cells is called a microglial star. Sometimes lymphocytes and macrophages of the usual type are mixed with the microglial cells and altered monocytes. Clusters of this sort are called gliomesenchymal nodules. If frank necrosis develops, inflammatory cells accumulate in greater number around the focus of necrosis. Large macrophages filled with lipid are prominent. Microglial cells also accumulate around foci of edema and rarefaction, though the reaction is slight. Activation of astrocytes is usually evident only in regions in which destruction of tissue is extensive.

Inclusion bodies are often found in viral encephalitides. The intracytoplasmic Negri bodies are found in 70% of patients dying of rabies and are diagnostic of rabies. In other viral encephalitides, the inclusions are usually intranuclear. Intranuclear inculsions of type A occupy most of the nucleus, often with a halo around the inclusion. The inclusion may

be homogeneous or granular and usually is brightly eosinophilic. Type A inclusions are found in infections with herpesviruses or cytomegaloviruses and in subacute sclerosing panencephalitis. Type B intranuclear inclusions are smaller, about the size of the nucleolus. There may be more than one in a nucleus. They are found in many conditions, poliomyelitis among them.

Most viral infections of the central nervous system cause meningitis, with an exudate of inflammatory cells in the leptomeninges. Neutrophils are numerous in the earliest stages of the infection but are soon replaced by lymphocytes, plasma cells, and macrophages.

In the majority of viral infections of the central nervous system, the pressure of the cerebrospinal fluid is normal or a little increased. The number of cells in the fluid usually increases, though rarely to more than 200×10^6/L (200/mm^3). Early in the infection, 50% of the cells may be neutrophils, but lymphocytes, plasma cells, and macrophages soon become predominant. Occasionally some of the lymphocytes are atypical. The pleocytosis causes a slight increase in the

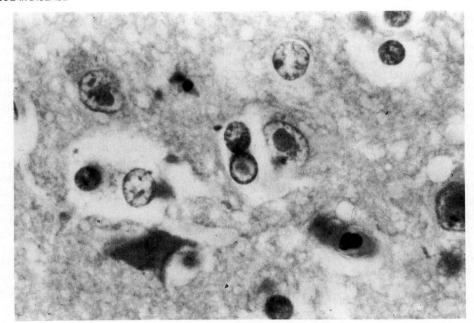

Fig. 57-6. Type A inclusions in the nuclei of neurons and glial cells in a patient with encephalitis caused by the Herpes simplex virus. (Courtesy of Dr. J. H. N. Deck)

concentration of protein in the cerebrospinal fluid. The concentrations of glucose and chloride remain normal.

HERPES ZOSTER. Viral infections of the central nervous system may involve the ganglia on the cranial and spinal nerves. The ganglia show changes like those in the brain, with an exudate predominantly of lymphocytes, sometimes necrosis of neurons, and neuronophagia. The prime example of a viral infection of the ganglia of the cranial or spinal nerves is herpes zoster, which is the most important of these infections.

Parasitic Infections

Protozoal infections such as congenital toxoplasmosis, amebic meningoencephalitis sleeping sickness, and Chagas' disease, can damage the central nervous system. Occasionally a brain abscess is caused by Entamoeba histolytica. These infections are described in Chapter 20.

Injury to the nervous system is common in cysticercosis and may occur in coenurosis or echinococcosis. Schistosomiasis, especially that caused by S. japonicum, paragonimiasis, trichinosis, filariasis, and other metazoal infections occasionally damage the brain. Metazoal infections are discussed in Chapter 21.

VASCULAR DISEASE

In most countries, 15% of deaths result from a cerebrovascular accident. Every year 100 people in every 100,000 die of cerebrovascular disease. In Japan and in American blacks, the death rate is even higher. Some 200 people in every 100,000 die every year of cerebrovascular disease.

The morbidity caused by cerebrovascular disease is even greater. Each year, 400 people in every 100,000 suffer a cerebrovascular accident. The risk of a cerebrovascular accident is low in people under 50 years of age, but then increases steadily as age increases. Every year, 500 people in every 100,000 between 55 and 74 years old and 1500 in every 100,000 over 75 years old develop cerebrovascular insufficiency.

The three most common forms of vascular disease of the central nervous system are occlusion or severe narrowing of one or more of the arteries that supply the brain and spinal cord; hemorrhage into the substance of the brain or, less often, into the spinal cord; and hemorrhage into the subarachnoid space. In most of the world, 60% of people dying of cerebrovascular disease die of obstruction of one of the arteries that supply the brain; 30% die of hemorrhage into the substance of the brain; and 10% die of hemorrhage into the subarachnoid space. In Japan, 80% of people dying of cerebrovascular disease die of hemorrhage into the substance of the brain. Thrombosis of a sinus in the dura mater, thrombosis of a cerebral vein, malformation of the cerebral vasculature, arteritis, and other diseases of the intracranial vessels are much less frequent. Hypoxia and hypertension can damage the brain and spinal column.

ARTERIAL OBSTRUCTION. Obstruction of one or more of the arteries supplying the central nervous system causes disease by inducing transient or permanent ischemia in part of the brain or spinal cord. Atherosclerosis is the cause of the ischemia in 60 to 90% of the patients. In most of the rest, it is caused by an embolus or emboli. Only in a small minority of patients is cerebral ischemia caused by arteritis, narrowing of the carotid arteries by a dissecting aneurysm, fibromuscular dysplasia of the arteries in the neck like that seen in the renal arteries, compression of an artery by the tentorium cerebelli or some other structure, thrombotic thrombocytopenic purpura, sickle cell disease, or polycythemia vera. Oral contraceptives increase five times the risk of developing serious ischemia of the brain.

Lesions. Atherosclerosis and cerebral emboli will be discussed first, then the lesions they cause in the brain and spinal cord.

Atherosclerosis. Atherosclerosis can affect any of the arteries that supply the central nervous system, from the great vessels in the mediastinum to the small arteries within the brain and spinal cord. The lesions are like those of atherosclerosis in other parts of the body, but especially in the smaller arteries they cause considerable narrowing as the atherosclerotic plaques extend around the

lumen of the vessel and bulge into its lumen. As in other parts of the body, atherosclerosis of the arteries that supply the central nervous system is more likely to be severe in people with hypertension or diabetes mellitus. Patients with severe atherosclerosis of the arteries supplying the brain are usually elderly. About 70% are men.

Often overlying thrombus adds to the narrowing caused by atherosclerosis or leads to complete occlusion. If a cerebral artery is completely occluded, thrombus is nearly always present. The occlusion of a cerebral artery by atherosclerosis and overlying thrombus is frequently called cerebral thrombosis. The thrombus is often recent, but sometimes is partially organized.

In many patients, infarction of the brain is caused when an artery narrowed by atherosclerosis is occluded by thrombus. In others,

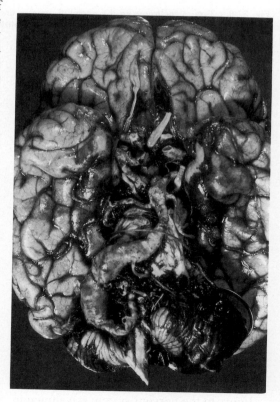

Fig. 57-7.   The base of a brain, showing the tortuosity and ectasia of the basilar artery caused by atherosclerosis. (Courtesy of Dr. J. H. N. Deck)

atherosclerosis alone is sufficient to cause infarction or less serious ischemia, especially if the blood flow to the brain is reduced by hypotension, or when it falls during sleep or exercise. In these people, secondary thrombus can develop at the site of obstruction if the narrowing is in one of the cerebral arteries.

The effect of occlusion or severe narrowing of one of the arteries supplying the central nervous system depends on the size of the vessel affected and the adequacy of the anastomotic channels available to bypass the obstruction. If the occlusion or narrowing is in one of the carotid or vertebral arteries, the outcome depends in large part on the state of the other carotid and vertebral arteries. If the blood flow in the other arteries is good and there are wide anastomoses between them and the occluded artery, even complete occlusion of one of these vessels produces little or no injury. If the flow in the other vessels is poor and anastomoses sparse, major infarction of the brain can result. The circle of Willis is particularly important. If its anastomotic channels are large, occlusion of one of the more proximal vessels is unlikely to cause dangerous ischemia.

When the obstruction is in an internal carotid artery, anastomoses develop between the facial and superficial temporal branches of the external carotid artery and the ophthalmic artery on the obstructed side. The flow through the anastomoses can become sufficiently large to reverse the flow in the ophthalmic artery, bringing blood to the internal carotid artery beyond the point of obstruction.

Anastomoses between the cerebral arteries are never good. Occlusion of one of these vessels by atherosclerosis and thrombosis is likely to cause serious ischemia.

Hypotension can precipitate cerebral ischemia in a person with severe cerebral atherosclerosis. The narrowed arteries can maintain oxygenation of the brain when the blood pressure is normal, but not when it falls. Occasionally anemia precipitates cerebral ischemia in a person with severe cerebral atherosclerosis, or mild hypoxia causes serious injury to the brain.

The ischemia caused by narrowing of the arteries supplying the brain often develops in the watersheds where the regions supplied by the anterior and middle or middle and posterior cerebral arteries meet. These regions are at the limit of the circulation and are easily made ischemic by a reduction in the blood flow in one or more of the cerebral arteries.

When atherosclerosis of a carotid artery causes cerebral injury, the narrowing is most often in the first part of the internal carotid artery, less frequently in its interosseous siphon. Atherosclerosis is often severe in the first 5 cm of the common carotid artery, but narrowing or occlusion at this site does not usually cause cerebral ischemia. The ischemia usually develops in the distribution of the ipsilateral middle cerebral artery. The internal capsule is often affected. Sometimes the lesions appear at the watershed between the middle and the anterior or posterior cerebral artery. Less often, a lesion appears in the distribution of the anterior or posterior cerebral artery. Occasionally the contralateral side of the brain is affected.

Insufficiency of the basilar circulation is most often caused by atherosclerosis of the vertebral or basilar arteries, often with overlying thrombosis. The narrowing is most often in the interosseous portion of the arteries or at the origin of a vertebral artery. Occasionally basilar insufficiency results from severe atherosclerosis of a subclavian or innominate artery proximal to the origin of the vertebral artery. Ischemia is most common in the distribution of the paramedian perforating branches of the basilar artery, but can develop in the distribution of the short circumferential arteries, the posterior cerebral artery, or the superior or anterior inferior cerebellar arteries.

In the subclavian steal syndrome, atherosclerotic narrowing of the subclavian or innominate artery proximal to the origin of the left vertebral artery causes anastomoses to develop between the proximal part of these arteries and the left vertebral artery. If the narrowing is sufficient to reduce seriously the blood flow to the arm, the increased demand for blood when the arm is exercised reverses the direction of blood flow in the vertebral artery to help meet the need of the arm. Cerebral ischemia sometimes results, but is rarely severe.

Atherosclerosis of the middle cerebral

artery is usually confined to the region proximal to its first bifurcation. The atherosclerosis or overlying thrombus may occlude the stem of the artery or may obstruct the lenticulostriate arteries that arise from it. The whole or part of the region supplied by the artery is rendered ischemic.

Narrowing of the anterior cerebral artery is most common in its proximal part. Obstruction proximal to the entry of the anterior communicating artery rarely causes ischemia if the communicating artery is widely patent and able to maintain the circulation. If the anterior communicating artery is atretic, or atheromatous lesions are more distal in the anterior cerebral artery, ischemia develops in the distribution of the artery.

Atherosclerosis of the posterior cerebral artery is usually confined to the proximal part of the vessel. It can cause ischemia in the distribution of the artery or obstruct its circumferential branches that supply the midbrain.

Embolism.   Emboli to the central nervous system are divided into large and small types. The large emboli usually lodge in the middle cerebral artery, less often in some other of the major vessels supplying the brain and spinal cord. Small emboli lodge in small arteries or arterioles within the brain or spinal cord. Small emboli are the more common.

Large emboli nearly always come from the heart and consist of thrombus. The patient has atrial fibrillation or some other cardiac arrhythmia, myocardial infarction with mural thrombus, thrombosis on a valve prosthesis, infective endocarditis, nonbacterial thrombotic endocarditis, or has undergone cardiac surgery. Less often a large thromboembolus comes from one of the large arteries supplying the brain. Occasionally a fragment of a calcified heart valve breaks off during an operation and lodges as an embolus in one of the cerebral arteries. Occasionally a fragment of a cardiac prosthesis serves as an embolus to the brain.

Large emboli to the central nervous system are usually single, though if the patient survives, there is risk of another. Emboli carried in the carotid artery lodge most often in the middle cerebral artery, but any of the major arteries supplying the central nervous system can be occluded by an embolus.

The sudden occlusion of a major artery to the brain by a large embolus is more dangerous than the slow occlusion of the same vessel by atherosclerosis. The slow evolution of atherosclerosis allows collateral vessels to open, and the blood flow through these anastomoses may be sufficent to reduce or overcome the effect of the occlusion. With a sudden embolus, no anastomoses can develop, and the tissue supplied by the occluded artery is suddenly rendered ischemic.

Small emboli are most often thrombi. Less often, a small embolus to the brain consists of a fragment of an atheromatous plaque, a clump of tumor cells, or some foreign material that gains entry to the circulation. Often the origin of the emboli is not apparent. A few small emboli do no harm, but often small emboli are multiple and together cause considerable damage. Sometimes showers of little emboli occur. Sometimes one or two lodge from time to time as months pass until many of the small arteries in the brain are obstructed.

Fat embolism, air embolism, and the emboli of decompression sickness are considered in Chapter 8. An infected embolus or infected emboli are likely to produce an abscess or abscesses in the brain or spinal cord, rather than the ischemic lesions that result from uninfected emboli.

Infarction.   If part of the brain or spinal cord is rendered severely ischemic by atherosclerosis and thrombosis or by an embolus, an infarct is likely to develop. Less severe ischemia that does not persist more than 10 minutes or so can cause temporary loss of function without causing necrosis or permanent injury.

An infarct can develop in any part of the brain—the cerebral hemispheres, basal ganglia, brain stem, or cerebellum. Infarction of the spinal cord is less common. In the brain, an infarct can involve much of a cerebral hemisphere or be less than 1 cm across. The infarct usually abuts against the surface of the brain, but can develop within it. Some are confined to the gray matter. Most extend to involve also the white matter. A few are confined to the white matter.

Two kinds of infarction of the central nervous system are distinguished. In red, or hemorrhagic, infarcts, the necrotic tissue is

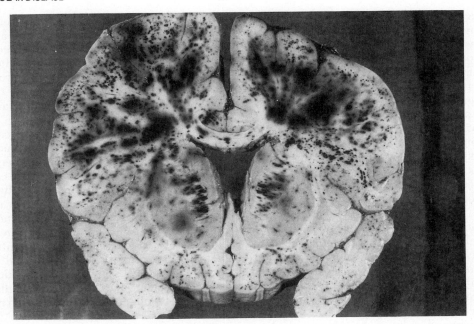

Fig. 57-8. Fat embolism, showing the numerous hemorrhagic infarcts caused by the droplets of fat in the blood. (Courtesy of Dr. J. H. N. Deck)

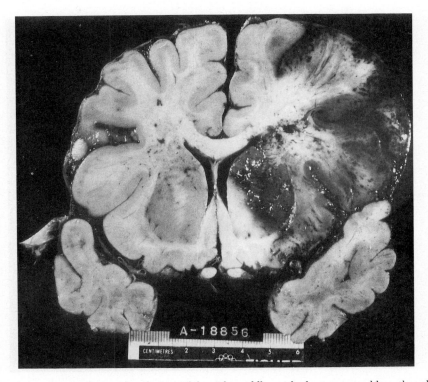

Fig. 57-9. A hemorrhagic infarct in the territory of the right middle cerebral artery caused by a thromboembolus lodged in the artery. (Courtesy of Dr. J. H. N. Deck)

flecked with foci of hemorrhage. In white, or anemic, infarcts, the necrotic tissue remains pale, without macroscopic evidence of hemorrhage.

Infarcts of the brain caused by large emboli are often hemorrhagic. Probably the embolus causes spasm in the artery in which it lodges, and after a few hours the spasm relaxes, allowing blood to pass the embolus and enter the infarct. In other patients, the embolus breaks up after some hours, allowing blood to enter the infarcted tissue.

Infarcts caused by atherosclerosis, with or without superadded thrombosis, are usually pale. In some patients, the infarct is hemorrhagic around its margins as anastomotic vessels allow blood to leak into the infarct. Occasionally an infarct caused by atherosclerosis is entirely hemorrhagic.

An infarct in the brain becomes evident macroscopically within a few hours. The infarcted area is well defined and softer than the surrounding brain. An infarct of the brain

is often called a softening. After three or four hours, the infarcted tissue is swollen and is becoming gelatinous. As the days pass, edema increases in and around the infarcted tissue. The infarct becomes more and more swollen. After three or four days, the necrotic tissue becomes brittle, crumbly, and fatty, as the infarcted tissue begins to break down.

In an anemic infarct, the swelling reaches its maximum after about two weeks, and the infarct then begins to shrink, as the necrotic tissue is removed. Often an irregular cavity appears in the center of the infarct. By the third week, the infarcted tissue is again about its normal volume. Shrinkage continues as the weeks pass, and the necrotic tissue and fluid are resorbed from the infarct. Eventually the patient is left with a shrunken glial scar, or a cyst with glial scarring round about.

Hemorrhagic infarcts behave similarly, though the swelling is often greater and more prolonged.

In the first few days, an infarct of the brain

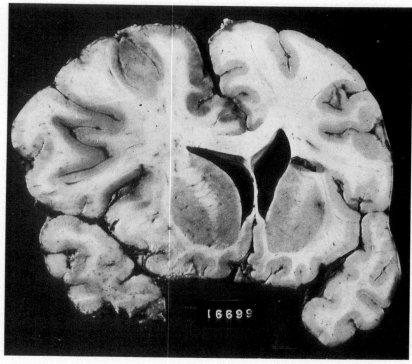

Fig. 57-10. A recent anemic infarct in the territories of the left anterior and middle cerebral arteries. The affected white matter is discolored by the infarct, and the left hemisphere is swollen. (Courtesy of Dr. J. H. N. Deck)

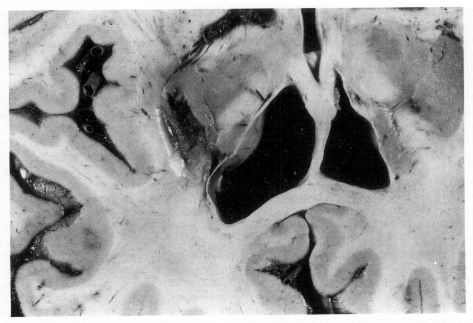

Fig. 57-11. An old, cystic infarct of the internal capsule. (Courtesy of Dr. J. H. N. Deck)

shows microscopically coagulative necrosis, with death of all elements of the brain in the central part of the infarct. The neurons and glial cells become structureless and pyknotic. The axons and their myelin sheaths swell and fragment. At the margin of the infarct, the necrosis is less complete, and the tougher cells survive, first the endothelial cells, then the microglia, and then the astrocytes. Acute inflammation develops at the margin of the infarct, with congestion, edema, and an exudate of neutrophils.

After three or four days, edema increases in the center of the infarct, and the dead cells begin to break down. At the margin of the infarct, the neutrophils have been replaced principally by macrophages, which become increasingly numerous. Many are distended by fatty debris from the infarcted tissue. The macrophages are derived in large part from monocytes that escape from the blood, but in part from microglial cells, which become swollen and show occasional mitoses. The endothelial cells lining the blood vessels at the margin of the infarct are swollen, increase in number, and show occasional mitoses. Hemosiderin is present in the macrophages and encrusts necrotic nerve cells at the mar-

gin of the infarct. In hemorrhagic infarcts, hemosiderin may be so abundant that the margin of the infarct looks brown.

After a week, macrophages distended with fat and debris surround the infarct and extend into it. The swelling of the endothelium in the blood vessels is still marked, and there are usually a few lymphocytes and plasma cells around the infarct. In the center of the infarct, the dead tissue is becoming liquefied, to form small cysts filled with clear fluid with a few lipophages floating in it. The astrocytes around the infarct are swollen, sometimes binucleate, and increase in number as they begin to form a mesh of glial fibers to encapsulate the infarct.

After several weeks, all the dead tissue is resorbed. The inflammatory cells go away. The infarcted area is small and shrunken. The patient is left either with a cyst filled with clear fluid and surrounded by a wall of gliosis or with a glial scar.

Tracts leading from an infarct undergo Wallerian degeneration. The axons of the infarcted neurons break up, and their myelin sheaths degenerate. Trans-synaptic degeneration may occur, as neurons that depend on the dead axons for their afferent stimuli become necrotic, and their axons break up.

Granular atrophy of the cortex occurs when small infarcts in the distribution of a cortical branch of a meningeal artery develop in the cerebral cortex. They are linear and perpendicular to the surface and do not extend beyond the gray matter. The infarcts heal, leaving a shrunken scar of gliosis. Usually these small cortical infarcts are few. Occasionally, they are so numerous that the surface of the affected part of the brain is pitted by glial scars, a condition called granular atrophy of the cortex. The surface of the part of the brain affected looks like the surface of a nephrosclerotic kidney.

Lacunar infarcts develop when one or more of the penetrating arteries that supply the deep part of the cerebral hemispheres, the basal ganglia, and the brain stem are occluded by atherosclerosis or thickening of the vessel wall. The patients all have hypertension. The infarct is less than 2 cm across and is often cystic. Commonly there is more than one. The infarcts are most frequent in the basal ganglia and adjacent white matter.

Clinical Presentation. The effect of narrowing or occluding an artery or arteries supplying the central nervous system depends on the site, severity, and duration of the ischemia that results. If the ischemia is mild, injury and dysfunction are not permanent. If it is more severe but short lived, a transient ischemic attack may occur. If it is still more severe and causes infarction, the patient suffers a stroke.

Transient Ischemic Attacks.   Transient ischemic attacks are common. The patient develops neurologic symptoms that persist for a few seconds to many hours and then disappear. Most attacks last from 5 to 10 minutes. Some patients suffer only one transient ischemic attack, or a few at long intervals. Some suffer many, sometimes several a day, all with the same symptoms. The nature of the symptoms indicates the part of the brain affected.

Repetitive transient ischemic attacks suggest that the ischemia is caused by atherosclerotic obstruction in an artery supplying the affected region. Often the obstruction is in a carotid or vertebral artery on the contralateral side of the neck, most often in the first part of the internal carotid artery or in its siphon. In some patients, a minor

increase in vascular tone or a reduction in blood flow too small to affect the perfusion of the brain in a normal person is sufficient to cause temporary ischemia in the brain, often in the watershed where the branches of the middle cerebral artery meet those of the anterior or posterior cerebral artery. In other patients, the ischemia is caused by repeated emboli from the atherosclerotic lesions in the contralateral vessel in the neck. Isolated attacks may be caused by reduction in blood flow, but are more likely to be due to emboli.

Transient ischemic attacks are more likely in people in whom the structure of the circle of Willis prevents the development of an anastomotic blood supply to the ischemic side of the brain. Severe narrowing of the basilar artery or severe, bilateral atherosclerosis in the neck also impairs or prevents the development of a collateral blood supply. Even complete occlusion of a carotid artery at its origin does not cause cerebral ischemia if the anastomotic circulation through the circle of Willis is good.

When the ischemia affects an eye, the slowing of the circulation is evident in the retinal vessels. Often small platelet thrombi are present in the retinal arteries. The thrombi may sometimes be the cause of the ischemia, but they are more likely to be secondary to the slowing of the blood flow.

In 80% of patients in whom infarction of the brain is caused by atherosclerosis and thrombosis, the infarct is preceded by one or more attacks of transient ischemia. There may be only one, or there may be hundreds. The infarct may follow a few hours after a transient attack, or transient attacks may continue for weeks or months before a more serious lesion develops. Nearly always, the infarct develops in the part of the brain indicated by the symptoms of the transient attacks.

Infarction is not an inevitable sequel of attacks of transient ischemia. In some patients, the attacks become less frequent and disappear altogether, even though no treatment has been given.

Stroke.   The neurologic dysfunction that results from infarction of the brain or hemorrhage into the brain is called a stroke. There is sharp distinction between a stroke and a transient ischemic attack. When a transient ischemic attack persists for many hours, the ischemia may well cause a small infarct, even though there is no permanent dysfunction.

When a stroke is caused by atherosclerosis and thrombosis, the symptoms sometimes develop rapidly, so that the stroke is fully established within a few minutes. More often, a stroke caused by atherosclerosis worsens slowly, often in steplike fashion over several hours or days. After the initial attack, the patient's condition becomes stable or improves, only to worsen after an interval, and again become stable. Often there are several exacerbations of this sort. Once a stroke is established, there is usually some recovery. Occasionally the improvement is dramatic, with almost complete restoration of function within hours or days. More often slow improvement continues for weeks or months.

The worsening of the symptoms of a stroke suggests that the infarct in the brain is enlarging. Early and rapid recovery is probably caused by improved perfusion in ischemic but not necrotic tissue around the infarct. The slow recovery seen in most patients is not caused by restoration of the infarct, but by the brain learning to use other pathways.

When a large embolus lodges in one of the arteries supplying the brain, the sudden ischemia causes a stroke that develops rapidly, but once established, progresses no further. Recovery of the circulation at the margin of the infarct sometimes brings rapid improvement. More gradual recovery often follows later.

Occasionally an infarct becomes so greatly swollen one or two weeks after its onset that it acts as a space-occupying lesion, like a tumor. In a few patients, tentorial herniation has brought death.

Syndromes. The symptoms caused by infarction or transient ischemia of the brain depend on the part of the brain affected. Each of the principal arteries supplying the central nervous system has its own syndrome. If only part of the territory supplied by the occluded artery is infarcted, the patient shows only some of the symptoms and signs produced by infarction of the whole of that artery's territory.

Ischemia in the distribution of the *middle cerebral artery* is the most common cause of transient ischemic attacks and cerebral infarction. About 40% of cerebral infarcts are caused by atherosclerosis of the middle cerebral artery or emboli that lodge in it. If the artery is obstructed near its origin, the patient develops contralateral hemiplegia and hemianesthesia. The paralysis is at first flaccid, but soon becomes spastic. If the dominant hemisphere is involved, aphasia is usual, and there may be agraphia or alexia. If the nondominant hemisphere is affected, the patient may lose consciousness of the paralyzed side of the body or may not realize that paralysis has developed. Homonymous hemianopsia and inability to conjugate gaze to the side away from the lesion are common. If the obstruction is more distal in the artery or less complete, the muscular weakness is less complete or involves only one limb. There may be dysphasia without paralysis or other more limited dysfunction.

Ischemia in the region supplied by the *anterior cerebral artery* causes 15% of strokes. If the whole of the region supplied by the artery is affected, the patient develops paralysis of the contralateral leg and sometimes weakness in the contralateral arm. Sensation is lost in the contralateral leg. Urinary incontinence is common. Disturbances of speech, impairment of gait, or dyspraxia can occur.

Less than 15% of infarcts develop in the region supplied by the *posterior cerebral artery*. The occlusion is most often caused by embolism, but can result from atherosclerosis with or without thrombosis, or from pressure by the tentorium cerebelli. If the obstruction is proximal to the entry of the posterior communicating artery, ischemia in the basal ganglia and brain stem may cause contralateral hemiplegia, contralateral ataxia, contralateral hemiballismus, a third nerve palsy and contralateral ataxia, a third nerve palsy and contralateral paralysis, contralateral loss of superficial and deep sensation, sometimes followed by severe pain in the affected region, or paralysis of upward gaze and inability to make a decision. If the obstruction is distal to the entry of the posterior communicating artery, ischemia in the occipital cortex commonly causes contralateral homonymous hemianopsia or some other disturbance of vision. Loss of memory sometimes develops. Visual agnosia or alexia can occur. If the posterior communicating artery is inadequate, proximal obstruction in the posterior cerebral artery gives both symptoms caused by ischemia of the basal ganglia and brain stem and those due to ischemia of the occipital cortex. Bilateral obstruction to the posterior cerebral arteries causes blindness or other serious ocular dysfunction, though the patient may not be aware of it.

Obstruction in a *vertebral artery* commonly causes transient ischemic attacks with temporary dizziness, vertigo, numbness in the ipsilateral face and contralateral limbs or disturbances in vision, speech, or swallowing. Paralysis is less common. If narrowing of a vertebral or the posterior inferior cerebellar artery causes more severe ischemia, the patients develop ipsilateral hemiparalysis of the tongue, contralateral hemiparesis, dysphagia, ipsilateral loss of sensation in the face, contralateral hemianesthesia in the limbs, loss of taste, Horner's syndrome, ataxis, or some combination of these manifestations.

Obstruction of the *basilar artery* causes transient ischemic attacks like those due to vertebral obstruction. More serious ischemia causes syndromes that reflect the dysfunction of the part of the brain rendered ischemic: ipsilateral ataxia; falling to the side of the lesion; dizziness; nausea; vomiting; ipsilateral nystagmus; ipsilateral tinnitus; ipsilateral deafness; paralysis of the ipsilateral eye muscles; ipsilateral paralysis of the face; contralateral paralysis of the limbs; myoclonic spasms involving the eyes, face, palate, pharynx, larynx, or respiratory muscles on the side of the lesion; loss of sensation in the ipsilateral or contralateral side of the face; loss of sensation in the contralateral limbs; or ipsilateral Horner's syndrome.

If a *carotid artery* is obstructed, transient ischemic attacks usually show evidence of dysfunction in the region supplied by the middle cerebral artery, less often signs of ischemia in the territory of the anterior or posterior cerebral artery. In 25% of the patients, ischemia of the optic nerve or retina causes transient blindness in one eye.

Lacunar infarcts cause syndromes reflecting the site of the infarct or infarcts. Among the more common are contralateral hemi-paresis, contralateral distortion of sensation, and contralateral ataxia with muscular weakness and dysarthria.

Treatment and Prognosis. Transient ischemic attacks are sometimes treated with heparin or other anticoagulants, especially when there is reason to think that increasing thrombosis might occlude a middle cerebral or a carotid artery. Aspirin and other antiplatelet drugs are often given to reduce the risk of thromboemboli. Endarterectomy benefits some patients with severe atherosclerosis of a carotid artery.

Heparin is sometimes given to patients with a small infarct in the hope of reducing or preventing its extension. Endarterectomy is at times helpful after a small infarct caused by narrowing of a carotid artery. Mannitol and other agents that reduce cerebral edema are of value if the swelling around an infarct causes dysfunction.

Multi-infarct Dementia. In 20% of elderly people with dementia, the dysfunction is caused by cerebral infarction. Another 15% have both cerebral infarcts and Alzheimer's disease. Most of the patients have multiple infarcts in the cerebral hemispheres. Some of the infarcts are large; most are small. Some are recent; most are old. The hemispheres shrink. Their sulci are widened and the ventricles are dilated.

Progressive Subcortical Encephalopathy. Progressive subcortical encephalopathy, called Binswanger's disease after the German physician who described it in 1894, develops in more than 1% of people over 60 years old. The patients have ill-defined foci of demyelination and axonal damage in the white matter of the cerebral hemispheres. More than 90% of them have lacunar infarcts in the internal capsule, centrum semiovale, basal ganglia, or cerebellum. Over 30% have cerebral infarcts. Almost all have hypertension, with hypertensive changes in the small cerebral vessels. Atherosclerosis is evident in the arteries at the base of the brain in 90% of the people affected. In 70% of the patients, symptoms develop slowly, with loss of memory followed by increasing dementia. Less often symptoms develop abruptly. In 90% of the patients with symptoms, there is evidence of mild pyramidal, extrapyramidal, or cerebellar dysfunction.

HEMORRHAGE INTO THE BRAIN OR SPINAL CORD. Hemorrhage into the brain or spinal cord can be secondary to trauma or can be caused by disease of the blood or blood vessels. Traumatic hemorrhage is discussed later in this chapter. Only the bleeding caused by disease of the blood or blood vessels is discussed in this section. Often this type of bleeding into the brain or spinal cord is called a spontaneous hemorrhage.

Except in Japan, less than 20% of strokes are caused by intracerebral hemorrhage. More than 80% of patients with spontaneous cerebral hemorrhage are hypertensive. Most are elderly. Men and women are equally affected.

Lesions. More than 50% of spontaneous hemorrhages involve the putamen and internal capsule. Less often the hemorrhage develops in the thalamus, pons, cerebellum, or beneath the cortex of the cerebral hemispheres. A subcortical intracerebral hemorrhage is sometimes called a lobar hemorrhage. Hemorrhage is uncommon in other parts of the brain and in the spinal cord. The bleeding is usually from a penetrating artery.

Within a few hours, the bleeding excavates an irregular cavity filled with a soft, red blood clot. In the basal ganglia, the cavity is usually over 3 cm across and can involve much of a hemisphere. Often there are petechiae in the edematous brain around the cavity. In the pons and cerebellum, the cavity is smaller. Subcortical lobar hemorrhages are commonly flattened. They may be less than 1 cm across or may extend round much of a hemisphere.

After a few days, the brain around the hemorrhage is swollen, edematous, and often is strained yellow by hemosiderin. As weeks pass, the cavity is surrounded by gliosis. The blood is resorbed until only a cyst remains, usually with its wall stained yellow or brown by hemosiderin.

Microscopically, in the first few hours edema and acute inflammation surround the cavity, and blood infiltrates into the surrounding tissue. The petechial hemorrhages in the surrounding tissue often show a necrotic arteriole in the center of the petechia. Often small arteries and arterioles around the lesion show hyaline arteriosclerosis of the sort seen in small vessels in other parts of the body in systemic hypertension.

After some days, macrophages accumulate

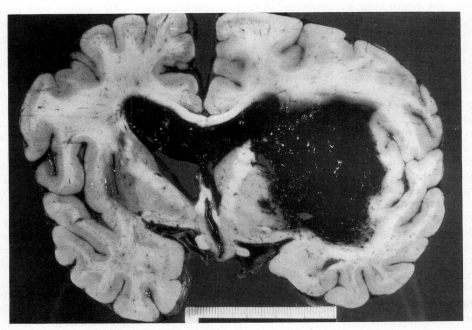

Fig. 57-12. Destruction of the right basal ganglia by a massive, recent hemorrhage that has ruptured into the ventricles. An old, slit hemorrhage is present in the putamen on the left. (Courtesy of Dr. J. H. N. Deck)

around the lesion and take up the fatty debris of the dead tissue and pigments derived from the breakdown of the red cells. Astrocytes adjacent to the lesion swell and begin to form a capsule of glial fibers. The reaction is similar to that around an infarct, except that hemosiderin is more abundant.

The swelling caused by hemorrhage into the brain and the edema around it acts as a space-occupying lesion. If the lesion is above the tentorium cerebelli, the increased cerebral pressure not uncommonly causes secondary hemorrhages in the midbrain and pons.

In 90% of patients with a large cerebral hemorrhage, the lesion ruptures into a ventricle. It rarely breaches the pia mater to enter the subarachnoid space. The bleeding into the cerebrospinal fluid may or may not increase the cerebrospinal fluid pressure. Usually only a limited quantity of blood escapes into the subarachnoid space.

Clinical Presentation. Symptoms and signs develop rapidly after a large hemorrhage into the brain, though it may be 24 hours before the extent of the neurologic deficit is clear. If signs continue to worsen after 24 hours, it is nearly always because of increasing edema around the lesion, not because of continuing hemorrhage. About 50% of the patients have severe headache. Some vomit or have a stiff neck.

The site and size of the hemorrhage determine the neurologic dysfunction it causes.

Putamen. If the hemorrhage is into the putamen, the face becomes flabby on the side distant from the lesion within a few minutes, speech becomes blurred, and the arm and leg on the side distant from the lesion become weak. The eyes tend to deviate away from the lesion. Sensation goes from the affected limbs. Flaccid paralysis and then spastic paralysis develop on the affected side. Sometimes compression of the brain stem causes coma or decerebrate rigidity.

Thalamus. Hemorrhage into the thalamus causes hemiparesis and hemianesthesia. The sensory defect is usually the more severe. If the lesion is on the dominant side, there may be aphasia; if on the nondominant, loss of conciousness of the paralyzed side. Homonymous hemianopia sometimes develops, but is usually transitory. Any of a variety of other eye signs may occur. Most often the eyes are deviated downwards and do not react to light.

Pons. Hemorrhage into the pons usually brings coma within a few minutes. Quadriplegia, decerebrate rigidity, and small pupils that react to light are usual. Hyperpnea, hypertension, and hyperhidrosis are less frequent.

Cerebellum. The symptoms of cerebellar hemorrhage frequently slowly worsen for several hours. Vomiting, inability to stand or walk, occipital headache, and vertigo are usual. Often the eyes are deviated to the contralateral side and cannot be turned to the side of the lesion. Dysarthria and dysphagia are sometimes prominent. Often the ipsilateral side of the face is weak. Occasionally there is quadriplegia or paraplegia.

Lobar Hemorrhage. Most lobar hemorrhages cause frontal headache. More than 50% of the patients are drowsy. Occipital lobar hemorrhages usually cause hemianopsia that worsens for some minutes. Temporal hemorrhages cause aphasia and delirium. A parietal hemorrhage usually causes contralateral loss of sensation. A frontal hemorrhage causes weakness in the contralateral arm.

Pathogenesis. In most patients with serious hemorrhage into the brain, the hemorrhage is due principally to hypertension. The penetrating arteries in the brain are weakened by hyaline arteriosclerosis and are ill-supported by the soft brain tissue. Some have found that small aneurysms are common in these vessels in people with systemic hypertension and suggest that the hemorrhage is caused by rupture of an aneurysm.

Hypertension is less frequent in patients with a lobar hemorrhage. In some of these people, the penetrating arteries are weakened by amyloid in the vessel wall. Some have an arteriovenous malformation or a bleeding diathesis. Petechiae are common in the brain in patients with thrombocytopenia and other disorders that cause excessive bleeding, but only occasionally do these people develop more serious hemorrhage.

Treatment and Prognosis. Nearly 80% of patients with major bleeding into the brain die within a month. Few with a pontine hemorrhage survive for more than a few days.

Only occasionally is surgical evacuation of the hematoma of value. Mannitol and other agents that reduce cerebral edema are sometimes helpful.

SUBARACHNOID HEMORRHAGE. Bleeding into the subarachnoid space is called subarachnoid hemorrhage. Each year 4 people in every 100,000 develop a subarachnoid hemorrhage. Over 80% of the patients are over 40 years old. More than 50% of them are hypertensive. About 60% of them are women.

Lesions. In more than 85% of the patients, a subarachnoid hemorrhage is caused by massive and sudden bleeding from a berry aneurysm on or near the circle of Willis. In 10% of patients, the bleeding comes from vascular malformation. Occasionally the hemorrhage is caused by a mycotic aneurysm or some other vascular lesion. Rarely, an intracerebral hemorrhage ruptures into the sub-arachnoid space. When an intracerebral hemorrhage ruptures into a ventricle, the quantity of blood reaching the subarachnoid space is not usually great.

In 50% of patients who bleed from a berry aneurysm and in most of those who bleed from a vascular malformation, the hemorrhage disrupts the substance of the brain around the lesion. In many, spasm of an artery irritated by the blood develops two days to two weeks after the hemorrhage and causes cerebral ischemia, most frequently in the region supplied by the middle or anterior cerebral artery. In 30% of the patients, the ischemia is severe enough to cause dysfunction or cerebral infarction.

The blood rapidly spreads throughout the subarachnoid space. There may be more than $1,000,000 \times 10^6/L$ $(1,000,000/mm^3)$ red cells in the cerebrospinal fluid. The pressure of

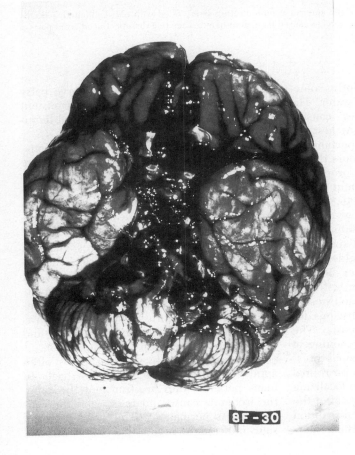

8F-30

Fig. 57-13. Extensive, subarachnoid hemorrhage caused by the rupture of a berry aneurysm filling the subarachnoid cisterns at the base of the brain with dark blood. (Courtesy of Dr. J. H. N. Deck)

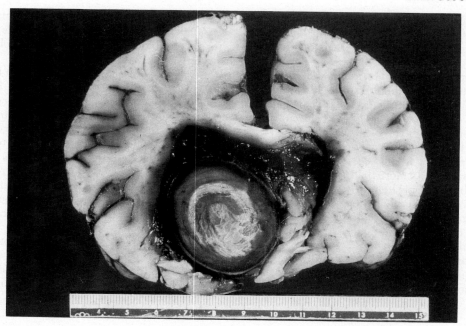

Fig. 57-14. A giant berry aneurysm of the anterior communicating artery filled with old, laminated, partially calcified thrombus. Leakage from the aneurysm has caused the recent hemorrhage that disrupts the adjacent parts of the brain. (Courtesy of Dr. J. H. N. Deck)

the cerebrospinal fluid rises abruptly, sometimes to as much as 1000 mm of water. The blood irritates the leptomeninges, causing edema and acute inflammation. At first the leukocyte count in the fluid is proportional to the red cell count, but after 48 hours the increasing meningitis increases the proportion of white cells. The leukocyte count in the cerebrospinal fluid can reach 3000×10^6/L (3000/mm^3). The blood usually shows a leukocytosis of about 15×10^9/L (15,000/mm^3).

Clinical Presentation. A massive subarachnoid hemorrhage causes sudden, violent, generalized headache. Over 50% of the patients become unconscious within a few minutes. In most the unconsciousness is transient, but 10% remain unconscious for several days. The headache persists. The neck becomes stiff because of the meningeal irritation. The increased intracranial pressure causes papilledema and often preretinal hemorrhages. Usually there are no localizing neurologic signs in the first few days after the rupture, though occasionally the disruption and edema of the brain caused by the hemor-

rhage induce a third or a sixth nerve palsy and occasionally ischemia causes transient dysfunction in the ipsilateral cerebral hemisphere.

Complications. In 20% of the patients, the aneurysm bleeds again within three weeks. The lesions and symptoms are similar to those of the first attack.

Hydrocephalus develops in some of the patients from four days to four weeks after the hemorrhage. It is usually caused by obstruction to the drainage of cerebrospinal fluid by blood clot in the basal cisterns. The hydrocephalus is often mild and transient, but in some patients causes drowsiness, impairment of eye movements, or urinary incontinence. In a few, fibrosis in the basal cisterns makes the hydrocephalus permanent and severe enough to require decompression.

Symptoms caused by vasospasm most often appear seven days after the hemorrhage. In many patients, they are transient. In some, the ischemia causes infarction and the dysfunction is permanent. The symptoms and signs indicate the region that is ischemic and are similar to those in other forms of cerebral ischemia.

Treatment and Prognosis. A patient with a subarachnoid hemorrhage is put at rest. In patients with a bleeding aneurysm, the aneurysm is usually clipped surgically after the patient's condition has become stable. Dopamine and other drugs that increase circulation to the brain are sometimes helpful if cerebral ischemia develops. Mannitol is valuable if cerebral edema is severe. The management and prognosis in a patient with a vascular malformation is discussed later in the chapter.

About 30% of patients with a bleeding berry aneurysm die within two days, another 20% within three months. The prognosis is worse if the patient bleeds a second time. Over 50% of those who survive are left with serious neurologic dysfunction.

VENOUS THROMBOSIS. Thrombosis of a venous sinus in the dura or of the veins in the meninges is uncommon. Primary venous thrombosis complicates a disease that involves principally some other part of the body. Secondary thrombosis is secondary to infection or some other injury to the vein thrombosed.

Primary thrombosis of a dural sinus is most common in children under two years old, though it can occur in older children or in adults. The affected infants are usually severely dehydrated, often malnourished, infected, or in heart failure. In adults, primary thrombosis occasionally complicates trauma, polycythemia rubra vera, or pregnancy. The superior longitudinal sinus is most commonly affected. Less often the lateral sinus, superior cerebral veins, or straight sinus is involved.

Secondary thrombosis of a dural sinus or meningeal vein is most often secondary to meningitis. The superior longitudinal sinus and the cerebral veins are the vessels most frequently involved. Otitis media and mastoiditis occasionally cause thrombosis of the lateral sinus. Infection of the face, sphenoid sinus, or ethmoid sinus can cause thrombosis of the cavernous sinus. Rarely, frontal sinusitis causes thrombosis of the superior longitudinal sinus. The thrombus may or may not be infected.

Thrombosis of an intracranial sinus or vein tends to extend along the vessel involved and into communicating veins and sinuses. The effect of the thrombosis depends on its site and extent. If the thrombus is short, anastomoses between veins may be sufficient to maintain the circulation. If it is more extensive, the thrombus often causes ischemia and infarction in the brain or congestion and edema of the tissues drained by the obstructed vessel. If the thrombus is infected, signs of infection are added to those caused by the obstruction.

Thrombosis of the superior longitudinal sinus or the cerebral veins causes hemorrhagic infarction in the underlying cerebral cortex. Considerable quantities of blood often leak into the subarachnoid space. The intracranial pressure rises, in part because of thrombosis of arachnoid granulations, in part because of edema around the infarct. Headache, confusion, contralateral hemiplegia, ocular pareses, and convulsions are common.

Thrombosis of the lateral sinus often causes venous congestion behind the ear, with pain and edema in this region. The cerebrospinal pressure is frequently raised, but infarction of the brain is unusual. Occasionally obstruction to the straight sinus causes infarction in the basal ganglia.

Thrombosis of a cavernous sinus obstructs the ophthalmic vein, bringing edema of the forehead and eyelids, chemosis, and proptosis. Pain in the eye or hyperesthesia of the forehead may result from involvement of the ophthalmic branch of the 5th nerve. Injury to the 3rd, 4th, and 6th cranial nerves can cause weakness of the ocular muscles. Papilledema and retinal hemorrhages are evident on the affected side.

The prognosis is bad if thrombosis of the venous sinuses or veins within the skull is extensive. In the patients who survive, the thrombus is organized and recanalized. Collateral vessels overcome the obstruction.

HYPERTENSIVE ENCEPHALOPATHY. Patients with severe hypertension sometimes develop severe headache, with nausea and vomiting. Hemiplegia, blindness, convulsions, and other neurologic signs often follow. They may be transient or permanent. The patient becomes stuperose and may lapse into coma. Increase in the cerebrospinal pressure causes papilledema and hemorrhages in the fundi of the eyes. The concentration of protein in the cerebrospinal fluid may exceed 1 g/L (100 mg/100 mL). Unless the blood pressure is reduced, death soon follows.

The blood vessels in the brain show severe arteriosclerosis and sometimes arteriolar necrosis. Perivascular petechial hemorrhages are common. Edema is usually severe but irregularly distributed. Often lacunar infarcts are present beside some of the tortuous arteries within the brain.

Spasm of the arteries of the brain seems to be the major cause of hypertensive encephalopathy. If the ischemia caused by the spasm is mild, it causes only edema. If it is more severe, there are petechial hemorrhages, increasing dysfunction, and infarction.

HYPOXIA. The brain and spinal cord are likely to be damaged in any condition in which there is severe hypoxia. Damage to the central nervous system becomes likely if a cardiac arrest persists for more than three or four minutes, if there is severe hypotension, if the oxygenation of blood in the lung fails, or if there is insufficient oxygen in the inhaled air. The severity of the injury to the nervous system depends principally on the severity and duration of the hypoxia.

Macroscopically, the brain is sometimes normal if the patient dies within one or two days of the onset of the hypoxia, but more often it is moderately or severely edematous. Potechial hemorrhages are especially common in the floor of the third and fourth ventricles.

After three or four days, laminar necrosis is often evident in the cerebral cortex, as the third and fourth layers of the cortex become necrotic. A band of brownish discoloration runs parallel to the surface of the cortex. Often it is most marked in the depths of the sulci. Sometimes similar necrosis discolors the caudate nucleus, putamen, globus pallidus, or the gray matter of the cerebellum.

After some weeks, the thalami and the amygdaloid nuclei shrink, and the brain stem flattens. If the hypoxia is severe, the brain atrophies. The meninges become opaque. The cerebral and cerebellar cortices are thin, with a granular surface. The hippocampus is shrunken, sometimes with a flattened cavity in Sommer's sector. The ventricles are dilated.

Microscopically, the neurons are the cells first and most severely affected. The oligodendroglia are less severely injured. The astrocytes, microglia, and blood vessels are usually little affected. Only if the hypoxia is severe is there almost complete infarction in the brain.

Within a few hours, the mitochondria of the neurons swell, and their endoplasmic reticulum dilates. Their cytoplasm becomes increasingly hyaline and their organelles disintegrate. The nuclei of the neurons shrink and become pyknotic. Small, polypoid excrescences called incrustations project from the surface of the neurons. The oligodendroglia are often swollen, but the other cells in the brain show little abnormality.

Within a few days, the dead neurons fragment and disappear. Astrocytes near the damaged neurons swell and divide. Microglial cells become rod shaped and are aligned perpendicular to the surface of the cortex. They take up the fatty debris of the dead neurons. Gliosis increases in the regions in which many neurons are lost.

The loss of neurons causes patchy demyelinization in the white matter. Occasionally, the demyelinization is more extensive than the loss of neurons. In the damaged regions, the necrotic debris of the axons and myelin sheaths is taken up by macrophages. The injury is repaired by gliosis.

Hypoxia does not affect all parts of the brain and spinal cord equally. The third and fourth layers of the cerebral cortex, Sommer's area in the hippocampus, and the Purkinje cells in the cerebellum are particularly susceptible and are often destroyed when neighboring neurons seem little affected. Neurons in the corpus striatum, thalamus, amygdaloid nucleus, and some of the nuclei in the brain stem are also susceptible, though in these regions some neurons are killed while others are little affected. In the cerebrum, the injury is sometimes greatest in the watersheds where the regions supplied by the cerebral arteries meet, presumably because hypoxia is most severe at this extreme limit of the circulation.

Mild hypoxia of the brain causes impairment of judgment, incoordination, and confusion, but leaves no permanent dysfunction. More severe hypoxia brings coma. If unconsciousness persists for more than 5 minutes, permanent injury to the brain is likely. Paralysis, visual defects, ataxia, and parkinsonism are among the more common defects. If the hypoxia is severe and prolonged, all cerebral functions may be lost, leaving only the motor centers that keep the body alive.

TRAUMA

Traumatic injuries of the nervous system are common, especially in young people who live an active life. The brain and peripheral nerves are often injured, the spinal cord less frequently. The different kinds of head injury will be considered first, then injury to the spinal cord, traumatic lesions of the peripheral nerves, and the various types of birth injury.

Head Injury

Each year, 1,000,000 people in the United States suffer a head injury severe enough to disable them for at least a day or two. Some 50,000 are left with some degree of permanent disability. More than 30,000 die primarily of the injury to the head.

Head injuries are divided into fractures of the skull; conditions that involve principally the meninges, extradural hemorrhage, subdural hemorrhage, and subarachnoid hemorrhage; and lesions of the brain, hemorrhage, contusion, laceration, tearing of nerve fibers, edema, infarction, and concussion. The different kinds of head injury are considered separately, though often the patient suffers more than one of these kinds of injury.

FRACTURE OF THE SKULL. A fracture of the skull may be linear, without separation or dislocation of the fragments; depressed, forming a saucer-like concavity that presses on the brain; comminuted, with fragments of bone driven into the tissues; or compound, with tearing of the skin overlying the fracture. Over 80% of fractures are of the linear type. In 70% of the patients, the patient also has injury to the meninges or brain. An inconspicuous linear fracture is commonly associated with major intracranial bleeding, but a more obvious depressed fracture often does little damage to the meninges and brain.

In addition to the injury done by the force causing the fracture, compound fractures increase considerably the risk of infection and occasionally allow air to enter the cranial cavity. Fractures through the middle ear, ethmoid bones, or frontal sinus also increase greatly the risk of intracranial infection and sometimes cause pneumocephalus or leakage of cerebrospinal fluid. A fractured temporal bone injures the facial nerve in 30% of patients, causing facial paralysis, and sometimes damages the inner ear. A fracture through the dorsum sellae can damage the optic, sixth, or seventh nerves.

In infants and young children, the meninges and part of the brain sometimes herniate through a fracture of the skull. If the defect is not repaired, the herniation enlarges to form a pulsatile mass under the skin of the head. In adults with a considerable defect in the skull caused by surgical procedures, the brain bulges little if the dura is intact. If the dura is torn, the brain herniates more extensively. The blood supply to the herniated brain may become constricted at the neck of the hernia, causing necrosis of the herniated brain. If the prolapse is allowed to continue, the herniated brain becomes fixed by adhesions to the tissues of the scalp, and cannot be reduced.

EXTRADURAL HEMORRHAGE. Extradural hemorrhage, or epidural hemorrhage as it is sometimes called, forms a hematoma between the dura mater and the overlying bone. Extradural hemorrhage occurs in 2% of head injuries. In fatal head injuries, an extradural hematoma is found in 15% of the patients.

Lesions. An extradural hemorrhage is most frequently under the convexity of the cranium, less often in the posterior fossa. The dura at the base of the skull is too firmly adherent to the bone to permit extradural bleeding. The hematoma is usually lens shaped, flattened between the tense dura and the overlying bone.

The hematoma usually enlarges rapidly. It presses the brain against the opposite side of the skull and increases the intracranial pressure. Symptoms develop when the hematoma contains 50 mL of blood. Often an extradural hematoma contains 400 or 500 mL.

An extradural hematoma heals in the usual way. The blood clot in the hematoma is organized. If the hematoma is small, only a dense scar remains. If it is larger, the lesion often becomes cystic, with a cavity bordered by a dense collagenous wall. Usually hemosiderin derived from the hemoglobin in the hemorrhage colors the scar or the wall of the cavity brown.

Clinical Presentation. Many of the patients are unconscious when first seen. In some, the hematoma develops more slowly, and there is an interval of from a few minutes to many hours before symptoms develop. If the hematoma overlies the cerebral cortex, drowsiness, confusion, headache, and vomiting progress to coma as the intracranial pressure rises. Pressure on the third nerve causes dilation of the pupil on the side of the lesion, less often dilation of the contralateral pupil. The contralateral cerebral peduncle is occasionally pressed against the tentorium cerebelli, causing ipsilateral hemiplegia, or other signs of compression of the brain are evident.

Somnolence and coma are less likely if the hematoma is below the tentorium. The midbrain and hypothalamus are not compressed as the intracranial pressure rises. Changes in the pupils are unlikely, for there is no pressure on the third nerves. Occasionally pressure on the cerebral peduncles causes quadriplegia.

Pathogenesis. Extradural hemorrhage is always caused by trauma. In almost all patients, it complicates a fracture of the skull, though often the fracture is linear, sometimes involving only the inner table of the cranium. In 70% of the patients, the bleeding results from rupture of the middle meningeal artery or one of its branches. Often the middle meningeal veins are also torn. The thin part of the temporal bone is easily fractured or distorted, tearing the underlying vessels.

Treatment and Prognosis. Once an extradural hematoma is large enough to cause symptoms, it must be drained surgically without delay. If drainage is prompt, recovery is usually complete. If it is delayed, permanent injury or death is inevitable. Overall, 20% of the patients die, often because of other serious injuries.

SUBDURAL HEMORRHAGE. Subdural hemorrhage forms a hematoma in the potential space between the dura mater and the arachnoid mater. If the lesion is detected soon after the hemorrhage, it is called an acute subdural hematoma. If it is detected only weeks or months later, it is called a chronic subdural hematoma. Subdural bleeding occurs in 5% of people with a head injury and is found in 50% of those dying of head injury.

Lesions. Most subdural hematomata develop over the frontoparietal cerebral cortex. Less often the bleeding is in the occipital region or in the middle fossa. Many of the hematomata are small, but some cover most of a cerebral or cerebellar hemisphere. Occasionally a subdural hematoma is bilateral. The force of a blow to one side of the head is easily transmitted through the brain and can tear a blood vessel on the other side.

The blood in a subdural hematoma clots and is organized in the usual way. The organization is principally from the dura. At the end of the first week, granulation tissue extends from the dura into the clot, but the arachnoid mater shows little or no reaction. By the second week, a little granulation tissue is formed from the arachnoid mater, but the response of the dura mater remains much greater.

The granulation tissue organizing the hematoma matures into dense collagen. As months pass, the collagen becomes increasingly sclerotic and is sometimes calcified. If a subdural hematoma is small, it is completely obliterated by dense scar tissue stained yellow by the hemosiderin remaining from the hemorrhage. If the hematoma is larger, a cyst is formed. The cyst has a wall of dense collagen containing many siderophages and contains clear, yellowish fluid.

Some subdural hematomata continue to grow larger as days or months pass. In some, continuing hemorrhage from the fragile vessels in the wall of the hematoma cause the enlargement. In some slow enlargement begins about two weeks after the hemorrhage and continues for weeks or months as the hypertonic fluid in the cyst draws water into the cavity.

Clinical Presentation. In an acute subdural hematoma, symptoms develop minutes or hours after the injury, as the hematoma presses on the brain and increases the intracranial pressure. Only in 30% of the patients is there a significant interval before symptoms appear. The patient is drowsy or comatose.

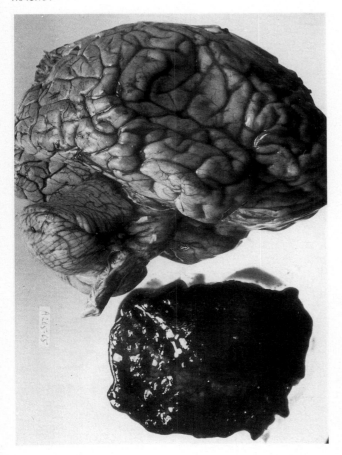

Fig. 57-15. Top, a depression of the anterior part of a brain caused by a recent subdural hematoma. Bottom, blood clot removed from the hematoma. (Courtesy of Dr. J. H. N. Deck)

Ipsilateral headache is common. The pupils are dilated on the side of the lesion in 90% of the patients; on the contralateral side in 10%. Hemiplegia and other localizing signs are uncommon and usually develop late in the course.

Symptoms of a chronic subdural hematoma develop weeks or months after the injury. Up to 30% of the patients can recall no injury to the head. The patient develops headache, confusion, changes in personality, seizures, or partial hemiplegia. The symptoms and signs sometimes worsen slowly, sometimes remain stationary or fluctuate in severity.

Pathogenesis. Subdural hematomata are caused by trauma, but the injury is sometimes slight. Only 50% of the patients have a fracture of the skull. In elderly patients in whom atrophy of the brain has caused a widening of the subdural space and in patients on anticoagulants, a minor blow on the head can cause bleeding into the subdural space. A whiplash injury or other sudden movement of the head, a fall in which the person lands on the feet or buttocks, and other minor injuries can cause a subdural hematoma.

Rupture of veins that cross the subdural space carrying blood from the brain to the dural sinuses is a common cause of subdural hemorrhage, especially when the injury causing the hemorrhage is minor. If the injury is more severe, the bleeding often comes from laceration of the dura or injury to the arachnoid mater. Less often, the hemorrhage is caused by rupture of an artery crossing the subdural space or by a tear in a dural sinus.

Treatment and Prognosis. A small, asymptomatic subdural hematoma needs no treatment. Most of the larger hemorrhages need surgical evacuation of the clot, though adreno-

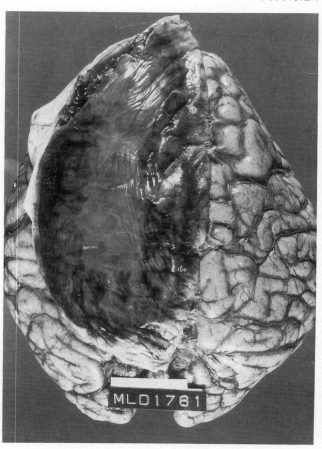

Fig. 57-16. A chronic subdural hematoma. The dura mater discolored by the hemorrhage has been folded back towards the midline to show the marked compression and distortion of the brain. (Courtesy of Dr. J. H. N. Deck)

cortical steroids control some chronic subdural lesions. If a chronic subdural hematoma continues to enlarge, craniotomy and removal of the membranes enclosing the cavity are sometimes needed. If the clot is evacuated promptly, the prognosis is good if there are no more serious cranial injuries. If diagnosis is delayed and the hematoma is large, permanent neurologic injury or death is likely.

SUBDURAL HYGROMA. In infants, the blood in a subdural hematoma is often resorbed quickly, leaving a cyst filled with clear fluid and bounded by a thin collagenous wall. The cyst is called a subdural hygroma, from the Greek for fluid and tumor. Rarely, a similar lesion develops in an adult when a tear in the arachnoid mater allows cerebrospinal fluid to enter the subdural space.

SUBARACHNOID HEMORRHAGE. Subarachnoid hemorrhage is common in severe head injuries. Small vessels in the leptomeninges are easily torn if the force of the injury makes the brain move within the skull. The bleeding is most common over the vertex of the brain where the movement of the brain within the skull is greatest, but it can occur in other parts of the subarachnoid space, even at the base of the brain like the subarachnoid hemorrhage caused by rupture of a berry aneurysm.

If the hemorrhage is small, the blood is diluted by cerebrospinal fluid and does not clot. In the course of a week or two, the red cells break down, and the cerebrospinal fluid is cleared by phagocytes. If the hemorrhage is larger, the lesions and symptoms are like those of a subarachnoid hemorrhage caused by rupture of a berry aneurysm. Fibrous adhesions may obliterate part of the subarachnoid space or interfere with the circulation of the cerebrospinal fluid.

HEMORRHAGE INTO THE BRAIN. A severe blow to the head or anything else that causes sudden acceleration or decleration of the head causes the brain to move or twist within the skull. Blood vessels within the brain are easily torn. Small hemorrhages in the pons, midbrain, or hypothalamus are nearly always found in severe head injuries and frequently are present in the corpus callosum or cerebral hemispheres. Larger hemorrhages are less common. Small hemorrhages cause no dysfunction unless the hemorrhage is in a critical region. Larger hemorrhages behave like the spontaneous hemorrhages considered earlier in the chapter. Occasionally injury to an artery causes thrombosis and infarction.

CONTUSION. The term *contusion* is used to describe injuries in which trauma causes a mixture of hemorrhage and necrosis in the brain. Most severe head injuries cause at least a slight contusion. A healed contusion of the brain is found in 2% of autopsies.

Two kinds of contusion of the brain are distinguished. A coup lesion occurs on the side of the injury. A contracoup lesion develops on the other side of the brain. Both terms come from the French word *coup*, meaning a blow.

If the head is struck by a blunt instrument, such as a club, the coup lesion is at the site of the injury. If a contracoup lesion develops, it is most often in the undersurface of the opposite frontal lobe, at the tip of the sylvian fissure, in the uncus or in the inferior or lateral part of the temporal lobe. Sometimes there is more than one contracoup lesion. The coup lesion results from the force of the blow. The contracoup lesion is caused by transmission of the force of the blow across the brain and by the twisting of the brain caused by the blow. The coup lesion is usually much the larger.

If a rapidly moving head strikes a stationary object, the injury to the brain is caused principally by the movement and twisting of the brain within the skull. Contracoup lesions are often multiple and are usually larger than the coup lesion.

If the head oscillates violently, but there is

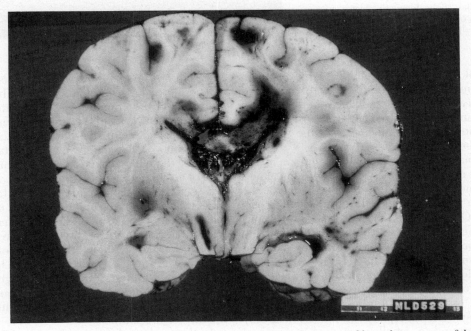

Fig. 57-17. Ruptured blood vessels and multiple intracerebral hemorrhages caused by violent rotation of the head in an accident. (Courtesy of Dr. J. H. N. Deck)

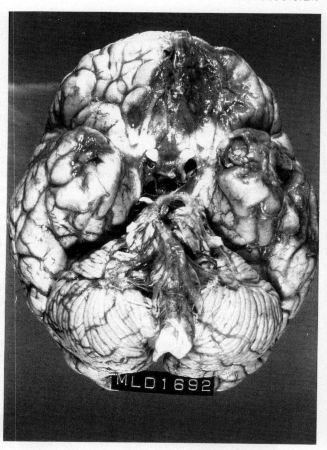

Fig. 57-18. Old contrecoup lesions resulting from a blow to the right occipital region. There is little evidence of injury at the site of the blow, the major injuries being on the left and anteriorly. (Courtesy of Dr. J. H. N. Deck)

no blow to the head, neither coup nor contracoup lesions develop. Instead, contusions are caused by the movement of the brain within the cranium. They are most common in the cerebral hemispheres at the vertex of the brain.

Small contusions are most common at the crest of the cerebral gyri. They are linear and extend 1 or 2 cm into the substance of the brain at right angles to the surface of the cortex. Often several adjacent gyri show lesions of this sort. Larger contusions are roughly pyramidal, with the base of the pyramid on the surface of the brain.

Microscopically, a contusion shows a mixture of hemorrhage and necrosis, sometimes with torn nerve bundles. Edema and inflammation develop around the lesion as they do around a small spontaneous cerebral hemorrhage. The lesion heals, leaving a glial scar, often stained yellow by hemosiderin.

The signs and symptoms produced by a contusion of the brain depend on its site and size and the severity of the edema around the lesion. A small contusion often produces no dysfunction. A large one may be fatal. In general, the effect of a contusion is similar to that of an infarct of similar location.

LACERATION. The injury caused by an object that penetrates into the brain is called a laceration. A rod or knife sometimes causes a small laceration in the brain. A cleaver or some other large object that lacerates the brain causes more extensive injury. A bullet sometimes penetrates into or through the brain. Fragments of bone are commonly driven into the brain from a comminuted fracture of the skull.

In the track of the laceration, the brain is destroyed. If the patient lives for a few hours, a zone of hemorrhagic necrosis 1 to 3 mm deep develops around the injury. Edema and inflammation likę that around an infarct follow. If the patient survives, the lesion heals by gliosis.

The caliber of a bullet wound in the brain is usually greater than that of the missile. A low velocity projectile is likely to tumble as it passes through the brain, and a high velocity bullet causes a large, pulsating cavity in the brain. The cavity collapses after a second or so, but leaves a track larger than the bullet. Occasionally the pressure of the cavity is sufficient to fragment the skull.

The effect of a laceration of the brain depends on the site of the injury and its extent. Anything from sudden death to a startling absence of symptoms can result.

TORN AXONS. In 70% of head injuries, axons are torn. The tearing results principally from the twisting and distortion of the brain caused by the trauma. If the injury is slight, only an occasional axon is affected. If it is severe, axons and bundles of axons are ruptured in many parts of the brain. The corpus callosum is usually the most severely affected. The anterior commissure, fornices,

sagittal strata of the occipital lobes, internal capsules, and pons are often involved.

After a few days, the ends of the ruptured axons swell. After five or six weeks, wallerian degeneration is evident as the damaged axons and their sheaths degenerate and fragment. The neurons involved show chromatolysis and, especially in the thalamus, sometimes become necrotic. The injury is repaired by gliosis. In infants, the lesions sometimes form smooth-walled cysts in the white matter. The dysfunction caused depends on the site and extent of the lesions.

Trauma sometimes divides one or more of the cranial nerves completely or partially. The injury is most often in the intraosseus part of the nerve, less often within the skull. The nerves most frequently injured are I, II, III, V, VII, and VIII.

EDEMA. In all kinds of head injury involving the brain, edema is a major cause of dysfunction. It increases the size of the lesions and tends to increase intracerebral pressure. Occasionally edema is the major feature of the injury. It sometimes is uncontrollable and brings death.

CONCUSSION. The transient loss of con-

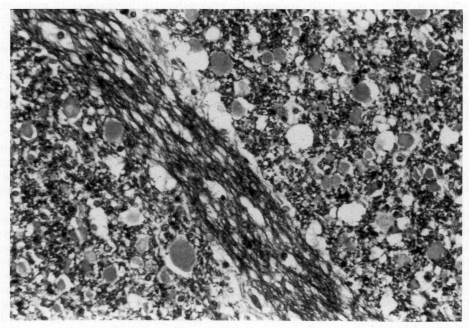

Fig. 57-19. A microscopic section from the pons, stained for myelin showing extensive disruption of axons caused by trauma. The round, gray bodies are the swollen remnants of the damaged axons. (Courtesy of Dr. J. H. N. Deck)

sciousness that often follows a blow to the head or sudden acceleration or deceleration is called concussion. The unconsciousness usually lasts only a few minutes, but can persist for several hours. When consciousness is regained, the patient cannot remember the injury or preceding events. Usually the amnesia extends for only a few minutes, but if the injury is severe, memory of the preceding weeks or months is lost in whole or part. Most patients have no other neurologic dysfunction. In a few, pallor, hypotension, bradycardia, or sluggish pupillary reactions are evident. Occasionally other reflexes are lost, and there is temporary paralysis or other more serious neurologic dysfunction.

Recovery is usually rapid and complete. In most patients, memory returns gradually in a few days or weeks. Any neurologic function disappears. Only occasionally do headache or episodes of dizziness continue.

Concussion is caused by movement of the brain within the skull. Probably the unconsciousness and loss of memory result from rotation of the cerebral hemispheres on the brain stem. In most patients, no permanent injury is caused. In some, torn axons or other minor effects of trauma are evident.

Boxers and others repeatedly concussed sometimes develop progressive neurologic disease, with incordination or dementia, the punch-drunk syndrome. Often the septum pellucidum is torn or cavitated. Neurofibrillary tangles like those of Alzheimer's disease are common in their neurons, especially in the temporal lobes, but the amyloid plaques of Alzheimer's disease are usually absent.

Injury to the Spinal Cord

Each year, trauma to the spinal cord renders 10,000 people in the United States paraplegic or quadriplegic. Less serious injuries are more common. In most patients, the injury is secondary to fracture or dislocation of the spine. Motor accidents, bullet wounds, and whiplash injuries are among its more common causes. Diseases that narrow the spinal canal and disorders such as rheumatoid arthritis that weaken the intervertebral joints add to the likelihood of injury to the cord.

The mildest of traumatic injuries to the spinal cord is called spinal concussion. A blow to the spine causes paralysis and loss of sensation below the level of the injury, but after a few hours or a few days the paralysis passes off, sensation is regained, and the victim is left with no residual dysfunction. The jarring caused by the blow causes edema of the spinal cord and perhaps a few small hemorrhages, but no permanent injury to the axons in the spinal tracts.

More serious injury to the spinal cord causes contusion or laceration, much as in the brain except that the lesions in the cord are usually less hemorrhagic. Still more severe injury tears the meninges or crushes the cord. Injury to the blood vessels supplying the spinal cord often adds to the damage. Occasionally cylindrical columns of partially necrotic tissue extend into the basal part of the dorsal horns or the ventral part of the dorsal columns for a few segments above or blow the lesion. This extension of the lesion is sometimes called traumatic hematomyelia, though bleeding is not often striking.

The cord reacts to injury as does the brain, first with edema and inflammation, later with gliosis as the lesions heal. Sometimes a cyst or cysts form in the glial scar. In some patients, a longitudinal cavity develops in the traumatic hematomyelia above the lesion.

If the meninges are torn, a dense collagenous scar binds the dura mater to the periosteum of the spine. At first, the subarachnoid space often persists, but as years pass, the scarring tends to obliterate the subarachnoid space and extend into the spinal cord.

Axons interrupted by the lesion show wallerian degeneration, and their neurons undergo chromatolysis. The axons in the spinal cord do not regenerate, but after several years axons from spinal nerves often grow into the fibrosis around the lesion in the cord.

The effect of injury to the spinal cord depends on the level of the injury and its severity. If the spinal cord is completely transected, immediate paralysis and loss of sensation below the level of the lesion, incontinence of urine and feces and loss of spinal reflexes follow. If the lower part of the cord is uninjured, the spinal reflexes will be regained within a few weeks, and reflex urination and defecation will develop. Transection above the fourth cervical vertebra brings respiratory paralysis and death.

Injury to Peripheral Nerves

Traumatic injury of a peripheral nerve is most often caused by continued or frequently repeated pressure. A crutch can compress the radial nerve in the axilla. A fracture, osteophyte, or prolapsed intervertebral disk can compress a spinal nerve. In the carpal tunnel syndrome, the median nerve is compressed as it passes beneath the flexor retinaculum in the wrist. In Morton's metatarsalgia, named after the American surgeon who described it in 1876, a metatarsal nerve is compressed between the heads of adjacent metatarsal bones. The ulna nerve is sometimes compressed as a workman leans on a bench.

Less often a peripheral nerve is cut by a knife, or by flying glass. An injection can damage a nerve. Sudden traction on a limb can avulse a nerve from the spinal cord. Cold can destroy a nerve.

In the mildest of injuries, a blow or compression causes temporary dysfunction in a nerve without causing disruption of its axons or leaving any permanent injury. Pins and needles in a leg is a familar example.

If the injury is more severe, some or many axons are destroyed, but the collagenous sheaths of the nerve are not breached. Wallerian degeneration follows, but as few if any of the Schwann cell columns around the broken axons are disrupted or displaced; regeneration is almost perfect and leaves no residual dysfunction.

If the injury is still more severe or is frequently repeated, the collagenous sheaths of the nerve are damaged. Collagen is laid down in and around the nerve, thickening and distorting it. Some of the regenerating axons are lost in the scarring and fail to find a Schwann cell column leading to their end organ. Some degree of dysfunction is inevitable.

Still less favorable is complete division of a nerve, even if the ends are carefully approximated surgically. Many of the regenerating axons from the proximal end of the nerve find a Schwann cell column leading to their end organ and again become functional, but many do not. Some degree of scarring in and around the nerve is inevitable.

TRAUMATIC NEUROMA. If the ends of a severed nerve are separated, the regenerating axons and Schwann cells from the proximal end of the nerve form a traumatic neuroma. Usually the neuroma is ovoid and 1 or 2 cm across. Occasionally it is tender. It consists of tangled bundles of axons and Schwann cells separated by collagen. A similar neuroma forms at the distal end of the nerve but contains only collagen and Schwann cells. Without surgical repair of the damaged nerve, function is not recovered.

TOMACULOUS NEUROPATHY. In a few kindred a defect inherited as an autosomal dominant character makes the nerves easily damaged by pressure. The axons in the peripheral nerves show sausage-like swellings up to 40 µm in diameter, usually due to excessive myelination, less often to duplication of the axon or the accumulation of debris from the breakdown of myelin between the axon and the myelin sheath. The condition is called tomaculous neuropathy, from the Latin for sausage, or hereditary liability to pressure palsy.

Birth injury

Injury to the brain sustained at the time of birth is responsible for the death of 1 infant in every 200 live-horn, and for the death of 1 in every 10 stillborn. The injury is due to mechanical trauma sustained during birth or the hypoxia common at that time.

Subdural hemorrhage caused by the distortion and molding of the head that occurs during birth is common. Compression of the head can tear the tentorium cerebelli, lacerating the straight sinus, the transverse sinus, the great vein of Galen, or its branches. Excessive overriding of the parietal bones can tear the veins entering the sagittal sinus or the sinus itself.

Subarachnoid hemorrhage is also common, but may be due to asphyxia rather than to direct mechanical trauma. Extensive intracerebral hemorrhage is unusual, but petechial hemorrhages and edema are frequent in the brain of these infants and may well be due to hypoxia rather than to mechanical injury.

Hypoxia causes the loss of neurons in the cerebral cortex, less often in the basal ganglia, thalamus, or elsewhere common in infants dying of birth injuries and the foci of hemorrhagic necrosis occasionally found along the watersheds where the regions supplied by two of the cerebral arteries meet. The foci of infarction occasionally found may be due to compression of one of the arteries supplying the brain.

Infants with birth injuries often do not show the neurologic signs found in adults with similar lesions. Instead, the child may be only listless and reluctant to eat. Because the blood volume is so small in the newborn child, the volume of blood lost in an intracranial hemorrhage may be enough to cause shock, and later the resorption of blood pigments may cause hyperbilirubinemia.

If the infant survives, the injuries are healed by gliosis. The cerebral cortices may show foci of granular atrophy, laminar necrosis, or more extensive lesions. In the white matter, gliosis is sometimes extensive in the centrum semiovale, often with a meshwork of cysts in the gliosis, a condition called cystic degeneration. The volume of the cerebral hemispheres and corpus callosum are sometimes greatly reduced, partially by the gliosis, partially because of impaired postnatal development.

Foci of gliosis and cystic degeneration cause shrinkage of the basal ganglia. Loss of neurons in the cerebral cortex causes secondary atrophy of the thalamus. Foci of gliosis with loss of neurons may be found in the cerebellum. Injury to the nuclei of a cranial nerve can cause weakness, paralysis, or atrophy of the muscles supplied. Probably birth injury is the usual cause of Möbius's syndrome, named after the German neurologist who described it in 1888, in which there is a combination of facial paralysis and ophthalmoplegia.

ULEGYRIA. Ulegyria, from the Greek for a scar and a ring, results from foci of cortical necrosis in the cerebrum or less often the cerebellum. It is caused by hypoxia at birth. A gyrus or group of adjacent gyri are shrunken, often with preservation of the crown of the gyrus, but severe shrinkage of its base. The affected gyri show gliosis, often with small

cysts. The myelinated fibers at the edge of the necrosis are usually compacted so that the margin seems overmyelinated. The white matter deep to the lesion shows demyelination because of the loss of neurons. At times there are in addition foci of granular atrophy of the cerebral cortex or laminar atrophy.

PERIVENTRICULAR LEUKOMALACIA. Periventricular leukomalacia is the name given to the foci of necrosis of the white matter, sometimes hemorrhagic, sometimes not, that are found in the cerebral hemispheres near the superior or lateral surfaces of the lateral ventricles in 20% of infants dying under one month of age. Macrophages take up the fatty debris of the dead tissue. Astrocytes proliferate, and the necrotic tissue is gradually replaced by gliosis, often with small cysts in the glial scar. Periventricular leukomalacia is due to hypoxia and is most common where the regions supplied by two of the cerebral arteries meet.

ÉTAT MARBRÉ. In état marbré, the myelinated nerve fibers in the corpus striatum and thalamus are aggregated into bundles considerably larger and coarser than is normal. In sections stained for myelin they form an irregular meshwork like the veins in marble, explaining the name état marbré given this condition from the French or status marmoratus if you prefer Latin. In état marbré, there is usually considerable loss of neurons and gliosis in the intervening parts of the affected nuclei. État marbré occurs only in infants and nearly always is due to birth injury. Rarely, it complicates meningitis or some other illness. The patients usually develop athetosis.

METABOLIC DISORDERS

The metabolic disorders of the nervous system are divided into the neuronal storage diseases, in which enzyme deficiency causes accumulation of a metabolic product or products in the neurons; the leukodystrophies, in which an enzyme deficiency damages principally the white matter of the nervous system; the injuries caused by poisoning; nutritional deficiencies; injuries caused by disease of other organs; and disorder of uncertain cause.

Neuronal Storage Diseases

Many kinds of enzyme deficiency result in the storage of a metabolic product or products in the neurons. Some of these disorders seriously injure the brain. Some cause only minor disability. Some injure principally the brain, with only minor changes in other organs. In some, the injury to the nervous system is overshadowed by injury to some other part of the body.

The neuronal storage diseases are all uncommon. Most result from the lack of a single lysosomal enzyme. Most are inherited as an autosomal recessive character. Most appear in infancy or childhood and progress inexorably. Most cause mental retardation, progressive dementia, repeated seizures, and increasing paralysis, usually bringing death within a few years.

SPHINGOLIPIDOSES. In the sphingolipidoses, lack of one or more lysosomal enzymes results in the storage of large quantities of sphingolipid, sometimes together with other lipids, in the lysosomes of the neurons and other cells. In Tay-Sachs disease, the lipid stored is principally the ganglioside G_{M2}. In Fabry's disease, it is mainly galactosylgalactosylglucosyl ceramide; in Gaucher's disease, glucosyl ceramide; in Niemann-Pick's disease, sphingomyelin; in G_{M1} ganglcosidosis, G_{M1} ganglioside; and in the extremely rare lactosyl ceramidosis, lactosyl ceramide.

Fabry's disease affects principally the kidneys and is discussed in Chapter 27. Niemann-Pick's disease and Gaucher's disease involve mainly the macrophages and are described in Chapter 51. Tay-Sachs disease, other forms of G_{M2} gangliosidosis, G_{M1} gangliosidosis, and lactosyl ceramidosis are most prominent in the brain and are considered in this section.

Tay-Sachs Disease. Tay-Sachs disease is named after the English ophthalmologist Tay who described it in 1881 and the American neurologist Sachs who discussed it in 1887. It is often called G_{M2} gangliosidosis, after the ganglioside that is the principal substance that accumulates in the affected cells. The G in G_{M2} stands for ganglioside; M is for mono, meaning that the ganglioside contains one residue of sialic acid; and 2 means that the molecule falls electrophoretically into the second group of gangliosides, those with three hexose residues. Formerly, the disease was called amaurotic family idiocy, from the Greek darkening or blinding.

Most patients with Tay-Sachs disease are Jewish. Among the Ashkenazi Jews in the United States, 1 child in every 6000 born alive develops the disease. In other races, only 1 child in 500,000 is affected. The disease is inherited as an autosomal recessive character. Heterozygotes suffer no disability. In the united States, 1 Jew in 30 carries the abnormal gene. In other Americans, 1 person in 300 harbors it.

Lesions. In Tay-Sachs disease, the brain may be of normal size, abnormally large, or abnormally small. Usually it is firm or indurated. There may be ulegyria. The gray matter of the cerebral cortex is thinned. The centrum ovale is often grayish and edematous. The cerebellum, brain stem, and optic nerves are often small and atrophic.

Microscopically, neurons in the brain, peripheral ganglia, and myenteric plexuses are distended by fine, cytoplasmic granules, which stain brightly with the periodic acid-Schiff reaction and with Luxol fast blue, stain strongly for acid phosphatase, are often metachromatic, and usually stain for fat. Electron microscopy shows the granules to be lysosomes. They are membrane bound, electron dense, and concentrically laminated. Chemical analysis shows that the granules contain G_{M2} ganglioside. Particularly in the cerebellum, there are often local swellings called torpedo bodies in the axons or dendrites of the affected neurons.

The affected neurons die and in the brain are replaced by gliosis, explaining the firmness of the brain. Demyelination occurs in the white matter around the axons of the dead neurons and excites further gliosis. Often the demyelination is greater than can be explained by the loss of neurons, suggesting that there is direct injury to the white matter as well as the secondary changes resulting from the loss of neurons. Macrophages take up the fatty debris of the degenerating myelin and dead neurons and phagocytose the G_{M2} ganglioside from the dead neurons.

A red spot is visible in the macula of the retina in many of the patients. Loss of neurons allows the choroid to shine through. Late in the disease, retinitis pigmentosa or more extensive degeneration of the retina sometimes develops.

Other tissues are little affected in G_{M2} gangliosidosis. A few macrophages in the liver or spleen may contain G_{M2} in their lysosomes, as may other cells. A few of the lymphocytes in the blood may be vacuolated. In tissue culture, fibrocytes store G_{M2}.

Clinical Presentation. The classic or infantile form of Tay-Sachs disease becomes evident when the child is about six months old. Lassitude, mental retardation, loss of vision, excessive reaction to noise, spasticity, paralysis, and often convulsions grow more severe. A cherry red spot is often present in the eyes. The head sometimes enlarges. Death usually comes before the child is three years old.

The juvenile form of the disease presents when the child is two to six years old. Increasing spasticity, difficulty with speech, dystonia, and seizures develop. Blindness follows. Death usually comes after about 10 years.

The adult form of Tay-Sachs disease causes muscular atrophy, incoordination, dystonia, and dysarthria. Intellect and vision are not impaired.

Pathogenesis. Tay-Sachs disease is caused by a lack of the enzyme hexosaminidase A. Both G_{M2} and G_{A2}, a similar cerebroside but lacking the sialic acid residue, accumulate in the affected neurons. The storage of G_{M2} is predominant, for it cannot be hydrolyzed by the hexosaminidase B still present. This enzyme can split G_{A2}.

Treatment and Prognosis. No treatment is available for Tay-Sachs disease. The missing enzyme cannot be replaced.

Because the concentration of hexosaminidase A in the serum is reduced in asymptomatic heterozygotes bearing the gene that causes Tay-Sachs disease, people carrying the gene can be warned of the danger that their children may develop the disease. The deficiency of hexosaminidase A can also be demonstrated in the amniotic fluid and amniotic cells during pregnancy if the fetus has the abnormal gene. If all such fetuses were detected during pregnancy and therapeutic abortions were performed, Tay-Sachs disease could be eradicated.

Other G_{M2} Sphingolipidoses. Other forms of G_{M2} sphingolipidosis are similar clinically to Tay-Sachs disease. In Sandler's disease, hexosaminidases A and B are both deficient. G_{M2} ganglioside, G_{A2} ganglioside, and globoside accumulate in the neurons, hepatocytes, renal tubular epithelial cells, pancreatic epithelium, and macrophages. In the AB variant of G_{M2} sphingolipidosis, lack of an activator renders hexosaminidases A and B inactive.

G_{M1} Sphingolipidosis. Lack of β-galactosidase causes the accumulation of G_{M1} ganglioside, glycoprotein, and keratin sulfate in neurons and other cells. When symptoms develop in infancy, the children are mentally retarded, with seizures, hepatosplenomegaly, macroglossia, and multiple bony lesions like those of Morquio's disease. Many have a cherry red spot in the retina. Death usually comes within a year. In the juvenile form of the disease, the lesions are less severe, but death comes within 10 years. When it occurs in adult life, bony lesions and corneal opacity are often predominant.

Lactosyl ceramidosis. Lactosyl ceramidosis is rare, affects the brain as does Tay-Sachs disease, causes similar symptoms, and brings death in a few years. Lactosyl ceramide and glucocerebroside accumulate in the liver and other organs as well as in the neurons. The disorder is closely related to Niemann-Pick disease.

MUCOPOLYSACCHARIDOSES. In the mucopolysaccharidoses, enzyme deficiency causes the accumulation of mucopolysaccharides and sometimes sphingolipids in the affected cells. Most of these disorders affect the brain, causing mental retardation, but they injure the bones more severely and are discussed with the diseases of bone (Chapter 59).

NEURONAL CEROID LIPOFUSCINOSIS. Neuronal ceroid lipofuscinosis is sometimes called Batten's disease after the English ophthalmologist who reported it in 1903. Ceroid and lipofuscin accumulate in cells throughout the body. The cause of the disease is unknown. In most patients, the disorder is inherited as an autosomal recessive character.

Neurons in the central and peripheral nervous systems are distended with granules of golden brown pigment that stains strongly with fat stains and with the periodic acid-Schiff reaction. Electron microscopy shows the pigment to be within lysosomes, sometimes forming lamellar structures, multivesicular bodies, or other patterns. In the brain, loss of neurons causes gliosis, demyelination, and cerebral atrophy. Similar pigment accumulates in macrophages, leukocytes, muscle, and other cells. The lymphocytes in the blood are vacuolated. Neutrophils are sometimes hypersegmented.

In infants, the disease causes dementia, convulsions, blindness, motor dysfunction, retinitis pigmentosa, and macular degeneration. The accumulation of pigment in other parts of the body causes little dysfunction. Death comes in a few years. In older children, the course is similar but less rapid. In adults, Batten's disease is less severe. The adult form of the disease may be identical with Kufs' disease, named after the German neurologist who described it in 1925.

ASPARTYLGLUCOSAMINURIA. In aspartylglucosaminuria, deficiency of aspartylglucosamine amidase causes aspartylglucosamine and glycopeptides to accumulate in the lysosomes of cells throughout the body. The patients excrete aspartylglucosamine in the urine. Many have acne or dermatitis caused by photosensitivity. Some have corneal opacities. Lymphocytes in the blood are vacuolated. The disease usually occurs in young adults and causes mental retardation.

FARBER'S DISEASE. Farber's disease, sometimes called lipogranulomatosis, is named after the American physician who described it in 1952. Ceramidase deficiency causes ceramide to accumulate in lysosomes in neurons and macrophages. Neurons are distended with ceramide. Subcutaneous nodules appear in the skin, especially near joints. Microscopically, the nodules consist of lymphocytes and macrophages. Many of the macrophages are distended with ceramide. Similar nodules appear in the synovium of joints and tendon sheaths. Large quantities of ceramide are stored in the liver, lungs, and kidneys. The concentration of protein in the cerebrospinal fluid is increased. Symptoms begin in infancy with hoarseness, arthritis, physical and sometimes mental retardation.

TYPE II GLYCOGEN STORAGE DISEASE. In Pompe's disease, described in Chapter 36, neurons throughout the body are distended with glycogen. There may be some loss of neurons with gliosis, but neurologic dysfunction is minor.

Leukodystrophies

The leukodystrophies are caused by deficiency of one of the enzymes needed for the formation or maintenance of myelin. All are uncommon. In most patients, the defect is inherited as an autosomal recessive character.

Symptoms of a leukodystrophy usually begin in infancy or childhood, less often in adults. Infants affected are often mentally retarded and show progressive ataxia and paralysis followed by seizures, dementia, blindness, deafness, and decerebrate rigidity. In older children and adults the disease is frequently milder, often dominated by behavioral changes, psychosis, or dementia. The diagnosis can be established in some of the leukodystrophies by demonstrating the enzyme deficiency in cultured fibrocytes or by other means. Death usually comes within a few years, though a few patients have survived for more than 20 years. No treatment is known.

SUDANOPHILIC LEUKODYSTROPHY. Sudanophilic leukodystrophy is the commonest of the leukodystrophies. Its cause is unknown. Cholesterol esters and other lipids accumulate in macrophages, astrocytes, and other cells. The lipid stains strongly with the Sudan dyes for fat, giving the condition its name.

Macroscopically, the brain is shrunken because of the reduction in the volume of the white matter. The ventricles are dilated. The gyri of the cerebral cortex are narrow. The inferior olives are prominent in the medulla. The core of the cerebral hemispheres feels hard beneath the soft cortex. On section, the white matter throughout the central nervous system is affected, with the exception of the arcuate fibers immediately beneath the cerebral cortex. The white matter is blue or gray, usually indurated, but sometimes rarefied. Occasionally cysts are scattered in the white matter.

Microscopically, demyelination is widespread throughout the central nervous system. Macrophages are full of fatty debris. Globules of fat lie free in the tissue fluid. Fat is abundant in hyperplastic astrocytes in and around the lesions. At first, the axons persist undamaged, and there is little or no change in the neurons. Later, axons are progressively destroyed, with secondary changes in their neurons. Neurons in the basal ganglia degenerate when the cortical axons that synapse with them are destroyed. As time passes, gliosis increases in the white matter, explaining its induration. The quantity of fat in the lesions becomes less.

Demyelination in the peripheral nerves is usually segmental. Myelin is lost from one node of Ranvier to the next, but is preserved in adjacent segments of the nerve fiber.

ADRENOLEUKODYSTROPHY. Adrenoleukodystrophy is inherited as an X-linked recessive character. The patients are boys or young men. Long chain fatty acid esters accumulate in the nervous system and adrenal glands. The urinary excretion of fatty acids having from 22 to 26 carbon atoms is increased. The nervous system shows widespread demyelination like that in sudanophilic leukodystrophy. In most patients, the brain is severely affected. In some, the neurologic lesions affect principally the peripheral nerves. Macrophages and other cells in lesions in the brain and peripheral nerves, the cells of the zona fasciculata of the adrenal glands, and, to a lesser degree, those of the zona reticularis, are distended with droplets of lipid. Electron microscopy shows parallel or twisted trilaminar lamellae in the affected cells. Progressive atrophy of the affected zones of the adrenal glands follows, often with an exudate of lymphocytes and fibrosis. The patients develop adrenal deficiency as well as increasing neurologic dysfunction. Death usually comes in a few years.

KRABBE'S DISEASE. Krabbe's disease, also called globoid cell leukodystrophy and galactosylceramide lipidosis, is named after the Danish neurologist who described it in 1916. A deficiency of galactosylceramide β-galactosidase inherited as an autosomal recessive character allows galactocerebroside to accumulate in globoid cells in the brain and in macrophages and Schwann cells in the peripheral nerves. The disease usually begins in infancy, with irritability, fever, and seizures. The concentration of protein in the cerebrospinal fluid is frequently increased. Death comes within two years.

Macroscopically, the brain is shrunken. Its white matter is indurated. Microscopically, the brain shows extensive demyelination, usually with considerable loss of axons. Often only the subcortical arcuate fibers remain intact. The peripheral nerves frequently show segmental demyelination.

Globoid cells accumulate in the lesions in the central nervous system. They are spheroidal and may have one or several nuclei. Most are 20 to 25 μm across. Some are larger. Their cytoplasm stains weakly with stains for fat, but strongly with the periodic acid-Schiff reaction. Electron microscopy shows tubular inclusions in their cytoplasm. The tubules vary from 10 to 100 nm in diameter. Most are free in the cytoplasm. Some are membrane bound. The globoid cells are probably altered macrophages. Often smaller macrophages called epithelioid cells are also present. Globoid cells are numerous only in Krabbe's disease, though an occasional cell of similar structure can be found in other conditions.

Globoid cells are not found in the peripheral nerves. Instead, material like that in the globoid cells is present in macrophages and Schwann cells in the demyelinated segments of the nerves. It stains as does the material in the globoid cells. By electron microscopy, the macrophages and Schwann cells contain tubular inclusions like those of the globoid cells.

METACHROMATIC LEUKODYSTROPHY. Metachromatic leukodystrophy, also called sulfatide lipidosis, occurs in 1 live birth in 40,000. Deficiency of arylsulfatase A inherited as an autosomal recessive character causes accumulation of galactosyl sulfatides in glial cells, neurons, Schwann cells, and in macrophages and epithelial cells throughout the body. Less often, deficiency of the sphingolipid activator protein 1 causes similar dysfunction. The disease usually begins in infancy with mental retardation and optic atrophy. Less often it causes psychosis or dementia in an older child or an adult.

The brain is usually small, but occasionally is of normal size or is enlarged. Extensive demyelination and gliosis in the brain spares the subcortical arcuate fibers. In some patients, the number of oligodendrocytes in the brain is reduced. Segmental demyelination in peripheral nerves is common.

In the demyelinated regions in the brain, granular bodies that stain metachromatically with dyes such as cresyl violet are present in the tissue fluid, macrophages, microglial cells, astrocytes, oligodendrocytes, and sometimes in neurons. In the tissue fluid, the metachromatic bodies are spheroidal and up to 30 μm across. In the cells they are smaller. The bodies are brown when stained with cresyl violet and stain strongly with Sudan black and with the periodic acid-Schiff reaction. Because the solvents used to prepare paraffin sections dissolve sulfatides, the metachromatic bodies are best seen in frozen sections. Electron microscopy shows flat or concentric lamellae in lysosomes.

In peripheral nerves, the metachromatic inclusions are present in macrophages and Schwann cells. The inclusions in the Schwann cells are best seen in segments in which the myelin is intact.

Irregularly shaped and variously sized granules of metachromatic sulfatides are present in the renal tubular epithelium and often in the epithelial cells of the liver, gallbladder, pancreas, adrenal glands, and ovaries. Renal tubular cells containing the inclusions can be detected in the urine. Metachromatic granules are present in macrophages in lymph nodes.

MULTIPLE SULFATASE DEFICIENCY. In multiple sulfatase deficiency, arylsulfatases A, B, and C and extralysosomal sulfatases are deficient. The disorder is inherited as an autosomal recessive character and causes metachromatic leukodystrophy, bony lesions like those of Hurler's disease, and ichthyosis. Gangliosides as well as sulfatides are stored in macrophages, glial cells, neurons, and epithelial cells. Neuronal and hepatic involvement is more extensive than in the usual form of metachromatic leukodystrophy. Often the neurons containing metachromatic bodies are ballooned. Macrophages filled with sulfatide are numerous in the spleen.

SPONGIFORM LEUKODYSTROPHY. Canavan's disease, also called spongiform leukodystrophy, is named after the American neurologist who reported a case in 1931. It is inherited as an autosomal recessive character, but the nature of the defect has not been determined. No abnormal material is stored in the brain or elsewhere. The patients are often Jewish. Symptoms usually begin in infancy or childhood. Dementia and enlargement of the head lead to spastic paralysis and death within a few years.

Demyelination is most extensive in the centrum semiovale, though other parts of the brain are affected. The subcortical arcuate fibers are usually destroyed. The affected white matter is severely edematous. Vacuoles and larger spaces are present between surviving axons and glial processes. The astrocytes with large, vesicular nuclei but little cytoplasm called Alzheimer II cells are prominent in the lesions, but there is little gliosis.

PELIZAEUS-MERZBACHER DISEASE. Pelizaeus-Merzbacher disease was reported by Pelizaeus from Germany in 1885 and by Merzbacher from Argentina in 1910. It occurs in boys and men and is probably inherited as an X-linked character. No enzyme deficiency has been identified. No abnormal product is stored. The course is more prolonged than in other forms of leukodystrophy. In infants, it causes nystagmus, tremor, ataxia, mental retardation, and eventually spastic paralysis. In adults, it causes psychoasis. Demyelination is extensive, but islands of well-preserved white matter persist in the demyelinated regions.

ALEXANDER'S DISEASE. Alexander's disease, which is named after the New Zealand pathologist who described it in 1949, does not seem to be a genetic disorder. Dementia, paralysis, and epilepsy begin in infancy or childhood. In infants, the head enlarges. The lesions are similar to those of spongiform leukodystrophy, but in addition irregular, elongated, hyaline structures called Rosenthal fibers after the German pathologist who described them in 1898 accumulate in the brain, especially around blood vessels in the white matter. The fibers stain strongly for myelin.

Poisoning

The poisons that affect the nervous system are discussed in Chapter 24. Among the more important are carbon monoxide, cyanides, and methanol, which interfere with cellular respiration and produce lesions like those of hypoxia. Mercury, lead, manganese, and carbon tetrachloride cause major injury to the brain. Lathyrism can destroy the long tracts in the spinal cord. Arsenic, lead, thallium, and anticholinesterases cause peripheral neuropathy. Hypervitaminosis A increases intracranial pressure.

Phenothiazines cause parkinsonism or retinopathy in 15% of patients treated. Hydantoins and other psychotropic drugs can cause loss of Purkinje cells. Vincristine, vinblastine, colchicine, aluminum, and lathyrogenic agents induce neurofibrillary tangles like those of Alzheimer's disease. Ergot causes degeneration of the posterior columns in the spinal cord, convulsions, or psychosis. Organic tin compounds induce focal edema in the myelin sheaths that resolves when the drug is withdrawn. Isoniazid and thalidomide sometimes cause peripheral neuropathy.

ETHANOL INTOXICATION. Little is known of the changes in the brain in acute ethanol intoxication. Probably the ethanol and acetaldehyde in the blood cause transient congestion and edema.

Chronic alcoholism sometimes causes thickening of the meninges, atrophy of the brain, and enlargement of the ventricles. Neurons are lost throughout the brain. Sometimes the loss is greatest in the parietal and frontal cortex, especially in the third layer. Sometimes it involves principally the granular cells and later the Purkinje cells in the cerebellum. If the gliosis induced by the loss of neurons in the cerebral cortex is unusually prominent, the condition is called laminar cortical sclerosis. The thiamine deficiency common in chronic alcoholics often causes Wernicke's syndrome or peripheral neuropathy.

Marchiafava-Bignami Disease. Marchiafava-Bignami disease, named after the Italian pathologists who described it in 1903, is an uncommon complication of chronic alcoholism found principally in those addicted to red wine. The brain shows demyelination of the central part of the corpus callosum and sometimes of other parts of the white matter. Axons in the lesions sometimes survive, sometimes are destroyed. The adventitia of the blood vessels in the lesions in thickened. Gliosis is slight. As years pass, the patients' intellect is increasingly impaired. Convulsions, hallucinations, dementia paralysis, in-

continence, and stupor sometimes progress to coma and death.

Central Pontine Myelinolysis. Central pontine myelinolysis is a rare complication of chronic alcoholism. It causes demyelination of the central part of the pons and loss of oligodendrocytes. The axons in the lesions are usually preserved.

Nutritional Deficiencies

The nutritional deficiencies are discussed in Chapter 22. Nicotinamide deficiency causes loss of neurons in the brain and demyelination of the long tracts in the spinal cord. Lack of vitamin K results in petechial hemorrhages in the brain. Lack of vitamin B_{12} causes subacute combined degeneration of the spinal cord. Pyridoxine deficiency and nicotinamide deficiency sometimes cause peripheral neuropathy.

Thiamine deficiency is common in alcoholics. It causes Wernicke's syndrome with loss of neurons in the mamillary bodies and elsewhere in the gray matter around the third ventricle and aqueduct. Peripheral neuropathy that begins peripherally and extends centrally is common in alcoholics and in beriberi.

Secondary to Disease of Other Organs

A number of diseases of other parts of the body cause metabolic derangements that damage the nervous system. In many of these conditions the damage to the nervous system is mild or is evident only in a minority of the patients. In some, the damage to the nervous system is great.

HYPOGLYCEMIA. If the blood sugar falls below 1.5 mmol/L (30 mg/100 mL), the patient often develops headache or becomes restless and confused, perhaps with visual disturbances. If it falls below 1.0 mmol/L (20 mg/100 ml), stupor, coma, and convulsions are likely. If severe hypoglycemia is allowed to persist or if attacks of hypoglycemia are repeated, permanent injury to the brain follows.

The injury to the brain caused by hypoglycemia is similar to that caused by hypoxia.

If oxidative metabolism in the neurons is interrupted for more than a few minutes, the more sensitive neurons begin to die. It makes little difference whether the interruption is due to lack of oxygen, lack of glucose, or to poisoning of the necessary enzymes by an agent such as cyanide. Hypoglycemia causes laminar necrosis in the cerebral cortex like that caused by hypoxia, and similar injury to the hippocampi, but usually damages the basal ganglia and the cerebellum less severely than does hypoxia. Rarely, hypoglycemia causes peripheral neuropathy.

HEPATIC FAILURE.   Hepatic failure, which is discussed in Chapter 36, causes the serious, even fatal injury to the brain called hepatic encephalopathy. The metabolic derangement caused by the liver disease can result in diffuse but patchy loss of neurons in the cerebral cortex, basal ganglia, and cerebellum, with a prominent proliferation of Alzheimer II astrocytes, with their large, vesicular nuclei surrounded by little or no cytoplasm. Vacuoles of glycogen are common in the nuclei of the astrocytes. Occasionally small cavities form in the cerebral cortex or basal ganglia.

HEPATOLENTICULAR DEGENERATION.   Hepatolenticular degeneration, or Wilson's disease, is described in Chapter 9. It causes serious loss of neurons in the corpus striatum, cerebral and cerebellar cortices, and nuclei of the brain stem. Often cysts develop in the putamen. Alzheimer II astrocytes are numerous in the injured regions. The Opalski cells peculiar to Wilson's disease are present in the thalamus and elsewhere. Fibrous gliosis is not prominent.

REYE'S SYNDROME.   The encephalopathy characteristic of Reye's syndrome, is described in Chapter 36. In spite of the severity of the dysfunction, the brain shows only severe edema and patchy loss of neurons, without inflammatory response.

KERNICTERUS.   Kernicterus is discussed in Chapter 9. If the concentration of unconjugated bilirubin in the plasma becomes very high in infants with hemolytic disease of the newborn or adults with the Crigler-Najjar syndrome, the blood-brain barrier is breached, allowing unconjugated bilirubin to escape into the basal ganglia. The bilirubin inhibits oxidative phosphorylation in the neurons, and necrosis of neurons in the basal ganglia

follows. The response to the necrosis is similar to that in hypoxia.

RENAL FAILURE.   The changes in the nervous system caused by renal failure are discussed in Chapter 27. Uremia often causes apathy, fatigue, or inability to concentrate, less frequently hallucinations, stupor, or twitching. The brain shows little abnormality, sometimes an increase in protoplasmic astrocytes. The movement of water into the brain during dialysis often causes headaches and sometimes more serious but temporary dysfunction. A few patients on dialysis develop dysarthria, myoclonus, seizures, and progressive dementia. Most of these people die within a year. The brain shows microcavitation throughout the cerebral cortices, probably caused by an excess of aluminum in the dialysate or given by mouth.

AMINOACIDURIA.   The aminoacidurias are discussed in Chapter 27. Hartnup disease, Lowe's syndrome, phenylketonuria, maple sugar disease, argininosuccinic aciduria, histidinemia, and hyperglycinemia can injure the brain, usually causing mental retardation. Galactosemia, described in Chapter 36 causes similar injury. Interference with the maturation of the brain causes focal or widespread demyelination, and sometimes focal necrosis with cysts in the gray or white matter.

CARCINOMA AND LYMPHOMA.   More than 5% of patients with carcinoma develop neurologic dysfunction, and occasionally a patient with lymphoma or multiple myeloma does so. Carcinomata of the lungs, especially oat cell carcinomata, are particularly likely to damage the nervous system, but carcinoma of the stomach, ovaries, and other organs can do so. Sometimes a patient with carcinoma or lymphoma develops more than one type of neurologic injury. The cause of the neurologic dysfunction is unknown. Neurologic dysfunction caused by a tumor is often called a paraneoplastic syndrome.

Peripheral neuropathy is one of the more common neurologic manifestations of carcinoma and can occur in lymphoma, multiple myeloma and Waldenström's macroglobulinemia. Segmental demyelination of the affected nerves often is accompanied by degeneration of the axons, to give a mixed sensory and motor neuropathy. The lesions are usually most severe in the lower limbs, but can be widespread. The cranial nerves are usually spared.

Degeneration of the cerebellar cortex causes cerebellar ataxia, at first with excitement and confusion, later with dementia. Purkinje cells and granular cells are lost. Gliosis increases in the damaged regions. Often perivascular cuffing with lymphocytes is prominent. Lymphocytes are frequently numerous in the overlying meninges. The direct spinocerebellar tracts in the spinal cord often show demyelination. The cerebrospinal fluid shows an excess of cells and protein.

Less often neurons are lost in the cingulate or orbital cortices, hippocampal formations, amygdaloid nuclei, brain stem, anterior horns of the spinal cord, or posterior root ganglia. The lesions are like those in the cerebellum, with secondary demyelination in the tracts or nerves affected. The dysfunction produced depends on the site of the lesion.

Probably related to these injuries to the nervous system is the polymyositis that sometimes causes muscular weakness in patients with carcinoma, a weakness that may antedate the discovery of the carcinoma by months or years, and conditions like myasthenia gravis or the Eaton-Lambert syndrome that sometimes develop in patients with cancer.

ACUTE PORPHYRIA. The porphyrias are discussed in Chapter 9. Peripheral neuropathy and mental changes are prominent in the acute hepatic form of the disease. The brain shows only hypoxic injury, sometimes with small infarcts, which may be caused by vascular spasm. The peripheral nerves affected show irregular, patchy demyelination, eventually with injury to the axons.

DIABETES MELLITUS. Peripheral neuropathy occurs in more than 30% of diabetics usually in people over 50 years old. It is most often mainly sensory, sometimes with hyperesthesia and attacks of severe pain. Less often there is diabetic amyotrophy, with wasting of the muscles of the upper anterior thigh, often with pain.

The affected nerves show segemental demyelination. At first, the axons are spared, and recovery of function is possible, but later the axons are destroyed. In most patients, the neuropathy is slowly progressive. The cause is uncertain. Some think diabetic neuropathy is due to vascular insufficiency. Others favor a direct metabolic injury to the nerves.

MALABSORPTION. Patients with adult celiac disease or Whipple's disease sometimes develop peripheral neuropathy or occasionally changes in the brain like those of Wernicke's syndrome. Both the neuropathy and the changes in the brain result from the complex metabolic derangement caused by the malabsorption.

Other Metabolic Disorders

A few diseases of the nervous system believed due to a metabolic derangement do not fit into any of the groups already discussed.

SUBACUTE NECROTIZING ENCEPHALOMYELOPATHY. Subacute necrotizing encephalomyelopathy, sometimes called Leigh's disease after the British physician who described it in 1951, usually occurs in infants and brings death within several months. Less often it follows a chronic course or begins in an adult. The infants fail to thrive and develop muscular spasticity or flaccidity, convulsions, loss of reflexes, ataxia, and often optic atrophy. Lactic acidosis, ketoacidosis, and hyperalaninemia are common. In some patients, the disease is probably inherited as an autosomal recessive character.

Lesions are most common in the thalamus, subthalamic nuclei, substantia nigra, and gray matter of the pons and medulla. Less often the corpus striatum, cerebral cortex, and posterior columns of the spinal cord are involved. The mamillary bodies are not often affected. The lesions show a patchy loss of neurons and hyperplasia of astrocytes and microglial cells. Proliferating capillaries are prominent in the lesions.

HALLERVORDEN-SPATZ DISEASE. Hallervorden-Spatz disease is named after the German physicians who described it in 1922. The patients are nearly always under 30 years of age, often children. They present with progressive rigidity, first in the lower limbs, then in the upper, and eventually in the face. Often there are choreiform or athetoid movements. Often there is mental deterioration. Some infants with Hallervorden-Spatz disease die in a few months; some live for several years. Older patients live from 1 to 30 years. Probably the disease is inherited as an autosomal recessive character.

The globus pallidus and reticular zone of the substantia nigra are stained brown by an increase in the iron-containing pigment normally present in these regions. Granules of pigment lie within neurons, astrocytes, and microglial cells, and are free in the extracellular space. They stain strongly with the periodic acid-Schiff reaction. In the pigmented regions, the loss of neurons is sometimes severe, sometimes slight, with demyelination and gliosis. Sometimes there is minor pigmentation or minor loss of neurons in other parts of the brain. The blood vessels in the pigmented regions are encrusted with iron and calcium. Often concretions containing calcium and iron lie free in the extracellular space.

Large, globular bodies called spheroids develop on axons, probably near their distal ends. They are most frequent in the lesions, but occur throughout the central nervous system. A spheroid is larger than a neuron. Its cytoplasm contains many organelles and neurofilaments. Often tubules 30 to 40 nm in diameter and smooth membranes are abundant in the spheroid. Similar structures occur in infantile neuroaxonal dystrophy and sometimes in encephalitis, around traumatic or ischemic lesions of the brain, or in old people without neurologic dysfunction. They are occasionally found in patients with diabetes mellitus, alcoholism, mucoviscidosis, or congenital biliary atresia.

INFANTILE NEUROAXONAL DYSTROPHY. In infantile neuroaxonal dystrophy, spheroids like those of Hallervorden-Spatz disease are numerous in the cerebrum, cerebellum, and brain stem. Focal destruction of neurons excites gliosis. Symptoms begin in infancy or childhood and progress to death in 1 to 10 years. The nature of the symptoms is determined by the site of the lesions.

TROPICAL NEUROMYELOPATHY. Tropical neuromyelopathy occurs in the Caribbean, West Africa, India, and Japan. The patients become weak and unsteady, with numbness and burning in the legs, and often become deaf or have impaired vision. Less often, muscular spasticity develops. The disorder is probably caused by drinking casava or some other toxic product.

Perivascular cuffing with lymphocytes, plasma cells, and macrophages is usually greatest in the gray matter of the spinal cord, but often involves less severely the brain stem, cerebellum, and cerebral cortex. Fibrosis sometimes develops around the inflamed vessels. Neurons are lost in the affected regions. Sometimes there is demyelination of the lateral pyramidal or spinocerebellar tracts, or the posterior columns. Peripheral nerves involved are inflamed and demyelinated.

KINKY HAIR DISEASE. Kinky hair disease, or Menkes' syndrome as it is called after the American pediatrician who described it in 1962, is inherited as an X-linked recessive character and occurs only in boys. In Melbourne, it occurs in 1 live birth in 35,000. The infant feeds poorly, gains weight poorly, and often has transient jaundice. Drowsiness and lethargy with seizures and progressive mental deterioration become evident at about four weeks of age. Death comes within a few years.

The patients have thick, pallid skin. Their hair is white or gray, stiff, erect, often sharply kinked, and breaks easily, leaving steely bristles. Malformation of collagen and elastin causes dissecting aneurysms, cardiac rupture, emphysema, and osteoporosis. The brain shows foci of neuronal loss in the cerebral cortex, basal ganglia, and cerebellum, with gliosis in these regions. The Purkinje cells have tortuous dendrites and show focal swelling of their dendrites and axons. The white matter shows secondary demyelination, with gliosis and sometimes small cysts.

Kinky hair disease is caused by disordered copper metabolism. The uptake of copper in the intestine is normal, and metal is present in normal or increased quantity in the intestine, kidneys, and dermis, but its concentration in the plasma, liver, and brain is low. The concentration of ceruloplasmin in the plasma is reduced. The activity of some copper containing enzymes is impaired.

CEREBROTENDINOUS XANTHOMATOSIS. *Cerebrotendinous xanthomatosis* is a rare familial disease in which defective synthesis of bile acids causes accumulation of cholesterol and cholestanol in macrophages throughout the body. It becomes evident during adolescence and causes mental retardation, slowly progressive cerebellar dysfunction, and myoclonus. It ends with bulbar or spinal paralysis.

Foci of demyelination are most severe in the cerebellum and superior cerebellar peduncles but occur throughout the brain and spinal cord. Macrophages filled with cholestanol are numerous in the lesions and are present in tendons, bones, the lungs, and other organs. The macrophages form clumps together with lymphocytes. They have foamy cytoplasm. Some are multinucleate. Often large, needle-shaped crystals are present between the macrophages. Similar clumps of macrophages form xanthelasmata on the eyelids.

DEMYELINATING DISEASES

Multiple sclerosis, Baló's concentric sclerosis, Schilder's disease, perivenous encephalomyelitis, and acute necrotizing hemorrhagic encephalomyelitis are grouped together as the demyelinating diseases. Demyelination is common and sometimes extensive in many other diseases and injuries of the central and peripheral nervous systems, but the term *demyelinating disease* has become restricted to these disorders. Foci of demyelination develop in the central nervous system, but the axons for the most part remain intact.

MULTIPLE SCLEROSIS. Multiple sclerosis, sometimes called disseminated sclerosis, is the commonest serious disease of the nervous system in North America, Europe, and Australasia. It is much less frequent in Japan, the East, and South Africa and is rare in central Africa. In North America, Europe, and Australasia, its frequency varies with the latitude. North of 40°N, which runs near New York and Madrid and south of 40°S, which runs between the North and South Islands of New Zealand and between the Australian continent and Tasmania, from 30 to 60 people in every 100,000 have multiple sclerosis. In the more southerly parts of Europe and North America and in the more northerly parts of Australia and New Zealand, the prevalence is 10 per 100,000. In the United States, the disease is equally frequent in black and white people.

Adults who move from a region in which the risk of developing multiple sclerosis is high to a place where the risk is low remain liable to develop the disease. Children who move from a high risk region to a low risk area are in no greater danger than the inhabitants of the low risk area.

Over 70% of patients with multiple sclerosis are between 20 and 40 years old when symptoms begin. The disease is rare in children under 10 years old and seldom begins in adults over 50 years old. Men and women are equally affected.

Lesions. In some patients dying of multiple sclerosis, the surfaces of the brain and spinal cord are normal macroscopically. In many, the brain is shrunken, with widening of the cerebral sulci and enlargement of the ventricles. In some, symmetrical, sharply defined depressions are present on the surface of the pons or spinal cord.

On sectioning the brain and spinal cord, lesions are usually numerous. Some are only a few millimeters across, often with a blood vessel in their center. Some are large and irregularly shaped. They are usually well defined. Recent lesions are pink or yellowish, soft, and gelatinous. Old lesions are brown or gray and firm. In most patients, both recent and old lesions are evident. The lesions are called plaques, though they are frequently spheroidal, not flat, as the name suggests.

If the brain is severely involved, lesions are usually extensive around the lateral ventricles and in the floor of the fourth ventricle. Both gray and white matter are involved, though the lesions in the gray matter are less obvious than those in the white matter. Lesions in the cerebral hemispheres often spare the fibers immediately under the cerebral cortex. Lesions in the cord commonly spare the fibers immediately under the arachnoid mater. The optic nerves are frequently involved. Occasionally the lesions are largely confined to the spinal cord and optic nerves.

Microscopically, a lesion a few days old shows bulging of the myelin sheaths and slight proliferation of microglial cells. Within a few weeks, the myelin sheaths in the lesion break down. Globules of fat and myelin lie free in the tissue fluid and are taken up by the microglial cells and by macrophages.

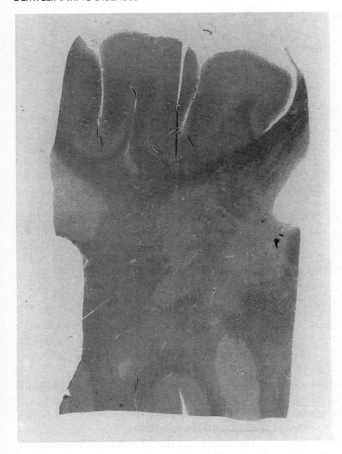

Fig. 57-20. Multiple sclerosis. A section stained for myelin shows several pale areas of demyelination. (Courtesy of Dr. J. H. N. Deck)

Plasma cells are common in and adjacent to the lesion. Axons in the lesion are irregularly thickened, but most remain intact. If there are neurons in the lesion, they are intact. The tissue adjacent to the lesion is edematous.

After several weeks, the myelin in the lesion is usually lost completely. The border between the lesion and the surrounding myelinated tissue is sharp. The concentration of nuclei in the lesion increases as astrocytes and microglial cells proliferate and macrophages accumulate. Oligodendrocytes disappear. Perivascular cuffs of lymphocytes are common around blood vessels in and near the lesion. As time passes, the cuffing becomes more prominent.

After six months, the quantity of fat in the lesion is much reduced. Lipophages are present only around blood vessels. Gliosis is well developed. The astrocytes are less pro-

minent. The edema around the lesion wanes. Eventually, the fat disappears, and only a mesh of glial fibers, with unmyelinated axons running among them, remains between the blood vessels in the lesion. Some axons are destroyed, but most survive. Neurons in the lesion survive. The lesion becomes quiescent and persists for the rest of the patient's life.

Especially in lesions in the brain stem, demyelination is not always complete. In some lesions, some fibers are demyelinated; others are spared. In some, all axons are involved, but are only partly demyelinated.

Occasionally the lesions progress more rapidly and are more severely inflamed. Many axons and sometimes neurons are destroyed. Blood vessels have thick cuffs of lymphocytes and plasma cells. Bizarre, multinucleated astrocytes appear. Some of the lesions in the optic nerves or spinal cord may

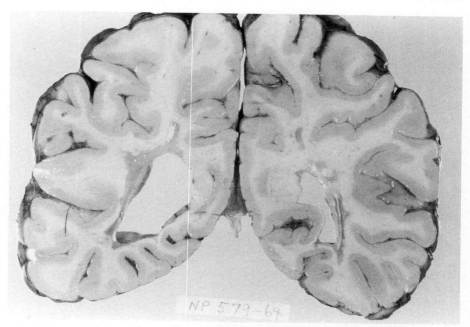

Fig. 57-21. Multiple sclerosis, showing several, well-defined, gray areas of demyelination in the white matter. The lesions are most prominent around the lateral ventricles. (Courtesy of Dr. J. H. N. Deck)

become necrotic. Edema and wallerian degeneration are prominent around the lesions.

In the cerebrospinal fluid, the concentration of protein is usually normal, but may be slightly elevated, rarely to more than 1 g/L (100 mg/100 mL). Especially late in the course of the disease the concentration of γ-globulin in the cerebrospinal fluid increases in 80% of the patients. Occasionally there is a slight lymphocytosis in the cerebrospinal fluid, nearly always less than 200×10^6/L (200/mm^3).

Late in the disease, the neurologic dysfunction caused by the lesions in the brain and spinal cord induces secondary changes in other organs. Flexion contractures in the limbs, emaciation, bedsores, cystitis, pyelonephritis, and repeated infections are common.

Clinical Presentation. In 70% of the patients, multiple sclerosis is episodic. Neurologic dysfunction worsens for a few days or weeks, then ameliorates or disappears in the course of a few weeks more. Occasionally the patient remains free of symptoms for years, but more often further attacks follow within weeks or months. Resolution is no longer

complete. As years pass, the patient becomes increasingly disabled. In the other 30% of the patients, the dysfunction worsens progressively, without remission.

The nature of the dysfunction depends on the site of the lesions. As new lesions develop, new symptoms and signs appear. Among the more common manifestations are unilateral impairment or loss of vision, nystagmus, dysarthria, ataxia, intention tremor, impairment or loss of sensation, muscular weakness, spastic paralysis, and urinary dysfunction. Late in the disease, seizures, changes in personality, and mental impairment sometimes become evident.

Pathogenesis. The pathogenesis of multiple sclerosis is obscure. Many theories have been advanced, but none has been proven. An immunologically mediated disorder and a viral infection are among the more popular suggestions.

The lesions in multiple sclerosis are similar to those of the allergic encephalomyelitis induced in mice by sensitization to myelin basic protein. Patients with multiple sclerosis are not sensitive to this antigen, but it is possible that they have been sensitized against some other component of myelin. Some have antibodies against myelin in their plasma. Increased numbers of activated T cells are present in the blood and cerebrospinal fluid of patients with multiple sclerosis. Suppressor T-cell function is reduced. An excess of gamma globulin is present in the cerebrospinal fluid in 80% of the patients.

A viral infection might precipitate an abnormal immunologic response like that in the allergic encephalomyelitis of mice, but no evidence of a viral infection has been found in the patients. Antibodies against the measles virus are present in the blood and cerebrospinal fluid in a higher proportion of the patients than in the general population, but the virus has not been found in the lesions.

Multiple sclerosis is 8 times as frequent in relatives of a patient with the disease as in the general population. A genetic predisposition on exposure of members of the family to similar environmental factors has been suggested as the cause. The HLA antigens B7 and DW2 occur more frequently in patients with multiple sclerosis than would be expected, and the prevalence of HLA-B12 is reduced.

Conduction of nervous impulses through the demyelinated axons in the lesions of multiple sclerosis is slowed. It is not known what causes the intermittent dysfunction common in the early stages of the disease.

Treatment and Prognosis. There is no treatment for multiple sclerosis. Adrenocortical steroids reduce the severe or acute attacks of neurologic dysfunction, but do not alter the ultimate outcome. Immunosuppressive agents are of uncertain value.

The prognosis is unpredictable. In most patients, the disease progresses slowly. Five years after the diagnosis, 70% of the patients are still at work. Ten years after diagnosis, 50% still work. Twenty years after diagnosis, 30% of the patients can work and 70% are able to walk. In a few patients, the disease brings death within a few months.

BALÓ'S CONCENTRIC SCLEROSIS. Baló's concentric sclerosis, named after the Hungarian pathologist who described it in 1928, is a rare form of multiple sclerosis. The lesions show concentric rings of demyelination separated by bands in which the myelin is preserved, or irregular blocks of well-preserved myelin surrounded by demyelination.

SCHILDER'S DISEASE. In 1912, the Austrian neurologist Schilder described a group of patients with extensive demyelination. Since that time, the term *Schilder's disease* has been applied to many different kinds of demyelination. It is sometimes used today to describe extensive demyelination in the cerebral hemispheres in children.

PERIVENULAR ENCEPHALOMYELITIS. Perivenular encephalomyelitis, also called acute disseminated encephalomyelitis, develops a few days after the rash appears in 1 person in 1000 with measles, and sometimes complicates chickenpox, less often rubella, mumps, or a mycoplasmal infection. It develops days or weeks after the first vaccination for smallpox in 1 person in 5000, but is uncommon after booster shots. It sometimes complicates smallpox. It developed in 1 person in 5000 when rabies vaccines containing brain tissue were used, but does not occur when more modern rabies vaccines are used. In some patients, it develops without a preceding infection or vaccination.

The lesions of perivenular encephalomyelitis are described in Chapter 18. Cylinders of demyelination develop around the blood vessels in many parts of the brain and spinal cord. Most of the axons and neurons in the lesions survive. An exudate of lymphocytes and plasma cells is present in the lesions and surrounds blood vessels adjacent to them. The damaged myelin is removed by macrophages. The lesions heal by gliosis.

The disease begins abruptly. The patients are feverish, confused, or somnolent. Headache and delirium are common. Convulsions, signs of meningeal irritation, and localizing signs that reflect the distribution of the lesions follow. About 20% of the patients die. Over 50% of those who survive are left with permanent neurologic dysfunction.

The similarity of the lesions in perivenular encephalomyelitis to those of experimental allergic encephalomyelitis suggest that perivenular encephalomyelitis is caused by sensitization to an antigen present in myelin. Sensitivity to myelin basic protein has been demonstrated in some patients.

ACUTE NECROTIZING HEMORRHAGIC ENCEPHALOMYELITIS. Acute necrotizing hemorrhagic encephalomyelitis is a rare form of perivenular encephalomyelitis in which much of the white matter of one or both cerebral hemispheres becomes necrotic. Hemorrhage into the necrotic tissue is common. A dense neutrophilic exudate is present in the lesions. The disease usually follows an upper respiratory infection. Death often comes within two days.

DEGENERATIVE DISEASES OF NEURONS

The degenerative diseases of neurons are conditions in which there is progressive loss of neurons in part of the central or peripheral nervous system. As years pass, the disease slowly worsens. Gliosis increases in the lesions, but there is little inflammatory reaction. The remainder of the nervous system is normal, except for secondary changes caused by the loss of neurons. The cause of these diseases is unknown. Many of them are inherited as an autosomal recessive or dominant character.

Some of the degenerative diseases of neurons have distinctive lesions that affect only part of the nervous system. In some, the lesions are less characteristic, and the disease is defined by the part of the nervous system involved. The disorders that affect principally the cerebral cortices will be discussed first, then the degenerative diseases of the basal ganglia, the spinocerebellar degenerations, the motor neuron diseases, and the diseases of peripheral nerves.

Diseases of the Cerebral Cortices

Alzheimer's disease is the principal degenerative disease of the cerebral cortical neurons. Other forms of senile dementia, Pick's disease, and progressive subcortical gliosis also affect cortical neurons.

ALZHEIMER'S DISEASE. Alzheimer's disease is named after the German neurologist who described it in 1907. It causes mental deterioration in the elderly. Except in patients with Down syndrome, most of whom develop Alzheimer's disease before they are 40 years old, it is uncommon in people under 50 years old, but becomes increasingly fre-

quent in older people. More than 20% of people over 80 years old have Alzheimer's disease. It is responsible for the mental deterioration in 60% of old people who suffer mental failure. From 1 to 10% of patients in psychiatric hospitals have Alzheimer's disease. About 70% of the patients are women. In a few kindred, Alzheimer's disease is familial, in some inherited as an autosomal dominant character. In most patients, there is no evidence of a genetic predisposition to the disease.

Lesions. At autopsy, the brain is small, often weighing about 1000 g instead of its normal 1200 g or more. Shrinkage and atrophy of the cerebral cortex are usually greatest in the frontal and temporal lobes, especially the hippocampi. In the affected areas, the gyri are narrowed, the sulci are widened, and the ventricles are dilated. The overlying meninges are often thickened. Atherosclerosis in the cerebral vessels is rarely severe.

Neurons are lost from the cerebral cortex. The loss is usually greatest in the 3rd or the 3rd and 5th layers, though all layers are affected. It is most severe in the frontal and temporal lobes. From 40 to 60% of neurons over 90 μm^2 in area disappear. Smaller neurons are little affected. The loss of neurons causes gliosis in the cortices, demyelination of their axons, and often secondary loss of neurons in the thalamus. The severely involved parts of the cortex become increasingly disorderly.

Other parts of the brain are spared or less severely affected. Loss of neurons is most often evident in the cholinergic nucleus basalis of Meynert, the noradrenergic locus ceruleus, the serotoninergic dorsal tegmentum, and the paramedial reticular nucleus.

Neurofibrillary tangles distort many of the neurons remaining in the cerebral cortices and are present in some of the neurons in the other central regions involved. The cytoplasm of the affected neurons is distended by tangled bundles and loops of fibers, which push the nucleus to one side. The tangles stain poorly with hematoxylin and eosin, but well with silver impregnation, the periodic acid-Schiff reaction, and with Congo red. They are birefringent when stained with Congo red, though no amyloid is present.

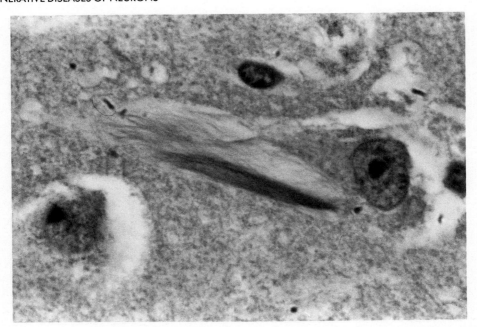

Fig. 57-22.   A prominent neurofibrillary tangle in a large, pyramidal neuron from the hippocampus of a patient with Alzheimer's disease. (Courtesy of Dr. J. H. N. Deck)

Electron microscopy shows that the fibers of the tangles are bifilar helices about 20 nm in diameter. They are not neurofilaments or microtubules.

Amyloid plaques, also called senile plaques, neuritic plaques, and argyrophilic plaques, are nearly always numerous in the cerebral cortices in Alzheimer's disease. The plaques have a spheroidal core of amyloid from 10 μm to 100 μm in diameter surrounded by thickened axons and dendrites. The plaques stain well with silver stains and with Congo red. By light microscopy, some have a dense core surrounded by a clear halo that is in turn surrounded by a dense periphery. Others are dense and homogeneous or appear granular. The molecular structure of the amyloid is unlike that of the amyloids found in other parts of the body. The structure of the amyloid found in old people differs slightly from that in patients with Down syndrome and is different from the amyloid in the familial form of Alzheimer's disease. Tubules like those in the neurofibrillary tangles are present in the neurites at the margin of the plaques.

Amyloid often thickens the walls of small blood vessels in the meninges and in the gray and white matter of the cerebral hemispheres, a condition called amyloid angiopathy or congophilic angiopathy. Vessels in other parts of the body are not affected. The molecular structure of the amyloid is the same as that of the amyloid in the plaques. Most patients with Alzheimer's disease have both amyloid plaques and amyloid angiopathy. Some have one but not the other.

In some patients, from 10 to 50% of the neurons in the hippocampus have in their cytoplasm one or more vacuoles 3 to 5 μm in diameter with a dense granule 1 μm across in the center of the vacuole. Occasionally a few neurons in the temporal cortices show similar granulovacuolar degeneration. Elongated, eosinophilic structures 10 to 15 μm across, called Hirano bodies after the American pathologist who described them in 1965, are present in the hippocampus in some patients. They form in neurites, consist of filaments 5 to 6 nm thick, and stain for actin.

The activity of acetyltransferase is reduced to 60 to 10% of normal in the brains of people with Alzheimer's disease. The concentration of acetylcholine is low. The receptors for

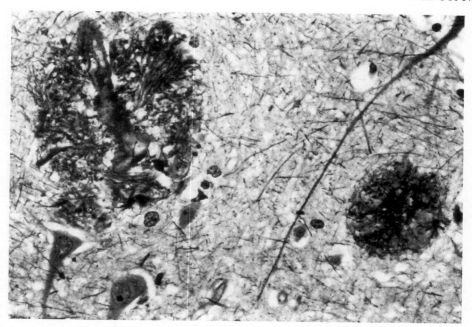

Fig. 57-23. Senile plaques in the cerebral cortex of a patient with Alzheimer's disease as shown in a section stained by silver impregnation. (Courtesy of Dr. J. H. N. Deck)

somatostatin are deficient, and the concentration of somatostatin in the brain is less than 50% of normal. Often glutamate binding is abnormal, the concentration of the corticotropin releasing factor is reduced, or the metabolism of serotonin, epinephrine, or dopamine is disturbed. Glucose utilization is low in the cerebral cortices.

Clinical Presentation. Alzheimer's disease causes slow but inexorable mental deterioration. In many patients, loss of memory, especially recent memory, is the first sign of the disease. Some patients become confused, emotionally unstable, depressed, or careless of dress and behavior. Some have delusions or hallucinations. As the dementia worsens, aphasia, dysarthria, agnosia, and apraxia are frequent. Late in the course, a shuffling gait is common as agonist and antagonist muscles contract simultaneously. Fecal or urinary incontinence or spasticity and hyperreflexia in the limbs may develop. Seizures are unusual. Eventually there is complete dementia, flexion contractures in the limbs, and decerebration.

Pathogenesis. The cause of Alzheimer's disease is unknown. Plaques and neuro-

fibrillary tangles are common in the brains of old people, though they are not as frequent as in Alzheimer's disease. Neurofibrillary tangles are found in boxers and others in whom the brain is injured, in postencephalic parkinsonism, the Guam parkinson-dementia complex, and scrapie. Suggestions that Alzheimer's disease is an abnormal form of aging, is secondary to an enzyme deficiency, is caused by infection with a virus or prion, is due to aluminum intoxication, results from the increased vascular permeability caused by vascular amyloidosis, or is due to a disturbance in neuroconduction have not been substantiated.

Treatment and Prognosis. No treatment benefits a patient with Alzheimer's disease. The speed at which the disease progresses varies considerably from one person to another. Most patients die about five years after the onset of symptoms, often from infection. Some die within a few months. Some live over 20 years.

PICK'S DISEASE. Pick's disease, named after the Czech psychiatrist who described it in 1892, is uncommon. It causes slowly progressive dementia, much as does Alzheimer's disease. Most patients are about 60 years old when symptoms appear. Some 60% are women. Most die within 10 years. The cause of the disease is unknown. In most patients, there is no genetic predisposition. In some, the disease is inherited as an autosomal dominant character.

Macroscopically, the brain shows atrophy of the frontal lobes, temporal lobes, or both. Occasionally it is unilateral. Both white and gray matter are involved. The basal ganglia, substantia nigra, and frontopontine tracts are shrunken. The demarcation between the atrophic part of the brain and the remainder is sharp. In the atrophic part of the brain, the gyri are thin and pointed, often yellowish brown or granular. The overlying meninges are thickened. The ventricles are dilated.

Microscopically, loss of neurons and gliosis are severe in the atrophic parts of the brain. Neuronal loss is less severe in other parts of the cortex and basal ganglia. Many of the surviving neurons in the cortex and basal ganglia are swollen. Tubules and fibrils 7 to 10 nm in diameter are present in their cytoplasm. In some neurons, the fibrils are widely dispersed and the cytoplasm is clear to light microscopy. In some, they are aggregated together to form a spheroidal inclusion called a Pick body. The bodies stain strongly with silver and are about the size of a nucleus. The fibrils and tubules are unlike those in Alzheimer's disease, but share antigens with the tubules of Alzheimer's disease. Granulovacuolar degeneration is sometimes present in the hippocampus, but neurofibrillary tangles and amyloid nodules do not occur.

PROGRESSIVE SUBCORTICAL GLIOSIS. Progressive subcortical gliosis is a rare condition that causes dementia like that of Alzheimer's disease or Pick's disease. It is characterized by gliosis immediately beneath the cerebral cortex, in the basal ganglia, thalamus, brain stem, and ventral horns of the spinal cord. The cerebral cortex is little affected.

Diseases of the Basal Ganglia

Parkinson's disease and Huntington's chorea are the most common neuronal degenerations of the basal ganglia. Less frequent are the Parkinson-dementia complex of Guam, progressive subnuclear palsy, and progressive familial myoclonic epilepsy.

PARKINSON'S SYNDROME. Parkinson's syndrome is named after the English physician who defined it in 1817. Three kinds of parkinsonism are distinguished. Most of the patients have the idiopathic form of the condition called Parkinson's disease or paralysis agitans. Postencephalitic parkinsonism developed in many of the patients who recovered from encephalitis lethargica, prevalent in Europe between 1915 and 1930.

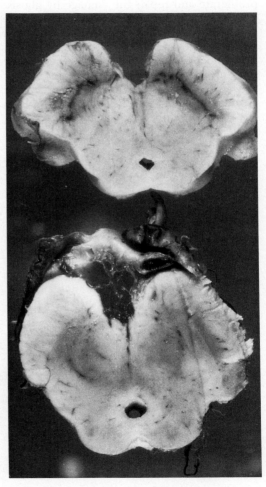

Fig. 57-24. Top, the prominent substantia nigra in a normal midbrain. Bottom, midbrain of a patient with idiopathic Parkinson's disease. The substantia nigra has almost entirely disappeared. (Courtesy of Dr. J. H. N. Deck)

Secondary parkinsonism is induced by a drug.

Parkinson's disease usually begins when the patient is between 50 and 65 years old. Men and women are equally affected. The disease occurs in all parts of the world. In a few kindred, the disease is familial.

Lesions. Patients with idiopathic Parkinson's disease show atrophy of the pigmented nuclei in the brain stem. The substantia nigra and locus ceruleus are the most severely affected.

Microscopically, many of the pigmented neurons in these nuclei are lost. Astrocytes proliferate and repair the damage by gliosis. Macrophages phagocytose melanin from the dead neurons. A few neurofibrillary tangles are sometimes present in the damaged nuclei. The concentration of dopamine in the caudate nucleus and putamen is reduced.

Many of the surviving neurons in the affected regions have in their cytoplasm large, eosinophilic inclusions called Lewy bodies after the German physician who described them in 1913. The bodies are sometimes concentrically laminated, sometimes are homogeneous. A clear halo often surrounds them. Electron microscopy shows that the halo around the Lewy bodies contains widely spaced, irregular filaments 7 to 20 nm in diameter. The core of the lesions is made of closely packed, linear profiles 7 to 8 nm thick intermixed with electron-dense granules 40 to 60 nm in diameter.

Postencephalitic parkinsonism causes more severe injury to the substantia nigra than does the idiopathic form of the disease. Neurofibrillary tangles are more numerous in the damaged nuclei, and are present in the cerebral cortex, basal ganglia, and thalamus. Lewy bodies are usually few. Glial scars caused by the encephalitis are numerous in other parts of the brain.

Secondary parkinsonism caused by a drug damages most severely the substantia nigra. The locus ceruleus is spared. Lewy bodies are few.

Clinical Presentation. Parkinsonism develops slowly and insidiously. The first sign is usually tremor, rigidity, or a tendency to stoop with the head flexed against the chest. The tremor usually affects first one hand, but later involves both arms and sometimes the head or lower limbs. It is abolished by

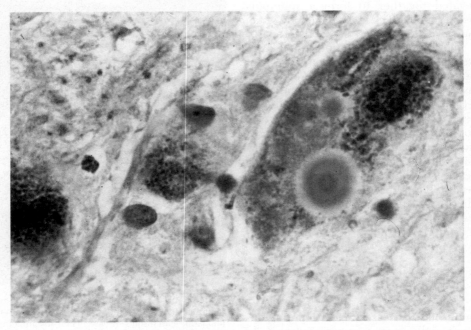

Fig. 57-25. A Lewy body in a pigmented neuron from the substantia nigra of a patient with Parkinson's disease. (Courtesy of Dr. J. H. N. Deck)

deliberate movements and disappears when the patient is asleep. The rigidity is most apparent in the face, which becomes fixed, masklike and expressionless, but eventually involves the whole body. As it increases, the patient tends to fall forward when walking and is forced to take short, rapid steps. Movements become jerky, often arrested in midcourse. The patient falls when sitting unsupported. Speech becomes monotonous and slow. The stiff, shaking mouth drools. In 30% of the patients, the intellect is eventually impaired.

Pathogenesis. The cause of idiopathic Parkinson's disease is unknown. Postencephalitic parkinsonism no longer occurs. Drugs such as reserpine that interfere with dopaminergic transmission cause secondary parkinsonism. Up to 15% of patients treated with a phenothiazine develop parkinsonism. Usually the dysfunction resolves when the drug is withdrawn, but in a few patients it has been permanent. The neurotoxin 1-methyl-1,2,5,6-tetrahydropyridine injected by drug abusers destroys neurons in the substantia nigra and causes parkinsonism. The locus ceruleus is spared.

Treatment and Prognosis. No treatment can replace the neurons lost in parkinsonism, but drugs relieve many of the effects of the disease. Stereotaxic surgery to produce a lesion in the thalamus or globus pallidus also brings relief, but is rarely needed.

Early in the disease, an anticholinergic drug such as trihexyphenidyl or benzotropine that blocks muscarinic receptors and reduces cholinergic transmission, the dopamine agonists amantadine or bromocriptine, a β-adrenergic antagonist such as propanolol or metopolol, or some combination of these agents usually gives relief. If the dysfunction is more severe, levodopa given together with a dopa-carboxylase inhibitor and sometimes one of the drugs used in the milder forms of the disease benefits 75% of the patients. Levodopa is converted to dopamine in the brain. The dopa-carboxylase inhibitor prevents its activation in the blood and other tissues, reducing the dose needed, and preventing nausea and other complications caused by dopamine in other tissues.

As the disease worsens, the drugs become less effective or bring benefit only intermit-tently, even if the dosage is increased. Weakness and immobility become more severe, often with involuntary movements. The patient becomes increasingly incapacitated and eventually is confined to bed or a chair. A few patients are incapacitated within five years of the onset. In most it is 10 or 20 years before disability becomes severe.

PARKINSONISM-DEMENTIA-AMYOTROPHIC LATERAL SCLEROSIS COMPLEX OF GUAM. About 10% of the Chamorro people living on Guam and other Mariana Islands develop amyotrophic lateral sclerosis, a combination of Parkinsonism and dementia, or both. The disease usually begins when the patient is between 40 and 60 years old. It frequently brings death within five years.

Loss of neurons and gliosis in the cerebral cortex, especially in the frontal and temporal lobes, and loss of neurons and melanin from the substantia nigra and locus ceruleus are found in patients with parkinsonism and dementia. Lesser numbers of neurons are lost in the globus pallidus, thalamus, hypothalamus, and brain stem. Neurofibrillary tangles like those of Alzheimer's disease are numerous. Amyloid plaques and Lewy bodies are few.

The patients with amyotrophic lateral sclerosis lose motor neurons as do other patients with amyotrophic lateral sclerosis. Neurofibrillary tangles are numerous in their neurons, even if there is no clinical evidence of parkinsonism or dementia.

HUNTINGTON'S CHOREA. Huntington's chorea, named after the American physician who described it in 1872, is inherited as an autosomal dominant character. The abnormal gene is on chromosome 4. The few cases without a family history are presumably due to a new mutation. In most of the world, 5 people in every 100,000 have the disease, and each year 1 person in 200,000 develops it. It is more common in parts of Scotland, Sweden, and Tasmania.

In most patients, symptoms develop when the patient is 35 to 50 years old. If symptoms appear in childhood or adolescence, the disease is usually severe. If symptoms appear only when the patient is over 50 years old, it is usually mild. Men and women are affected equally.

Lesions. At autopsy, the exterior of the

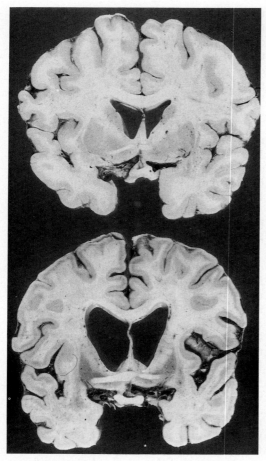

Fig. 57-26. Top, a normal brain. Bottom, the brain of a patient with Huntington's chorea, showing atrophy of the caudate nucleus and the putamen, with compensatory dilatation of the lateral ventricles. (Courtesy of Dr. J. H. N. Deck)

Aspiny neurons with few dendrites are spared. In the cerebral cortex, the loss of neurons is not great. It is most severe in the 3rd layer. The injury in the basal ganglia and cortex is repaired by gliosis.

The activity of the glutamic acid decarboxylase associated with the spiny neurons in the caudate nucleus, putamen, globus pallidus, and substantia nigra is low. The concentration of γ-butyric acid and other neurotransmitters associated with the spiny neurons is reduced. The stomatostatin and neuropeptide Y associated with the aspiny neurons is increased. The activity of choline acetyltransferase in the corpus striatum nucleus is reduced. The concentration of substance P is low in the striatonigral and striatopallidal pathways. Met-enkephalin, dynorphin, and cholecystokinin are reduced in the globus pallidus and substantia nigra.

Clinical Presentation. Huntington's disease develops insidiously. It causes involuntary movements, changes in personality, dementia, and sometimes rigidity. Involuntary grimaces, uncontrollable movements of the limbs, or difficulty with speech are usually the first sign of the disease. In children, rigidity is often the predominant feature in its early stages. The neurologic deterioration worsens slowly but inexorably. The patients become irritable and truculent. Some become paranoid. Some are depressed and slovenly. The involuntary movements become more violent. Dementia grows more severe.

Treatment and Prognosis. No treatment is known to benefit Huntington's chorea. Death usually comes in about 10 years, often from infection or suicide.

PROGRESSIVE SUPRANUCLEAR PALSY. Progressive supranuclear palsy, also called the Steele-Richardson-Olszecoski syndrome after the Canadian physicians who described it in 1964, is a rare condition most common in men. The patients are over 50 years old when they develop progressive paralysis of vertical eye movements, dysarthria, and muscular rigidity, most prominent in the neck. Death usually comes within five years.

Neurons are lost in the globus pallidus, subthalamic nucleus, red nucleus, substantia nigra, tectum, and periaqueductal gray matter. Neurofibrillary tangles, which to light

brain may be normal, but usually shows mild or moderate cerebral atrophy. On section, the caudate nucleus is severely shrunken. The putamen and thalamus are less affected. The cerebral cortex is often thin, especially in the frontal and parietal regions. The white matter in the cerebral hemispheres and corpus callosum is reduced. The ventricles are dilated.

Neurons are lost in the caudate nucleus and to a lesser degree in the other basal ganglia. Many of the neurons that survive are shrunken and contain much lipochrome pigment. The loss affects principally medium-sized spiny neurons with many dendrites.

microscopy look like those of Alzheimer's disease, are frequent in these regions, and in other parts of the brain stem. They consist of straight fibrils 15 nm in diameter, not the bifilar helices of Alzheimer's disease. The cerebral cortex is not affected. The amyloid plaques of Alzheimer's disease are not found. The injury is repaired by gliosis.

PROGRESSIVE FAMILIAL MYOCLONIC EPILEPSY. Progressive familial myoclonic epilepsy, sometimes called Lafora's disease after the Spanish neurologist who described it in 1911, is an uncommon disorder inherited as an autosomal recessive character. It begins in adolescence or early adult life with generalized seizures, myoclonic jerks, or both. The attacks increase in severity and frequency. Mental function becomes increasingly impaired. Death comes within 10 years, often from infection.

Cytoplasmic inclusions called Lafora bodies are most frequent in neurons in the thalamus, substantia nigra, and dentate nucleus, but are present in smaller numbers in neurons in the cerebral cortices, globus pallidus, and the nuclei in the brain stem. Their distribution varies from patient to patient. Neurons are lost throughout the brain, with slight gliosis.

The Lafora bodies are from 1 to 30 μm in diameter. A neuron may contain one or several. Some are concentrically laminated; some are homogeneous. Electron microscopy shows that the bodies consist of fibrils 6 to 7 nm in diameter running at random. Organelles and glycogen lie between the fibrils. Sometimes a body has an amorphous, electron-dense core. The fibrils consist of polyglucosans. Similar bodies are present in the myocardium, skeletal muscles, and liver.

Spinocerebellar Degenerations

The spinocerebellar degenerations are a group of diseases in which neurons are lost in the cerebellum, spinal cord, or dorsal root ganglia. More than 50 forms of spinocerebellar degeneration have been described. Most are inherited as an autosomal recessive character, some as an autosomal dominant trait. The patients present with some combination of ataxia, paralysis, sensory loss, blindness, dementia, or extrapyramidal signs.

Only the more common syndromes are described.

CEREBELLO-OLIVARY DEGENERATION. Cerebello-olivary degeneration is also called cerebellar cortical degeneration. It is usually inherited as an autosomal recessive character, though sporadic cases occur. Symptoms begin when the patient is over 40 years old. First comes an ataxic gait, which slowly worsens. Tremor of the head and limbs, dysarthria, and occasionally nystagmus often develop later. Mental acuity is not affected. Life is not shortened.

Purkinje cells are lost from the cerebellum, especially from the superior vermis. Loss of granular cells is less severe. Reactive gliosis repairs the damaged regions. The loss of the Purkinje cells causes secondary atrophy of the olivary bodies, loss of olivary neurons, and gliosis.

OLIVOPONTOCEREBELLAR DEGENERATION. The term *olivopontocerebellar degeneration* includes a group of conditions, some inherited as an autosomal dominant character, some as an autosomal recessive trait. The symptoms vary from patient to patient, even within a single kindred. Symptoms begin when the patient is over 40 year old, with some combination of slowly progressive cerebellar ataxia, dysmetria, tremor, inability to perform rapid movements, dysarthria, parkinsonism, impairment of vision, and dementia. Most patients are incapacitated within five years.

The brain shows atrophy of the ventral part of the pons, middle cerebellar peduncles, cerebellar cortex, and inferior olivary bodies. In the cerebellum, Purkinje cells are lost, inciting gliosis, but the granular cells are preserved. Myelin is lost from the cerebellar hemispheres and the middle cerebellar peduncles. The loss of the cerebellar neurons causes secondary loss of neurons and gliosis in the inferior olivary bodies. Sometimes there is gliosis in the dentate nuclei, though their neurons are preserved. In the patients with parkinsonism, neurons are lost in the substantia nigra and putamen. Retinal degeneration is present in the patients with visual impairment.

FRIEDREICH'S ATAXIA. Friedreich's ataxia, named after the German physician who described it in 1863, is one of the commoner neuronal degenerative diseases. It is usually inherited as an autosomal recessive character, sometimes as an autosomal dominant trait. Sporadic cases occur. Symptoms usually begin in childhood.

Lesions. Neurons in the dorsal root ganglia die and are replaced by proliferation of their capsular cells. The sensory fibers in the peripheral nerves involved degenerate and demyelinate. The large fibers are the most severely affected, and motor fibers remain intact.

In the spinal cord, the posterior columns atrophy. The fasciculus gracilis is almost completely destroyed, but the fasciculus cuneatus is less severely affected. The posterior spinocerebellar tract shrinks. The anterior spinocerebellar tract is less affected. The pyramidal tracts are severely damaged in the spinal cord, but are often intact in the brain stem. Axons and myelin sheaths disappear in the parts of the cord affected and are replaced by gliosis.

In the brain, changes vary from patient to patient. Because of the loss of their afferent fibers, the cuneate and gracile nuclei are gliotic and lose neurons. Other nuclei in the brain stem are sometimes gliotic and lose neurons. The sensory or motor tracks in the brain stem may be damaged.

Myocarditis, described in Chapter 26, causes foci of necrosis and fibrosis in the heart. Congestive heart failure and heart block are frequent. Mural thrombi in the heart sometimes give rise to emboli that lodge in the brain or elsewhere. Diabetes mellitus is common.

Clinical Presentation. Unsteadiness and clumsiness of gait is the first sign of Friedreich's ataxia. As the disease progresses, ataxia in the legs grows more severe and extends to the arms. Speech grows increasingly dysarthric. Position sense is lost, especially in the legs. The deep tendon reflexes are impaired, most severely in the lower limbs. There is an extensor plantar response. Muscular weakness increases, but there is no rigidity. Choreiform movements develop in some patients. Nystagmus is usual. Optic atrophy sometimes causes blindness. The weakness of the muscles often causes kyphoscoliosis or pes cavus.

Treatment and Prognosis. No treatment can change the course of the disease. Most patients are disabled within 5 or 10 years. They cannot move or feed themselves. Their speech is incomprehensible. Infection often causes death.

AUTONOMIC FAILURE. Degeneration of the autonomic neurons is called the Shy-Drager syndrome, after the American physicians who reported it in 1960. Neurons are lost in the peripheral autonomic ganglia, the intermediolateral column of the thoracic cord, the caudate nuclei, substantia nigra, locus ceruleus, olivary nuclei, dorsal vagal nuclei, and sometimes the cerebellum. The patients develop dizziness, urinary dysfunction, hypohidrosis, and postural hypotension. Later comes parkinsonism or ataxia. Most patients are disabled within five years.

HEREDITARY ATAXIA-TELANGIECTASIA. Hereditary ataxia-telangiectasia is a form of spinocerebellar neuronal degeneration, but because of the prominent immunologic deficiency in these patients it is described in Chapter 10.

Motor Neuron Disease

The term *motor neuron disease* is used to describe conditions in which motor neurons are lost from the spinal cord, the nuclei of the cranial nerves, or the cerebral cortex. Amyotrophic lateral sclerosis is the most common of these disorders. Less frequent are primary lateral sclerosis, Werdnig-Hoffmann disease, the form of amyotrophic lateral sclerosis that occurs on Guam, and other rare syndromes.

AMYOTROPHIC LATERAL SCLEROSIS. Amyotrophic lateral sclerosis is one of the commoner neuronal degenerations. In the United States, 3000 people develop the disease each year, and 10,000 suffer from it. The name describes the disease: *amyotrophic* because it causes muscular atrophy, *lateral sclerosis* because it causes gliosis in the lateral columns of the spinal cord. In 10% of the patients, amyotrophic lateral sclerosis is inherited as an autosomal dominant character. In the rest, no genetic disposition is evident. Over 60% of the patients are men. Most are over 40 years old when symptoms begin, but many are considerably older.

Lesions. Motor neurons are lost in the

spinal cord, some of the nuclei of the spinal nerves, and from the cerebral cortices. Most often, the loss is greatest and begins in the lumbar and cervical enlargements of the spinal cord and in the hypoglossal nuclei. The nuclei of the facial and trigeminal nerves and the nuclei ambigui are usually less severely involved, and the oculomotor, trochlear, and abducent nuclei are spared. Early in the disease, the loss of neurons may be largely confined to the basal ganglia or the spinal cord.

In the affected regions, motor neurons shrink and disappear. Especially in the cerebrospinal tracts, the degeneration seems to begin at the distal end of the axons and to spread centrally until the neuron becomes necrotic and disappears, a process called dying back. Often lipochromes accumulate in the cytoplasm of the neurons. Focal enlargements called spheroids develop on the motor axons and contain numerous neurofilaments. Occasionally neuronophagia is evident, but usually there is no reaction around the dying neurons. The injury is repaired by gliosis.

The pyramidal tracts in the spinal cord degenerate. Sometimes the demyelination extends into the cerebral hemispheres; sometimes it is confined to the lower part of the spinal cord or extends only into the medulla. Demyelination and gliosis in the anterior and lateral columns are prominent in most patients. The posterior columns are spared.

The muscles supplied by the lost motor neurons shrink. Microscopically, they show denervation atrophy.

Clinical Presentation. Amyotrophic lateral sclerosis usually first becomes evident in one limb, though it can appear first in any part of the body. The muscles affected become weak, waste, and sometimes show fasciculation. As time passes, the weakness extends, until most muscles supplied by the spinal nerves and many of those supplied by cranial nerves are affected. The muscles of respiration, chewing, and swallowing are all involved. Loss of the upper motor neurons sometimes causes spasticity, especially in the lower limbs, and an upgoing plantar response that persist until the increasing loss of lower motor neurons make movement impossible.

If the motor neurons in the spinal cord are first affected and the disease involves prin-cipally the muscles supplied by the spinal nerves, it is called spinal muscular atrophy. If involvement of the nuclei in the brain stem is predominant, it is called bulbar palsy. If emotional disturbances are striking, it is called pseudobulbar palsy.

Treatment and Prognosis. No treatment alters the progression of amyotrophic lateral sclerosis. The weakness extends and increases. More than 50% of the patients die within five years, usually of pulmonary infection caused by weakness of the respiratory muscles or secondary to aspiration caused by weakness of the muscles of swallowing. Rarely, the disease becomes stable or regresses.

PRIMARY LATERAL SCLEROSIS. Primary lateral sclerosis is an uncommon disorder that develops in elderly people. Loss of motor neurons in the precentral gyrus causes atrophy of the corticobulbar and corticospinal tracts. The lower motor neurons are not affected. The patients develop spasticity and weakness in the muscles. Most die within five years.

WERDNIG-HOFFMANN DISEASE. Werdnig-Hoffmann disease, named after the Austrian and German neurologists who described it in 1891 and 1893, is inherited as an autosomal recessive character. Generalized muscular weakness present at birth or appearing soon after birth brings death within a few months, from respiratory failure or aspiration. The infants show widespread loss of motor neurons in the spinal cord, nuclei ambigui, hypoglossal and facial nuclei. Neuronophagia is often prominent in the affected regions. The pyramidal tracts are intact.

Occasionally a similar condition inherited as a autosomal recessive character develops in infants or older children, but progresses slowly. In adults, a slowly progressive form of spinal muscular atrophy is inherited as an autosomal recessive, autosomal recessive dominant or X-linked character.

Diseases of Peripheral Nerves

The neuronal degenerations that involve principally the peripheral nerves are divided into the hereditary motor and sensory neuropathies in which the motor axons are the most severely affected, the hereditary sensory neuropathies that involve the sensory fibers and the neurons in the dorsal root ganglia, and giant axonal neuropathy that involves axons in the peripheral nerves and central nervous system.

HEREDITARY MOTOR AND SENSORY NEURO-PATHY. The hereditary motor and sensory neuropathies, also called Charcot-Marie-Tooth disease after the French and English physicians who reported them in 1886, and peroneal muscular atrophy because the muscles in the feet and lower legs are usually the most severely affected, are a group of conditions that cause degeneration or demyelination of the axons in the peripheral nerves. Most are inherited as an autosomal dominant character. Symptoms usually begin in childhood or adolescence, but sometimes not until the patient is an adult. Less frequently, the disease is inherited as an X-linked character, expressed in heterozygous girls as well as in boys, and begins in infants or young children.

Most often, the nerves involved show extensive, segmental demyelination. The motor fibers are the most severely affected, but sensory axons are also involved. Often the nerves are swollen, and in cross section show microscopically a concentric proliferation of Schwann cells and collagen around the demyelinated axons, a lesion called an onion bulb. Nerve conduction velocity is greatly reduced. Less frequently, the disease affects principally the axons, which die back from their distal end towards their neurons in the spinal cord or dorsal root ganglia. Nerve action potential is low, but nerve conduction velocity is only slightly reduced.

The severity of the dysfunction caused varies considerably from one patient to another, even in the same kindred. Motor weakness predominates. Muscular wasting, foot drop, pes cavus, and deformities of the hips are among the more common manifestations. In most patients, the disease worsens slowly. Often it is years or decades before serious dysfunction develops.

HEREDITARY SENSORY NEUROPATHY. The hereditary sensory neuropathies are a group of uncommon conditions in which neurons in dorsal root ganglia degenerate and sensation is lost in the regions supplied. Most frequently the disorder is inherited as an autosomal dominant character, less often as an autosomal recessive trait. The patients are children or young adults when symptoms begin.

The ganglion cells in the dorsal ganglia affected shrink and are lost. The capsular cells around them proliferate. The sensory fibers in the nerves involved degenerate. The severity of the dysfunction varies from patient to patient. If the disease is severe, trophic ulcers, unsteadiness of movement, defective lachrymation and sweating, defective temperature control, postural hypotension, and shooting pains in the limbs are common. Because of the loss of sensation, the hands and feet are easily mutilated.

GIANT AXONAL NEUROPATHY. Giant axonal neuropath is an uncommon disorder inherited as an autosomal recessive character. In the peripheral nerves, the number of myelinated axons is reduced. Segments of those that remain are enlarged, sometimes to more than 30 μm in diameter. The enlarged axons are filled with whorls and skeins of neurofilaments 10 nm across. Similar swellings are present on axons in the spinal cord. Masses of Rosenthal fibers, like those in Alexander's disease, form nodules that bulge into the ventricles. Vimentin fibers are abnormally abundant in fibrocytes, endothelial cells, and melanocytes.

Symptoms begin in childhood. Often the children have scoliosis or deformed feet or hands. Clumsiness of gait and weakness in the legs become increasingly severe as the muscles in the lower limbs atrophy. Signs of cerebellar dysfunction are common. Some patients develop mental retardation, extensor plantar responses, or dysfunction of the urinary bladder.

PERIPHERAL NEUROPATHY

Disease of the peripheral nerves is called peripheral neuropathy or peripheral neuritis. If it involves a single nerve, it is called a mononeuropathy. If several nerves in different parts of the body are affected, it is called mononeuropathy multiplex. If the involvement of nerves is widespread, it is called polyneuropathy. Autonomic neuropathy affects principally the autonomic system.

The lesions, clinical presentation, treatment and prognosis are similar in all kinds of peripheral neuropathy and will be discussed first. The Guillain-Barré syndrome, and the types of peripheral neuropathy caused by disease of other organs, poisoning, or trauma are then considered. The peripheral neuropathies caused by neuronal degeneration have already been discussed.

Lesions. Peripheral neuropathy causes demyelination, axonal degeneration, or both. Demyelination is sometimes segmental, extending from one node of Ranvier to the next. Sometimes much or all the nerve is involved. Remyelination is often evident in some segments while demyelination continues in others.

In the affected regions, macrophages take up the debris of the myelin. Schwann cells proliferate. If the axons are damaged, they shrink and fragment. Often axonal degeneration begins at the distal end of the fiber, and the axon dies back towards its neuron. If local injury is severe, reparative fibrosis distorts or interrupts the nerve.

Secondary changes develop in the tissues supplied by the nerves involved if peripheral neuropathy is severe. Muscles waste and show denervation atrophy. Bones become osteoporotic. Joints show the disorganization sometimes called a Charcot's joint. Trophic changes and often trophic ulcers appear on the skin. Lack of sensation results in multiple injuries and increasing deformity.

Clinical Presentation. Symptoms of peripheral neuropathy sometimes develop acutely, reaching a maximum within a few days. More often the disorder develops subacutely, over the course of several weeks. Still more frequently it is chronic and slowly worsens for months, years, or decades.

The symptoms depend on the distribution and function of the nerve or nerves involved and on whether the disorder affects motor axons, sensory axons, or both. Loss of motor axons causes weakness or flaccid paralysis in the muscles involved and later denervation atrophy. Involvement of sensory fibers causes pain, paresthesia, anesthesia, trophic ulcers in the skin, and other manifestations of sensory loss. Injury to the autonomic system causes postural hypotension, fainting, hypohidrosis, lack of tears, dysfunction of the urinary bladder, constipation, and impotence and less often systemic hypertension, hyperhidrosis, or diarrhea.

Treatment and prognosis. Peripheral neuropathy is treated by controlling the disease or other agent causing the neuropathy. Little can be done to change the course of the idiopathic forms of the disorder. If the process is arrested and the axons are intact, recovery comes within several weeks. If the axons are damaged but the Schwann sheaths in the nerve remain intact, the axons regenerate, but it is often months before function is restored. If the continuity of the nerve is disrupted or interrupted by fibrosis, repair is imperfect or impossible.

GUILLAIN-BARRÉ SYNDROME. The Guillain-Barré syndrome is named after the French neurologists who described it in 1916. In North America, 1 person in 100,000 develops the syndrome each year. In 70% of the patients, the syndrome develops 10 to 20 days after a viral infection, most often a cytomegaloviral infection or infectious mononucleosis. In 10% of the patients, it follows a surgical procedure. Less often it complicates a lymphoma, systemic lupus erythematosus, or follows vaccination against rabies or influenza.

The affected nerves show segmental demyelination and an exudate of lymphocytes, though the inflammatory response may not be great. The axons are for the most part intact, even in nerves in which there is severe impairment of conduction of nerve impulses. The affected muscles show denervation atrophy. If the intraspinal part of the spinal nerves is involved, the protein in the cerebrospinal fluid often increases without increase in pressure. Usually there is no pleocytosis in the cerebrospinal fluid; sometimes there is an increase in lymphocytes.

Patients with the Guillain-Barré syndrome develop weakness and then flaccid paralysis. Symptoms usually worsen rapidly for several days or weeks and then become stationary and remain so for several weeks, before beginning to recede. The disease often begins in the legs and ascends to involve the trunk, arms, and head, a syndrome called Landry's ascending paralysis after the French physician who described it in 1859. Paralysis of the respiratory muscles and urinary retention are common. Over 25% of the patients need assisted respiration. Paresthesia and other sensory changes are commonly present, but are overshadowed by the paralysis.

The cause of the Guillain-Barré syndrome is unknown. The similarity of the lesions to those of experimental allergic neuritis and the presence of lymphocytes in the lesions suggest that it is immunologically mediated.

Over 85% of patients with the Guillain-Barré syndrome recover completely. The dysfunction slowly resolves over several weeks or months. Some are left with minor muscular weakness. In a few, the disorder persists, with repeated exacerbations and remissions. Less than 3% of the patients die. If the disease is severe, plasmapheresis is beneficial.

SECONDARY NEUROPATHY. Table 57-1 shows the diseases that cause secondary peripheral neuropathy. Diabetes mellitus is the most common cause, followed by far advanced carcinoma. In most forms of secondary peripheral neuropathy, the disease develops slowly.

Diabetes Mellitus. Diabetic neuropathy complicates long-standing hyperglycemia. Patients with juvenile onset diabetes mellitus are usually over 30 years old when the neuropathy develops. Those with adult onset diabetes are over 50 years old. Most often the disease is symmetrical, with both demyelination and axonal injury, and affects mainly the sensory and autonomic axons. Pain is sometimes a prominent symptom. Less often the neuropathy is asymmetrical, causing third or sixth nerve palsy on one side, pain in the distribution of one or more intercostal nerves on one side, or motor weakness in one quadriceps femoris, iliopsoas, or adductor magnus. If the diabetes is controlled, slow recovery is usual.

Paraproteinemia. Peripheral neuropathy develops in a minority of patients with paraproteinemia. Usually both sensory and motor axons are involved. About 5% of patients with multiple myeloma who have lytic lesions develop peripheral neuropathy, and sometimes it develops in patients with benign monoclonal gammopathy, macroglobulinemia, cryoglobulinemia, or plasmacytoma. Nearly 50% of the 3% of patients with multiple myeloma who have sclerotic lesions develop peripheral neuropathy. The neuropathy is predominantly axonal in the patients with the lytic type of multiple myeloma, benign monoclonal IgG or IgA gammopathy, macroglobulinemia, or cryoglobulinemia, but in the sclerotic form of myeloma, plasmacytoma, and benign monoclonal IgM gammopathy the nerves show both axonal lesions and demyelination. IgM directed against the myelin associated protein is present in the nerves in some patients with benign monoclonal IgM gammopathy.

Neoplasia. In patients with carcinoma, axonal degeneration is most common late in the disease and affects principally the sensory axons. Less often axonal degeneration de-

TABLE 57-1.   Diseases That Cause Secondary Peripheral Neuropathy

Disease	Lesion		Dysfunction	
	Axonal	Demyelinating	Motor	Sensory
Acromegaly	+			+
Amyloidosis	+	+		+
Diabetes mellitus	+	+	+	+
Diphtheria		+	+	+
Fabry's disease	+			+
Hypothyroidism		+		+
Liver disease		+	+	+
Malabsorption	+		+	+
Neoplasia	+	+	+	+
Paraproteinemia	+	+	+	+
Porphyria	+		+	
Uremia	+		+	+
Vitamin deficiency	+		+	+

TABLE 57-2. Toxic Neuropathy

Toxin	Lesion		Dysfunction	
	Axonal	Demyelinating	Motor	Sensory
Acrylamide	+		+	+
Amiodarone	+	+	+	+
Arsenic	+		+	+
Carbon Disulfide	+	+	+	+
Dapsone	+		+	
Diketone hexacarbons	+	+	+	+
Dimethylaminopropionitrile	+		+	+
Gold	+	+	+	+
Isoniazid	+		+	+
Lead	+		+	+
Metronidazole	+			+
Misonidazole	+			+
Organophosphate	+		+	+
Perhexilene	+	+	+	+
Phenytoin	+		+	+
Platinum	+			+
Pyridoxine	+			+
Thalidomide	+		+	+
Thallium	+		+	+
Vinca alkaloids	+		+	+

velops earlier in the disease, especially in patients with carcinoma of a lung, and causes a mixed motor and sensory neuropathy, sometimes with autonomic dysfunction, or a carcinoma causes demyelination affecting both sensory and motor axons. Lymphomata cause both axonal injury and demyelination, usually with both motor and sensory dysfunction.

Amyloid. Amyloid is deposited in peripheral nerves principally in the endoneurium and destroys mainly unmyelinated nerve fibers and to a lesser degree small myelinated fibers. The result is a slowly progressive neuropathy, which is mainly sensory, with pain, paresthesias, and muscular tenderness.

TOXIC NEUROPATHY. Table 57-2 lists some of the more common forms of toxic neuropathy. In most, the dysfunction develops slowly, though arsenic and other agents given in large dose can cause acute peripheral neuropathy. Alcohol is a common cause of peripheral neuropathy but is not listed here because the injury to the nerves is caused by vitamin deficiency.

TRAUMATIC NEUROPATHY. Traumatic neuropathy can result from direct injury to a nerve or from pressure on a nerve by some adjacent structure. Pressure from a crutch can injure the radial nerve in the axilla. Pressure in the carpal tunnel is a common cause of median neuropathy. Pressure at the elbow can damage the ulna nerve. Compression of a nerve by the head of a metatarsal gives rise to Morton's neuroma, named after an American surgeon (1835–1903). Usually traumatic neuropathy involves only one nerve, and both motor and sensory axons are affected. Often there is scarring at the site of the lesion. The dysfunction depends on the nerve involved and the severity of the injury.

EPILEPSY

Epilepsy is the term used to describe a group of conditions in which the patients have repeated seizures, usually all much alike. If the cause of the seizures is known, the patient is said to have secondary epilepsy. If the cause is unknown, the patient has cryptogenic or idiopathic epilepsy. Between 500 and 2000 people in every 100,000 have epilepsy. A relative of a patient with epilepsy is more likely to develop epilepsy than is the general population. The seizures can begin at any age.

The term *epilepsy* is not applied to isolated

seizures that develop in children or adults. Up to 5% of infants and young children develop seizures if they become feverish, but if the seizure is short-lived and generalized, and there are no abnormalities in the electroencephalogram between attacks, there is little risk that the child will have epilepsy later in life. In older people, uremia, hepatic failure, hypocalcemia, hypercalcemia, hypoglycemia, hyperglycemia, hyponatremia, and hypernatremia are among the causes of isolated seizures.

Lesions. Epileptic seizures are caused by a rhythmic and highly synchronized discharge of many neurons. Often the abnormal discharge begins in a localized focus. Frequently it spreads to neighboring neurons or to neurons joined by synapses to those in the original focus, increasing the severity of the seizure. The concentration of potassium in the extracellular fluid rises in the regions involved, and the concentration of calcium falls. Neurotransmitters are released in large quantity.

In secondary epilepsy, lesions in the brain initiate the abnormal discharge. In idiopathic epilepsy, lesions in the brain are common, but are unrelated to the epilepsy or caused by it.

Secondary Epilepsy. In infants and children, secondary epilepsy is most often precipitated by birth injuries, hypoxia, ischemia, intracranial infection, hypoglycemia, hypocalcemia, or a congenital anomaly. The local lesion in the brain determines the site of the abnormal neuronal discharge.

In adolescents and young adults, head injury is the most common cause of secondary epilepsy. If the dura is torn or amnesia persists for more than 24 hours, over 40% of the patients develop epilepsy. About 10% of patients with cerebral contusion without breach of the dura develop epilepsy. An arteriovenous aneurysm or withdrawal of drugs or alcohol sometimes precipitates epilepsy in people of this age.

In 30% of people who develop epilepsy when between 30 and 50 years old, a brain tumor is responsible. Most often the tumor is a meningioma that presses on the cerebral cortex or is a slow-growing glioma. In people over 50 years old, ischemia or hemorrhage caused by cerebrovascular disease is the most common cause of secondary epilepsy. Over 10% of patients with a cerebrovascular accident have at least one seizure. Primary or secondary brain tumors are another common cause of secondary epilepsy in people over 50 years old. Some 5% of patients with multiple sclerosis develop epilepsy. Neuronal degenerative and demyelinating diseases can cause epilepsy.

Idiopathic Epilepsy. In 70% of adults and 50% of children with epilepsy no cause for the dysfunction is found. The lesions in the brain are thought to be caused by the epilepsy. Lesions like those of hypoxia are present in the hippocampi in 50% of the patients. In 45% of the patients, the loss of Purkinje cells and a lesser degree granular cells from the cerebellum causes gliosis. The dentate nuclei are similarly involved. Lesions are present in other parts of the cerebral cortex in 25% of the patients, in the thalamus in 25%, and in the amygdaloid nuclei in 25%.

About 25% of patients with epilepsy have cerebral contusions caused by falling during a seizure. Some have in the cerebral cortex small foci of malformed neurons and bizarre astrocytes. Some have one or more nodules up to 2 cm across in the cerebral cortex or white matter of the cerebral hemispheres. Microscopically, the nodules consist of a proliferation of abnormal astrocytes, oligodendrocytes, or both. They are probably hamartomatous, not neoplastic.

Clinical Presentation. If the seizure involves motor functions, the patient has a convulsion. If not, the patient suffers a sensory, autonomic, cognitive, or emotional seizure, manifest by abnormal sensations, abnormal autonomic discharge, confusion of thought, or temporary psychiatric derangement.

In a focal or partial seizure, the abnormal discharge is confined to one part of the cerebral cortex. Often the attack begins in a hand and extends to involve the arm. The attack usually lasts a few minutes. In a simple seizure, the patient remains conscious and aware of the environment. In a complex seizure, consciousness is lost, or the patient is no longer aware of the surroundings. When the seizure is over, a patient with a complex seizure does not remember what happened during the seizure.

Generalized seizures, often called grand mal seizures from the French for great evil, are the most common form of epileptic attack. Some grand mal attacks are preceded by a focal seizure or a prodromal phase, but most start abruptly. The patient suddenly loses consciousness and falls. For some seconds, spasms of the muscles hold the body rigid in opisthotonos. Breathing may stop. Then come a series of convulsive contractions and relaxations of the muscles that last for a second or minutes. As the convulsion ends, the muscles relax. The patient remains unconscious for some minutes longer and then gradually returns to consciousness. Urinary and fecal incontinence are common during the seizure. Often the tongue is bitten. Less often, a patient suddenly becomes rigid, but does not develop the convulsive movements of a grand mal attack.

Absence or petit mal seizures, from the French for small evil, begin in childhood, rarely in adult life. The patient suddenly ceases all activity for a few seconds or minutes, with only minor if any motor manifestations. Full consciousness is regained immediately. Sometimes a child has more than 100 such attacks a day. Sometimes the attacks are so short that they go undetected for months.

In status epilepticus, seizures follow one another without interval. In some patients, seizures occur only in relation to the menstrual cycle, when the patient is touched, or are triggered by exposure to light, certain kinds of music, or reading.

Treatment and Prognosis. In 70% of patients with epilepsy, the seizures can be controlled by anticonvulsive drugs. In secondary epilepsy, surgical removal of the lesion causing the seizures often brings cure. If the focus originating the attack in idiopathic epilepsy can be localized in a temporal lobe, removal of the focus ameliorates the condition in 70% of the patients and brings cure in 30%. The tissue removed often shows ischemic changes or a hamartoma.

In status epilepticus with grand mal attacks, 10% of the patients die, and 20% are left with permanent neurologic damage. Other patients with epilepsy have a normal life span. In some, behavioral changes become prominent.

DISTURBANCES IN HYDRATION

This section considers cerebral edema, increased intracranial pressure, hydrocephalus, and hydromyelia.

EDEMA. Most lesions in the brain cause edema in the surrounding tissue. Edema around a tumor, abscess, or hemorrhage is often sufficiently severe to increase considerably the size of the lesion. Edema is usual around infarcts, injuries, and infections. Many of the demyelinizing and metabolic diseases of the central nervous system cause edema. Poisoning with lead, carbon monoxide, or methanol, hypoxia, and diabetic ketoacidosis cause widespread cerebral edema.

Two kinds of cerebral edema are distinguished. In one, increased vascular permeability increases quantity of fluid in the extracellular space. In the other, fluid accumulates in the processes of astrocytes and oligodendrocytes because of a disturbance in the mechanisms governing ion transport across their membranes. In most forms of cerebral edema, both mechanisms are involved. Fluid accumulates both in the extracellular space and in the glial cells.

Edema of the brain or spinal cord affects principally the white matter. The affected part of the white matter is swollen and on section is damp or yellowish. The edematous region is ill-defined and merges vaguely with the surrounding white matter. Because of the increased volume of the edematous tissue, the overlying gyri are thickened and flattened. The ventricles may be distorted.

Microscopically, the cells and fibers in the white matter are separated by fluid. Myelin sheaths and later axons become swollen and beaded and eventually break down, though there is little microglial or macrophage reaction. Proliferation of astrocytes is often so profuse that the lesion resembles a glioma. Eventually, loose, fine gliosis surrounding little spaces and microcysts filled with edema fluid repair the injury.

INCREASED INTRACRANIAL PRESSURE. Anything that increases the volume of the brain, the intracranial meninges or the cerebrospinal fluid increases the intracranial pressure. The intracranial tissues can do little to make room for anything that takes up space. Once its sutures have closed, the skull is rigid and cannot expand. The ventricles contain 40 mL of cerebrospinal fluid, and there are a few mL of fluid in the subarachnoid space. The rest of the cranium is filled with the incompressible brain and its meninges. A sudden increase of 80 mL in the intracranial volume brings death. A lesion that grows slowly can become larger, for it allows time to adjust the position of the brain, and often atrophy of white matter to accommodate the mass.

Among the more common focal lesions that increase the intracranial pressure are tumors of the brain or meninges, intracranial hematomata, abscesses, and infarcts. Cerebral edema, local or generalized, causes increased intracranial pressure. The increase in the volume of the cerebrospinal fluid in meningitis or benign intracranial hypertension raises the intracranial pressure.

Lesions. Increased intracranial pressure causes papilledema, as edema of the head of the optic nerve is called. The papilledema is due in part to the increased pressure in the prolongations of the subarachnoid space along the optic nerves, in part to the venous congestion caused by the increased intracranial pressure.

The increased cranial pressure compresses veins and capillaries in the brain, reducing the blood flow to the brain and causing hypoxia. The systemic blood pressure rises in an attempt to maintain the oxygenation of the brain, but often is unable to do so. The hypoxia causes more edema, raising further the intracranial pressure. The ventricles are pressed flat. Often the brain is pressed against the skull, compressing the subarachnoid space. Its gyri are flattened and thickened. The sulci are obscured.

If a lesion above the tentorium cerebelli makes the pressure above the tentorium greater than that in the occipital fossa, the upper part of the brain stem and the medial parts of one or both temporal lobes are pushed down through the incisura. If the supratentorial lesion is unilateral, the herniation is greater on the side of the lesion. Frequently pressure of the incisura forms a groove in the herniated temporal lobe.

The compression of the brain stem as it is forced through the incisura of the tentorium cerebelli obstructs its arterial and venous blood flow. Foci of hemorrhagic necrosis develop in the midbrain and upper pons, especially in the reticular nuclei and the

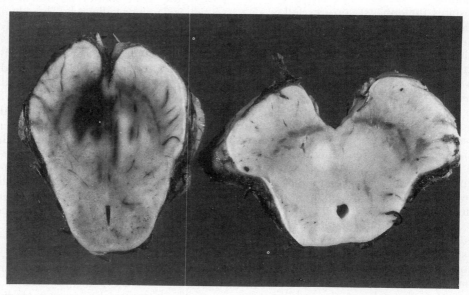

Fig. 57-27. Left, distortion of the midbrain, with focal, hemorrhagic necroses, caused by bilateral herniation of the temporal lobes through the incisura of the tentorium. The patient had a supratentorial mass. Right, a normal midbrain. (Courtesy of Dr. J. H. N. Deck)

nuclei of the upper cranial nerves. Compression of the herniated part of a temporal lobe sometimes causes ischemia and necrosis in the herniated part of the lobe. Sometimes the posterior cerebral artery is stretched against the edge of the tentorium cerebelli, causing hemorrhagic infarction of the medial part of the occipital lobe. Frequently the third nerve is stretched around a displaced posterior cerebral artery, causing a third nerve palsy.

If a supratentorial lesion causing herniation through the tentorium cerebelli is unilateral, the opposite cerebral peduncle is sometimes pressed against the margin of the tentorium, causing necrosis of the pyramidal tracts on the side of the supratentorial lesion. The indentation caused by pressure on the peduncle is called Kernohan's notch, after the American pathologist who described it in 1929.

If the pressure in the posterior cavity increases sufficiently, the lower part of the medulla and the inferior part of the cerebellum are forced down through the foramen magnum. The pressure of the foramen often produces prominent grooves in the cerebellar tonsils. Sometimes the herniated tonsils show foci of hemorrhagic necrosis. Fragments of

the herniated cerebellum are occasionally shed into the cerebrospinal fluid. Lumbar puncture in a patient with increased intracranial pressure can precipitate herniation of the medulla and cerebellum into the foramen magnum by suddenly reducing the pressure in the spinal canal.

Less often, a tumor in the cerebellum causes herniation of the cerebellum upwards through the tentorium cerebelli, compressing the midbrain and impairing its blood supply. Sudden reduction of the supratentorial pressure during ventriculography can induce this kind of herniation.

A space-occupying lesion in one cerebral hemisphere pushes the midline structures towards the other side. Sometimes the cingulate gyrus herniates beneath the falx cerebri. The gyrus sometimes becomes necrotic.

Clinical Presentation. The clinical signs caused by increased intracranial pressure depend on the site and severity of the injury to the brain. As the pressure increases, traction on the intracranial vessels causes headache. The more rapid the increase in intracranial pressure, the more severe the headache. Examination of the eyes reveals papilledema. Pressure on the third nerves or injury to their nuclei causes temporary con-

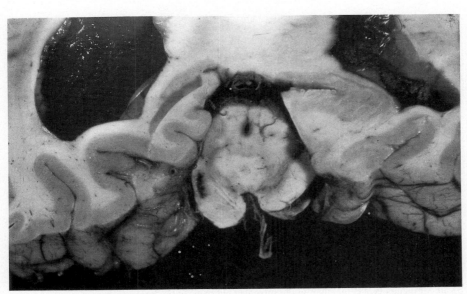

Fig. 57-28. Herniation of the right temporal lobe through the incisura and the tentorium, distorting the left cerebral peduncle and producing a left Kernohan's notch caused by a right intracerebral hemorrhage, with rupture into the lateral ventricle. (Courtesy of Dr. J. H. N. Deck)

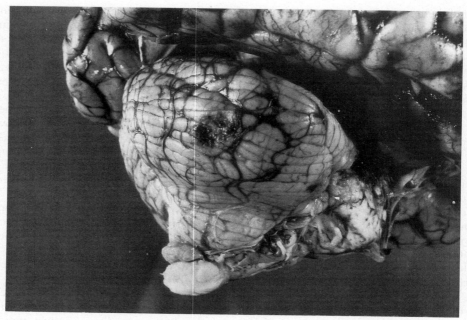

Fig. 57-29. Conical compression and distortion of the cerebellum caused by herniation of the cerebellar tonsils through the foramen magnum. (Courtesy of Dr. J. H. N. Deck)

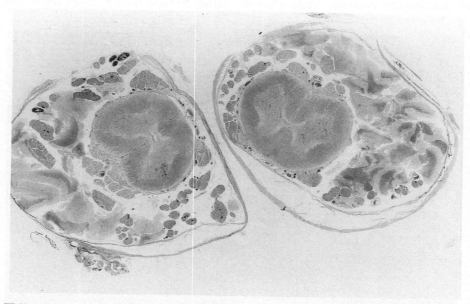

Fig. 57-30. Fragments of cerebellum in the subarachnoid space in the lumbar region of a patient with increased intracranial pressure and herniation of the cerebellum through the foramen magnum. The herniation caused necrosis and disruption of the cerebellum, shedding fragments of cerebellar tissue into the cerebrospinal fluid. (Courtesy of Dr. J. H. N. Deck)

striction of the pupils and then the fixed, dilated pupils common in increased intracranial pressure. Only occasionally is there loss of visual acuity. Compression of a cerebral peduncle causes pyramidal signs on the side of a supratentorial lesion. Herniation of the cingulate gyrus causes no dysfunction.

Confusion and coma develop when increased intracranial pressure damages the brain stem or causes cerebral ischemia. Cheyne-Stokes breathing and other disorders of respiration may appear. Decorticate posturing sometimes develops. The eyes may be divergent and roving or fixed.

Treatment and Prognosis. The treatment of increased intracranial pressure depends largely on its cause. Reducing the P_{CO_2} in the plasma to below 30 mm Hg and dehydration with mannitol help lower the pressure. If it cannot be reduced to less than 20 mm Hg (300 mm water), the prognosis is poor. The damage to the medulla caused by herniation through the foramen magnum and the infarcts and hemorrhages in the brain stem caused by herniation through the tentorium cerebelli often cause death. About 50% of people with a severe head injury die from increased intracranial pressure.

BENIGN INTRACRANIAL HYPERTENSION. Benign intracranial hypertension is a rare condition, most often found in young women. The cerebrospinal fluid pressure rises to between 20 and 45 mm Hg, (300 and 600 mm water), without other detectable abnormality. The condition usually resolves in a few months, though occasionally the papilledema causes optic atrophy. A similar increase in cerebrospinal fluid pressure occasionally complicates hypoparathyroidism, Addison's disease, adrenal corticosteroid therapy, and tetracycline therapy. Thiazide diuretics can often reduce the intracranial pressure sufficiently to control the symptoms.

HYDROCEPHALUS. The term *hydrocephalus* is derived from the Greek words for water and head, and is used to describe the conditions in which the quantity of cerebrospinal fluid in the cranium is greatly increased. If only the ventricles are dilated, the disorder is called an internal hydrocephalus. In a communicating hydrocephalus, cerebrospinal fluid flows freely between dilated ventricles and the spinal canal. A localized collection of cerebrospinal fluid in the subarachnoid space is called an external hydrocephalus. Hydrocephalus caused by shrinkage of the brain is called hydrocephalus ex vacuo.

Most often, hydrocephalus is caused by obstruction to the flow of cerebrospinal fluid from the ventricles to the subarachnoid space at the base of the brain. Less often, the obstruction is in the aqueduct, at the foramina of Luschka and Magendie, the incisura of the tentorium cerebelli, or in the subarachnoid space over the surface of the cerebral hemispheres.

Adhesions caused by meningitis or a subarachnoid hemorrhage are among the more common causes of hydrocephalus. In children, congenital malformations often cause hydrocephalus, most frequently by obstructing the aqueduct or as part of the Arnold–Chiari syndrome. A tumor and other lesions can obstruct the aqueduct or some other part of the ventricular system. Occasionally thrombosis of the venous sinuses causes hydrocephalus by preventing the resorption of cerebrospinal fluid by the subarachnoid villi. Any condition that causes shrinkage of part of the brain causes hydrocephalus ex vacuo as the ventricles or the subarachnoid space enlarge to fill the space.

If hydrocephalus develops before the cranial sutures have closed, the head enlarges, often greatly. The cranial bones are widely separated. The eyes are displaced downwards. The ventricles become enormously dilated, reducing the cerebral cortex to a thin rind. The brain stem is usually preserved. The cerebral atrophy causes progressive mental deterioration. Papilledema sometimes causes optic atrophy and blindness. Injury to the corticospinal tracts sometimes causes spastic paraplegia.

In older children and in adults, the cranial sutures have closed, and the head cannot enlarge. The pressure of the cerebrospinal fluid proximal to the obstruction rises. The ventricles dilate, as the continuing pressure causes progressive atrophy of the white matter of the cerebral hemispheres. The cerebral cortex and the basal ganglia are well preserved, and there is usually no mental change. The symptoms are those of increased intracranial pressure.

In many patients, hydrocephalus becomes

stationary, ceases to enlarge, and causes no serious disability. If the hydrocephalus is more severe and continues to increase, it is managed by establishing a shunt proximal to the site of obstruction to drain away the excess cerebrospinal fluid and reduce the intracranial pressure. Without treatment, 50% of children with progressive hydrocephalus die within two years.

NORMAL PRESSURE HYDROCEPHALUS. Patients with normal pressure hydrocephalus gradually lose memory and as months pass become slowly demented. Movements become slowed, usually with abnormalities in gait. Incontinence is common. The patients have a communicating hydrocephalus with widely dilated ventricles and increasing destruction of the white matter in the cerebral hemispheres. The intracranial pressure is normal. The cause of the disorder is unknown. In over 60% of the patients, a shunt to drain cerebrospinal fluid from the ventricles arrests the disease and improves function.

HYDROMYELIA. Dilatation of the central canal in the spinal cord is called hydromyelia, from the Greek for water and marrow. It sometimes develops in patients with hydrocephalus, in infants with a meningomyelocele, people with bony deformity of the neck, or occasionally extends for a few segments in people otherwise normal. Hydromyelia is rarely of importance clinically.

CONGENITAL ANOMALIES

Nearly 1% of infants have a congenital anomaly of the nervous system. In the United States, 500 infants in every 100,000 born alive have cerebral palsy. In many of the children affected, there are also anomalies in other organs.

In 60% of the infants, the cause of the anomaly is unknown. In 25% a genetic abnormality is responsible, acting alone or with an environmental factor. In 5%, a chromosomal abnormality is present. In 10%, a toxin injures the fetus. Congenital anomalies are more common in children born of older mothers.

Among the more common causes of congenital defects in the nervous system are the trisomies 21, 17, and 13. Rubella, cyto-

megaloviral infections, and toxoplasmosis are among the infections most likely to injure the fetus. Thalidomide, cytotoxic agents, and organic mercury are some of the drugs that cause fetal anomalies. Irradiating the fetus is dangerous, especially during the first four months of pregnancy. Diabetes mellitus, phenylketonuria, hypoxia, excess or deficiency of vitamin A, and other nutritional or metabolic disorders can cause anomalies of the nervous system.

Spinal Cord

The congenital anomalies that affect principally the spinal cord are caused by malformation of the neural tube. They are often associated with malformation of the vertebrae in the region involved. Bony faults of this sort have been reported in from 2 to 25% of people, but only in 1 person in 1000 has an anomaly in the spinal cord or its meninges.

RACHISCHISIS. Failure of the closure of the vertebral arches is called rachischisis, from the Greek for the backbone and a cleft. It may or may not be associated with anomalies in the spinal cord or its meninges. Several types of rachischisis are distinguished.

Spina Bifida Occulta. Spina bifida occulta, from the Latin for the spine, split in two, and hidden, is the commonest and least severe form of rachischisis. The arches of one or more vertebrae, usually in the lumbar region, are partially or completely absent. The spinal cord and its meninges are usually normal, but occasionally an adhesion binds the cord to the edge of the defect. In 40% of the infants, diastomatomyelia is present above or below the lesion. Often a tuft of hair in the skin overlies the defect. Less often, the overlying soft tissues are thickened by an angioma, a lipoma, or a firm plaque of collagenous tissue. Occasionally a dermoid cyst, perhaps with a sinus to the surface of the skin, is present over the lesion. Spina bifida occulta usually causes no disability.

Meningocele. In a meningocele, the meninges in the spinal cord herniate through the defect in the vertebral arches, usually in the thoracic or lumbar region. Usually the sac of the meningocele is closed, but sometimes there is a fistula to the surface. Occasionally the sac contains islands of aberrant glial tissue containing a few neurons. About 80% of infants with a meningocele have hydrocephalus or some other neurologic anomaly. If the meningocele is the only defect and is closed, it usually causes no disability.

Meningomyelocele. In a meningomyelocele, both the spinal cord and its meninges are present in the sac that herniates posteriorly through the defect in the vertebral arches. Meningomyeloceles occur more frequently than meningoceles. In some patients, the cord is attached to the spine anteriorly, but its central canal is greatly dilated, allowing the posterior part of the cord to herniate. In others, the cord loses contact with the vertebral bodies and is distorted as it is pulled backwards into the sac. Often isolated islands of glial tissue containing neurons are present in the sac. Most of the patients have other neurologic anomalies, most often hydrocephalus, syringomyelia, or diastomatomyelia. The dysfunction produced depends on the severity of the injury to the spinal cord and the spinal nerves.

Myelocele. In a myelocele, the spinal canal fails to close in the part of the spinal cord involved. The cord remains as a flat plate with its posterior surface covered at least in part with ependyma. The posterior part of the vertebrae fails to form in the region affected. Often the cord is covered posteriorly only by a thin layer of granulation tissue. Usually the cord and spinal nerves are malformed. Ectopic nervous tissue is common. Most of the patients are anencephalic or have other major neurologic abnormalities.

Filum Terminale. In some patients with rashischisis, the filum terminale is short and thick. Often tubules lined by ependyma lie between the thickened fila, or hamartomatous nodules of cartilage, bone, or adipose tissue are present.

Ventral Defects. Ventral defects in the vertebrae are uncommon. Often they are associated with cysts, most often enterogenous cysts, in the cervical or thoracic region.

DIASTEMATOMYELIA. Diastematomyelia, from the Greek words for an interval and marrow, is a deformity in which the lower part of the spinal cord is split in two antero-posteriorly, with one anterior horn and one posterior horn in each half. The central canal bifurcates, with a branch in each half of the cord. Sometimes each part of the cord has its own meningeal sheath, and the two limbs are separated by a fibrous or bony septum. The division rarely extends above the midthoracic region. More than half the patients have spina bifida. Diastematomyelia causes no disability.

SYRINGOMYELIA. Syringomyelia is a condition in which a longitudinal cavity develops in the spinal cord parallel to the spinal canal. The name comes from the Greek words for tube or pipe and marrow. Syringomyelia is often a congenital anomaly, but sometimes is caused by trauma, cavitation of a tumor, or myelitis. In patients with the congenital form of the disease, the Arnold-Chiari anomaly and other malformations of the nervous system are common.

The cavity in syringomyelia usually begins in the gray matter of the spinal cord near the midline, dorsal to the central canal. The longitudinal extent of the cavity varies from one patient to another. Most frequently, it extends from the lower or midthoracic region to the upper cervical region. In most patients, the cavity is largest in the lower cervical region, where it is tubular, expands the cord, and replaces much of its substance. At its upper and lower limits, the cavity is often transversely flattened and involves only the gray matter. Sometimes the cavity is unilateral, or two cavities combine near the midpart of the lesion. Sometimes the cavity communicates with the central canal. In the medulla, the cavity of syringobulbia is slitlike and may or may not be associated with syringomyelia.

The cavity is usually surrounded by a glial capsule 1 or 2 mm thick. Sometimes part of the cavity is lined by collagenous tissue. If the cavity communicates with the spinal canal, it is frequently lined in part by ependyma. Occasionally the wall consists of ragged, degenerating neural tissue.

The cavity slowly enlarges. Symptoms usually begin in adolescence, but may not appear until the patient is 60 or 70 years old. The nature of the symptoms depends on the site of the cavity. Wasting and weakness of the muscles of the arms and shoulders are common because of destruction of the motor neurons in the cervical cord. Often a high thoracic kyphoscoliosis develops. Destruction of the spinothalamic fibers crossing to the other side frequently causes loss of pain and temperature sensation. The anesthesia is often complicated by injuries to the extremities and degenerative changes in the joints. Trophic changes in the skin are common. Touch, vibration sense, and deep sensation are preserved because they are transmitted by uncrossed fibers. Pressure on the cerebrospinal tracts can cause spastic paraplegia.

If the patient has syringobulbia, weakness in the face, tongue, palate, throat, and vocal cords is likely. Nystagmus and dizziness are common. Involvement of the autonomic system can cause Horner's syndrome.

In most patients, the symptoms slowly worsen as years pass. Often the progression is intermittent, with long periods in which there is little change. Eventually, more than 50% of the patients become confined to a chair. Surgical decompression to prevent further enlargement of the cavity is sometimes of value.

Brain

Many congenital anomalies affect the brain. Among the more common are anencephaly, the Arnold-Chiari malformation, and tuberous sclerosis.

ANENCEPHALY. Anencephaly, from the Greek for without and brain, is not compatible with life for more than one or two days. In different parts of the world, from 1 infant in 2000 to 1 in 250 is born with anencephaly. The defect is caused in part by failure of the upper part of the neural tube to close, in part by destruction of the parts of the midbrain and cerebral hemispheres that are formed. Major malformations in other organs are common.

Occasionally the brain and spinal cord are completely absent, though the peripheral nerves are formed. More often, all that remains of the brain is a highly vascular plate of glial tissue containing a few neurons that covers the base of the skull. An atrophic anterior pituitary gland is often present, though the neurohypophysis is absent. In a few patients, the cerebellum and brain stem persist.

The bones of the vault of the skull are largely or completely absent. The face and eyes are formed, though the optic nerves are often absent. If the scalp is present, it collapses over the base of the skull. In more than 50% of the patients, there is extensive craniorachischisis, with loss of skin and bone from the posterior part of the skull and spine, leaving the cranial cavity and spinal cord exposed. The base of the skull is small. The number of cervical vertebrae is reduced. The fetal zone of the adrenal cortex is absent.

ENCEPHALOCELE. Herniation of the brain through a defect in the skull is an uncommon defect called an encephalocele. In 90% of the patients, the defect is in the occipital bone. In some it is confined to the squamous part of the bone. In some, it extends into the foramen magnum, and the posterior arch of the atlas is deficient. Less often, the herniation is anterior and distorts the face, extends into a nasal cavity, or bulges into an orbit.

If the defect in the bone is small, only the meninges herniate. If it is larger, the posterior fossa is often enlarged and the skull is distorted. Up to half of one or both cerebral hemispheres prolapse into the hernia and sometimes into part of the cerebellum or brain stem. Pressure on blood vessels often causes infarction or hemorrhage in the herniated tissue. Obstruction to the drainage of cerebrospinal fluid can cause hydrocephalus in the hernia. Islands of ectopic nervous tissue are often present in the hernia. The meninges are intact, but injury to the overlying skin can easily cause meningitis.

NARROWING OF THE AQUEDUCT. Four types of congenital stenosis of the aqueduct cause hydrocephalus. In some infants, two stenoses in the aqueduct are separated by a dilated segment. In some kindred, this malformation is inherited as an autosomal recessive character. In other infants, the aqueduct divides into two narrow channels, often with many blind branches from the posterior channel. One or both of the channels may be blind. Sometimes a septum closes the aqueduct. Sometimes gliosis around the aqueduct causes stenosis.

ARNOLD-CHIARI MALFORMATION. The Arnold-Chiari malformation, named after the

German pathologist Arnold who described it in 1894 and Chiari of the German University in Prague who classified a number of conditions of this sort in 1891, is one of the more common neurologic anomalies. The term is used to describe a group of similar malformations. Nearly 50% of children with hydrocephalus have the Arnold-Chiari syndrome. Almost all the patients have other anomalies in the nervous system and in the bones of the spine and skull.

The medulla and part of the cerebellum herniate through the foramen magnum into the cervical canal. The medulla is usually elongated, with part of the fourth ventricle in the cervical canal. Often the medulla partially overlies the cervical cord and makes an S-shaped bend to pass back upwards to join with the spinal cord. Much of the cerebellar hemispheres herniate with the medulla. The deformed vermis forms a prolongation overlying the elongated fourth ventricle. Often the structure of the vermis is abnormal or there are gliosis and loss of neurons in the herniated part of the medulla and cerebellum. Adhesions often bind the displaced medulla and cerebellum to the cervical canal.

Hydrocephalus is almost invariably present. In some patients, the cerebellum is corked so tightly in the foramen magnum that it obstructs the flow of the cerebrospinal fluid, and a communicating hydrocephalus results. In some, stenosis of the aqueduct or obstruction to the foramina of Luschka and Magendie by the abnormal vermis or by thickening of the roof of the fourth ventricle couses an internal hydrocephalus. Sometimes there is a combination of these abnormalities.

Almost all patients with the Arnold-Chiari malformation have rachischisis, most often a meningomyelocele. In many, the base of the skull is flattened, a condition called platybasia. In some, the odontoid process of the axis projects into the posterior fossa, an abnormality called basilar impression. Reduction in the number of cervical vertebrae is common. Some patients have subluxation of the axis. In some, one or more cervical vertebrae are fused, or the atlas is fused to the skull. Some of the patients with fusion and a reduced number of cervical vertebrae have the short, stiff neck, hypoplastic posterior fossa, and low hairline of the Klippel-Feil

deformity, named after the French physicians born in 1858 and 1884. Some patients with the Arnold-Chiari malformation have polygyria, microgyria, or other deformities of the cerebral hemispheres.

If the herniation of the brain is severe, the hydrocephalus caused by the Arnold-Chiari malformation becomes evident in childhood. The prognosis is poor. If the anomaly is less severe, symptoms begin in adult life, often with episodes of dizziness or weakness, sometimes with signs of injury to the medulla, cerebellum, or lower cranial nerves, less often with hydrocephalus.

DANDY-WALKER SYNDROME. The Dandy-Walker syndrome is an unusual condition named after the American surgeons who described it in 1914 and 1942. Malformation of the vermis of the cerebellum allows a cystic dilation of the fourth ventricle to bulge between the cerebellar hemispheres. Often the foramina of Luschka and Magendie are obliterated. Many of the patients have hydrocephalus with dilation of all ventricles. The posterior fossa is often enlarged, causing distortion and anteroposterior elongation of the skull. Other deformities of the brain and other organs are often present.

PROSENCEPHALY. In the most severe form of prosencephaly, the cerebral hemispheres are fused. The corpus callosum and septum pellucidum are absent. The basal ganglia are fused. The patient has a single ventricle surrounded by a rudimentary cerebral cortex. The cortex may be so thin that the ventricle is a thin-walled sac. The pyramidal tracts are absent. The olfactory bulbs are absent. The brain stem and cerebellum remain intact. Many of the patients have a single, central eye, a condition called cyclopia after the cyclopes, the one-eyed giants of Greek mythology. The face is deformed, often with a rudimentary nose superior to the single eye.

If the condition is less severe, the cerebral hemispheres are separate except anteriorly. The corpus callosum is often absent. Instead, the hemispheres are sometimes joined by a plate of gray and white matter. The olfactory system is completely or partially absent. The face is usually deformed.

COMMISURAL ANOMALIES. Occasionally the corpus callosum fails to develop, though the cerebral hemispheres are otherwise well formed. The septum pellucidum is absent or deformed. In some of the patients, the anterior commissure is absent. If there is no other abnormality in the brain, the patients develop normally and are of normal intelligence.

ARHINENCEPHALY. In arhinencephaly, the olfactory structures fail to develop. The anterior commissure is absent. The corpus callosum is small or absent.

MALFORMATION OF THE SEPTUM PELLUCIDUM. Persistence of the cavum in the septum pellucidum is not uncommon. At times it becomes dilated, either because of congenital malformation or because of trauma or other disease. The dilated cavum is called a fifth ventricle. Most persistent cava cause no dysfunction, but occasionally one is large enough to obstruct the foramina of Munro, causing hydrocephalus. Less often the posterior part of the septum pellucidum persists and gives rise to a cyst called the cavum vergae, or the sixth ventricle. Occasionally the septum pellucidum is fenestrated or absent.

MICROCEPHALY. If the brain weighs less than 900 g, the person is said to have microcephaly, from the Greek for small and head, or microencephaly, from the Greek for small and brain. Often the brain weighs as little as 200 g. Its convolutions are simplified. The cortical neurons are often arranged in columns perpendicular to the surface of the brain. The basal ganglia and cerebellum are less affected and seem disproportionably large. The face is normal, but the cranium is small with premature fusion of its sutures. In some kindred, the anomaly is inherited as an autosomal recessive character.

In a few patients with microcephaly, an abnormal glycoprotein is deposited in the cerebral cortex, corpus striatum, dentate nuclei, and other parts of the brain, and the regions involved are massively calcified. There are gliosis and loss of neurons in these regions.

MEGALENCEPHALY. In megalencephaly, or macrencephaly, the brain weighs over 1600 g, and may reach as much as 2800 g. In many of the patients, the enlargement of the brain is due to overgrowth of glial cells, often with distortion of the neuronal pattern or with ectopic clumps of neurons in the white matter. In some, the structure of the brain is

normal. The patient is sometimes mentally defective, sometimes of normal intelligence.

PORENCEPHALY. The term *porencephaly*, from the Greek for path and brain, was introduced to describe conditions in which there was a passage through the brain from the subarachnoid space to a ventricle, but is often used loosely to describe any condition in which a cystic space or spaces develop in the brain in a young person. The lesion may be congenital or acquired after birth.

In one form of porencephaly, symmetrical clefts are present in the line of the primary fissures. The clefts are lined by pial and ependymal tissue. Often the walls of the clefts fuse. The gray matter at the margins of the cleft is thick and unlaminated. Nests of primitive cells and abnormal neurons are sometimes present.

More often, a large cyst develops in each hemisphere, often replacing much of the frontal and parietal lobes. At the surface of the brain, the walls of the cysts consist only of a thin membrane. The cysts are lined by ependyma. Islands of ectopic neurons are often present in the white matter.

ARACHNOID CYST. An arachnoid cyst is a form of localized, external hydrocephalus caused by malformation of the meninges. The cyst presses on the underlying brain, indenting its surface.

HYDRENCEPHALY. In hydrencephaly, from the Greek for water and brain, the part of the brain supplied by the carotid arteries is reduced to a thin-walled sac. The basal ganglia may or may not be present. The brain looks as if the lateral ventricles were enormously dilated, but the lining of the cavities consists only of thinned pia mater and gliosis, without neurons or ependyma.

PACHYGYRIA. Pachygyria, from the Greek for thick and a ring, also called lissencephaly, from the greek for smooth and brain, is a condition in which the number of gyri in the cerebral hemispheres is reduced. Often the condition is unilateral. At its most severe, only the sylvian fissures remain, and the surface of the hemispheres is smooth. More often, the number of gyri is reduced in part of the cerebral cortex, and those that remain are thicker than normal. In the regions involved, the structure of the cortex is disordered, with gliosis and large, atypical neurons. Ectopic clumps of neurons are present in the white matter. The dysfunction produced depends on the region involved and the extent of the lesion. If the motor cortex is affected, spastic paralysis is common.

MICROGYRIA. Microgyria, also called micropolygyria, from the Greek for small, much, and ring, is a congenital defect in which there are many small gyri in the affected part of a cerebral hemisphere or hemispheres. From the surface, the affected gyri look large, but on section large numbers of little sulci can be seen to branch from the walls of the major sulci. In the affected region, the architecture of the cerebral cortex is disrupted. Involvement of the motor cortex can bring spastic paralysis.

CEREBELLAR MALFORMATIONS. Congenital cerebellar atrophy is often secondary to malformation of the cerebral cortex. Both Purkinje and granular cells are lost, causing gliosis. Often the thalamus and the pontine and dentate nuclei are also atrophied.

Primary malformations of the cerebellum sometimes affect principally the Purkinje cells, sometimes the granular cells. In the regions affected, the cerebellar cortex loses its gyri or shows microgyria. The structure of the cerebral cortex is disrupted. Islands of neurons are often present in the white matter of the cerebellum. The vermis may fail to develop, allowing the cerebellar hemispheres to separate.

TUBEROUS SCLEROSIS. In tuberous sclerosis hamartomata develop in one or more organs. About 1 person in 100,000 has the disease. It is familial in 50% of the patients, inherited as an autosomal dominant character. In the others, it is caused by a new mutation. Men and women are affected equally.

Lesions. Usually tuberous sclerosis involves only one or a few organs. The brain is frequently but not always involved.

When the brain is involved, hard nodules up to 2 cm across develop in the cerebral cortex, widening and hardening the affected gyri. Similar nodules often project into the ventricles, especially the lateral ventricles. Some resemble the guttering of a candle. Smaller nodules are frequently present in the white matter of the cerebral hemispheres or in the brain stem or cerebellum.

Microscopically, the tubers, as the nodules are called, are ill-defined. They consist of dense gliosis, with a much increased number of astrocytic nuclei. Large, atypical astrocytes and neurons are usually present in the lesions. Some of the large cells are multinucleated. Often they have glycogen-filled vacuoles in their cytoplasm. Occasionally some of the abnormal neurons contain inclusions like those of Pick's disease, fibrillary tangles like those of Alzheimer's disease, or granulovacuolar degeneration of the sort seen in Alzheimer's disease. The axons in the tubers are coiled and tangled, often demyelinated. Amyloid bodies like those of Alzheimer's disease are often present in the lesions. Calcospherites are common, and sometimes the lesions become massively calcified. Sometimes clumps of the large cells are present without gliosis, or small nodules of gliosis develop without atypical cells. Occasionally, there is widespread gliosis with scattered atypical cells.

If the retina is involved, hamartomata form nodules in the head of the optic nerve or small, or flattened masses elsewhere in the retina. The term phakoma, from the Greek for a lentil and a lump is used to describe the lesions. Microscopically, the lesions consist of gliosis with large, atypical cells like those in the tubers in the brain. Calcification or ossification may occur. An angiomatous malformation of the choroid is sometimes present.

In the skin, adenoma sebaceum is the most common manifestation of tuberous sclerosis. The adenomata appear on the face during childhood and form multiple pink or yellowish nodules up to 1 cm across. Often angiofibromata appear beneath the nails of the fingers or toes, a patch of roughened shagreen skin develops in the lumbosacral region, or patches of depigmentation become evident. About 50% of the patients have a rhabdomyoma in the heart. Some have an angiomyolipoma in a kidney. Occasionally angiomyomata develop in the lungs, or a fibroma or angiofibroma occurs in bone, the pancreas, or elsewhere. These lesions are discussed with the diseases of the organ principally involved.

Clinical Presentation. When tuberous sclerosis involves the brain, it usually causes epilepsy and mental impairment. Seizures begin in childhood. Frequently adenomata sebacea are present on the face. In the 30% of patients in whom the lesions in the brain are not extensive, intelligence is normal. The symptoms depend on the site of the lesion or lesions.

Treatment and Prognosis. The lesions in the brain and other parts of the body slowly enlarge as years pass. Some of the cerebral lesions become malignant, progressing to become an astrocytoma or glioblastoma multiforme. Few patients with severe involvement of the brain live more than 30 years.

Vascular Malformations

Telangiectases are common in the brain. Larger vascular malformations are infrequent. Occasionally the brain is involved in Sturge-Weber disease or the von Hippel-Lindau syndrome.

TELANGIECTASES. Small vascular hamartomata like the hemangiomata in other parts of the body are present in the central nervous system in 1 autopsy in about 500. They are most frequent in the cerebral hemispheres, cerebellum, and pons. Not uncommonly they are multiple. Microscopically, the lesions are cavernous or capillary hemangiomata, like those in other parts of the body. They rarely cause any dysfunction, but occasionally they cause hemorrhage or serve as a focus for epilepsy.

ARTERIOVENOUS MALFORMATIONS. Larger vascular malformations in the central nervous system are called arteriovenous aneurysms, or cirsoid aneurysms, from the Greek for varix. About 3% of intracranial tumors, using the word loosely to include all kinds of tumor-like masses, are arteriovenous aneurysms.

The aneurysms consist of a tangle of large, thin-walled vessels mixed with well-formed veins and arteries. They are most common in the cerebral hemispheres, less frequent in the cerebellum and parts of the brain or spinal cord. The aneurysm may be less than 1 cm across or may replace much of a cerebral hemisphere or the cerebellum. Often the aneurysm is pyramidal, with its base on the surface of the cerebral hemisphere. It is surrounded by a zone of gliosis. Most arteriovenous aneurysms are supplied by a dilated middle cerebral artery, but if the aneurysm is large, it often draws blood from more than one artery.

An arteriovenous aneurysm of the brain enlarges slowly as the years pass. Some rupture, causing major hemorrhage into the brain or into the subarachnoid space. Even a small aneurysm can cause fatal hemorrhage. Less often, the slow enlargement of the aneurysm produces neurologic signs like those of a tumor. Sometimes an aneurysm serves as a focus of irritation and causes epilepsy.

STURGE-WEBER DISEASE. Sturge-Weber disease is named after the British physicians who described it in 1879 and 1922. The affected children are born with a port wine nevus in the distribution of the ophthalmic branch of the trigeminal nerve and malformation of the vessels in the pia mater overlying the occipital or the occipital and parietal lobes on the same side. Some have an angioma in the retina on that side. The disease is not familial and is not inherited.

In the affected part of the pia mater, large numbers of congested, tortuous, small veins are mixed with large muscular vessels. The meningeal arteries often have subintimal calcification. The vessels in the cerebral cortex are little or not affected.

The superficial layers of the cerebral cortex beneath the malformed pia are atrophied, with extensive calcification that becomes evident radiographically as a linear shadow when the child is one or two years old. The deeper layers of the cerebral cortex and the subjacent white matter are less affected, though there may be occasional calcospherites or calcification of vessels.

Many of the children show only some of the lesions of this syndrome. If the meninges are involved, epilepsy is likely to begin in childhood. Spastic paralysis on the side opposite the lesions is common. Often there is a visual defect on the side of the lesion, or glaucoma on that side causes blindness. Mental retardation is usual.

VON HIPPEL-LINDAU SYNDROME. In the von Hippel-Lindau syndrome, called after the German ophthalmologist von Hippel who described it in 1904 and the Swedish pathologist Lindau who described the lesions in the brain in 1926, the patients have vascular lesions in the retina and the brain. Often there are also angiomata in the liver and other organs; cysts in the liver, pancreas, or kidneys; an adenoma or carcinoma in a

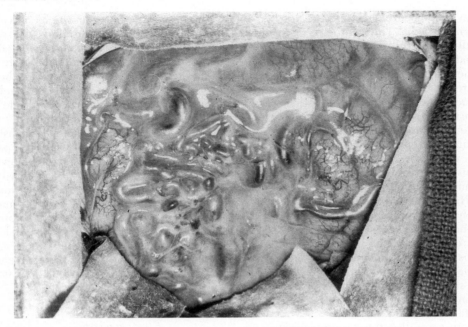

Fig. 57-31. An arteriovenous malformation as seen at craniotomy, showing the tangle of abnormal vessels in and below the subarachnoid membrane. The opacity of the membrane suggests that the malformation has been leaking, causing irritation and thickening of the membrane. (Courtesy of Dr. J. H. N. Deck)

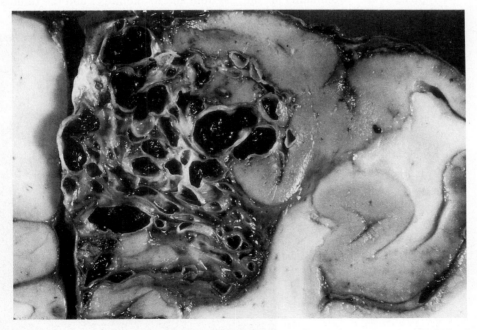

Fig. 57-32. A cross section of an arteriovenous malformation in the brain showing the labyrinth of intertwining blood vessels making up the lesion. The brain adjacent to the malformation is infarcted, because the blood flow through the malformation was so great that it stole blood away from the nearby normal tissue. (Courtesy of Dr. J. H. N. Deck)

kidney; a pheochromocytoma; polycythemia; or syringomeylia. The disorder is inherited as an autosomal recessive character. Many of the patients have only the lesion in the brain or the lesions in the eyes, without other features of the syndrome. Some have only a phaeochromocytoma or some other of the inconstant features of the disorder.

The lesion in the brain in the von Hippel-Lindau syndrome is called a hemangioblastoma. Less than 2% of intracranial tumors are of this type. Only 10% of people with a hemangioblastoma show other features of the von Hippel-Lindau syndrome. The tumor is usually in the cerebellum, frequently in the midline, but can occur in other parts of the brain or in the spinal cord. Sometimes the lesions are multiple. The tumor is attached to the meninges, but lies within the cerebellum or in some other part of the central nervous system. In the cerebellum, hemangioblastomata are often cystic.

Microscopically, the tumor consists of a proliferation of large capillaries like those of other hemangiomata, though with thicker, more active-looking endothelium. Large, fat-filled macrophages are prominent in the connective tissue between the blood vessels. In the cystic cerebellar tumors, the cyst is lined by gliosis. The tumor is confined to a small nodule that bulges into the cyst.

The lesions in the retina are like those in the brain, with similar capillary channels and lipophages. They are usually multiple. The retinal lesions are solid, not cystic.

In the patients with a hemangioblastoma, symptoms usually develop when the patient is 15 to 30 years old. The patient develops the symptoms and signs of a cerebellar tumor or less often shows evidence of a tumor in some other part of the central nervous system. In some patients, other features of the syndrome suggest the nature of the lesion. Complete resection of the tumor cures. Incomplete resection leads to recurrence in 15% of the patients. Coagulation usually controls the retinal lesions.

TUMORS

Primary tumors of the nervous system are divided into the lesions of the central nervous system and its meninges and the tumors that

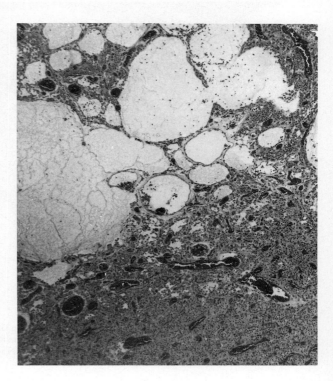

Fig. 57-33. A hemangioblastoma of the cerebellum, showing the large vascular spaces seen in this condition.

arise from the nerves and peripheral ganglia. In the central nervous system, tumors arise from glial cells, neurons, meninges, and blood vessels, rarely from the collagenous tissue within the brain. In the nerves and peripheral ganglia, they arise from Schwann cells, neurons, and the collagenous tissue within the nerves. Table 57-3 shows a classification of these tumors.

Each year, 5 people in every 100,000 develop a primary tumor of the central nervous system. They cause 2 or 3% of deaths from neoplasia. Most arise in children or in people over 50 years old. Tumors of the peripheral nervous system are more common, but most of them are benign.

Glial Tumors

Tumors of the astrocytes, oligodendrocytes, and ependyma are called gliomata. A tumor of astrocytes is called an astrocytoma, a tumor of oligodendrocytes an oligodendroglioma, and a tumor of ependyma an ependymoma. An anaplastic tumor of the glial cells is usually called a glioblastoma multiforme. Most glioblastomata arise from astrocytes, but originate from oligodendrocytes or the ependyma. The tumors of the choroid plexus, the lesion called an subependymal glioma, and the cysts of the third ventricle are considered with the glial tumors.

In adults, carcinomata are 50 times more frequent than gliomata, and hematopoietic tumors are 4 times as frequent. In children only hematopoietic tumors are more common than tumors of the central nervous system, and 60% of the tumors of the nervous system are gliomata.

Over 95% of gliomata arise in the brain. About 40% of intracranial tumors are gliomata. Some 25% of intracranial tumors are metastases, and 15% are meningiomata. Only 15% of tumors of the spinal cord are gliomata. Schwannomata on the spinal nerves, meningiomata, and metastases are the common tumors in the spinal canal. Rarely, a glioma arises in the nose or in the sacral region. A glioma can develop at any age. Gliomata are a little more frequent in boys and men than in girls and women.

All gliomata tend to invade and by the

TABLE 57-3.   Tumors of the Nervous System

CENTRAL NERVOUS SYSTEM

Tumors of glial cells
   Tumors of astrocytes
      Astrocytoma   (Astrocytoma grade I)
      Astroblastoma   (Astrocytoma grade II)
      Glioblastoma multiforme (Astrocytoma grades III & IV)

   Tumors of oligodendrocytes
      Oligodendroglioma

   Tumors of ependyma
      Ependymoma
      Papilloma of the choroid plexus
      Subependymal glioma
      Colloid cyst of the third ventricle

Tumors of neurons
      Medulloblastoma
      Medulloepithelioma
      Neuroblastoma
      Ganglioneuroma
      Ganglioglioma
      Dysplastic gangliocytoma

Tumors of the meninges
      Meningioma
      Malignant meningioma
      Meningeal hemangiopericytoma
      Meningeal sarcoma

Tumors of the blood vessels
      Hemangioblastoma
      Telangiectasis
      Lymphoma

Secondary Tumors
      Carcinoma
      Leukemia
      Lymphoma

PERIPHERAL NERVOUS SYSTEM

Tumors of Schwann cells
      Schwannoma
      Neurofibroma
      Granular cell myoblastoma

Tumors of Neurons
      Neuroblastoma
      Ganglioneuroma
      Ganglioneuroblastoma

Sarcoma of nerves
      Neurofibrosarcoma

Secondary tumors

von Recklinghausen's disease

usual criteria should be considered to be malignant. However, the term *malignant* is often reserved for the more anaplastic gliomata. Sometimes a well-differentiated glioma is said to have become malignant if it becomes more anaplastic.

ASTROCYTOMA. In the past, the tumors of the astrocytes were divided into a number of subgroups and given names that described the microscopic appearence of the tumor cells, often comparing them to cells seen at various stages of the development of the nervous system in utero. This system is no longer used, but some of the names are still employed to describe the microscopic appearance of the tumors.

A more simple classification of the tumors of the astrocytes divides them into four grades. Many centers have adopted this classification, but it has failed to win general acceptance. Those who use it call the most highly differentiated tumors of the astrocytes an astrocytoma grade I, and divide the less well-differentiated tumors into astrocytomata grade II, III, and IV.

Other centers prefer to reserve the term *astrocytoma* for the astrocytomata of grade I, use the term *astroblastoma* for astrocytomata of grade II, and group astrocytomata of grades III and IV together as glioblastoma multiforme. This usage will be adopted here. About 25% of gliomata are well-differentiated tumors of grade I.

Lesions. An astrocytoma, or an astrocytoma of grade I if that terminology is preferred, can arise in any part of the central nervous system. In adults, most originate in one of the cerebral hemispheres. In children and adolescents, they are more common below the tentorium cerebelli, in the cerebellum, brain stem, or around the third ventricle. Rarely, there is more than one astrocytoma.

In adults, an astrocytoma of the cerebral hemispheres usually forms an ill-defined mass, more or less spheroidal, usually 5 to 10 cm in diameter. Occasionally the tumor replaces much of a hemisphere or even more of the brain. The tumor has no clear margin, but merges vaguely with the surrounding tissues. Usually the tumor is firmer than the surrounding brain, but sometimes it is soft and pulpy. Occasionally a few small cysts are present within the astrocytoma.

In children, the astrocytomata below the tentorium cerebelli are usually more clearly defined. In the cerebellum, an astrocytoma is often cystic and is particularly well demarcated. Often the cyst makes up most of the mass, with only a small nubbin of solid tumor in the wall of the cyst. The cyst contains clear or yellowish fluid and may be lined by tumor or by reactive gliosis. Astrocytomata that infiltrate widely also occur in the cerebellum in children, less often in the pons, and other parts of the brain stem.

Microscopically, an astrocytoma can show any of a variety of patterns or a combination of these patterns. The fibrillary pattern is the most common. The bulk of the tumor consists of a dense meshwork of glial fibers. The bodies of the tumor cells may be small and regular or larger, more irregular in size and often stellate. Mitoses are rare. The intertwining processes of the tumor cells contain many glial filaments and microtubules. At times a biopsy of such a tumor is hard to distinguish from reactive gliosis.

Less common is the protoplasmic type of astrocytoma. The tumor cells are plump and swollen, with short processes and few glial filaments. They are separated by filmy, eosinophilic material.

In a pilocytic astrocytoma, from the Latin for a hair, the tumor cells are elongated and often lie more or less parallel to one another. Their nuclei are spindle shaped and tend to lie side by side. Glial filaments are numerous in the long extensions of the pilocytic cells. In children, though rarely in adults, the tumor cells in a pilocytic astrocytoma are often concentrated around the blood vessels, and the parts of the tumor distant from the vessels become loose and cystic. Rosenthal fibers like those in Alexander's disease are sometimes prominent.

A gemistocytic astrocytoma, from the Greek for laden, has large, globoid tumor cells with short processes and hyaline, eosinophilic cytoplasm. The nuclei are small and eccentric. The tumor cells are closely packed. Their cytoplasm contains variable numbers of mitochondria with more or less endoplasmic reticulum and a few lysosomes. Glial filaments

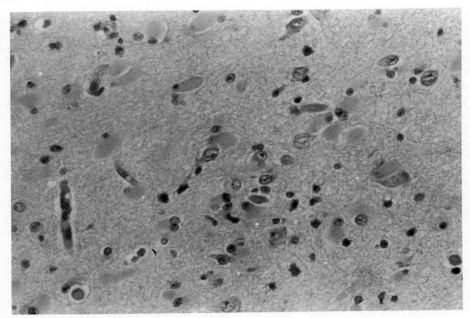

Fig. 57-34. A well-differentiated astrocytoma, showing tumor cells with abundant cytoplasm scattered in an otherwise well-preserved cerebral cortex. (Courtesy of Dr. J. H. N. Deck)

are present only at the periphery of the gemistocytes.

Occasional calcified spherules like psammoma bodies are present near blood vessels or elsewhere in an astrocytoma. Occasionally the endothelium in the blood vessels is hyperplastic.

Cerebral astrocytomata are usually predominantly of the fibrillary form, though often with some admixture of pilocytic or gemistocytic regions. Occasionally a tumor is principally of the pilocytic or gemistocytic pattern. The tumors contain not only neoplastic astrocytes, but also a considerable proliferation of oligodendrocytes, though whether the oligodendrocytes are neoplastic is uncertain.

Cerebellar tumors frequently show a mixture of compact areas of pilocytic pattern and loose regions with stellate astrocytes concentrated around the many blood vessels. Only an occasional protoplasmic or pilocytic astrocyte is present in the loose tissue between the vessels. Less often, a cerebellar astrocytoma shows only the juvenile pilocytic pattern or is an infiltrating fibrillary tumor.

Astrocytomata in the region of the third ventricle are most often of the juvenile pilocytic type. Tumors of the pons and brain stem are usually fibrillary, but may be of the juvenile pilocytic type.

The concentration of protein in the cerebrospinal fluid often increases in a patient with an astrocytoma. The cellularity of the fluid remains normal.

Behavior. An astrocytoma usually grows slowly. Most invade to some degree, some to a considerable extent. Only the cerebellar tumors in children are relatively well contained. The astrocytoma pushes in among the surrounding tissue elements, distorting and displacing them, but for a long time leaving them intact. Both the surrounding brain and the overlying meninges are invaded. Metastases to other parts of the subarachnoid space are rare.

A cystic astrocytoma in the cerebellum sometimes enlarges rapidly. The tumor remains well defined and does not increase in size, but fluid is attracted into the cyst, which becomes increasingly swollen.

As years pass, many astrocytomata show one or more foci in which the tumor has become more anaplastic. More than 80%

of cerebral astrocytomata eventually show anaplastic changes. Only astrocytomata of the cerebellum rarely become anaplastic. In the anaplastic regions, the astrocytoma becomes more cellular, more pleomorphic, with atypical cells, and proliferation and hyperplasia of the blood vessels, much as in a glioblastoma multiforme. Macroscopically, the anaplastic areas often show foci of necrosis and hemorrhage.

Clinical Presentation. An astrocytoma is often present for many years before the patient comes for treatment. Often epilepsy is the first sign of a cerebral astrocytoma and persists with little change for several years before other signs of cerebral dysfunction or signs of increased intracranial pressure develop. A sudden worsening of symptoms usually indicates progression of part of the tumor to a more anaplastic form.

A tumor near the third ventricle sometimes causes diabetes insipidus, obesity, emaciation, or other evidence of hypothalamic dysfunction, which persists with little change for years. An astrocytoma of the pons causes slowly progressive injury to the nuclei of the cranial nerves and to the long motor and sensory tracts. If a cerebellar astrocytoma enlarges rapidly, it causes symptoms and signs like those of other rapidly expanding cerebellar lesions.

Treatment and Prognosis. If possible, an astrocytoma is excised. Irradiation is valuable if surgical resection is impossible. If the astrocytoma is in a cerebral hemisphere, 70% of the patients survive for one year and 50% for two years. About 30% are alive after five years and are probably cured. Resection is less likely to leave serious neurologic dysfunction if the tumor is in the nondominant hemisphere. If the tumor is in the cerebellum, most patients survive over 20 years and are cured. The prognosis is better if the tumor is cystic. The prognosis for an astrocytoma of the third ventricle or pons is bad, though some patients have survived for several years. Sometimes a shunt to relieve hydrocephalus is helpful. People with an astrocytoma of the spinal cord usually survive 10 years or more.

ASTROBLASTOMA. Astroblastomata or astrocytoma grade II, make up 2% of gliomata. They are most common in young adults, but can occur in children. Foci that have the structure of an astroblastoma are sometimes present in an astrocytoma or a glioblastoma multiforme. A tumor should not be called an astroblastoma unless its structure is predominantly that of an astroblastoma.

Most astroblastomata arise in the cerebral hemispheres. A few occur in the cerebellum, rarely elsewhere in the central nervous system. The tumor forms a well-defined gray or pink mass, usually 5 to 10 cm in diameter. The tumor sometimes contains cysts or foci of necrosis.

Microscopically, an astroblastoma is highly vascular. The collagenous walls of the vessels are thick. Sometimes a few lymphocytes are present in the vessel wall. The majority of the tumor cells are clustered around the blood vessels, with the nuclei and cell bodies of the neoplastic astrocytes separated from the vessel by long astrocytic processes, often called pseudorosettes, that extend radially from the vessel. The foot plates of the processes encase the vessel. The nuclei of the tumor cells are even and regular. Mitoses are rare. Between the pseudorosettes, the structure of the tumor is loose, with scattered stellate tumor cells with nuclei like those of the cells in the rosettes. Blepharoplasts are not present.

Astroblastomata tend to grow more rapidly than astrocytomata. Some progress to glioblastoma multiforme. The treatment is excision, if possible, and irradiation.

GLIOBLASTOMA MULTIFORME. About 50% of patients with a glioma have a glioblastoma multiforme. The patients are usually over 40 years old, often older. In people over 60 years old, 90% of gliomata are of this type.

Most glioblastomata arise from astrocytes, but some are anaplastic tumors of other glial cells. With so anaplastic a tumor, it is not always possible to determine its cell of origin. A distinction is sometimes drawn between a glioblastoma multiforme, in which the whole tumor is anaplastic, and a malignant astrocytoma, in which part of the tumor is anaplastic like a glioblastoma multiforme, but part remains better differentiated, like an astrocytoma.

Lesions. Almost all glioblastomata arise in the white matter of the cerebral hemispheres, most often in the anterior part of the

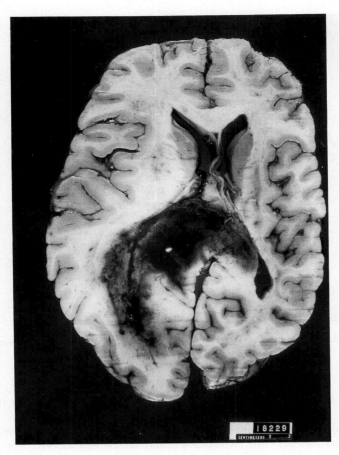

Fig. 57-35. A glioblastoma multiforme involving the splenium of the corpus callosum. (Courtesy of Dr. J. H. N. Deck)

brain. They form a fairly well-demarcated mass, often spheroidal and 5 to 10 cm in diameter, but at times larger. Sometimes a glioblastoma multiforme involves both hemispheres, growing in a butterfly pattern. The cut surface of the tumor is variegated, with yellowish areas of necrosis and red areas of hemorrhage widespread in the soft, pinkish-gray tumor. Often a few small cysts containing yellowish fluid are present in the tumor. In 2% of the patients, there are more than one glioblastoma.

Microscopically, a glioblastoma is highly cellular, with many mitoses. Its appearance varies considerably from one part of the tumor to another. In some regions, there are sheets of large, polygonal cells varying in size and shape and sometimes multinucleated.

Elsewhere, the cells may be spindle shaped, in interweaving bundles. Often the tumor cells form a palisade around a small patch of necrosis, with long processes extending in towards the necrosis. There may be pseudo-rosettes like those of an astroblastoma. In areas, gemistocytes or fibrillary astrocytes may be prominent. Occasionally the whole tumor consists of large, pleomorphic, bizarre giant cells, which tend to surround blood vessels. Rarely, the tumor consists of elongated cells with the nuclei lined up in rows, a variety of glioblastoma sometimes called a polar spongioblastoma.

Changes in blood vessels, are often prominent, especially at the margin of the tumor. Nearly every glioblastoma multiforme shows some change of this sort.

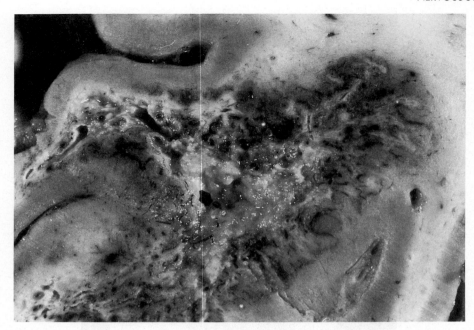

Fig. 57-36. Cut surface of a glioblastoma multiforme, showing multiple foci of necrosis and hemorrhage. (Courtesy of Dr. J. H. N. Deck)

Small, thin-walled, tortuous, capillaries sometimes form clumps like a renal glomerulus. Often some of the capillaries have plump, swollen endothelial cells, which are often several layers thick, with frequent mitoses. Sometimes the endothelial proliferation completely occludes the vessel.

The adventitia of the blood vessels is often thickened. Reticulin fibers increase in the adventitia. The fibrocytes in the adventitia may be atypical.

In 5% of glioblastomata, the adventitial cells become malignant in part of the tumor. They grow as a fibrosarcoma, occasionally with cartilagenous or osteoid metaplasia. Rarely, the sarcoma contains an admixture of rhabdomyoblasts.

Thrombosis is common in vessels around a glioblastoma. The vessels are abnormally permeable. Radioactive markers, which normally do not pass the blood-brain barrier when given intravenously, leak into the tumor.

The concentration of protein in the cerebrospinal fluid is often over 1 g/L (100 mg/ 100 mL). A pleocytosis of more than 100 × 10^6/L (100/mm^3) cells, mostly lymphocytes, sometimes occurs.

Behavior. Glioblastomata grow rapidly and invade extensively. For a time, adjacent structures survive in the tumor. Often the tumor reaches a ventricle and extends into it. The overlying leptomeninges are invaded extensively. Often the tumor is adherent to the dura. Occasionally it penetrates the dura and invades or penetrates the cranial bones.

Metastases in the ventricles or subarachnoid space develop in less than 10% of the patients. Sometimes numerous, tiny implants develop in the ventricles. Occasionally nodules or sheets of glioblastoma grow in the leptomeninges. Tumor sometimes covers the brain stem or cerebellum. In the spinal canal, nodules of tumor are most frequent on the spinal nerves and the corda equina. The metastases sometimes invade the adjacent part of the brain, spinal cord, or nerves.

Metastases outside the central nervous system are rare. They are most common in patients in whom a glioblastoma has extended into the soft tissues of the scalp through a defect left by a craniotomy. The lymph

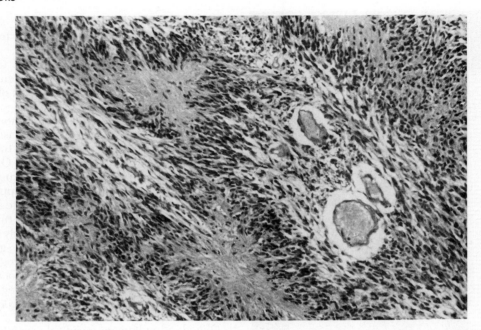

Fig. 57-37. A glioblastoma multiforme, showing the palisading of tumor cells around foci of necrosis. (Courtesy of Dr. J. H. N. Deck)

nodes, bones, and kidneys are the organs most often involved.

The tumors containing both glioblastoma multiforme and fibrosarcoma behave as do other glioblastomata. If metastases develop, they may contain either element or both elements. A few such tumors have metastasized to the lungs or lymph nodes, with both elements evident in the metastases.

Clinical Presentation. Headache is the first sign of the tumor in 50% of patients with a glioblastoma. Other signs of increased intracranial pressure follow. Seizures occur in 20% of the patients. Localizing signs develop in many of the patients: motor or sensory changes if the tumor involves the motor or sensory areas, disturbances of mentation if it is in a frontal lobe, changes in personality if a temporal lobe is involved, signs and symptoms suggesting the part of the brain affected if the brain stem or cerebellum is involved.

Treatment and Prognosis. A glioblastoma multiforme is treated surgically if possible; if surgical treatment is not possible, it is treated by irradiation. Most patients die within a few months. Only 10% are alive two

years after the diagnosis. Most die of increased intracranial pressure.

OLIGODENROGLIOMA. The 5% of gliomata that arise from the oligodendrocytes are called oligodendrogliomata. An oligodendroglioma may occur at any age, but most of the patients are 30 to 50 years old.

Lesions. Most oligodendrogliomata arise in or near the cerebral cortex. Some originate more deeply in the cerebral hemispheres, near the third ventricle, in the cerebellum, or spinal cord. The tumor is usually spheroidal, 5 to 10 cm in diameter, well demarcated, and grayish-pink. Sometimes it is gelatinous. Foci of necrosis and small cysts are rarely extensive. The tumor is often calcified, especially at its periphery.

Microscopically, most oligodendrogliomata consist of sheets of uniform, small cells, supported by a delicate, vascular stroma. The tumor cells have a small, dark, central nucleus; pale, empty cytoplasm; and a clear cell border. Mitoses may or may not be numerous. At the margin of the tumor, the tumor cells often form clumps, sometimes around neurons, with little between the

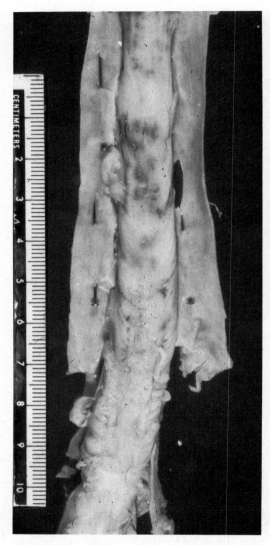

Fig. 57-38. Implants of a cerebral glioblastoma multiforme on the spinal cord and its meninges. (Courtesy of Dr. J. H. N. Deck)

clumps except the filmy processes of the tumor cells. In these clumps the tumor cells are smaller, with unobtrusive cytoplasm.

In the gelatinous tumors, clumps of tumor cells are widely separated by mucus containing a sulfated acid mucopolysaccharide. Swollen tumor cells often contain mucus.

The calcification common in oligodendrogliomata begins near the blood vessels. Calcospherites appear first. They often fuse to form considerable masses, even bone. About

70% of oligodendrogliomata contain some calcium. In 40%, there is enough to be evident radiologically.

Often large, atypical cells believed to be astrocytes are present within an oligodendroglioma. Occasionally a glioma is in part oligodendroglioma, in part astrocytoma.

Behavior. Most oligodendrogliomata grow slowly, changing little as years pass. In some patients, epilepsy caused by the tumor persists unchanged for 10 or 20 years. Other oligodendrogliomata grow rapidly, bringing death within months. The histologic appearance of the tumor does little to indicate how it will behave. A well-differentiated tumor sometimes grows rapidly, and a poorly differentiated oligodendroglioma can grow slowly. Some oligodendrogliomata progress to a more anaplastic form, with foci of glioblastoma multiforme mixed with regions that preserve the structure of an oligodendroglioma.

Oligodendrogliomata invade the overlying leptomeninges. Occasionally the tumor becomes attached to the dura. At times, the tumor in the meninges excites a desmoplastic reaction, forming so much collagenous tissue that the part of the tumor in the meninges resembles a meningioma.

About 10% of oligodendrogliomata metastasize to the subarachnoid space. The metastases sometimes grow slowly, causing fibrosis of the involved part of the leptomeninges, sometimes are widespread and rapidly growing. Rarely, usually after craniotomy, metastases develop in the lungs, lymph nodes, bones, or elsewhere.

Clinical Presentation. The signs and symptoms caused by an oligodendroglioma are similar to those of other gliomata. They depend on its position and on the rapidity of its growth.

Treatment and Prognosis. An oligodendroglioma is usually treated by a combination of surgery and radiation. The tumor recurs in 50% of the patients. On the average, the patients live five years after surgery.

EPENDYMOMA. Tumors arising from the ependymal epithelium are called ependymomata. In the brain, they make up 7% of gliomata. In the spinal cord, 60% of gliomata are of this type. In spite of this difference, gliomata are so much more common in the

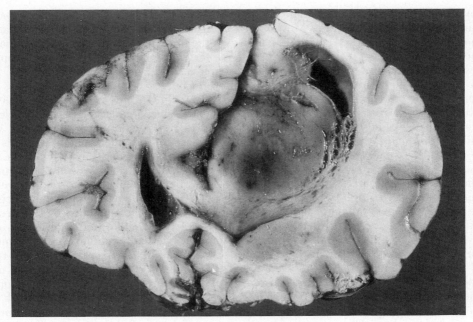

Fig. 57-39. An oligodendroglioma with cysts at the margin of the tumor. (Courtesy of Dr. J. H. N. Deck)

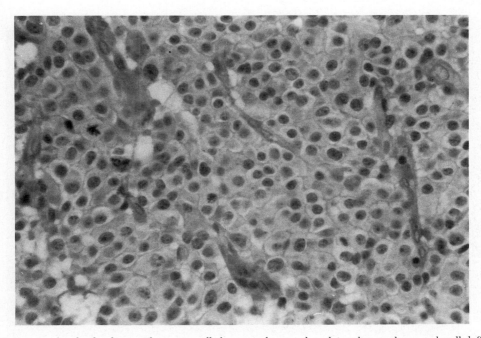

Fig. 57-40. An oligodendroglioma. The tumor cells have regular round nuclei, pale cytoplasm, and well-defined margins. (Courtesy of Dr. J. H. N. Deck)

brain than in the spinal cord that 70% of ependymomata are in the brain. Most ependymomata arise in children or adolescents. Some occur in adults.

Lesions. In the brain, most ependymomata arise in the fourth ventricle. Some originate in one of the other ventricles or in a cerebral hemisphere remote from a ventricle. In the spine, 60% develop in the region of the filum terminale. Most of the other 40% arise within the spinal cord. Occasionally an ependymoma arises anterior to the spine in the hollow of the sacrum.

Ependymomata arising in the fourth ventricle are sometimes rounded or lobulated as the tumor bulges into the ventricle, sometimes soft and papillary. Some protrude through the foramen of Luschka into the cerebellopontine angle.

Ependymomata of the spine and cerebral hemispheres usually form spheroidal masses, often partly or largely cystic. Ependymomata of the spinal cord are often associated with syringomyelia, with the tumor somewhere along the course of the syrinx.

Microscopically, an ependymoma, shows a

cellular, epithelial or myxopapillary pattern of growth. Many tumors show more than one of the these patterns. The cellular pattern is the most common. Most myxopapillary tumors arise in the region of the filum terminale.

The cellular tumors consist of sheets of cuboidal or columnar cells. Their nuclei are small, dark, regular, and spheroidal. Their cytoplasm is ill-defined. The tumor cells form pseudorosettes around blood vessels. The cells forming the pseudorosette surround the vessel, but their nuclei and bodies are separated from it by long protoplasmic processes. The processes do not have foot plates like those of the pseudorosettes of an astroblastoma. They usually contain no glial filaments.

In an epithelial ependymoma, the tumor cells are like those of the cellular form of the tumor and form similar sheets. Blepharoplasts are often evident in the cells, though they are not common in other kinds of ependymoma. Some of the tumor cells surround small cavities, forming rosettes. Sometimes the nucleus and body of the cells forming the rosette are separated from the cavity by

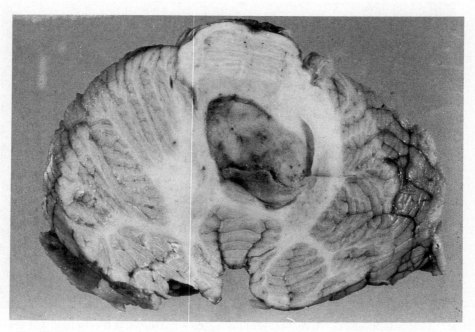

Fig. 57-41.   An ependymoma occupying the fourth ventricle. (Courtesy of Dr. J. H. N. Deck)

long protoplasmic processes like those of a pseudorosette. Sometimes the cavity is larger, and the cells lining it look more like epithelial cells. Often astrocytes lie among the tumor cells. Sometimes clumps of tumor cells are supported by a glial stroma.

In the myxopapillary form of ependymoma, the tumor cells line fronds that project into cystic spaces. The tumor cells are cuboidal or columnar. They have regular, vesicular nuclei. Their cytoplasm is homogeneous or finely granular. The tumor cells are supported by a collagenous stroma. Often the stroma is loose with abundant, mucoid intercellular substance. Often some of the tumor cells contain droplets of mucus.

Electron microscopy shows that the cells of an ependymoma are joined by desmosomes. Blepharoplasts and cilia are present in all types of ependymoma. Often glial filaments are evident in the tumor cells. Microrosettes, small cavities lying between two or more cells, are often filled by a complex interdigitation of microvilli. Occasionally a cilium projects into the cavity. In the myxopapillary type of ependymoma, a basement membrane separates the tumor cells from their collagenous stroma.

Behavior. Most ependymomata grow slowly. Metastases to the subarachnoid space are rare, and when they occur they are few and small. The tumor sometimes grows through a craniotomy defect into the adjacent soft tissues. In a few patients, a tumor that has reached the extraneural tissues has metastasized to a lung or elsewhere. Rarely, an ependymoma becomes anaplastic and resembles a glioblastoma multiforme.

Clinical Presentation. An ependymoma projecting into a ventricle often obstructs the flow of the cerebrospinal fluid and causes hydrocephalus. Symptoms and signs of hydrocephalus are sometimes the first evidence of the tumor. In other patients, the dysfunction caused by the tumor is similar to that of other gliomata and depends on its site and rate of growth.

Treatment and Prognosis. An ependymoma is treated by surgical excision followed by radiation. Often it is impossible to remove the tumor completely. Ependymomata in the brain frequently cause symptoms for more than a year before the patient comes to

surgery. On the average, patients live five years after surgery. If the tumor is in the spinal cord, most patients live more than 10 years after the removal of the tumor. If it is in the region of the filum terminale, the average survival is over 15 years.

PAPILLOMA OF THE CHOROID PLEXUS. Papillomata of the choroid plexus make up 1% of gliomata. Over 50% of the patients are under 20 years old, though the tumor can arise at any age.

In adults, papillomata of the choroid plexus are most common in the fourth ventricle. In children, they are most frequent in the lateral ventricles, especially on the left. Overall, about 50% of the tumors originate in the fourth ventricle. The tumor forms a globoid mass usually 1 or 2 cm across. Its surface is ridged. Often the tumor is partially calcified.

Microscopically a papilloma of the choroid plexus resembles a myxopapillary ependymoma. It consists of fine fronds with a vascular, collagenous core covered by regular, cuboidal tumor cells. The tumor cells rest on a basement membrane, are joined by desmosomes, have microvilli, and occasionally a cilium. In children, they sometimes contain much glycogen. Occasionally a tumor cell contains mucus. Calcospherites are sometimes present in the stroma.

Most papillomata of the choroid plexus grow slowly and do not invade. Some metastasize to the subarachnoid space, where the metastases grow slowly and do not invade. Only rarely does a papilloma of the choroid plexus grow rapidly, invade extensively, and metastasize widely in the subarachnoid space. Some of the rapidly growing tumors extend through a craniotomy defect and metastasize to the lungs or other organs. Some are pigmented with melanin.

The symptoms caused by a papilloma of the choroid plexus depend on its site. Some cause hydrocephalus. Surgical excision usually eradicates the tumor.

SUBEPENDYMAL GLIOMA. Subependymal gliomata, or subependymomata as they are sometimes called, are uncommon. Usually they produce no symptoms and are found only at autopsy. Occasionally one is large enough to cause hydrocephalus.

Subependymal gliomata are most common

in the fourth ventricle. Less often a subependymal glioma arises elsewhere in the
ventricles or in the spinal cord. Sometimes
there is more than one. The tumor forms a
small nodule, that bulges into the ventricle.
Microscopically, it is a well differentiated
fibrillary astrocytoma containing clumps of
ependymal cells that sometimes form rosettes
or pseudorosettes.

The nature of subependymal gliomata is in
question. Some may be hamartomata; some
are slow growing astrocytomata or astrocytomata whose growth has become arrested;
some foci of gliosis are caused by inflammation.

COLLOID CYST OF THE THIRD VENTRICLE.
Colloid cysts of the third ventricle make up
less than 1% of intracranial tumors. Sometimes they are called paraphyseal cysts,
though it is unlikely that more than a small

minority of them are derived from the
paraphysis.

The cyst arises from the anterior wall of the
third ventricle. It is smoothly rounded and
usually 0.3 to 3.0 cm in diameter. Sometimes
the cyst adheres to the wall of the ventricle.
The cyst has a collagenous wall and is lined
by cuboidal or columnar epithelium. Often
the epithelial cells are ciliated or contain
mucus. It is filled with inspissated material.

Colloid cysts of the third ventricle are
probably congenital malformations, not neoplasms. They become evident only in adult
life when the cyst blocks one or both foramina
of Munro, causing hydrocephalus. Sometimes the obstruction is intermittent. Movement of the head can make the cyst temporarily obstruct one of the foramina, causing
headache. Excision cures.

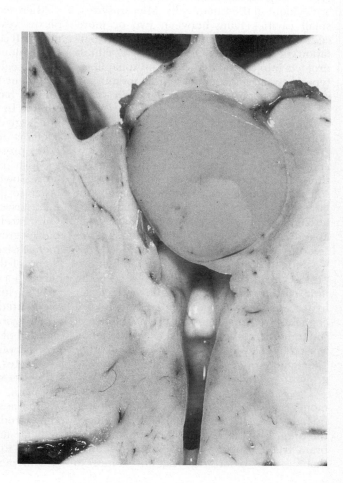

Fig. 57-42. A colloid cyst at the anterior end of the third ventricle, showing
its proximity to the foramina of Monro.
(Courtesy of Dr. J. H. N. Deck)

Neuronal Tumors

Tumors of neurons are sometimes called neuroepithelial neoplasms. They are most common in the peripheral nervous system. A neuroblastoma is the most anaplastic and most frequent of the neuronal tumors of the peripheral nervous system. Less often a ganglioneuroblastoma or ganglioneuroma arises in the peripheral nervous system. A medulloblastoma is the most common neuro-epithelial tumor in the central nervous system. Occasionally a medulloepithelioma, dysplastic gangliocytoma, ganglioglioma, one of the neuronal tumors more frequent in the peripheral nervous system, or some other form of neuroepithelial tumor is found in the brain. A tumor of the neurons in the retina is called a retinoblastoma.

NEUROBLASTOMA. About 80% of neuroblastomata become evident during the first year of life. Occasionally the tumor is present at birth, or is detected in a fetus in utero. Almost all the rest develop in children under 8 years old. A neuroblastoma rarely is found in an adult. It is the most common tumor in infancy, but less than 10% of malignant tumors in older children are neuroblastomata.

In infants, almost all neuroblastomata arise in the medulla of an adrenal gland, the left more often than the right. In older children, some arise in an adrenal gland, some in an autonomic ganglion elsewhere in the body. Rarely, a neuroblastoma develops in a cerebral hemisphere.

Lesions. Macroscopically, a neuroblastoma forms a soft, lobulated mass. Usually the tumor is large, with extensive invasion of neighboring tissues. If it is small, it may appear encapsulated. The cut surface of the tumor is gray or white, often with foci of hemorrhage or necrosis. Fine calcification is frequently evident throughout the tumor radiologically, but is not evident macroscopically.

Microscopically, a neuroblastoma consists of small, spheroidal cells like lymphocytes. The cells are packed closely together in masses separated by fine collagenous septa containing many blood vessels. The tumor cells have a dense, hyperchromatic nucleus and scant cytoplasm. They occasionally con-

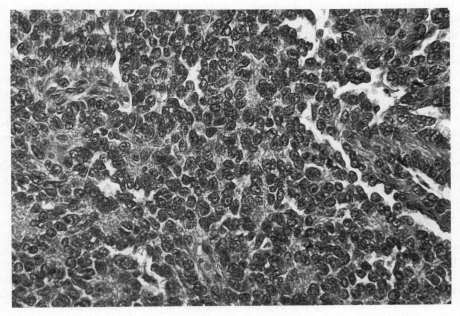

Fig. 57-43.   A neuroblastoma, showing the small cells and fibrillary processes characterizing this tumor. (Courtesy of Dr. J. H. N. Deck)

tain a few neurosecretory granules. Some have short processes like axons. Some have more than one nucleus. Mitoses are few.

Pseudorosettes are present in 50% of the tumors. In a pseudorosette, the tumor cells surround a small lumen filled with fibrillary material. Less often, true rosettes are present, with tumor cells surrounding an empty lumen.

The neuroblastomata of the brain are more variable microscopically. In 50% of the patients, differentiation to ganglion cells is recognizable in places. In 70% of the children, a collagenous stroma is present in part or all of the tumor, dividing the tumor cells into clumps or surrounding individual tumor cells.

Most neuroblastomata secrete excessive quantities of catecholamines, their precursors, or their metabolities. The urinary excretion of vanillylmandelic acid and metanephrine are almost always increased. An excess of dopa and dopamine is often found in the urine.

Behavior. Neuroblastomata metastasize early and widely. In many of the children, metastases are present when the tumor is discovered. The tumor spreads by the lymphatics to the regional lymph nodes and by the blood stream throughout the body. Hematogenous metastases are often multiple and large. The liver, bones, and lungs are frequently involved. Metastases to the skull sometimes cause proptosis or hemorrhage around the eyes. Metastases to bone can cause anemia. Sometimes the bony metastases are symmetrical. If the metastases are most prominent in the liver, the patient is said to have Pepper's syndrome, named after an American physician (1874–1947). If the metastases are principally in the bones, the child has Hutchison's syndrome, named after the English pediatrician Sir Robert Hutchison (1871–1960).

In a few children, a neuroblastoma has become more differentiated, changing to a ganglioneuroblastoma or ganglioneuroma. In a few, the tumor has regressed spontaneously.

Clinical Presentation. In most children with a neuroblastoma, the tumor is discovered when a parent finds the primary tumor or one of its metastases. Abdominal distention,

weight loss, pathologic fractures, and masses bulging from the skull are among its more common manifestations.

Less often, the patient develops a syndrome like the carcinoid syndrome, with diarrhea, flushing of the skin, hypokalemia, and fever. Probably the syndrome is caused by kinins produced by the tumor or by the prostaglandins that are present in large quantity in these tumors and in the plasma of the patients. Occasionally, a patient develops hypertension, because of the catecholamines produced by the tumor or Cushing's syndrome.

Treatment and Prognosis. A neuroblastoma is treated by a combination of surgery, radiotherapy, and chemotherapy. About 30% of the children survive for more than 18 months and are probably cured.

GANGLIONEUROBLASTOMA. Ganglioneuroblastomata are less common than neuroblastomata. They occur in older children and adolescents. Most arise in the posterior mediastinum or an adrenal gland.

Most ganglioneuroblastomata are large, spheroidal or bosselated, and apparently encapsulated. The tumor is firmer and more homogeneous than a neuroblastoma. Foci of hemorrhage and necrosis are infrequent. Fine calcification is often evident radiologically.

Microscopically a ganglioneuroblastoma sometimes consists of moderate sized spindle-shaped cells with vesicular nuclei. Fine processes like axons extend from the poles of the cells. In other patients, the tumor shows a mixture of cells like those of a neuroblastoma, spindle cells, and more highly differentiated neurons of the kind found in a ganglioneuroma.

A ganglioneuroblastoma grows more slowly than a neuroblastoma. About 20% of the tumors metastasize, often widely. A ganglioneuroblastoma is treated by surgery, radiation and chemotherapy, like a neuroblastoma.

GANGLIONEUROMA. A ganglioneuroma is an uncommon tumor most often found in adolescents or young adults, though it can arise at any age. Most arise in the posterior mediastinum. Some originate in a peripheral ganglion in some other part of the body. Rarely, a patient has multiple, subcutaneous ganglioneuromata and pigmentation of the

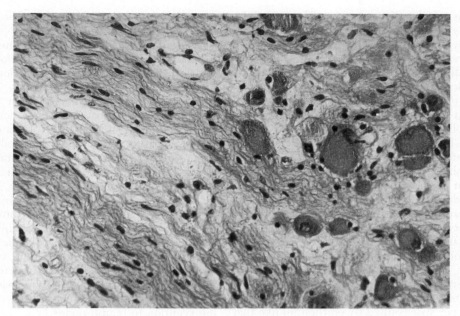

Fig. 57-44. A ganglioneuroma, showing well-differentiated neurons and their axons.

overlying skin. Rarely, a ganglioneuroma arises in the brain, most often in the floor of the third ventricle or in the hypothalamus.

A ganglioneuroma is usually spheroidal, firm, and well defined. Some bulge through a spinal foramen forming a dumbbell-shaped mass, partly in the mediastinum, partly in the spinal canal. Some weigh less than 20 g; some more than 200 g.

Microscopically, large neurons, like those in normal peripheral ganglia are scattered singly or in small groups among the fine collagen bundles that make up most of the tumor. The axons of the neurons wind among the collagen fibers. Foci of calcification are common.

In the brain, a ganglioneuroma contains in addition glial tissue. Sometimes the glial proliferation is the principal feature of the tumor, with only a few ganglion cells present.

Ganglioneuromata secrete catecholamines. The urinary excretion of vanillylmandelic acid and metanephrine is increased in most of the patients. An excess of norepinephrine is sometimes present in the urine.

Most ganglioneuromata are benign. They grow slowly, if at all. Most produce symptoms only because of their size and position.

A few cause a carcinoid-like syndrome. Rarely, a well-differentiated ganglioneuroma has metastasized. The metastases have been equally well differentiated.

GANGLIOGLIOMA. A ganglioglioma is a rare tumor of the brain. It grows like a ganglioneuroma of the brain, but the glial element in the tumor is neoplastic.

MEDULLOBLASTOMA. Most medulloblastomata arise in children, 50% of them in children under 10 years old. Few of the patients are more than 30 years old. Nearly 60% of them are boys. If medulloblastomata are grouped together with intracranial gliomata in children, 25% of the tumors are medulloblastomata. Only astrocytomata are more common.

Lesions. Medulloblastomata occur only in the cerebellum. In children, 80% of them develop in the midline, in the vermis. In adults, they often involve one of the cerebellar hemispheres. Usually the tumor is roughly spheroidal, 5 to 10 cm in diameter, soft and friable, pinkish-gray or purplish. Hemorrhage into the tumor and cystic changes are unusual. Less often, the tumor is firm or is flattened forming a plaque over the surface of one of the cerebellar hemispheres. The tumor invades the surrounding brain and the overlying leptomeninges extensively. Often it bulges into the fourth ventricle and may fill it, invading the floor of the ventricle. Occasionally it extends into the subdural space.

Microscopically, a medulloblastoma consists of closely packed cells with little cytoplasm and small, dark, spheroidal, or ovoid nuclei. Mitoses are often numerous. Sometimes fine fibrils can be distinguished between the tumor cells. Sometimes only a fine mesh of thin-walled blood vessels supports the tumor cells, or there is gliosis between them. Pseudorosettes like those in a neuroblastoma are present in 30% of the tumors.

Occasionally parts of the tumor resemble an astrocytoma, oligodendroglioma, or glioblastoma multiforme. Pseudorosettes like those of an astroblastoma are sometimes present in the glial part of the tumor. Rarely, part of medulloblastoma consists of tubules or larger spaces lined by epithelium like that of a papilloma of the choroid plexus, with melanin in the tumor cells lining the tubules and spaces.

By electron microscopy, most of the tumor cells show few organelles. Sometimes intercellular junctions are present between the tumor cells. Rarely, neurosecretory granules are present in a few of them, or rudimentary synaptic junctions can be identified. Rarely, glial fibers are present in some of the tumor cells.

In the meninges, the tumor excites the formation of a collagenous stroma. The tumor cells form columns separated by bundles of collagen or masses surrounded by collagenous septa.

Behavior. Medulloblastomata grow rapidly and invade extensively. Metastases in the subarachnoid space develop in over 50% of the patients. Often there are numerous nodules of tumor in the meninges, the tumor forms a sheet that covers a large part of the brain or encases the spinal cord. The tumor in the metastases invades the adjacent tissues extensively. Metastases to lymph nodes, bones, and other organs are most common after a craniotomy, but sometimes occur in patients who have not undergone surgery.

Clinical Presentation. The symptoms and signs of medulloblastoma are increased intracranial pressure or cerebellar dysfunc-

tion. Hydrocephalus is common. The symptoms worsen rapidly.

Treatment and Prognosis. A medulloblastoma is usually treated by excision of as much of the tumor as is possible, followed by radiation and chemotherapy. Up to 75% of the patients are alive five years later.

MEDULLOEPITHELIOMA. A medulloepithelioma is a rare tumor found in infants and young children, usually in a cerebral hemisphere. The tumor consists of branching tubules lined by cuboidal or columnar cells like those of the medullary plate in the developing embryo and supported by a fine collagenous stroma. The cells are limited by a membrane both on their basal and their luminal surfaces. Usually parts of the tumor show evidence of differentiation towards neurons, ependymal cells, or astrocytes. The tumor grows rapidly, metastasizes widely to the subarachnoid space, and after surgical intervention to lymph nodes.

DYSPLASTIC GANGLIOCYTOMA. A dysplastic gangliocytoma thickens and enlarges the folia in part or much of the cerebellar cortex. Less frequently, it involves the cerebral cortex. The lesion has a rind of nerve fibers with a disorderly arrangement of large neurons within. The condition becomes evident during adult life. The lesions slowly enlarge.

Meningeal Tumors

A benign tumor of the meninges is usually called a meningioma. Its malignant form is called a malignant meningioma, or a meningeal sarcoma. Hemangiopericytomata of the meninges are occasionally confused with meningiomata.

MENINGIOMA. About 15% of intracranial tumors are meningiomata and 25% of intraspinal tumors, though intracranial tumors are so much more frequent than intraspinal tumors that 90% of meningiomata are intracranial. Most are found in people between 20 and 60 years old. About 70% of intracranial meningiomata and 80% of intraspinal meningiomata arise in women.

Lesions. Meningiomata most often arise in regions in which arachnoid villi are numerous. In the cranium, 50% of them occur near the sagittal sinus, usually in its middle third, either lateral to the sinus or in the falx cerebri. The sphenoid ridge is a common site. Sometimes meningiomata arise from the tuberculum sellae, olfactory groove, ponto-cerebellar angle, or the petrous ridge of the temporal bone in relation to the tentorium cerebelli. An intraventricular meningioma can arise from the tela choroidea or the choroid plexus. In the spine, they are most common in the thoracic region, usually in relation to a spinal nerve. Rarely, a meningioma arises from the sheath of the optic nerve within the orbit, within the petrous bone, or from some other extension of the meninges. Occasionally, a patient has more than one meningioma.

Macroscopically, a meningioma is usually a well-circumscribed spheroidal or hemispheroidal mass, often flattened where it abuts against the bone. Less often, the tumor causes a flat, plaque-like thickening in the meninges, is dumbbell shaped, or distorted by the falx cerebri or some other hard structure. The tumor is usually 1 to 10 cm across. The surface of the tumor may be smooth or bosselated. Its cut surface is firm and fibrous, sometimes with foci of calcification or soft yellowish areas.

As a meningioma enlarges, it distorts and compresses the underlying brain or spinal cord. Sometimes a meningioma bulges into the brain and is almost completely surrounded by it, or a spinal meningioma surrounds and compresses the cord. Meningiomata are firmly attached to the dura, but the leptomeninges usually remain intact between the meningioma and the underlying brain or spinal cord, so that the tumor is easily separated from the brain or cord.

In 5% of patients with an intracranial meningioma, the bone overlying the tumor is thickened, dense, and sclerotic. Less often, a meningioma erodes and destroys the overlying bone. Bony changes are less common with spinal tumors.

Microscopically, meningiomata are divided into meningotheliomatous, transitional, fibroblastic, and angioblastic types. Over 60% of meningiomata show some variant of the meningotheliomatous or transitional pattern.

In a meningotheliomatous meningioma, the tumor consists of sheets and whorls

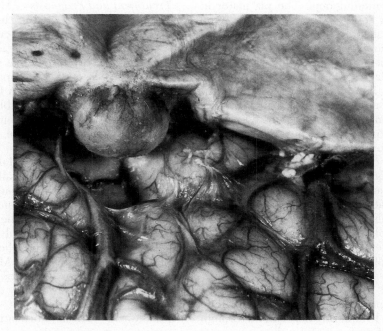

Fig. 57-45. A meningioma arising in the parasagittal region. The tumor is firmly attached to the meninges, but has caused a depression in the underlying brain. (Courtesy of Dr. J. H. N. Deck)

of large, polygonal cells, with large, pale, spheroidal, central nuclei and abundant homogeneous or granular cytoplasm. The clumps and sheets of tumor cells are supported by a collagenous stroma, which divides the tumor into irregular lobules.

In a transitional meningioma, the whorling is more pronounced, often with a small vessel in the center of the whorl, and the tumor cells tend to become elongated and crescent shaped. Often many psammoma bodies are present. At least some of the psammoma bodies result from calcification of whorls of tumor cells.

Less often, a meningioma is of the fibroblastic type, with intertwining bundles of long spindle-shaped cells, with collagen or reticulin fibers between them, much as in a fibroma.

An angioblastic meningioma resembles a hemangiopericytoma. It is highly cellular, with numerous capillaries between the tumor cells. Some of the capillaries are widely dilated. Many are collapsed. The tumor cells are cuboidal, with ill-defined cytoplasm, and ovoid nuclei. Sometimes mitoses are frequent. They are rare in other types of mesothelioma.

Macrophages filled with lipid are often present in a meningioma. The pia mater in the posterior fossa of the skull and in the upper cervical spine is normally pigmented, and meningiomata from this region sometimes have melanin in their cells. Metaplastic bone or cartilage sometimes can be found in a meningioma. Rarely, there is overproduction of intercellular substance, so that the tumor shows myxomatous degeneration. Occasionally the tumor cells become multinucleated and bizarre, or the tumor contains nodules of lymphocytes or plasma cells.

By electron microscopy, the cells of a meningioma are joined by desmosomes. They have elaborately interdigitated cell membranes. Fibrils 10 nm in diameter are present in the cytoplasm. They do not show the myofibrils, hemidesmosomes, and basement membranes of a hemangiopericytoma.

Behavior. Meningiomata grow slowly. They invade the dura mater, often extensively. Commonly they compress or occlude a dural sinus. Frequently they extend through the pores of the overlying bone into its marrow space. Occasionally the tumor ex-

tends through the whole thickness of the bone into the overlying soft tissue. Often invasion of the bone is associated with hyperostosis, but hyperostosis can occur without invasion and invasion can occur without hyperostosis. The tumor does not invade the leptomeninges, brain, or spinal cord, though it frequently compresses and distorts them.

Metastases are rare. Occasionally a meningioma spreads to lymph nodes or the lungs after incomplete removal. Less frequently metastases develop in the subarachnoid space.

Clinical Presentation. A meningioma often remains asymptomatic for months or years. Eventually signs of increased intracranial pressure slowly develop, or the patient gradually develops localizing signs that indicate the position of the tumor. Parasagittal tumors eventually cause seizures or paralysis. Tumors of the sphenoid ridge cause unilateral exophthalmos or unilateral blindness. A meningioma of the olfactory groove causes unilateral anosmia or unilateral blindness. Tumors in the spinal column compress the spinal cord or spinal nerves. In some patients, the concentration of protein in the cerebrospinal fluid exceeds 2 g/L (200 mg/100 mL).

Treatment and Prognosis. Meningiomata are treated surgically. If the tumor is completely removed, the patient is cured, though in 15% of patients with an intracranial meningioma and 5% of those with a spinal tumor in whom the resection was apparently complete, the tumor recurs within five years. If complete removal is impossible, radiation helps prevent recurrence. Even if complete removal is impossible, 50% of the patients are relieved of symptoms.

MALIGNANT MENINGIOMA. Malignant meningiomata are rare. Occasionally a meningioma is more anaplastic than usual and grows more rapidly than most meningiomata. Such tumors often invade the underlying brain or spinal cord, though only to a limited extent. Sometimes extensive gliosis develops around the region invaded. Metastases to extraneural organs or less often to the subarachnoid space are more likely than with the usual types of meningioma.

MENINGEAL HEMANGIOPERICYTOMA. Hemangiopericytomata of the meninges tend to behave like a malignant meningioma, with local invasion of the underlying brain or spinal cord. Metastases are common, especially after surgical excision has been attempted.

MENINGEAL SARCOMA. Meningeal sarcomata are rare. They usually occur in infants or young children. The tumor sometimes arises from the meninges. Sometimes it begins within the brain, presumably from the extension of the meninges around the blood vessels. Meningeal sarcomata are bulky tumors, often with foci of necrosis and hemorrhage.

Microscopically, some of these tumors are well-differentiated fibrosarcomata. Others are more anaplastic, with spindle cells. Some are highly pleomorphic. Rarely, a myxosarcoma, a chondrosarcoma, or an embryonal rhabdomyosarcoma arises in the meninges.

Sarcomata of the meninges invade the surrounding brain and other neighboring tissues, but metastases are uncommon. Only occasionally they spread to the subarachnoid space like a glioblastoma multiforme or metastasize to extraneural organs. Rarely, there is widespread sarcomatosis of the meninges without a clear primary tumor.

Vascular Tumors

Most of the tumor-like lesions of blood vessels in the nervous system are malformations. They are described earlier in the chapter.

Tumors of Nerves

Four kinds of tumor arise from the Schwann cells of peripheral nerves: schwannoma, neurofibroma, granular cell tumor, and neurofibrosarcoma. In von Recklinghausen's disease, the patients have multiple neurofibromata or schwannomata. Some develop a neurofibrosarcoma.

SCHWANNOMA. A schwannoma is named after the German anatomist (1810–1882) who described the Schwann cells. Less often it is called a neurilemoma, after the neurilemal sheath. Except in von Recklinghausen's disease, the patients are usually adult, though the tumor can arise at any age.

Lesions. About 8% of intracranial tumors are schwannomata. Most arise on an auditory nerve. A few arise from a trigeminal nerve. Other intracranial nerves are rarely affected. A schwannoma of an auditory nerve is called an auditory neuroma or auditory neurinoma. As the tumor enlarges, it distorts the brain stem and cerebellum. Often the tumor extends into the auditory foramen, which becomes enlarged and funnel-shaped. Adjacent cranial nerves are stretched over the tumor.

Nearly 30% of intraspinal tumors are schwannomata. Most arise on a posterior root, most frequently in the lumbar region. The tumor distorts the spinal cord and sometimes erodes adjacent vertebrae. Some spinal schwannomata are shaped like an hour glass, with part of the tumor within the spinal canal, a narrow neck in an intervertebral foramen, and part of the tumor outside the spine.

In the peripheral nerves, a schwannoma can arise on any sensory, motor, or autonomic nerve that has a sheath of Schwann cells. Most arise on one of the larger nerves, most frequently in the posterior mediastinum. The tumor is spheroidal and encapsulated and does not adhere to adjacent structures. Most are less than 5 cm across. On section, the tumor is firm, grayish-white, and rubbery. Often the cut surface has a whorled pattern. Occasionally the tumor is lobulated, contains soft yellowish regions, or is cystic.

Microscopically, schwannomata have a collagenous capsule. The tumor expands the affected nerve, with almost all the nerve fibers running round the margin of the tumor, though a few wander through it. Within the mass, two patterns of growth are distinguished, called Antoni A and Antoni B, after the Swedish neurologist who described them in 1920. Most schwannomata show both patterns. The Antoni A and Antoni B regions are usually sharply demarcated.

In the Antoni A regions, a schwannoma consists of intertwining bundles of long, spindle-shaped cells, with little between the cells except a few reticulin fibers. Sometimes the nuclei of the spindle cells are lined up in rows side by side, an arrangement called palisading. Sometimes the spindle cells are arranged in whorls or resemble a Verocay body.

In the Antoni B regions, the tumor cells

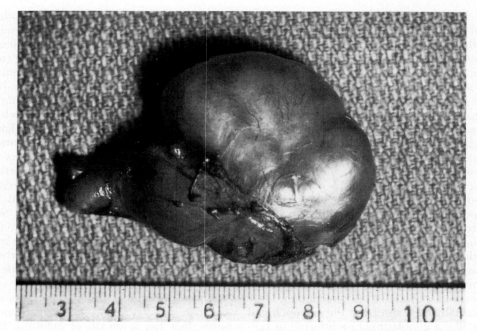

Fig. 57-46. A schwannoma of a peripheral nerve, showing the well-circumscribed, encapsulated tumor.

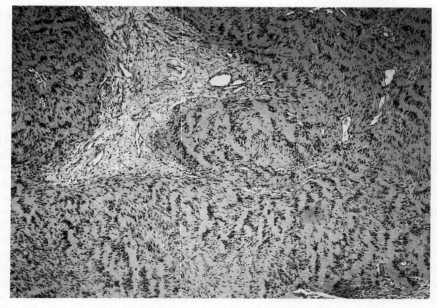

Fig. 57-47. A schwannoma showing the more cellular Antoni A and the looser Antoni B regions. The palisading in the Antoni A regions is unusually prominent.

are plumper, vaguely defined, and are separated by large quantities of faintly eosinophilic intercellular substance in which reticulin fibers are few and irregularly distributed. Microcysts are common in Antoni B regions. They coalesce to form the larger cysts sometimes found in schwannomata, or clumps of fat-filled macrophages are frequently present. The blood vessels in the Antoni B regions often are ectatic, show hyalinization or fibrinoid change, or are thrombosed. Sometimes hemosiderin gives evidence of old hemorrhage. Occasionally some of the nuclei in the Antoni B regions are large and bizarre.

In 5% of schwannomata, some tumor cells resemble epithelial cells. They form cords or sheets separated by the collagenous stroma.

The fine structure of the tumor cells in a schwannoma is like that of normal Schwann cells. The tumor cells have fine, interdigitating processes and are surrounded by a basement membrane. The tumor cells in the Antoni B regions have more mitochondria, lysosomes, and fat droplets than do those in the Antoni A regions. In many of the reticulin fibers in the tumor the periodicity of the cross banding of the collagen is from 130 to 150 nm, instead of the normal 64 nm. The tumor cells stain for the protein S-100 and sometimes for the myelin basic protein.

Behavior. Schwannomata are benign. They grow slowly but do not invade. They rarely become malignant.

Clinical Presentation. Most schwannomata cause no dysfunction until the tumor is big enough to press on an adjacent structure or to increase intracranial pressure. They seldom cause pain or motor dysfunction in the distribution of the affected nerve. An acoustic neuroma frequently causes tinnitus, deafness, and vertigo that persist for years before pressure on the bone causes pain, increases the intracranial pressure, or increases the concentration of protein in the cerebrospinal fluid.

Treatment and Prognosis. Excision of a schwannoma cures. If the tumor is intracranial or intraspinal, resection may be difficult or impossible. If an acoustic neuroma cannot be completely removed, it recurs in 25% of the patients.

NEUROFIBROMA. A cutaneous neurofibroma arises in the skin. Rarely, a similar tumor is found in another organ. A plexiform neurofibroma thickens a major nerve.

Cutaneous Neurofibroma. A single cutaneous neurofibroma is often found in a person who has no evidence of von Recklinghausen's disease. If a patient has more than 6 cutaneous neurofibromata, other lesions of von Recklinghausen's disease are probably present or will develop. Most patients with a solitary neurofibroma are 20 to 30 years old.

A cutaneous neurofibroma forms a soft rubbery mass that bulges above the surface of the skin or is polypoid. Most are about 1 cm across. Rarely, the lesion involves much of the skin of the head or neck, a condition called a diffuse neurofibroma. On section, a neurofibroma arises in the dermis. It is circumscribed but not encapsulated. The larger tumors extend into the subcutaneous fat.

Microscopically, the tumor consists principally of elongated Schwann cells separated by fine collagen. A basement membrane surrounds the Schwann cells. The periodicity of the collagen is normal. Twisted axons run through the tumor. Many of them are enclosed in the neoplastic Schwann cells. Fibrocytes lie among the Schwann cells but are not numerous. Often a few lymphocytes, macrophages, and mast cells are present in the tumor. Occasionally part of a cutaneous neurofibroma is more cellular and resembles an Antoni A region of a schwannoma, part of the tumor has abundant intercellular substance and resembles a myxoma, or the tumor forms structures that resemble a Pacinian or Meissner's corpuscle.

In patients with one or a few cutaneous neurofibromata, excision cures. If cutaneous neurofibromata are numerous, they are overshadowed by the other lesions of von Recklinghausen's disease.

Plexiform Neurofibroma. Plexiform neurofibromata occur only in von Recklinghausen's disease. They involve the larger nerves and are nearly always multiple. The lesions are most common on peripheral nerves, but can involve the intracranial or intraspinal nerves.

The affected nerves are irregularly thickened, soft and rubbery. Often the lesion extends along the nerve for 10 cm or more. On palpation, the lesion feels like a bag of worms. The overlying skin is loose and myxomatous, often hanging in redundant folds. Sometimes it is pigmented. The underlying bones are often thickened and distorted.

Microscopically, a plexiform neurofibroma begins with an increase in the intracellular matrix of the affected nerve, followed by a proliferation of the Schwann cells. The nerve bundles are separated by the increased intercellular matrix and proliferation of Schwann cells, but usually remain intact. Many of the neurites are ensheathed by the tumor cells. As the lesion ages, the Schwann cells become elongated and separated by fine collagen. The structure of the nerve is increasingly distorted. Fibrocytes persist within the lesion, often with a few lymphocytes, macrophages, or mast cells. Mitoses are few. Collagen is deposited at the margin of the nerve and extends into the surrounding tissue.

A plexiform neuroma grows slowly as years pass. The deformity caused by the mass and the overlying excess of redundant skin is often considerable. In less than 5% of the patients, one or more of the lesions becomes malignant, progressing to a neurofibrosarcoma.

GRANULAR CELL TUMOR. The benign tumor of Schwann cells called a granular cell tumor, granular cell myoblastoma, or granular cell schwannoma is discussed in Chapter 31.

NEUROFIBROSARCOMA. The malignant tumor of Schwann cells called a neurofibrosarcoma, neurosarcoma, or malignant schwannoma, makes up 10% of the malignant tumors of the soft tissues. About 50% of them arise in patients with von Recklinghausen's disease. In 10% of the patients, the tumor is induced by irradiation. The patients are usually between 20 and 50 years old. Some 80% of the patients with von Recklinghausen's disease who develop a neurofibrosarcoma are men. In people without von Recklinghausen's disease, men and women are affected equally.

The sarcoma forms a spheroidal mass that thickens one of the larger nerves. Often the mass is more than 5 cm in diameter. Frequently it is attached to the surrounding tissues. Microscopically, some tumors resemble the Antoni A region of a schwannoma, though the tumor cells are more pleomorphic

and have irregular, hyperchromatic nuclei. Mitoses are often numerous. Foci of necrosis with tumor cells palisaded around them are common. In other patients, the sarcoma resembles a fibrosarcoma, though the nuclei of the tumor cells are more irregular. Some tumors have myxomatous regions. Some become highly anaplastic, with large, bizarre tumor cells.

Electron microscopy shows that most of the tumor cells are Schwann cells. Some are more like fibrocytes. In up to 90% of neurofibrosarcomata, the tumor cells stain for the protein S100. In 50% of the tumors, they stain for the myelin basic protein. Some of the collagen in the tumor is of the long spaced type.

Some neurofibrosarcomata grow slowly, invade only to a limited extent, and do not metastasize. Others grow rapidly, invade extensively, and metastasize widely. The tumor is treated by amputation or radical local excision. In patients with von Recklinghausen's disease, 80% of the tumors recur and 60% metastasize, most often to the lungs, liver, subcutaneous tissues, and bones. Only 20% of the patients survive for five years. In patients without von Recklinghausen's disease, the sarcoma is often less aggressive. Nearly 50% of the patients are alive five years after resection of the sarcoma.

VON RECKLINGHAUSEN'S DISEASE. von Recklinghausen's disease is named after the German pathologist who described it in 1882. Often it is called neurofibromatosis, because of the neurofibromata prominent among its lesions. Two forms of von Recklinghausen's disease are distinguished, neurofibromatosis 1 or peripheral von Recklinghausen's disease and neurofibromatosis 2 or central von Recklinghausen's disease.

Both types of von Recklinghausen's disease are inherited as an autosomal dominant character. One child in every 4000 born alive has neurofibromatosis 1. New mutations are responsible for 50% of the cases. One child in 50,000 has neurofibromatosis 2. The abnormal gene is in the pericentric region of chromosome 17 in neurofibromatosis 1, on the long arm of chromosome 22 in neurofibromatosis 2. In many of the patients with neurofibromatosis 2, the long arm of one of the chromosomes 22 is partly or completely absent, perhaps allowing unopposed action of the abnormal allele on the other chromosome 22.

Neurofibromatosis 1. The severity of neurofibromatosis 1 varies from one patient to another. In some, it causes major deformity or death. In others, the lesions are minor. A patient is said to have neurofibromatosis 1 if any two of the following manifestations of the disease are present.

1. More than 6 café-au-lait spots in the skin. Before puberty, the lesions must be more than 0.5 cm across, after puberty more than 1.5 cm across. In a café-au-lait spot, increase in the melanin in the basal layers of the epidermis of the skin causes a well-defined, ovoid patch of pigmentation in the skin, like a large freckle. Often giant melanosomes are present in the lesions. Café-au-lait spots are most common on the trunk. Many normal people have one or a few small lesions. Over 90% of patients with neurofibromatosis 1 have more than 6; many have hundreds.

2. A plexiform neurofibroma, two or more schwannomata on peripheral nerves, or more than two cutaneous neurofibromata. In many of the patients, plexiform neurofibromata are multiple and cause great deformity. In some, tens or hundreds of cutaneous neurofibromata are present.

3. Freckles or café-au-lait spots in the axillae or groins.

4. Bowing of the long bones caused by thinning of their cortex or dysplasia of the wings of the sphenoid bone. Sometimes a fracture in a weakened long bone causes a pseudarthrosis. About 40% of patients with neurofibromatosis 1 have some bony abnormality.

5. A glioma on an optic nerve.

6. More than 2 of the pigmented retinal hamartomata called Lisch nodules. More than 90% of people with neurofibromatosis 1 have 2 or more of these lesions.

7. A parent or sibling with neurofibromatosis 1.

Less frequently a patient with neurofibromalformed vertebrae, syringomeylia, gigantism of a limb, a pheochromocytoma, honeymalformed vertebrae, syringomeylia, gigantism of a limb, a pheochromocytoma, honeycombing in the lungs, stenosis of a renal artery, enlarged breasts, the Sturge-Weber syndrome, the von Hippel-Lindau syndrome, or mild mental retardation. In some patients, the concentrations of the nerve growth factor and the glial growth factor in the plasma are increased.

Plexiform neurofibromata are usually present at birth. They grow as the years pass, causing increasing deformity. Cutaneous neurofibromata and café-au-lait spots often appear or enlarge during adolescence or pregnancy, suggesting that endocrine stimulation may be important in their development.

Most patients with neurofibromatosis 1 need no treatment or need treatment only for cosmetic reasons. In the others, the more disabling lesions are excised, and bony defects are repaired. In less than 5% of the patients, a neurofibrosarcoma develops in one or more of the plexiform neurofibromata.

Neurofibromatosis 2. If bilateral auditory neuromata are present, the patient almost certainly has neurofibromatosis 2. The diagnosis is also made if a parent or sibling has neurofibromatosis 2 and the patient has a unlilateral auditory neuroma or two of the following: a glioma, a meningioma, a plexiform neurofibroma, more than one schwannoma, multiple cutaneous neurofibromata, multiple café-au-lait spots, a juvenile posterior subcapsular lenticular opacity.

The auditory neuromata in neurofibromatosis 2 usually appear during childhood. In some patients, they grow slowly and for many years cause no disability. In some, they enlarge rapidly. Most of the gliomata that develop in neurofibromatosis 2 are well-differentiated astrocytomata that become stationary or grow slowly. Some are glioblastomata. Some patients have more than one glioma or more than one meningioma. Extensive involvement of the peripheral nerves or more than a few neurofibromata or café-au-lait spots in the skin is unusual. When necessary, the lesions are excised.

Lymphoma

Primary lymphoma of the brain is rare except in people who are immunodeficient. About 10% of people with a renal transplant develop a lymphoma in the brain. Lymphoma of the brain is common in people with the acquired immune deficiency syndrome. The tumor is usually a poorly differentiated B cell lymphoma.

Secondary Tumors

About 20% of tumors in the brain are metastatic. Almost all are carcinoma caused by emboli carried to the brain in the blood. In nearly 50% of the patients, the primary carcinoma is in a lung; in 25% in a breast. Less often a carcinoma of a kidney, the alimentary tract, a malignant melanoma, a chorioepithelioma, or some other tumor metastasizes to the brain. Occasionally metastatic Hodgkin's disease or non-Hodgkin's lymphoma involves the brain. One or more metastases are present in the brain in 5% of patients dying of cancer. Occasionally leukemic cells obstruct blood vessels in the brain causing foci of edema, hemorrhage, or infarction.

Metastases in the brain are often multiple. They are most common in the cerebral hemispheres, though any part of the brain can be affected. Often a metastasis begins at the junction between the cerebral cortex and the underlying white matter. The metastasis usually forms a well-defined, firm, spheroidal mass, often with considerable edema in the surrounding brain. As it enlarges, the metastasis invades the adjacent brain and the meninges. Microscopically, the metastasis usually resembles the primary tumor from which it arose.

If a carcinoma reaches the subarachnoid space, the tumor can spread in the cerebrospinal fluid and implant in other parts of the meninges. If metastases to the leptomeninges are extensive, the patient is said to have carcinomatous meningitis. About 50% of children dying of acute lymphoid leukemia have involvement of the leptomeninges, sometimes with invasion of the underlying brain, spinal cord, or nerves. Other acute leukemias involve the meninges less frequently. Lymphomata and multiple myeloma rarely involve the leptomeninges, but sometimes form extradural deposits that compress the spinal cord or a spinal nerve.

Metastases rarely form in the spinal cord, but the spinal cord is sometimes damaged by compression or invasion from a metastases in the leptomeninges or a vertebra. About 25% of tumors that damage the cord are metastatic. Both lymphomata and carcinomata can damage the spinal cord in this way.

Metastases to the peripheral nervous system are rare, if direct invasion of nerves and ganglia by an adjacent tumor are excluded.

BIBLIOGRAPHY

General

Adams, J. H., Corsellis, J. A. N., and Duchen, L. W. (Eds.): Greenfield's Neuropathology, 4th Ed. London, Edward Arnold, 1984.
Adams, J. H., and Graham, D. I.: An Introduction of Neuropathology. Edinburgh, Churchill Livingstone, 1988.
Burger, D., and Vogel, S.: Surgical Pathology of the Nervous System and its Coverings, 2nd Ed. New York, John Wiley and Sons, 1982.
Davis, R. I., and Robertson, D. M. (eds.): Textbook of Neuropathology. Baltimore, Williams & Wilkins, 1985.
Hughes, J. T.: Pathology of the Spinal Cord. London, Lloyd-Luke, 1978.
Leibowitz, S., and Hughes, R. A. C.: Immunology of the Nervous System. London, Edward Arnold, 1983.
Okazaki, H., and Sheithauer, B. W.: Atlas of Neuropathology. Philadelphia, Lippincott, 1988.

Infection

Anders, K. H., et al.: The neuropathology of AIDS. Am. J. Pathol., 124:537, 1986.
Anderson J. R.: Viral encephalitis and its pathology. Curr. Top. Pathol., 76:23, 1988.
Barnes, D. W., and Whitley, R. S.: CNS diseases associated with varicella zoster virus and herpes simplex virus infection. Neurol. Clin., 4:265, 1986.
Berger, J. R., Kaszovitz, B., Post, M. J., and Dickinson, G.: Progressive multifocal leukoencephalopathy associated with human immunodeficiency virus infection. Ann. Intern. Med., 107:78, 1987.
Burger, P. C.: Surgical pathological considerations in inflammatory and transmissible diseases of the central nervous system. Am. J. Surg. Pathol., 11(Supple. 1):38, 1987.
Chapman, P. H., and Borges, L. F.: Shunt infections. Clin. Neurosurg., 32:652, 1985.
Davanipour, Z., Alter, M., and Sobel, E.: Creutzfeld-Jakob disease. Neurol. Clin., 4:415, 1986.
Dee, R. R., and Lorber, B.: Brain abscess due to Listeria monocytogenes. Rev. Infect. Dis., 8:968, 1986.
Delisle, M. B., Bouissou, H., and Saidi, A.: What's new

in cerebral pathology in acquired immune deficiencies? Pathol. Res. Pract., *181*:85, 1986.

Elder, G. A., and Sever, J. L.: Neurologic disorders associated with AIDS retrovirus infection. Rev. Infect. Dis., *10*:286, 1988.

Epstein, L. G., Sharer, L. R., and Goudsmit, J.: Neurological and neuropathological features of human immunodeficiency virus infection in children. Ann. Neurol., *23*(Suppl.):S19, 1988.

Fischer, P. A., and Enzensberger, W.: Neurological complications in AIDS. J. Neurol., *234*:269, 1987.

Gabuzda, D. H., and Hirsch, M. S.: Neurologic manifestations of infection with human immunodeficiency virus. Ann. Intern. Med., *107*:383, 1987.

Gray, F., Gherardi, R., and Scaravilli, F.: The neuropathology of the acquired immune deficiency syndrome. Brain, *111*:245, 1988.

Harris, A. A., Segreti, J., and Levin, S.: Central nervous system infection in patients with the acquired immune deficiency syndrome (AIDS). Clin. Neuropharmacol., 8:201, 1985.

John, D. T.: Primary amebic meningoencephalitis and the biology of Naegleria fowleri. Annu. Rev. Microbiol., 36:101, 1982.

Jordan, M. C., Jordan, G. W., Stevens, J. G., and Miller, G.: Latent herpesviruses in humans. Ann. Intern. Med., *100*:866, 1984.

Lasker, B. R., and Harter, D. H.: Cervical epidural abscess. Neurology, 37:1747, 1987.

Loeser, J. D.: Herpes zoster and postherpetic neuralgia. Pain, 25:149, 1986.

Lyons, R. W., and Andriole, V. T.: Fungal infections of the CNS. Neurol. Clin., 4:159, 1986.

Marks, W. A., and Bodensteiner, J. B.: Anterior cervical epidural abscess with pneumococcus in an infant. J. Child Neurol., 3:25, 1988.

McArthur, J. C.: Neurologic manifestations of AIDS. Medicine, 66:407, 1987.

Naidich, T. P., McLone, D. G., and Radkowski, M.A.: Intracranial arachoid cysts. Pediatr. Neurosci., *12*:112, 1985–86.

Neilsen, H.: Cerebral abscess. Dan. Med. Bull., 32:170, 1985.

Patrick, C. C., and Kaplan, S. L.: Current concepts in the pathogenesis and management of brain abscesses in children. Pediatr. Clin. North Am., 35:625, 1988.

Prusiner, S. B.: Prions causing degenerative neurological diseases. Annu Rev. Med., 38:381, 1987.

Prusiner, S. B.: Prion disease and central nervous system degeneration. Clin. Res., 35:177, 1987.

Prusiner, S. B.: Prions and neurodegenerative diseases. N. Engl. J. Med., *317*:1571, 1987.

Prusiner, S. B., Gabizon, R., and McKinley, M. P.: On the biology of prions. Acta Neuropathol., 72:299, 1987.

Quagliarello, V. J., and Scheld, W. M.: Recent advances in the pathogenesis and pathophysiology of bacterial meningitis. Am. J. Med. Sci., 292:306, 1986.

Seidel, J.: Primary amebic meningoencephalitis. Pediatr. Clin. North Am., 32:881, 1985.

Sheller, J. R., and Des Prez, R. M.: CNS tuberculosis. Neurol. Clin., 4:143, 1986.

Simon, M. W., and Wilson, H. D.: The amebic meningoencephalitides. Pediatr. Infect. Dis., 5:562, 1986.

Southwick, F. S., Richardson, E. P., Jr., and Swartz, M. N.: Septic thrombosis of the dural venous sinuses. Medicine, 65:82, 1986.

Wispelwey, B., and Scheld, W. M.: Brain abscess. Clin. Neuropharmacol., *10*:483, 1987.

Yogev, R.: Suppurative intracranial complications of upper respiratory tract disease. Pediatr. Infect. Dis. J., 6:324, 1987.

Vascular Disease

Babikian, V., and Ropper, A. H.: Binswanger's disease. Stroke, *18*:2, 1987.

Benson, M. D., and Rebar, R. W.: Relationship of migraine headache and stroke to oral contraceptive use. J. Reprod. Med., *31*:1082, 1986.

Blass, J. P.: Circulatory and degenerative dementias. J. Am. Geriatr. Soc., 35:1127, 1987.

Brann, A. W., Jr.: Hypoxic ischemic encephalopathy (asphyxia). Pediatr. Clin. North Am., 33:451, 1986.

Brust, J. C. M.: Dementia and cerebrovascular disease. Adv. Neurol., *38*:131, 1987.

Buckingham, et al. Traumatic cerebral aneurysms in childhood. Neurosurgery, *22*:398, 1988.

Cahill, B. E., and Kerstein, M. D.: Ischemic neuropathy. Surg. Gynecol. Obstet., *165*:469, 1987.

Caplan, L. R., Gorelick, P. B., and Hier, D. B.: Race, sex and occlusive cerebrovascular disease. Stroke, *17*:648, 1986.

Caplan, L. R., and Pressin, M. S.: Symptomatic carotid artery disease and carotid endarterectomy. Annu. Rev. Med., *39*:273, 1988.

Cerebral Embolism Task Force: Cardiogenic brain embolism. Arch. Neurol., *43*:71, 1986.

Dobkin, D. H.: Management of transient ischemic attacks. Hosp. Pract., *22*(3):113, 1987.

Fahn, S.: Posthypoxic action myoclonus. Adv. Neurol., *43*:157, 1986.

Firsching, R., Frowein, R. A., and Thun, F.: Intracerebeller haematoma. Neurochirugia, *30*:182, 1987.

Gaehtgens, P., and Marx, P.: Hemorheological aspects of the pathophysiology of cerebral ischemia. J. Cereb. Blood Flow, 7:259, 1987.

Gillum, R. F.: Stroke in blacks. Stroke, *19*:1, 1988.

Grotta, J. C., Manner, C., Pettigrew, L. C., and Yatsu, F. M.: Red blood cell disorders and stroke. Stroke, *17*:811, 1986.

Henrich, J. B.: The association between migraine and cerebral vascular events. J. Chronic Dis., *40*:329, 1987.

Hindman, B. J.: Perioperative stroke. Int. Anesthesiol. Clin., *24*(4):101, 1986.

Hopkins, L. N., et al.: Vertebrobasilar insufficiency, Pt. 2. J. Neurosurg., 66:662, 1987.

Hosoda, Y.: Pathology of so-called "spontaneous occlusion of the circle of Willis". Pathol. Annu., *19*(Pt. 2):221, 1984.

Jackson, A. C.: Neurologic disorders associated with mitral valve prolapse. Can. J. Neurol. Sci., *13*:15, 1986.

Johansson, B. B., and Fredriksson, K.: Cerebral arteries in hypertension. J. Cardiovasc. Pharmacol., 7(Suppl. 2):S90, 1985.

Kapelle, L. J., and van Gijn, J.: Lacunar defects. Clin. Neurol. Neurosurg., 88:3, 1986.

Kaplan, J., Dimlich, R. V., Biros, M. H., and Hedges, J.: Mechanisms of ischemic cerebral injury. Resuscitation, 15:149, 1987.

Kase, C. S.: Intracerebral hemorrhage: non-hypertensive causes. Stroke, 17:590, 1986.

Leipzig, T. J., and Dohrmann, G. J.: The tortuous or kinked carotid artery, pathogenesis and clinical considerations. Surg. Neurol., 25:478, 1986.

Levine, M., and Hirsh, J.: Hemorrhagic complications of long-term anticoagulant therapy for ischemic vascular disease. Stroke, 17:111, 1986.

Malmgren, R., Warlow, C., Bamford, J., and Sandercock, P.: Geographic and secular trends in stroke incidence. Lancet, 2:1196, 1987.

Meyer, F. B., Sundt, T. M., Jr., Yanagihara, T., and Anderson, R. E.: Focal cerebral ischemia. Mayo Clin. Proc., 62:35, 1987.

Nedergaard, M.: Mechanisms of brain damage in focal cerebral ischemia. Acta Neurol. Scand., 77:81, 1988.

O'Hare, T. H.: Subarachnoid hemorrhage. J. Emerg. Med., 5:135, 1987.

Quandt, C. M., Talbert, R. L., and de los Reyes, R. A.: Ischemic cerebrovascular disease. Clin. Pharm., 6:292, 1987.

Ross, R. T.: Spinal cord infarcts in disease and surgery of the aorta. Can. J. Neurol. Sci., 12:289, 1985.

Rothman, S. M., and Olney, J. W.: Glutamate and the pathophysiology of hypoxic-ischemic brain damage. Ann. Neurol., 19:105, 1986.

Shaywitz, B. A.: The sequellae of hypoxic-ischemic encephalopathy. Semin. Perinatol., 11:180, 1987.

Solomon, R. A. and Fink, M. E. Current stratagems for the management of aneurysmal subarachnoid hemorrhage. Arch. Neurol., 4:769, 1987.

Spetzler, R.F., et al.: Vertebrobasilar insufficiency. Pt 1. J. Neurosurg., 66:648, 1987.

Wolf, P. A., and Sila, C. A.: Cerebral ischemia with mitral valve prolapse. Am. Heart J., 113:1308, 1987.

Trauma

Adams, J. H.: Autopsy in fatal non-missile head injuries. Curr. Top. Pathol., 76:1, 1988.

Adams, J. H., and Graham, D. I.: Diffuse brain damage in non-missile head injury. Rec. Adv. Histopathol., 12:241, 1984.

Allan, W. C., and Volpe, J. J.: Periventricular-intraventricular hemorrhage. Pediatr. Clin. North Am., 33:47, 1986.

Bell, C. C.: Coma and the etiology of violence. J. Natl. Med. Assoc., 79:79, 1987.

Dowling, G., and Curry, B.: Traumatic basal subarachnoid hemorrhage. Am. J. Forensic Med. Pathol., 9:23, 1988.

Enzmann, D., et al.: The natural history of subependymal germinal matrix hemorrhage. Am. J. Perinatol., 2:123, 1985.

Hayes, R. L., et al.: Metabolic and neurophysiologic sequelae of brain injury. Cent. Nerv. Syst. Trauma, 3: 163, 1986.

Lehman, L. B.: Nervous system sports-related injuries. Am. J. Sports Med., 15:494, 1987.

Ment, L. R., Duncan, C. C., and Ehrenkranz, R. A.: Intraventricular hemorrhage of the preterm neonate. Semin. Perinatol., 11:132, 1987.

Ment, L. R., Duncan, C. C., and Ehrenkranz, R. A.: Perinatal cerebral infarction. Semin. Perinatol., 11: 142, 1987.

Ment, L. R., Duncan, C. C., and Stewart, W. B.: Perinatal cerebral insults, hemorrhage and ischemia. Pediatr. Neurosci., 12:168, 1985–1986.

Perkins, R. P.: Perspective on perinatal brain damage. Obstet. Gynecol., 69:807, 1987.

Rorke, L. B.: Pathology of Perinatal Brain Injury. New York, Raven Press, 1982.

Metabolic Disorders

Alfrey, A. C.: Dialysis encephalopathy. Clin. Nephrol., 24(Suppl. 1):S15, 1985.

Anderson, N. E., Cunningham, J. N., and Posner, J. B.: Autoimmune pathogenesis of paraneoplastic neurological syndromes. Crit. Rev. Neurobiol., 3:245, 1987.

Arieff, A. I.: Aluminum and the pathogenesis of dialysis encephalopathy. Am. J. Kidney Dis., 6:317, 1985.

Auer, R. N.: Hypoglycemic brain damage. Stroke, 17:699, 1986.

Berkovic, S. F., et al.: Kuf's disease. Brain, 111(Pt. 1):27, 1988.

Biasioli, S., et al.: Uremic encephalopathy. Clin. Nephrol., 25:57, 1986.

Bode, J. C., and Schäfer, K.: Pathophysiology of chronic hepatic encephalopathy. Hepatogastroenterology, 32: 259, 1985.

Chad, D. A., and Recht, L. D.: Neurological paraneoplastic syndromes. Cancer Invest., 6:67, 1988.

Ede, R. J., and Williams, R.: Hepatic encephalopathy and cerebral edema. Semin. Liver Dis., 6:107, 1986.

van Erven, et al.: Leigh syndrome. Clin. Neurol. Neurosurg., 89:217, 1987.

Fraser, C. L., and Arieff, A. I.: Hepatic encephalopathy. N. Engl. J. Med., 313:865, 1985.

Fraser, C. L., and Arieff, A. I.: Nervous system complications in uremia. Ann. Intern. Med, 109:143, 1988.

Glen-Bott, A. M.: Aspirin and Reye's syndrome. Med. Toxicol., 2:161, 1987.

Glew, R. H., Basu, A., Prence, E. M., and Remaley, A. T.: Lysosomal storage diseases. Lab. Invest., 53:250, 1985.

Gocht, A., and Colmant, H. J.: Central pontine and extrapontine myelinolysis. Clin. Neuropathol., 6:262, 1987.

Goldstein, G. W., Robertson, P., and Betz, A. L.: Update on the role of the blood-brain barrier in damage to the immature brain. Pediatrics, 81:732, 1988.

Hall, S. M.: Reye's disease and aspirin. J. R. Soc. Med., 79:596, 1986.

Hansen, T. W. R., and Bratlid, D.: Bilirubin and brain toxicity. Acta Pediatr. Scand., 75:513, 1986.

Heubi, J. E., Partin, J. C., Partin, J. S., and Schubert,

W. K.: Reye's syndrome. Hepatology, 7:155, 1987.

Jones, E. A., and Schafer, D. F.: Hepatic encephalopathy: a neurochemical disorder. Prog. Liver Dis., 8:525, 1986.

Kelley, R. I., et al: Neonatal adrenoleukodystrophy. Am. J. Med. Genet., 23:869, 1986.

Kornfeld, S., and Sly, W. S.: Lysosomal storage defects. Hosp. Pract., 20(8):71, 1985.

Leonard, B. E.: Ethanol as a neurotoxin. Biochem. Pharmacol., 36:2055, 1987.

Leone, A.: Metallothionein gene regulation in Menke's disease. Horiz. Biochem. Biophys., 8:207, 1986.

Levade, T., Salvayre, R., and Douste-Blazy, L.: Sphingomyelinases and Niemann-Pick disease. J. Clin. Chem. Clin. Biochem., 24:205, 1986.

Libert, J.: Diagnosis of lysosomal storage diseases. Pathol. Annu., 15(Pt. 1):37, 1980.

MacMath, T. L., and Pons, P. T.: Hepatic encephalopathy. J. Emerg. Med., 3:401, 1985.

Martin, P. R., et al.: Alcoholic organic brain disease. Prog. Neuropsychopharmacol. Biol. Psychiatry, 10:147, 1986.

Moser, H. W., Naidu, S., Kumar, A. J., and Rosenbaum, A. E.: The adrenoleukodystrophies. CRC Crit. Rev. Clin. Neurol., 3:29, 1987.

Mowat, A. P.: Reye's disease. Adverse Drug React. Acute Poisoning, 6:211, 1987.

Norenberg, M. D.: The role of astrocytes in hepatic encephalopathy. Neurochem. Pathol., 6:13, 1987.

Ojeda, V. J., and Walters, M. N-I.: Spinal cord disorders in patients with cancer. Pathol. Annu., 19 (Pt. 2):63, 1984.

Patchell, R. A., and Posner, J. B.: Neurologic complications of systemic cancer. Neurol. Clin., 3:729, 1985.

Peiffer, J.: Encephalomyelopathies associated with extracranial malignant tumors. Pathol. Res. Pract., 182:585, 1987.

Powers, J. M., Moser, H. W., Moser, A. B., and Schaumburg, H. H.: Fetal adrenoleukodystrophy. Hum. Pathol., 13:1013, 1982.

Rossi-Fanelli, et al.: Amino acids and hepatic encephalopathy. Prog. Neurobiol., 28:277, 1987.

Salmon, D. P., and Butters, N.: The etiology and neuropathology of alcoholic Korsakoff's syndrome. Recent Dev. Alcohol., 5:27, 1987.

Savazzi, G. M.: Pathogenesis of cerebral atrophy in uremia. Nephron, 49:94, 1988.

Siesjö, B. K.: Hypoglycemia, brain metabolism and brain damage. Diabetes Metab. Rev., 4:113, 1988.

Sohal, R. S., et al.: Lipofuscin: characteristics and significance. Progr. Brain Res., 70:171, 1986.

Thomas, P. K.: Alcohol and disease: central nervous system. Acta Med. Scand. (Suppl.), 703:251, 1985.

Trompeter, R. S., Polinsky, M.S., Andreoli, S. A., and Fennell, R. S.: Neurologic complications of renal failure. Am. J. Kidney Dis., 7:318, 1986.

Walker, P. G.: Neonatal bilirubin toxicity. Clin. Pharmacokinet., 13:26, 1987.

Watkins, P. A., Naidu, S., and Moser, A. W.: Adrenoleukodystrophy: biochemical procedures in diagnosis, prevention and treatment. J. Inherited Metab. Dis., 10(Suppl. 1):46, 1987.

Zieve, L.: The mechanism of hepatic coma. Hepatology, 1:360, 1981.

Demyelinating Diseases

Arnason, B. G. W.: Multiple sclerosis, allied central nervous system diseases and immune-mediated neuropathies. In The Autoimmune Diseases. Edited by Rose, N. R., and Mackay, I. R. Orlando, Academic Press, 1985.

Arnason, B. G. W.: Autoimmune neuropathies. Ann. N.Y. Acad. Sci., 505:313, 1987.

Barna, B. P.: Multiple sclerosis: neuroimmunologic puzzle. Clin. Lab. Med., 6:103, 1986.

Baumheffner, R. W., and Tourtellotte, W. W.: Cellular immunity in multiple sclerosis. Concepts Immunopathol., 2:151, 1985.

Birk, K., and Rudick, R.: Pregnancy and multiple sclerosis. Arch. Neurol., 43:719, 1986.

Dalgleisch, A. G., Fazakerley, J. K., and Webb, H. E.: Do human T-lymphotropic viruses (HTLVs) and other enveloped viruses induce autoimmunity in multiple sclerosis? Neuropathol. Appl. Neurobiol., 13:241, 1987.

Dick, G., and Gay, D.: Multiple sclerosis—autoimmune or microbial? J. Infect., 16:25, 1988.

Dore-Duffy, P., Ho, S.-Y., and Longo, M.: The role of prostaglandins in altered leukocyte function in multiple sclerosis. Springer Semin. Immunopathol., 8:305, 1985.

Glass, J. P., Lee, Y.-Y., Bruner. J., and Fields, W. S.: Treatment-related leukoencephalopathy. Medicine, 65:154, 1986.

Gordon, N.: Peroxisomal disorders. Brain Dev., 9:571, 1987.

Larner, A. J.: Aetiological role of viruses in multiple sclerosis. J. R. Soc. Med., 79:412, 1986.

Ludwig, S. K.: Remyelination in demyelinating diseases of the central nervous system. Crit. Rev. Neurobiol., 3:1, 1987.

Macchi, G.: Experimental patterns related to multiple sclerosis pathology. Riv. Neurol., 57:145, 1987.

McDonald, W. I.: The pathogenesis of multiple sclerosis. J. R. Coll. Physicians Lond., 21:287, 1987.

O'Gorman, M., and Oger, J.: Cell-mediated immune functions in multiple sclerosis. Pathol. Immunopathol. Res., 6:241, 1987.

Paterson, P. Y., Koh, C. S., and Kwaan, H. C.: Role of the clotting system in the pathogenesis of neuroimmunologic disease. Fed. Proc., 46:91, 1987.

Poser, C. M.: Pathogenesis of multiple sclerosis. Acta Neuropathol., 71:1, 1986.

Poser, C. M.: The peripheral nervous system in multiple sclerosis. J. Neurol. Sci., 79:83, 1987.

Rosenthal, A.: The cerebrospinal fluid proteins in multiple sclerosis. Clin. Lab. Med., 6:457, 1986.

Rutledge, S. L., and Snead, O. C., III.: Neurologic complications of immunizations. J. Pediatr., 109:917, 1986.

Sayetta, R. B.: Theories of the etiology of multiple sclerosis. J. Clin. Lab. Immunol., 21:55, 1986.

Srensen, K. V.: Somatostatin in multiple sclerosis. Acta Neurol. Scand., 75:161, 1986.

Waxman, S. G.: Clinical course and electrophysiology of multiple sclerosis. Adv. Neurol., 47:157, 1988.

Weinshenker, B. G., and Ebers, G. C.: The natural

history of multiple sclerosis. Can. J. Neurol. Sci., *14*:255, 1987.

Whitaker, J. N., and Snyder, D. S.: Studies of autoimmunity in multiple sclerosis. CRC Crit. Rev. Clin. Neurobiol., *1*:45, 1984.

Wisniewski, H. M., et al.: Pathogenetic aspects of multiple sclerosis and experimental models of inflammatory demyelination. Concepts Immunopathol., *2*: 128, 1985.

Zweiman, B., and Levinson, A. I.: Immunologic aspects of neurologic diseases. I. General responses and demyelinating diseases. J. Allergy Clin. Immunol., *81*:1067, 1988.

Zweiman, B., and Lisak, R. P.: Cell-mediated immunity in neurologic disease. Hum. Pathol., *17*:234, 1986.

Degenerative Diseases of Neurons

Agid, Y., and Blin, J.: Nerve cell death in degenerative diseases of the central nervous system. Ciba Found. Symp., *126*:3, 1987.

Agid, Y., Taquet, H., Cesselin, F., and Javoy-Agid, F.: Neuropeptides and Parkinson's disease. Prog. Brain Res., *66*:107, 1986.

Allen, Y. S., Bloom, S. P., and Polak, J. M.: The neuropeptide Y immunoreactive neuronal system. Hum. Neurobiol., *5*:227, 1986.

Beal, M. F., and Growdon, J. H.: CSF neurotransmitter markers in Alzheimer's disease. Prog. Neurophyschopharmacol. Biol. Psychiatry, *10*:259, 1986.

Berkovic, S. F., Anermann, F., Carpenter, S., and Wolfe, L. S.: Progressive myoclonus epilepsies. N. Engl. J. Med., *315*:296, 1986.

Bertholf, R. L.: Aluminum and Alzheimer's disease. CRC Crit. Rev. Clin. Lab. Sci., *25*:195, 1987.

Broder, E.: Ataxia-telangiectasia. KROC Found. Ser., *19*:1, 1985.

Brooks, B. R. (ed.): Amyotrophic lateral sclerosis. Neurol. Clin., *5*:1, 1987.

Castano, E. M., and Frangione, B.: Human amyloidosis, Alzheimer's disease and related disorders. Lab. Invest., *58*:122, 1988.

Chamberlain, S., Worrall, C., and Williamson, R.: Attempts to identify the chromosomal location of the Friedreich's ataxia locus. Adv. Neurol., *48*:257, 1988.

Chozick, B.: The nucleus basalis of Meynert in neurological dementing disease. J. Neurosci., *37*:31, 1987.

Coleman, P. D., and Flood, P. G.: Neuron numbers and dendritic extent in normal aging and Alzheimer's disease. Neurobiol. Aging, *8*:521, 1987.

Collerton, D.: Cholinergic function and intellectual decline in Alzheimer's disease. Neuroscience, *19*:1, 1986.

Cosi, V., et al. (eds.): Amyotropic lateral sclerosis. Adv. Exp. Med. Biol., *209*:1, 1987.

Coyle, J. T., Oster-Granite, M. L., and Gearheart, J. D.: The neurobiologic consequences of Down syndrome. Brain Res. Bull., *16*:773, 1986.

Crapper McLachlan, D. R., and Farnell, B. J.: Cellular mechanisms of aluminium toxicity. Ann. Inst. Super. Sanita, *22*:697, 1986.

Cummings, J. L.: Subcortical dementia. Br. J. Psychiatry, *149*:682, 1986.

Davies, I.: Aluminium, neurotoxicity and dementia. Rev. Environ. Health, *6*:251, 1986.

Davies, P.: The genetics of Alzheimer's disease. Neurobiol. Aging, *7*:459, 1986.

Davies, P., and Wolozin, B. L.: Recent advances in the neurochemistry of Alzheimer's disease. J. Clin. Psychiatry, *48*(Suppl.):23, 1987.

Davison, A. N.: The ageing brain and dementia. Br. J. Clin.. Prac., *39*(Symp. Suppl.):3, 1985.

Davison, A.N.: Pathophysiology of the ageing brain. Gerontology, *33*:129, 1987.

De Estable-Puig, R. F., et al.: On the pathogenesis and therapy of dementia of the Alzheimer type. Prog. Neuropsychopharmacol. Biol. Psychiatry, *10*:355, 1986.

Deutsch, S. I., and Morihisa, J. M.: Glutamatergic abnormalities in Alzheimer's disease. Clin. Neuropharmacol., *11*:18, 1988.

Duvoisin, R. C.: Etiology of Parkinson's disease. Clin. Neuropharmacol., *9*(Suppl. 1):S3, 1986.

Emson, P. C.: Neuropeptides and the pathology of Huntington's disease. Prog. Brain Res., *66*: 91, 1986.

Feldman. R. G.: Parkinson's disease: individualizing therapy. Hosp. Pract., *20*(12):80A, 1985.

Gibb, W. R. G.: Idiopathic Parkinson's disease and the Lewy body disorders. Neuropathol. Appl. Neurobiol., *12*:223, 1986.

Glenner, G. G.: On causative theories in Alzheimer's disease. Hum. Pathol., *16*:433, 1985.

Harrison, P. J.: Pathogenesis of Alzheimer's disease. J. R. Soc. Med., *79*:347, 1986.

Hefti, F., and Weiner, W. J.: Nerve growth factor and Alzheimer's disease. Ann. Neurol., *20*:275, 1986.

Heston, L. L.: Clinical genetics of dementing illness. Neurol. Clin., *4*:439, 1986.

Hollander, E., Mohs, R. C., and Davis, K. L.: Antemortem markers of Alzheimer's disease. Neurobiol. Aging, *7*:367, 1986.

Hoyer, S.: Senile dementia and Alzheimer's disease. Prog. Neuropsychopharmacol. Biol. Psychiatry, *10*: 447, 1986.

Jankovic, J.: Progressive supranuclear palsy. Neurol. Clin., *2*:473, 1984.

Janota, I.: Pathology of dementia. Rec. Adv. Histopathol., *11*:49, 1981.

Jellinger, K.: Quantitative changes in some subcortical nuclei in aging, Alzheimer's disease and Parkinson's disease. Neurobiol. Aging, *8*:556, 1987.

Kopin, I. J.: MPTP: an industrial chemical and contaminant of illicit narcotics stimulates a new era in research on Parkinson's disease. Environ. Health Perspect., *75*:45, 1987.

Krigman, M. R., Bouldin, T. W., and Mushak, P.: Metal toxicity in the nervous system. Monogr. Pathol., *26*:58, 1985.

Kwentus, J. A., et al. Alzheimer's disease. Am. J. Med., *81*:91, 1986.

Langston, J. W.: MPTP: insights into the etiology of Parkinson's disease. Eur. Neurol., *26*(Suppl. 1):2, 1987.

Lewis, D. A., and Bloom, F. E.: Clinical perspectives on neuropeptides. Annu. Rev. Med., *38*:143, 1987.

Mann, D. M. A.: The neuropathology of Alzheimer's disease. Mech. Ageing Dev., *31*:213, 1985.

Mann, D. M. A.: Alzheimer's disease and Down's syndrome. Histopathology, 13:125, 1988.

Mann, D. M. A., and Yates, P. O.: Neurotransmitter defects in Alzheimer's disease and other dementing disorders. Hum. Neurobiol., 5:147, 1986.

Martin, J. B., and Barchas, J. D. (eds.): Neuropeptides in neurologic and psychiatric disease. New York, Raven Press, 1986.

Martin, J. B., and Gusella, J. F.: Huntington's disease. N. Engl. J. Med., 315:1267, 1986.

Masters, C. L., and Beyruther, K.: Neuronal origin of cerebral amyloidogenic proteins and their role in Alzheimer's disease and unconventional viral diseases. Ciba Found. Symp., 126:49, 1987.

McDonald, K. C., and Valmassy, R. L.: Cerebral palsy. J. Am. Podiatr. Med. Assoc., 77:471, 1987.

McGeer, P. L., McGeer, E. G., Itagaki, S., and Mizukawa, K.: Anatomy and pathology of the basal ganglia. Can. J. Neurol. Sci., 14(3 Suppl.):363, 1987.

McLachlan, D. R.: Aluminum and Alzheimer's disease. Neurobiol. Aging, 7:525, 1986.

McLachlan, D. R., and Van Berkum, M. F. A.: Aluminum: a role in degenerative brain disease associated with neurofibrillary tangles. Progr. Brain Res., 70:399, 1986.

Jellinger, K.: Neuropathological substrates of Alzheimer's disease and Parkinson's disease. J. Neurol. Transm. (Suppl.), 24:109, 1987.

Jenden, D. J., and McIntyre, H. B. (Eds.): Workshop on early diagnosis in Alzheimer's disease. Bull. Clin. Neurosci., 50:1, 1985.

Jorm, A. F., Korten, A. E., and Henderson, A. S.: The prevalence of dementia. Acta Psychiatr. Scand., 76:465, 1987.

Karlinsky, H.: Alzheimer's disease in Down's syndrome. J. Am. Geriatr. Soc., 34:728, 1986.

Katzman, R.: Alzheimer's disease as an age-dependant disorder. Ciba Found. Symp., 134:68, 1988.

Katzman, R. N.: Alzheimer's disease. N. Engl. J. Med., 314:964, 1986.

Kisilevsky, R.: From arthritis to Alzheimer's disease: current concepts on the pathogenesis of amyloidosis. Can J. Physiol. Pharmacol., 65:1805, 1987.

McLachlan, D. R. C., Kruck, T. P. A., and Van Berkum, M. F. A.: Aluminum and neurodegenerative disease. Am. J. Kidney Dis., 6:322, 1985.

Mozar, H. N., Bal, D. G., and Howard, J. T.: Perspectives on the etiology of Alzheimer's disease. J.A.M.A., 257:1503, 1987.

Myers, R. H., Schoenfeld, M., and Bird, E. D.: Huntington's disease: genetics, chemical pathology, and management. Prog. Med. Genet., 6:277, 1985.

Nakanishi, T. (ed.): Symposium on a long time clinical cure of Parkinson's disease. Eur. Neurol., 26(Suppl. 1):1–55, 1987.

Paller, A. S.: Ataxia-telangiectasia. Neurol. Clin., 5:447, 1987.

Pendlebury, W. W., Munoz-Garcia, D., and Perl, D. P.: Cytoskeletal pathology in neurodegenerative disease. Adv. Exp. Med. Biol., 221:427, 1987.

Perl, D. P., and Pendelbury, W. W.: Neuropathology of dementia. Neurol. Clin., 4:355, 1986.

Petit, T. L.: Aluminum in human dementia. Am. J. Kidney Dis., 6:313, 1985.

Pitt, B.: Dementia. Edinburgh, Churchill Livingstone, 1987.

Plum, F.: Cerebral changes in Alzheimer's disease. Prog. Brain Res., 66:135, 1986.

Price, D. L.: New perspectives on Alzheimer's disease. Annu. Rev. Neurosci., 9:489, 1986.

Price, D. L., et al.: Dysfunction and death of neurons in human degenerative neurological diseases and experimental models. Ciba Found. Symp., 126:30, 1987.

Price, D. L., et al.: Neurobiological studies of transmitter systems in aging and in Alzheimer-type dementia. Ann. N.Y. Acad. Sci., 457:35, 1985.

Price, D.L., Whitehouse, P. J., and Struble, R. G.: Alzheimer's disease. Annu. Rev. Med., 36:349, 1985.

Quinn, N. P., Rossor, N. P., and Marsden, C. D.: Dementia and Parkinson's disease. Br. Med. Bull., 42:86, 1986.

Radouco-Thomas, C., et al.: Senile dementia and Alzheimer's disease. Prog. Neuropsychopharmacol. Biol. Psychiatry, 10:247, 1986.

Rapin, I.: Myoclonus in neuronal storage and Lafora diseases. Adv. Neurol., 43:65, 1986.

Rapoport, S. I.: Brain evolution and Alzheimer's disease. Rev. Neurol., 144:79, 1988.

Roth, M., and Iversen, L. L. (eds.): Alzheimer's disease and related disorders. Br. Med. Bull., 42:1, 1986.

Sanberg, P. R., and Coyle, J. T.: Scientific approaches to Huntington's disease. CRC Crit. Rev. Clin. Neurobiol., 1:1, 1984.

Saper, C. B., Wainer, B. H., and German, D. C.: Axonal and transneuronal transport in the transmission of neurological disease. Neuroscience, 23:389, 1987.

Schoenberg, B. S.: Epidemiology of Alzheimer's disease and other demyelinating illnesses. J. Chronic Dis., 39:1095, 1986.

Scholtz, C. L.: Dementia in middle and late life. Curr. Top. Pathol., 76:105, 1988.

Schultz, W.: MPTP-induced parkinsonism in monkeys. Gen. Pharmacol., 19:153, 1988.

Selkoe, D. J.: Altered structural proteins in plaques and tangles. Neurobiol. Aging, 7:425. 1986.

de Souza, E.: CRH defects in Alzheimer's and other neurologic diseases. Hosp. Pract., 23(9):59, 1988.

Spencer, P. S.: Guam ALS/parkinsonism-dementia. Can. J. Neurol. Sci., 14(3 Suppl.):347, 1987.

Stewart, J. T.: Huntington's disease. Am. Fam. Physician, 37(5):105, 1988.

Struble, R. G., et al.: Neuropeptidergic systems in plaques of Alzheimer's disease. J. Neuropathol. Exp. Neurol., 46:567, 1987.

Swaab, D. F., et al. (eds.): Aging of the brain and Alzheimer's disease. Prog. Brain Res., 70:1, 1986.

Symposium: Research advances in Alzheimer's disease and related neurodegenerative disorders. Can. J. Neurol. Sci., 13(4 Suppl.):381, 1986.

Tandan, R., and Bradley, W. G.: Amyotrophic lateral sclerosis: Part 2. Ann. Neurol., 18:419, 1985.

Tandan, R., et al.: Childhood giant axonal neuropathy. J. Neurol. Sci., 82:205, 1987.

Timme, T. L., and Moses, R. E.: Diseases with DNA damage-processing defects. Am. J. Med. Sci., 295:40, 1988.

Verity, M. A., and Wechsler, A. F.: Progressive

subcortical gliosis of Neumann. Arch. Gerontol. Geriatr., 6:245, 1987.

Vinters, H. V.: Cerebral amyloid angiopathy. Stroke, 18:311, 1987.

Vogel, F. S.: Dementia. Adv. Pathol., 1:177, 1988.

Weber, M.: Alzheimer's disease and the cytoskeleton. Biochemie, 68:593, 1986.

Whitehouse, P. J.: Understanding the etiology of Alzheimer's disease. Neurol. Clin., 4:427, 1986.

Whitehouse, P. J., et al.: Alzheimer's disease and related dementias. Neurobiology, 1:319, 1985.

Willis, G. L.: Amine accumulation in Parkinson's disease and other disorders. Neurosci. Biobehav. Rev., 11:97, 1987.

Wisniewski, H. M., and Rabe, A.: Discrepancy between Alzheimer-type neuropathology and dementia in persons with Down's syndrome. Ann. N.Y. Acad. Sci., 477:247, 1986.

Zweig, R. M., and Hedreen, J. C.: Brain stem pathology in cranial dystonia. Adv. Neurol., 49:395, 1988.

Peripheral Neuropathy

Aldskogius, H., Arvidson, J., and Grant, G.: The reaction of primary sensory neurons to peripheral nerve injury with particular emphasis on transganglionic changes. Brain Res., 357:27, 1985.

Alexander, I. J., Johnson, K. A., and Parr, J. W.: Morton's neuroma. Orthopedics, 10:103, 1987.

Antti-Poika, M.: Symptoms and signs in solvent exposed populations. Prog. Clin. Biol. Res., 220:255, 1986.

Baker, E. L., and Fine. L. J.: Solvent neurotoxicity. J. Occup. Med., 28:126, 1986.

Baker, E. L., Jr., Smith, T. J., and Landrigan, P. J.: The neurotoxicity of industrial solvents. Am. J. Ind. Med., 8:207, 1985.

Ehle, A. L.: Lead neuropathy. Neurotoxicology, 7:203, 1986.

Gregson, N. A., and Liebowitz, S.: IgM paraproteinaemia, polyneuropathy and myelin-associated glycoprotein (MAG). Neuropathol. Appl. Neurobiol., 11:329, 1985.

Jakobsen, J., and Sidenius, P.: Nerve morphology in experimental diabetes. Clin. Physiol., 5(Suppl. 5):9, 1985.

Juntunen, J.: Occupational solvent poisoning. Prog. Clin. Biol. Res., 220:265, 1986.

Kelly, J. J., Jr.: Peripheral neuropathies associated with monoclonal proteins. Muscle Nerve, 8:138, 1985.

Legha, S. S.: Vincristine neurotoxicity. Med. Toxicol., 1:421, 1986.

Leonard, B. E.: Ethanol as a neurotoxin. Biochem. Pharmacol., 36:2055, 1987.

Meier, C.: Polyneuropathy in paraproteinemia. J. Neurol., 232:204, 1985.

Mora, J. S., Bradley, W. G., and Berkman, E. M.: Acute and chronic polyneuropathies. Int. J. Neurol., 15:231, 1981.

Niakan, E., Harati, Y., and Comstock, J. P.: Diabetic autonomic neuropathy. Metabolism, 35:224, 1986.

Ochoa, J.: Recognition of unmyelinated fiber disease. Muscle Nerve, 1:375, 1978.

Quarles, R. H., Ilyass, A. A., and Willison, H. J.: Antibodies to glycolipids in demyelinating diseases of the human peripheral nervous system. Chem. Phys. Lipids, 42:235, 1986.

Román, G. C.: Tropical myelopathies and myeloneuropathies. Bull. Pan Am. Health Organ., 21:293, 1987.

Sabin, T. D.: Classification of peripheral neuropathy. Muscle Nerve, 9:711, 1986.

Sanders, E. A. C. M., Peters. A. C. B., Gratana, J. W., and Hughes, R. A. C.: Guillian-Barré syndrome after varicella-zoster infection. J. Neurol., 234:437, 1987.

Seppäläinen, A. M.: Solvents and peripheral neuropathy. Prog. Clin. Biol. Res., 220:247, 1986.

Steck, A. J., et al. Peripheral neuropathy associated with monoclonal IgM autoantibody. Ann. Neurol., 22:764, 1987.

Steiner, I., and Abramsky, O.: Immunology of Guillain-Barré syndrome. Springer Semin. Immunopathol., 8:165, 1985.

Stewart, S. S., and Appel, S. H.: Trophic factors in neurological disease. Annu. Rev. Med., 39:193, 1988.

Tabor, E.: Guillian-Barré syndrome and other neurologic syndromes in hepatitis A, B, and non-A, non-B. J. Med. Virol., 21:207, 1987.

Thomas, P. K.: Clinical aspects of PNS regeneration. Adv. Neurol., 47:9, 1988.

Zito, G., Cook, S. D., and Dowling, P. C.: Acquired demyelinating neuropathies. Int. J. Neurol., 15:254, 1981.

Epilepsy

Anderson, V. E., and Hauser, W. A.: The genetics of epilepsy. Prog. Med. Genet., 6:9, 1985.

Bleck, T. P.: Epilepsy. Dis. Mon., 33:601, 1987.

Blume, H. W., and Schomer, D. L.: Surgical approaches to epilepsy. Annu. Rev. Med., 39:301, 1988.

Bradford, H. F., and Peterson, D. W.: Current views on the pathobiochemistry of epilepsy. Mol. Aspects Med., 9:119, 1987.

Bruyn, G. W.: Migraine and epilepsy. Funct. Neurol., 1:315, 1986.

Delgado-Escueta, A. V., Ward. A. A. Jr., Woodbury, D. M., and Porter, R. J. (eds.): Basic mechanisms of the epilepsies. Adv. Neurol., 44:1, 1986.

Dichter, M. A., and Ayala, G. F.: Cellular mechanisms of epilepsy. Science, 237:157, 1987.

Ingvar, M.: Cerebral blood flow and metabolic rate during seizures. Relationship to epileptic brain damage. Ann. N.Y. Acad. Sci., 462:194, 1986.

Majkowski, J.: Kindling: a model for epilepsy and memory. Acta Neurol. Scand., Suppl., 109:97, 1986.

McNamara, J. O., et al.: The kindling model of epilepsy. CRC Crit. Rev. Clin. Neurobiol., 1:341, 1985.

Meldrum, B. S.: Neuropathological consequences of chemically and electrically induced seizures. Ann. N.Y. Acad. Sci., 462:186, 1986.

Mirsky, A. F., Duncan, C. C., and Myslobodsky, M. S.: Petit mal epilepsy. J. Clin. Neurophysiol., 3:179, 1986.

Pedley, T. A. (ed.): Pediatric aspects of epilepsy. Epilepsia, 28 (Suppl. 1):S1, 1987.

Sander, J. W. A., and Shorvon, S. D.: Incidence and prevalence studies in epilepsy and their methological problems. J. Neurol. Neurosurg. Psychiatry, 50:829, 1987.

Schmutz, M.: Relevance of kindling and related processes to human epileptogenesis. Prog. Neuropsychopharmacol. Biol. Psychiatry, 11:505, 1987.

Siesjö, B. K., Ingvar, M., and Wieloch, T.: Cellular and molecular events underlying epileptic brain damage. Ann. N.Y. Acad. Sci., 462:207, 1986.

Snead, O. C., III: Neuropeptides and seizures. Neurol. Clin., 4:863, 1986.

Disturbances in Hydration

Bartowski, H. M.: Peritumoral edema. Prog. Exp. Tumor Res., 27:179, 1984.

Ede, R. J., and Williams, R.: Hepatic encephalopathy and cerebral edema. Semin. Liver Dis., 6:107, 1986.

Joó, F.: A unifying concept on the pathogenesis of brain oedemas. Neuropathol. Appl. Neurobiol., 13:161, 1987.

Klatzo, I.: Blood-brain barrier and ischaemic brain oedema. Z. Kardiol., 76(Suppl. 4):67, 1987.

Rosenblum, W. I.: Aspects of endothelial malfunction and function in cerebral microvessels. Lab. Invest., 55:252, 1986.

Weiss, M. H.: Cerebral edema. Acute Care, 11:187, 1985.

Yarnitsky, D., Honigman, S., Hemli, J. A., and Bental, E.: Normal pressure hydrocephalus associated with spinal cord tumor. Acta Neurol. Scand., 78:302, 1987.

Zimmerman, A. W.: Hormones and epilepsy. Neurol. Clin., 4:853, 1986.

Congenital Anomalies

Barth, P. G.: Disorders of neuronal migration. Can. J. Neurol. Sci., 14:1, 1987.

Bauman, M. L.: Neuroembryology. Semin. Perinatol., 11:74, 1987.

Bender, B. L., and Yunis, E. J.: The pathology of tuberous sclerosis. Pathol. Annu., 17(Pt. 1):339, 1982.

Buchfelder, M., Fahlbusch, R., Huk, W. J., and Thierauf, P.: Intrasphenoidal encephaloceles. Acta Neurochr., 89:10, 1987.

Campbell, L. R., Dayton, D. H., and Sohal, G. S.: Neural tube defects. Teratology, 34:171, 1986.

Choi, B. H.: Methylmercury poisoning of the developing nervous system. Neurotoxicology, 7:591, 1986.

Cohen, F. J.: Neural tube defects. J. Obstet. Gynecol. Neonatal. Nurs., 16:105, 1987.

Cowie, V.A.: Microcephaly: a review of genetic implications in its causation. J. Ment. Defic. Res., 31:229, 1987.

Farhood, A. I., Morris, J. H., and Bieber, F. R.: Transient cysts of the choroid plexus. Am. J. Med. Genet., 27:977, 1987.

Friede, R. L.: Developmental Neuropathology. Wien, Springer-Verlag, 1975.

Gooskens, R. H., Williemse, J., Bijlsma, J. B., and

Hanlo, P. W.: Megalencephaly. Brain Dev., 10:30, 1988.

Hanno, R., and Beck, R.: Tuberose sclerosis. Neurol. Clin., 5:531, 1987.

Hassler, W.: Hemodynamic aspects of cerebral angiomas. Acta Neurochir. (Suppl.), 37:1, 1986.

Leech, R. W., Bowlby, L. S., Brumback, R. A., and Schaeffer, G. B., Jr.: Agnathia, holoprosencephaly and situs inversus. Am. J. Med. Genet., 29:483, 1988.

Leech, R. W., and Shuman, R. M.: Holoprosencephaly and related midline cerebral anomalies. J. Child Neurol., 1:3, 1986.

Lemire, R. J.: Neural tube defects. J.A.M.A., 259:558, 1988.

Liptak, G. S., et al.: The management of children with spinal dysraphism. J. Child Neurol., 3:3, 1988.

Lobato, R. D., Perez, C., Rivas, J. J., and Cordobes, F.: Clinical, radiological and pathological spectrum of occult intracranial vascular malformations. J. Neurosurg., 68:518, 1988.

Nager, G. T.: Cephaloceles. Laryngoscope, 97:77, 1987.

Noterman, J., Georges, P., and Brotchi, J.: Arteriovenous aneurysm associated with multiple aneurysms of the posterior fossa. Neurosurgery, 21:387, 1987.

Ouvrier, R., and Billson, F.: Optic nerve hypoplasia. J. Child Neurol., 1:181, 1986.

Rifkinson-Mann, S., Sachdev, V. P., and Huang, Y. P.: Congenital fourth ventricle midline obstruction. J. Neurosurg., 67:595, 1987.

Sarnat, H. B.: Cerebral dysgeneses and their influence on fetal muscle development. Brain Dev., 8:495, 1986.

Seller, M. J.: Nutritionally induced congenital defects. Proc. Nutr. Soc., 46:227, 1987.

Steiger, H.-J., Markwalder, T.M., and Reulen, H.J.: Clinicopathological relationships of cerebral cavernous angiomas. Neurosurgery, 21:879, 1987.

Stone, D.H.: The declining prevalence of anencephalus and spina bifida. Dev. Med. Child. Neurol., 29:541, 1987.

Weinblatt, M. E., Kahn, E., and Kochen, J.: Renal cell carcinoma in patients with tuberose sclerosis. Pediatrics, 80:898, 1987.

Williams, B.: Progress in syringomyelia. Neurol. Res., 8:130, 1986.

Tumors

Al-Mefty, O., et al.: Medulloblastomas: a review of modern management. Surg. Neurol., 24:606, 1985.

Alvord, E. C., Jr., and Lofton, S.: Gliomas of the optic nerve or chiasm. J. Neurosurg., 68:85, 1988.

Ariel, A. M.: Tumors of the peripheral nervous system. Semin. Surg. Gynecol., 4:7, 1988.

Becker, L. E., and Halliday, W. C.: Central nervous system tumors of childhood. Perspect. Pediatr. Pathol., 10:86, 1987.

Bigner, S. H., Bjerkvig, R., and Laerum, O. D.: DNA content and chromosomal composition of malignant human gliomas. Neurol. Clin., 3:769, 1985.

Bigner, S. H., and Schold, S. C.: The diagnosis of metastases to the central nervous system. Pathol.

Annu., *19* (Pt. 2):89, 1984.

Bonnin, J. M., and Garcia, J. H.: Primary malignant non-Hodgkin's lymphoma of the central nervous system. Pathol. Annu., *22* (Pt. 1):353, 1987.

Boylan, S. E., and McCunniff, A. J.: Recurrent meningioma. Cancer, *61*:1447, 1988.

Bruner, J. M.: Oligodendroglioma: diagnosis and prognosis. Semin. Diagn. Pathol., *4*:251, 1987.

Bruner, J. M.: Peripheral nerve tumors of the head and neck. Semin. Diagn. Pathol., *4*:136, 1987.

Collins, V. P.: Biochemical and immunologic diagnosis of cancer. Central nervous system tumors. Tumour Biol., 8:147, 1987.

Collins, V. P., and Gordon-Cardo, C. L.: Biochemical and immunologic diagnosis of cancer. Neuroblastoma. Tumour Biol., 8:143, 1987.

Crawford, A. H., Jr., and Bagamery, N.: Osseous manifestations of neurofibromatosis in childhood. J. Pediatr. Orthop., 6:72, 1986.

Dehner, L.P.: Peripheral and central primitive neuroectodermal tumors. Arch. Pathol. Lab. Med., *110*:997, 1986.

DiSimone, R. E., Berman, A. T., and Schwentker, E. P.: The orthopedic manifestations of neurofibromatosis. Clin. Orthop., *230*:277, 1988.

Dolman, C. L.: Ultrastructure of Brain Tumours and Biopsies. New York, Praeger Publishers, 1984.

Duffner, P. K., Cohen, M. E., and Freeman, A. I.: Pediatric brain tumors. CA, 35:287, 1985.

Dunn, D. W.: Neurofibromatosis in children. Curr. Probl. Pediatr., 17:445, 1987.

Ehret, M., Jacobi, G., Hey, A., and Segerer, S.: Embryonal brain neoplasms in the neonatal period and early infancy. Clin. Neuropathol., 6:218, 1987.

Elandson, R. A.: Peripheral nerve sheath tumors. Ultrastruct. Pathol., 9:113, 1985.

Eng, L. F., De Vellis J., and Skoff, R. P.: Recent studies of the glial fibrillary acid protein. Ann. N.Y. Acad. Sci., *455*:525, 1985.

Epstein, F.: Spinal cord astrocytomas of children. Prog. Exp. Tumor Res., 30:135, 1987.

Erlandson, R. A.: Peripheral nerve sheath tumors. Ultrastruct. Pathol., 9:113, 1985.

Evans, A. E., D'Angio, G. J., Knudson, A. G., and Seeger, R. C. (eds.): Advances in neuroblastoma research. Prog. Clin. Biol. Res., *271*:1, 1988.

Ferrante, L., Acqui, M., Mastronardi, L., and Nucci, F.: Familial meningiomas. J. Neurosurg. Neurosci., *31*:145, 1988.

Finklestein, J. Z.: Neuroblastoma. Hematol. Oncol. Clin. North Am., *1*:675, 1987.

Franks, A. J.: Diagnostic Manual of Tumours of the Central Nervous System. Edinburgh, Churchill Livingstone, 1988.

Goebel, H. H., Schlie, H., and Eng, L. F.: Immunohistopathologic spectrum of glial fibrillary acidic protein in neurooncology. Acta Histochem. (Suppl.), *34*:81, 1987.

Goffin, J.: Estrogen- and progesterone-receptors in meningiomas. J. Clin. Neurol. Neurosurg., *88*:169, 1986.

Gonzalez-Crussi, F.: Extragonadal Teratomas. Washington D. C., Armed Forces Institute of Pathology, 1982.

Gonzalez-Crussi, F., and Hsueh, W.: Bilateral adrenal ganglioneuroblastoma with neuromelanin. Cancer, *61*:1159, 1988.

Hajdu, S. I.: Pathology of Soft Tissue Tumors. Philadelphia, Lea & Febiger, 1979.

Hays, D. M.: Malignant solid tumors of childhood. Curr. Probl. Surg., *23*:161, 1986.

Henson, R. A., and Urich, H.: Cancer and the Nervous System. Oxford, Blackwell Scientific Publications, 1982.

Hochberg, F. H., and Miller, D. C.: Primary central nervous system lymphoma. J. Neurosurg., *68*:835, 1988.

Hoffman, H. J.: Congenital spinal cord tumors in children. Neurosurgery., *14*:175, 1986.

Holt, G. R.: Von Recklinghausen's neurofibromatosis. Otolaryngol. Clin. North Am., *20*:179, 1987.

Hoshino, T.: Proliferative potential of pediatric brain tumors. Prog. Exp. Tumor Res., *30*:31, 1987.

Ilgren, E. B., Kinnier-Wilson, L. M., and Stiller, C. A.: Gliomas in neurofibromatosis. Pathol. Annu., *20* (Pt. 1):331, 1985.

Ilgren, E. B., and Stiller, C. A.: Cerebellar astrocytomas. Clin. Neuropathol., *6*:185, 1987.

Jaeckle, K. A.: Assessment of tumor markers in cerebrospinal fluid. Clin. Lab. Med., 5:303, 1985.

Jennings, M. T., Gelman, R., and Hochberg, F.: Intracranial germ-cell tumors. J. Neurosurg., *63*:155, 1985.

Kessler, E., and Brandt-Rauf, P. W.: Occupational cancers of brain and bone. State Art Rev. Occup. Med., 2:155, 1987.

Kleihues, P., Kiessling, M., and Janzer, R. C.: Morphological markers in neuro-oncology. Curr. Top. Pathol., 77:307, 1987.

Korf, B. R.: The neurofibromatoses. Postgrad. Med., 83(2):79, 1988.

Ladisch, S.: Tumor cell gangliosides. Adv. Pediatr., *34*:45, 1987.

Laerum, O. D., Bjerkvig, R., Steinsväg, S. K., and de Ridder, L.: Invasiveness of primary brain tumors. Cancer Metastasis Rev., 3:223, 1984.

Lapras, C., Patet, J. D., Mottolese, C., and Vitale, G.: Cerebellar astrocytomas in children. Prog. Exp. Tumor Res., *30*:128, 1987.

Lesch, K. P., Engl, H. G., Schott, W., and Gross, S.: Immunoreactive estrogen receptor protein in meningiomas. Zentralbl. Neurochir., *48*:124, 1987.

Levine, S. A., and Greenberg, S. H.: Primary cerebellar glioblastoma multiforme. J. Neurooncol., 5:231, 1987.

Lewis, A. J.: Sarcoma metastatic to the brain. Cancer, *61*:593, 1988.

Lipkin, A. F., Coker, N. J., Jenkins, H. A., and Alford, B.R.: Intracranial and intratemporal facial neuroma. Otolaryngol. Head Neck Surg., 96:71, 1987.

Lusk, M. D., Kline, D. G., and Garcia, C. A.: Tumors of the branchial plexus. Neurosurgery, *21*:439, 1987.

Manz, H. J.: Neuropathology of systemic malignant neoplasia. Pathobiol. Ann., *12*:233, 1982.

Martuza, R. L., and Eldridge, R.: Neurofibromatosis 2. N. Engl. Med. J., *318*:684, 1988.

Mattox, D. E.: Vestibular schwannomas. Otolaryngol. Clin. North Am., *20*:149, 1987.

McComb, R. D., and Burger. P. C.: Pathologic analysis

of primary brain tumors. Neurol. Clin., *3*:711, 1985.

Milbouw, G., et al.: Clinical and radiological aspects of dysplastic gangliocytoma (Lhermitte-Duclos disease). Neurosurgery, *22*:124, 1988.

Mizumo, J., et al.: Ganglioneuroma of the cerebellum. Neurosurgery, *21*:584, 1987.

Reifenberger, G., Szymas, J., and Wechsler, W.: Differential expression of glial- and neuronal-associated antigens in human tumors of the central nervous system. Acta Neuropathol., *74*:105, 1987.

Riccardi, V. M.: Von Recklinghausen neurofibromatosis. N. Engl. J. Med., *305*:1617, 1981.

Riccardi, V. M.: Neurofibromatosis. Neurol. Clin., *5*:337, 1987.

Rimm, I. J., et al.: Brain tumors after cranial irradiation for childhood acute lymphoblastic leukemia. Cancer, *59*:1506, 1987.

Roelvink, N. C. A., Kamphorst, W., van Alphen, H. A. M., and Rao, B. R.: Pregnancy-related primary brain and spinal tumors. Arch. Neurol., *44*:209, 1987.

Romansky, S. G., and Crocker, D. W.: Neuroblastoma. Prog. Surg. Pathol., *5*:67, 1983.

Ross, D. A., Edwards, M. S., and Wilson, C. L. B.: Intramedullary neurilemomas of the spinal cord. Neurosurgery, *19*:458, 1986.

Rubinstein, L. J.: Embryonal central neuroepithelial tumors. J. Neurosurg., *85*:795, 1985.

Rubinstein, L. J.: The correlation of neoplastic vulnerability with central neuroepithelial cytogeny and glioma differentiation. Neurooncol., *5*:11, 1987.

Rubinstein, L. J., Herman, M. M., and Vanden Berg, S. R.: Differentiation and anaplasia in central neuroepithelial tumors. Prog. Exp. Tumor Res., *27*:32, 1984.

Saleman, M.: The morbidity and mortality of brain tumors. Neurol. Clin. *3*:229, 1985.

Scheithauer, B. W.: Neuropathology of pineal region tumors. Clin. Neurosurg., *32*:351, 1985.

Scheithauer, B. W., and Bruner, J. M.: Central nervous system tumors. Clin. Lab. Med., *7*:157, 1987.

Scheithauer, B. W., and Bruner, J. M.: The ultrastructural spectrum of astrocytic neoplasms. Ultrastruct. Pathol., *11*:535, 1987.

Schiffer, D., Giordana, M. T., Mauro, A., and Migheli, A.: Immunohistochemistry in neuro-oncology. Basic Appl. Histochem., *30*:253, 1986.

Schmidek, H. H.: The molecular genetics of nervous system tumors. J. Neurosurg., *67*:1, 1987.

Schneider, S. L., Sasaki, F., and Zeltzer, P. M.: Normal and malignant neural cells: a comprehensive survey of human and murine nervous system markers. CRC Crit. Rev. Oncol. Hematol., *5*:199, 1985.

Shapiro, W. R. (ed.): Brain tumors. Semin. Oncol., *13*:1, 1986.

Shaw, A., and Konrad, P. N.: Update on Wilms' tumor, neuroblastoma and rhabdomyosarcoma. Curr. Probl. Cancer, *8*(10):1, 1984.

Stokes, R. W.: Neurofibromatosis. J. Am. Osteopath. Assoc., *86*:49, 1986.

Takakura, K.: Intracranial germ cell tumors. Clin. Neurosurg., *32*:429, 1985.

Tally, P. W., Laws, E. R. Jr., and Scheithauer, B. W.: Metastases to central nervous system neoplasms. J. Neurosurg., *68*:811, 1988.

deTribolet, N., Frank, E., and Mach, J. P.: Monoclonal antibodies: their application in the diagnosis and treatment of CNS tumors. Clin. Neurosurg., *34*:42, 1988.

Ushio, Y., et al.: Malignant recurrence of childhood cerebellar astrocytoma. Neurosurgery, *21*:251, 1987.

Van Landegem, W., Vakaet, A., De Paepe, A., and Verschraegen-Spae, M. R.: Familial meningioma. Clin. Neurol. Neurosurg., *90*:61, 1988.

Vandenberg. S. R., Herman, M. M., and Rubinstein, L. J.: Embryonal central neuroepithelial tumors. Cancer Metastasis Rev., *5*:343, 1987.

Werner, B. H., and Schold, S. C. Jr.: Primary intracranial neoplasms in the elderly. Clin. Geriatr. Med., *3*:765, 1987.

Westermark, B., Nister, M., and Heldin, C.-H.: Growth factors and oncogenes in human malignant glioma. Neurol. Clin., *3*:785, 1985.

Yates, A. J., and Stephens, R. E.: Biology of human gliomas. Perspect. Pediatr. Pathol., *10*:135, 1987.

Zülch, K.: Brain Tumors, 3rd Ed. Berlin, Springer Verlag, 1986.

58

Skeletal Muscles

THE diseases of the skeletal muscles are divided into the inflammatory disorders called myositis, the diseases grouped together as muscular dystrophy or myopathy, neuromuscular disorders; vascular disorders, the different forms of periodic paralysis, congenital anomalies, and tumors.

MYOSITIS

Inflammation of the muscles is sometimes caused by infection. The disease called polymyositis or dermatomyositis causes serious inflammation in the muscles. Focal nodular myositis causes a tumor-like inflammation in the muscle involved. Fibromyositis is common. Focal myositis often complicates disease of other organs. Myositis ossificans causes ossification in the muscles. Inclusion-body myositis is rare.

INFECTION. Bacterial infection of the muscles is uncommon. The infection usually spreads to the muscle from an ulcer or an abscess in an adjacent tissue. Occasionally anaerobic or microaerophilic streptococci cause widespread myositis and cellulitis, or clostridia cause gas gangrene. Occasionally a tuberculous abscess of the spine tracks along the psoas muscle towards the skin.

Several of the parasitic diseases discussed in Chapters 20 and 21 involve the muscles. Trichinosis occurs wherever poorly cooked pork, bear meat, or horse meat is eaten. Cysticercosis, toxoplasmosis, Chagas' disease, and sarcosporidiosis are all common in parts of the world.

Pleurodynia caused by a coxsackievirus is the commonest of the viral diseases of muscle. Fungi rarely infect muscles, though occasionally actinomycosis or some other fungus spreads into a muscle from a lesion nearby.

POLYMYOSITIS AND DERMATOMYOSITIS. Poly-myositis and dermatomyositis cause widespread inflammation in the skeletal muscles. If the disease is confined to the muscles, it is called polymyositis. If it involves both skin and muscles, it is called dermatomyositis. The names come from the Greek words for many, muscle, and skin.

About 5 people in every 100,000 have polymyositis or dermatomyositis. Fewer than 1 person in every 200,000 develops the disease in any one year. Nearly 70% of the patients are women. The disease can develop at any age, but most patients are 40 to 60 years old when it first becomes evident. In over 50% of the patients, the disease is confined to the muscles. In the rest, both muscles and skin are involved.

Lesions. Polymyositis and dermatomyositis affect the muscles similarly. The severity of the disease varies considerably from one muscle to another, and from one part of a muscle to another. Even in a single muscle fiber, the disease is often segmental. Macroscopically, the more severely involved muscles are pale, yellowish, or gray. Some are soft and friable; some are firm and rubbery. The less involved muscles are of normal size and appearance.

In most patients, the myositis worsens slowly as weeks and months pass. Increasing numbers of muscle fibers are lost and are replaced with fibrosis, though there is little evidence of degeneration or regeneration in the muscle fibers. Often islands of adipose tissue are present within the muscles. The surviving muscle fibers differ in size. The smaller fibers often have many sarcolemmal nuclei. Sometimes 3 or 4 small fibers are tightly clustered together. Only a sparse, focal exudate mainly of lymphocytes is present.

Less often a patient with slowly worsening polymyositis or dermatomyositis shows extensive degeneration of muscle fibers. Macro-

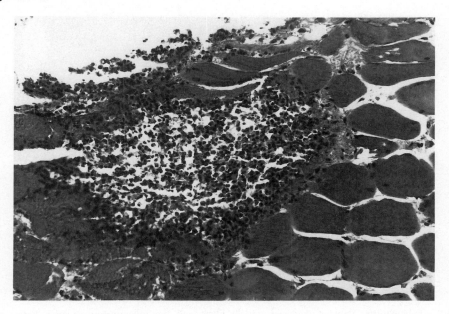

Fig. 58-1.   A pyogenic abscess in a skeletal muscle. (Courtesy of Dr. W. C. Halliday)

phages accumulate around the damaged fibers. A diffuse exudate of lymphocytes and plasma cells is present. Occasionally the muscle fibers at the periphery of the fasciculi are lost or shrunken, but those in the core of the fasciculi are swollen and vacuolated, a change called vacuolar myopathy.

In the minority of patients in whom the disease develops rapidly, the muscles show widespread degeneration and necrosis. In the most severely involved regions, almost every muscle fiber is affected, though the severity of the injury varies from one fiber to another. Even in the most severely involved muscles, a few normal fibers remain. The degenerating muscle fibers are often swollen and hyaline, with loss of their myofibrils, but they may be granular, vacuolated, or fragmented. In some fibers, the number and size of the sarcolemmal nuclei increase. Sometimes a multinucleated bud of sarcoplasm bulges from the end of a broken fiber. Macrophages accumulate around the injured muscle fibers, phagocytose the debris, and sometimes fill sarcolemmal sheaths. An exudate of lymphocytes and plasma cells, sometimes with a few neutrophils, is often extensive, but sometimes is focal and principally perivenous. In the most severely involved muscles, almost all muscle fibers are lost within a few weeks, and the muscle is replaced by cellular collagenous tissue. In the less severely damaged muscles, the lesions come to resemble those of the more chronic form of the disease.

About 50% of children who develop polymyositis or dermatomyositis, have vasculitis, most often polyarteritis nodosa. The vasculitis is prominent in the muscles, but also affects other organs. Often the muscles show foci of infarction.

The sensory and motor nerves that supplied the lost muscle fibers persist in the fibrosis. They are often attenuated, have bulbous thickenings, or end in a bulbous enlargement.

The leakage of enzymes from the damaged muscle fibers is usually sufficient to increase in the plasma the activity of aspartate aminotransferase, aldolase, and creatine phosphokinase. If the destruction of muscle fibers is extensive, neutrophilia, an increased erythrocyte sedimentation rate, increased urinary excretion of creatine and decreased urinary excretion of creatinine are common. About 60% of the patients have hypergamma-

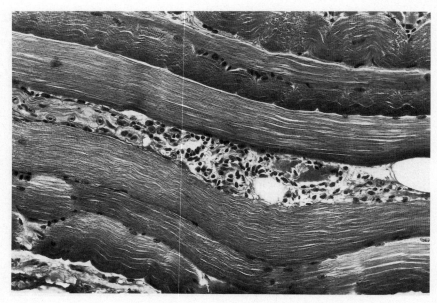

Fig. 58-2. Polymyositis, showing damaged muscle fibers and the inflammatory reaction between them. (Courtesy of Dr. W. C. Halliday)

globulinemia; 50% have rheumatoid factors in the plasma; in 5% the LE cell test is positive.

In the skin, the disease often begins on the face. A dusky, erythematous rash appears in butterfly distribution on the nose and cheeks. Later it extends to the neck and trunk. Often the upper eyelids become a peculiar heliotrope color. Red, scaly thickening is common over pressure points. Hyperemia at the bases of the finger nails and tight, shiny skin over the hands are common. Calcification of the subcutaneous tissues occurs particularly in children. Occasionally there is widespread, exfoliative dermatitis.

Microscopically, the erythematous rash in the skin is like that of systemic lupus erythematosus. The epidermis is thinned. Its basal layer is vacuolated. The dermis is edematous, with a patchy exudate of lymphocytes with a few plasma cells and macrophages. Sometimes there is a focal increase in ground substance in parts of the dermis, or material that stains with the periodic acid-Schiff reaction is deposited around blood vessels in the superficial dermis. Occasionally lesions like those in the dermis are present in the subcutaneous fat.

Related Diseases. Over 20% of patients with polymyositis or dermatomyositis have also rheumatoid arthritis, scleroderma, mixed connective tissue disease, or systemic lupus erythematosus. Indeed, polymyositis and dermatomyositis are sometimes considered to be collagen diseases. People with dermatomyositis are more likely to have another collagen disease than are those with polymyositis.

About 10% of patients with dermatomyositis have a malignant tumor. The risk of an underlying malignancy is particularly great in people with dermatomyositis who are over 50 years old. People without changes in the skin are less likely to have a malignant tumor. The tumor is most often a carcinoma of the stomach, breast, lung, or ovary, but other kinds of carcinoma, lymphoma, leukemia, or sarcoma may be found. In some patients, the dermatomyositis regresses when the tumor is removed.

Clinical Presentation. Polymyositis and dermatomyositis may be acute, chronic, or subacute.

The acute form of the disease is uncommon. Widespread and profound weakness develops in the course of a few days. The affected muscles are painful and tender. Destruction of muscle fibers causes an increase in the activity of the muscle enzymes in the plasma. Myoglobinemia and myoglobinuria are common. The patient has high fever, malaise, arthralgia, often edema of the face and limbs, and sometimes renal failure.

In most patients, increasing muscular weakness develops slowly as weeks pass. Usually, the weakness is evident first in the muscles of the pelvis and thighs or in the shoulder girdle. After some weeks, the patient may find it difficult to rise from a chair or hard to reach a high shelf. Aching or tenderness in the affected muscles is sometimes evident. The tendon reflexes are often preserved. Involvement of the muscles in the neck often brings dysphagia or dysarthria. The ocular muscles are rarely affected. There may be arthralgia or Reynaud's phenomenon. Sometimes the myocardium is involved, with arrhythmias or heart failure.

Patients with dermatomyositis usually have the subacute form of the disease. The muscular weakness can be profound, and the changes in the skin minor, or the changes in the skin can be severe, with only minor muscular weakness. The changes in the skin sometimes appear before muscular weakness is evident; sometimes the muscular changes are well developed.

The chronic form of polymyositis is unusual. The skin is rarely involved. Muscular weakness worsens slowly, as years pass. Often the distal muscles are involved, as well as those of the hip and shoulder girdles.

Pathogenesis. The pathogenesis of polymyositis and dermatomyositis is unknown. The most popular theory is that they result from an immunologic derangement, like the other collagen diseases. A disease like polymyositis can be induced in animals by sensitizing them against muscle. Lymphocytes from patients with polymyositis or dermatomyositis can sometimes destroy muscle fibers in vitro. Rheumatoid arthritis or one of the other collagen diseases is present in many of the patients with polymyositis or dermatomyositis. Probably the injury is cell mediated, with activated lymphocytes attacking the muscle. Antibodies against antigens in muscle are present only in a minority of patients with polymyositis or dermatomyositis.

In most patients with polymyositis or dermatomyositis, the cause of the immunologic disorder is not clear. In the patients with cancer, it may well be that the disease of the muscles is initiated in some way by the cancer. In a few patients, bodies like a picornavirus or a myxovirus have been found in muscle and other cells. Perhaps the virus initiates the disorder.

Prognosis and Treatment. Without treatment, polymyositis and dermatomyositis cause incapacitation and death in 50% of the patients. Death usually comes from pulmonary, renal, or cardiac complications. About 25% recover completely. In the rest, the disease sooner or later becomes stationary, leaving the patient with some disability.

Adrenocortical steroids ameliorate the disease in most patients. If they fail, immunosuppressive drugs are sometimes successful. More than 75% of patients so treated are alive five years after diagnosis. About 50% of them are symptom free and have ceased treatment. In 30%, the disease is quiescent, but muscle weakness remains. In 20%, steroids or immunosuppressive drugs must be continued.

FOCAL NODULAR MYOSITIS. Occasionally a localized mass like a neoplasm or a more diffuse induration develops in a muscle. The mass is often tender or painful. Sometimes the lesion seems due to trauma.

Microscopically, the lesion shows degenerating and regenerating muscle fibers. Usually there is an exudate of macrophages, lymphocytes, and plasma cells. Frequently proliferating capillaries and young fibrocytes extend between the muscle fibers. Occasionally the lesion is so cellular and some of the cells are so atypical that it mimics a sarcoma.

After several weeks or months, the lesion resolves. The damaged muscle is replaced by scar tissue. Often the muscle involved is shortened and contracted.

FIBROMYOSITIS. Fibromyositis is a common condition in which cold or fatigue causes stiffness and aching in a group of muscles. Occasionally tender nodules up to some centimeters in diameter can be palpated in the affected muscles. Biopsy shows no lesion. Presumably the stiffness and the nodules are due to muscle spasm. Time brings resolution.

FOCAL MYOSITIS. Focal myositis is common in rheumatoid arthritis, systemic lupus erythematosus, and scleroderma. It sometimes occurs in myasthenia gravis, cirrhosis of the liver, systemic hypertension, and cancer. The lesions are too small to be evident macroscopically or to cause dysfunction.

Clumps of lymphocytes called lymphorrhages are scattered in the muscles. Usually a few plasma cells and macrophages are mixed with the lymphocytes. Less often neutrophils or eosinophils are present in the lymphorrhages. The clumps are from 50 to 300 μm across. They are often adjacent to a small blood vessel. The muscle fibers adjacent to the clumps are sometimes hyaline, vacuolated, shrunken, or degenerate. Less often increased numbers of sarcolemmal nuclei are present in them, or multinucleated buds of sarcoplasm are present. Similar lymphorrhages are sometimes present in tendons or in nerves supplying the skeletal muscles.

Myositis Ossificans. Myositis ossificans is a disorder that causes ossification of a muscle or its tendon. Two kinds of myositis ossificans are distinguished, traumatic myositis ossificans and generalized myositis ossificans.

Traumatic Myositis Ossificans. Traumatic myositis ossificans is usually caused by repeated, minor trauma to a muscle or its tendon. The rider's bone that develops in the adductor muscles of the thighs in horsemen is an example. Less often the ossification follows a single injury that causes hemorrhage into a muscle. Bone develops as the hematoma resolves.

In most patients, granulation tissue repairs the injury to the muscle or tendon. Spicules of bone are deposited in the granulation tissue and mature to well-formed bony trabeculae. Eventually, much of the affected muscle of tendon may be replaced by bone, usually with a collagenous rather than a fatty marrow. Less often, cartilage forms in the damaged tissue and subsequently ossifies, or injury to the periosteum causes periosteal new bone formation. In some patients, the granulation tissue and the osteoblasts around the newly formed bony spicules are atypical and have a high mitotic rate; bizarre, multinucleated giant cells are formed from the dying muscle fibers. Sometimes the lesion is sufficiently atypical to suggest that it is malignant.

In most patients, traumatic myositis ossificans becomes quiescent as the bone matures. If the dysplastic bone is within a muscle, it

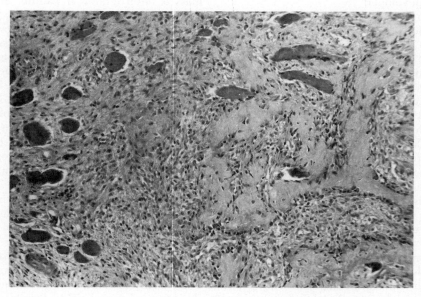

Fig. 58-3. Traumatic myositis ossificans. Bony trabeculae are present in the the collagenous tissue that repairs the damaged muscle.

causes little dysfunction. If it involves the tendons of an elbow or some other joint, the disability can be great. In a few patients, the lesion has been reported to have become malignant.

Generalized Myositis Ossifications. Generalized myositis ossificans is a rare disorder in which there is widespread ossification in the muscles, tendons, ligaments, fasciae, and skin. The disease usually first becomes evident when the patient is about 10 years old. A soft or a firm mass develops in one of the muscles of the back or the neck. After a few days or weeks, the mass may shrink or disappear before being converted into bone. Often the overlying skin is reddened. Usually the mass is painless.

Other such masses appear and ossify as months and years pass. Almost any muscle can be affected, though most of the lesions are in the back or the proximal muscles of the limbs. The palmar and plantar aponeuroses sometimes ossify. Often tendons and ligaments ossify where they insert into bone. Occasionally the diaphragm, tongue, ocular muscles, or heart is affected.

The ossified muscles become bound together by bony bridges. Ossification of the masseters may fix the jaws. Ossification of tendons and ligaments ankyloses joints. Some of the bony masses may ulcerate through the skin. Death usually comes from respiratory embarrassment as the intercostal and other respiratory muscles ossify.

In the early stages of the disease, the masses consist of collagenous tissue. The involved muscles are compressed and atrophy. Spicules of bone develop in the collagenous tissue and mature to trabecular bone, or plates of cartilage form in the fibrosis and ossify.

More than 70% of the patients with generalized myositis ossificans have a congenital defect in their great toes or thumbs. Often the patients have other congenital defects, most often absence of ear lobes, absence of the upper incisors, or spinal bifida.

The cause of generalized myositis ossificans is unknown. It does not seem to be inherited, though many of the congenital malformations with which it is associated are inherited as an autosomal dominant character. Trauma seems to play no part, except perhaps to localize some of the lesions. No abnormality in the metabolism of calcium or phosphorus is evident.

INCLUSION-BODY MYOSITIS. Inclusion-body myositis is uncommon. Progressive, widespread muscular weakness, sometimes with dysphagia, develops slowly. Biopsy shows occasional degenerating or necrotic muscle fibers, with an interstitial infiltrate principally of lymphocytes. Some of the muscle fibers contain even, eosinophilic, hyaline inclusions in the sarcoplasm. Some have lysosomes filled with the concentric whorls of membranes called myelin figures. Some of the muscle fibers contain tubular structures in the nucleus and cytoplasm. The tubules resemble a myxovirus but have not been proved to be viral. The disease does not respond to adrenocortical steroids.

GRANULOMATOUS MYOSITIS. Rarely, a giant cell myositis develops in the skeletal muscles in a patient with giant cell myocarditis. The term granulomatous myositis is also used to describe the lesions in muscles involved by sarcoidosis, tuberculosis, and other granulomatous inflammations.

MUSCULAR DYSTROPHY

The muscular dystrophies are a group of hereditary diseases in which a group or groups of muscles become weak, and the weakness steadily worsens and extends as time passes. Because they inevitably become worse, these diseases are often called the progressive muscular dystrophies.

The muscular dystrophies are divided into groups in which the disease presents similarly, progresses similarly, and is inherited similarly (Table 58-1). In some of these groups, the presentation and progression of the disease differ from one kindred to another, though in any one kindred the disease is usually much the same.

The nature of the dysfunction in the muscular dystrophies is unknown. The structure or enzymatic activity in the cell wall may be defective, but this has not been established. In most of the muscular dystrophies, no treatment slows the progression of the disorder.

The lesions in the muscles are similar in all forms of muscular dystrophy. They will be

TABLE 58-1. TYPES OF MUSCULAR DYSTROPHY

X-Linked recessive inheritance
 Severe X-linked muscular dystrophy (Duchenne)
 Benign X-linked muscular dystrophy (Becker)

Autosomal recessive inheritance
 Limb-girdle dystrophy

Autosomal dominant inheritance
 Facioscapulohumeral dystrophy
 Myotonic dystrophy
 Distal muscular dystrophy
 Progressive dystrophic ophthalmoplegia
 Oculopharyngeal dystrophy

described first; then the different types of muscular dystrophy will be considered.

Lesions. The muscular dystrophies cause a gradual loss of muscle fibers. The muscles involved are replaced by adipose tissue and fibrosis. Often the disease is more widespread microscopically than the clinical findings suggest, with minor lesions in apparently unaffected muscles.

Macroscopically, the affected muscles are sometimes enlarged and look yellowish because of the large quantities of adipose tissue within them. In other patients, the muscles are shrunken. They are yellowish if they contain fat, gray if they are replaced mainly by collagenous tissue.

In the most severely affected muscles, few muscle fibers remain. The muscle is replaced almost entirely by collagenous and adipose tissue.

If the disease is less severe, the surviving muscle fibers lie in clumps or singly, separated by collagenous and adipose tissue. Often the fat cells form orderly columns between the muscle fibers, which vary greatly in size, with large and small fibers haphazardly jumbled together. The largest fibers are over 200 µm in diameter and often are hyaline, with indistinct myofibrils. Electron microscopy shows that they have lost their plasma membrane and are confined only by the basement membrane. The smallest muscle fibers are often only 10 µm in diameter and look tortuous. Sometimes a large fiber splits into five or more small fibers, which lie closely packed together. In both the large and the small fibers, the number of sarcolemmal nuclei is frequently increased, and the nuclei are larger and more pleomorphic than usual.

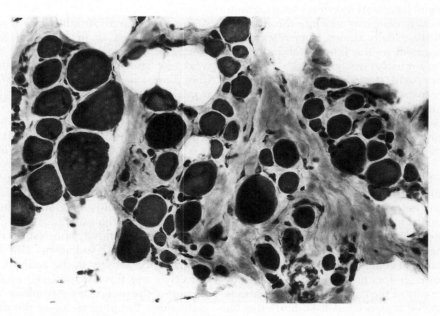

Fig. 58-4. A late stage of Duchenne's severe X-linked muscular dystrophy showing the variation in size of the muscle fibers and the adipocytes and collagenous tissue between them. (Courtesy of Dr. W. C. Halliday)

Often the nuclei lie centrally in the muscle fibers. Occasionally all that remains of a muscle fiber is a line of nuclei enclosed in a shrunken sarcolemmal sheath. The neuromuscular junctions extend over 10 mm, rather than the normal 0.5 mm.

Nerves that have lost their muscle fibers lie in the connective tissue. In the more active forms of muscular dystrophy, macrophages accumulate around dying muscle fibers, perhaps with a few lymphocytes. Otherwise, there is little inflammation. The blood vessels in the connective tissue sometimes have thick walls.

Necrosis of muscle fibers is most prominent in the Duchenne, Becker, and limbgirdle forms of muscular dystrophy. It is usually less striking in facioscapulofacial dystrophy, distal muscular dystrophy, and myotonic dystrophy and is uncommon in the ocular dystrophies. In facioscapulofacial dystrophy and distal muscular dystrophy, atrophy of muscle fibers is usually more prominent than is necrosis.

In myotonic dystrophy, displacement of the nuclei into the center of the muscle fibers is particularly marked. Sometimes a muscle fiber contains a chain of more than 100 central nuclei. The displacement of the nuclei may be the only abnormality seen in a biopsy. Sometimes the myofibrils are concentrated in the center of the fiber, leaving a clear ring of sarcoplasm at the margin of the fiber. The shrinkage of type 1 fibers is greater than the shinkage of type 2 fibers.

In the ocular dystrophies, some of the muscle fibers have central nuclei. Some show autophagic vacuoles. There are often crytalloids in the mitochondria.

If the myocardium is involved, it usually shows only irregular fibrosis. Occasionally the size of the myocardial fibers varies, or degenerating myocardial fibers are present.

If muscular dystrophy causes severe reduction in the total muscle mass, excretion of creatinine in the urine is reduced, and excretion of creatine is increased. In the more active forms of muscular dystrophy, the activity in the plasma of creatine phosphokinase, aldolase, aspartate aminotransferase, and other intracellular enzymes that leak into the plasma from the damaged muscle fibers increases considerably. Often the activity of creatine phosphokinase is increased 10 or more times. In the more chronic forms of muscular dystrophy, in which the destruction of muscle is less active, the activity of these enzymes is normal or only slightly increased.

SEVERE X-LINKED MUSCULAR DYSTROPHY. Severe X-linked muscular dystrophy is called Duchenne's muscular dystrophy or Duchenne's pseudohypertrophic muscular dystrophy after a French neurologist (1806–1875) who wrote extensively on the muscular dystrophies. It is inherited as an X-linked recessive character. The abnormal gene is in the Xp21 region of the short limb of the X chromosome. The patients are almost all boys, though female heterozygotes sometimes show some features of the disease. New mutations are common. In 30% of the patients, no family history of the disease can be discovered. It is the commonest of the muscular dystrophies. One boy in every 5000 born alive is affected.

Severe X-linked muscular dystrophy becomes evident when the boy affected is three to five years old. It begins with weakness of the muscles of the pelvis and thigh. The child has a waddling gait and often falls. Often it is difficult for him to rise from a chair or to climb stairs. Running becomes impossible, as the boy cannot raise his knees. As the years pass, the weakness becomes more severe and more extensive. The muscles of the shoulders and upper arms become weak. Later the distal parts of the limbs are involved. The muscles of the trunk progressively become weak, eventually with severe weakness of the respiratory muscles. By the time the patient is 20 years old, he is likely to be completely paralyzed from the neck down. The muscles of the head are rarely affected.

Early in the disease, the affected muscles often contain so much adipose tissue that they are considerably enlarged, explaining why it is called pseudohypertrophic muscular dystrophy. Later they become small and shrunken. Sometimes they are shrunken from the outset. The limbs become flaccid. Tendon reflexes are lost. Contractures are common, causing flexion deformities or kyphoscoliosis. Mental retardation is frequent. In 30% of the patients the intelligence quotient is less than 75%. Myocardial involvement is usual, but severe cardiac dysfunction is uncommon. Death usually comes when the patient is betwen 20 and 30 years old, most often from respiratory failure or pneumonia.

BENIGN X-LINKED MUSCULAR DYSTROPHY. Benign X-linked muscular dystrophy is called Becker's muscular dystrophy after the German geneticist who described it in 1955. It is inherited as an X-linked recessive character. The abnormal gene is on the short arm of the X chromosome at or near the site of the gene for Duchenne's muscular dystrophy. Becker's disease is less common than Duchenne's disease.

Symptoms begin in late boyhood or adolescence and are similar to those of severe X-linked muscular dystrophy except that they progress more slowly. The muscles affected are often markedly enlarged. Some patients die of respiratory dysfunction when they are over 40 years old. Some live longer and are only partially disabled.

LIMB-GIRDLE DYSTROPHY. Limb-girdle muscular dystrophy is inherited as an autosomal recessive character. It is equally common in boys and girls. Some 5 people in every 100,000 have this kind of muscular dystrophy; 2 infants in every 100,000 are born with it. New mutations are common.

The disease begins in adolescence or early adult life usually with weakness in the pelvis and thighs, sometimes with weakness in the shoulders and upper arms. Sooner or later, all four limbs are involved, often with enlargement of some of the affected muscles. Some patients become disabled after 20 years or so. In others, the disease progresses more slowly. Few live out a normal life span. Most die of respiratory or cardiac failure.

FACIOSCAPULOHUMERAL DYSTROPHY. Facioscapulohumeral muscular dystrophy is inherited as an autosomal dominant character. New mutations are common. Only 1 person in every 100,000 has this form of muscular dystrophy.

The disease most often begins when the patient is 20 to 40 years old, but can begin at any age. Weakness in the shoulders and upper arms makes it difficult to raise the arms. Weakness of the muscles of the trunk makes the scapulae prominent and may eventually lead to scoliosis. Sometimes the muscles of the pelvis or calf are also weak.

The muscles of the face are always affected, though the patient may not be aware of it. There may be difficulty in pursing the lips, the lower lip may protrude, or the patient may be unable to close the eyes completely, even when asleep. Enlargement of the affected muscles is unusual.

In some people, facioscapulohumeral muscular dystrophy is so mild that the patient is unaware of it. Even when facioscapulohumeral dystrophy is more severe, the patient usually lives a normal life. Often the disease becomes arrested after a few years and persists without change for the rest of the patient's life.

Myotonic Dystrophy. Myotonic muscular dystrophy is inherited as an autosomal dominant character. The abnormal gene is on chromosome 19. New mutations are uncommon. About 10 people in every 100,000 have this kind of muscular dystrophy.

The disease usually first becomes evident in adolescents and young adults, but can begin in children. It starts with weakness in the hands or peroneal muscles and wasting of the affected muscles. The muscles of the face are always affected. Ptosis, facial weakness, and wasting and weakness of the muscles of mastication are common. The mouth tends to hang open. The sternomastoid muscles are weak and shrunken, giving a swan neck. There may be dysarthria or dysphagia. Myotonia, so that the patient has difficulty in letting go after grasping something or in relaxing after some other muscular contraction, occurs at some time in most patients with myotonic dystrophy, but is not usually present at the onset and often passes off as the years pass. Occasionally it is the first sign of the disease.

The weakness worsens slowly and may extend to more proximal muscles. The heart is often affected, with dysrhythmias or congestive heart failure. Cataracts develop in most of the patients and occasionally are the only evidence of the disease. Sometimes there is mental retardation. The basal metabolic rate is often low, though thyroid function is normal. In men, frontal baldness and testicular atrophy are common, though the testicular atrophy may become evident only after the patient has fathered children.

DISTAL MUSCULAR DYSTROPHY. Distal

muscular dystrophy may be inherited as an autosomal dominant or an autosomal recessive character. Both forms are uncommon.

Distal muscular dystrophy usually first becomes evident when the patient is 30 to 50 years old. It begins with weakness and wasting of the small muscles of the hands or feet, sometimes with weakness in the forearms or lower legs. The disease is slowly progressive. In some patients the proximal muscles in the arms are not affected until 40 years after the onset. In some forms of the disorder, cardiomyopathy is common.

OCULAR DYSTROPHIES. Progressive dystrophic ophthalmoplegia is a rare form of muscular dystrophy, which is inherited as an autosomal dominant character. It usually begins in adolescents or young adults with weakness of the levatores palpebrarum superiores and the external ocular muscles. Occasionally other facial muscles are weak. The patients present with ptosis and gradual loss of eye movements. Progressive dystrophic ophthalmoplegia is slowly progressive, but may become arrested at any time.

In another rare and slowly progressive form of muscular dystrophy called oculopharyngeal dystrophy, weakness of the levatores palpebrarum causes ptosis, and weakness of the pharyngeal muscles causes dysphagia. Usually the disease becomes evident after the patient is 50 years old.

CONGENITAL MYOPATHY

The congenital myopathies are rare hereditary diseases that cause structural or enzymatic abnormalities in the muscles affected. In most patients, the disease causes weakness in a group or groups of muscles, but after a time becomes stationary and worsens little, if at all, as years pass. In some, the weakness continues to worsen.

The principal forms of congenital myopathy are central core myopathy, nemaline myopathy, centronuclear myopathy, multicore disease, and congenital fiber type disproportion. In a few patients, the muscles affected have shown fingerprints, reducing bodies, myofibrillar inclusions, or other abnormalities.

CENTRAL CORE MYOPATHY. Central core myopathy is inherited as an autosomal dominant character. Occasionally a new mutation occurs. Symptoms usually begin in infancy, but sometimes the muscular weakness is first detected in an adult. Pectus excavatum, scoliosis, congenital dislocation of the hips, and pes cavus are common.

The disease causes moderate weakness of the muscles of the face and limbs, usually most severe in the legs. The patients find it difficult to rise from a chair, climb stairs, or to run. Some patients are prone to develop malignant hyperthermia.

The muscles affected are of normal size. In most of their fibers, the central part of the fiber is hyalinized. In some fibers, more than one hyaline core is present. The cores stain with the periodic acid-Schiff reaction and often stain blue with a trichrome stain. Because mitochondria are absent in the cores, they lack oxidative and phosphorylase activity. Adenine phosphatase may or may not be deficient. The myofibrils in the cores sometimes have distorted Z bands or have lost the thin filaments of the I bands. The peripheral part of the fibers is normal.

NEMALINE MYOPATHY. Nemaline myopathy, also called rod myopathy, is usually inherited as an autosomal dominant character, less often as an autosomal recessive trait. Occasionally a new mutation occurs. The disease frequently becomes evident in infancy, but is sometimes detected only in an adult. The patients are slender, with a long face and high arched palate. Many have pectus excavatum, kyphoscoliosis, or pes cavus.

Nemaline myopathy causes muscular weakness and wasting principally in the muscles of the face, trunk, and limb girdles. In some patients, the disease becomes stationary. In some, it progresses, confining the patient to a chair or causing respiratory failure.

Microscopically, the affected muscles contain large numbers of rods about 3 μm long that look like bacilli. The name *nemaline* comes from the Greek for a thread and refers to these rods. Electron microscopy suggests that the rods are derived from the Z bands. They are usually most numerous immediately under the sarcolemma or in the center of the muscle fibers and are most common in type 1 fibers. Occasionally a similar rod can be found in other conditions.

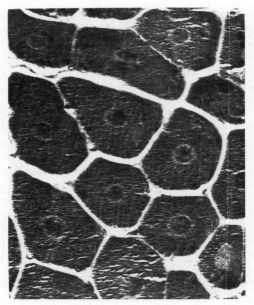

Fig. 58-5. Central core myopathy, showing the hyaline cores in the center of the muscle fibers. (Courtesy of Dr. W. C. Halliday)

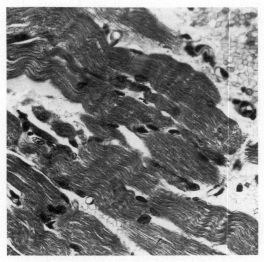

Fig. 58-6. Nemaline myopathy. Numerous tiny rods are present in the muscle fibers. (Courtesy of Dr. W. C. Halliday)

Rare patients with congenital myopathy have both nemaline rods and central cores in the affected muscle fibers. In one kindred, some had central cores; others, nemaline rods.

CENTRONUCLEAR MYOPATHY. Centronu-clear myopathy is sometimes called myotu-bular myopathy because the abnormal muscle fibers resemble the myotubular stage of em-bryonic myogenesis. In many patients, the disease results from a new mutation. In some, it is inherited as an autosomal domi-nant, autosomal recessive, or X-linked reces-sive character. In some patients, the disease causes weakness in infancy. In others, it first becomes evident in adult life. Many of the patients have a long face, pectus excavatum, scoliosis, or pes cavus.

Centronuclear myopathy causes wide-spread muscular weakness and wasting. Ex-ternal ophthalmoplegia is common. In some patients, the weakness is mild or moderate. In some, it progresses to cause major dis-ability or death.

In the affected muscles, the nuclei are in the center of the cells in from 25 to 95% of the muscle fibers. The nuclei are surrounded by a small, clear zone. The proportion of type 1 fibers in the muscles is increased. In some kindred, the type 1 fibers become atrophic.

MULTICORE DISEASE. Multicore disease is probably inherited as an autosomal recessive character. It begins in infancy with weakness, hypotonia, and a reduction in the size of the muscles.

Microscopically, the muscle fibers show numerous small, ovoid foci in which the myofibrils are blurred. Electron microscopy shows disruption of the normal fibrillar pat-tern in these foci. The proportion of type 1 fibers in the muscles is increased. Usually the type 1 fibers are abnormally small, and the type 2 fibers are larger than normal.

CONGENITAL FIBER-TYPE DISPROPORTION. Congenital fiber-type disproportion is prob-ably inherited as an autosomal dominant character. It begins in infancy with muscular weakness, hypotonia, and often muscular contractures. Pectus excavatum, scoliosis, and pes cavus are common. In most patients, the weakness lessens as the patient grows older. In some, it worsens.

Microscopically, the muscles show an ex-cess of type 1 fibers. Often the type 1 fibers are small, and the type 2 fibers are slightly enlarged. Electron microscopy shows that the myofibrils in the type 1 fibers are less clearly separated than is normal, and their Z bands zigzag.

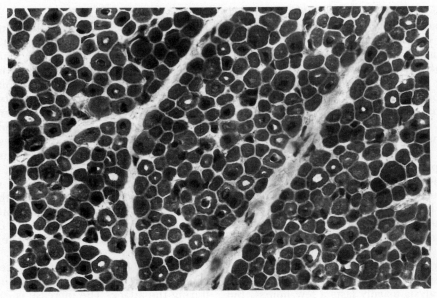

Fig. 58-7. Centronuclear myopathy, showing the central nuclei surrounded by a clear zone. (Courtesy of Dr. W. C. Halliday)

OTHER MYOPATHIES

This section includes a group of unrelated disorders that affect the skeletal muscles. They include myotonia congenita, familial periodic paralysis, paroxysmal myoglobinuria, glycogen storage diseases, carnitine deficiency, mitochondrial myopathies, and malignant hyperthermia.

MYOTONIA CONGENITA. Two forms of myotonia congenita are distinguished. Both are rare. One is inherited as an autosomal dominant character, the other as an autosomal recessive trait. The autosomal dominant form is called Thomsen's disease, after the Danish physician who suffered from it and described it in 1876. The autosomal dominant form usually begins in childhood, though sometimes not until adult life. The autosomal recessive form usually begins when the patient is three or four years old and is more severe that the autosomal dominant form.

People with myotonia congenita cannot relax after a voluntary muscular movement. They remain fixed in position by spasm of the muscles used in the movement. If a movement is repeated, the spasm that follows each movement gradually lessens until the mus-

cles relax normally. If the patient rests for a few minutes, the spasm induced by the movement returns. The temporary relief gained by repeated movement affects only the muscles involved in that movement. If another movement is attempted, the muscles involved go into spasm. All the skeletal muscles react to movement in this way, though the muscles in the legs are usually the most severely affected.

The muscles often become hypertrophied in people with myotonia congenita, so that the patient looks like Hercules. Microscopically, the muscles are usually normal, except for hypertrophy of their fibers. Only when the disease is severe, do the muscle fibers vary in size or a few fibers become degenerate.

The cause of myotonia congenita is unknown. The fault is in the muscles. The nerves supplying the muscles and the motor end-plates are normal, but the muscle fibers respond to stimulation abnormally. The disease can be controlled by quinine, phenytoin, and other drugs.

FAMILIAL PERIODIC PARALYSIS. Familial period paralysis is a rare disease in which the patients suffer repeated attacks of flaccid paralysis. Three types are distinguished. Most patients are hypokalemic during an attack; some are hyperkalemic; some are normokalemic.

Hypokalemic Periodic Paralysis.

Hypokalemic periodic paralysis is inherited as an autosomal dominant character, but penetrance is more complete in men than in women, so that 70% of the patients are men. Less than 1 person in 100,000 has the disease.

The patient is usually 15 to 20 years old when the disease begins. Often after a day of strenuous activity, the patient wakes up with all four limbs weak or paralyzed. The weakness usually begins in the trunk and extends to the limbs. The affected muscles are flaccid without tendon reflexes and do not respond to electrical stimulation. The cranial muscles and muscles of respiration are usually spared. The paralysis usually lasts a few hours , but may persist for a week. It passes off gradually, and the affected muscles usually return to normal. Only after repeated attacks does permanent weakness with atrophy of the muscles sometimes develop. The interval between attacks varies, from a few days to months or years. Eating too much carbohydrate, or sodium, drinking alcohol, emotional stress, and the injection of insulin or epinephrine can precipitate an attack. Often an attack can be aborted if the patient exercises mildly when the first symptoms are detected.

During the attack, the concentration of potassium in the plasma calls falls sharply, though usually not below 2.9 mmol/L (2.9 mEq/L). The fall is caused by the movement of potassium into cells throughout the body. The excretion of potassium decreases. The cause of the redistribution of potassium is unknown.

Vacuoles up to 400 μm across are often present in some of the skeletal muscle fibers. The vacuoles sometimes contain amorphous material, sometimes look empty. Tubular aggregates of long straight tubules 40 to 80 nm in diameter are sometimes present in the vacuolated fibers. Both the vacuoles and the tubules are probably dilated segments of the sarcoplasmic reticulum.

Administration of potassium salts relieves the paralysis. Acetazolamide can often prevent attacks.

Hyperkalemic Periodic Paralysis.

Hyperkalemic periodic paralysis is inherited as an autosomal dominant character. It usually begins when the patient is a child. The attacks often occur when the child is resting after exercise. They can be precipitated by hunger, ingestion of potassium salts, or the administration of adrenocortical steroids. In most patients, the attacks are milder than those of hypokalemic periodic paralysis. They last minutes or hours and may occur several times a day. Weakness begins in the legs and spreads to the arms, with loss of reflexes. Often the child is myotonic during the attack and cannot relax after a muscular contraction. Permanent weakness sometimes develops after repeated attacks of hyperkalemic periodic paralysis.

In many of the patients, the concentration of potassium in the plasma is increased during the attack. The increase is caused by movement of potassium from the cells into the extracellular fluid. In some, the concentration of potassium in the plasma remains normal or is low. Hyperkalemic periodic paralysis differs from the hypokalemic form of the disease principally in that administration of potassium to the patient induces the hyperkalemic but not the hypokalemic form of the disease, and administration of insulin induces hypokalemic but not hyperkalemic periodic paralysis.

The lesions in the muscles are similar to those of hypokalemic periodic paralysis. Vacuoles and tubular arrays are prominent. Dilation of the sarcoplasmic reticulum is evident in less severely affected fibers.

An attack of hyperkalemic periodic paralysis is controlled by giving glucose. Thiazide diuretics and acetazolamide prevent attacks.

Normokalemic Periodic Paralysis.

Normokalemic periodic paralysis is inherited as an autosomal dominant character. Many consider it a form of hyperkalemic periodic paralysis. It has a similar onset, similar symptoms and signs, and similar lesions. In most patients, an attack can be induced by administering potassium salts.

PAROXYSMAL MYOGLOBINURIA. In paroxysmal myoglobinuria, destruction of skeletal muscle fibers causes episodes of myoglobinuria. Two kinds of paroxysmal myoglobinuria are distinguished. In children, the myolysis is often precipitated by infection. In adolescents and young adults, it is caused by deficiency of carnitine palmityltransferase.

In the form of myoglobinuria caused by carnitine palmityltransferase deficiency, the patients are usually boys or young men. Often the attack begins a few hours after severe exertion, with pain in the muscles exercised. The muscles involved become weak, swollen, and tender. The urine becomes pink and deepens to dark red as myoglobinuria becomes more severe. In the plasma, the activity of aspartate transferase, aldolase, and other muscular enzymes increases and the concentration of creatine rises. After a few days, the attack subsides and the patient is left without disability. Only after repeated attacks do the muscles involved sometimes become permanently weak and wasted.

In the children in whom infection causes myolysis, the cause of the abnormality is unknown. The changes in the muscles and the myoglobinuria are similar to those in patients with carnitine palmityltransferase deficiency. Renal tubular injury and renal failure are more frequent in children with myoglobinuria than in older patients.

During the attack, some of the muscle fibers in the affected muscles undergo segmental, hyaline necrosis. They sometimes fragment or become calcified. Usually there is only a mild inflammatory exudate of lymphocytes and macrophages.

CARNITINE DEFICIENCY. Two kinds of carnitine deficiency occur. One affects only the muscles; the other involves tissues throughout the body. Probably both are inherited as an autosomal recessive character.

In the form of carnitine deficiency affecting only the muscles, generalized muscular weakness usually becomes evident in childhood. The heart is sometimes involved. The concentration of carnitine in the plasma is normal, but its concentration in the skeletal muscles is reduced. The addition of carnitine to the diet is often beneficial. In some patients, prednisone reduces the weakness.

The generalized type of carnitine deficiency causes similar muscular weakness, but in addition causes episodes of hepatic encephalopathy that often lead to death. The concentration of carnitine in the plasma as well as in the muscles is low in some patients because of decreased synthesis of carnitine, in some because of increased urinary excretion. The addition of carnitine to the diet or the administration of adrenocortical steroids sometimes ameliorates the disorder.

In both forms of carnitine deficiency, the muscle fibers contain droplets of triglyceride. Type 1 fibers are more severely affected than type 2 fibers. In the generalized form of the disease, similar fatty change sometimes occurs in the liver, heart, and kidneys.

MITOCHONDRIAL MYOPATHY. The mitochondrial myopathies are a group of unusual conditions in which the mitochondria in the skeletal muscles are abnormal. The patients develop muscular weakness, sometimes with ophthalmoplegia or disturbance of cardiac conduction. Some of the patients are of short stature; have gonadal defects; develop lactic acidosis, encephalopathy, paralysis, or seizures; or become blind.

The number of mitochondria in the skeletal muscle fibers is usually increased. Many of the mitochondria have distorted cristae. Some contain crystalline inclusions. In a trichrome stain, the muscle fibers stain red and are ragged.

GLYCOGEN STORAGE DISEASE. The glycogen storage diseases are discussed in Chapter 36. The muscles are involved in types II, III, IV, V, VII, VIII, IX, and X. Muscular weakness and cramps after exercise usually begin in childhood, but sometimes not until adult life. In most of the glycogen storage diseases, involvement of the muscles is not severe, but in Pompe's disease, type II, muscular dysfunction is severe and progressive. In McArdle's disease, type V, overexertion causes myocytolysis, myoglobinuria, and sometimes renal failure.

MALIGNANT HYPERTHERMIA. The term *malignant hyperthermia* is used to describe a group of inherited muscular disorders in which the administration of an anesthetic such as halothane, methoxyflurane, cyclopropane, or a muscle relaxant such as succinylcholine causes the skeletal muscles to contract. The body temperature increases rapidly to as much as 44°C (113°F). About 1 person in 50,000 has some form of the disorder.

One type of malignant hyperthermia is inherited as an autosomal dominant character. About 50% of the patients are normal between

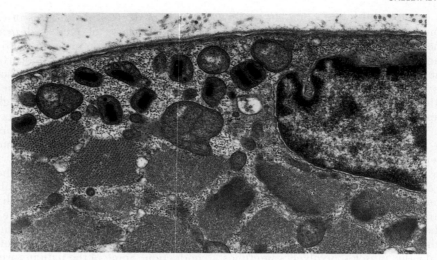

Fig. 58-8. Mitochondrial myopathy, showing the abnormal mitochondria.

attacks. In 50%, the activity of creatine phosphokinase in the plasma is increased. Caffeine, halothane, or hexamethonium in a concentration too low to affect normal muscle causes contraction of muscles in these patients. In some, weakness or wasting of the muscles eventually develops. Another form of the disease is inherited as a recessive trait. It affects boys more often than girls. The patients are short, with low-set ears, an antimongoloid slant to the eyes, ptosis, a small chin, a webbed neck, winged scapulae, pectus excavatum, kyphosis, lordosis, and undescended testes. The activity of creatine phosphokinase in the plasma is high between attacks. Sometimes malignant hyperthermia complicates Duchenne's muscular dystrophy, central core disease, or myotonia

Microscopically, the muscles are sometimes normal between attacks, sometimes show foci of degeneration with a lymphocytic exudate, have abnormally sized muscle fibers, or show the lesions of some other myopathy. The activity of phosphorylase A and adenylate cyclase is frequently increased. During an attack, extensive hyaline necrosis occurs in skeletal muscle fibers throughout the body. Myoglobin escapes into the blood and the urine. The activity of creatine phosphokinase and other muscular enzymes in the plasma increases.

The muscular contraction and pyrexia are caused by abnormal release of calcium from the sarcoplasmic reticulum. The concentration of calcium in the striated muscle cells rises, activating myosin adenosine triphosphatase and phosphorylase kinase, uncoupling oxidative phosphorylation, and inhibiting troponin. The muscles contract and release heat.

The hyperpyrexia is likely to prove fatal unless the patient is rapidly cooled. Dantrolene sodium helps lower the concentration of calcium in the muscles.

NEUROLEPTIC MALIGNANT SYNDROME. In the neuroleptic malignant syndrome, a therapeutic dose of haloperidol, thiothixine, or some other neuroleptic drug causes muscular contraction, pyrexia, and often coma. Autonomic dysfunction causes sweating, tachycardia, dyspnea, and incontinence. The leukocyte count rises to more than 15×10^9/L (15,000/mm^3). The activity of creatine phosphokinase in the plasma rises. The dysfunction persists for 5 to 10 days and then subsides. About 20% of the patients die. Less often, the syndrome is caused by the sudden withdrawal of DOPA in a patient with idiopathic parkinsonism or occurs spontaneously in a patient with schizophrenia. The cause of the disorder is unknown, but its similarity to malignant hyperthermia suggests that it may be due to muscular dysfunction.

NEUROMUSCULAR DISORDERS

In myasthenia gravis, the Eaton-Lambert syndrome, congenital myasthenia, and toxic myasthenia, dysfunction of the motor end-plates makes the muscles weak and easily fatigued. In denervation atrophy, loss of the nerves supplying a muscle causes wasting.

MYASTHENIA GRAVIS. Myasthenia gravis is an autoimmune disorder that damages the acetylcholine receptors in the motor end-plates of the muscles. The name comes from the Greek words for muscle and weakness, and the Latin for serious. It causes weakness and easy fatigability first in the ocular muscles. In most patients, it later becomes generalized, involving muscles in other parts of the body. Nearly 70% of the patients have hyperplasia of the thymus gland, and 10% have a thymoma. About 10% of the patients have hyperthyroidism, systemic lupus erythematosus, Sjögren's syndrome, rheumatoid arthritis, or some other autoimmune disease.

About 4 people in every 100,000 have myasthenia gravis. Each year, 1 person in 200,000 to 500,000 develops the disease. Myasthenia gravis can begin at any age. In men, most patients are 50 to 70 years old when symptoms develop. In women, most are between 20 and 30 years old. About 60% of the patients are women.

Lesions. Macroscopically, the muscles are normal in most patients with myasthenia gravis. Only late in the disease do the muscles severely involved sometimes become wasted.

By light microscopy, the muscles involved usually contain a few clumps of lymphocytes, called lymphorrhages, near small blood vessels. In less than 50% of the patients, are there a few degenerating muscle fibers. More severe necrosis like that in polymyositis is unusual. Late in the disease, the affected muscles sometimes show denervation atrophy.

Electron microscopy shows that presynaptic vesicles containing acetylcholine are present in normal numbers in the nerves supplying the affected muscles. The synaptic area of the motor axons is reduced by 30 to 40%. The synaptic clefts are widened. Ill-defined, granular material accumulates in the clefts. The elaborate folds of the underlying sarcolemma are reduced to a few stubby fingers.

The number of receptors for acetylcholine in the motor end-plate is greatly reduced. Immune complexes are deposited in the end-plates, especially in the less severely injured plates. The complexes contain IgG and complement. The whole complement sequence is activated in the complexes, including its terminal cytolytic complex.

Antibodies against the receptors for acetylcholine in the end-plates are present in the plasma of over 85% of adults with generalized myasthenia gravis. They are detectable in less than 20% of the patients with disease confined to the ocular muscles.

Nearly 30% of patients with generalized myasthenia gravis and 10% of those with disease confined to the ocular muscles have antinuclear antibodies in the plasma; 10% of those with generalized disease and 40% of those with occular disease have antibodies against the thyroid gland; 5% of patients have antibodies against the parietal cells of the stomach.

Nearly 90% of patients with myasthenia gravis who have a thymoma have in the plasma antistriational antibodies against the myofibrils of skeletal muscle. Antistriational antibodies are present in 45% of patients without a thymoma who develop myasthenia gravis after they are 40 years old, and 5% of those without a thymoma who develop myasthenia gravis before the age of 40 years. They occur in 20% of patients without myasthenia gravis who are threated with D-penicillinamine.

The frequency of the HLA antigens is normal in patients with a thymoma who develop myasthenia gravis. Except in Japan, the HLA antigens A3, B7, and DRw2 are unduly common in patients without a thymoma who develop myasthenia gravis after they are 40 years old, and the HLA antigens A1, B8, and DRw3 are unduly frequent in those who develop myasthenia gravis before the age of 40 years. HLA-B10 is more frequent than would be expected in Japanese without a thymoma who develop myasthenia gravis after the age of 40, and HLA-B12 in Japanese who develop myasthenia before that age.

Clinical Presentation. In 90% of the patients, myasthenia gravis involves first the ocular muscles. In 10%, it begins in a limb or some other part of the body. In 85% of the patients, it spreads to involve other muscles within a year; in 40% of the patients within a month. Most often the disease spreads from the ocular muscles to those innervated by the cranial nerves and then to the trunk and limbs. In 15%, it remains confined to the ocular muscles.

The muscles involved are weak and easily become fatigued. Involvement of the ocular muscles causes ptosis or diplopia on one or both sides. Dysarthria, dysphagia, and aspiration or regurgitation of food are common. The masseters are sometimes so weak that the patient must prop up the lower jaw with a hand. It becomes difficult to perform repeated movements, to comb the hair, climb stairs, or walk. The weakness and fatigability of the respiratory muscles often cause dyspnea.

The severity of the symptoms usually varies from hour to hour and week to week. Remissions that last for weeks or months, occasionally longer, occur in 50% of the patients in the first years of the disease. In some patients, the disease progresses slowly. In most, it inexorably worsens as years pass. Crises in which the severity of the weakness suddenly worsens occur in 25% of the patients and may cause respiratory paralysis. Often a crisis is precipitated by infection, the trauma of an operation, or some other stress.

Pathogenesis. In myasthenia gravis, the antibodies against the receptors for acetylcholine in the motor plates bind to the receptors and destroy them. The destruction is due in part to activation of the lytic complex of complement, which lyses both the receptors and the folds of sarcolemma that bear them, in part to internalization and destruction of receptors linked by antibody. New receptors are formed but are insufficient to compensate for the destruction. Less important are blocking antibodies that prevent acetylcholine from binding to its receptor.

The relationship of the abnormalities in the thymus found in 80% of patients with myasthenia gravis to the abnormal antibodies is uncertain. T cells in the thymus may become sensitized and stimulate the production of the antireceptor antibodies by the B cells.

Treatment and Prognosis. The symptoms and signs of myasthenia gravis are ameliorated by neostigmine, pyridostigmine, and other anticholinesterases. The dose of the drug must be adjusted carefully. It will not bring complete remission and, if given in excess, causes increased muscular weakness, abdominal pain, nausea, vomiting, lachrymation, and increased bronchial secretion.

Thymectomy brings improvement in 70% of patients with myasthenia gravis who have follicular hyperplasia of the thymus. Neither the changes in the thymus nor the nature of the myasthenia give any indication of which patients are likely to benefit from the operation. Sometimes the improvement is delayed, becoming evident only months or years after the operation. Thymectomy ameliorates the symptoms in only 25% of patients with a thymoma. In the people who enjoy a remission, the production of antibody against the receptors for acetylcholine falls, and the number of receptors in the motor end-plates increases.

Prednisone induces a remission in over 50% of the patients, though it is three months or more before the improvement becomes evident. Azathioprine is equally effective but also takes several months to bring relief. Plasmapheresis brings rapid improvement by reducing the concentration of antireceptor antibodies.

EATON-LAMBERT SYNDROME. The Eaton-Lambert syndrome is an uncommon condition named after the American physicians who described it in 1957. Muscular weakness and fatigability develop in the proximal muscles of the limbs and in the torso. Tendon reflexes are depressed. In 50% of the patients, autonomic dysfunction causes a dry mouth, reduced sweating, or impotence.

Men and women are affected equally. In 70% of the men and 30% of the women, the patient has a carcinoma, in 80% of the patients a small cell carcinoma of a lung. Sometimes the muscular dysfunction develops up to three years before the carcinoma is detected.

Electron microscopy shows distortion of the presynaptic region of the motor axons. The axons fail to release acetylcholine in adequate quantity, though the stores of acetylcholine in the axons are normal. The motor plates are normal, and the muscle fibers respond normally to the acetylcholine that does reach them.

The Eaton-Lambert syndrome is probably

an autoimmune disease. Adrenocortical steroids, immunosuppressive drugs, and plasmapheresis relieve the symptoms. Guanidine hydrochloride and 3, 4-diaminopyridine enhance the strength of the muscles.

CONGENITAL MYASTHENIA. The congenital myasthenias are a group of rare conditions that cause muscular weakness. In familial infantile myasthenia, inherited as an autosomal recessive character, acetylcholine is not delivered normally to the end-plates. In congenital end-plate acetylcholinesterase deficiency, acetylcholinesterase is deficient in the end-plate. In the slow channel syndrome inherited as an autosomal dominant character, slow closure of the acetylcholine receptor ion channel causes dysfunction. In congenital end-plate receptor deficiency, inherited as an autosomal recessive character, the number of acetylcholine receptors is reduced. No antireceptor antibodies are present.

SECONDARY MYASTHENIA. The antireceptor antibodies in myasthenia gravis cross the placenta and cause transient neonatal myasthenia in infants born of a mother with myasthenia gravis. The muscular weakness passes as the infant ages and the antibodies are destroyed.

Occasionally a tetracycline, aminoglycoside, beta-adrenergic blocking agent, phenothiazine, or other drug causes myasthenia. Insecticides containing anticholinesterases can do so. In a small proportion of patients, D-penicillamine induces the formation of antireceptor antibodies and myasthenia gravis. The symptoms resolve when the drug is withdrawn.

DENERVATION ATROPHY. If a muscle or part of a muscle is deprived of its motor nerves, the affected muscle fibers atrophy. After a week or two, the sarcolemmal nuclei of the affected muscle fibers swell. Some of them move centrally, among the myofibrils. After a month, the affected muscle fibers are rounded and smaller than normal. After two months, most are less than half their normal size, though there is considerable variation from one muscle fiber to another. After four months, the shrunken fibers are only 10 to 15 μm in diameter. If the denervation of the muscle is not complete, the contrast between the groups of shrunken, denervated muscle fibers and the plump, normal, or even hypertrophic fibers that retain their innervation is striking.

As the denervated muscle fibers shrink, myofibrils are progressively lost from the periphery of the cells. Cross striations are preserved. If a denervated muscle fiber is cut in cross section and stained for adenosinetriphosphatase, the center of the fiber often fails to stain, then comes a ring of dense staining, and normal staining is seen at the periphery of the fiber.

After four months, the rate of shrinkage of the denervated fibers slows, but the fibers continue to shrink and to lose their myofibrils. Their sarcolemmal nuclei aggregate into clumps. Eventually cross striations are lost, and only clumps of nuclei remain in a shrunken sarcolemma. Finally even these remnants of the denervated muscle fibers break up and disappear.

If a considerable proportion of the muscle fibers in a muscle are denervated, they are replaced by adipose tissue and fibrosis. The appearance of the muscle is similar to that in the end stage of muscular dystrophy or polymyositis.

If some of the motor axons in a partially denervated muscle survive, they branch and can reinnervate up to 5 denervated muscle fibers. The reinnervated muscle fibers regain their normal size, forming a clump of plump fibers among the shrunken denervated fibers. The innervating axon determines whether the reinnervated muscle fibers are type 1 or type 2. All the muscle fibers in a clump of reinnervated fibers are of the same type.

If only the motor axons are lost, the muscle spindles survive. If the sensory axons are lost, the muscle spindles atrophy.

VASCULAR DISORDERS

The principal vascular disorders that affect the skeletal muscles are gangrene, Volkmann's ischemic contracture, the anterior tibial syndrome, and polyarteritis nodosa.

GANGRENE. Gangrene, described in Chapter 4, is a common cause of muscular necrosis in the elderly. It results from ischemia and causes necrosis of all elements in the ischemic region. Unless the necrotic tissue becomes infected, inflammation in the adjacent viable tissue is not usually great.

VOLKMANN'S ISCHEMIC CONTRACTURE. Volkmann's ischemic contracture is named after the German surgeon von Volkmann who described it in 1872. It most often complicates a fracture of a forearm, less often an injury to a leg. Some of the muscles in the injured limb become ischemic. The ischemia is sometimes caused by injury to a blood vessel, but more often results from pressure on the muscles caused by too tight a cast that does not allow room for the swelling caused by the injury. Sometimes a traumatized muscle trapped in an unexpandable space bounded by bone or fasciae becomes ischemic when increasing edema increases the pressure in the space so greatly that it cuts off the blood supply to the muscle.

If the ischemia is allowed to persist, some or most of the muscle fibers in the ischemic muscles are destroyed. They are replaced by collagenous tissue, leaving only a few surviving muscle fibers and sometimes multinucleated clumps of sarcoplasm formed in an attempt at regeneration. Inflammation is not marked. The fibrosis binds the damaged muscles firmly to the surrounding structures.

As the collagen in the fibrosis matures and shortens, it causes increasing deformity.

The ischemia causes pain. If the forearm is involved, the hand becomes swollen, cyanotic, or pale. The radial pulse weakens or disappears. Often the fingers are cool. Within a few days, irreparable damage can occur.

ANTERIOR TIBIAL SYNDROME. The anterior tibial syndrome usually occurs in young men and is brought on by unaccustomed exercise, running, jumping, or walking when the patient is out of condition. Within a few hours, the anterior tibial muscles become swollen and ache. The muscles may feel hot. Any attempt to flex or extend the ankle causes pain in the anterior tibial compartment. Sometimes the activity of creatine phosphokinase and aldolase in the plasma increases. Within a few days the symptoms subside and do not recur.

If the anterior tibial syndrome is more severe, the skin overlying the anterior tibial muscles becomes erythematous, edematous, and tense. The pain in the muscles becomes more severe. The tibialis anterior, extensor digitorum longus, and extensor hallucis longus may be weakened or paralyzed. Sometimes sensation is lost in the distribution of

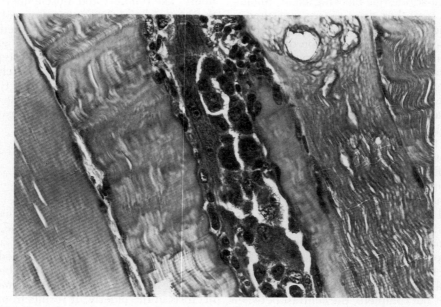

Fig. 58-9.   Traumatic injury to a muscle, showing the degenerating muscle fibers. (Courtesy of Dr. W. C. Halliday)

the anterior tibial nerve. Usually improvement occurs within a few days. In some patients, the paralysis persists and becomes permanent. Rarely, a patient with the anterior tibial syndrome has myoglobinuria or renal failure.

Probably the anterior tibial syndrome results from edema in the muscles caused by the release of metabolites in large quantity during exercise. In most muscles, the edema can easily leak away into the surrounding tissues, and the tissue pressure within the muscle does not rise unduly. The anterior tibial muscles are confined in a rigid space, bordered by bone and fasciae, and the edema cannot escape. As the muscles become edematous, the tissue pressure rises, circulation is impaired, and the muscles become ischemic.

If it is severe, the anterior tibial syndrome is treated surgically. If the pressure on the muscles is relieved by decompression of the anterior tibial compartment before serious ischemic injury has occurred, the patient is cured.

POLYARTERITIS NODOSA. The muscles are involved in many patients with polyarteritis nodosa. The diagnosis can often be establish-ed by taking a random biopsy of an apparently normal muscle. The lesions in the muscles are like those in other parts of the body. There is a similar arteritis, sometimes with foci of infarction caused by the obliteration of some of the arteries. Other types of vasculitis less frequently involve the muscles.

CONGENITAL ANOMALIES

Occasionally a child is born with a muscle or group of muscles absent or paralyzed. More often, a congenital contracture of a muscle or group of muscles causes club foot, congenital torticollis, or less frequently some other deformity. Rarely, malformation of the skeletal muscles causes the multiple deformities of arthrogryphosis multiplex congenita.

CONGENITAL ABSENCE OF MUSCLES. Rarely, a muscle or group of muscles is absent or fails to develop normally. The pectoral muscles are the most commonly affected. The defect is usually unilateral, but can be bilateral.

CONGENITAL PALSIES. Congenital palsies cause weakness or paralysis of a muscle or group of muscles. Ptosis is a common mani-

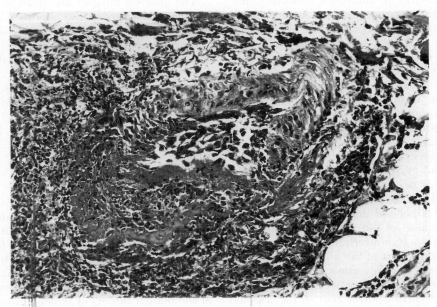

Fig. 58-10. Polyarteritis nodosa in a skeletal muscle. (Courtesy of Dr. W. C. Halliday)

festation. In many of these infants, the injury is probably to the nerve supplying the affected muscle but in some the muscle itself is malformed.

CLUBFOOT. In 1 infant in every 500 born alive, the feet show some form of the deformity called clubfoot or talipes, from the Latin for ankle. In talipes equinus, the feet are fixed in plantar flexion, like the feet of a horse. In talipes calcaneus, they are held in dorsiflexion, so that the infant stands on the os calcis. In talipes varus, they are inverted and adducted. In talipes valgus, they are everted and abducted. Nearly 80% of the infants affected have the combination of talipes equinus and talipes varus called talipes equinovarus.

In most infants with clubfoot, injury in utero causes weakness of the anterior tibial or peroneal muscles. At birth, the muscle fibers in the muscles affected are 5 to 6 μm across rather than the normal 7.5 μm. As the child ages, the atrophy increases, and adipose tissue replaces the shrinking muscle fibers. The antagonists of the weak muscles become shortened, fixing the feet in their abnormal position. The bones of the feet are distorted. The capsules of the unused joints become thick and stiff.

In 10% of infants with talipes, the deformity is inherited as an autosomal dominant character with low penetrance and less frequently as an X-linked recessive trait. Occasionally clubfoot is caused by shortening and contracture of a muscle or group of muscles, by injury to the nerves supplying the weakened muscles, or is one feature of a widespread muscular disorder. Surgical correction is usually required to overcome the deformity.

CONGENITAL TORTICOLLIS. Wryneck, or congenital torticollis from the Latin for twisted and neck, causes shortening of one sternomastoid muscle. The deformity is present at birth or becomes evident within the first few weeks of life. Because of the shortening, the head is inclined and rotated to the affected side. Because of the abnormal tension, the face is often asymmetrical.

The upper part of the affected sternomastoid muscle remains normal, but the lower part is progressively replaced by collagenous tissue. Often the lower part of the affected muscle is swollen and tender during the first few weeks of life and shows active proliferation of fibrocytes and destruction of muscle fibers. Later the fibrosis becomes less cellular as the collagen matures. The muscle becomes increasingly shortened. It adheres to adjacent structures. Often the insertion of the muscle into the clavicle becomes calcified or ossified.

Congenital torticollis is ascribed to injury in utero. Sometimes the loss of muscle and the scarring result from ischemia, as in Volkmann's contracture. If the condition is recognized early, the affected muscle can be stretched by physiotherapy, and the deformity avoided. If the torticollis becomes established, surgical correction is needed.

ARTHROGRYPOSIS MULTIPLEX CONGENITA. Arthrogryposis multiplex congenita, or amyoplasia congenita as it is sometimes called, is an uncommon condition in which many of the muscles in the limbs fail to develop normally. The name comes from the Greek for a joint and curved. Because of the unopposed action of the antagonists of the affected muscles, the limbs are held stiffly, usually in extension, like the limbs of a wooden doll. Usually the hands are flexed. Often there are bilateral clubfeet. Because of the failure of development of many of the muscles, the limbs are thin, and the joints are unduly prominent.

The affected muscles are small or absent. The muscle fibers in the abnormal muscles are small and vary considerably in size. Adipose tissue often replaces the missing muscle fibers. Often there is considerable fibrosis around the joints involved.

In most infants with arthrogryposis multiplex congenita neurons fail to develop in the anterior columns of the spinal cord, and the affected muscles are not innervated. In other infants, the fault is in the muscles.

TUMORS

Both primary and secondary tumors are uncommon in the skeletal muscles. A benign mesenchymal tumor occasionally is found in a skeletal muscle. The malignant tumor of skeletal muscle is called a rhabdomyosarcoma.

BENIGN. A hemangioma is the commonest of the benign tumors of skeletal muscle. Occasionally a lipoma or some other mesenchymal tumor occurs. Rarely, a rhabdomyoma arises in a muscle in the head or neck, less often elsewhere.

RHABDOMYOSARCOMA. A primary malignant tumor of skeletal muscle is called a rhabdomyosarcoma. The name comes from the Greek words for a rod and muscle. Three kinds of rhabdomyosarcoma are distinguished, pleomorphic rhabdomyosarcoma, alveolar rhabdomyosarcoma, and botryoid rhabdomyosarcoma. The botryoid and alveolar forms of the tumor are sometimes called embryonal rhabdomyosarcomata.

All kinds of rhabdomyosarcoma are uncommon. Less than 0.1% of malignant tumors arise from the soft tissues. In adults 10% of them are rhabdomyosarcomata. In children, rhabdomyosarcomata are the commonest of the malignant tumors of the soft tissues.

Pleomorphic Rhabdomyosarcoma.
Most alveolar rhabdomyosarcomata develop in people over 40 years old. More than 50% of them arise in a lower limb. Macroscopically, the tumor forms a fairly well-circumscribed mass of soft, whitish tissue, often with foci of hemorrhage and necrosis. Frequently the sarcoma is more than 15 cm across when it is discovered.

Microscopically, the tumor cells vary considerably in size and shape. Some are large and rounded, with abundant eosinophilic cytoplasm and often several nuclei. Others are elongated, sometimes with two or more nuclei in a row. Some are racquet-shaped, with a tapering tail and bulbous body. Some are vacuolated, with the nucleus supported only by thin strands of cytoplasm. Still others are smaller, spindle shaped, and less bizarre. Cross striations are often difficult to find, though they are present in a few of the tumor cells.

Pleomorphic rhabdomyosarcomata invade beyond the apparent limit of the tumor. Local excision is usually followed by recurrence. Metastases are usually hematogenous. If radical excision of the sarcoma is possible, 30% of the patients survive for more than five years. Overall, 5% of the patients are free of disease five years after the operation. Most patients die a few years after the sarcoma was discovered.

Alveolar Rhabdomyosarcoma.
Nearly 60% of patients with an alveolar rhabdomyosarcoma are less than 20 years old when the tumor is discovered. Few are over 30 years old. Over 70% of the patients are boys or men.

The tumor arises in a skeletal muscle, most often in a limb. The tumor forms a small mass. Sometimes it is painful. Usually the sarcoma is well defined. Some are as hard as cartilage; some are soft and gelatinous.

Microscopically, the tumor is divided into spaces called alveoli by fine, collagenous septa. The tumor cells in the spaces are sometimes small and resemble lymphocytes, sometimes are larger with more cytoplasm, like the cells of a lymphoma. The cells that abut on a collagenous septum are often polypoid, with a thin stalk joining them to the septum. The cells within the spaces seem to float free. Only occasionally can cross striations be found.

An alveolar rhabdomyosarcoma invades locally and metastasizes by the blood stream. Over 80% of the patients die within three years with widespread metastases.

BOTRYOID RHABDOMYOSARCOMA. More than 70% of botryoid rhabdomyosarcomata arise in children less than 10 years old. More than 90% develop before the age of 20 years. About 70% of the patients are boys. The tumor takes its name from the Greek for a bunch of grapes.

Few botryoid rhabdomyosarcomata arise in a skeletal muscle. The tumor is most common in the head and neck, especially in the orbit and nasopharynx. Some arise in the urinary bladder, prostate, vagina, or elsewhere in the genitourinary system. Less often a botryoid rhabdomyosarcoma arises in a bile duct, the retroperitoneum, or a limb. The sarcoma usually forms edematous, glistening masses that bulge from a mucosal surface. The more common botryoid sarcomata are discussed in more detail with the tumors of the organ they involve.

Microscopically, a botryoid sarcoma consists of widely separated round or stellate cells in an abundnt, mucoid intracellular matrix. The cells show little atypicality. Beneath the overlying mucosa, the sarcoma is often more cellular, and the tumor cells are larger and more pleomorphic. Cross striations can sometimes be demonstrated in the tumor cells in this part of the tumor.

Botryoid sarcomata invade extensively. Local recurrence is common. Hematogenous metastases are not uncommon. A combination of radical surgery, irradiation, and chemotherapy allows 70% of the children to survive for more than five years.

SECONDARY TUMORS. Metastases in the skeletal muscles are found in less than 1% of people dying of cancer. More often, a skeletal muscle is invaded by extension of tumor from some neighboring organ. Occasionally metastatic carcinoma in a muscle grows inside an intact sarcolemmal sheath.

BIBLIOGRAPHY

General

Carpenter, S., and Karpati, G.: Pathology of Skeletal Muscle. New York, Churchill Livingstone, 1984.

Kelsey, J. L., and Hochberg, M. C.: Epidemiology of chronic musculoskeletal disorders. Annu. Rev. Public Health, 9:379, 1988.

Korényi-Both, A. L.: Muscle Pathology in Neuromuscular Disease. Springfield, IL, Charles C Thomas, 1983.

Mastaglia, F. L., and Walton, J.: Skeletal Muscle Pathology. Endinburgh, Churchill Livingstone, 1982.

Weller, R. O.: Muscle biopsy and the diagnosis of muscle disease. Rec. Adv. Histopathol., 12:259, 1984.

Myositis

Armbrustmacher, V. W., and Griffin, J. L.: Pathology of inflammatory and metabolic myopathies. Pathol. Annu., 16(Pt. 1):15, 1981.

Behan, W. M., and Behan, P. O.: Immunological features of polymyositis/dermatomyositis. Springer Semin. Immunopathol., 8:267, 1985.

Callen, J. P.: Dermatomyositis. Neurol. Clin., 5:379, 1987.

Callen, J. P.: Dermatomyositis. Dis. Monogr., 35:237, 1987.

Carpenter, S., and Karpati, G.: The major inflammatory myopathies of unknown cause. Pathol. Annu., 16(Pt. 2):205, 1981.

Dawkins, R. L., and Garlepp, M. J.: Autoimmune diseases of muscle: myasthenia gravis and myositis. In The Autoimmune Diseases. Edited by Rose, N. R., and Mackay, I. R. Orlando, FL, Academic Press, 1985.

Fudman, E. J. and Schnitzer, T. J.: Clinical and biochemical characteristics of autoantibody systems in polymyositis and dermatomyositis. Semin. Arthritis Rheum., 15:255, 1986.

Giorno, R., and Ringel, S. P.: Analysis of macrophages, activated T cell subsets in inflammatory myopathies using monoclonal antibodies. Pathol. Immunopathol. Res., 5:491. 1986.

Hochberg, M. C., Feldman, D., and Stevens, M. B.: Adult onset polymyositis/dermatomyositis. Semin. Arthritis Rheum., 15:168, 1986.

Kagen, L. J.: Dermatomyositis and polymyositis. Clin. Exp. Rheumatol., 2:271, 1984.

Mimori, T.: Scleroderma-polymyositis overlap syndrome. Int. J. Dermatol., 26:419, 1987.

Müller, W.: The fibrositis syndrome. Scand. J. Rheumatol. (Suppl), 65:40, 1987.

Naylor, C. D., Jevnikar, A. M., and Witt, N. J.: Sporadic viral myositis in two adults. Can. Med. Assoc. J., 137:819, 1987.

Pachman, L. M.: Juvenile dermatomyositis. Pediatr. Clin. North Am., 33:1097, 1986.

Peiffer, J.: Classification of myositis. Pathol. Res. Pract., 182:141, 1987.

Smith, R., and Triffitt, J. T.: Bones in muscles: the problem of soft tissue ossification. Q. J. Med., 61:985, 1986.

Wolfe, S. M., Pinals, R. S., Aelion, J. A., and Goodman, R. E.: Myopathy in sarcoidosis. Semin. Arthritis Rheum., 16:300, 1987.

Yunis, M. B.: Diagnosis, etiology and management of fibromyalgia syndrome. Compr. Ther., 14:8, 1988.

Yunis, M. B., Kalyan-Raman, U. P., and Kalyan-Raman, K.: Primary fibromyalgia syndrome: clinical features and muscle pathology. Arch. Phys. Med. Rehabil., 69:451, 1988.

Muscular Dystrophy

Armbrustmacher, V. W.: Pathology of the muscular dystrophies and the congenital nonprogressive myopathies. Pathol. Annu., 15(Pt. 1):301, 1980.

Brook, J. D., Shaw, D. J., and Meredith, A. L.: Myotonic dystrophy and gene mapping on human chromosome 19. Biotechnol. Genet. Eng. Rev., 3:311, 1985.

Davies, K. E., et al.: Molecular analysis of human muscular dystrophies. Muscle Nerve, 10:191, 1987.

Duranceau, A. C., Beauchamp, G., Jamieson, G. G., and Barbeau, A.: Oropharyngeal dysphagia and oculopharyngeal muscular dystrophy. Surg. Clin. North Am., 63:825, 1983.

Harper, P. S.: The genetics of muscular dystrophies. Prog. Med. Genet., 6:53, 1985.

Jaffe, R., Mock, M., Abramowicz, J., and Ben-Aderet, N.: Myotonic dystophy and pregnancy. Obstet. Gynecol. Surv., 41:272, 1986.

McComas, A. J., Preswick, G., and Garner, S.: The sick motoneurone hypothesis of muscular dystrophy. Prog. Neurobiol., 30:309, 1988.

Romeo, G., et al.: X-linked muscular dystrophies. Adv. Neurol., 48:31, 1988.

Walton, J. N., and Mastaglia, F. L. (eds.): The muscular dystrophies. Br. Med. Bull., 36:105, 1980.

Worton, R. G.: Molecular analysis of Duchenne and Becker muscular dystrophy. Bioessays, 7:57, 1987.

Congenital Myopathy

Armbrustmacher, V. W.: Pathology of the muscular dystrophies and the congenital nonprogressive myopathies. Pathol. Annu., 15(Pt. 1):301, 1980.

Korényi-Both, A., and Korényi-Both, I.: Congenital myopathies with "diagnostic" pathological features. J. Med. Clin. Exp. Theor., 18:93, 1987.

Tomé, F. M. S., and Fardeau, M.: Nuclear changes in muscle disorders. Methods Achiev. Exp. Pathol., 12:261, 1986.

Other Myopathies

Angelini, C., et al.: Clinical varieties of carnitine and carnitine palmitoyltransferase deficiency. Clin. Biochem., 20:1, 1987.

Appell, H. J.: Skeletal muscle atrophy during immobilization. Int. J. Sports Med., 7:1, 1986.

Armbrustmacher, V. W., and Griffin, J. L.: Pathology of inflammatory and metabolic myopathies. Pathol. Annu., 16(Pt. 1):15, 1981.

Carpenter, S., and Karpati, G.: Lysosomal storage in human skeletal muscle. Hum. Pathol., 17:683, 1986.

DiMauro, S., et al.: Mitochondrial myopathies. J. Inherited Metab. Dis., 10(Suppl. 1):113, 1987.

DiMauro, S., Bresolin, N., and Hays, A. P.: Disorders of glycogen metabolism in muscle. Clin. Neurobiol., 1:83, 1984.

DiMauro, S., et al.: Biochemical and molecular aspects of cytochrome C oxidase deficiency. Adv. Neurol., 48:93, 1988.

Fahn, S., Marsden. C. D., and Van Woort, M. H.: Myoclonus. Adv. Neurol., 43:1, 1986.

Garcia Silva, M. T., Aicardi, J., Goutières, F., and Chevrie, J. J.: The syndrome of myoclonic epilepsy with ragged-red fibers. Neuropediatrics, 18:200, 1987.

Gibb, W. R., and Lees, A. J.: The neuroleptic malignant syndrome. Q. J. Med., 56:421, 1985.

Halliday, A. M.: Evolving ideas on the neurophysiology of myoclonus. Adv. Neurol., 43:339, 1986.

Herbison, G. J., Ditunno, J. F., and Jaweed, J. M.: Muscle atrophy in rheumatoid arthritis. J. Rheumatol., 14(Suppl. 15):78, 1987.

Herbison, G. J., and Talbot, J. M.: Muscle atrophy during space flight. Physiologist, 28:520, 1985.

Hopkins, L. C., and Rosing, H. S.: Myoclonus and mitochondrial myopathy. Adv. Neurol., 43:105, 1986.

Kellam, A. M.: The neuroleptic malignant syndrome. Br. J. Psychiatry, 150:752, 1987.

O'Brien, P. J.: Etiopathogenetic defect of malignant hyperthermia. Vet. Res. Commun., 11:527, 1987.

Ruderman, M. I., and Zito, G.: Metabolic myopathies. N. J. Med., 83:36, 1986.

Rush, P., Baron, M., and Kapusta, M.: Cliofibrate myopathy. Semin. Arthritis Rheum., 15:226, 1986.

Stadhouders, A. M., and Stengers, R. C.: Morphological observations in skeletal muscle in patients with a mitochondrial myopathy. J. Inherited Metab. Dis., 10(Suppl. 1):105, 1987.

Stengers, R. C., and Stadhouders, A. M.: Secondary mitochondrial pathology. J. Inherited Metab. Dis., 10(Suppl. 1):98, 1987.

Symposium: Malignant hyperthermia. Br. J. Anaesth., 60:251, 1988.

Takamiya, S., et al.: Mitochondrial myopathies involving the respiratory chain. Ann. N.Y. Acad. Sci., 488:33, 1986.

Turnbull, D. M., and Sherratt, H. S.: Metabolic studies using isolated skeletal muscle. Baillière's Clin. Endocrinol. Metab., 1:967, 1987.

Neuromuscular Disorders

Ashizawa, T., and Appel, S. M.: Immunopathologic events at the endplate in myasthenia gravis. Springer Semin. Immunopathol., 8:177, 1985.

Bailey, R. O., Dunn, H. G., Rubin, A. M., and Ritaccio, A. L.: Myasthenia gravis with thymoma and pure red cell hypoplasia. Am. J. Clin. Pathol., 89:687, 1988.

Dawkins, R. L., and Garlepp, M. J.: Autoimmune diseases of muscle: myasthenia gravis and myositis. In The Autoimmune Diseases. Edited by Rose, N. R., and Mackay, I. R. Orlando, FL, Academic Press, 1985.

De Baets, M. H., and van Breda Vriesman, P. J. C.: Autoimmunity to cell membrane receptors. Surv. Synth. Pathol. Res., 4:185, 1985.

Drachman, D.B. (ed.): Myasthenia gravis: biology and treatment. Ann. N. Y. Acad. Sci., 505:1, 1987.

Editorial: Autoantibody activity in Lambert-Eaton myasthenia syndrome. Lancet, 1:920, 1988.

Engel, A. G., and Lambert, A. H.: Congenital myasthenic syndromes. Electroencephalogr. Clin. Neurophysiol. (Suppl.), 39:91, 1987.

Harrison, L. C.: Antireceptor antibodies. In The Autoimmune Diseases. Edited by Rose, N. R., and Mackay, I. R. Orlando, FL, Academic Press, 1985.

Lefvert, A. K.: Auto-anti-idiotypic immunity and acetylcholine receptors. Concepts Immunopathol., 3:285, 1986.

Lefvert, A. K.: Idiotypes and antiidiotypes of human antibodies to the acetylcholene receptor in myasthenia gravis. Monogr. Allergy, 22:57, 1987.

Levinson, A. I., Lisak, R. P., Zweiman, B., and Kornstein, M.: Phenotypic and functional analysis of lymphocytes in myasthenia gravis. Springer Semin. Immunopathol., 8:209, 1985.

Levinson, A. I., Zweiman, B., and Lisak, R. P.: Immunopathogenesis and treatment of myasthenia gravis. J. Clin. Immunol., 7:187, 1987.

Lindstrom, J.: Immunobiology of myasthenia gravis, experimental autoimmune myasthenia gravis, and Lambert-Eaton syndrome. Annu. Rev. Immunol., 3:109, 1985.

Lindstrom, J., Shelton, D., and Fujii, Y.: Myasthenia gravis. Adv. Immunol., 42:233, 1988.

Lisak, R. P., Levinson, A. I., and Zweiman, B.: Autoimmune aspects of myathenia gravis. Concepts Immunopathol., 2:65, 1985.

Schlumberger, H. D., and Cohen, M. S.: Epidemiology of myasthenia gravis. Monogr. Allergy, 21:246, 1987.

Wekerle, H., and Müller-Hermelink, H. K.: The thymus in myasthenia gravis. Curr. Top. Pathol., 75:179, 1986.

Whitaker, J. N.: Myasthenia gravis and autoimmunity. Adv. Intern. Med., 26:489, 1981.

Whitaker, V. P.: The structure and function of cholinergic synaptic vesicles. Biochem. Soc. Trans., 12:561, 1984.

Zweiman, B., and Lisak, R. P.: Cell-mediated immunity in neurologic disease. Hum. Pathol., 17:234, 1986.

Congenital Anomalies

Ruymann, F. B., et al.: Congenital anomalies associated with rhabdomyosarcoma. Med. Pediatr. Oncol., *16*:33, 1988.

Sarnat, H.B.: Cerebral dysgeneses and their influence on fetal muscle development. Brain Dev., 8:495, 1986.

Tumors

Agamanolis, D. P., Dasu, S., and Krill, S. E., Jr.: Tumors of skeletal muscle. Hum. Pathol., *17*:778, 1986.

Bell, J., Averette, H., Davis, J., and Toledano, S.: Genital rhabdomyosarcoma. Obstet. Gynecol. Surv., *41*:257, 1986.

Fletcher, C. D., and McKee, P. H.: Sarcomas: a clinicopathological guide with particular reference to cutaneous manifestations. II. Malignant nerve sheath tumour, leiomyosarcoma and rhabdomyosarcoma. Clin. Exp. Dermatol., *10*:201, 1985.

Hajdu, S. I.: Pathology of Soft Tissue Tumors. Philadelphia, Lea & Febiger, 1979.

Hays, D. M., et al.: Raga clinical staging and treatment results in rhabdomyosarcoma of the female genital tract among children and adolescents. Cancer, *61*: 1893, 1988.

Hertler, A. A., and Moore, J. O.: Sarcomas in the elderly. Clin. Geriatr. Med., *3*:781, 1987.

Otto, H. F., Berndt, R., Schwechheimer, K., and Möller, P.: Mesenchymal tumor markers: special proteins and enzymes. Curr. Top. Pathol., 77:179, 1987.

Renick, B., Clark, R. M., and Feldman, L.: Embryonal rhabdomyosarcoma: presentation as a parotid gland mass. Oral Surg., *65*:575, 1988.

Rosen, G.: Bone and soft part sarcomas. Surg. Annu., *20*:121, 1988.

Ruymann, F. B.: Rhabdomyosarcoma in children and adolescents. Hematol. Oncol. Clin. North Am., *1*:621, 1987.

Sim, F. H.: Musculoskeletal oncology. Orthopedics, *10*:1673, 1987.

Sund, S., et al.: Large intramuscular spindle cell lipoma. Acta Pathol. Microbiol. Immunol. Scand., *96*:347, 1988.

59

Bones

SOME disease of the skeleton affect principally the bones. Others are secondary to disease of other organs or involve other organs as well as the bones. The disorders can be divided into infections, physical and chemical injuries, metabolic disorders, conditions in which there is increased production of bone, aseptic necroses, congenital anomalies, tumor-like conditions, and tumors.

INFECTION

An infection in a bone is called osteomyelitis, from the Greek words for bone and marrow and the ending that implies inflammation. Unless otherwise qualified, osteomyelitis means a bacterial infection.

BACTERIAL OSTEOMYELITIS. In most patients with bacterial osteomyelitis, the infection is caused by staphylococci. Streptococci, gram-negative bacilli, and brucellae are found less frequently. Pseudomonas aeruginosa is a common cause of osteomyelitis in addicts who take drugs intravenously. Salmonellar osteomyelitis is particularly frequent in people with sickle cell disease. Hemodialysis increases the risk of developing osteomyelitis. Tuberculous and syphilitic osteomyelitis are now uncommon in most of the world.

The bacteria can be carried to the bone in the blood, can extend into the bone from an infection in a contiguous structure, or be introduced into the bone by an injury that breaches the skin. Hematogenous osteomyelitis used to be common, especially in children, but since the introduction of antibiotics has become less frequent. Bacterial osteomyelitis still complicates trauma, especially compound fractures, and sometimes complicates surgical procedures that involve the bones, especially the implantation of prostheses. If often complicates gangrene in a limb, especially in diabetics.

In children, hematogenous osteomyelitis is most common in the long bones, especially the femora and the tibiae. Usually, the infection beings in the metaphysis of the bone. In adults, it is most common in the vertebrae. Presumably the richness of the blood supply in these regions determines the site of infection. Some 80% of children with osteomyelitis are boys, perhaps because they are more likely to suffer a minor injury that helps establish the infection. In many patients, the origin of the infection is not apparent.

Lesions. The bacteria cause acute inflammation in the cavity of the bone involved. In the early stages of the infection, congestion, edema, and an exudate of neutrophils develop at the site of infection. Because the bone cannot expand, the tension in the marrow cavity rises. The infection spreads along the marrow cavity and into the haversian and Volkmann's canals. Often it reaches the subperiosteal space, forming one or more subperiosteal abscesses, or extends into the surrounding soft tissues. Sinuses from the bone may drain onto the skin. Sometimes the infection extends to a joint, causing septic arthritis.

The increased pressure in the marrow cavity compresses the blood vessels and impairs the blood supply to the cortical bone. The cortical bone may be eroded or thinned. Often parts of the cortical bone overlying the lesion are infarcted. The infarcted bone is called a sequestrum. It often becomes detached from the bone and lies free. The word *sequestrum* means placed apart.

As weeks pass, new bone is sometimes formed beneath the periosteum overlying the infected bone. The new bone forms an incomplete and often perforated capsule that surrounds the inflamed region. It is called an involucrum, from the Latin word meaning to involve.

If the infection is not controlled, it continues for months or years. The bone involved shows a mixture of chronic inflammation and continuing acute inflammation. Often there is fibrosis and new bone formation. The sequestra become densely calcified and highly radiopaque. Frequently fragments of dead bone lie in pockets of pus. The involucrum slowly enlarges. Sinuses often continue to drain on the skin. The destruction of the bone and the deformity increase.

Chronic Sclerosing Nonsuppurative Osteomyelitis of Garré. Rarely, osteomyelitis forms a small, localized lesion that is surrounded by a dense osteosclerosis, a condition called chronic sclerosing nonsuppurative osteomyelitis of Garré, after the Swiss surgeon who described it in 1893.

Brodie's Abscess. Occasionally osteomyelitis becomes encapsulated, forming a well-demarcated abscess. The abscess is often 1 to 3 cm across. It is frequently at the lower end of a tibia. This form of osteomyelitis is called a Brodie's abscess, after the English surgeon Sir Benjamin Brodie who described it in 1832. Some patients have two symmetrical Brodie's abscesses, one on each side. The abscess sometimes contains pus, sometimes glairy material showing few inflammatory cells. Its wall consists of granulation tissue that matures into collagen. Often the surrounding bone is sclerotic.

Clinical Presentation. In children with acute osteomyelitis in a limb, the lesion is painful and tender. Usually fever, leukocytosis, and malaise become severe within 48 hours. Without treatment with antibiotics, the symptoms worsen rapidly. In adults with vertebral osteomyelitis, the onset is usually less abrupt. Pain is the principal symptom. Fever and leukocytosis are often slight or absent. Occasionally osteomyelitis is not discovered until it has become chronic. Patients with a Brodie's abscess or Garré's osteomyelitis often have few symptoms. When osteomyelitis develops around a prosthesis, it often does not become apparent for 3 to 12 months.

Complications. In a few patients, a squamous cell carcinoma or a sarcoma has arisen in a sinus draining chronic osteomyelitis. When osteomyelitis commonly persisted for many years, it frequently gave rise to AA amyloidosis.

Treatment and Prognosis. Antibiotics cure most patients with acute osteomyelitis. Surgical stabilization is necessary if the infection has caused serious erosion of the bone, and sometimes an abscess must be drained. Chronic osteomyelitis and traumatic osteomyelitis require surgical debridement of the lesion, which is allowed to heal slowly. If a prosthesis is infected, it usually must be removed.

Tuberculous Osteomyelitis. In the last century, 1 person in 1000 had tuberculous osteomyelitis. In most of the world, it is now rare. The infection of bone is now most frequently caused by hematogenous extension from a lung. Tuberculosis of the spine is called Pott's disease, after an English surgeon (1714–1788).

Tuberculous osteomyelitis is most common in the lower thoracic and lumbar vertebrae. Often two or more adjacent vertebrae are involved. Less often, the disease develops in a long bone. The infected bone or bones are slowly eroded by the granulomatous inflammation caused by the tubercle bacilli. Often the intervertebral disks between affected vertebrae are destroyed. The eroded vertebrae collapse, often with sharp posterior angulation of the spine. Pus from the lesion tracks out into the surrounding tissues. If the osteomyelitis is in the lumbar region, it extends along the sheath of the psoas muscle, forming a psoas abscess. Occasionally the abscess points in the groin. Usually chemotherapy and surgical correction of the deformity control the disease.

FUNGAL OSTEOMYELITIS. Fungal osteomyelitis is uncommon. In the western United States and in Mexico, Coccidioides immitis occasionally spreads from the lungs to cause acute osteomyelitis in the end of a long bone, often with involvement of the adjacent joint. In Africa, Histoplasma duboisii sometimes causes necrotizing osteomyelitis of the vertebrae, skull, or long bones. Occasionally Cryptococcus neoformans, Blastomyces dermatitidis, Histoplasma capsulatum, or the fungus-like Actinomyces israelii infects a bone.

PARASITIC INFECTION. A hydatid cyst develops in a bone in 10% of patients with echinococcosis. Other parasitic infections of the bones are rare.

VIRAL INFECTION. Smallpox used to cause focal necroses in the bones and subperiosteal new bone formation. Other viral infections rarely involved the bones.

PHYSICAL AND CHEMICAL INJURY

The bones can be injured by mechanical trauma, by radiation, and by toxic substances.

TRAUMA. A fracture of a bone is the commonest of serious injuries. Young active people who engage in dangerous activities and elderly people with fragile tissues are especially likely to break a bone.

Nearly always, a fracture of a bone is associated with injury to the adjacent soft tissues. The extent of the injury to the soft tissues varies from one patient to another. With a hairline fracture of the skull, it is negligible. A massive crushing injury not only breaks one or more bones, but causes extensive necrosis and hemorrhage in the soft tissues.

Types. A number of different kinds of fracture are distinguished. In a closed fracture, the skin overlying the lesion is not broken. In an open fracture, the skin over the lesion is torn. In a simple fracture, a single fracture line divides the bone into two parts. In a comminuted fracture, the bone is broken into more than two fragments. A complete fracture divides the bone into two or more parts. An incomplete fracture extends only part way through the bone, leaving part of its surface intact. A pathologic fracture occurs in a bone weakened by some other disease.

In an overriding fracture, one end of a fractured bone slides past the other. In an impacted fracture, one end of the bone is driven into the other. In an angulated fracture, the bone is bent at the line of fracture. In a rotated fracture, one or both ends of the bone are twisted out of their normal position.

A fracture line may be transverse, oblique, or spiral. An avulsion fracture is caused by violent muscular contraction that tears away the part of the bone into which the muscle or its tendon is inserted.

In young children, the long bones are less rigid than in adults and may suffer a greenstick fracture in which the bone is bent, with an incomplete fracture on the convex aspect of the angulation, but preservation of the cortex on its concave aspect. A young child sometimes suffers a buckle fracture of a long bone, in which longitudinal compression of the bone fractures the bony trabeculae in the medulla of the bone, causing shortening of the bone. The cortex remains intact and bulges out at the site of the fracture. In children, a fracture through the metaphysis can cause complete or partial separation of the epiphysis from the diaphysis.

In a compression fracture, a vertebra or some other bone is compresed or shortened. A vertebra may become wedge-shaped or flattened into a disk about 1 cm thick. In a hairline fracture, the fracture line is so thin that it is difficult to detect.

Lesions. A fracture of a bone usually causes hemorrhage between the bone ends. Granulation tissue forms, and as it matures, osteoid and sometimes cartilage are laid down to form the primary callus in the way described in Chapter 6. As weeks pass, the irregular trabeculae of woven bone are replaced by haversian bone, and the trabeculae are remodelled to meet the stresses of the part.

Most compression fractures of a vertebra are due principally to weakening of the bone caused by osteoporosis or tumor. The weakened bone is unable to meet the normal stresses on the spine and slowly becomes distorted and flattened. There are little or no evidence of healing and little or no new bone formation. Other pathological fractures often show a similar lack of callus.

Complications. If a fracture is not well immobilized, healing is likely to be slow and imperfect. Often cartilage is deposited in the callus and ossifies only slowly. Sometimes the ends of the fractured bone are joined only by collagenous tissue in what is called a fibrous union. Occasionally a false joint called a pseudarthrosis forms between the bone ends.

If the nutrient vessels to the bone are damaged by the fracture, ischemia delays healing or causes necrosis of bone. When the neck of a femur is fractured, injury to the blood vessels that run along its neck sometimes causes infarction of the head of the femur.

Emboli of bone marrow to the lungs occur in most fractures, but are rarely large or numerous enough to cause dysfunction. Fat emboli are also common, but rarely cause symptoms. Occasionally they cause serious injury to the brain or lungs, as described in Chapter 8.

Treatment and Prognosis. In most patients, a fractured bone can be restored to full function by restoring the bone ends to their normal position and immobilizing the part until bony union is achieved.

OSGOOD-SCHLATTER DISEASE. Osgood-Schlatter disease is a form of partial avulsion of an anterior tibial tuberosity. It is named after the American and Swiss surgeons who described it independently in 1903. Osgood-Schlatter disease occurs in children 8 to 15 years old. In most parts of the world 80% of the patients are boys. In 20% or more of the patients, both tibiae are affected.

Pain tenderness, and swelling develop in the affected region when a sudden muscular contraction avulses part of the patella tendon from the bone, carrying part or all of the tibial tuberosity with it. Scar tissue soon develops between the torn end of the tendon and the bone and usually soon binds the avulsed part of the tuberosity firmly to the underlying bone, and the tuberosity reforms. The separated fragment of the tuberosity often persists in the tendon as a small sesamoid bone. Sometimes it becomes necrotic.

RADIATION OSTEITIS. The injury to bone caused by ionizing radiation is called radiation osteitis. The radiation may be from an external source or from radioactive isotopes incorporated in the bone.

If the dose of radiation is large, the osteocytes, osteoclasts, and hematopoietic cells in the bone marrow die. The bony trabeculae in the dead bone persist for sometime without resorption or new born formation. Eventually, collagenous tissue grows in from the edges of the lesion, and resorption of the dead bone begins. Often the collagen in the lesion is heavily calcified. Radiologically, the lesions are radiopaque.

If a growing epiphyseal plate is damaged by the radiation, the chondrocytes swell and degenerate. Growth slows or stops, causing stunting and distortion of the bone.

Osteomyelitis sometimes complicates radiation osteitis, especially in the jaws. The irradiated bone is fragile and easily fractured. The fracture heals slowly and poorly. Occasionally an osteogenic sarcoma, fibrosarcoma, chondrosarcoma, or giant cell tumor develops in the irradiated bone. The sarcoma rarely appears less than three years after the irradiation; sometimes not for more than 20 years.

POISONING. Lead, bismuth, and other heavy metals are stored in the bones. In growing children, both induce osteosclerosis in the metaphyses. Yellow phosphorus causes necrosis of the jaw bones. Fluoride poisoning causes osteosclerosis, especially in the spine and pelvis, ossification of tendons and ligaments, and multiple exostoses. These disorders are discussed in Chapter 24.

METABOLIC BONE DISEASE

Among the metabolic disorders that affect the bones are osteoporosis, rickets, osteomalacia, hyperparathyroidism, renal osteodystrophy, the mucopolysaccharidoses, the mucolipidoses, and other enzyme deficiencies.

OSTEOPOROSIS. The term *osteoporosis* is used to describe any condition in which there is loss of bony substance from one or more bones. The name comes from the Greek words for bone and a passage.

Most elderly people have osteoporosis. After the age of 40 to 50 years, bony substance is lost from the bones. Women tend to be affected sooner and more severely than are men. In one series of people from 63 to 95 years old, 20% of men and 30% of women had osteoporosis severe enough to have caused a compression fracture in one or more vertebrae.

Many conditions favor the development of osteoporosis or are often associated with it (Table 59-1). In most of these disorders, the osteoporosis develops in younger people. The term *idiopathic osteoporosis* is reserved for osteoporosis that develops in otherwise healthy children or young adults.

Lesions. In most forms of osteoporosis, the rarefaction of the bones first becomes evident and is most severe in the vertebrae, heads of the metatarsals, and the necks of the

Idiopathic
  In the elderly
    Type I
    Type II
  In children and young adults
    Idiopathic osteoporosis

Secondary
  Endocrine dysfunction
    Acromegaly
    Cushing's syndrome
    Hyperparathyroidism
    Hypogonadism
    Thyrotoxicosis

  Hereditary disorders
    Ehler-Danlos syndrome
    Homocystinuria
    Hypophosphatasia
    Marfan's syndrome
    Menke's disease
    Osteogenesis imperfecta

  Other
    Alcoholism
    Calcium deficiency
    Chronic obstructive lung disease
    Diabetes mellitus
    Epilepsy
    Heparin
    Immobilization
    Malabsorption
    Malnutrition
    Mastocytosis
    Multiple myeloma
    Primary biliary cirrhosis
    Rheumatoid arthritis
    Scurvy
    Space flight

femora. Other bones are involved later and less severely. The skull is usually spared.

Osteoporosis in the elderly is divided into types I and II. In type I, the patients are elderly women. Bony substance is lost from the medullary trabeculae, but the cortices of the bones are less affected. Type II is more common and affects both men and women. Both the medullary trabeculae and the cortices of the bones are thinned. Most of the disorders listed in Table 59-1 also cause thinning of both the trabeculae and the cortices.

In the spine, the lower thoracic and upper lumbar vertebrae are usually the most severely affected. Because the cortices of the vertebrae are normally thin, the loss of substance from the trabeculae is harmful. The trabeculae gradually become thinner, until many of them are lost altogether. The transverse trabeculae are lost first, but eventually the longitudinal trabeculae are also lost. The loss of bony substance causes no reaction. The feeble trabeculae that remain lie widely separated by normal fatty or hematopoietic marrow.

The intervertebral disks swell and bulge into the weakened vertebrae, which become biconcave. Often compression fractures develop in several adjacent vertebrae. The collapse of the vertebrae reduces the patient's stature, bringing the ribs closer to the pelvis. Often the collapse is greatest in the anterior part of the vertebrae, which become wedge-shaped, causing a rounded kyphosis. Often the marrow in the collapsed vertebrae becomes fibrotic, and sometimes a little osteoid is formed, but repair is always inadequate.

In the long bones, both cortex and trabeculae are thinned. The haversian canals are widened, making the cortex increasingly porous. If the weakened bone is fractured, healing is slow and often imperfect.

Clinical Presentation. In many elderly patients with osteoporosis, the disease causes no disability or only aching in the back. Sometimes sudden collapse of a vertebra caused by minor trauma causes more severe pain that subsides after some days or weeks. In elderly women with type I disease, vertebral collapse and fracture of one of the bones in a wrist are common complications. In people with type II disease, vertebral lesions and fractures of the neck of a femur, humerus, tibia, and pelvis are common. In younger people with osteoporosis associated with some other disorder or with idiopathic osteoporosis, the disease causes few or no symptoms unless one of the weakened bones is fractured.

Pathogenesis. The cause of the osteoporosis common in the elderly is unknown. The balance between the resorption of bone and the deposition of new bone is disturbed, causing the slow thinning of the bones. The concentrations of calcium and phosphorus in the plasma are usually normal. The level of parathyroid hormone in the plasma is sometimes low in women with type I disease and sometimes is slightly increased in people with type II disease. The concentration of 1, 25-dihydroxycholecalciferol in the plasma is normal or low.

In some of the conditions associated with osteoporosis, the cause of the osteoporosis is known. In Cushing's syndrome, the excess of glucocorticoids depresses bone formation and increases bone resorption. Glucocorticoids potentiate the parathyroid hormone and 1, 25-dihydroxycholecalciferol and reduce collagen synthesis. Hyperthyroidism increases the resorption of bone. Acromegaly causes a negative calcium balance and sometimes osteoporosis. Large doses of heparin increase the lysis of collagen. In multiple myeloma, the osteoclast activating factor increases resorption of bone. In other disorders, the cause of the osteoporosis is not understood. Immobilization causes rapid loss of substance from the bones affected. Astronauts become osteoporotic. Osteoporosis sometimes develops in insulin-dependent diabetics or complicates obstructive lung disease.

Treatment and Prognosis. Little can be done to treat osteoporosis in the elderly or in young people with idiopathic osteoporosis. Estrogens in women and androgens in men sometimes slow the course of the disease in older people. Calcium often causes a temporary improvement in the deposition of bone and reduces its resorption. The value of fluorides and combinations of fluoride with other agents remains to be established.

When idiopathic osteoporosis develops in a child, it is often temporary and the patient recovers within a few years. In adults, it usually persists and worsens. In patients with secondary osteoporosis, the bones revert to normal if the underlying condition is controlled.

RICKETS. Rickets is a disease of children caused by lack of vitamin D or resistance to its action. The deficiency can be due to inadequate intake of the vitamin or to any other of the factors listed in Table 59-2. The name *rickets* is probably a distortion of the Greek word for disease of the spine.

Rickets is uncommon in the sunny parts of the world. Sunlight converts the 7-dehydrocholesterol present in the skin to cholecalciferol in sufficient quantity to meet

TABLE 59-2. CAUSES OF RICKETS AND OSTEOMALACIA

Vitamin D deficiency
  Inadequate intake
  Lack of solar synthesis

Malabsorption
  Celiac disease
  Hepatobiliary disease
  Surgery

Renal disease
  Dialysis
  Renal failure
  Tubular disorders

Hereditary
  α-Hydroxylase deficiency
  Deficient vitamin D receptors

Other
  Acidosis
  Anticonvulsant therapy
  Hypophosphatasia
  Hypophosphatemia
  Tumor

the body's needs. In less sunny countries, rickets was common at the end of last century, especially in towns and among the poor. The intake of vitamin D was low, and there was insufficient sunlight to activate enough 7-dehydrocholesterol. Supplementation of the diet with vitamin D has made rickets much less common, but minor forms of the disorder still occur. The disease usually becomes evident when the child is 6 to 18 months old.

Lesions. If rickets is severe, the metaphyseal growth zones in the long bones become up to 1 cm thick and extend laterally, increasing the diameter of the metaphysis. The enlargement of the metaphyses is usually most marked in the wrists, knees, and ankles.

The epiphyseal plates consist of irregular tongues of cartilage separated by vascular collagenous tissue. The chondrocytes in the cartilage are arranged in a disorderly pattern. Some blood vessels penetrate far into the metaphyseal plates, but others scarcely enter them. Osteoid is deposited around the vessels invading the cartilage, but fails to calcify. Broad bands of osteoid and altered cartilage surround the vessels.

The trabeculae in the shafts of the long bones are poorly mineralized and are surrounded by a coat of unossified osteoid. The cortices of the long bones are sometimes thin, with wide haversian canals lined by a layer of unossified osteoid sometimes thickened by subperiosteal deposition of woven bone.

In some long bones, the epiphysis becomes angulated or is displaced laterally. Fractures through the shaft of the long bones are common, but usually fail to breach the periosteum. Callus forms but does not ossify. Especially in the lower limbs, the long bones often become bent, so that the patient is knock-kneed or bowlegged. The tibia sometimes bends forward to give a saber shin. Distortion of the neck of a femur sometimes causes coxa vara. Frequently the longitudinal growth of the long bones is reduced, especially in the lower limbs.

Often the first sign of rickets is the swelling of the costochondral junctions of the ribs called a rickety rosary. The ribs are softened and frequently distorted. Some children have a furrow parallel to the sternum, pigeon breast, or funnel breast. Often there is a groove along the line of insertion of the diaphragm. Sometimes the pelvis is also distorted.

The bones of the skull are usually involved early in the disease. The fontanelles, especially the anterior fontanelle, fail to close. Craniotabes, from the Greek for skull and the Latin for wasting, often appears when the child is three or four months old. It causes asymmetrical areas of thinning and flattening in the posterior and posterolateral parts of the skull. The hair over the lesions is thin. The lesions resolve when the child is eight or nine months old. Deposition of subperiosteal new bone often causes thickening or bossing over the frontal or parietal eminences.

The eruption of the teeth is delayed. Often the deciduous teeth appear in an abnormal sequence. Defects in the enamel and premature caries are common.

Muscular weakness is often severe. Many children with rickets have a pot belly. Some find it hard to walk or difficult to rise from the ground.

The concentration of calcium in the plasma is at the lower limit of normal in most children with rickets. The concentration of phosphorus is often 0.6 mmol/L (2 mg/100 mL) or less. The activity of alkaline phosphatase in the plasma is usually increased, sometimes considerably. The concentration of 25-hydroxycholecalciferol is low.

Clinical Presentation. Children with rickets are often listless and irritable. Muscular weakness grows more severe, and the bony malformations more prominent. If the deficiency of vitamin D is unusually severe, hypocalcemia causes tetany or seizures.

Pathogenesis. Lack of vitamin D reduces absorption of calcium from the intestine and the mobilization of calcium from the bones. The concentration of calcium in the plasma tends to fall, stimulating the secretion of the parathyroid hormone. The parathyroid hormone increases resorption of calcium in the kidneys, increasing the concentration of calcium in the plasma, but causes increased loss of phosphate in the renal tubules and hypophosphatemia. If the phosphorus level in the extracellular fluid becomes low enough, mineralization of the bones cannot continue.

Malabsorption sometimes reduces the uptake of vitamin D sufficiently to cause rickets. Occasionally rickets is caused by a deficiency of the α-hydroxylase that converts 25-hydroxycholecalciferol to the active 1, 25-dihydroxycholecalciferol inherited as an autosomal recessive character, a lack of the receptors for vitamin D, or some other impediment to its action. Patients with a deficiency of α-hydroxylase are said to have vitamin D-dependent rickets type I, and those lacking receptors to have vitamin D-dependent rickets type II. Anticonvulsant drugs increase the catabolism of vitamin D. Anything that causes severe hypophosphatemia or severe acidosis can damage the bones. Occasionally rickets develops in a patient with a nonossifying fibroma of a bone, sclerosing hemangioma, giant cell tumor, or some other mesenchymal tumor. Renal osteodystrophy is discussed later in the chapter.

The increased secretion of the parathyroid hormone enhances the conversion of 25-hydroxycholecalciferol to the active of 1, 25-dihydroxycholecalciferol in the kidneys, to make best use of what vitamin D is available. Hypophosphatemia also favors the formation of 1, 25-dihydroxycholecalciferol in the kidneys.

Treatment. Rickets should be prevented by ensuring that there is an adequate intake of vitamin D in the diet. If the disease does develop, administration of vitamin D brings prompt arrest of the changes in the bones in most patients. The seams of uncalcified osteoid are mineralized. Centers of ossification appear in the cartilage. Orderly endochondral calcification is resumed. Resorption and remodeling restore the bones to normal, provided that there is no severe deformity.

In children with renal tubular disease, treatment is more difficult. Even large doses of vitamin D are often only partially effective. Phosphorus given together with the vitamin enhances healing.

OSTEOMALACIA. Osteomalacia, from the Greek for bone and soft, is caused when deficiency of vitamin D or resistance to its action develops in an adult after metaphyseal bone growth has ceased. It can be caused by any of the mechanisms listed in Table 59-2.

Its pathogenesis is similar to that of rickets. Severe osteomalacia is unusual, but minor degrees of the disorder are common, especially in elderly people.

Lesions. Osteomalacia affects first the vertebrae, pelvis, and other bones of the trunk. The long bones are affected later and less severely. The new bone that is formed as the bones are resorbed and remodeled is not ossified. The trabeculae in the medulla have a thin core of ossified bone surrounded by unossified osteoid. The cortices of the bones are thinned. The haversian canals enlarge. Seams of uncalcified osteoid appear at the margin of the cortices and in the haversian canals. The concentrations of calcium and phosphorus in the plasma are usually low. The activity of alkaline phosphatase is increased.

If osteomalacia is severe, the bones are soft and pliable. They become misshapen and deformed, especially in the thorax and pelvis. Compression fractures of the vertebrae and fractures of the long bones are

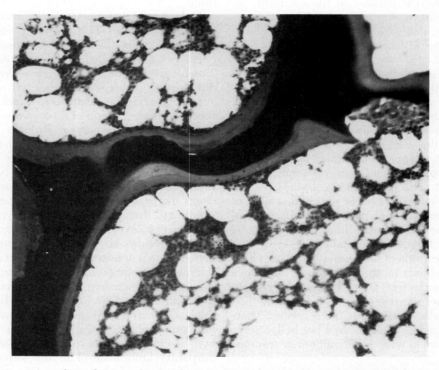

Fig. 59-1. Osteomalacia, showing pale osteoid surrounding the more darkly stained calcified core of a trabeculum in a vertebra.

common. Callus forms, but is not calcified.

Clinical Presentation. Mild osteomalacia causes no symptoms and no disability. More severe involvement causes pain and tenderness in the bones. Any movement that stresses the bones is avoided. Muscular weakness often increases the disability.

Treatment and Prognosis. Osteomalacia is treated like rickets. In many patients, full recovery is achieved.

HYPOPHOSPHATASIA. In hypophosphatasia alkaline phosphatase is deficient throughout the body. One person in 100,000 born alive has the disorder. In some patients, symptoms begin in childhood, and the disorder is inherited as an autosomal recessive character. In some, symptoms appear in adult life, and the condition is inherited as an autosomal dominant trait with variable expressivity.

The children develop rickets and the adults osteomalacia. Craniotabes is often extensive in the children. The concentrations of calcium and phosphate in the plasma are in the high normal range or greater. Nephrocalcinosis is not uncommon. The activity of alkaline phosphatase is low. The urinary excretion of phosphoryl ethanolamine is increased.

HYPERPARATHYROIDISM. Hyperparathyroidism is discussed in Chapter 48. Only the bony lesions that complicate the disease are considered here.

An excess of parathyroid hormone increases the resorption of bone. Osteoclasts become more numerous and more active. If the supply of calcium is good, as it usually is today, reossification keeps pace with the increased resorption, and the bones show little abnormality other than the increase in osteoclasts.

If the calcium balance is less favourable, osteoporosis develops. The cortices of the bones are thinned, and their haversian canals enlarge. The trabeculae in the medulla are often thinned. Increased osteoclastic activity is evident. Sometimes the bone marrow becomes fibrotic. Radiologically, the erosion of bone is often evident first in the phalanges of the hands. More serious erosion often begins in the vertebrae and mandible.

Osteitis Fibrosa Cystica. Osteitis fibrosa cystica, called von Recklinghausen's disease

of bone after the German surgeon who described neurofibromatosis, is uncommon. It occurs only if severe hyperparathyroidism persists for months or years in a person with a strongly negative calcium balance.

The lesions are most severe in the long bones, though all bones are affected. Osteoporosis is severe. The activity of the osteoclasts is greatly increased. The bone marrow is fibrotic. Often part of a bone is replaced by collagenous tissue in which there are fragments of newly formed woven bone and many multinucleated cells like osteoclasts. Sometimes a bone is expanded by one or more soft, brown or reddish, spheroidal masses called brown tumors that consist of similar fibrosis and new bone formation, with many multinucleated osteoclasts. Sometimes a bone contains cysts filled with clear or bloody fluid and lined by collagenous tissue.

Osteitis fibrosa cystica used to cause serious deformities. The long bones were shortened and deformed. Collapsed vertebrae caused kyphosis. Distortion of the pelvis was common. The skull was sometimes so soft that it could be cut with a knife. The lamina dura around the teeth eroded, and the teeth fell out. Improved management of hyperparathyroidism has made such deformities rare.

RENAL OSTEODYSTROPHY. Renal osteodystrophy is a term used loosely to describe disease of the bones that complicates renal disease or develops in a patient on dialysis because of renal failure. About 10% of patients in renal failure have symptoms of bone disease. Over 35% have roentgenologic evidence of bony injury. Nearly 90% have histologic lesions in the bones. Rickets or osteomalacia is likely to develop in any patient in whom tubular disease causes loss of phosphorus and hypophosphatemia. The rickets caused by renal tubular dysfunction responds poorly to vitamin D and is often called vitamin D-resistant rickets.

Lesions. In renal failure, the bones show some combination of lesions induced by hyperparathyroidism, rickets, osteomalacia, osteoporosis, and osteosclerosis. In children, rickets is often predominant, sometimes with stunted growth so that the child is a renal dwarf. In adults, either osteomalacia or hyperparathyroidism may be predominant, though there is usually evidence of both. Osteoporosis is often generalized. Foci of osteosclerosis are most common in the vertebrae. Sometimes dense plates of sclerotic bone develop beneath the intervertebral disks and contrast sharply with the osteoporortic bodies of the vertebrae.

Children with renal tubular dysfunction causing hypophosphatemia develop rickets; adults develop osteomalacia. Often the insertions of tendons and adjacent parts of the capsules of joints become calcified or ossified.

Pathogenesis. In renal failure, the damaged kidneys are unable to excrete phosphorus adequately, and the concentration of phosphate in the plasma rises. In consequence, the concentration of calcium in the plasma falls, and secondary hyperparathyroidism develops. The injury to the bones is often complicated by the inability of the failing kidneys to convert adequately 25-hydroxycholecalciferol to 1, 25-dihydroxycholecalciferol, adding vitamin D deficiency and rickets or osteomalacia to the hyperparathyroidism. The acidosis common in renal failure increases the injury. In patients on dialysis, aluminum from the dialysate is sometimes deposited in the bones in sufficient quantity to prevent calcification, increasing the severity of the rickets or osteomalacia.

The rickets or osteomalacia caused by renal tubular disease most often results from a defect inherited as an X-linked dominant character that causes increased excretion of phosphorus and hyperglycinuria. Less often it is due to hypophosphatemia caused by the Fanconi syndrome or proximal renal tubular acidosis. The concentration of 25-hydroxycholecalciferol and 1, 25-dihydroxycholecalciferol in the plasma are in the normal range, but the concentration of 1, 25-dihydroxycholecalciferol is less than is appropriate. The bone disease caused by the X-linked form of hypophosphatemia usually becomes evident in childhood and is severe, but sometimes is first detected in adult life and is associated with muscular weakness.

Treatment and Prognosis. In patients with chronic renal failure, transplantation overcomes the osteodystrophy. If this is not possible, restriction of the intake of phosphorus together with large doses of vitamin D or small doses of 1, 25-dihydroxycholecalciferol benefits most patients. If an excess of aluminum is present in the bones, it can be removed with the chelating agent deferoxamine. The rickets and osteomalacia caused by renal tubular dysfunction are controlled by giving phosphorus and 1, 25-dihydroxycholecalciferol.

MUCOPOLYSACCHARIDOSIS. In the mucopolysaccharidoses, deficiency of a lysosomal

TABLE 59-3   MUCOPOLYSACCHARIDOSES

Type	Name	Deficiency	Products stored
IH	Hurler's syndrome	α-L-iduronidase	Dermatan sulfate Heparan sulfate
IS	Scheie's syndrome	α-L-iduronidase	Dermatan sulfate Heparan sulfate
IH/S	Hurler-Scheie syndrome	α-L-iduronidase	Dermatan sulfate Heparan sulfate
II	Hunter's syndrome	Iduronosulfate sulfatase	Dermatan sulfate Heparan sulfate
IIIA	Sanfilippo's syndrome A	Heparan N-sulfatase	Heparan sulfate
IIIB	Sanfilippo's syndrome B	N-acetylglucosaminidase	Heparan sulfate
IIIC	Sanfilippo's syndrome C	Acetyl-CoA; α-glucosaminide N-acetyltransferase	Heparan sulfate
IIID	Sanfilippo's syndrome D	N-acetylglucosamine-6-sulfate sulfatase	Heparan sulfate
IV	Morquio's syndrome	N-acetylgalactosamine 6-sulfate sulfatase	Keratan sulfate
VI	Maroteaux-Lamy syndrome	Arylsulfatase B	Dermatan sulfate
VII		β-Glucuronidase	Dermatan sulfate Heparan sulfate

enzyme needed for the catabolism of mucopolysaccharides causes lesions in the bones and other tissues. Dermatan sulfate, heparan sulfate, or keratan sulfate accumulates in the cells involved and is excreted in the urine. Table 59-3 lists the different types of mucopolysaccharidosis.

Hurler's syndrome. Hurler's syndrome, or mucopolysaccharidosis IH, is the most severe of the mucopolysaccharidoses. It is named after the Austrian pediatrician who described it in 1919. It affects 1 child in every 40,000 born alive. Deficiency of α-L-iduronidase is inherited as an autosomal recessive character. Dermatan sulfate and heparan sulfate accumulate in the affected cells.

Hurler's syndrome becomes evident during the first year of life and worsens progressively. The head grows large. occipital and frontal hyperostoses and other deformities of the skull are common. The features become coarse and ugly. The bulging eyes are widely spaced. The corneae are clouded. A saddle nose has flaring nostrils. A big, thick mouth hangs open to show a big tongue. The ears are coarse and low set. The neck is short. Often collapse and angulation of the vertebrae make the patient kyphotic. The limbs are short and distorted, frequently with coxa vara, genu valgum, talipes equinovarus, or other deformities. The hands are broad with stubby fingers. The skin is coarse with lanugo hairs on the trunk and rough, adult hair on the limbs. The abdomen is protuberant. The liver and spleen enlarge. Inguinal and umbilical hernias are common. The heart is large, often with valvular lesions. Dementia grows increasingly severe. The term *gargoylism* is sometimes used to describe the condition.

The bones are thick and greasy when cut. Ossification in cartilage is slow, with inactive cartilage around the ossification centers and in the epiphyseal plates. Some of the chondrocytes are distended by mucopolysaccharide. Often a thin plate of bone separates the epiphysis from the diaphysis. Trabeculae of osteoid or woven bone are usually present within the bones. The marrow is fibrotic. Clumps of macrophages distended with dermatan and keratan sulfate are present in the marrow. The macrophages have vacuolated cytoplasm and stain metachromatically.

Their lysosomes are large and numerous. By electron microscopy, the lysosomes contain granular material or are striped.

In the liver, hepatocytes and Kupffer cells are distended with mucopolysaccharide. Sometimes the liver becomes fibrotic. Macrophages in the spleen, skin, and elsewhere are filled with mucopolysaccharide. It is present in smaller quantities in fibrocytes and in the white cells in the blood. In the eyes, cells filled with mucopolysaccharide accumulate beneath the epithelium of the corneae. In the heart, the endocardium is often thickened and fibrotic. The chordae tendineae are shortened. The valves are thickened and distorted. The coronary arteries are frequently narrowed by intimal thickening.

The brain is sometimes normal macroscopically, sometimes is shrunken, with thick, opaque meninges. Dermatan sulfate and heparan sulfate accumulate in the lysosomes of the neurons and sometimes in astrocytes. Neurons are lost. Gliosis increases. Often a well-defined zone of rarefaction surrounds the blood vessels, with a few macrophages filled with mucopolysaccharide in the loose perivascular tissue.

Heparan sulfate and dermatan sulfate are excreted in the urine. The deficiency of α-L-iduronidase can be demonstrated in cultured fibrocytes. No treatment is available. Most of the children die before they are 10 years old.

Scheie's Syndrome. Scheie's syndrome, or mucopolysaccharidosis IS, is also due to deficiency of α-L-iduronidase inherited as an autosomal recessive character. It affects 1 child in every 500,000 born alive. The abnormal gene is allelic with the gene that causes Hurler's syndrome. Dermatan sulfate and heparan sulfate accumulate in the affected cells. The patients have stiff joints, corneal clouding, and often aortic incompetence and the carpal tunnel syndrome, but are of normal intelligence and survive into adult life.

Hurler-Scheie Syndrome. Some patients with α-L-iduronidase deficiency have a condition intermediate between Hurler's syndrome and Scheie's syndrome, called the Hurler-Scheie syndrome or mucopolysaccharidosis IH/S. These people may have the allele for Hurler's syndrome on one of the pair of chromosomes involved, the allele for Scheie's syndrome on the other.

Hunter's Syndrome. Hunters syndrome, or mucopolysaccharidosis II, named after the Canadian physician who described it in 1917, is inherited as an X-linked recessive character. One boy in 15,000 born alive is affected. The enzyme iduronosulfate sulfatase is deficient. Dermatan sulfate and heparan sulfate accumulate in the cells. The severe form of the disease begins in childhood and resembles Hurler's syndrome, though clouding of the corneae is unusual and mental deterioration is slower. Deafness, nodular thickening of the skin, cardiomegaly, and pulmonary hypertension are often present. A milder form of Hunter's syndrome allows survival into adult life. The diagnosis is established by demonstrating iduronosulfate sulfatase deficiency in cultured fibrocytes.

Sanfilippo's Syndrome. Sanfilippo's syndrome, mucopolysaccharidosis III, named after the American physician who described it in 1962, has four forms. One child in 100,000 born alive has the disease. In Sanfilippo's syndrome A, mucopolysaccharidosis IIIA, heparan N-sulfatase is deficient; in mucopolysaccharidosis IIIB, N-acetyl-α-glucosaminidase; in mucopolysaccharidosis IIIC, acetyl-CoA:α-glucosaminide N-acetyltransferase; and in mucopolysaccharidosis IIID, N acetylglucosamine 6-sulfate sulfatase. All forms of the disease are inherited as an autosomal recessive character. Heparan sulfate accumulates in cells throughout the body. Somatic changes are not prominent, but mental deterioration is severe. The diagnosis is made by determining the nature of the enzyme deficiency in cultured fibrocytes.

Morquio's Syndrome. Morquio's syndrome, or mucopolysaccharidosis IV, is named after the Uraguayan pediatrician who described it in 1929. One child in 40,000 born alive is affected. Deficiency of N-acetylgalactosamine 6-sulfate sulfatase is inherited as an autosomal recessive character. Keratan sulfate is stored in the cells affected and is usually abundant in the urine. The disease becomes evident when the child is a few years old. The neck is short. The odontoid process is often hypoplastic, making dislocation of the cervical spine easy. Compression of the spinal cord or medulla is not infrequent. The vertebrae are progressively flattened, causing scoliosis and kyphosis. The acetabula and long bones are distorted. Corneal clouding, enlargement of the liver, and aortic regurgitation are common. Mental deterioration does not occur.

Maroteaux-Lamy Syndrome. Maroteaux-Lamy syndrome, mucopolysaccharidosis VI, called after the French physicians who described it in 1963, is rare. Deficiency of arylsulfatase B is inherited as an autosomal recessive character. The condition varies in severity. Usually bony changes like those of Hurler's syndrome and corneal clouding are severe, but intelligence is normal.

Mucopolysaccharidosis VII. In a few kindred, deficiency of β-glucuronidase inherited as an autosomal recessive character has caused severe deformities like those of Hurler's syndrome. In other kindred, the disease is milder, resembling Scheie's syndrome. Dermatan sulfate and heparan sulfate accumulate in cells and are excreted in the urine.

MUCOLIPIDOSIS. The mucolipidoses are uncommon disorders inherited as an autosomal recessive character in which a defect in the posttranslational processing of lysosomal enzymes causes skeletal and bodily changes like those of the mucopolysaccharidoses and mental retardation. Glycoproteins and glycolipids accumulate in the cells involved.

OTHER ENZYME DEFICIENCIES. Bony changes are prominent in G_{M1} gangliosidosis and in multiple sulfatase deficiency, described in Chapter 57. The bones are often involved in Gaucher's disease and Niemann-Pick disease, described in Chapter 51.

HYPEROSTOSIS

The hyperostoses are conditions in which an excess of bone is formed. They include Paget's disease of bone, hypertrophic osteoarthropathy, pachydermoperiostitis, hyperostosis frontalis interna, leontiasis ossea, and infantile cortical hyperostosis.

PAGET'S DISEASE OF BONE. Paget's disease of bone, or osteitis deformans as Paget called it, is named after the English surgeon Sir James Paget, who described it in 1877. It bears no relation to Paget's disease of the nipple, also called after Sir James.

Paget's disease is rare in people under 40 years old, but becomes increasingly common as age increases until 10% of people over 90 years old have one or more foci of Paget's disease in their bones. At autopsy, 3% of people over 40 years old have Paget's disease. Radiologically, it is demonstrable in 1% of the adult population in the United Kingdom, United States, and Australia. It is less frequent in Japan, Asia, Africa, and Scandinavia. About 60% of the patients are men.

Lesions. In over 95% of people with Paget's disease, the lesions are small and involve only one or a few bones. In a few, they are widespread, involving much of the skeleton.

The lesions are most common in the skull, pelvis, vertebrae, and long bones of the lower limbs. The short tubular bones of the hands and feet are rarely involved. In the localized form of the disease, the lesions are sharply demarcated, and usually 1 to 3 cm across. In the disseminated form of the disease, the lesions are larger and involve much or all of the bones involved.

Paget's disease first causes rarefaction of the part or parts of the bone or bones affected. Numerous osteoclasts erode the bony trabeculae and the cortex. Often some of the osteoclasts are large with 100 or more nuclei. Frequently the surfaces of the trabeculae and the cortex are scalloped by the lacunae of the osteoclasts. The marrow within the lesion is replaced by highly vascular collagenous tissue. The blood flow through the lesion may be 20 times that in normal bone.

As months or years pass, the haversian bone in the trabeculae and cortex is slowly destroyed and replaced by irregular plates of coarse, woven bone, with prominent cement lines between them. The trabeculae and cortex become thicker, as more woven bone is deposited and resorption slows. Eventually, the lesion consists of coarse trabeculae of woven bone that merge with the thickened cortex. The trabeculae are sometimes numerous and closely packed, sometimes few. Microscopically, the cement lines between the plates of woven bone that make up the thickened trabeculae and cortex form the mosaic pattern typical of Paget's disease. The collagenous tissue between the trabeculae gradually becomes less vascular as it matures and the collagen bundles coarsen.

An early lesion is radiolucent and macro-

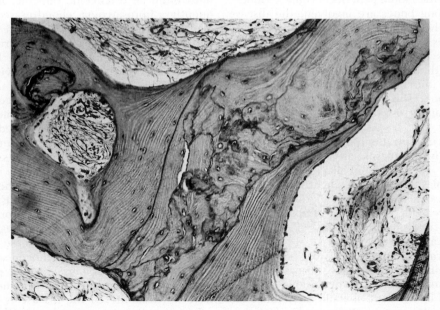

Fig. 59-2. Paget's disease of bone showing in the center of the trabecula the irregular plates of bone and prominent cement lines typical of Paget's disease, with more normal bone peripherally. The bone marrow is fibrotic.

scopically appears purple because the great vascularity of the medulla shows through the thinned cortical bone. As a lesion ages, it become radiopaque as the trabeculae grow thicker and the cortex thickens. A localized lesion often consists almost entirely of coarse bony trabeculae that merge with the thick overlying cortex. Occasionally the bone in the lesions is dense like ivory. More often it is soft and crumbly like pumice stone.

If Paget's disease is widespread, it causes serious deformity. In the lytic stage of the disease, the softened bones are easily bent or distorted. In its sclerotic stage, fractures add to the deformity. Frequently, there are multiple lesions in the skull. At first the lesions are radiolucent, a condition called osteoporosis circumscripta cranii. As they merge and are ossified, the skull becomes up to 2 to 3 cm thick. Both the inner and the outer tables are thickened, and the diploë is filled by thickened trabeculae. The thick skull enlarges the head and sometimes compresses the brain. Vertebrae involved often become biconcave as the intervertebral disks compress the softened bones. Sometimes the intervertebral disks disappear and adjacent vertebrae fuse. Often the periphery of the vertebrae becomes sclerotic while the core is still porotic. Some patients become kyphotic. If the long bones are involved, the disease nearly always begins at one or both ends and advances along the shaft. Often the medulla contains only a few misshapen trabeculae, though the cortex is greatly thickened. Frequently the bones are swollen, bent, and misshapen. The distortion of the long bones often causes osteoarthritis in the adjacent joints.

The concentrations of calcium and phosphorus in the plasma are normal in Paget's disease. The activity of alkaline phosphatase in the plasma increases, slightly if there are only focal lesions, greatly if the disease is widespread. If the activity of alkaline phosphatase is high, the activity of acid phosphatase also increases.

Clinical Presentation. Most people with the localized form of Paget's disease have no symptoms. The lesion or lesions are discovered by accident, if at all. Sometimes the skin overlying an early vascular lesion is warm.

If the lesions are more extensive, they frequently cause pain or discomfort. In some patients, headache, pain in the back, or the deformity of a long bone is the first sign of the disease. In some, distortion and thickening of the skull compresses the brain stem or causes dementia. Collapse or fracture of a vertebra can compress the spine. Involvement of the auditory ossicles or pressure on the eighth nerve sometimes causes deafness.

The syndrome described by Paget is not often seen. His patients had a large head, bald in men, thin-haired in women; kyphosis caused by disease of the vertebrae; and bandy and bowed legs, often with prominently curved and thickened tibiae.

Complications. If more than 30% of the skeleton is involved, the increased blood flow in the lesions occasionally increases the cardiac output sufficiently to cause heart failure. Fractures are common in the diseased bones and often result from minor trauma. The incidence of renal stones is slightly increased.

Sarcoma develops in less than 1% of people with Paget's disease, usually in patients with extensive disease. About 5% of people with widespread involvement of many bones develop a sarcoma. The tumor is most often an osteogenic sarcoma, less frequently a fibrosarcoma, chondrosarcoma, or giant cell tumor of bone. In 20% of the patients, the tumor is multicentric. The tumors are most common in the femora, humeri, skull, facial bones, and pelvis. They rarely involve the vertebrae.

Pathogenesis. The cause of Paget's disease of bone is unknown. No metabolic derangement has been demonstrated. Electron microscopy has shown structures like the virus of measles or a respiratory syncytial virus in the nuclei of the osteoclasts in some patients with osteitis deformans. Their relevance is uncertain. In one study in England, people with Paget's disease were more likely to own a dog than were controls, suggesting the distemper or some other disease of dogs might be important in its pathogenesis.

Treatment and Prognosis. Most patients with Paget's disease need no treatment and have no disability. If the disease is severe, calcitonin, the cytotoxic drugs plicamycin and dactinomycin and etidronate and other diphosphonates often give lasting improvement. Surgical correction of deformities is sometimes needed.

HYPERTROPHIC OSTEOARTHROPATHY. Hypertrophic osteoarthropathy takes its name from the Greek words for bone, joint, and suffering or disease. It causes clubbing of the fingers and toes, deposition of subperiosteal new bone, and swelling and tenderness of the joints. Most patients have only clubbing. Some have both clubbing and subperiosteal new bone formation or only subperiosteal new bone formation. Occasionally arthropathy is added to one or both of these conditions.

In adults, hypertrophic osteoarthropathy is usually secondary to disease of the lungs. Most adults who have only clubbing have bronchiectasis, a lung abscess, empyema, or some other chronic inflammatory disease of the lungs; idiopathic pulmonary fibrosis, asbestosis, or some other kind of diffuse pulmonary fibrosis; or a tumor of a lung or the pleura. Occasionally clubbing develops in an adult with infective endocarditis, cirrhosis of the liver, or chronic inflammatory bowel disease. Occasionally it occurs in a person who has no other disease. Over 95% of adults who have both clubbing and the subperiosteal deposition of bone have a pulmonary or pleural neoplasm. In children, hypertrophic osteoarthropathy most often complicates a congenital anomaly of the heart, lungs, or liver.

Lesions. Clubbing makes the tips of the fingers and toes swollen and bulbous. The nails curve longitudinally as well as transversely to conform with the swollen ends of the digits. The angle between the nail and the cuticle is lost. Often the clubbed digits are cyanotic. Microscopically, the swelling is due principally to edema, but there are fibrosis and increased vascularity in the lesions. The number of arteriovenous anastomoses increases. Often there is a sparse, chronic inflammatory exudate. The distal phalanges are thickened early in the disorder, but later become thinned.

The subperiosteal deposition of bone in hypertrophic osteoarthropathy is most common in the distal part of the tubular bones of the limbs. The radii, ulnae, tibiae, and fibulae are the most commonly involved.

The metacarpals and metatarsals are more severely involved than the phalanges. Occasionally, the clavicles, scapulae, ribs, pelvis, or other bones are affected. In the regions involved, the periosteum becomes edematous and congested, with an exudate of lymphocytes and plasma cells. New bone is deposited beneath the periosteum, increasing the diameter of the bone. Often bone is resorbed from the endosteal side of the cortex.

The metacarpophalangeal and metatarsophalangeal joints, wrists, ankles, and knees are the joints most frequently involved. The affected joints are swollen and tender. Their synovium is thickened and edematous, with an exudate of lymphocytes and plasma cells. The quantity of fluid in the joints increases. The fluid contains fewer than 500 mononuclear cells per mL.

Clinical Presentation. The lesions of hypertrophic osteoarthropathy develop slowly over weeks or months. Sometimes they precede the discovery of the underlying pulmonary or other disease. Often the lesions ache or are tender. Elevation of the extremity usually relieves the discomfort.

Pathogenesis. The cause of hypertrophic osteoarthropathy is unknown. It is suggested that a vasodilator elaborated in the lungs increases the blood flow through the regions affected, but that much of the blood passes through arteriovenous shunts and the ischemia that results causes the swelling of the fingertips and the changes in the bones and joints. No such vasodilator has been isolated. Division of the vagus nerve causes the lesions of hypertrophic osteoarthropathy to regress, suggesting that a neurovascular mechanism is involved.

Treatment and Prognosis. If the lesion causing hypertrophic osteoarthropathy is controlled, the changes in the digits, bones, and joints regress, leaving the patient with no disability.

PACHYDERMOPERIOSTITIS. Pachydermoperiostitis is a rare disorder inherited as an autosomal dominant character with variable expressivity. The name comes from the Greek words for thick, skin, around, and bone. The disorder becomes evident in adolescence with severe clubbing of the fingers and toes, extensive subperiosteal bone deposition in the extremities, and coarsening and thickening of the skin of the face. The hands and feet enlarge. The face is greasy. Sweating is excessive in the palms and soles.

Pachydermoperiostitis worsens slowly for years, then usually becomes stationary, and persists with little change for many years. Eventually, ossification of the articular capsules often causes ankylosis of the small joints in the hands and feet. The costochondral junctions ossify. Pressure on spinal nerves caused by the deposition of new bone sometimes causes neurologic symptoms.

HYPEROSTOSIS FRONTALIS INTERNA. Hyperostosis frontalis interna is common in elderly women but rare in men. Often it is associated with obesity and virilism. In one study, it was found in 60% of women in an old-age home.

Smooth or bosselated thickenings develop on the inner surface of the frontal bones, most often in their squamous part. The lesions are usually less than 1 cm across. In the affected regions, the diploë is coarse and sclerotic, but both inner and outer tables are thinned. In pregnancy, similar thickenings sometimes develop on the inner surface of the frontal bones. They disappear after delivery.

LEONTIASIS OSSEA. Leontiasis ossea, from the Greek for lion and the Latin for bony, is an uncommon condition in which the facial bones become thickened and distorted. Sometimes the thickened bones cause nasal or lachrymal obstruction or compress the optic nerves. Sometimes leontiasis ossea is caused by slowly progressive periostitis that causes subperiosteal bone deposition. Sometimes it results from fibrous dysplasia, cherubism, neoplasia, or Paget's disease of bone.

INFANTILE CORTICAL HYPEROSTOSIS. Infantile cortical hyperostosis becomes evident in the first few months of life. A few or many bones become thickened and tender. The mandible, clavicles, scapulae, ribs, and long bones are the most frequently affected. The overlying tissues are indurated. The infant is irritable and feverish and usually has an increased erythrocyte sedimentation rate and neutrophilia. In the early stages of the disease, the periosteum of the bones involved is edematous with an exudate predominantly of neutrophils. Later, increasing subperiosteal bone deposition thickens their cortex. After a few weeks or months, the condition becomes stationary. The excess of bone is resorbed. After months or years, the bones revert to normal.

ASEPTIC NECROSIS

Infarction of part of a bone is called aseptic necrosis. It is particularly common in the head of the femur. The different forms of aseptic necrosis that develop in children are called the osteochondroses. Infarction of the ossification center in the head of a femur causes Legg-Perthes disease. Infarction of the tarsal navicular bone causes Köhler's disease, infarction in metatarsal Freiberg-Köhler disease, infarction of a lunate bone Kienböck's disease, and infarction in vertebrae Scheuermann's disease. Necrosis of fragments of subarticular bone is called osteochondritis dissecans. Diseases of other organs sometimes cause secondary infarction in one or several bones.

ASEPTIC NECROSIS OF THE FEMORAL HEAD. Aseptic necrosis of the femoral head is most common in elderly people. More than 50% of the patients are over 70 years old. Nearly 80% of them are women. In most, the ischemia that causes the infarction results from trauma.

Lesions. The changes in the femoral head in aseptic necrosis develop slowly. Months often pass before the injury is evident radiologically and a year or more before distortion of the head of the femur becomes evident.

Macroscopically, aseptic necrosis of the femoral head is most common in the weight-bearing region. The infarct is well demarcated and yellowish in its early stages. It is usually pyramidal, with its base on the articular cartilage. At first the shapes of the head of the femur and the articular cartilage are intact. They sometimes remain so if the infarct heals without distortion. If not, the cartilaginous surface of the head becomes flattened as the necrotic bone collapses. The overlying cartilage is buckled, thin and, cracked. If the infarct is large, the head of the femur becomes greatly distorted. Osteoarthritis caused by the distortion of the head adds to the disability.

Microscopically, the first evidence of infarction is necrosis of the hematopoietic and connective tissues in the bone marrow. The osteocytes persist in the lacunae of the bony trabeculae for three or four weeks, then disappear. The acellular bony trabeculae persist with little change for weeks or months, separated by the necrotic debris of the bone marrow. Occasionally some of the dead trabeculae break, but excite no reaction.

Repair begins after weeks or months. Blood vessels grow in from the margin of the infarct and revascularize the infarct. The dead bone in the vascularized part of the infarct is resorbed and replaced. As new bone is deposited, the lesion becomes radiopaque. Often deposition of bone is predominant in parts of the lesion, while resorption and fibrosis are extensive in other parts, so that radiologically the lesion is mottled. Often the surrounding viable bone becomes sclerotic, adding to the radiopacity. In children, healing is brisk, but in adults it is slow, in old people very slow. Especially in old people, healing is often imperfect, and the unhealed necrotic bone in the center of the infarct collapses.

Clinical Presentation. Recent aseptic necrosis of the head of the femur causes few symptoms. It is overshadowed by the effects of the fracture or other injury that causes the ischemia. Later, symptoms and dysfunction develop only if the necrosis causes deformation of the femoral head.

Pathogenesis. The commonest cause of aseptic necrosis of the head of the femur is fracture of the neck of the femur. The arteries ascending the neck are torn, and ischemia of the head results. Infarction of greater or lesser degree probably occurs in the femoral head in every fracture of the neck of the femur, though in many of the patients the infarct heals and does not cause serious distortion of the head.

Dislocation of the hip, posterior dislocation in 90% of the patients, is another common result of trauma, particularly in motor accidents. The dislocation jeopardizes the blood supply to the head of the femur, and aseptic necrosis may follow, especially if reduction is delayed for more than six hours,

if the head of the femur is fractured or if the acetabulum is seriously injured.

The blood supply to the head of the femur is occasionally obstructed by air emboli in caisson disease, by thromboemboli in heart or vascular disease, or by the distorted red cells in sickle cell anemia. Necrosis of the head of the femur can complicate Gaucher's disease and other conditions that infiltrate the marrow of the femur. Prolonged therapy with high doses of adrenocortical steroids occasionally causes aseptic necrosis of the femoral head, often on both sides. Aseptic necrosis of the head of the femur is unduly common in alcoholics. Occasionally aseptic necrosis of the head of the femur is found in a person in whom no cause is evident.

Treatment and Prognosis. Early aseptic necrosis of the head of the femur is managed by treating the disease that caused the injury. The late effects of the necrosis are treated like other forms of osteoarthritis.

LEGG-CALVÉ-PERTHES DISEASE

Legg-Calvé-Perthes disease, sometimes called Legg-Perthes disease, is named after the American, French, and German surgeons who described it independently in 1910. It is caused by infarction of the ossification center for the head of the femur in childhood. The distortion of the femoral head usually becomes evident when the child is between 3 and 10 years old. In 85% of the patients, the disease is unilateral. About 80% of the patients are boys. Legg-Calvé-Perthes disease is uncommon in black children.

Lesions. The loss of the blood supply to the head of the femur causes necrosis of the cells in part or all of the ossification center and in adjacent bony trabeculae and bone marrow. The superficial part of the cartilaginous femoral head is nourished by the synovial fluid and remains healthy or becomes thicker than normal.

When revascularization begins, granulation tissue forms around the blood vessels growing into the infarcted region. The dead ossification center is heavily but irregularly calcified. The infarcted bony trabeculae are resorbed and replaced by soft, malleable woven bone. Unless the head of the femur is protected, weight bearing flattens and distorts it. The neck of the femur becomes short and thick. A fracture through the weight-bearing area or subluxation of the joint often increases the deformity. After many years, osteoarthritis adds to the disability.

The woven bone in the infarcted region is slowly replaced by haversian bone that is remodeled to meet the stresses of the part. If deformity is avoided, the head of the femur becomes almost normal. If the head is distorted, the deformity becomes fixed and irreparable.

Clinical Presentation. Legg-Calvé Perthes disease causes few symptoms and little or no disability in its early stages. Only if a fracture through the articular cartilage involves the joint is there likely to be pain or an effusion. Later, the deformity of the joint produces increasing pain and malfunction.

Pathogenesis. The cause of Legg-Calvé-Perthes disease is not usually apparent. The condition is most common in active children, and presumably some minor injury interrupts the blood supply to the head of the femur.

Treatment and Prognosis. Legg-Calvé Perthes disease is treated by preventing pressure on the infarcted head of the femur to avoid deformity. In children under five years of age, the outlook is good. In older children, residual deformity is more likely. The prognosis is better if only part of the ossification center is necrotic.

KÖHLER'S DISEASE. Aseptic necrosis of the tarsal navicular bone is called Köhlers disease after the German physician who described it in 1908. It occurs in children three to seven years old. Over 80% of the patients are boys. It causes few symptoms, perhaps a little pain or tenderness, and nearly always heals without deformity.

FREIBERG-KÖHLER DISEASE. Aseptic necrosis of the head of one of the metatarsals, usually the second, is called Freiberg-Köhler disease after the American physician who described it in 1914 and the German physician who reported it in 1920. It occurs most frequently in girls 12 to 18 years old, sometimes in older women, but is uncommon. The infarction causes pain and tenderness. It heals with some deformity. Osteoarthritis in the joint affected is usual. High-heeled shoes

and a second metatarsal long in relation to the first favor the development of Freiberg-Köhler disease.

KIENBÖCK'S DISEASE. Infarction of a lunate bone is called Kienböck's disease after the Austrian radiologist who described it in 1910. It is fairly common. The patients are usually men 20 to 40 years old who work as riveters, carpenters, or in some other occupation that causes repeated, minor injuries to the wrists. It is most frequent on the right side. The aseptic necrosis of the lunate causes pain, tenderness, and swelling. Osteoarthritis usually develops in the injured wrist and causes permanent dysfunction.

SCHEUERMANN'S DISEASE. Aseptic necrosis in one or more vertebrae is called Scheuermann's disease after the Danish surgeon who described it in 1921. The condition usually becomes evident when the patient is 13 to 17 years old. Usually 3 or 4 adjacent vertebrae in the lower thoracic region are involved. Sometimes the disease is more extensive; sometimes it is confined to a single vertebra.

In the vertebrae involved, the cartilaginous plates on the upper and lower surfaces of the vertebrae that are responsible for their growth are eroded. The growth of the vertebrae is slowed, especially in their anterior part, making the vertebrae wedge-shaped. The patients often become round-shouldered or kyphotic. The intervertebral disks adjacent to the damaged vertebrae swell, making the vertebrae biconcave. Sometimes an intervertebral disk herniates through the cartilaginous plate into the body of a vertebra, a protrusion called a Schmorl's node after the German pathologist who described it in 1930. When the growth of the vertebrae stops, Scheuermann's disease ceases to progress, but the deformity persists for the rest of the patient's life.

OSTEOCHONDRITIS DISSECANS. In osteochondritis dissecans, a fragment of subarticular bone becomes necrotic, and the overlying cartilage degenerates. The patients are usually men 15 to 25 years old. In 90% of the patients, the lesion is in a knee, most frequently in the medial condyle of the femur. Less often, an elbow, hip, ankle, or shoulder is affected. Occasionally the disease is familial.

The lesion is usually less than 2 cm across.

Often deposition of calcium makes the necrotic bone radiopaque. In some patients, the lesion heals in one or two years, leaving no deformity. In some, the necrotic bone collapses, distorting the joint and causing osteoarthritis. In some, the necrotic bone and overlying cartilage separate and become a loose body in the joint.

SECONDARY ASEPTIC NECROSIS. Caisson disease, thromboemboli, sickle cell anemia, and large doses of adrenocortical steroids sometimes cause foci of infarction in one or more bones. Sometimes vascular insufficiency in a limb or the fat necrosis of pancreatitis causes one or more foci of aseptic necrosis in the bones. The lesions are similar to those of aseptic necrosis of the head of a femur and heal in similar fashion. If a joint is involved, osteoarthritis is likely.

CONGENITAL ANOMALIES

Many congenital anomalies cause malformation of the skeleton. Among them are achondroplasia, achondrogenesis, osteopetrosis, pyknodysostosis, osteogenesis imperfecta, melorheostosis, osteopoikilosis, diaphyseal dysplasia, nonmelic medullary osteosclerosis, chondrodysplasia punctata, congenital dislocations, deformities of the feet, malposition of a scapula, hypoplasia of a bone or bones, hyperplasia of a bone or bones, and deformity caused by trauma in utero.

ACHONDROPLASIA. Achondroplasia takes its name from the Greek words for without, cartilage, and to mould or form. Endochondral ossification fails. The bones formed in cartilage are small and abnormal. The membranous bones develop normally. One child in 10,000 live-born has achondroplasia. Dachshunds and basset hounds have a similar disease.

Achondroplasia is inherited as an autosomal dominant character. Few achondroplastics bear children. In most patients, achondroplasia results from a new mutation, and the child's parents do not have the disease. Most of the patients are heterozygotes. In homozygotes, the disease is more severe and often causes death in utero. A milder form of achondroplasia inherited as an auto-somal dominant character allelic with achondroplasia is called hypochondroplasia.

Achondroplastic adults have a big head, a trunk of normal size, and short arms and legs. Most are less than 1.3 m in stature. The lower limbs are often less than half the normal length. The arms are less severely affected. The hands and feet are short. The fingers are of equal length. The face has a saddle nose and is small in relation to the calvarium. Maldevelopment of the base of the skull makes the foramen magnum small. Lumbar lordosis and thoracic kyphosis are common. Occasionally distortion of the spine or herniation of an intervertebral disk compresses a spinal nerve. The pelvis is small and distorted.

In children with achondroplasia, the proliferation of chondrocytes in the cartilaginous ossification centers is reduced and disorderly. The ingrowth of vessels is less than normal. Calcification is impaired. The vertebrae remain cartilaginous longer than is normal. In the long bones, longitudinal growth is slow, but subperiosteal deposition of bone continues, so that the cortices are disproportionally thick. Often the long bones are bowed or deformed.

Apart from the skeletal deformities, patients with achondroplasia have no disability. Most reach adult life and have a normal life span.

ACHONDROGENESIS. The two forms of achondrogenesis are rare conditions inherited as an autosomal recessive character. Achondrogenesis I causes stillbirth or death in infancy. Failure of enchondral ossification gives the child short limbs, a trunk that is nearly as wide as it is long, and a broad pelvis. Achondrogenesis II allows survival to adult life, but distortion of enchondral ossification causes major deformity of the limbs, hands, and feet, often with polydactyly.

OSTEOPETROSIS. Osteopetrosis, from the Greek words for bone and stone, is also called marble bone disease and Albers-Schönberg's disease, after the German radiologist who described it in 1904. The bones are stony hard and densely radiopaque.

Several different disorders cause osteopetrosis. In infants, several types of osteoclastic dysfunction inherited as an autosomal recessive character cause a severe form of the disease. In adults, a milder disorder is inherited as an autosomal dominant character. Some kindred with deficiency of carbonic anhydrase II inherited as an autosomal recessive character have both osteopetrosis and renal tubular acidosis.

Macroscopically, the bones are usually of normal size and shape, except that the epiphyses are enlarged. The bones are heavy. Their cortices are thickened; sometimes the marrow cavity is obliterated. The bone is dense, but crumbles easily. In the severe forms of the disease, all bones are involved, the bones that form in cartilage more severely than the membranous bones. In its milder forms, the long bones are most affected. Often the phalanges and skull are spared. The abnormal bones fracture easily and heal poorly. Multiple fractures sometimes cause deformity.

Microscopically, both the deposition and resorption of bone are abnormal. In children, the epiphyseal cartilages of the long bones are thickened. The chondrocytes proliferate normally, but the calcified cartilage is not resorbed and in places persists unchanged for years. Both in children and in adults, the trabeculae in the bones have a core of heavily calcified cartilage surrounded by irregular, woven bone. In the mild forms of the disease, the trabeculae are little thickened. In the severe forms, they are confluent or nearly so, obliterating the marrow space and merging with the thickened cortex. Osteoblasts and osteoclasts may be few or numerous and are sometimes atypical. The osteoclasts sometimes lack their ruffled membranes. The concentrations of calcium and phosphorus in the plasma are normal. In some patients, the activity of alkaline phosphatase in the plasma is increased.

In 50% of patients with the mild, adult form of osteopetrosis, the disease causes no symptoms and is discovered by accident when a roentgenogram is taken for some other reason. In some, fractures draw attention to the disorder.

In the severe, infantile form of osteopetrosis, replacement of the bone marrow causes anemia. Extramedullary hematopoiesis enlarges the spleen, liver, and lymph nodes. Distortion of the base of the skull sometimes compresses one or more cranial nerves, causing blindness, deafness, facial palsy, or other malfunction. Hydrocephalus is common. The risk of osteomyelitis is increased, especially in the mandible. Many of the patients die in childhood, often from infection. In some, bone marrow transplantation to provide normal osteoclasts has ameliorated the disease. In some, large doses of 1, 25-dihydroxycholecalciferol have been beneficial.

PYKNODYSOSTOSIS. Pyknodysostosis is an uncommon condition inherited as an autosomal recessive character. The patients are short, often less than 1 m in stature in adult life. Their bones are thickened and fragile. The terminal phalanges are hypoplastic. The fontanelles in the skull do not close. Often other abnormalities of the skull are present. The mandible is small. The inner parts of the clavicles are sometimes absent. The bones are easily fractured, but otherwise the disorder causes no disability. The patients have a normal life span.

OSTEOGENESIS IMPERFECTA. Osteogenesis imperfecta, or fragilitas ossium, is a term used to describe a group of conditions in which the bones are abnormally fragile. One person in 20,000 has some form of the disease.

Four types of osteogenesis imperfecta are distinguished. Type I is inherited as an autosomal dominant character but is mild. Type II is inherited as an autosomal recessive character with many new mutations and is the most severe form of the disorder. Type III is also severe and is inherited as an autosomal recessive character. Type IV is of variable severity and is inherited as an autosomal dominant character.

In the bones formed in cartilage, the ossification centers develop normally but fail to ossify. Their cortex is thin. Their medullary trabeculae are few and weak. In severely affected infants, the skull is fibrous, with only small plates of bone. In adults, the skull is usually complete, but sometimes is formed in part by a mosaic of small, wormian bones joined by irregular sutures.

In type I osteogenesis imperfecta, the changes in the bones are sometimes so slight that they pass unnoticed. In other patients with type I disease, multiple fractures occur. In type II, fractures of the long bones and vertebrae are numerous and severe usually bringing death in utero or within a few weeks of birth. In types III and IV, multiple fractures stunt growth and distort the bones. Minor trauma, even a sudden muscular contraction, is often able to fracture the fragile bones. In many patients, the fractures become less frequent after puberty. Pregnancy increases the risk of fracture. Fractures become more frequent after the menopause. The fractures usually heal with little callus, but at times the callus is so exuberant that it suggests a tumor.

Malformation of the teeth, called dentinogenesis imperfecta, occurs in all types of osteogenesis imperfecta but is not present in all patients. The enamel of the teeth is normal, but the dentine is abnormal, giving the teeth a brownish or bluish color. If the enamel is fractured, erosion of the abnormal dentine follows rapidly.

The sclerae of the eyes are blue in osteogenesis imperfecta of types I and II, sometimes in children with type III, but not in those with type IV. Distortion of the ossicles in the ears causes deafness in many patients with type I osteogenesis imperfecta, but is not common in the other types of the disease. In some patients, bluing of the sclerae or deafness is the only sign of the disease. In some, the joints are lax and hypermotile. In others, the skin is thin and translucent. Some patients have a floppy mitral valve or some other defect in the valves of the heart, hyperthermia, increased secretion of thyroid hormones, or hyperhidrosis.

Osteogenesis imperfects is caused by malformation of type I collagen. In the minority of kindreds in which the abnormality has been characterized, type I procollagen molecules are abnormal and easily degraded. The nature of the abnormality differs from one kindred to another. The disease affects principally the bones, sclerae, and teeth because type I collagen is abundant in these organs.

No treatment benefits osteogenesis imperfecta. In the less severe forms of the disease, careful management of the fractures reduces deformity and allows a normal life.

MELORHEOSTOSIS. Melorheostosis is a rare condition that takes its name from the Greek words for a limb, to flow, and bone. Usually only one limb is affected. Occasionally more than one limb or some other part of the skeleton is involved.

In the affected limb and the adjacent part of the hip or shoulder girdle, the bones are thickened by an irregular deposition of subperiosteal new bone, which forms roughly longitudinal streaks, like the guttering of a wax candle. The condition begins in childhood, with pain and restriction of movement in the affected limb, and progresses slowly. Eventually endosteal new bone is laid down, and ossification of the para-articular tissues restricts movement.

OSTEOPOIKILOSIS. Osteopoikilosis, from the Greek for bone and spotted, affects 1 person in 17,000. It is inherited as an autosomal dominant character. Many of the bones have in their medulla foci of well-differentiated haversian bone less than 1 cm across. Roentgenologically, the abnormal foci appear as spots of increased density. Less often the abnormal bone is deposited in longitudinal streaks, a condition called osteopathia striata. About 30% of the patients have collagenous nodules less than 1 cm across in the dermis, a condition called dermatofibrosis lenticularis. Osteopoikilosis causes no symptoms and no dysfunction. It is found by accident when the bones are X-rayed.

DIAPHYSEAL DYSPLASIA. Diaphyseal dysplasia is inherited as an autosomal dominant character. The diaphysis of the long bones, base of the skull, and less often other bones are enlarged by increased deposition of periosteal and endosteal bone of normal structure. The condition begins in childhood and often becomes stationary in adult life. Pain in the affected bones and muscular wasting are prominent. In some patients the activity of alkaline phosphatase in the plasma is increased. Some have hypocalcemia, hyperphosphatemia, anemia, leukopenia, or an increased erythrocyte sedimentation rate. Glucocorticoids often relieve the symptoms and improve function.

MONOMELIC MEDULLARY OSTEOSCLEROSIS Monomelic medullary osteosclerosis affects a single limb. The bones in the limb are iregularly thickened by endosteal formation of new bone.

CHONDRODYSPLASIA PUNCTATA. The term *chondrodysplasia punctata* describes a number of conditions that cause patchy calcification of the epiphyses in children. Some are inherited as an autosomal recessive character, some as an autosomal dominant trait. Often the children have short limbs, scoliosis, depression of the bridge of the nose, cataracts, and ichthyosis. Some die in infancy. Some are mentally retarded. Some have a normal life span and are of normal intelligence.

CONGENITAL DISLOCATIONS. Many children are born with a congenital dislocation of one or more bones. Congenital dislocation or subluxation of one or both hips occurs in 1 child in every 700 born alive. Less often the head of a radius is displaced laterally, a knee is dislocated anteriorly, a patella is displaced laterally, or some other bone is dislocated.

Nearly 90% of the children with a dislocation of a hip are girls. In 50%. both hips are affected. The hip joint is unusually lax. When the femur is extended and adducted, its head comes to lie on the rim of the acetabulum or above it. If the condition is recognized in infancy, and the joint is maintained in flexion and abduction for a few months, the hip becomes stable, and the femur and acetabulum develop normally. If the dislocation is not recognized, the acetabulum becomes distorted, and the neck of the femur increasingly anteverted. The iliopsoas and adductor muscles shorten. The patient develops a limp as the limb shortens. The longer the dislocation persists, the more difficult it is to restore normal function. Osteoarthritis caused by the deformity of the joint adds to the disability.

DEFORMITY OF THE FEET. One child in 500 is born with adduction and supination of all five metatarsals in one or both feet, an anomaly called metatarsus varus. Less common is metatarsus primus varus, in which the first metatarsal is adducted in relation to the others. If it is not corrected, it often causes hallux valgus during adolescence. Not uncommonly the fifth toe is dislocated on one or both sides and overrides the fourth toe.

MALPOSITION OF A SCAPULA. Sometimes one of the scapulae fails to descend normally. The misplaced scapula is smaller than normal and rotated downwards, limiting abduction at the shoulder. It is bound to the adjacent spinous processes by a ligament that often ossifies.

HYPOPLASIA. Hypoplasia of one or more bones is uncommon. Cleidocranial dysplasia, from the Greek for clavicle and cranium, is one of its better known forms. The lateral parts of the clavicles are absent, allowing the shoulders almost to meet in the midline. The frontal bones and sometimes other cranial bones are separated by wide, collagenous sutures. The malformation causes no disability.

Less often a radius and the bones on the radial side of the wrist and hand are partly or completely absent, and the muscles on the radial side of the arm are ill-formed. Hypoplasia of the neck of a femur sometimes causes coxa vara. Occasionally a tibia or fibula is absent. Hypoplasia of one side of one or more vertebrae is an uncommon cause of scoliosis.

HYPERPLASIA. Occasionally one side of the body is bigger than the other, a condition called hemihypertrophy. Occasionally a child is born with one or more accessory fingers or toes, a deformity called polydactyly. Usually the accessory digits are ill-formed. More often, two or more fingers or toes are joined by a fleshy web. Sometimes an additional tarsal navicular bone or some other accessory bone is formed.

In a tarsal coalition, two of the tarsal bones are bound together, first by a cartilaginous and then by a bony bridge. The fixation of the bone causes osteoarthritis in the joints affected. Occasionally the radius and ulna are joined at their proximal end on one or both sides by a bony bridge, a malformation that causes little disability.

TRAUMA IN UTERO. A constricting collagenous band can cause amputation of a limb or limbs in utero or less serious injury. Occasionally injury to a tibia causes a pseudarthrosis.

TUMOR-LIKE CONDITIONS

A number of non-neoplastic lesions of bone resemble a neoplasm. Some of the non-neoplastic lesions are inherited disorders. Some result from injury in utero or in infancy. Often the distinction between these lesions and benign tumors is arbitrary. Table 59-4 shows the classification of tumor-like lesions and neoplasms used in this textbook.

TABLE 59-4.   PRIMARY TUMORS AND TUMOR-LIKE LESIONS OF BONE

Tumor-like	Benign	Malignant
	Cartilaginous	
	Chondroblastoma	Chondrosarcoma
	Chondromyxoid fibroma	Clear cell
	Enchondroma	Dedifferentiated
	Enchondromatosis	Mesenchymal
	Osteochondroma	
	Osteochondromatosis	
	Subperiosteal chondroma	
	Bony	
	Osteoblastoma	Osteogenic sarcoma
	Osteoid osteoma	Parosteal
	Osteoma	
	Collagenous	
Central reparative granuloma	Periosteal desmoid tumor	Desmoplastic fibroma
Cherubism		Fibrosarcoma
Fibrous cortical defect		
Fibrous dysplasia		
Nonossifying fibroma		
Solitary bone cyst		
Subchondral bone cyst		
	Vascular	
Aneurysmal bone cyst	Glomus tumor	Hemangiosarcoma
	Hemangioma	Hemangiopericytoma
	Hemangiomatosis	
	Lymphangioma	
	Mesenchymal	
Lipoma		Leiomyosarcoma
Synovial cyst		Liposarcoma
	Notochordal	
Ecchordosis		Chordoma
	Epithelial	
Epidermal cyst		Adamantinoma
	Hematopoietic	
Histiocytosis X		Leukemia
		Lymphoma
		Multiple myeloma
	Other	
	Schwannoma	Ewing's tumor
		Giant cell tumor
		Malignant fibrous histiocytoma

FIBROUS DYSPLASIA. Fibrous dysplasia is one of the more common tumor-like lesions of bone. One or more collagenous masses containing bony trabeculae develop in a bone or bones. Their cause and pathogenesis are unknown.

Three kinds of fibrous dysplasia are distin-

guished. About 70% of the patients have the monostotic form of the disease in which only one bone is involved. Nearly 30% have the polyostotic form, with lesions in more than one bone. Less than 5% have polyostotic fibrous dysplasia, pigmentation of the skin, and sexual precocity, a disorder called Albright's syndrome after the American physician who described it in 1937.

Most patients with monostotic fibrous dysplasia are between 20 and 30 years old when the diagnosis is made. The polyostotic form of the disease and Albright's syndrome are usually detected in childhood. Over 70% of the patients with Albright's syndrome are girls. In the other forms of fibrous dysplasia, boys and girls are affected equally.

Lesions. The monostotic form of fibrous dysplasia most often involves a rib, femur, tibia, the mandible, maxilla, one of the bones of the skull, or a humerus. The polyostotic forms involve several bones. In 25% of the patients, more than 50% of the skeleton is involved. The skull, facial bones, ribs, vertebrae, and long bones of the limbs are the bones most frequently affected. In 50% of patients with polyostotic fibrous dysplasia, there are one or more lesions in the cranial or facial bones. In some patients, the lesions are confined to one side of the body. In some, only one limb is involved, or the lesions are confined to one arm and that side of the head.

The lesions are usually 2 to 5 cm across, occasionally much larger. In children, they spare the epiphyses, but in adults the epiphyses are often involved. The lesions are well demarcated with a scalloped margin. Especially in the smaller bones, they frequently expand the bone. The cortex overlying a lesion is usually thin and smooth, but intact. On section, a lesion is firm, white, fibrous, and gritty. Occasionally it contains thin-walled cysts filled with serous or bloody fluid. In a roentgenogram, bony ridges extending into a lesion from the cortex often give it a multilocular appearance.

Microscopically, the lesion consists of fine collagenous tissue in which there are small, often hooked trabeculae of woven bone. The collagenous tissue is vascular and moderately cellular. The bony trabeculae sometimes show little osteoblastic activity; sometimes they are lined by plump osteoblasts. Often they show a mosaic of prominent cement

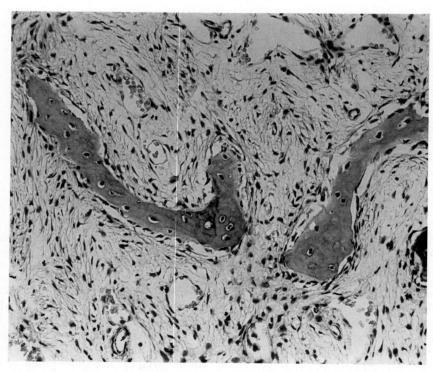

Fig. 59-3. Fibrous dysplasia, showing spicules of bone in fine collagenous tissue.

lines. Multinucleated cells like osteoclasts are sometimes numerous in relation to the trabeculae or free in the collagenous tissue. The quantity of bony trabeculae varies considerably from one lesion to another and in different parts of the same lesion. Sometimes the lesion is almost entirely collagenous. Sometimes ossification is extensive. Particularly in the more collagenous areas, there are often foci of degeneration, with microcysts or collections of foam cells. In 10% of patients, there are islands of cartilage within the lesion.

If the lesions are extensive and active, the activity of alkaline phosphatase in the plasma is increased. If they are few and inactive, it is usually normal. The concentrations of calcium and phosphorus in the plasma are normal. If the lesions are active, the urinary excretion of hydroxyproline increases.

Pigmentation of the skin is unusual in patients with monostotic fibrous dysplasia, but occurs in some patients with the polyostotic form of the disease and in most with Albright's syndrome. Increase in the quantity of melanin in the basal layers of the epidermis causes patches of yellowish brown discoloration that are often confined to one side of the body. The patches vary from 0.5 cm to over 10 cm across. They are sharply defined, usually with a jagged, irregular border. There are usually fewer than six. Sometimes the pigmentation overlies the bony lesions.

The sexual precocity in Albright's syndrome causes premature development of secondary sexual characters and early closure of the metaphyses, so that the patients are short in stature. The cause of the dysfunction is uncertain. The ovaries and pituitary gland are normal. Less often polyostotic fibrous dysplasia is complicated by hyperthyroidism, Cushing's syndrome, acromegaly, hyperparathyroidism, or pleuriglandular dysfunction.

Clinical Presentation. The monostotic form of fibrous dysplasia is often asymptomatic. Occasionally a pathologic fracture draws attention to the lesion. In the polyostotic forms of the disease, the lesions are sometimes painful. Fractures through the lesions often cause deformity. Lesions in the head cause headache and occasionally deafness or leontiasis ossea.

Complications. In 0.5% of patients with polyostotic fibrous dysplasia, an osteogenic sarcoma, chondrosarcoma, or fibrosarcoma develops in one of the lesions. In some of these people, the lesion had been previously irradiated. Rarely, the lesions of fibrous dysplasia are sufficiently vascular to increase the cardiac output and cause heart failure.

Treatment and Prognosis. In many patients with fibrous dysplasia, the lesion or lesions enlarge during childhood, but then become quiescent. In most, they remain so, often becoming sclerotic. In some, they enlarge again after years of quiescence. Curettage and surgical excision can usually control the lesions and prevent deformity. Calcitonin is beneficial if the lesions are numerous and active.

CHERUBISM. Cherubism is an uncommon disorder probably inherited as an autosomal dominant character. When a child affected is two or three years old, symmetrical, bilateral swelling of the posterior part of the mandible or maxilla makes the face round, like that of a cherub. As the child grows older, the lesions slowly enlarge, interfering with dentition. The lesions are like those of fibrous dysplasia. Multinucleated cells like osteoclasts are often numerous in them. Sometimes they contain remnants of tooth buds. Growth of the lesions usually stops at puberty. Plastic surgery can repair the deformity.

CENTRAL REPARATIVE GRANULOMA. A central reparative granuloma is a lesion of the jaws, most common in the anterior part of the mandible. Most of the patients are children or young adults. A well-defined, radiolucent lesion erodes and often expands the bone. Adjacent teeth are displaced. Microscopically, the lesion consists of vascular granulation tissue. Multinucleated giant cells are frequent, especially adjacent to the blood vessels. Often there are foci of hemorrhage or hemosiderin. Curettage cures, though the lesion may recur if not completely eradicated.

FIBROUS CORTICAL DEFECT. One or more fibrous cortical defects are demonstrable in 30% of children. Boys and girls are equally affected. Nearly 50% of the children have more than one. Often the lesions are bilateral. They probably are caused by minor injury to the developing bones.

Lesions. Epiphyseal cortical defects are most common in the lower end of a femur, the proximal end of a tibia, and in a fibula. The lesions are always close to an epiphyseal plate, though as the bone grows they move away from the plate. They are 1 to 4 cm across, sharply demarcated by a scalloped plate of sclerotic bone, and always abut on the cortex. The overlying cortex is smooth. Sometimes a lesion bulges from the surface of the bone.

Microscopically, a fibrous cortical defect consists of swirling or interwoven bundles of moderately cellular collagenous tissue. Often multinucleated cells that resemble osteoclasts are numerous in the lesions. In 50% of the lesions, clumps of fat-filled macrophages are present. Often deposits of hemosiderin are present. No bony trabeculae are present in the lesions.

Clinical Presentation. In most children, a fibrous cortical defect causes no symptoms and no disability. The lesion is discovered by accident when a bone is X-rayed for some other reason.

Treatment and Prognosis. Most fibrous cortical defects persist for a few years, then disappear. Occasionally a nodule of sclerotic bone persists at the site of the lesion. No treatment is needed.

NONOSSIFYING FIBROMA. A nonossifying fibroma is similar to a fibrous cortical defect except that it occurs within a bone and is usually larger. It is a response to minor injury, not a neoplasm.

Nonossifying fibromata are most frequent in the long bones. They are always adjacent to an epiphysis. The lesions are sharply defined, scalloped, and often thin the overlying cortex. They are usually 5 to 10 cm across. Microscopically, the lesions consist of interweaving bundles of collagenous tissue, like those in a fibrous cortical defect.

Many nonossifying fibromata cause no symptoms and slowly resolve. Some cause pain. Occasionally a fracture occurs through the lesion. The fracture heals normally. Lesions that cause symptoms can be curetted or excised.

SOLITARY BONE CYST. A solitary bone cyst, also called a unicameral bone cyst, is fairly common. Most patients are between 3 and 13 years old when the cyst is discovered. Some 70% of them are boys.

In 50% of the patients, the cyst is in the shaft of a femur. In most of the rest, it is in the shaft of one of the other long bones. The cyst is in the medulla of the bone. Usually it is 3 to 10 cm across when discovered. It expands the bone and thins the overlying cor-

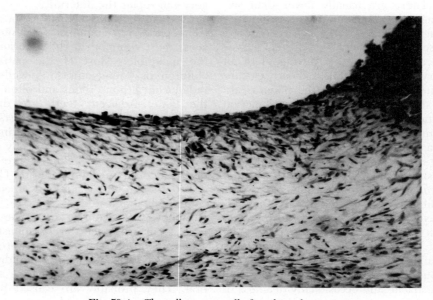

Fig. 59-4. The collagenous wall of a solitary bone cyst.

tex. At first, its upper margin is close to the epiphyseal plate, but does not breach the plate. As the child grows, the cyst becomes separated from the plate.

The cyst is unilocular. Often bony or collagenous septa project into the cyst and roentgenographically make it seem multiloculated. It has a smooth lining and a thin wall of collagenous tissue. Sometimes a few small trabeculae of newly formed woven bone are present in the wall. Frequently multinucleated giant cells like osteoclasts, clumps of macrophages filled with fat, or deposits of hemosiderin are present in the wall. Unless it has been injured, the cyst is filled with clear serous fluid.

During childhood, a solitary bone cyst enlarges slowly. It does not affect the growth of the bone. In adult life, the cyst becomes stationary, but unless treated or injured persists throughout life.

Most solitary bone cysts cause no symptoms until a fracture through the cyst draws attention to it. Some cause discomfort or ache. A fracture through a solitary cyst heals normally. The cyst is treated by curettage and packing with bone chips. About 20% of them recur.

SUBCHONDRAL BONE CYST. A subchondral bone cyst is rare. It is like a solitary bone cyst, except that it involves the epiphysis and abuts on the articular cartilage.

ANEURYSMAL BONE CYST. An aneurysmal bone cyst distends the bone in which it occurs. The "aneurysmal" in the name of the condition refers to the distention of the bone, not to the blood spaces that comprise the lesion. Most of the patients are 10 to 30 years old when the lesion is discovered. About 60% of them are girls or women.

Aneurysmal bone cysts are most common in the long bones, especially the femur, and in the vertebrae. In the long bones, the lesion is usually near one end of the shaft and bulges eccentrically from the bone. Most lesions are about 5 cm across when discovered. Some are smaller; some are more than 20 cm in greatest dimension.

The lesion consists of large blood spaces separated by thin collagenous septa. Many of the spaces are lined by endothelium. Some are lined by vascular granulation tissue. Deposits of hemosiderin and multinucleated giant cells that resemble osteoclasts are often prominent in the septa. Sometimes occassional trabeculae of woven bone or osteoid are present in the septa. The cortex overlying the lesion is smooth but thin.

Some aneurysmal bone cysts change little as years pass. Some enlarge rapidly, causing

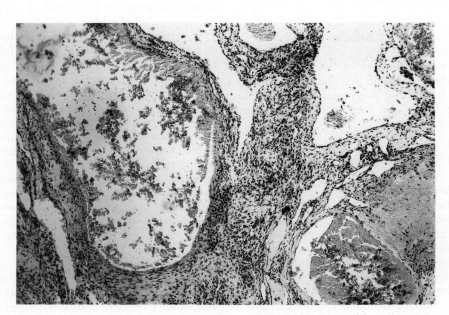

Fig. 59-5. An aneurysmal bone cyst, showing large vascular spaces separated by collagenous septa.

tenderness and pain. A pathologic fracture may occur through the lesion. Occasionally an aneurysmal bone cyst in a vertebra compresses a spinal nerve or the spinal cord.

An aneurysmal bone cyst is treated by curettage and packing with bone chips. About 20% of the lesions recur. If the cyst is inoperable, irradiation slows its growth and sometimes brings cure.

EPIDERMAL CYST. Epidermal cysts in bone are uncommon. They are nearly always in the calvarium or in a terminal phalanx of a finger. The cyst is spheroidal and sharply demarcated. Most are 1 to 2 cm across. The cyst is lined by stratified squamous epithelium and is filled with keratin. It arises from epidermis embedded in the bone by trauma or included during organogenesis.

SYNOVIAL CYST. Rarely, a synovial cyst like those of osteoarthritis is found in one of the long bones of a patient in whom there is no evidence of disease in the neighboring joint.

HISTIOCYTOSIS X. Histiocytosis X is discussed in Chapter 51. Bone can be affected in all three types of histiocytosis X, eosinophilic granuloma, Hand-Schüller-Christian disease, and Letterer-Siwe disease. Unifocal eosinophilic granuloma is its most common manifestation.

TUMORS

The benign tumors of bone will be discussed first, then the malignant tumors arising in bone, the hematopoietic tumors involving bone, and tumors of other organs metastatic to bone.

Benign

As mentioned earlier, the distinction between benign neoplasms of bone and tumor-like lesions is often arbitrary. Some of the lesions considered here are hamartomata or are a non-neoplastic response to injury and might be better considered with the tumor-like lesions. The tumors that are principally collagenous—the osteochondroma chondroma, chondroblastoma, and chondromyxoid fibroma—are considered first; then those

that form bone, the osteoma, osteoid osteoma, and osteoblastoma; the periosteal desmoid tumor; and the angiomata of bone. Rarely, a Schwannoma, lipoma, or some other benign mesenchymal tumor arises in a bone.

OSTEOCHONDROMA. An osteochondroma takes its name from the Greek words from bone and cartilage. It consists of a body spur or knob that projects from a bone and is covered by cartilage. Sometimes the lesion is called an exostosis, from the Greek for out of and bone. Two kinds of osteochondroma are distinguished. Patients with a solitary osteochondroma have only one lesion. Patients with multiple osteochondromatosis have many.

An osteochondroma is the commonest of bone tumors. Many of them are never removed, but nearly 15% of bone tumors that are removed or subjected to biopsy are of this type. Nearly 50% of benign bone tumors removed surgically are osteochondromata. In 90% of the patients, the tumor is solitary. The patient is usually between 10 and 20 years old when the tumor is discovered. Boys and girls are affected equally.

Solitary Osteochondroma. An osteochondroma can arise from any bone formed in cartilage. Most are near the metaphyseal region of one of the long bones. Over 40% of them arise from the lower end of a femur or the upper end of a tibia.

An osteochondroma forms a flattened or pedunculated mass that protrudes from the bone. Most are 1 to 10 cm in greatest dimension. The basal part of the lesion consists of well-formed haversian bone. Its cortex is continuous with the cortex of the bone from which it arises, and its medullary cavity is continuous with the medullary cavity of the bone. The surface of the tumor is covered by a smooth plate of articular cartilage, usually less than 3 mm thick. The periosteum covering the lesion is continuous with that of the underlying bone. The underlying bone is often widened at the site of the tumor, but shows no other deformity. Often a bursa overlies the lesion.

Most solitary osteochondromata enlarge during childhood and adolescence as new bone is formed from the cartilaginous cap. The tumors become stationary during adult life. Often the cartilaginous cap is partially or completely lost. Less than 1% of solitary osteochondromata become malignant, giving rise to a chondrosarcoma or rarely an osteogenic sarcoma.

Probably most solitary osteochondromata are hamartomata, caused by displacement of a fragment of articular cartilage. Some, especially those that arise under the nails, are a response to trauma.

Many solitary osteochondromata cause no symptoms and need no treatment. If the tumor is painful or causes dysfunction, it should be removed. Occasionally a solitary osteochondroma recurs after removal, probably because part of the articular cartilage was left behind.

Multiple osteochondromatosis. Patients with multiple osteochondromatosis have numerous osteochondromata and sometimes other bony anomalies. The condition is inherited as an autosomal dominant character. Sometimes it is called diaphyseal achalasia.

Individually, the lesions of multiple osteochondromatosis are similar to a solitary osteochondroma. They are most common near the metaphyses of the long bones, often with several lesions on a single bone. Often the ribs or vertebrae are involved. Frequently the bones formed in cartilage are shortened or deformed.

The lesions in multiple osteochondromatosis behave like solitary osteochondromata, growing until puberty and then becoming stationary. A chondrosarcoma or rarely an osteogenic sarcoma develops in from 10 to 20% of the patients. Usually multiple osteochondromata are too numerous to allow prophylactic removal of all the lesions. Those that cause symptoms or show any suggestion of abnormal growth should be removed.

CHONDROMA. A benign tumor of cartilage is called a chondroma. Three kinds of chondroma arise in the bones. A solitary enchondroma, from the Greek for in and cartilage, arises within a bone. A periosteal chondroma arises between the periosteum and the bone. In multiple enchondromatosis, the patient has numerous chondromata in the bones.

Many chondromata remain untreated. Those removed or subjected to biopsy make up 5% of bone tumors, 15% of benign bone tumors. Nearly 85% of the patients have only one lesion. Most are enchondromata. Most of the patients are between 10 and 40 years old when the lesion is recognized. Men and women are affected equally.

Solitary Enchondroma. An enchondroma can arise in any bone formed in cartilage. Nearly 40% of them arise in the hands and 5% in the feet.

An enchondroma nearly always lies centrally in the diaphysis of the bone. The tumor is often close to a metaphyseal plate, but does not extend into the diaphysis until enchondral growth has ended. Rarely, an enchondroma is confined to a diaphysis. Most enchondromata are small, though in the bones of the hands and feet the tumor often occupies much of the shaft of a metacarpal, metatarsal, or phalanx. The tumor is poorly defined. It consists of lobules of translucent cartilage usually less than 1 cm across. Occasionally an enchondroma is mucoid or partially calcified. In the small bones, the tumor often expands the bone and thins the overlying cortex.

Microscopically, an enchondroma consists of lobules of cartilage separated by thin fibrovascular septa. The chondrocytes in the lesions are small, with small nuclei that vary little in size. Multinucleated cells and cells with large nuclei are few. Mitoses are absent. Usually there is only one chondrocyte in a lacuna, though occasionally several chondrocytes are present in large, oblong lacunae like those in a growing metaphyseal plate. The chondrocytes are usually separated by well-formed cartilage. Occasionally part of the tumor is myxoid, with stellate cells separated by abundant intercellular substance, is calcified, or is ossified. Foci of degeneration and necrosis are sometimes present. In the small bones of the hands, the lesions are often highly cellular, but in other bones a solitary enchondroma is not more cellular than is articular cartilage.

Solitary enchondromata grow slowly during childhood and adolescence. Growth usually stops in adult life, and the lesion becomes stationary. A solitary enchondroma in a hand or foot rarely becomes malignant, but occasionally a solitary enchondroma in a long bone develops into a chondrosarcoma.

Enchondromata are usually considered to be neoplasms, though most of them are

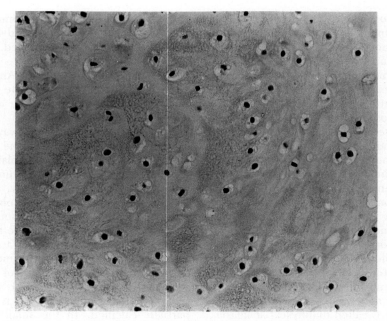

Fig. 59-6.   An enchondroma showing the well-differentiated cartilage found in these tumors.

probably hamartomata. The lesion is caused by some fault of ossification in cartilage.

Many solitary enchondromata cause no symptoms and need no treatment. Sometimes an enchondroma in a hand or foot is big enough to cause deformity, the lesion aches or is painful. Occasionally a pathologic fracture draws attention to the chondroma. If treatment is required, curettage and filling with bone chips is usually curative, though occasionally an enchondroma recurs.

Subperiosteal Chondroma. Subperiosteal chondromata, also called juxtacortical chondromata, are not common. They are most frequent in the upper part of the humerus. The tumor is up to 5 cm across and lies beneath the periosteum in a depression in the thinned cortex of the bone. Microscopically the lesion is like an enchondroma, but is often so atypical that it is hard to distinguish from a chondrosarcoma.

Multiple Enchondromatosis. Multiple enchondromatosis is uncommon. It is not a hereditary disorder. The patients have multiple enchondromata. Often the lesions are confined to one limb, one hand, or one side of the body. Especially when it is confined to one side of the body, multiple enchondromatosis is sometimes called Ollier's

disease, after the French surgeon who described it in 1900. Most of the patients are under 30 years old when the disease is discovered. Over 60% of them are men or boys.

Often the bones affected by multiple enchondromatosis contain several enchondromata, some large, some small. In some patients, some of the chondromata are big enough to cause deformity. Frequently the growth of the bones involved is slowed, and the bones are bowed or distorted. Microscopically, the lesions are like a solitary enchondroma, but are more likely to be cellular and atypical.

About 20% of people with multiple enchondromatosis have multiple cavernous hemangiomata in the skin and internal organs. Such people are said to have Maffucci's syndrome, named after the Italian physician who reported it in 1889. Sometimes the hemangiomata are present only in the limb or limbs involved. Phleboliths are frequently present in the hemangiomata.

Some patients have a combination of multiple enchondromatosis and fibrous dysplasia. Especially in the femur, they have lesions that are in part enchondromatosis, in part fibrous dysplasia. Such people sometimes have pigmented lesions in the skin like those of fibrous dysplasia.

The lesions in multiple enchondromatosis enlarge until puberty and then usually become stationary. A chondrosarcoma develops in 30% of the patients, usually after the age of 40 years. Rarely, one of the lesions becomes an osteogenic sarcoma.

CHONDROBLASTOMA.   Less than 2% of bone tumors are chondroblastomata. The tumor is often called a benign chondroblastoma, but some invade and some metastasize. Most patients are between 10 and 20 years old when the tumor is discovered. Nearly 70% of the patients are men or boys.

A chondroblastoma can develop in any bone formed in cartilage. It is most common in the epiphyses of the long bones. Nearly 50% of chondroblastomata take origin in the upper end of a humerus, lower end of a femur, or upper end of a tibia. The tumor arises within the bone. It is well defined and 1 to 7 cm across. Frequently it is surrounded by a thin rim of sclerotic bone. On section, a chondroblastoma consists of gritty, yellowish cartilage. Foci of hemorrhage and cysts less than 1 cm across are often present. The tumor often abuts on the metaphyseal cartilage, but rarely invades it. Occasionally it breaches the cortex and invades the surrouding tissues.

Microscopically, a chondroblastoma usually consists mainly of closely packed, fairly uniform, polyhedral cells of moderate size. The cells have spheroidal or ovoid nuclei that are often indented. Their cytoplasm is clear. Usually the cell membrane is clearly evident. Mitoses are present. Scattered among the tumor cells are large, multinucleated cells with from 5 to 40 nuclei.

In parts of the tumor, the tumor cells are separated by chondroid material that sometimes resembles cartilage, sometimes is less differentiated. Some of these regions are degenerate and calcified. Often the calcification forms fine, interlacing bands.

Occasionally part of a chondroblastoma resembles a giant cell tumor of bone or a chondromyxoid fibroma. Sometimes part or much of the tumor is like an aneurysmal bone cyst. Sometimes part of the tumor undergoes osteoid or bony metaplasia.

Most chondroblastomata grow slowly and remain localized. Pain is often the principal symptom. Often discomfort in the bone has been present for months or years before the tumor is diagnosed. A few of the tumors invade the surrounding tissues. A few metastasize to the lungs or more widely. The metastases usually grow sluggishly like the primary tumor. Rarely, a chondroblastoma becomes a chondrosarcoma. In most patients, local excision or curettage and packing with bone chips cures. If the chondroblastoma is incompletely removed, it is likely to recur.

CHONDROMYXOID FIBROMA.   Less than 1% of bone tumors are chondromyxoid fibromata. Most of the patients are 10 to 39 years old. About 70% of them are men or boys.

A chondromyxoid fibroma can arise in any bone formed in cartilage. Nearly 70% of them occur in a lower limb, most often in the metaphysis of a long bone near a knee or ankle. The tumor is within the bone. It is sharply demarcated, sometimes with a thin capsule of sclerotic bone. Most are less than 5 cm across. On section, the lesion is gray or tan, sometimes lobulated, firm, and rubbery.

Microscopically, most chondromyxoid fibromata consist principally of ill-defined lobules of mxyoid tissue. The tumor cells are stellate or spindle shaped, with prominent spheroidal, ovoid, or spindle-shaped nuclei. Mitoses are rare. Near the margin of the lobules, the tumor is often more cellular and more atypical. Multinucleated giant cells are usually present in the septa between the lobules. Occasionally the septa contain macrophages filled with fat, deposits of hemosiderin, or a sparse exudate of lymphocytes and plasma cells.

In many chondromyxoid fibromata, the tumor cells in some lobules are like fibrocytes and are separated by collagenous tissue or resemble chondrocytes and are separated by a chondroid stroma. In some tumors, collagenous or chondroid differentiation is predominant. Often the tumor cells in parts of the tumor are larger, irregularly shaped, and vary in size. Some of them may be multinucleated. Often parts of the tumor are calcified. Occasionally part of a chondromyxoid fibroma resembles a chondroblastoma.

Chondromyxoid fibromata grow slowly. Pain or swelling draws attention to the tumor. Local excision cures. About 25% of tumors treated by curettage recur because of the difficulty of eradicating the tumor com-

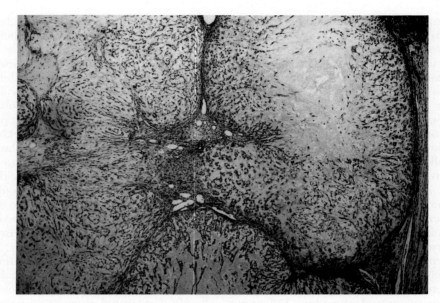

Fig. 59-7. A chondromyxoid fibroma showing the lobules of myxoid tissue usual in this tumor.

pletely. Malignant transformation of a chondromyxoid fibroma is rare.

OSTEOMA. The term *osteoma* is used to describe benign, bony lesions of the membranous bones of the skull and face. Roentgenographically, 1 person in 200 has an osteoma. Most of the patients are over 40 years old. About 70% of them are men.

Osteomata are most common in the frontal and ethmoid sinuses, less so in the jaws, facial bones, and calvarium. Occasionally there is more than one. The lesion is a stony hard, rounded mass 1 to 5 cm across that bulges from the underlying bone. It consists of closely packed trabeculae of lamellar bone covered by a thin cortex.

Most osteomata are hamartomata or result from injury. Most cause no symptoms. If necessary, the lesion can be excised.

OSTEOID OSTEOMA. About 3% of bone tumors, over 10% of benign bone tumors, are osteoid osteomata. Nearly 90% of the patients are between 5 and 25 years old. Over 70% of them are boys or men.

An osteoid osteoma can arise in any bone. It is most common in the long bones. More than 50% of them arise in a femur or tibia. Most osteoid osteomata develop in the cortex of the bone, but the tumor can occur in the medulla or beneath the periosteum.

An osteoid osteoma has a spheroidal nidus usually less than 1.5 cm across. The nidus is sharply demarcated, reddish, or gray. It may be soft and friable or stony hard. The nidus is embedded in sclerotic bone. When the tumor is in the cortex, the sclerosis often extends for more than 5 cm. When the tumor is in the medulla, it is less extensive.

Microscopically, the nidus of an osteoid osteoma is sharply demarcated. It consists of closely packed, anastomosing trabeculae of osteoid separated by vascular collagenous tissue. Normal appearing osteoblasts and osteoclasts line the trabeculae. Often some of the trabeculae are calcified, especially in the center of the lesion. Occasionally some of them are ossified and consist of immature, woven bone. The sclerotic bone around the nidus is normal, except for its thickness and density.

An osteoid osteoma causes pain. At first the discomfort is slight and intermittent. It gradually worsens and is often most severe at night when the patient is in bed. In many of the patients, aspirin relieves the pain. The cause of the pain is uncertain. It may be due to tension in the nidus or to the high concentration of prostaglandins in the nidus. Occasionally an osteoid osteoma is tender, or the skin overlying the tumor is warm. Occa-

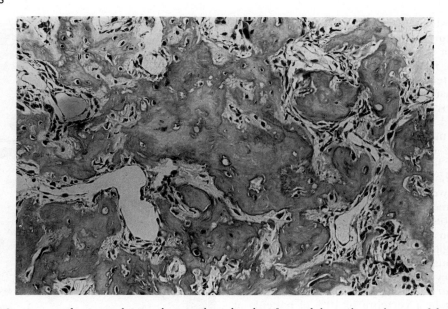

Fig. 59-8. An osteoid osteoma showing the irregular trabeculae of osteoid that make up the core of the lesion.

sionally an osteoid osteoma impairs the growth of the bone involved or causes an effusion into an adjacent joint.

Most consider an osteoid osteoma a neoplasm. Some have suggested that it might be a form of sclerosing osteomyelitis caused by infection. The tumor grows slowly. If left untreated, it persists with little change for years. Complete excision of the nidus cures. If the nidus is not completely removed, the tumor is likely to recur.

OSTEOBLASTOMA. An osteoblastoma, often called a benign osteoblastoma or giant osteoid osteoma, is similar to an osteoid osteoma. Sometimes it is hard to decide whether a lesion should be called an osteoid osteoma or an osteoblastoma. Less than 1% of bone tumors are of this type. Over 80% of the patients are under 30 years old when the tumor is discovered. Over 70% of them are boys or men.

Nearly 40% of osteoblastomata arise in a vertebra or the sacrum, 30% in a long bone, and 20% in the skull or jaws. The tumor usually arises in the medulla of the bone, but occasionally is eccentric and seems to arise beneath the periosteum. As it enlarges, the tumor expands the bone or bulges from it. The overlying cortex is thin. Occasionally it is defective, and the tumor is limited only by

the periosteum. The internal surface of the tumor is sometimes limited by a thin plate of bone, but the massive osteosclerosis that surrounds an osteoid osteoma does not occur. On section, the tumor is hemorrhagic, friable, and gritty.

Microscopically, an osteoblastoma is sharply demarcated. It consists of anastomosing trabeculae of osteoid, usually more widely separated by a highly vascular collagenous stroma than are the trabeculae in an osteoid osteoma. The trabeculae are continuous with normal trabeculae in the adjacent parts of the bone. The osteoblasts lining the trabeculae are often large and prominent, but remain regular. Often multinucleated cells like osteoclasts are scattered throughout the lesion. Often some of the trabeculae are calcified. Occasionally part of the tumor resembles an aneurysmal bone cyst. Occasionally an osteoblastoma is multifocal, consisting of several islands of tumor separated by normal bone.

An osteoblastoma causes pain that slowly worsens as months pass. The pain is not worse at night and is not relieved by aspirin. Occasionally the patient notices a mass, or the tumor is tender. Occasionally an osteoblastoma in the spine compresses a spinal nerve.

An osteoblastoma is considered to be a neoplasm. The tumor slowly enlarges, but does not invade or metastasize. Curettage is curative in most patients. If the tumor is not completely eradicated, it may recur, Malignant change in an osteoblastoma is rare.

PERIOSTEAL DESMOID TUMOR. A periosteal desmoid tumor is an uncommon lesion that occurs most often in relation to the medial condyle of a femur. If forms a firm mass usually less than 3 cm across. Microscopically, the tumor consists of interwoven bundles of well-differentiated collagenous tissue. The tumor is benign. Excision cures.

ANGIOMA. Solitary hemangiomata are common in bones. In hemangiomatosis, hemangiomata are numerous. Occasionally a lymphangioma, glomus tumor, or hemangiopericytoma arises in a bone.

Solitary Hemangioma. A hemangioma is present in a vertebra in 10% of patients at autopsy. Less frequently a hemangioma is found in the skull, mandible, or some other bone. Most of the lesions are small and cause no dysfunction. Only occasionally is a hemangioma large enough to weaken or distort the bone. Most hemangiomata in bone consist of cavernous blood vessels lined by endothelium and separated by collagenous septa. Less often a capillary hemangioma develops in a bone. Especially in the skull, new bone deposited between the vascular channels sometimes makes the lesion hard.

Hemangiomatosis. Hemangiomatosis is an uncommon condition in which numerous hemangiomata are present in a bone or several contiguous bones. Often hemangiomata are also present in the overlying soft tissues. In some of the patients, the bones or bones involved increase in length and circumference. A limb affected may become 10 cm too long. In others, the hemangiomata gradually destroy the bone, a condition called massive osteolysis.

Malignant

Several types of malignant tumor arise in the bones: chondrosarcoma, osteogenic sarcoma, fibrosarcoma, hemangiosarcoma, malignant fibrous histiocytoma, giant cell tumor of bone, Ewing's tumor, chordoma,

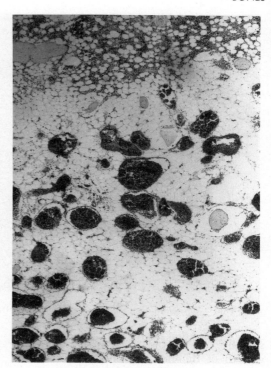

Fig. 59-9. A solitary hemangioma of a bone, showing large blood vessels in the bone marrow.

and adamantinoma. Less often a hemangiopericytoma, liposarcoma, leiomyosarcoma, or some other malignant tumor of the connective tissues arises in a bone. Malignant tumors of the hematopoietic system often involve the bones. Metastases to the bones are common. All primary tumors of the bones are uncommon. Less than 0.3% of malignant tumors arise in a bone.

CHONDROSARCOMA. About 20% of malignant tumors primary in bone are chondrosarcomata. Most patients are over 30 years old when the tumor is discovered. Over 60% of them are men.

Lesions. Over 85% of chondrosarcomata are central tumors that arise within a bone. Most of the rest are peripheral tumors that develop beneath the periosteum. Rarely, an extraosseus chondrosarcoma arises in the soft tissues.

Nearly 80% of central chondrosarcomata arise in the trunk, a shoulder girdle, or the upper end of a humerus or femur. Less than 3% arise in the hands or feet. Over 50% of peripheral chondrosarcomata arise in an osteo-chondroma of the pelvis or upper end of a femur. Most of the rest arise from an osteochondroma in some other part of the skeleton. Extraosseus chondrosarcomata are most common in the lower limbs, especially in the synovium. Occasionally an extraosseus chondrosarcoma arises in a lung or from the cartilage in the nasal cavity.

Central osteochondromata destroy and enlarge the bone involved. At first, the tumor is confined to the medulla, and the cortex overlying the tumor is thickened. Often new bone is deposited beneath the periosteum. As the tumor enlarges, the cortex is thinned or breached, allowing the sarcoma to invade the adjacent tissues. On section, the sarcoma forms a lobulated mass of rubbery, bluish cartilage. Often the tumor is 5 to 10 cm across. Foci of necrosis, cysts, and calcification are common. Occasionally part of much of the tumor is soft and myxomatous.

A peripheral chondrosarcoma arising in an osteochondroma thickens the cartilaginous

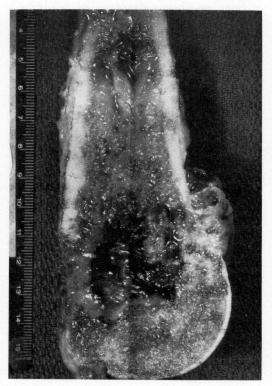

Fig. 59-10. A chondrosarcoma that has breached the cortex of the bone and extends along the medulla.

cap overlying the exostosis and makes its surface irregular or bosselated. If the cartilage overlying an exostosis is more than 1 cm thick, the lesion is likely to be malignant. The rare peripheral chondrosarcomata that arise from the surface of a bone resemble a periosteal chondroma. Most periosteal chondromata are less than 3 cm across. Most peripheral chondrosarcomata arising from the surface of a bone are more than 5 cm across. As a peripheral chondrosarcoma enlarges, it invades the surrounding tissues and the underlying bone, becoming indistinguishable from a central tumor.

An extraosseus chondrosarcoma forms a well-demarcated, lobulated mass that on section is similar to other types of chondrosarcoma.

Microscopically, most chondrosarcomata consist of well-differentiated cartilage. Often it is difficult to determine whether the lesion is a chondrosarcoma or an enchondroma. Lesions that are highly cellular, have many chondrocytes with plump nuclei, more than an occasional chondrocyte with two nuclei, or giant chondrocytes with one or more nuclei with coarse chromatin are likely to be malignant. Foci of myxomatous change suggest malignancy. Often parts of the tumor are calcified or are replaced by trabeculae of woven bone.

Dedifferentiated Chondrosarcoma. In 10% of chondrosarcomata, part or much of the tumor consists of more obviously malignant tissue. Such lesions are called dedifferentiated chondrosarcomata. Macroscopically, much of the mass often consists of soft, gray tissue, with only small parts of the tumors preserving its cartilaginous appearance. Microscopically, the anaplastic regions resemble an osteogenic sarcoma, fibrosarcoma, or occasionally a malignant fibrous histiocytoma. The transition between the cartilaginous part of the sarcoma and the more anaplastic regions is sharp.

Clear Cell Chondrosarcoma. In 2% of chondrosarcomata, part or all the tumor consists of well-defined clear cells, like those of chondroblastoma. Often some of the tumor cells are calcified, and trabeculae of osteoid or bone are present in the tumor. Multinucleated cells like osteoclasts are present in the tumor singly or in small clumps.

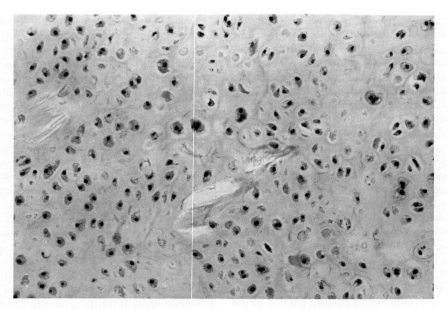

Fig. 59-11. A chondrosarcoma showing the moderately atypical cartilage that consistutes the tumor.

Mesenchymal Chondrosarcoma. In 2% of chondrosarcomata, the tumor consists in part of well-differentiated cartilage, in part of small round or spindle-shaped cells. Nearly 80% of the patients are between 10 and 40 years old. About 30% of the tumors arise in the soft tissues.

Behavior. Most chondrosarcomata grow slowly. Often the tumor is present for several years before it is removed. The sarcoma often appears to push the surrounding soft tissues aside, but does invade them. Hematogenous metastases develop in 20% of the patients, usually after the sarcoma has been present for several years. They are most common in the lungs, liver, kidneys, and brain. Metastases to lymph nodes are rare. Only the dedifferentiated and mesenchymal forms of the tumor are likely to grow more rapidly and to metastasize soon and widely.

Clinical Presentation. Pain or the discovery of a mass causes most patients with a chondrosarcoma to seek treatment.

Pathogenesis. About 10% of chondrosarcomata arise in an osteochondroma. Less than 2% develop in a patient with multiple enchondromatosis. Malignant change in a solitary enchondroma is rare. Rarely, an osteochondroma complicates Paget's disease

of bone or fibrous dysplasia or arises in a bone irradiated some years earlier.

Treatment and Prognosis. Complete excision cures most well-differentiated chondrosarcomata. The sarcoma invades beyond its apparent limits, and wide excision is needed to eradicate it completely. If part of the tumor remains, it is likely to recur, though it may be 5 or 10 years before the recurrence is evident. In 10% of the patients, the recurrent tumor becomes more anaplastic. The risk of metastasis increases after the tumor has recurred one or more times.

Most of the patients with a dedifferentiated chondrosarcoma or a mesenchymal chondrosarcoma die of the tumor within five years. Clear cell chondrosarcomata probably behave as does the usual type of chondrosarcomata.

Osteogenic Sarcoma. Osteogenic sarcoma, or osteosarcoma, is the must common primary malignant tumor of bone. About 40% of primary malignant tumors of bone are of this type. Some 75% of the patients are 10 to 25 years old. Few are over 40 years old, unless the patient has Paget's disease of bone. About 60% of the patients are men or boys.

Lesions. Over 95% of osteogenic sarcomata arise within a bone. Less than 5% arise beneath the periosteum. Rarely, an osteogenic sarcoma arises in the soft tissues.

Over 75% of osteogenic sarcomata develop in a long bone, most often near one end of the bone, 35% of them in the lower end of a femur, 15% in the upper end of a tibia, and 8% in the upper end of a humerus. Nearly 10% arise in the pelvis or sacrum, over 5% in the jaws. Rarely, an osteogenic sarcoma originates in the soft tissues. Less than 0.2% of patients have more than one osteogenic sarcoma.

The central osteogenic sarcomata destroy and replace the bone. The sarcoma extends along the medulla, usually 1 to 3 cm beyond its apparent margin. It penetrates the cortex and grows beneath the periosteum. The expanding tumor strips the periosteum from the bone, but for a time the periosteum remains intact. Often non-neoplastic new bone fills the space between the elevated periosteum, the margin of the tumor, and the underlying bone. In 50% of the patients, the tumor between the cortex and the periosteum forms bony trabeculae that radiate perpendicular to the surface of the bone, giving the tumor a sunburst pattern roentgenologically. Eventually, the periosteum is breached, and the tumor extends into the surrounding soft issues. The sarcoma rarely damages or penetrates the articular cartilage.

By the time it is discovered, most central osteogenic sarcomata are more than 10 cm across. Many of them are stony hard and calcified, though usually the growing margin of the tumor remains soft. Some are partially cartilaginous. A few are soft, friable, and gritty with foci of necrosis and hemorrhage. A few are partially collagenous.

The periosteal osteogenic sarcomata form a mass between the cortex and the periosteum. Some of the tumors invade extensively like most central osteogenic sarcomata; some grow sluggishly and invade only slowly.

Microscopically, most osteogenic sarcomata are pleomorphic and differ considerably in structure from one region to another. In its most anaplastic regions, the tumor often consists of large, bizarre tumor cells with large, atypical nuclei and well-defined, eosinophilic cytoplasm. Some of the tumor cells have more than one nucleus. Mitoses are numerous and often atypical. Frequently small deposits of osteoid are present between the tumor cells or form trabeculae lined by the tumor cells. At the margins of the sarcoma, neoplastic new bone sometimes surrounds preexisting trabeculae. In some of

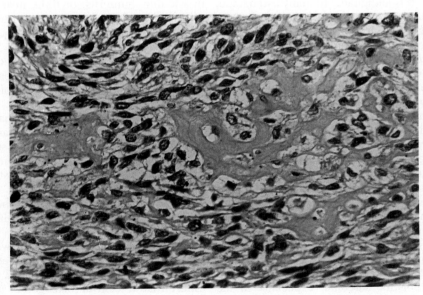

Fig. 59-12.   An osteogenic sarcoma showing the spicules of bone formed by the poorly differentiated tumor cells.

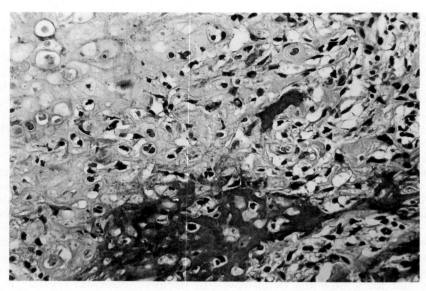

Fig. 59-13.   An osteogenic sarcoma showing the ill-differentiated cartilage often present in these tumors.

the tumors multinucleated cells like osteo-clasts are present.

In the center of many osteogenic sarco-mata, the bony trabeculae are better dif-ferentiated, calcified, or ossified. The tumor cells lining them are smaller and less atypical. In 1% of osteogenic sarcomata, the whole tumor is so well differentiated that it is hard to be sure it is malignant. In many osteogenic sarcomata, part or much of the tumor consists of cartilage. The tumor cells in the cartilag-inous regions are sometimes atypical, some-times resemble the well-differentiated chondrocytes of a chondrosarcoma. Other parts of an osteosarcoma sometimes resemble a fibrosarcoma or a malignant fibrous his-tiocytoma. Occasionally the tumor is almost entirely fibrosarcomatous, with only a few ill-formed trabeculae of osteoid to show that it is an osteogenic sarcoma. Occasionally part of an osteogenic sarcoma resembles an aneurys-mal bone cyst.

In over 50% of osteogenic sarcomata, the formation of osteoid and bone is predominant in the tumor. In 25%, the tumor is mainly cartilaginous. In 25%, it is predominantly collagenous.

The activity of alkaline phosphatase is high in an osteogenic sarcoma, especially in its actively growing peripheral region. In 50% of

the patients, the activity of the enzyme in the plasma is increased to twice its normal value. The concentrations of calcium and phos-phorus in the plasma are normal.

Parosteal Osteogenic Sarcoma. About 80% of periosteal osteogenic sarcomata, 4% of all osteogenic sarcomata, are of the par-osteal type. The tumor almost always arises in a femur, humerus, or tibia, near one end of the bone. It forms a subperiosteal mass, occasionally with a cartilaginous cap beneath the periosteum. Microscopically, the sar-coma consists of well-differentiated trabec-ulae of lamellar or woven bone separated by slightly atypical spinal cells. Foci of cartilag-inous differentiation are common. Invasion of the medullary cavity is unusual except after incomplete resection of the sarcoma.

Behavior. Most osteogenic sarcomata grow rapidly and invade the adjacent tissues extensively. Hematogenous metastases are often present before the primary tumor is detected. The lungs and other bones are their most common site. Lymph nodes are rarely involved.

Osteogenic sarcomata of the jaws usually grow slowly and are unlikely to metastasize. Parosteal osteogenic sarcomata and the well-differentiated central osteogenic sarcomata grow slowly, invade slowly, and usually metastasize only after several unsuccessful attempts to remove the tumor.

Clinical Presentation. Pain is often the first sign of an osteogenic sarcoma. Frequently the mass can be felt.

Pathogenesis. About 3% of osteogenic sarcomata complicate Paget's disease of bone. Another 3% arise in a bone that has been irradiated. Beryllium causes osteogenic sarcoma in animals, but is not known to do so in man.

Treatment and Prognosis. Osteogenic sarcoma is treated by radical excision of the tumor, often by amputation, combined with radiation and chemotherapy. If necessary, metastatic lesions in the lungs are excised. In up to 80% of the patients, the combined treatment brings cure.

FIBROSARCOMA. About 5% of malignant tumors primary in bone are fibrosarcomata. Most patients are between 20 and 70 years old. Men and women are affected equally.

More than 50% of fibrosarcomata primary in bone arise in the long bones, 15% of them in the lower end of the femur and 10% in the upper end of the tibia. About 20% arise in the pelvis or sacrum and 10% in the jaws.

Most primary fibrosarcomata of bone arise within a bone. The tumor destroys the bone as it enlarges, erodes the cortex, and invades the surrounding tissues. Less often fibrosarcoma arises from the periosteum and forms a mass that bulges from the bone with little invasion of the underlying cortex. On section the tumor is firm and fleshy. Occasionally myxoid regions are evident. Occasionally there are foci of necrosis or hemorrhage.

Most fibrosarcomata of bone are moderately differentiated and consist of interweaving bundles of collagen with moderately atypical tumor cells. A few are highly differentiated and resemble a benign lesion. A few are anaplastic. The tumor forms no osteoid and no bony trabeculae. If any osteoid or any trabeculae are present, the lesion is an osteogenic sarcoma.

The moderately differentiated fibrosarcomata grow more slowly than an osteogenic sarcoma and are less likely to metastasize. When metastases do occur, they are usually to the lungs. The anaplastic fibrosarcomata behave like an osteogenic sarcoma.

More than 10% of fibrosarcomata primary in bone develop in giant cell tumor of bone, usually after the giant cell tumor has been irradiated. Another 10% develop in a bone irradiated for some other reason. In 3% of patients, the fibrosarcoma complicates Paget's disease; less often it complicates fibrous dysplasia or a bone infarct.

A fibrosarcoma of a bone causes pain and often a detectable mass. The tumor is treated surgically. About 30% of the patient are well five years later, but some of them die later of local recurrence of the sarcoma or metastases.

Desmoplastic Fibroma. A desmoid fibroma is a rare tumor that occurs within a bone. It is usually 2 or 3 cm across when discovered. The fibroma slowly invades the bone and sometimes penetrates the cortex and extends into the adjacent tissue. Microscopically it is similar to a desmoid tumor of the soft tissues and consists of interwoven bundles of well-differentiated collagenous tissue. Complete excision cures. If part of the tumor remains, it is likely to recur.

HEMANGIOSARCOMA. About 1% of malignant tumors primary in bone are hemangiosarcomata. The patients are usually adult. Men and women are affected equally. In 30% of the patients, the tumor is in a long bone; in 15%, in a vertebra. In 30%, there is more than one tumor. The tumors are similar to hemangiosarcomata in other organs. Bone sometimes forms between the neoplastic blood vessels. Over 95% of patients with well-differentiated lesions survive more than five years, but less than 20% of those with anaplastic tumors.

MALIGNANT FIBROUS HISTIOCYTOMA. A malignant fibrous histiocytoma primary in bone is similar to the malignant fibrous histiocytomata that occur in the soft tissues. Less than 1% of primary bone tumors are of this type. The lesions resemble those in the soft tissues and behave similarly.

GIANT CELL TUMOR. A giant cell tumor of bone is often called an osteoclastoma because of the multinucleated cells like osteoclasts prominent in the lesion. Sometimes it is called a benign giant cell tumor, though the lesions often recur and occasionally metastasize. Less than 15% of malignant tumors primary in bone are of this type. Over 80% of the patients are over 20 years old when the tumor is discovered, 65% of them between 20 and 40 years old. Nearly 60% of the patients are women.

Lesions. Nearly 80% of giant cell tumors of bone arise in a long bone, usually near the end of the bone. Almost 30% of them are in the lower end of a femur, 20% in the upper end of a tibia, 15% in the lower end of an ulna or radius, and 10% in the sarcum. Rarely, a patient has more than one giant cell tumor.

Giant cell tumors of bone arise within the bone. As they enlarge, they destroy and replace the bony tissue, forming an ill-defined mass without surrounding osteosclerosis. Often the tumor is eccentric and bulges from one side of the bone. The overlying cortex is thinned or destroyed, but the periosteum usually remains intact, even when the tumor is large. Most are 5 to 10 cm

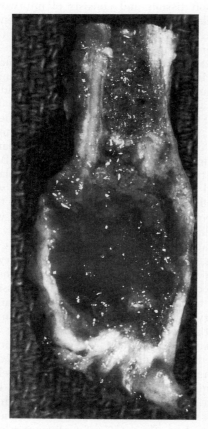

Fig. 59-14. A giant cell tumor of the ulna, showing the expansion and destruction of the bone caused by the tumor.

across when discovered. The tumor frequently abuts on the articular cartilage and sometimes destroys it. On section, a giant cell tumor is soft and friable, gray or reddish. Cysts and foci and hemorrhage or necrosis are unusual except in recurrent tumors where they are sometimes extensive.

Microscopically, a giant cell tumor of bone consists of plump, spindle-shaped or ovoid tumor cells. The tumor cells have a single large, spheroidal or ovoid nucleus with even chromatin. Their cytoplasm is sparse and ill-defined. They are closely packed with little intercellular material between them. The cells and their nuclei vary little in size or shape. A few mitoses are usually evident. Occasionally they are numerous. Small blood vessels run among the tumor cells. No bone or collagen is present within the tumor, except in regions in which the tumor has been injured and sometimes at the margin of the lesion.

Numerous multinucleated giant cells are scattered among the mononuclear tumor cells in most parts of most giant cell tumors of bone. The giant cells are well defined, often with 50 or more nuclei and abundant cytoplasm. Their nuclei are similar to those of the mononuclear tumor cells.

Like osteoclasts, the giant cells have a ruffled cytoplasmic border, many mitochondria, and little endoplasmic reticulum and contain abundant acid phosphatase, β-glucuronidase and succinic dehydrogenase. In the mononuclear tumor cells, the activity of these enzymes is low, mitochondria are few, and the endoplasmic reticulum is better developed.

Behavior. Giant cell tumors of bone grow slowly. If not removed, they become large, but usually remain localized. Incomplete excision is followed by recurrence. The recurrent tumor grows slowly, but invades the soft tissues, making its complete removal increasingly difficult. Hematogenous metastases develop in less than 2% of patients with an uncomplicated giant cell tumor of bone. They resemble the primary tumor and grow slowly.

In 10% of patients with a giant cell tumor of bone, a fibrosarcoma, osteogenic sarcoma, or malignant fibrous histiocytoma develops in the tumor. In 80% of these people, the

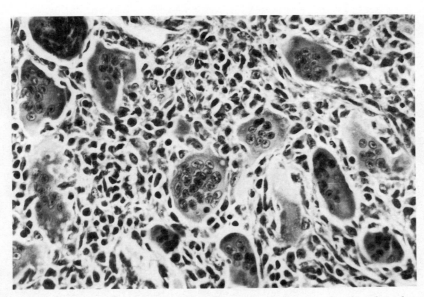

Fig. 59-15.   A giant cell tumor of bone showing the small tumor cells intermixed with multinucleated cells that resemble osteoclasts.

change to a more malignant lesion occurs in a giant cell tumor that has recurred after incomplete excision. In 75% of them, the giant cell tumor was irradiated, usually 10 or more years before the appearance of the more malignant lesion. When the more dangerous neoplasm appears, the tumor begins to grow more rapidly. The more malignant tumor invades and metastasizes in its usual fashion.

Clinical Presentation.   Most giant cell tumors of bone cause pain. Sometimes the patient notices the mass. Occasionally a pathologic fracture draws attention to the tumor.

Pathogenesis.   The origin of the spindle cells that are the principal feature of a giant cell tumor of bone is unknown. The multinucleated giant cells in the tumor are probably osteoclasts, but there is little evidence that the mononuclear cells are derived from osteoclasts. Occasionally a giant cell tumor arises in a patient with Paget's disease of bone.

Treatment and Prognosis.   Giant cell tumors of bone are treated by curettage or by local excision. Before the risk of inducing a more malignant neoplasm was realized, they were often irradiated. About 50% of giant cell

tumors recur. Progression to a more malignant tumor can occur up to 30 years after the original lesion was first discovered.

EWING'S TUMOR.   Ewing's tumor is called after the American pathologist who described it in 1921. About 10% of malignant tumors primary in bone are of this type. Nearly 90% of the patients are between 10 and 30 years old. About 60% of the patients are boys or men.

Lesions.   Over 50% of Ewing's tumors arise in a long bone, 10% of them in the upper end of a humerus, 10% in the upper end of a femur, 10% in the shaft of a femur, and 5% in the lower end of a femur, and 5% in the upper end of a tibia. Less than 10% arise in a rib, 5% in the sacrum, and 5% in the short bones of a foot. Rarely, a similar tumor arises in the soft tissues.

A Ewing's tumor arises within the bone. It extends along the marrow cavity, eroding and destroying the bone. Usually the tumor in the medulla extends far beyond its apparent margin. The overlying cortex is thinned and often expanded. Sometimes concentric rings of subperiosteal bone are deposited around the tumor. Frequently the tumor breaches the periosteum and invades the soft tissues extensively. On section, the

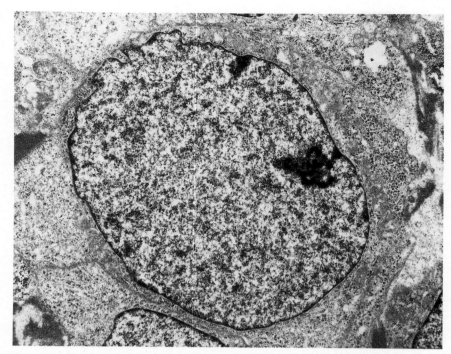

Fig. 59-16. A Ewing's tumor showing the sparse cytoplasm of the tumor cells with few organelles. (Courtesy of Dr. Y. Bédard)

tumor is soft, glistening, grayish. Often it is largely necrotic or hemorrhagic. Sometimes it is almost liquid, like pus.

Microscopically, a Ewing's tumor consists of sheets of closely packed round or spindle-shaped tumor cells. The cells have regular, spheroidal, or ovoid nuclei about twice the diameter of the nucleus of a lymphocyte. The nuclei have fine, granular nucleoplasm and often one or more nucleoli. Mitoses are usually few. The cytoplasm of the tumor cells is sparse and ill defined. Often it contains glycogen and stains with the periodic acid-Schiff reaction. Necrosis is frequently extensive. In the necrotic regions, the tumor cells are often smaller and have more clearly demarcated cytoplasm. In places, only the tumor cells surrounding small blood vessels survive. Sometimes neutrophils are present in the necrotic regions. Occasionally the tumor cells form structures like the rosettes of a neuroblastoma. Electron microscopy shows that the tumor cells are much simplified, with few organelles.

Behavior. A Ewing's tumor grows rapidly and metastasizes soon and widely. Hematogenous metastases are present in the lungs and bones in more than 50% of the patients and are often numerous. Other organs are commonly involved. Metastases in lymph nodes are present in 20% of the patients.

Clinical Presentation. Pain often draws attention to a Ewing's tumor. The pain is at first intermittent, but increases in severity. Sometimes a mass is the first sign of the tumor. Many of the patients have a fever of 38°C, mild anemia, an increased erythrocyte sedimentation rate, and a mild leukocytosis.

Pathogenesis. The origin of a Ewing's tumor is unknown. The tumor cells do not have the markers of a lymphoma or any other kind of hematopoietic tumor. They do not stain for desmin, vimentin, or keratin like mesenchymal tumors. They do not contain neurosecretory granules or stain for neuron-specific esterase or other markers of neural tumors.

Treatment and Prognosis. Radiation and chemotherapy allow 40% of patients with a

Ewing's tumor to survive more than five years, including some with metastases. Some patients seem to have been cured.

Chordoma. A chordoma is derived from remnants of the notochord. About 5% of primary malignant bone tumors are chordomata. The patients are usually over 30 years old. Over 60% of them are men.

Chordomata arise in the midline. Over 50% of them originate in the sacrococcygeal region and 35% in the spheno-occipital region. The rest arise in a vertebra. Small rests of notochordal tissue called ecchordoses are common in these regions.

A chordoma erodes the bone in which it arises and protrudes from it. A sacrococcygeal chordoma usually destroys much of the sacrum and coccyx and forms a well-defined mass 5 to 10 cm across that bulges from the anterior surface of the sacrum into the pelvis. A spheno-occipital chordoma is usually about 5 cm across and bulges into the cranial cavity, distorting the base of the brain. Occasionally a cranial chordoma bulges into a nasal sinus or the nasopharynx. The tumor bulging from the bone is usually covered by intact periosteum. On section, the tumor is lobulated. It consists of firm, translucent material like cartilage or of slimy, mucoid tissue. Foci of hemorrhage are common. Occasionally part of the tumor is calcified.

Microscopically, a chordoma consists of lobules of tumor separated by collagenous septa. Often the structure of the tumor differs from one lobule to another. Frequently much of the tumor consists of ill-defined strands of tumor cells separated by abundant mucinous intercellular substance. Often part resembles a chondrosarcoma, with tumor cells separated by cartilage-like material. Usually cells distended by droplets of mucus in their cytoplasm, called physaliphorous cells, from the Greek words for bubble and bearer, are present in some part of the tumor. Occasionally some of the lobules consist of closely packed tumor cells with little or no mucus in their cytoplasm and little intercellular substance. In some chordomata, the tumor cells vary in size and shape. In some, a few mitoses are present.

Most chordomata grow slowly. They press on adjacent structures, but only late in the course do they breach the periosteum and invade it. Hematogenous metastases are present in 10% of the patients when the tumor is discovered and become more likely if the tumor recurs after incomplete removal. Often the metastases are in unusual sites.

Pain is usually the first symptom in patients with a sacrococcygeal chordoma. Occasionally pressure on nerve roots or constipation caused by the extension of the tumor into the pelvis draws attention to the lesion. Spheno-occipital chordomata are usually discovered when the enlarging tumor presses on the optic nerves or other intracranial nerves or compresses the pituitary gland. The first manifestation of a vertebral chordoma is commonly compression of a spinal nerve.

Chordomata are treated by excision or irradiation. If the tumor is not completely eradicated, it is likely to recur. Partial

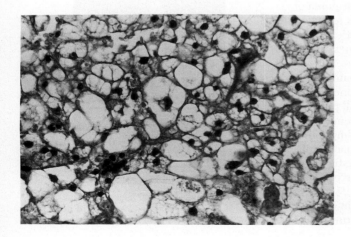

Fig. 59-17. A chordoma showing the physaliphorous cells often present in these tumors.

removal often relieves the symptoms for several years, but eventually local complications caused by the slow growth of the tumor are likely to cause death. Over 50% of patients with a spheno-occipital chordoma that is partly or largely chondroid are alive 15 years after the discovery of the tumor, but few patients with other types of cranial chordoma survive 10 years.

ADAMANTINOMA OF A LONG BONE. Less than 0.5% of malignant tumors primary in a bone other than a maxilla or mandible are epithelial lesions. The tumor presumably arises from eipthlium implanted in the bone. It is called an adamantinoma, because the lesion is often similar to an adamantinoma or ameloblastoma of a jaw. Most patients are between 10 and 50 years old when the tumor is discovered. Men and women are affected equally.

Extraoral adamantinomata are always in a long bone. Over 90% of them are in a tibia. Rarely, a similar tumor arises in the soft tissues adjacent to a long bone. The tumor is usually over 5 cm in greatest dimension when it is discoverd. It destroys and distorts the bone. Macroscopically, it is well demarcated, sometimes soft, sometimes hard, often cystic. Microscopically, many adamantinomata of a long bone resemble an ameloblastoma of the jaws. Some are more like a basal cell carcinoma of the skin. Some contain clumps of cells that resemble a squamous cell carcinoma.

Most adamantinomata of a long bone grow slowly. Many years often pass before the tumor becomes painful or the patient notices a mass. Radical excision of an adamantinoma of a long bone cures. Local excision is followed by recurrence in 70% of the patients. In some, metastases to the lungs, bones, liver, or lymph nodes has caused death.

HEMATOPOIETIC TUMORS. Hematopoietic tumors frequently involve the bones. The bone marrow is affected in almost all patients with multiple myeloma or leukemia and frequently in patients with lymphoma. Myelofibrosis, Waldenström's macroglobulinemia, and other non-neoplastic proliferations of hematopoietic cells involve the bones.

Occasionally a lymphoma arises in a bone. About 5% of primary malignant tumors of bone are lymphomata. Most of the patients are adult. Over 60% of them are men. Any bone can be involved. The lymphoma erodes the bone, often destroying much of it. It erodes or thickens the cortex. Usually the tumor has extended into the surrounding soft tissues by the time it is discovered. Microscopically, most lymphomata primary in bone are poorly differentiated B cell tumors. Formerly, they were called reticulum cell sarcomata. The lymphoma is treated with radiation and chemotherapy, like other lymphomata. Nearly 50% of the patients are alive five years after the tumor is discovered.

SECONDARY TUMORS. Metastases in the bones are found in over 25% of patients dying of cancer and are often multiple. They are more than 50 times more frequent than are primary malignant tumors of bone. Car-

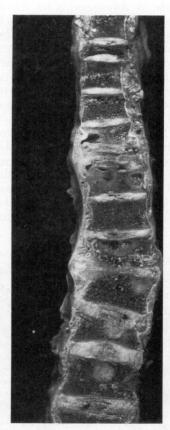

Fig. 59-18. Metastatic carcinoma, showing the destruction of some vertebrae and spheroidal deposits of tumor in others.

cinomata of the breasts, lungs, kidneys, prostate, and intestine are among the cancers that most commonly spread to the bones.

Most bony metastases are caused by tumor cells that reach the bones in the arterial blood or in the venous blood of the paravertebral plexus. The vertebrae, pelvis, ribs, skull, sternum, and upper ends of the femora are the bones most often involved. Most bony metastases are lytic and destroy bone. Some, especially metastatic carcinoma of the prostate, cause new bone formation and osteosclerosis. Occasionally bony metastases cause leukoerythroblastic anemia or hypercalcemia. Pain caused by bony metastases sometimes develops before the metastases are demonstrable radiologically. In most patients, the structure of the metastases is similar to that of the primary tumor.

BIBLIOGRAPHY

General

Frisch, B., Lewis, S. M., Burkhardt, R., and Bartl, R: Biopsy Pathology of Bone and Bone Marrow. London, Chapman and Hall, 1985.

Kelsey, J. L., and Hochberg, M. C.: Epidemiology of chronic musculoskeletal disorders. Annu. Rev. Public Health, 9:379, 1988.

Revell, P. A.: Pathology of Bone. New York, Springer-Verlag, 1986.

Infection

Emslie, K. R., and Nade, S: Pathogenesis and treatment of acute hematogenous osteomyelitis. Rev. Infect. Dis., 8:841, 1986.

Fink, C. W., and Nelson, J. D.: Septic arthritis and osteomyelitis in children. Clin. Rheum. Dis., 12:423, 1986.

Green, N. E., and Edwards, K.: Bone and joint infections in children. Orthop. Clin. North Am., 18:555, 1987.

Karlin, J. M.: Osteomyelitis in children. Clin. Podiatr. Med. Surg., 4:37, 1987.

Physical and Chemical Injury

Bikle, D. D.: Effects of alcohol on bone. Compr. Ther., 14:16, 1988.

Black, J.: Metallic ion release and its relationship to oncogensis. Hip. 199, 1985. (Review)

Krishnamachari, A.K.: Skeletal fluorosis in humans. Prog. Food Nutr. Sci., 10:279, 1986.

Michel, L. J.: Traction apophysitises. Clin. Sports Med., 6:389, 1987.

Parfitt, A.M.: Trabecular bone architecture in the pathogenesis and prevention of fractures. Am. J. Med., 82(1B):68, 1987.

Peck, W. A.: Falls and hip fracture in the elderly. Hosp. Pract., 21(12):72A, 1986.

Riggs, B. L., and Melton, L. J., III: Osteoporosis and age-related fracture syndromes. Ciba Found. Symp., 134:129, 1988.

Smith, G. E.: Fluoride, teeth and bone. Med. J. Aust., 143: 283, 1985.

Metabolic Bone Disease

Angus, R. M., and Eisman, J. A.: Osteoporosis: the role of calcium intake and supplementation. Med. J. Aust., 148:630, 1988.

Bauer, T. W., Licata, A. A., and Stulberg, B. N.: Skeletal pathology in endocrine disease. In Diagnosis and Pathology of Endocrine Diseases. Edited by G. Mendelsohn. Philadelphia. J. B. Lippincott, 1988.

Bauwens, S. F., Drinka, P. J., and Boh, L. E.: Pathogenesis and management of primary osteoporosis. Clin. Pharm., 5:639, 1986.

Brautbar, N., and Gruber, H. E.: Magnesium and bone disease. Nephron, 44:1, 1986.

Chan, J. C., Alon, U., and Hirschman, G. M.: Renal hypophosphatemic rickets. J. Pediatr., 106:533, 1985.

Chesney, R. W., et al.: Renal osteodystrophy in children: the role of vitamin D. phosphorus, and the parathyroid hormone. Am. J. Kidney Dis., 7:275, 1986.

Coburn, J. W., and Henry, D. A.: Renal osteodystrophy. Adv. Intern. Med., 30: 387, 1984.

Coburn, J. W., Norris, K. C., and Nebeker, H. G.: Osteomalacia and bone disease arising from aluminum. Semin. Nephrol., 6:68, 1986.

Compston, J. E.: Hepatic osteodystrophy. Gut, 27: 1073, 1986.

Cummings, S. R., Kelsey, J. L., Nevitt, M. C., and O'Dowd, K. J.: Epidemiology of osteoporosis and osteoporotic fractures. Epidemiol. Rev., 7:178, 1985.

Cundy, T., et al. Hyperparathyroid bone disease in chronic renal failure. Ulster Med. J., 54(Suppl.): S334, 1985.

Cushner, H. M., and Adams, N. D.: Renal osteodystrophy—pathogenesis and treatment. Am. J. Med. Sci., 291:264, 1986.

Dequeler, J.: The relationship between osteoporosis and osteoarthritis. Clin. Rheum. Dis., 11:271, 1985.

Doppelt, S. H.: Vitamin D, rickets and osteomalacia. Orthoped. Clin. North Am., 15:671, 1984.

Eastell, R., and Riggs, B. L.: Calcium homeostasis and osteoporosis. Endocrinol. Metab. Clin. North Am., 16:829, 1987.

Ellis, H. A.: Metabolic bone disease. Rec. Adv. Histopathol., 11:185, 1981.

Eriksen, E. F.: Normal and pathological remodelling of human trabecular bone. Endocr. Rev., 7:379, 1986.

Felsenfeld, A., and Llach, F.: Vitamin D and metabolic bone disease. Pathol. Annu., 17(Pt. 1):383, 1982.

Frost, H. M.: The pathomechanics of osteoporoses.

Clin. Orthop., *200*:198, 1985.

Glew, R. H., Basu, A., Prence, E. M., and Remaley, A.T.: Lysosomal storage disease. Lab. Invest., *53*:250, 1985.

Gruber, H. E., and Singer, F. R.: The spectrum of pathology of osteomalacia. Appl. Pathol., *5*:160, 1987.

Hayward, M., and Fielder-Nagy, C. L.: Mechanisms of bone loss: rheumatoid arthritis, periodontal disease and osteoporosis. Agents Action, *22*:251, 1987.

Heaf, J. G.: Hepatic osteodystrophy. Scand. J. Gastroenterol., *20*:1035, 1985.

Hodgson, S. F.: Skeletal remodelling and renal osteodystrophy. Semin. Nephrol., *6*:42, 1986.

Klein, G. L., and Coburn, J. W.: Metabolic bone disease associated with total parenteral nutrition. Adv. Nutr. Res., *6*:76, 1984.

Kornfeld, S., and Sly, W. S.: Lysosomal storage defects. Hosp. Pract., *20*(8):71, 1985.

Lane, J. M., Cornell, C. N., and Healy, J. H.: Osteoporosis: the structural and reparative consequences. Instr. Course Lect., *36*:71, 1987.

Lane, J. M., and Vigorita, V. J.: Osteoporosis. Orthop. Clin. North Am., *15*:711, 1984.

Lane, J. M., Werntz, J.., Healey, J. H. and Vigorita, V. J.: Metabolic bone disease and Paget's disease in the elderly. Part I. Metaoblic bone disease. Clin. Rheum. Dis., *12*:48, 1986.

Lee, D. B., Goodman, W. G., and Coburn, J. W.: Renal osteodystrophy. Am. J. Kidney Dis., *11*:365, 1988.

Liberman, U. A., Eil, C., and Marx, S. J.: Clinical features of hereditary resistance to 1, 25-dihydroxyvitamin D (hereditary hypocalcemic vitamin D resistant rickets type II). Adv. Exp. Med. Biol., *196*:391, 1986.

Lindsay, R.: Osteoporosis. Clin. Geriatr. Med., *4*:411, 1988.

Lloyd, C. W., and Johnson, C. E.: Management of hypophosphatemia. Clin. Pharm., *7*:123, 1988.

McKenna, M. J., and Frame, B.: Hormonal influences on osteoporosis Am. J. Med., *82*:(1B):61, 1987.

Marks, S. C., Jr: Osteoporosis—multiple pathways for the interception of osteoclastic function. Appl. Pathol., *5*:172, 1987.

Muenzer, J.: Mucopolysaccharidoses. Adv. Pediatr., *33*:269, 1986.

Mundy, G. R.: Osteopenia. Dis. Mon., *33*:537, 1987.

Nebeker, H. G., and Coburn, J. W.: Aluminum and renal osteodystrophy. Annu. Rev. Med., *37*:79, 1986.

Nordin, B.E.C., Need, A. G., Morris, H. A., and Horowitz, M.: New approaches to the problems of osteoporosis. Clin. Orthop., *200*:181, 1985.

Norris, K. C., et al.: Iliac crest biopsy for diagnosis of aluminum toxicity. Semin. Nephrol., *6*(4 Suppl. 1):27, 1986.

Orwoll, E. S., and Belsey, R. E.: The laboratory evaluation of osteopenia. Clin. Lab. Med., *4*:763, 1984.

Raisz, L. G.: Local and systemic factors in the pathogenesis of osteoporosis. N. Engl. J. Med., *318*:818, 1988.

Reeve, J., and Zanelli, J. M.: Parathyroid hormone and bone. Clin. Sci., *71*:231, 1986.

Riggs, B. L., and Melton, L. J., III: Involutional osteoporosis. N. Engl. J. Med., *314*:1676, 1986.

Riggs, B. L., and Melton, L. J., III: Osteoporosis and age-related fracture syndromes. Ciba Found. Symp., *134*:129, 1988.

Rodysill, K. J.: Postmenopausal osteoporosis. Chronic Dis., *40*:743, 1987.

Rush, P. J., et al.: The musculoskeletal manifestations of cystic fibrosis. Semin. Arthritis Rheum., *15*:213, 1986.

Savory, J., Berthoff, R. L., and Wills, M. R.: Aluminium toxicity in chronic renal insufficiency. Clin. Endocrinol. Metab., *14*:681, 1985.

Schaafsma, G., van Beresteyn, E.C.H., Raymakers, J. A., and Duursma, S. A.: Nutritional aspects of osteoporosis. World Rev. Nutr. Diet., *49*:121, 1987.

Selby, P. L., and Francis, R. M.: Endocrinology and osteoporosis. J. Endocrinol., *117*:1, 1988.

Sherrard, D. J.: Renal osteodystrophy. Semin. Nephrol., *6*:56, 1986.

Silberberg, R.: The skeleton in diabetes mellitus. Diabetes Res., *3*:329, 1986.

Silverberg, S. J., and Lindsay, R.: Postmenopausal osteoporosis. Med. Clin. North Am., *71*:41, 1987.

Smith, R.: Osteoporosis: cause and management. Br. Med. J., *294*:329, 1987.

Spranger, J: Inborn errors of complex carbohydrate metabolism. Am. J. Med. Genet., *28*:489, 1987.

Sterrett, J. D.: The osteoclast and periodontitis. J. Clin Periodontol., *13*:258, 1986.

Stulberg, B. N., Licata, A. A., Bauer, T. W., and Belhobek, G. H.: Hyperparathryoidism, hyperthyroidism and Cushing's disease. Orthop. Clin. North Am., *15*:697, 1984.

Teitelbaum, S. L.: Renal osteodystrophy. Hum. Pathol., *15*:306, 1984.

Vick, K. E., and Johnson, C. A.: Aluminum-related osteomalacia in renal-failure patients. Clin. Pharm., *4*:434, 1985.

Vigorita, V. J.: Osteoporosis: a diagnosable disorder? Pathol. Annu., *23*(Pt. 2):185, 1988.

Wasserman, S.H.S., and Barzel, U. S.: Osteoporosis. Semin. Nuc. Med., *17*:283, 1987.

Westrich, B. J.: Effect of physical activity on skeletal integrity and its implications for calcium requirement studies. Nutr. Health, *5*:53, 1987.

Hyperostosis

Altman, R. D.: Paget's disease of bone. Bull. Rheum. Dis., *34*(3):1, 1984.

Avioli, L. V.: Paget's disease. Clin. Ther., *9*:567, 1987.

Freeman, D. A.: Paget's disease of bone. Am. J. Med. Sci., *295*:144, 1988.

Hansen-Flaschen, J., and Nordberg, J.: Clubbing and osteoarthropathy. Clin. Chest Med., *8*:287, 1987.

Kerkow, R. L., and Lane, J. M.: Metabolic bone disease and Paget's disease in the elderly. Part II. Paget's disease. Clin. Rheum. Dis., *12*:70, 1986.

Kruger, G. D., Rock, M. G., and Munro, T. G.: Condensing osteitis of the clavicle. J. Bone Joint Surg. (Am), *69*:550, 1987.

Merkow, R. L., and Lane, J. M.: Current concepts of Paget's disease of bone. Orthop. Clin. North Am., *15*:747, 1984.

Outwater, E., and Oates, E.: Condensing osteitis of

the clavicle J. Nucl. Med., 29:1122, 1988.

Pinenda, C. J., et al.: The skeletal manifestations of clubbing. Semin. Arthritis Rheum., 14:263, 1985.

Rebel, A. (Ed.): Paget's disease. Clin. Orthop., 217:2, 1987.

Resnik, C. S., Waters, B. K., and Wilkin, J. K.: Sternoclavicular hyperostosis. South. Med. J., 80:577, 1987.

Rothschild, B. M.: Diffuse idiopathic skeletal hyperostosis. Compr. Ther., 14:65–69, 1988.

Talab, Y. A., and Mallouh, A.: Hyperostosis with hyperphosphatemia J. Pediatr. Orthop., 8:338, 1988.

Utsinger, P. D.: Diffuse idiopathic skeletal hyperostosis. Clin. Rheum. Dis., 11:325, 1985.

Aseptic necrosis

Alexander, A. H., and Lichtman, D. M.: Keinböck's disease. Orthop. Clin. North Am., 17:461, 1986.

Calder, I. M.: Bone and joint diseases in workers exposed to hyperbaric conditions. Curr. Top. Pathol., 71:103, 1982.

Cruess, R. L.: Osteonecrosis of bone. Current concepts as to etiology and pathogenesis. Clin. Orthop., 208:30, 1986.

Gemne, G., and Sarasate, H.: Bone and joint pathology in workers using hand-held vibrating tools. Scand. J. Work Environ. Health, 13:290, 1987.

Hungerford, D. S., and Lennox, D. W.: The importance of increased intraosseous pressure in the development of osteonecrosis of the femoral head. Orthop. Clin. North Am., 16:635, 1985.

Jones, J. P., Jr.: Fat embolism and osteonecrosis. Orthop. Clin. North Am., 16:595, 1985.

Kaklamanis, P.: Osteoarticular manifestations of sickle-cell disorders. Clin. Rheumatol., 3:419, 1984.

Lotke, P. A., and Ecker, M. L.: Osteonecrosis of the knee. J. Bone Joint Surg. (Am.), 70:470, 1988.

Palmer, A. J.: Kienbock's disease. J. Hand Surg. (Br.), 12:291, 1987.

Seale, J. P., and Compton, M. R.: Side-effects of corticosteroid agents. Med. J. Aust., 144:139, 1986.

Thomson, G. H., and Salter, R. B.: Legg-Calvé-Perthes Disease. Clin. Symp., 38(3):1, 1986.

Weinstein, S. L.: Legg-Calvé-Perthes disease: results of long-term follow-up. Hip. p 28–37, 1985 (Review).

Congenital anomalies

Benson, D. R.: Idiopathic scoliosis. Orthopedics, 10:1691, 1987.

Borochowitz, Z., et al.: Achondrogenesis type I. J. Pediatr., 112:23, 1988.

Bradway, J. K., Klassen, R. A., and Peterson, H. A,: Blount disease. J. Pediatr, Orthop., 7:472, 1987.

Carty, H.: Brittle or battered. Arch. Dis. Child., 63:350, 1988.

Eteson, D. J., and Stewart, R. E.: Craniofacial defects in the human skeletal dysplasias. Birth Defects, 20:19, 1984.

Frost, H. M.: Osteogenesis imperfecta. Clin. Orthop., 216:280, 1987.

Gilbert, E. F., et al.: Pathologic changes of osteochon-

drodysplasia in infancy. Pathol. Annu., 22(Pt. 2): 283, 1987.

Goldberg, M. J., and Bartoshesky, L. E.: Congenital hand anomaly. Hand Clin., 1:405, 1985.

Hall, J. G., Dorst, J. P., Rotta, J., and McKusick, V. A.: Gonadal mosaicism in pseudoachrondroplasia. Am. J. Med. Genet., 28:143, 1987.

Jacobson, R. I.: Abnormalities of the skull in children. Neurol. Clin., 3:117, 1985.

Johnson, J., and Omer, G. E., Jr.: Congenital ulnar deficiency. Hand Clin., 1:499, 1985.

Kalen, V., Burwell, D. S., and Omer, G. E.: Macrodactyly of the hands and feet. J. Pediatr. Orthop., 8:311, 1988.

Kling, T. F., Jr.: Angular deformities of the lower limbs in children. Orthop. Clin. North Am., 18:513, 1987.

Kornreich, L., et al.: Osteopathia striata, cranial sclerosis with cleft palate and facial nerve palsy. Eur. J. Pediatr., 147:101, 1988.

Lachman, R. S., Rimoin, D. L., and Spranger, J.: Metaphyseal chondrodysplasia, Schmid type. Pediatr Radiol., 181:93, 1988.

Lamesch, A. J., and Jaquemart, J.: Dysplasia epiphysealis hemimelia. Bull. Soc. Sci. Med. Grand Duché Luxemb., 125(Spec. No): 84, 1988.

Langer, L. O., Jr., et al.: Thanatophoric dysplasia and cloverleaf skull. Am. J. Med. Genet. (Suppl.), 3:167, 1987.

Lin, A. E., and Perloff, J. K.: Upper limb malformations associated with congenital heart disease. Am. J. Cardiol., 55:1576, 1985.

Pyeritz, R. E.: Interitable defects in connective tissue. Hosp. Pract., 22(2):153, 1987.

Root, L.: The treatment of osteogenesis imperfecta. Orthop. Clin. North Am., 15:775, 1984.

Silman, A. J.: Musculo-skeletal disorders in childhood. Br. Med Bull., 42:196, 1986.

Simmons, B. P.: Polydactyly. Hand Clin., 1:545, 1986.

Stanescu, V., Stanescu, R., and Maroteaux, P.: Pathogenic mechanisms in osteochrondrodystrophies. J. Bone Joint Surg., A66:817, 1984.

Stanescu, V., Stanescu, R., and Maroteaux, P.: Articular degeneration as a sequella of osteochrondrodysplasias. Clin. Rheum. Dis., 11:239, 1985.

Taitz, L. S.: Child abuse and osteogenesis imperfecta. Br. Med. J., 295:1082, 1987.

Thomas, R. L., Hess, L. W., and Johnson, T. R.: Prepartum diagnosis of limb-shortening defects associated with hydramnios. Am. J. Perionatol., 4:293, 1987.

Udell, J., Schumacher, H. R., Jr., Kaplan. F., and Fallon, M. D.: Idiopathic familial acroosteolysis. Arthritis Rheum., 29:1032, 1986.

Yabut, S. M., Jr., Kenan, S., Sissons, H. A., and Lewis, M. M.: Malignant transformation of fibrous dysplasia. Clin. Orthop., 228:281, 1988.

Younai, F., Eisenbud, L., and Sciubba, J. J.: Osteopetrosis. Oral Surg., 65:214, 1988.

Tumor-like conditions

Danon, M., and Crawford, J. D.: The McCune-Albright syndrome. Ergeb. Inn. Med. Kinderheilkd., 55:81, 1987.

Forssell, K., Forssell, H., Happonen, R.-P., and Neva, M.: Simple bone cyst. Int. J. Oral. Maxillofac. Surg., 17:21, 1988.

Moule, I: Unilateral multiple solitary bone cysts. J. Oral Maxillofac. Surg., 46:320, 1988.

Nigrisoli, M.: Monostotic fibrous dysplasia of the spine. Ital. J. Orthop. Traumatol., 13:273, 1987.

Osband, M. E.: Histiocytosis X. Hematol. Oncol. Clin. North Am., 1:737, 1987.

Osband, M. E., and Pochedly, C. (Eds.): Histiocytosis X. Hematol. Oncol. Clin. North Am., 1:1, 1987.

Patel, S. C., and Sanders, W. P.: Synovial cyst of the cervical spine. Am. J. Neuroradiol., 9:602, 1988.

Riccardi, V. M.: Neurofibromatosis and Albright's syndrome. Dermatol. Clin., 5:193, 1987.

Rosenblum, B., et al.: Monostotic fibrous dysplasia of the thoracic spine. Spine, 12:939, 1987.

Unni, K. K., McLeod, R. A., and Dahlin, D. C.: Conditions that simulate primary neoplasms of bone. Pathol. Annu., 15(Pt. 1):91, 1980.

Tumors

Altmannsberger, W., and Osborn, M.: Mesenchymal tumor markers: intermediate filaments. Curr. Top. Pathol., 777:155, 1987.

Bramwell, V. H., et al.: Review of the clinical trials activity of the soft tissue and bone sarcoma group of the European Organization for Research and Treatment of Cancer. Semin. Surg. Oncol., 4:45, 1988.

Carter, J. R., and Abdul-Karim, F.W.: Pathology of childhood osteosarcoma. Perspect. Pediatr. Pathol., 9:133, 1987.

Carter, R. L.: Patterns and mechanisms of localized bone invasion by tumors: studies with squamous cell carcinoma of the head and neck. CRC Crit. Rev. Clin. Lab. Sci., 22:275, 1985.

Coleman, R. E., and Rubens, R. D.: Bone metastases and breast cancer. Cancer Treat. Rev., 12:251, 1985.

Crawford, A. H., Jr., and Bagamery, N.: Osseous manifestations of neurofibromatosis in childhood. J. Pediatr. Orthop., 6:72, 1986.

Dahlin, D. C., and Unni, K. K.: Bone Tumors. 4th Ed. Springfield, Charles C Thomas. 1986.

Dehner, L. P.: Mesenchymal neoplasms in childhood. Am. J. Surg. Pathol., 10(Suppl. 1): 32, 1986.

Eckardt, J. J., and Grogan, T. J.: Giant cell tumor of bone. Clin. Orthop., 204:45, 1986.

Ein, S. H., Mancer, K., and Adeyemi, S. D.: Malignant sacrococcygeal teratoma. J. Pediatr. Surg., 20:473, 1985.

Elte, J. W., et al.: Osteolytic bone metastasis in breast carcinoma. Eur. J. Cancer Clin. Oncol., 22:493, 1986.

Fletcher, C. D., and Krausz, T.: Cartilagenous tumors of soft tissue. Appl. Pathol., 3:208, 1988.

Fletcher, C. D., and McKee, P. H.: Sarcomas: a clinicopathological guide with particular reference to cutaneous manifestations. IV. Extraskeletal osteosarcoma, extraskeletal chrondrosarcoma, alveolar soft part sarcoma, clear cell carcinoma. Clin. Exp. Dermatol., 10:523, 1985.

Foucher, G., Lemarechal, P., Citron, N., and Merle, M.: Osteoid osteoma of the terminal phalanx. J. Hand Surg. (Br.), 12:382, 1987.

Freiberg, T. A.,: Hembree, S. L., and Laine, W.: Periosteal chondroma. J. Foot Surg., 25:54, 1986.

Fujii, N., and Eliseo, M.L.T.: Chondromyxoid fibroma of the maxilla. J. Oral Maxillofac. Surg., 46:235, 1988.

Garrington, G. E., and Collet, W. K.: Chondrosarcoma. J. Oral Pathol., 17:1, 1988.

Gill, M., McCarthy, M., Murrells, T., and Silcocks, P.: Chemotherapy for the primary treatment of osteosarcoma. Lancet, 1:689, 1988.

Goldring, S. R. et al: Characterization of cells from human giant cell tumors of bone. Clin. Orthop., 204:59, 1986.

Goorin, A. M., Abelson, H. T. and Frei, E. III: Osteosarcoma. N. Engl. J. Med., 313:1637, 1985.

Hajdu, S. I.: Differential Diagnosis of Soft Tissue and Bone Tumors. Philadelphia, Lea & Febiger, 1986.

Harsanyi, B. B., and Larsson, A.: Xanthomatous lesions of the mandible. Oral Surg., Oral Med., Oral Pathol., 65:551, 1988.

Hertler, A. A., and Moore, J. O.: Sarcomas in the elderly. Clin. Geriatr. Med., 3:781, 1987.

von Hochstetter, A. R., Hättenschwiler, J., and Vogt, M.: Primary osteosarcoma of the liver. Cancer, 60:2312, 1987.

Huebner, G. R., Brenneise, C. V., and Ballenger, J.: Central ossifying fibroma of the anterior maxilla. J. Am. Dental. Assoc., 116:507, 1988.

Huvos, A. G.: Surgical pathology of bone sarcomas. World J. Surg., 12:284, 1988.

Johnston, A. D.: Giant cell lesions of bone. Prog. Surg. Pathol., 4:217, 1982.

Kespi, Y. P., Leving, T. M., and Oppenheimer, R.: Skull base chordomas. Otolaryngol. Clin. North Am., 19:797, 1986.

Kessler, E., and Brandt-Rauf, P. W.: Occupational cancers of brain and bone. State Art Rev. Occup. Med., 2:155, 1987.

Kochersberger, G. G., and Lyles, K. W.: Skeletal disorders in malignant disease. Clin. Geriatr. Med., 3:561, 1987.

Krespi, J. P., Levine, T. M., and Oppenheimer, R.: Skull base chordomas. Otolaryngol. Clin. North Am., 19:797, 1986.

Lewis, M. M., Sissons, H.A., Norman. A., and Greenspan, A.: Benign and malignant cartilage tumors. Instr. Course Lect., 36:87, 1987.

Llombart-Bosch, A., Blache, R., and Peydro-Olaya, A.: Round-cell sarcomas of bone. Pathol. Annu., 17(Pt. 2):113, 1982.

Mankin, H. J., and Gebhardt, M. C.: Advances in the management of bone tumors. Clin. Orthop., 200:73, 1985.

Meyers, P. A.: Malignant bone tumors in children: osteosarcoma. Hematol. Oncol. Clin. North Am., 1:655, 1987.

Meyers, P. A.: Malignant bone tumors in children: Ewing's tumor. Hematol. Oncol. Clin. North Am., 1:667, 1987.

Miller- Breslow, A., and Dorfman, H. D.: Dupuytren's (subungual) exostosis. Am. J. Surg. Pathol., 12:368, 1988.

Mirra, J. M.: Bone Tumors. Philadelphia. J. B. Lippincott Co., 1980.

Mirra, J. M., Kameda, N., Rosen, G., and Eckardt, J.: Primary osteosarcoma of toe phalanx. Am. J. Surg. Pathol., 12:300, 1988.

Otto, H. F., Berndt, R., Schwechheimer, K., and Möller, P.: Mesenchymal tumor markers: special proteins and enzymes. Curr. Top. Pathol., 77:179, 1987.

Paterson, A. H.: Bone metastases in breast cancer, prostate cancer and myeloma. Bone, 8(Suppl. 1):S17, 1987.

Poleduak, A. P.: Human biology and epidemiology of childhood bone cancers. Hum. Biol., 57:1, 1985.

Povyšil, C.: Histopathology and ultrastructure of tumours and tumour-like lesions of bone. Acta Univ. Carol. (Med. Monogr.), 116:1, 1986.

Raymond, A. K., et al: Osteosarcoma: chemotherapy effect. Semin. Diagn. Pathol., 4:212, 1987.

Reiman, H. M., and Dahlin, H. C.: Cartilage-and bone-forming tumors of the soft tissues. Diagn. Pathol., 3:288, 1986.

Robinson, E., Neugut, A. I., and Wylie, P.: Clinical aspects of postirradiation sarcoma. J. Natl. Cancer Inst., 80:233, 1988.

Roessner, A., and Grundmann, E.: Electron microscopy in bone tumor diagnosis. Curr. Top. Pathol., 71:153, 1982.

Rosen, G.: Bone and soft part sarcomas. Surf. Annu., 20:121, 1988.

Schajowicz, F.: Tumors and tumorlike lesions of bone and joints. New York, Springer-Verlag, 1981.

Scher, H. I., and Yagoda, A: Bone metastases. Am. J. Med., 82(2A):6, 1987.

Schubiner, J. M., and Simon, M.A.: Primary bone tumors in children. Orthop. Clin. North Am., 18:577, 1987.

Shankman, S., Green span, A., Klein, M. J., and Lewis, M. M: Giant cell tumor of the ischium. Skeletal Radiol., 17:46, 1988.

Sim. F. H.: Musculoskeletal oncology. Orthopedics, 10:1673, 1987.

Singh, W., and Kaur, A.: Nasopharyngeal chordoma presenting with metastases. J. Laryngol. Otol., 101:1198, 1987.

Spjut, H. J., Dorfman, H. D., Fechner, R. E., and Ackerman, L. V.: Tumors of Bone and Cartilage. Washington D. C., Armed Forces Institute of Pathology, 1971.

Spjut, H. J., Fechner, R. E., and Ackerman, L. V.: Tumors of Bone and Cartilage, Supplement. Washington D. C., Armed Forces Institute of Pathology, 1981.

Unni, K. K. (Ed.): Bone tumors. Contemp. Issues Surg. Pathol., 11:1, 1988.

Wold, L. E., Swee, R. G., and Sim, F. H.: Vascular lesions of bone. Pathol. Annu., 20(Pt. 2):101, 1985.

Wu, K. K.: Chondrosarcoma of the foot, J. Foot Surg., 26:449, 1987.

Yunis, E. J.: Ewing's sarcoma and related small round cell neoplasms in children. Am. J. Surg. Pathol., 10(Suppl. 1):54, 1986.

Yunis, E. J., and Barnes, L.: The histologic diversity of osteosarcoma. Pathol. Annu., 21(Pt. 1):121, 1986.

Zachariades, N., Vairaktaris. E., Mezitis, M., and Triantafyllou, D.: Chondrosarcoma of the orofacial region. Rev. Stomatol. Chir. Maxillofac., 88:382, 1987.

60

Joints and Tendons

INFLAMMATION of the joints is called arthritis, or less often arthropathy. Sometimes the joints are damaged by trauma. Cysts are common in and around the joints. Inflammation can injure the tendons and their sheaths. Proliferative lesions distort the aponeuroses. Tumors arise in the joints, tendons, and aponeuroses.

ARTHRITIS

The term *arthritis* is derived from the Greek for a joint. Rheumatoid arthritis and osteoarthritis are common. Gout, ankylosing spondylitis, infective arthritis, and other forms of arthritis are less frequent or less disabling.

RHEUMATOID ARTHRITIS. Rheumatoid arthritis is one of the collagen diseases. It affects principally the joints and tendons. The name was coined to distinguish rheumatoid arthritis from rheumatic arthritis. Both terms are derived from the Greek for a flowing stream or river.

In the temperate countries, 1% of the population has rheumatoid arthritis. It is less frequent in tropical regions. Over 80% of the patients are between 30 and 50 years old when the disease begins. Over 70% of them are women.

Lesions. The lesions in the joints and tendons will be discussed first, then the rheumatoid nodules common in the subcutaneous tissues, the lesions in other organs, and the rheumatoid factors present in the plasma.

Joints and Tendons. The severity of rheumatoid arthritis varies from one patient to another. It usually involves first and most severely the proximal interphalangeal and metacarpophalangeal joints in the hands, the small joints in the feet, the wrists, ankles,

elbows, and knees. The cervical spine is commonly affected, but the lumbar spine is spared. Frequently the sacroiliac, temporomandibular, and cricoarytenoid joints are involved. Other joints are involved less commonly and usually less severely. In most patients, the disease is symmetrical.

Rheumatoid arthritis begins with acute inflammation in the joints involved. The synovium is congested. Its blood vessels are dilated with an exudate of neutrophils in their walls. Some of the vessels contain thrombi. Occasional small perivascular hemorrhages are present.

Most of the lymphocytes in the exudate are T cells. Helper cells are more numerous than suppressor cells. Many of the T cells have HLA-DR antigens on their surface and secrete interleukin 2, γ-interferon, and other lymphokines. Activated macrophages form interleukin 1 and other monokines. B cells present in the exudate produce the rheumatoid factors and other immunoglobulins.

The acute reaction is soon replaced by chronic inflammation. The synovial membrane of the joints involved continues to be edematous and congested. Swollen synovial villi bulge into the joint cavity. Sometimes they are pinched between the bone ends, adding to the injury. A prominent exudate of lymphocytes, plasma cells, and macrophages is present in the synovium. Often some of the lymphocytes are aggregated into clumps around blood vessels. Occasionally germinal centers are present. Sometimes a few of the macrophages are multinucleate. The synovial cells lining the joint hypertrophy. Frequently the synovium is 6 to 10 cells thick rather than the normal 1 to 3. Often a plug of fibrin overlies a region in which the synovial cells are lost, or granulation tissue with an exudate of neutrophils forms beneath the damaged synovium. The inflammation extends into the

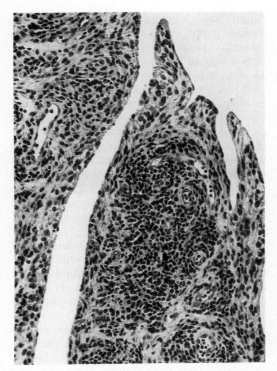

Fig. 60-1. Rheumatoid arthritis, showing inflamed synovium. Hyperplasia of the synovial cells lining the joint is not present in this picture.

capsule of the joints and into adjacent ligaments, tendons, and tendon sheaths.

The joints involved are distended by an increased quantity of turbid synovial fluid. It is less viscous than normal. The concentration of protein in the fluid is increased. Sometimes it contains enough fibrinogen to clot. The concentration of mucopolysaccharides is low, and the mucin clot that forms on acidification is small. The concentration of glucose is frequently lower than in the plasma. The fluid contains from 5 to 50,000 cells per mm^3, most of them neutrophils.

In most patients, rheumatoid arthritis is episodic, with repeated exacerbations and remissions. During the remissions, the inflammation lessens. When an exacerbation occurs, the synovium again becomes congested, edematous, and severely inflamed.

As years pass, the affected joints are damaged ever more severely. The articular cartilages and intraarticular menisci are eroded, narrowing the joint space. The loss

of cartilage is caused in part by an extension of the inflamed synovium called pannus, from the Latin for cloth, that grows across the surface of the articular cartilages and destroys them. In parts of some joints, the articular cartilage may be lost altogether, and the bone is covered only by pannus. Inflammation extends into the subchondral bone. The marrow near the joints involved becomes fibrotic. The bones become increasingly osteoporotic. The capsules of the joints and the ligaments around them become lax. Fibrosis thickens the loosened capsules of the joints and the sheaths of adjacent tendons. Bursae near the rheumatic joints are frequently inflamed, with changes in their synovium like those in the joints.

The weakening and disorganization of the joints causes subluxation, dislocation, and deformity. Muscular weakness caused by the disease adds to the deformity and further restricts function. Often the joints involved are enlarged and distorted. Radial deviation at the wrists, ulnar deviation of the fingers, and palmar subluxation of the metacarpophalangeal joints are common. Hyperextension of the proximal and flexion of the distal interphalangeal joints or flexion of the proximal and extension of the distal interphalangeal joints are common. Eversion of the feet, plantar subluxation of the heads of the metatarsal bones, hallux valgus, and lateral deviation of the toes are frequent. Damage to the diarthrodial joints can make the spine rigid. Rarely, atlantoaxial subluxation compresses the spinal cord.

Late in the disease, osteoarthritis adds to the disorganization of the joints. Adhesions between plates of pannus in a joint sometimes ossify, causing intra-articular ankylosis. Ossification of a thickened joint capsule sometimes causes extra-articular ankylosis. Adhesions often bind a tendon to its sheath, or the sheath of the tendon is narrowed, restricting its movement. A weakened tendon may stretch or rupture. Tenosynovitis sometimes compresses the medial nerve in the carpal tunnel.

Rheumatoid Nodules. One or more subcutaneous rheumatoid nodules develop in 20% of patients with rheumatoid arthritis. They are usually adjacent to a joint or bursa, often over a pressure point or in a region that suffers repeated minor trauma. Less often a rheumatoid nodule is found in a lung, in the connective tissues near the heart, in the meninges, or in some other internal organ.

Most rheumatoid nodules are between 0.2 and 2 cm across. Subcutaneous nodules cause a dome-shaped elevation in the skin. They are at first soft, but become firm. Some are slightly tender. Microscopically, the nodules have a core of fibrinoid necrosis. Often the core is stellate or irregularly shaped. The core is bordered by a palisade of macrophages that merge with dense surrounding collagenous tissue. Frequently a few lymphocytes or plasma cells are present among the macrophages. Occasionally an adjacent blood vessel shows fibrinoid necrosis or vasculitis.

Rheumatoid nodules usually cause no symptoms and no disability. Most persist with little change for years, though some eventually disappear. Similar nodules occasionally develop in people with no evidence of rheumatoid arthritis, but are usually in the dermis rather than the subcutaneous tissue.

Extra-articular Lesions. The muscles in patients with severe rheumatoid arthritis are usually weak and atrophic. The small clumps of lymphocytes called lymphorrhages are often present in them, together with a few plasma cells and macrophages. Sometimes a few of the muscle fibers show degenerative changes. Similar clumps of lymphocytes are sometimes present in nerves and tendons.

Hypersensitivity vasculitis is common in patients with rheumatoid arthritis who have a high concentration of rheumatoid factors in the plasma. In the skin, it causes brown spots in the nail beds or occasionally ischemic ulcers. In nerves, it causes sensory neuropathy or occasionally mononeuropathy multiplex. Rarely, it is severe enough to cause gangrene of fingers or toes or severe polyneuropathy or to involve the lungs, intestine, liver, or other internal organs.

Lesions in other organs are discussed with the diseases of the organ principally affected. In the lungs, rheumatoid arthritis often causes pleurisy, less frequently interstitial pneumonitis, interstitial fibrosis, Caplan's nodules, or vasculitis. Nearly 50% of the patients have pericarditis, rarely aortic regurgitation or a conduction defect. About 15% of them develop Sjögren's syndrome.

About 10% develop splenomegaly and enlarged lymph nodes. Psoriasis is unduly common. Less than 1% develop scleritis or episcleritis in the eyes. A few develop AA amyloidosis.

When rheumatoid arthritis is active, the erythrocyte sedimentation rate is high, and the concentrations of C-reactive protein and ceruloplasmin in the plasma increase. Normocytic, normochromic anemia caused by ineffective erythropoiesis is common. Occasionally there is mild leukocytosis or mild leukopenia. In the blood, the ratio of helper to suppressor T cells increases, and the number of activated T cells that express HLA-DR antigens grows.

Rheumatoid Factors. The rheumatoid factors are antibodies that react with the Fc fragment of IgG. Some rheumatoid factors are IgM, some IgG, some IgA. The tests commonly used detect principally the IgM antibodies.

Rheumatoid factors are present in the plasma in over 70% of patients with rheumatoid arthritis, more frequently and in higher titer in patients with severe, active disease. They are always present in patients with rheumatoid nodules or vasculitis and in the synovial fluid in inflamed joints. Immune complexes containing rheumatoid factors are present in the neutrophils in the fluid. The low concentration of complement in the synovial fluid suggests fixation of complement by the complexes.

Rheumatoid factors are often present in the plasma of patients with systemic lupus erythematosus, Sjögren's syndrome, liver disease, pulmonary fibrosis, sarcoidosis, leukemia, lymphoma, infective endocarditis, mononucleosis, tuberculosis, syphilis, leprosy, malaria, schistosomiasis, and other infections. The titer of the factors is usually lower than in active rheumatoid arthritis. About 5% of normal people have rheumatoid factors in the plasma; over 10% of people are over 65 years old.

Over 30% of patients with rheumatoid arthritis have antinuclear antibodies in the plasma and synovial fluid. Many of them have other autoantibodies in the blood.

Clinical Presentation. In 70% of the patients, rheumatoid arthritis develops insidiously. Often the patient feels ill, is easily tired, and has vague aches and a poor appetite for weeks or months before evidence of arthritis appears. In 30% of the patients, at first only one or a few joints are involved. In most, the disease is symmetrical from the beginning. In 10% of the patients, the onset is acute, with widespread and severe polyarthritis, fever, splenomegaly, and lymphadenopathy.

The joints affected are swollen, painful, and tender. Movement increases the pain. The overlying skin is often dusky or feels warm. The joints are stiff, especially in the morning after inactivity during the night. As the disease worsens, the joints become increasingly deformed, and their movements are increasingly limited. Injury to tendons often adds to the disability.

Lesions in extra-articular organs cause symptoms in a minority of the patients. The involvement of the lungs or heart is rarely severe enough to cause dysfunction. Occasionally vasculitis causes lesions in the skin or neuropathy, or a patient develops Sjögren's disease, lesions in the eyes, or splenomegaly.

Pathogenesis. Immunologic reactions play a major role in the pathogenesis of rheumatoid arthritis. The inflammatory reaction in the joints is similar to that in delayed hypersensitivity reactions. It seems likely that the lymphokines and monokines formed by the lymphocytes and macrophages in the inflamed joints initiate the inflammation and are a major cause of the fibrosis and damage to cartilage. Interleukin 1 is believed to be of particular importance. Chemotactic factors attract the neutrophils into the synovial fluid. The phagocytosis of immune complexes by the neutrophils in the joint fluid and the synovial cells releases lysosomal enzymes and further damages the articular cartilages and synovium. Activation of complement adds to the injury. Collagenases formed in the pannus erode the underlying cartilage. Prostaglandins help cause inflammation and osteoporosis. Circulating immune complexes formed with the rheumatoid factors are responsible for the vasculitis and the rheumatoid nodules.

The cause of the abnormal immunologic reaction is unknown. It is not known if it is a reaction to an external factor such as a virus or is due to a fault in the immune system that leads to the production of abnormal auto-antibodies, such as the rheumatoid factors.

Genetic factors are important in the causation of rheumatoid arthritis. The HLA antigen DR4 is present in 70% of Caucasian and Japanese patients with rheumatoid arthritis, in less than 30% of the control population. The association between HLA-DR4 and rheumatoid arthritis is less striking or absent in other races. Rheumatoid arthritis is four times as frequent in close relatives of patients with the disease as in the general population.

Treatment and Prognosis. In most patients, rheumatoid arthritis is mild and progresses slowly. In over 50% of the patients, it is never severe enough to restrict activity. About 25% of the patients are severely affected, but maintain a normal life. Less than 10% become completely disabled.

Aspirin and other nonsteroidal anti-inflammatory drugs are sufficient to control the pain and discomfort in most patients. If the disease is more severe, gold salts, D-penicillamine, and antimalarial drugs bring benefit in 70% of the patients, though their mode of action is uncertain. Immunosuppressive drugs also relieve 70% of the patients, but are more dangerous, especially in predisposing the patient to cancer. Glucocorticoids relieve the symptoms, but are dangerous when given for a prolonged period. Surgery is helpful in managing the deformities caused by the disease and in excising redundant synovium.

Felty's Syndrome. Felty's syndrome is named after the American physician who described it in 1924. It develops in 1% of patients with rheumatoid arthritis, usually in people with long-standing and severe disease. The patients develop splenomegaly and neutropenia. Often they have anemia and thrombocytopenia. The titer of rheumatoid factors in the plasma is usually high. Many of the patients have circulating antinuclear antibodies. Subcutaneous nodules and other manifestations of extra-articular rheumatoid disease are common. In some patients the cytopenias are due to hypersplenism. In some, splenectomy does not improve the condition. Antibodies against the neutrophils or the activation of complement by immune complexes bound to the neutrophils may be responsible for the neutropenia in these people. The lack of neutrophils and the defective function of those that remain make the patients subject to infection.

Juvenile Rheumatoid Arthritis. In 5% of people with rheumatoid arthritis, the disease develops before the patient is 16 years old. These patients are said to have juvenile rheumatoid arthritis.

In 25% of children with juvenile rheumatoid arthritis, the disease begins with a sudden onset of fever of over 39°C, severe malaise, a morbilliform rash; often generalized lymphadenopathy, hepatomegaly, and splenomegaly; and sometimes a pericardial effusion, pleural effusion, myocarditis, or pneumonitis. These symptoms persist for weeks or months before polyarthritis becomes evident. This acute form of juvenile rheumatoid arthritis is called Still's disease, after the English physician Sir George Still who described it in 1897. Less frequently, the term *Still's disease* is applied to all forms of juvenile rheumatoid arthritis or is used to describe rheumatoid arthritis in adults that evolves with a similar acute prodrome.

The lesions in juvenile rheumatoid arthritis are like those in adults, except that the growth of the affected bones is sometimes slowed or distorted. In 30% of children, the disease is confined to one or a few joints, most often a knee or ankle. Over 10% of these children develop iridocyclitis, but other extra-articular manifestations of the disease are unusual. In the other children with rheumatoid arthritis, the lesions are symmetrical and most severe in the hands and feet. The cervical spine is involved in 50% of the children, in some with lesions like those of ankylosing spondylitis.

The IgM rheumatoid factors detected by the usual tests are found in only 10% of children with rheumatoid arthritis. IgG and IgA rheumatoid factors are present in 50% of the children. Antinuclear antibodies are more common than in adults. Often there is a leukocytosis of over $15 \times 10^9/L$ (15,000/mm^3).

In over 50% of children with juvenile rheumatoid arthritis, the arthritis subsides leaving no residual disability. In another 25%, the disease remains mild. Children with involvement of only one or a few joints do especially well. In many of those with symmetrical disease, the arthritis continues into adult life. Those with an acute onset do particularly badly.

OSTEOARTHRITIS. Osteoarthritis, also called osteoarthrosis, takes its name from the Greek words for bone and joint. It is caused by degeneration of the articular cartilage in the joints involved. Some consider degeneration of the intervertebral disks a form of osteoarthritis; some prefer to call it spondylitis or spondylosis, from the Greek for a vertebra. The term *degenerative joint disease* includes both osteoarthritis of the diarthrodial joints and degenerative disease of the intervertebral disks. In this chapter, degeneration of the intervertebral disks is considered to be a form of osteoarthritis.

Two kinds of osteoarthritis are distinguished. In primary osteoarthritis, the cause of the degeneration of the cartilage or intervertebral disk is unknown. In secondary osteoarthritis, the degeneration is caused by an injury or disease of the joint.

Osteoarthritis is uncommon in young people. It usually begins after a person is 40 or more years old. By the age of 60 years, almost everyone has osteoarthritis. It is almost universal in the spine. More than 80% of people over 60 years old have radiologic evidence of osteoarthritis in one or both knees and 30% in one or both hips. Over 30% of elderly women have osteoarthritis in the interphalangeal joints of the hands. Except in the hands, men and women are affected equally, though the lesions often appear at a younger age in men. Only 3% of elderly men have primary osteoarthritis in the hands.

Lesions. Osteoarthritis is common in the knees and hips, the interphalangeal joints of the hands, and the diarthrodial joints and synchondroses of the spine. It is unusual in other joints.

Diarthrodial Joints. When osteoarthritis develops in a diarthrodial joint, the articular cartilage in the joint degenerates. At first, only part of the cartilage is affected. In the regions involved, the cartilaginous matrix and the chondrocytes swell. The proteoglycans in these regions are smaller than normal. The proportion of chondroitin sulfate falls, and the proportion of keratan sulfate rises. Metachromatic staining is not as strong as in normal cartilage. The change in the character of the proteoglycans exposes the collagen fibers in the cartilage. Poorly formed type I collagen tends to replace the type II collagen normal in cartilage.

In the degenerating regions, small fissures develop in the cartilage. The fissures separate irregular fronds of cartilage 20 to 150 μm long that project perpendicular to the articular surface, a change called fibrillation. Clumps of chondrocytes are often present near the clefts. Blood vessels sometimes grow into the deeper part of the degenerate cartilage, or its basal part becomes calcified or ossified. Macroscopically, the abnormal cartilage often looks brownish and feels velvety. It flakes off when the surface of the cartilage is rubbed.

As years pass, much or all of the articular cartilage is slowly worn away. In places, it is lost altogether. Eventually, only irregular patches of degenerating cartilage remain on the articular surfaces of the bones. The exposed bone in the articular surface often becomes thickened by layers of new lamellar bone. Its surface is frequently smooth and polished, a change called eburnation, from the Latin for ivory.

The bone marrow in the subarticular bone is replaced by collagenous tissue. Sometimes a few macrophages filled with hemosiderin or a few lymphocytes and plasma cells are present. Occasionally small nodules of cartilage are present in the subarticular bone. Frequently the bones affected become osteoporotic.

Small cysts often develop beneath the exposed bone in the articular surfaces, especially in the hips. In the regions involved, the bony trabeculae in the subarticular bone become necrotic and are replaced by loose, myxomatous tissue. The cysts form in the myxoid tissue. They are lined by collagenous tissue, sometimes with a thin rim of new bone. The cysts frequently communicate with the joint space by a narrow neck.

Osteophytes frequently form in or around osteoarthritic joints. They take their name from the Greek words for bone and plant or growth. Internal osteophytes are formed by ossification of the basal part of the degenerating articular cartilage. They make the articular surface of the bone bumpy or ridged. Occasionally ossification in the midpart of the articular cartilage forms an internal osteophyte that has a basal layer of cartilage, then a layer of bone, and then a superficial layer of

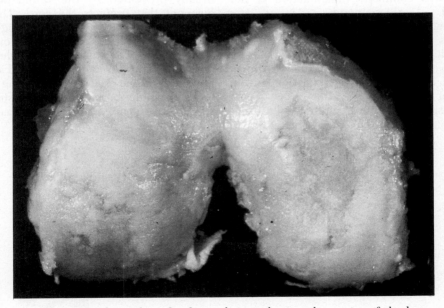

Fig. 60-2. The lower articular surface of a femur showing the irregular erosion of the bone caused by osteoarthritis.

cartilage. External osteophytes are irregular masses of bone that bulge outward from the margins of the joints, less often from the surface of the bone a short distance from an osteoarthritic joint. The cortex and medulla of the osteophyte are continuous with the cortex and medulla of the underlying bone. Many external osteophytes have a cap of articular cartilage.

External osteophytes are particularly striking in patients with osteoarthritis of the finger joints. They are often numerous and large around the terminal interphalangeal joints, especially on their dorsal surface, where they are called Heberden's nodules after the English physician who described them in 1802. Similar osteophytes around the proximal interphalangeal joints are called Bouchard's nodes after a French physician (1837–1915).

The synovium is little affected in the early stages of osteoarthritis. When the disease becomes severe, the synovial villi become large and coarse. Often cartilage or adipose tissue develops in some of the villi. Occasionally a villus is crushed between the bones of the disordered joint. The capsule of the joint becomes increasingly fibrotic. Calcification at the points of insertion of ligaments and tendons is common. Inflammation is not marked.

The synovial fluid in an osteoarthritic joint remains normal until late in the disease, when it increases in volume. Crystals of calcium pyrophosphate, calcium hydroxyapatite, or both are present in the fluid in many of the patients.

Occasionally a villus, often a villus con-taining a nodule of cartilage, breaks off and becomes a loose body within an osteoarthritic joint. The loose body remains viable, nourished by the joint fluid. It is called a joint mouse.

Synchondroses.   Degenerative disease of the synchondral joints of the spine is often called disk disease. It is most common in the lumbar synchondroses and in the cervical spine.

In the joint or joints affected, the nucleus pulposus loses water. It becomes smaller and less resilient and often is fissured or calcified. Chondroitin sulfate is lost from the nucleus. Keratan sulfate and collagen accumulate in it. The thin cartilaginous plates that separate the intervertebral disk from the vertebrae degenerate, becoming fissured or fibrillated like the articular cartilages in osteoarthritic diarthrodial joints. Often the nucleus pulposus herniates through the cartilaginous plate into one or both of the adjacent vertebrae. The herniated part of the nucleus pulposus is usually 1 to 2 cm across and is called a Schmorl's node after the German pathologist who described it in 1930. The annulus fibrosus of the disk is weakened, allowing the disk to bulge anteriorly and laterally. Posterior protrusion of the disk is usually prevented by the strong posterior ligament that protects the cord. The joint space is narrowed. Often narrowing of the spinal foramina compresses one or more spinal nerves. Occasionally the nucleus pulposus herniates through a weakened annulus fibrosus causing sudden narrowing of an intervertebral foramen, compressing the spinal cord, or compressing the corda equina.

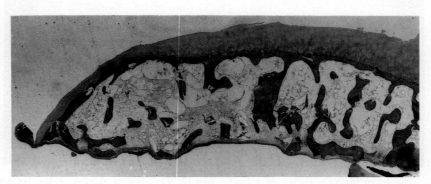

Fig. 60-3.   A joint mouse found free in an osteoarthritic joint.

The bulging intervertebral disk lifts the periosteum from the adjacent vertebrae. Shelflike osteophytes form around the lateral and anterior edges of the joint. The osteophytes curve round the capsule of the joint. Sometimes they fuse, causing ankylosis of the adjacent vertebrae. As their ends enlarge, the affected vertebrae become bobbin-shaped.

Clinical Presentation. Minor degrees of osteoarthritis cause no symptoms and no disability, at the most the minor stiffness and creaking seen in old people. When symptoms do develop, they are usually confined to one or a few joints, even in people in whom other joints are equally severely involved.

In the large joints of the limbs, aching or pain is often the principal symptom. Movement increases the pain. Rest relieves it. Changes in the weather sometimes accentuate the pain. Often the joint is stiff, especially when the patient wakes in the morning. If osteoarthritis is severe, crepitation or crunching is sometimes evident in the disordered joint. A joint mouse sometimes causes a knee joint suddenly to lock. Sometimes a severely damaged joint is subluxated or deformed.

In the hands, osteoarthritis causes pain, stiffness, and swelling. Often Heberden's nodes are a major cause of disability. Sometimes the skin overlying the nodes is red and tender. If fusion of the nodes causes ankylosis, symptoms cease.

In the cervical spine, osteoarthritis in the diarthrodial joints causes pain when the neck is turned or bent. Compression of a cervical nerve by a disk or by osteophytes often causes sudden pain referred to the occiput, shoulder, or arm. Occasionally the osteophytes compress a vertebral artery. Rarely, the spinal cord is compressed. In the lumbar spine, instability of an intervertebral joint or joints often causes stiffness or pain in the back and spasm of the spinal muscles. Herniation of a nucleus pulposus into a vertebra causes no symptoms, but herniation through the annulus fibrosus causes sudden and severe pain and spasm of the spinal muscles. Often a bulging disk or herniated nucleus pulposus compresses a spinal nerve, causing pain in the distribution of the nerve or sensory loss. Occasionally degenerative disease of a lumbar disk causes compression of the spinal cord or of the corda equina.

Pathogenesis. Anything that causes continuing distortion of a joint or causes excessive and repeated stress is likely to cause secondary osteoarthritis. Among its causes are trauma, the repeated minor injuries suffered by athletes, congenital dislocation of a hip, Legg-Calvé-Perthes disease, avascular necrosis of the head of a femur, rheumatoid arthritis, gout, infective arthritis, hemophilia, the repeated injuries that occur when sensation in a limb is impaired, and ochronosis.

Little is known of the cause of primary osteoarthritis. Probably repeated minor injuries cause minor, focal degeneration in the articular cartilages of the joint affected. The progression of the disease is caused in part by the factors that initiated it, in part by the increasing deformation of the joint caused by the disease. Genetic factors may be important in osteoarthritis of the hands in women. The disease is more common in mothers and sisters of the patients than in the general population.

Treatment and Prognosis. In many patients with mild osteoarthritis, protection of the joint or joints affected is all that is required. The disease slowly worsens, but may never become disabling. If pain is prominent, it can usually be controlled with nonsteroidal anti-inflammatory drugs. Intra-articular injection of adrenocortical steroids relieves pain and swelling in a severely affected joint, but the effect is temporary and the injections cannot be frequently repeated. If the disease is severe, surgical replacement of a hip or knee usually restores good function. The symptoms caused by degeneration of an intervertebral disk can frequently be controlled by rest and exercise. If not, surgical removal of the disk with stabilization of the spine when necessary often brings cure.

GOUT. Gout is caused by the precipitation of crystals of monosodium urate in joints, soft tissues, and the kidneys. The name is from the Latin for a drop, because in the Middle Ages it was thought that gout was caused by drops of some toxic substance that accumulated in the joints affected. The theory is true: the toxic substance is monosodium urate.

Gout figures prominently in history and

literature. It was described by Hippocrates and has afflicted many of the wise and the famous. Having gout was at one time considered a sign of intellectual superiority. It was a sign of superior social status. The association of gout with high living, rich food, and ample to drink has been known for centuries.

In North America and Europe, 1 person in 300 has gout. About 5% of patients treated for arthritis have gout. Most of the patients are over 40 years old, though occasionally the disease begins in a child. Almost 95% of them are men. When the disease occurs in a woman, it nearly always appears after the menopause. In the Maoris in New Zealand, 1 man in 10 has gout. In Japan, it has become increasingly common as the intake of protein in the diet has increased.

Lesions. In 80% of patients with gout, the first sign of the disease is gouty arthritis. In 20%, nephrolithiasis is its first manifestation. Lesions in the soft tissues are rare except in patients who have gouty arthritis.

Gouty Arthritis. In many patients with gouty arthritis, the first attack of gout involves the metatarsophalangeal joint of one big toe. Gouty arthritis is often called podagra, from the Greek for a foot and a trap. Less often the first attack involves some other joint in the foot, ankle, knee, wrist, finger, or elbow. Sometimes a prepatellar or olecranon bursa is affected. In less than 10% of the patients, more than one joint is involved.

The joint affected is acutely inflamed. Its synovium is edematous and congested, with an exudate of neutrophils. The overlying skin is red and hot. The joint is distended by serous fluid containing up to 25,000/mm^3 leukocytes, over 70% of them neutrophils. Deposits of urate are not visible macroscopically, but crystals of monosodium urate are abundant microscopically. Over 90% of them are in the phagosomes of neutrophils. If the attack is severe, the inflammation persists for three or four days, then slowly subsides over two or three weeks.

The first attack of gouty arthritis leaves no residual injury. If treatment is not instituted, a second attack follows in over 90% of the patients, in 60% of them within a year, sometimes within a few weeks. Similar acute inflammation develops, sometimes in the same joint, sometimes in another joint, often in several joints.

After several acute attacks, the synovial membrane of the joint is scarred and thickened. Coarse synovial villi project into the joint. An exudate of lymphocytes, plasma cells, and macrophages persists in the synovium. The quantity of fluid in the joint is increased and contains many neutrophils with crystals of sodium urate in their phagosomes. Crystals of sodium urate too large to be phagocytosed by neutrophils precipitate in the synovium. They form nodules 0.3 to 3 cm across. In the acellular core of the nodules, the crystals are bound together by a proteinaceous substance. At the margin, the crystals excite a prominent foreign body reaction with many large multinucleated macrophages. When an acute attack occurs, acute inflammation is superimposed on the persisting chronic inflammation.

Urate crystals are deposited in the articular cartilage where they excite no cellular reaction. The deposits in the cartilage are at first small and near its junction with the synovium, but as time passes they increase in size, and more of the articular cartilage is involved. Some of the deposits become large enough to erode the underlying bone. The articular cartilage is gradually destroyed. Sometimes synovium grows over the peripheral part of the damaged cartilage, like pannus. Fragments of the articular cartilage often break off and float free within the joint.

Tophi. Before gout could be controlled, large deposits of urate crystals called tophi, from the Latin for porous rock, appeared in the soft tissues in 60% of patients with gout. Less frequently, small tophi were found within bones. When gout is well managed, tophi are uncommon and small.

Tophi are most frequent around the affected joints, especially in the insertion of a tendon or ligament. They are common on the ulnar surface of the forearms, in the olecranon bursae, Achilles tendons, helices of the ears, and over pressure points. Macroscopically, a tophus resembles a rheumatoid nodule. Microscopically, it has an acellular core of urate crystals with a foreign body reaction and fibrosis at the margin. Occasionally a large tophus causes inflammation of the overlying skin or ulcerates, releasing the chalky or pasty mass of crystals in its core.

Renal Lesions. The renal lesions of gout are discussed in Chapter 27. More than 70% of the patients have deposits of urate in the kidneys. More than 20% have uric acid stones. Over 20% have proteinuria or mild azotemia.

Clinical Presentation. Gouty arthritis usually begins abruptly. A man who was well when he went to bed is awakened by severe pain in the joint affected. Chills and fever follow. The pain grows increasingly severe. The joint becomes swollen, red, and hot. The patient cannot bear the least pressure on the joint or the least movement. If the attack is severe, the leukocyte count and erythrocyte sedimentation rate increase. A mild attack subsides within several hours. A severe attack lasts two or three days, and it is often weeks before symptoms disappear. Without treatment, subsequent attacks slowly become more frequent and more severe. Usually tophi do not become apparent until 10 or more years after the onset of arthritis.

Pathogenesis. Almost all patients with gout have hyperuricemia. Usually arthritis or nephrolithiasis develops only after the hyperuricemia has persisted for 20 or 30 years. The greater the concentration of urate in the plasma, the greater the risk and the sooner the disease is likely to develop.

In the United States, less than 1% of men followed for 12 years in whom the concentration of urate in the plasma did not exceed 350 μmol/L (6 mg/100 mL) developed gouty arthritis; 6% of those in whom the concentration was between 350 and 415 μmol/L (6 and 7 mg/100 mL); 20% of those between 420 and 475 μmol/L (7 and 8 mg/100 mL); 40% of those between 475 and 540 μmol/L (8 to 9 mg/100 mL); and 90% of men with a concentration of more than 540 μmol/L (9 mg/100 mL). In 75% of the men who developed gouty arthritis, the highest concentration of urate in the plasma was between 350 and 475 μmol/L (6 and 8 mg/100 mL). On the average, the first attack occurred before the patient was 40 years old in men with more than 540 μmol/L (9 mg/100 mL) of urate in the plasma, after the age of 55 years in those with less than 415 μmol/L (7 mg/100 mL).

The plasma is fully saturated with urate when its concentration reaches 415 μmol/L (7 mg/100 mL). It is not known why the supersaturated solution in the tissues of people with hyperuricemia persists many years for some and then suddenly precipitates in the urine or why it precipitates in one joint and not another. In some patients, an attack of gouty arthritis seems to be precipitated by unusual exercise, excessive intake of alcohol, or the stress of a surgical procedure. In many, no such precipitating factor is evident.

Hyperuricemia. In 90% of patients with hyperuricemia, the increased concentration of urate in the plasma is caused by renal disease that impairs the excretion of urate. In 10%, it results from increased production of urate in the body. In some patients, there are both increased production and defective excretion. Excessive intake of purines in the diet and reduced excretion of urate in the bile alone do not change the concentration of urate in the plasma sufficiently to cause hyperuricemia. Rarely, deficiency of the globulin that binds urate in the plasma is inherited as an autosomal recessive character. The patients develop tophi, though the concentration of urate in the plasma is normal.

Both overproduction of urate and defective excretion are divided into primary and secondary forms. In the primary forms, hyperuricemia is the principal feature of the disorder. In the secondary forms, the hyperuricemia is secondary to some other disease or is a minor feature of the disorder.

In the kidneys, urate is filtered by the glomeruli, resorbed in the proximal tubules, excreted by a more distal part of the proximal tubules, and again partially resorbed. Primary renal hyperuricemia results from dysfunction of these tubular mechanisms. In men, the concentration of urate in the plasma rises after puberty and remains high throughout life. In women, the concentration does not reach similar levels until after the menopause.

Secondary renal hyperuricemia is caused by any condition that impairs sufficiently glomerular filtration or causes sufficient damage to the renal tubules. It occurs in many chronic renal diseases that reduce glomerular filtration or injure the tubules. Acidosis, Bartter's syndrome, beryllium poisoning, Down syndrome, hyperparathyroidism, hypertension, hypoparathyroidism, hypothyroidism, hypovolemia, lead poisoning, maple sugar disease, myxedema, nephrogenic diabetes insipidus, pseudohypoparathyroidism, sarcoidosis, and sickle cell anemia are among conditions sometimes associated with reduced renal excretion of urate. Diuretics impair the excretion of urate. Ethanol does so. Aspirin, ethambutol, nicotinic acid, pyrazinamide, and other drugs sometimes do so.

In most patients with primary hyperuricemia due to overproduction of purines, the overproduction is caused by a polygenetic derangement that has not been characterized. In 15% of the patients, it is caused by increased activity of 5-phosphoribosyl-1-pyrophosphate synthetase or by partial deficiency of hypoxanthine-guanine phosphoribosyltransferase, enzymes active in the metabolism of purines. Both the increased activity and the partial deficiency are inherited as X-linked recessive characters. In these people, the concentration of urate in the plasma is high during childhood and remains high throughout life.

Most patients with secondary overproduction of urate have increased catabolism of nucleic acids caused by a malignant tumor, myeloproliferative, or lymphoproliferative disease. Carcinoma, Gaucher's disease, some hemoglobinopathies, infectious mononucleosis, leukemia, lymphoma, multiple myeloma, pernicious anemia, polycythemia rubra vera, secondary polycythemia, severe psoriasis, thalassemia and other hemolytic anemias, and Waldenström's macroglobulinemia are among the conditions that can cause hyperuricemia in this way. Treatment of lymphoma, leukemia, or some other tumor by chemotherapy sometimes causes massive breakdown of nucleic acids and hyperuricemia.

In a minority of patients with secondary overproduction of urate, the malfunction is caused by the glucose-6-phosphatase deficiency of type I glycogen storage disease inherited as an autosomal recessive character, or by almost complete deficiency of hypoxanthine-guanine phosphoribosyltransferase inherited as an X-linked recessive character, a disorder that causes the Lesch-Nyhan syndrome of mental retardation, choreoathetosis, spasticity, selfmutilation, impairment of growth, and hyperuricemia.

Inflammatory Response. The precipitation of monosodium urate in the tissues causes acute inflammation that attracts neutrophils. The neutrophils phagocytose the small crystals of monosodium urate first formed. They release chemotactic factors that attract more neutrophils and lysosomal products that damage the tissues. The crystals activate the Hageman factor and so the enzymes that form kinins. The concentration of bradykinin increases in gouty joints. Activation of complement adds to the chemotaxis of neutrophils and to the inflammation.

If the crystals of monosodium urate remain in the tissues, they become too large to be phagocytosed by neutrophils. They aggregate together and excite the foreign body reaction that occurs around aggregates of urate in the synovium, soft tissues, and kidneys.

Treatment and Prognosis. Colchicine given by mouth or intravenously relieves the pain of an acute attack of gouty arthritis within 12 hours in 75% of the patients, though gastrointestinal or neurologic side effects are often severe. Indomethacin and other nonsteroidal anti-inflammatory agents control most acute attacks of gouty arthritis and are less likely to cause serious side effects. If necessary, glucocorticoids are given systemically or intra-articularly to reduce the inflammation and relieve the pain. The renal calculi that develop in gout are managed as are other urinary calculi.

Once the acute attack has been overcome, the risk of gouty arthritis and nephrolithiasis is reduced by giving allopurinol to decrease the synthesis of urate or a drug such as probenecid or sulfinpyrazone to increase its excretion. In most patients, further attacks are prevented, and deformity or dysfunction in the joints does not occur.

CHONDROCALCINOSIS. Chondrocalcinosis is caused by the precipitation of calcium pyrophosphate dihydrate in the joints. It is often called pseudogout, because the acute form of the disease is similar to gout. At autopsy, up to 5% of the population have crystals of calcium pyrophosphate in the knee joints, but in North America only one person in 1000 has symptoms caused by the disease. Most of the patients are over 50 years old when symptoms begin. Men and women are both affected.

Lesions. In 25% of the patients with symptoms, chondrocalcinosis causes acute arthritis. The attack is usually confined to a single joint, most often a knee, less often an ankle, wrist, elbow, hip, vertebral joint, or the metatarsophalangeal joint of a big toe. Involvement of other joints may follow. Usually the inflammation perists for several days, then resolves. The joint affected is painful, swollen, and hyperemic. Its synovium is congested and edematous, with an exudate predominantly of neutrophils. Neutrophils are numerous in the joint fluid. Crystals of calcium pyrophosphate are present in the phagosomes of the neutrophils.

In most of the patients with symptoms, the arthritis is chronic. It is symmetrical and involves several joints. The knees, wrists, metacarpophalangeal joints, hips, shoulders, elbows, and ankles are the most frequently involved. Crystals of calcium pyrophosphate are deposited in the articular cartilages midway between their articular and bony surfaces and throughout menisci within the joint. The cartilage degenerates. The crystals surround the chondrocytes and accumulate around foci of degenerate cartilage. They escape into the synovial fluid. The joints become chronically inflamed. Crystals of calcium pyrophosphate are present in the synovium and capsule of the joint, but are few. They are often more numerous in adjacent ligaments and tendons. The calcium in the cartilages and ligaments can be demonstrated roentgenographically. In 50% of patients, acute attacks are superimposed on the chronic arthritis.

In 5% of the patients, chondrocalcinosis resembles rheumatoid arthritis. In some, the disease becomes severe in one or several joints, causing destruction like that of neuropathic arthropathy.

Clinical Presentation. Acute chondrocalcinosis resembles gout. The diagnosis is made by demonstrating crystals of calcium pyrophosphate in the synovial fluid and by showing that urates and organisms that might cause a similar acute arthritis are not present. Sometimes crystals of calcium pyrophosphate are present in the synovial fluid in a patient with gout or septic arthritis.

Chronic chondrocalcinosis is similar to osteoarthritis. It is often difficult to distinguish between chondrocalcinosis and osteoarthritis. Many patients show features of both.

Pathogenesis. In a few patients, chondrocalcinosis is inherited. In some it complicates primary hyperparathyroidism or hemochromatosis, less often gout, hypermagnesemia, hypophosphatasia, hypothyroidism, ochronosis, or Wilson's disease. In most, it is idiopathic.

The relationship between chondrocalcinosis and osteoarthritis is obscure. Calcium pyrophosphate is present in the synovial fluid in many patients with osteoarthritis, and changes like those of osteoarthritis are present in many patients with chronic chondrocalcinosis. In some patients the disorganization of the joints caused by chondrocalcinosis may cause osteoarthritis; in others injury to the cartilage caused by osteoarthritis may result in the precipitation of calcium pyrophosphate.

In all forms of chondrocalcinosis, the disease is initiated by the precipitation of calcium pyrophosphate in the articular cartilages. The inflammation is caused by the release of the crystals from the cartilages into the synovial fluid and into the synovium. An acute attack can be provoked by inducing the release of crystals by reducing the concentration of calcium or pyrophosphate ions in the synovial fluid or by trauma or inflammation that damages the cartilage and releases crystals of pyrophosphate. The crystals are phagocytosed by neutrophils and cause inflammation by the mechanisms active in gout.

Treatment and Prognosis. The deposition of crystals of calcium pyrophosphate in the joints of people with chondrocalcinosis cannot be prevented or reversed. Indomethacin and other nonsteroidal anti-inflammatory drugs control an acute attack of chondrocalcinosis. Chronic chondrocalcinosis is managed as is osteoarthritis.

HYDROXYAPATITE ARTHROPATHY. Hydroxyapatite arthropathy is similar to chondrocalcinosis, though less common. Crystals of calcium hydroxyapatite precipitate in the joints affected, most often a knee or shoulder. The crystals are too small to be detected by light microscopy, but are evident by electron microscopy. In some patients, both calcium hydroxyapatite and calcium pyrophosphate are precipitated in the joints.

ANKYLOSING SPONDYLITIS. Ankylosing

spondylitis is a form of arthritis that affects the spine and other joints, frequently causing ankylosis. The name comes from the Greek words for crooked and a vertebra. Ankylosing spondylitis is sometimes called Marie-Strümpell disease, after the French physician Marie (1853–1940) and the German physician von Strümpell (1853–1925), or Bekhterev's disease, after a Russian neurologist (1857–1927). It is sometimes grouped with psoriatic arthritis, Reiter's disease, enteropathic arthropathy, and perhaps Behçet's disease as the seronegative arthritides, because in none of these conditions are rheumatoid factors detectable in the plasma and in all the HLA-B27 antigen is more frequent than in the general population. In the United States, 1 white person in 2000 develops ankylosing spondylitis. It is less common in black people. Over 90% of the patients are men. Most are 15 to 30 years old when symptoms begin.

Lesions. Ankylosing spondylitis often begins in the sacroiliac joints. As months pass, it extends up the spine, involving both the diarthrodial joints and the synchondroses. Part or all of the spine may be affected. In 30% of the patients, the hips are involved; in some the joints of the shoulder girdle, only occasionally other peripheral joints. The disease in the hips and shoulders usually begins after the involvement of the spine, but in some patients both the spinal and the peripheral joints are involved from the outset, or the first sign of the disease is arthritis in a peripheral joint or joints.

In the diarthrodial joints, the lesions are at first like those of rheumatoid arthritis. Similar inflammation thickens the synovium. The exudate of lymphocytes, plasma cells, and macrophages is like that in rheumatoid arthritis. Germinal centers are commonly present. The inflammation is particularly marked where the capsule of the joint, ligaments, and tendons joins the bone. In the later stages of the disease, the synovium becomes increasingly fibrotic. Granulation tissue like pannus extends over the articular cartilages, destroying them and eroding the underlying bone. The denuded bone ends become fixed together, first by fibrosis and then by bony ankylosis. Eventually, ankylosis may almost entirely obliterate the joint cavity.

In the synchondroses, the outer parts of the sacroiliac joints and symphysis pubis are inflamed and replaced by granulation tissue that erodes the adjacent bone. New bone deposited in the granulation tissue forms a bony union between the adjacent bones. In the intervertebral disks, similar inflammation of the outer part of the annulus fibrosus causes ankylosis. Often the interspinous, costovertebral, and anterior longitudinal ligaments ossify.

The destruction of the spinal joints makes the spine increasingly rigid. Usually the lumbar spine is straight, but often the thoracic spine is fixed in flexion. The destruction of the costovertebral joints makes movement of the ribs impossible. The stiffness of the thoracic cage reduces the vital capacity to about 70% of normal.

The erythrocyte sedimentation rate is elevated in most patients with active ankylosing spondylitis. Rheumatoid factors are not detectable in the plasma.

Clinical Presentation. Most often, the first symptom of ankylosing spondylitis is pain in the lower back that sometimes radiates in the distribution of the sciatic nerves. As the disease advances up the spine, the pain ascends to higher parts of the back or involves the ribs. Often the affected joints are tender. When ankylosis prevents movement of the joints, the pain ceases. If the peripheral joints are involved, they cause symptoms and dysfunction like those of osteoarthritis. In some patients, the arthritis in the hips is the most disabling feature of the disease.

Complications. Iridocyclitis develops in 20% of patients with ankylosing spondylitis. In 5%, the deformity of the aortic valve and aorta described in Chapter 25 causes aortic incompetence. Some have a disturbance in cardiac conduction. About 5% develop amyloidosis. In some patients a vertebral or sacroiliac lesion compresses a spinal nerve root or rarely the cauda equina. Occasionally fibrosis at the apices of the lungs mimics tuberculosis.

Pathogenesis. Genetic factors are of major importance in the causation of ankylosing spondylitis. About 90% of patients with ankylosing spondylitis have the HLA antigen B27. In the general population, less than 7%

of white people are positive for HLA-B27. About 50% of close relatives of patients with ankylosing spondylitis who are positive for HLA-B27 also have the HLA-B27 antigen. About 20% of them have ankylosing spondylitis.

It has been suggested that people who carry the HLA-B27 antigen have a defective immunologic system that makes them unduly susceptible to an infection that causes ankylosing spondylitis. The nature of the defect and the nature of the infective agent are unknown.

Treatment and Prognosis. Most patients with ankylosing spondylitis live a normal life. No treatment alters the course of the disease. Nonsteroidal anti-inflammatory agents can control the pain in most patients. Careful maintenance of an erect posture reduces the spinal deformity. In some patients, surgical correction of a spinal deformity or replacement of a hip is necessary.

PSORIATIC ARTHRITIS. If patients with rheumatoid arthritis who have rheumatoid arthritis with rheumatoid factors in their blood are excluded, about 5% of patients with psoriasis have arthritis. These people are said to have psoriatic arthritis. Most are between 20 and 40 years old when psoriatic arthritis begins. Men and women are affected equally. About 85% have had psoriasis for months or years before arthritis appears. In 15%, the arthritis precedes the psoriasis.

In 70% of patients with psoriatic arthritis, only 2 or 3 joints are involved. Usually the involvement is asymmetrical. Proximal joints in the hands or feet are the most frequently involved. In 15% of the patients, several joints are affected. The involvement is symmetrical and indistinguishable from rheumatoid arthritis except that rheumatoid factors are not detectable in the plasma. In 10%, the arthritis is confined to some of the terminal interphalangeal joints. Usually the adjacent nail shows psoriatic changes. In a few patients, the arthritis involves many joints and is severe and mutilating.

The arthritis is at first acute, but as it becomes chronic, it resembles mild rheumatoid arthritis. Ankylosis is more common than in rheumatoid arthritis. Periostitis in the shaft of the bones affected sometimes makes the phalanges involved swollen and sausage-shaped. Only in the uncommon mutilating form of the disease does psoriatic arthritis cause destruction of the joints, deformity, loss of bone, and telescoping of the fingers. Rheumatoid factors are not detectable in the plasma.

In 20% of patients with psoriatic arthritis, changes like those of ankylosing spondylitis are present in the sacroiliac joints and spine. Some of the patients have one of the forms of peripheral psoriatic arthritis. In some the disease is confined to the spine.

Genetic factors are important in the causation of psoriatic arthritis. It occurs with increased frequency in close relatives of patients with the disease. About 50% of patients with psoriatic spondylitis have the HLA-B27 antigen.

In most patients, psoriatic arthritis is mild and intermittent. Occasionally long remissions occur. If nonsteroidal anti-inflammatory drugs are insufficient, gold is helpful. Methotrexate and other immunosuppressive agents control both the psoriasis and the arthritis.

REITER'S SYNDROME. Reiter's syndrome is named after the German physician who described a case in 1916. The patients have urethritis, conjunctivitis, and arthritis. In developed countries, Reiter's syndrome is most common in men 20 to 40 years old with chlamydial or mycoplasmal urethritis. In developing countries, it involves men and women equally and usually follows a shigellar, salmonellar, yersinial, or campobacterial infection of the intestine. About 2% of men with nongonococcal urethritis and 2% of people with a severe intestinal infection develop Reiter's syndrome.

In both forms of the syndrome, urethritis is usually the first manifestation. It is usually mild. Often it passes unnoticed. Conjunctivitis develops a few days or weeks later. It too is usually mild and lasts only a few days or weeks. Rarely it causes uveitis and blindness.

Arthritis develops days or weeks after the onset of the urethritis. It is usually asymmetrical and involves only a few joints. The knees, ankles, and small joints of the feet are the most frequently affected. The joints involved are swollen, red, and painful. Their synovium is hyperemic and edematous, with an exudate of neutrophils. The joint fluid contains more than 1,000/mm^3 cells, 70% of them neutrophils. The inflammation usually reaches a peak within two weeks, and then begins to subside. In 70% of the patients, there is little permanent injury to the joint. In 30%, the inflammation becomes chronic and persists for months or recurs. In some patients, recrudescence of the arthritis follows reinfection of the urethra. In 20% of the patients, the disease causes permanent deformity of the feet.

In some patients, lesions like those of ankylosing spondylitis occur in the sacroiliac or vertebral joints. Inflammation of the plantar fasciae and Achilles' tendons is common. Frequently the disease involves tendons or bursae. Periostitis often develops in the phalanges involved, causing a sausage-like swelling of the fingers or toes affected.

In 30% of the patients, painless vesicles develop on the glans penis, in the mouth, or on the palms and soles. They ulcerate, but heal within a few days. In 30% of people in whom the syndrome is caused by nongonococcal urethritis, but not in those in whom it follows an intestinal infection, scaling papules develop on the glans penis, palms, and soles, less often elsewhere in the skin, a condition called keratoderma blennorrhagica. Macroscopically and microscopically, the papules resemble psoriasis. Subungual cornified material sometimes lifts and distorts the nails. Occasionally a lesion like that of ankylosing spondylitis distorts the aortic valve or a conduction defect develops in the heart.

Nearly 90% of the patients express the HLA-B27 antigen. Presumably the arthritis and other lesions are caused by the interaction of the infection with some factor associated with the HLA-B27 locus. Reiter's syndrome is treated symptomatically.

ENTEROPATHIC ARTHROPATHY. About 20% of patients with Crohn's disease and 10% of those with ulcerative colitis develop arthritis in the peripheral joints. Nearly 5% of them develop spondylitis. Another 10% have radiologic evidence of disease in the sacroiliac joints but no symptoms. In Crohn's disease, involvement of the joints is more common in people with lesions in the colon. In ulcerative colitis, it is most common in people with extensive disease. In both Crohn's disease and ulcerative colitis, the arthritis usually begins six months or more after the onset of the bowel disease, but occasionally is the first sign of the disease.

The peripheral arthritis usually involves a single joint. A knee, ankle, proximal interphalangeal joint, elbow, shoulder, or wrist is most often affected. Sometimes asymmetrical involvement of three or four other joints follows. The joints involved are acutely inflamed. The inflammation reaches a peak in about 24 hours and then usually subsides within a few weeks. Most patients recover completely.

The spondylitis that occurs in patients with Crohn's disease or ulcerative colitis is like ankylosing spondylitis. In many of the patients, it progresses to ankylosis of much or all the spine. Over 70% of the patients with spondylitis express the HLA-B27 antigen. In people with asymptomatic arthritis of the sacroiliac joints or peripheral arthritis, the HLA-B27 antigen is no more frequent than in the general population.

About 30% of patients with a jejunocolic or jejunoileal bypass develop fleeting arthralgias, and some develop arthritis, most often in the knees, ankles, wrists, or shoulders. The arthritis begins months or years after the operation. It is usually acute, but in some patients becomes chronic. It rarely causes permanent disability. Antibodies against Escherichia coli and other bacteria that proliferate in the blind loop formed by the bypass circulate in the blood and form immune complexes. The arthritis is probably caused by the deposition of the immune complexes in the joints.

Nearly 70% of patients with Whipple's disease have repeated attacks of acute arthritis. Commonly the arthritis begins months or years before intestinal disease becomes evident. The arthritis usually lasts only a few days. It is most common in the knees, ankles, fingers, hips, shoulders, elbows, and wrists. In most patients, no permanent injury is caused. In a few, the inflammation persists and becomes chronic. Some patients have radiologic changes like those of ankylosing spondylitis in the sacroiliac joints. The exudate in the synovium of the acutely inflamed joints and in the synovial fluid is predominantly of neutrophils, but macrophages containing the organisms that cause Whipple's disease are present in the inflamed joints and sometimes in the synovial fluid.

RELAPSING POLYCHONDRITIS. Relapsing polychondritis is an uncommon condition that causes destruction of cartilage and damages the eyes and cardiovascular system. The patients are usually between 40 and 60 years old. Men and women are affected equally.

The cartilages of the ears and nose are involved in 80% of the patients. During an attack, the affected region becomes red, swollen, and painful. The tissues around the cartilages involved are congested and edematous. An exudate of lymphocytes and plasma cells develops adjacent to the cartilage. The matrix of the cartilage loses mucopolysaccharides and becomes less metachromatic. Some of the chondrocytes die. Granulation tissue invades the cartilage and replaces it with collagenous tissue. Occasionally the collagenous tissue becomes calcified or ossified. The attack subsides after days or months, but recurs in the same or another region months or years later. In many of the patients, the ears become floppy and deformed, and the bridge of the nose collapses.

Less often involvement of the eustachian tubes causes otitis media, distortion of the larynx and trachea causes hoarseness or respiratory obstruction, or collapse of bronchi causes respiratory failure or obstructive pneumonitis. Involvement of the articular cartilages sometimes causes arthritis.

Over 60% of the patients have conjunctivitis, episcleritis, scleritis, or iritis. Dilation of the aortic valve ring or distortion of the aortic valve causes aortic insufficiency in 25% of the patients. Other cardiac valves are affected less frequently. Some of the patients have arteritis, focal proliferative glomerulonephritis, rheumatoid arthritis, systemic lupus erythematosus, or some other collagen disease.

Circulating immune complexes, rheumatoid factors, or antinuclear antibodies are present in the plasma in some of the patients. The erythrocyte sedimentation rate is usually elevated. Often there is mild leukocytosis or mild anemia.

Presumably relapsing polychondritis is immunologically mediated. In most patients, prednisone suppresses the attack. In some cyclophosphamide or azathioprine is needed.

INFECTIVE ARTHRITIS. Acute bacterial arthritis, often called septic arthritis, is uncommon. Most frequently it results from hematogenous infection by Neisseria gonorrhoeae, Staphylococcus aureus, a streptococcus, haemophilus, or gram-negative bacillus. Less commonly the infection is caused by trauma that breaches the skin, instrumentation, or extension from osteomyelitis.

Immunosuppression, misuse of intravenous drugs, alcoholism, hypogammaglobulinemia, cancer, diabetes mellitus, and liver disease make infection of a joint easier. Rheumatoid arthritis, other forms of chronic arthritis, and a prosthesis in a joint increase the risk of developing bacterial arthritis.

Usually only one joint is involved. In 50% of the patients, it is a knee, less often a hip, shoulder, wrist, ankle, elbow, sternoclavicular, or sacroiliac joint. The joint is painful, swollen, red, and hot. Its synovium is edematous and congested, with an exudate predominantly of neutrophils. Often small abscesses develop in the synovium or in the adjacent soft tissues or bones. The cavity of the joint is distended with fluid under increased pressure. Usually the fluid contains more than $50,000/mm^3$ cells, 90% of them neutrophils. The concentration of glucose in the fluid is often less than 50% of that in the plasma. If the infecting organism is a staphylococcus, the fluid contains much fibrin and may be pus. If the infection is not rapidly overcome, the increased pressure in the joint and the enzymes released by the neutrophils cause erosion of the articular cartilage and often serious injury to the underlying bone and adjacent soft tissues. Healing often brings fibrous or bony ankylosis.

Less often a bacterium of low virulence causes less severe acute or chronic infection, often in a joint containing a prosthesis or damaged by rheumatoid arthritis. In Lyme disease, Borrelia burgdorferi causes mild, acute arthritis in 60% of the patients. A joint is involved in 1% of patients with tuberculosis, most often a vertebral or sacroiliac joint, hip, knee, wrist, or ankle. Mycobacterium kansasii, M. marinum, or M. avium sometimes infects a joint. Syphilis involves joints in its secondary and tertiary stages.

A joint is sometimes infected in a patient

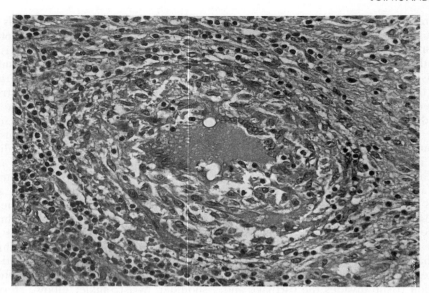

Fig. 60-4. A tuberculous granuloma in a patient with tuberculous arthritis.

with blastomycosis, candidiasis, coccidi-oidomycosis, cryptococcosis, histoplasmosis, or sporotrichosis. Actinomycosis sometimes involves a joint.

A mild arthropathy that causes no permanent injury occurs in 30% of patients with rubella, most often in the fingers, wrists, and knees. Similar arthropathy is frequent in hepatitis B. It is common in chikungunya fever, o'nyong-nyong fever, Ross river disease, and other arboviral infections, less frequent in adenoviral infections, infectious mononucleosis, mumps, and varicella.

HEMARTHROSIS. Hemorrhage into a joint is called a hemarthrosis, from the Greek for blood and joint. Among its more frequent causes are trauma, bleeding diseases such as hemophilia, and overdose of anticoagulant drugs.

The blood distends the joint. The synovium and surrounding tissues become edematous, hyperemic, and acutely inflamed. The joint is painful and is held still in the position that reduces the pressure in the joint to a minimum. Fever and leukocytosis are common. If the hemorrhage does not continue, the blood is absorbed in three to six weeks. The synovium and the articular cartilages are stained brown by hemosiderin, but there is rarely any residual dysfunction.

Repeated bleeding into a joint causes severe arthritis. The blood often clots in the joint cavity. Fibrin often coats parts of the articular cartilages or synovium. The synovium becomes increasingly hyperplastic. Long, thin villi project into the joint. often one of the villi is pinched between the bone ends, adding to the injury. An exudate of lymphocytes and plasma cells is present in the synovium. Massive accumulations of hemosiderin in macrophages turn the synovium dark brown. The synovium becomes increasingly scarred and fibrotic.

Changes like those of osteoarthritis add to the injury. The articular cartilages show foci of fibrillary degeneration. As portions of the articular cartilages are lost, the underlying bone ends become eburnated. The bones grow increasingly porotic. Often subchondral cysts like those of osteoarthritis develop. The bone ends become flattened and widened. Osteophytes develop around the joint. The joint becomes increasingly disorganized. Collagenous or bony ankylosis sometimes follows.

NEUROARTHROPATHY. The arthritis that develops in joints in which sensation is lost is called neuroarthropathy or neuropathic joint disease. Tabes dorsalis, diabetic neuropathy, syringomyelia, meningocele, alcoholic neuropathy, leprosy, and amyloidosis are among its more frequent causes. Repeated intra-articular injections of a glucocorticoid cause similar changes. Particularly when it is due to tabes dorsalis, neuroarthropathy is often called Charcot's joint, after the French neurologist who described it in 1868.

The distribution of the loss of sensation determines the joints involved. In tabes dorsalis, the knees, hips, and ankles are most frequently affected; in diabetic neuropathy, the samll joints of the feet; in syringomyelia, the joints of the shoulders and arms. The disease usually begins in a single joint, but later involves other joints.

Swelling of the affected joint is the first sign of neuroarthropathy. The joint is not painful and is not inflamed. Usually the effusion into the joint resolves, and little permanent injury remains.

After several episodes of this sort, the synovium becomes chronically inflamed. The effusion into the joint persists and increases. The articular cartilages degenerate and are largely or completely lost. The articular surface of the bones is in part eburnated, in part is covered by collagenous tissue or new formed fibrocartilage. The ends of the bones become increasingly distorted by erosion and fractures. Usually the bone ends become flattened and widened. Large osteophytes form around the joint. Fragments of cartilage or bone split from the articular surface lie free in the synovium or in the joint cavity. Masses of metaplastic bone sometimes form in the synovium. The ligaments and tendons around the joint stretch and grow lax. Subluxation or dislocation often adds to the deformity. The end is a greatly swollen joint that is distorted and unstable. The joint crunches when it is moved, as the irregular fragments of bone rub together.

The destruction of the joint in neuroarthropathy usually develops slowly, but in some patients occurs within a few weeks. It is due in part to multiple minor injuries and more serious fractures that go unnoticed because of the loss of sensation, in part to trophic factors. The damage cannot be repaired. Splints and braces help overcome the dysfunction.

PIGMENTED VILLONODULAR SYNOVITIS. Pigmented villonodular synovitis is uncommon. The patients are usually young adults.

Men and women are affected equally. Usually only one joint is affected, most often a knee, less often a hip, ankle, elbow, or one of the small joints in a hand or foot.

The affected joint becomes swollen and painful. Its synovium is inflamed and hyperplastic, with large villi that fuse to form nodules within the joint. It is usually brown. The inflamed synovium erodes the articular cartilages. Often it bulges into the subchondral bone or into the periarticular tissues. Microscopically, the synovial cells lining the joint are hyperplastic. A dense exudate of macrophages with smaller numbers of lymphocytes and plasma cells is present in the synovium. Some of the macrophages are multinucleate. Many contain hemosiderin. Many contain droplets of fat. The synovial fluid is hemorrhagic and dark.

The cause of pigmented villonodular synovitis is unknown. Most think that it is an inflammation. Some suggest that it may be neoplastic. If left untreated, it slowly worsens as months and years pass. Complete synovectomy cures. If part of the synovium is left behind, the disease recurs.

TIETZE'S SYNDROME. Tietze's syndrome, sometimes called costochondritis, is named after the German surgeon who described it in 1921. Two forms of the disease are distinguished. In people under 40 years old, a painful swelling develops in one or more of

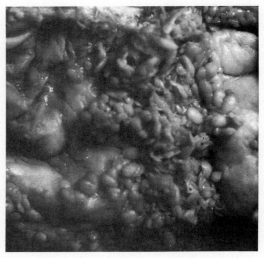

Fig. 60-5. Pigmented villous synovitis, showing irregular hyperplasia of the synovial villi.

the costochondral joints. Men and women are affected equally. In people over 40 years old, similar pain develops in one or more of the costochondral joints without swelling. Women are affected more frequently than men. In both forms of the disease, the pain is sometimes severe, mimicking myocardial infarction. It lasts some weeks, then subsides. Some patients suffer more than one attack. The cause of the arthritis and the changes in the joints affected are unknown. The disorder is treated with analgesics or by infiltration with a local anesthetic.

FLEETING ARTHROPATHY. Mild arthritis that lasts for only a few days is common in many conditions. It may affect one joint or several joints. Frequently it affects now one joint or group of joints, now another. Behçet's syndrome, Crohn's disease, gonorrhea, Henoch-Schönlein purpura, hypogammaglob-ulinemia, Mediterranean fever, rheumatic fever, sarcoidosis, serum sickness, systemic lupus erythematosus, ulcerative colitis, vas-culitis, and Whipple's disease are among the conditions in which it is frequent.

In the mildest form of the condition, called arthralgia, the joint is painful but shows no inflammation. If the arthropathy is more severe, the joint is swollen or hyperemic.

The cause of this type of arthritis is uncertain. Probably in most patients it is mediated immunologically, perhaps by the precipitation of circulating immune complexes.

TENDONS AND APONEUROSES

The principal non-neoplastic diseases of the tendons and aponeuroses are tenosynovi-tis, sclerosing tenosynovitis, the degenera-tive diseases of tendons, and Dupuytren's contracture.

TENOSYNOVITIS. Inflammation of a tendon sheath is called tenosynovitis, or sometimes tenovaginitis, from the Greek for a tendon, and the Latin for a sheath. Many of the diseases that affect the synovium of joints affect also the tendon sheaths. Rheumatoid arthritis causes changes in tendon sheaths like those in the joints, with pain and swelling and sometimes weakening or rupture of the tendons. Transient inflammation of tendon sheaths is common in gonorrhea. Tuberculosis of tendon sheaths still occurs. Occasionally other diseases of the synovium of the joints affect the adjacent tendon sheaths. Repeated minor injuries often cause inflammation in a tendon sheath without involving the adjacent joints.

The inflammation makes the affected tendon sheath swollen and tender. Some-times crepitus can be felt when the tendon moves through the inflamed segment of the sheath. In the carpal tunnel syndrome, swollen tendon sheaths in the carpal tunnel compress the median nerve, causing pain or paresthesia in the hand and sometimes in the arm. Less often a similar syndrome occurs in the tarsal tunnel. Inflammation around the insertion of the extensor tendons into the lateral epicondyle of a humerus causes tennis elbow.

Rest often relieves tenosynovitis. Local injection of adrenocortical steroids does so. Division of the transverse carpal ligament is needed if the carpal tunnel syndrome persists.

SCLEROSING TENOSYNOVITIS. Stenosis of the common sheath of the abductor pollicis longus and the extensor pollicis brevis at the wrist is common, especially in women. It is called de Quervain's disease, after a Swiss surgeon (1968–1940). Repeated minor trauma causes chronic inflammation in the sheath. Scarring narrows the sheath and causes pain and tenderness. Local injection of adrenocortical steroids often relieves the condition. In some patients, surgical division of the sheath is needed.

Similar stenosis of the sheath of a flexor tendon in a finger prevents re-extension of the finger after it is flexed. The stenosis is sometimes caused by rheumatoid arthritis; more often it results from trauma. Congenital stenosis of the sheath of the flexor pollicis longus sometimes causes trigger thumb in infants.

DEGENERATION. Degenerative changes in tendons are most common in the supraspina-tus tendons, the rotator cuffs of the shoulders, and the biceps tendons.

Calcification of a supraspinatus tendon is demonstrable radiologically in 3% of adults, but in most of these people causes no symptoms and no disability. Less often, some other tendon is involved. When symptoms develop, the patient is usually a man over 50 years old. In the part of the tendon involved, its collagen bundles are separated and partially replaced by pultaceous material like that in an atheromatous plaque. Often the material is calcified. The degeneration sometimes causes pain or discomfort, especially when the arm is abducted, pressing the diseased tendon against the subacromial bursa. Aspiration and injection of adrenocortical steroids often relieves the symptoms. In some patients, surgical repair is necessary.

Small tears are present in the rotator cuffs of the shoulders in 25% of old people. Usually they cause no symptoms. Occasionally there is pain or discomfort when the arm is abducted. A more extensive tear makes the glenoid fossa communicate with the subacromial bursa. It causes more severe pain. Often the patient cannot abduct the arm or hold it in abduction. Occasionally adhesions between the head of a humerus and the joint capsule limit the movement of the joint.

Degeneration of the tendon of the long head of the biceps causes pain or discomfort. Tenosynovitis in its sheath causes similar symptoms. Occasionally the tendon ruptures, and the long head contracts into a ball.

DUPUYTREN'S CONTRACTURE.   Dupuytren's contracture, or palmar fibromatosis, is named after the French surgeon Baron Dupuytren who described it in 1832. It grows increasingly common after the age of 40 years. Over 25% of people over 60 years old have some thickening of the plantar fasciae. Over 85% of the patients are men.

In 50% of the patients, the disease is bilateral, though unequal. In some, there is a similar lesion in the plantar fascia in one or both feet. A painless nodule or less frequently a diffuse thickening develops in the ulnar part of the palmar fascia. In most patients, the disease slowly extends as years pass. In a few, usually in younger people, it evolves rapidly. Often the fascia becomes attached to the skin. As the lesion ages, the fascia is shortened. The fifth finger, often the fourth finger, sometimes the third finger, become fixed in flexion. The capsules of the joints in the immobilized fingers shrink. Their articular cartilages are eroded. Eventually the process becomes stationary. The deformity is permanent.

In the early stages of the disease, the thickened fascia is highly cellular. It consists of swirling, intertwining bundles of spindle-shaped fibrocytes. Electron microscopy shows that many of them contain myofibrils. Often the lesion extends into the surrounding fatty tissues or becomes attached to the overlying dermis. As years pass, increasing quantities of collagen are deposited, and the lesion becomes less cellular. Eventually it consists of broad bundles of hyaline collagen with few cells remaining.

Some consider Dupuytren's contracture neoplastic. Most think it is a non-neoplastic reaction to injury. The nature of the injury is unknown. The disease does not seem to be a response to trauma. In 60% of the patients, Dupuytren's contracture is familial. Nearly 50% of men and 25% of women with epilepsy have Dupuytren's contracture. Alcoholism, diabetes mellitus, and pulmonary tuberculosis increase the risk of developing palmar fibromatosis. Prolonged intake of barbiturates may do so.

Dupuytren's contracture is treated by excision or division of the diseased palmar fascia. It frequently recurs. Repeated operations are sometimes needed to maintain function.

TRAUMA

This section considers the injury to intra-articular menisci caused by trauma and traumatic rupture of tendons. The importance of trauma in the causation of osteoarthritis, neuroarthropathy and tenosynovitis is discussed earlier in the chapter.

TORN MENISCUS.   A meniscus in a knee is frequently damaged in athletes and others who subject their knees to sudden stress. In 85% of the patients, the medial meniscus is affected. Often there has been earlier injury to the ligaments in the joint affected. The meniscus involved is displaced toward the center of the joint, where it is crushed between the ends of the bones. Most frequently the meniscus is split longitudinally for part of its length. Less often the tear is transverse. The injury to the meniscus causes instability in the knee and often prevents its complete extension. Sometimes an increase

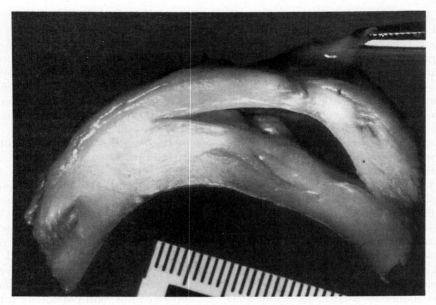

Fig 60-6. A longitudinal tear in a meniscus from a knee joint.

in synovial fluid causes swelling of the joint. The damaged meniscus is removed surgically.

In the congenital anomaly called a discoid lateral meniscus, the lateral meniscus of the knee is unusually thick and more or less disk shaped. It extends into the center of the joint where it is likely to be trapped between the articular surfaces of the femur and tibia. Often crushing of the abnormal meniscus causes pain in childhood and necessitates its removal.

TORN LIGAMENT. Trauma can cause complete or partial rupture of one or more ligaments in a joint. The knees and ankles are the most often affected. In a sprain, only a few fibers in the ligament are affected. The injury causes pain and sometimes an effusion into the joint, but little or no permanent dysfunction. If the injury to the ligament is more severe, it may cause hemorrhage into the joint. Often the joint becomes unstable. Surgical repair may be needed.

RUPTURED TENDON. Sudden trauma sometimes causes rupture of a tendon, usually at its junction with the muscle. Rheumatoid arthritis, degeneration of the biceps tendon, and other disorders weakening tendons make rupture more likely. Among the muscles and tendons most often ruptured are the pectora-

lis major, rectus abdominis, patellar tendon, and Achilles' tendon. The injury causes local hemorrhage, edema, and often spasm of the muscle involved. Surgical repair is usually needed.

CYSTS

Among the cysts associated with the joints are ganglia, popliteal cysts, the swelling caused by bursitis, and the cysts of the semilunar cartilages.

GANGLION. A ganglion takes its name from the Greek for a swelling under the skin. Ganglia are common on the dorsal aspect of the wrists, on the fingers, and on the dorsal aspect of the feet. The lesion is cystic, usually 1 to 4 cm across and roughly spheroidal. It lies in the tissues adjacent to a joint or tendon. Occasionally it is joined to the joint or tendon by a narrow channel. The ganglion has a thick collagenous wall and contains mucoid fluid.

Microscopically, a ganglion has a wall like that of a joint or bursa. It is sometimes lined by synovium, sometimes by a thin layer of necrotic tissue.

Most ganglia persist with little change for

months or years. Some disappear spontaneously. Many resolve if their content is aspirated and an adrenocortical steroid is injected into the lesion. Some must be removed surgically. If ruptured, a ganglion is likely to recur.

SYNOVIAL CYST. Synovial cysts are most common in the popliteal spaces, where they are called Baker's cysts, after a British surgeon who described various kinds of cyst in 1877. In children, a Baker's cyst is usually a distended bursa or ganglion. Often the lesion is bilateral. It causes few symptoms and usually regresses spontaneously. In adults, a Baker's cyst is nearly always a herniation of the synovium of the knee joint. Most arise in patients with osteoarthritis, rheumatoid arthritis, a torn meniscus or some other joint disease. Often the cyst is large, extending into the upper part of the calf. The cyst is sometimes lined by synovium, but more often has a thin, collagenous wall lined by flattened cells. It communicates with the joint through a narrow channel. If troublesome, a Baker's cyst is excised.

Synovial cysts of other joints are unusual except in rheumatoid arthritis. Occasionally trauma causes a synovial cyst of a hip or some other joint.

BURSITIS. Inflammation of a bursa is called bursitis. The name comes from the Greek for a hide or wineskin.

Repeated minor trauma is the most common cause of bursitis. The bursa becomes swollen. Its wall is thickened and fibrous, usually with a sparse exudate mainly of lymphocytes and plasma cells. Several types of traumatic bursitis have special names. Traumatic bursitis of the bursa overlying the first metacarpophalangeal joint is called a bunion. Housemaid's knee is bursitis of the prepatellar bursa. Inflammation of the olecranon bursa is called student's elbow. Relief from the irritation, nonsteroidal anti-inflammatory drugs, or local injections of an adrenocorticosteroid usually control traumatic bursitis. Occasionally the bursa must be excised.

Less often bursitis is caused by hematogenous or direct infection or develops in a patient with rheumatoid arthritis or gout. In these conditions, the changes in the bursa or bursae involved are similar to those in the joints affected.

CYSTS OF SEMILUNAR CARTILAGES. Cysts sometimes develop in one of the menisci in the knee, usually in the anterior end of the lateral meniscus. They contain mucinous fluid. Some are lined by synovium; some by frayed fibrocartilage.

TUMORS

Tumors of the joints, tendons, and aponeuroses are uncommon. Almost all are primary.

Benign

The benign tumors and tumor-like proliferations arising in the joints, tendon sheaths, and aponeuroses are synovial chrondromatosis, nodular synovitis, and the juvenile aponeurotic fibroma. Less often a hemangioma, lipoma, or some other benign connective tissue tumor arises in a joint, tendon, or aponeurosis.

Synovial Chondromatosis. Synovial chondromatosis is an uncommon condition in which nodules of cartilage develop in the synovium of the affected joint or rarely in a tendon sheath or bursa. Usually only a single joint is affected, most often a knee, less frequently a hip, elbow, or shoulder. The patient is usually a young adult, more often a man than a woman.

The synovium of the affected joint usually shows dozens or hundreds of small nodules of cartilage, most less than 0.5 cm across. Less often, the nodules of cartilage are fewer and up to 3 cm across. Some of the nodules are within the synovium; some hang from fine pedicles. Often some of the nodules are free in the joint. Microscopically, the nodules consist of well-differentiated cartilage, sometimes with a few plump or binucleated chondrocytes. Frequently some of the nodules are calcified or ossified.

Some patients remain asymptomatic. Some have episodes of pain, an effusion into the joint, or limitation of movement. In some, the loose bodies free in the joint cause it to lock. Often symptoms continue for years before the patient seeks treatment.

Synovial chondromatosis is probably not

neoplastic. It is probably a type of metaplasia. Excision of the involved part of the synovium cures.

Nodular Synovitis. Nodular synovitis has many names. Giant cell tumor of tendon sheath is one of the more common. Some call it nodular pigmented villonodular synovitis. Others prefer names such as xanthofibroma or benign synovioma. The patient is usually over 40 years old. Women are affected more often than men.

Nodular synovitis is most common in the tendon sheaths of the fingers, wrists, ankles, and feet. Occasionally it develops in a knee, rarely in another joint. In a tendon, the lesion is a well-defined, spheroidal mass from 0.3 to 3 cm across. On section, it is firm, rubbery, gray, or brown, often flecked with yellow. Frequently a lesion in a tendon extends into the adjacent soft tissues or erodes bone. In a knee, the lesion is similar but often forms one or more pedunculated masses.

Microscopically, the lesion varies from one patient to another and in different parts of the same lesion. Usually, the mass is divided into ill-defined lobules by collagenous septa. Within the lobules are many small mononuclear cells, mainly lymphocytes or small macrophages. With them are mixed lipophages and macrophages containing hemosiderin. The lipophages are sometimes the dominant feature of the lesion; sometimes they are few. Giant, multinucleated macrophages are usually present and may be numerous. Often small slits lined with synovium are present within the mass. Sometimes part of a lesion becomes hyalinized and consists of little but coarse collagen.

In a tendon sheath, nodular synovitis rarely causes pain or limitation of movement.

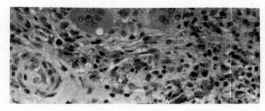

Fig. 60-7. A giant cell tumor of tendon showing the giant cells and macrophages usually prominent in this form of nodular synovitis.

Often the lesion has been present for many years before the patient seeks help. In a knee, nodular synovitis sometimes causes a mild effusion into the joint, locking, or restriction of movement.

Nodular synovitis is probably a nonneoplastic reaction to injury, though some consider it a benign neoplasm of the synovium. Many think it is a localized form of pigmented villonodular synovitis. Complete excision cures. Partial excision is often followed by recurrence.

JUVENILE APONEUROTIC FIBROMA. A juvenile aponeurotic fibroma is an uncommon condition most frequent in the palmar or plantar fascia of young children. Occasionally it arises in an aponeurosis or fascia elsewhere in the body or in an older child or adult. A mass develops in the affected aponeurosis or fascia. It sometimes extends into neighboring structures. Microscopically, the lesion consists of a proliferation of spindle-shaped or ovoid fibrocytes, with little collagen between them. Foci of chondroid differentiation are common and often are calcified. The chondroid foci are frequently more extensive when the lesion develops within the body.

A juvenile aponeurotic fibroma is probably a neoplasm near the borderline of a malignancy. It invades but does not metastasize. Complete excision cures. Incomplete excision is usually followed by recurrence.

Malignant

The malignant tumors primary in the joints, tendons, and aponeuroses are the synovioma and the closely related epithelioid sarcoma, clear cell sarcoma, and chordoid sarcoma. Many consider that these tumors are forms of synovioma. Often a metastasis of one of the other types of sarcoma has the structure of a synovioma, and occasionally a metastasis of a synovioma resembles one of the other types of sarcoma.

Secondary tumors of joints, tendons, and aponeuroses are uncommon. Occasionally a tumor of bone or the soft tissues invades a joint or tendon. Rarely, a metastatic tumor develops in the synovium of a joint or in a tendon.

SYNOVIOMA. A synovioma is often called a

malignant synovioma, a synovial sarcoma, or a tenosynovial sarcoma. Less than 10% of malignant tumors of the soft tissues are of this type. Over 50% of the patients are between 20 and 40 years old. Nearly 60% of them are men.

Lesions. Most synoviomata arise near a joint, but do not involve it. Nearly 20% of synoviomata arise in the thigh, 20% in a foot, 10% near a knee, 10% near a shoulder, and 5% in a forearm. Occasionally a synovioma arises in a buttock, the pelvis, back, retroperitoneal space, pharynx, an orbit, or elsewhere.

Usually a synovioma forms a well-defined, spheroidal mass, from 1 to 20 cm in diameter. Less often it infiltrates the surrounding tissues or extends along a tendon sheath. On section, it is soft and gray with areas of necrosis and hemorrhage. Foci of calcification are often present. Occasionally the tumor is cystic.

Microscopically, most synoviomata consist of uniform, closely packed, spindle-shaped cells with sparse, ill-defined cytoplasm and ovoid nuclei. The spindle cells form sheets or bundles. Usually there is little or no intercellular substance between them. Mitoses are few. Rarely, broad bands of collagen divide the spindle cells into clumps. In some tumors, often in only part of the tumor, slits or spaces lined by cuboidal or columnar cells are present among the spindle cells. Sometimes slits or spaces are lined by the spindle cells. Solid clumps of epithelioid cells like the cuboidal cells lining the spaces may be present. Occasionally, a synovioma is predominantly of glandlike spaces lined by cuboidal or columnar cells. Foci of calcification are often present in the tumor.

The spindle-shaped cells have prominent endoplasmic reticulum and many microfilaments. They stain for vimentin. Some of them stain for cytokeratin. The cuboidal cells lining the spaces have many mitochondria, less prominent endoplasmic reticulum, and few microfilaments. They are often joined by desmosomes and rest on a basement membrane. They stain strongly for cytokeratin but not for vimentin. Forms intermediate between the two types of cell are sometimes present.

Behavior. A synovioma invades the adjacent tissues more extensively than is apparent macroscopically. In 15% of the patients it involves an adjacent bone. After local excision, more than 50% of synoviomata recur. In 70% of the patients, the tumor metastasizes to the lungs, in 20% to the regional lymph nodes, and in 15% to the bones.

Clinical Presentation. Most synoviomata grow slowly. The lesion is detected when the patient discovers the mass. Pain is unusual.

Treatment and Prognosis. A synovioma is treated by radical local excision or amputation, usually followed by chemotherapy. About 60% of the patients are alive five years after the resection, 50% 10 years afterwards. Over 75% of patients with a tumor less than 5 cm in diameter and only 25% of those with a larger tumor survive more than 5 years. The prognosis is better in children and old people. It is better in women than in men. A synovioma on a hand or foot has a better prognosis than a more proximal tumor. A synovioma that contains glandlike spaces has a better prognosis than a lesion that consists entirely of spindle cells.

EPITHELIOID SARCOMA. An epithelioid sarcoma is an uncommon tumor that arises in tendons and aponeuroses. The patients are usually young adults. The sarcoma is most common in the hands, wrists, forearms, and lower legs. One or more masses develop in the tendon or aponeurosis involved. Sometimes the lesion ulcerates through the skin. Microscopically, the tumor consists of clumps of cuboidal or polygonal cells separated by a collagenous stroma. The tumor cells have little endoplasmic reticulum and few mitochondria. Necrosis is often extensive. Frequently a prominent inflammatory or granulomatous reaction is present at the margin of the clumps of tumor cells.

An epithelioid sarcoma is treated like a synovioma. If not widely removed, the sarcoma recurs. Metastases are most common in the regional lymph nodes, but also occur in the lungs and bones. Over 50% of the patients survive more than five years.

CLEAR CELL SARCOMA. A clear cell sarcoma is a rare tumor of tendons and aponeuroses. It is most common in the tendons and fasciae of the feet and knees. The tumor usually forms a mass less than 5 cm in diameter that grows slowly. Microscopically, it consists of clumps of large round cells with abundant clear cytoplasm and vesicular nuclei with prominent nucleoli. Glycogen is abundant in the cytoplasm. The clumps of tumor cells are separated by a scanty collagenous stroma. In some patients, a tumor first thought to be a clear cell sarcoma has proved to be a melanoma. A clear cell sarcoma recurs if not completely removed. It frequently metastasizes to the regional lymph nodes and to the lungs.

CHORDOID SARCOMA.   A chordoid sarcoma is a rare lesion most common in the hands and wrists. Most patients are middle-aged. The sarcoma forms a gray, gelatinous mass that often extends along tendons or into a bursa. Microscopically, it consists of small round or polygonal cells with sparse, dense cytoplasm. The tumor cells have prominent nucleoli. They are separated by abundant mucoid stroma. Small nodules of cartilage are often present. The sarcoma grows slowly. It metastasizes in 30% of the patients.

BIBLIOGRAPHY

General

Berry, C. L. (Ed.): Bone and joint disease. Curr. Top. Pathol., 71:1, 1982.

McCarty, D. J. (Ed.): Arthritis and Allied Conditions. Philadelphia, Lea & Febiger, 1989.

Arthritis

Adams, M. E., and Billingham, M. E. J.: Animal models of degenerative joint disease. Curr. Top. Pathol., 71:265, 1982.

Agenlli, M., and Wahl, S. M.: Cytokines and fibrosis. Clin. Exp. Rheumatol., 4:379, 1986.

Ahlquist, J.: On the structural and physiological basis of the influence of exercise, movement and immoblization in inflammatory joint diseases. Ann. Chir. Gynaecol., 74(Suppl. 198):10, 1985.

Aho, K., Leirisalo-Repo, M., and Repo, H.: Reactive arthritis. Clin. Rheum. Dis., 11:25, 1985.

Alarcón, G. S., Bocanegra, T. S., Gotuzzo, E., and Espinoza, L. R.: The arthritis of brucellosis. J. Rheumatol., 14:1083, 1987.

Allen, R. C., and Ansell, B. M.: Juvenile chronic arthritis. Postgrad. Med. J., 62:821, 1986.

Alpert, S. D., Koide, J., Takada, S., and Engelman, E. G.: T cell regulatory disturbances in the rheumatic diseases. Rheum. Dis. Clin. North Am., 13:431, 1987.

Altman, R. D., and Gray, R.: Inflammation in osteoarthritis. Clin. Rheum. Dis., 11:353, 1985.

Ansell, B. M.: Juvenile arthritis. Clin. Rheum. Dis., 10:657, 1984.

Arenzana-Seisdedos, F., Teyton, L., and Virelizier, J. L.: Immunoregulatory mediators in the pathogenesis of rheumatoid arthritis. Scand. J. Rheumatol., Suppl. 66:13, 1987.

Arnett, F. C.: Seronegative spondyloarthropathies. Bull. Rheum. Dis., 37:1, 1987.

Baty, B. J., Cubberley, D., Morris, C., and Carey, J.: Prenatal diagnosis of arthrogryphosis. Am. J. Med. Genet., 29:501, 1988.

Benedek, T. G.: Neoplastic associations of rheumatic diseases and rheumatic manifestations of cancer. Clin. Geriatr. Med., 4:333, 1988.

van den Berg, W. B.: Influence of joint inflammation on chondrocyte function. Int. J. Tissue React., 10:17, 1988.

Black, J.: Metallic ion release and its relationship to oncogenesis. Hip, (Review). 199–213, 1985.

Bogoch, B. R.: Silicone synovitis. J. Rheumatol., 14:1986, 1987.

Bora, F. W., Jr., and Miller, G.: Joint physiology, cartilage metabolism and the etiology of osteoarthritis. Hand Clin., 3:325, 1987.

Brandt, K. D.: Osteoarthritis. Clin. Geriatr. Med., 4:279, 1988.

Brandt, K. D., and Fife, R. S.: Ageing in relation to the pathogenesis of osteoarthritis. Clin. Rheum. Dis., 12:117, 1986.

Brown, K. A.: The polymorphonuclear cell in rheumatoid arthritis. Br. J. Rehumatol., 27:150, 1988.

Brown, R. A., and Weiss, J. B.: Neovascularization and its role in the osteoarthritis process. Ann. Rheum. Dis., 47:881, 1988.

Bruneau, C., et al.: Seronegative spondyloarthropathies and IgA glomerulonephritis. Semin. Arthritis Rheum., 15:179, 1986.

Bullough, P. G., DiCarlo, E. F., Hansraj, K. K., and Neves, M. C.: Pathologic studies of total joint replacement. Orthop. Clin. North Am., 19:611, 1988.

Butler, R. C., Thompson, J. M., and Keat, A. C. S.: Paraneoplastic rheumatic disorders. J. R. Soc. Med., 80:168, 1987.

Calin, A.: Ankylosing spondylitis. Clin. Rheum. Dis., 11:41, 1985.

Calin, A.: Pathogenesis of ankylosing spondylitis. Br. J. Rheumatol., 27(Suppl. II):106, 1988.

Carson, D. A., et al.: Molecular basis for the cross-reactive idiotypes on human anti-IgG antibodies (rheumatoid factors). Ciba Found. Symp., 129:123, 1987.

Cavender, D., et al.: Pathways to chronic inflammation in rheumatic synovitis. Fed. Proc., 46:113, 1987.

Chang-Miller, A., et al.: Renal involvement in relapsing perichondritis. Medicine, 66:202, 1987.

Charron, D., and Teyton, L.: Autoimmunity in rheumatoid arthritis. Concepts Immunopathol., 4:200, 1987.

Chen, P. P., Fong, S., and Carson, D. A.: Rheumatoid factor. Rheum. Dis. Clin. North Am., 13:545, 1987.

Cooke, T. D. V.: Pathogenetic mechanisms in polyarticular osteoarthritis. Clin. Rheum. Dis., 11:203, 1985.

Davis, M. A.: Epidemiology of osteoarthritis. Clin. Geriatr. Med., 4:241, 1988.

Dayer, J. M., and Demczuk, S.: Cytokines and other mediators in rheumatoid arthritis. Springer Semin. Immunol., 7:387, 1984.

Dieppe, P. A., and Doherty, M.: The role of particles in the pathogenesis of joint disease. Curr. Top. Pathol., 71:199, 1982.

Dieppe, P., and Watt, I.: Crystal deposition in osteoarthritis. Clin. Rheum. Dis., 11:367, 1985.

Doherty, M., and Dieppe, P.: Crystal deposition disease in the elderly. Clin. Rheum. Dis., 12:97, 1986.

Dorner, R. W., Alexander, R. L., Jr., and Moore, T. L.: Rheumatoid factors. Clin. Chem. Acta, 167:1, 1987.

Duff, G. W.: Arthritis and interleukins. Br. J. Rheumatol., 27:2, 1988.

Edwards, J. C. W.: Pathophysiology of chronic synovitis. Br. J. Rehumatol., 27(Suppl. II):116, 1988.

Ellman, M. H., and Curran, J. J.: Causes and management of shoulder arthritis. Compr. Ther., 14:29, 1988.

Emery, P., Williamson, D. J., and Mackay, I. R.: Role of cytokines in rheumatological inflammation. Concepts Immunopathol., 4:171, 1987.

Espinoza, L. R.: Rheumatoid arthritis: etiopathogenetic considerations. Clin. Lab. Med., 6:27, 1986.

Eulderink, F.: The synovial biopsy. Curr. Top. Pathol., 71:25, 1982.

Fantini, F.: Infection and arthritis. Scand. J. Rheumatol., Suppl. 66:93, 1987.

Fassbender, H. G.: Role of chondrocytes in the development of osteoarthritis. Am. J. Med., 83(5A):17, 1987.

Fergusson, C. M.: The aetiology of osteoarthritis. Postgrad. Med. J., 63:439, 1987.

Fink, C. W.: Reactive arthritis. Pediatr. Infect. Dis. J., 7:58, 1988.

Fink, C. W., and Nelson, J. D.: Septic arthritis and osteoarthritis in children. Clin. Rheum. Dis., 12:423, 1986.

Firestein, G. S., Tsai, V., and Zvaifler, N. J.: Cellular immunity in the joints of patients with rheumatoid arthritis. Rheum. Dis. Clin. North Am., 13:191, 1987.

Firestein, G. S., and Zvaifler, N. J.: Reactive arthritis. Annu. Rev. Med., 38:351, 1987.

Firestein, G. S., and Zvaifler, N. J.: The pathogenesis of rheumatoid arthritis. Rheum. Dis. Clin. North Am., 13:447, 1987.

Fong, S., et al.: The diversity and idiotypic patterns of rheumatoid factors in disease. Concepts Immunopathol., 5:168, 1988.

Fong, S., et al.: Rheumatoid factors in human autoimmune disease. Pathol. Immunopathol. Res., 5:305, 1986.

Ford, D. K.: Reactive arthritis. Clin. Rheum. Dis., 12:389, 1986.

Franssen, M. J., Boerbooms, A. M., and Van de Putte, L. B.: Polychondritis and rheumatoid arthritis. Clin. Rheumatol., 6:453, 1987.

German, D. C., and Holmes, E. W.: Hyperuricemia and gout. Med. Clin. North Am., 70:419, 1986.

Glickstein, S. L., and Nashel, D. J.: Mycobacterium kansasii arthritis complicating rheumatoid arthritis. Semin. Arthritis Rheum., 16:231, 1987.

Goldenberg, D. L., and Reed, J. I.: Bacterial arthritis. N. Engl. J. Med., 312:764, 1985.

Goldstein, R., and Arnett, F. C.: The genetics of rheumatic disease in man. Rheum. Dis. Clin. North Am., 13:487, 1987.

Gordon, S. C., and Lauter, C. B.: Mumps arthritis. Rev. Infect. Dis., 6:338, 1984.

Gran, J. T.: The epidemiology of rheumatoid arthritis. Monogr. Allergy, 21:162, 1987.

Gravallese, E. M., and Kantrowitz, F. G.: Arthritic manifestations of inflammatory bowel disease. Am. J. Gastroenterol., 83:703, 1988.

Green, N. E., and Edwards, K.: Bone and joint infections in children. Orthop. Clin. North Am., 18:555, 1987.

Gregersen, P. K., Gallerstein, P., Jaffe, W., and Enlow, R. W.: Valvular heart disease associated with juvenile onset ankylosing spondylitis. Bull. Hosp. Jt. Dis. Orthop. Inst., 42:103, 1982.

Hall, J. G.: Diagnostic approaches and prognosis in arthrogryphosis. Pathologica, 78:701, 1986.

Hamerman, D.: Osteoarthritis. Orthop. Rev., 17:353, 1988.

Hamerman, D., and Klagsbrun, M.: Osteoarthritis. Am. J. Med., 78:495, 1985.

Harris, E. D., Jr.: Synovial inflammation in rheumatoid arthritis. Hosp. Pract., 21(9):71, 1986.

Haskard, D.: Lymphocyte traffic, endothelium, and rheumatoid arthritis. Ann. Rheum. Dis., 46:881, 1987.

Hayward, M., and Fielder-Nagy, C. L.: Mechanisms of bone loss: rheumatoid arthritis, periodontal disease and osteoporosis. Agents Actions, 22:251, 1987.

Healey, L. A.: Rheumatoid arthritis in the elderly. Clin. Rheum. Dis., 12:173, 1986.

Helliwell, P., and Wright, V.: Seronegative spondyloarthritides. Bailière's Clin. Rheumatol., 1:491, 1987.

Henderson, B., and Pettipher, W. R.: The synovial lining cell. Semin. Arthritis Rheum., 15:1, 1985.

Henderson, B., Pettipher, E. R., and Higgs, G. A.: Mediators of rheumatoid arthritis. Br. Med. Bull., 43:415, 1987.

Henderson, B., Revell, P. A., and Edwards, J. C.: Synovial lining cell hyperplasia in rheumatoid arthritis. Ann. Rheum. Dis., 47:348, 1988.

Herbison, G. J., Ditunno, J. F., and Jaweed, J. M.: Muscle atrophy in rheumatoid arthritis. J. Rheumatol., 14(Suppl. 15):78, 1987.

Heymer, B., Spanel, R., and Haferkamp, O.: Experimental models of arthritis. Curr. Top. Pathol., 71:123, 1982.

Hochberg, M. C.: Osteoarthritis: pathophysiology, manifestations, management. Hosp. Pract., 19(12):41, 1984.

Hough, A. J., Jr., and Webber, A. J.: Aging phenomena and osteoarthritis. Ann. Clin. Lab. Sci., 16:502, 1986.

Huaux, J. P., Vanderbroucke, J. M., and Noël, H.: Amyloidosis 1970-1985 with special reference to amyloid arthropathy. Acta Clin. Belg., 42:365, 1987.

Hull, R. G.: Outcome in juvenile arthritis. Br. J. Rheumatol., 27(Suppl. 1):66, 1988.

Husby, G.: Amyloidosis and rheumatoid arthritis. Clin. Exp. Rheumatol., 3:173, 1985.

Jasin, H. E.: Intra-articular antigen-antibody reactions. Rheum. Dis. Clin. North Am., 13:179, 1987.

Johansson, N. A.: Endocrine arthropathies. Clin. Rheum. Dis., 11:297, 1985.

Jolly, D. J.: The role of the HPRT gene in human disease. Horiz. Biochem. Biophys., *8*:123, 1986.

Keat, A. N.: Reiter's syndrome and reactive arthritis. N. Engl. J. Med., *309*:1606, 1983.

Kim, S. K.: Mycoplasma hominis arthritis. Ann. Plast. Surg., *20*:163, 1988.

Kimberly, R. P.: Immune complexes in rheumatic diseases. Rheum. Dis. Clin. North Am., *13*:583, 1987.

Kirwan, J. R., and Silman, A. J.: Epidemiological, sociological and environmental aspects of rheumatoid arthritis and osteoarthritis. Baillière's Clin. Rheumatol., *1*:467, 1987.

Klareskog, L., Holmdahl, R., Goldschmidt, T., and Björk, J.: Immunoregulation in arthritis. Scand. J. Rheumatol., Suppl. *64*:7, 1987.

Klareskog, L., et al.: Synovial class II antigen expression and immune complex expression in rheumatoid arthritis. Acta Med. Scand., Suppl. *715*:85, 1987.

Klareskog, L., and Johnell, O.: Induced expression of class II transplantation antigens in the pannus in RA. Br. J. Rheumatol., *27*(Suppl. II):141, 1988.

Klein, R. S.: Joint infection, with consideration of the underlying disease and source of bacteremia in hematogenous infection. Clin. Geriatr. Med., *4*:375, 1988.

Koss, P. G.: Disseminated gonococcal infection. The tenosynovitis-dermatitis and suppurative arthritis syndromes. Cleve. Clin. Q., *52*:161, 1985.

Kouri, T.: Etiology of rheumatoid arthritis. Experentia, *41*:434, 1985.

Krane, S. M., and Simon. L. S.: Rheumatoid arthritis: clinical features and pathogenetic mechanisms. Med. Clin. North Am., *70*:263, 1986.

Lanchbury, J. S. S.: Molecular genetics of the HLA-D region component of inherited susceptibility to rheumatoid arthritis. Br. J. Rheumatol., *27*:171, 1988.

Lane, N. E., and Fries, J. F.: Relationship of running to osteoarthritis and bone density. Compr. Ther., *14*:7, 1988.

Laurent, M. R.: Psoriatic arthritis. Clin. Rheum. Dis., *11*:61, 1985.

Leak, A. M.: Autoantibody profile in juvenile chronic arthritis. Ann. Rheum. Dis., *47*:178, 1988.

Leicht, M. J., Harrington, T. M., and Davis, D. E.: Cricoarytenoid arthritis. Ann. Emerg. Med., *16*:885, 1987.

Leirisalo-Repo, M.: Yersinia arthritis. Contrib. Microbiol. Immunol., 9:145, 1987.

Levinson, A. I., and Martin, J.: Rheumatoid factor: Dr. Jekyll or Mr. Hyde? Br. J. Rheumatol., *27*:83, 1988.

Lydyard, D. M., and Irving, W. L.: Is there a role for Epstein-Barr virus in the aetiology of rheumatoid arthritis? Br. J. Rheumatol., 27 (Suppl. II):120, 1988.

McCarty, D. J.: Arthritis associated with crystals containing calcium. Med. Clin. North Am., *70*:437, 1986.

McCarty, D. J.: Arthropathies associated with calcium-containing crystals. Hosp. Pract., *21*(10):109, 1986.

McCarty, D. J.: Intractable gouty arthritis. Hosp. Pract., *22*(6):191, 1987.

McCarty, D. J. (Ed.): Crystaline deposit diseases. Rheum. Dis. Clin. North Am., *14*:253, 1988.

McCarty, G. A.: Autoantibodies and their relation to rheumatic diseases. Med. Clin. North Am., *70*:237, 1986.

McDaniel, D. O., et al.: Analysis of restriction fragment length polymorphisms in rheumatic diseases. Rheum. Dis. Clin. North Am., *13*:353, 1987.

McDuffie, F. C. (Ed.): Neoplasms in rheumatoid arthritis. Am. J. Med., *78*(1A):1, 1985.

McGuigan, L. E., Geczy, A. F., and Edmonds, J. P.: The immunopathology of ankylosing spondylitis. Semin. Arthritis Rheum., *15*:81, 1985.

McKenna, F.: Clinical and laboratory assessment of outcome in rheumatoid arthritis. Br. J. Rheumatol., 27 (Suppl. 1):12, 1988.

Macy, N. J., Lieber, L., and Haberman, E. T.: Arthritis caused by Clostridium septicum. J. Bone Joint Surg. (Am), *68*:465, 1986.

Mainardi, C. L.: Biochemical mechanisms of articular destruction. Rheum. Dis. Clin. North Am., *13*:215, 1987.

Maini, R. N., Plater-Zyberk, C., and Andrew, E.: Autoimmunity in rheumatoid arthritis. Rheum. Dis. Clin. North Am., *13*:319, 1987.

Mankin, H. J., and Treadwell, B. V.: Osteoarthritis: a 1987 update. Bull. Rheum. Dis., *36*:1, 1986.

Mannik, M., and Nardella, F. A.: IgG rheumatoid factors and self-association of the antibodies. Clin. Rheum. Dis., *11*:552, 1985.

March, L. M.: Dendritic cells in the pathogenesis of rheumatoid arthritis. Rheumatol. Int., 7:141, 1987.

Martini, A.: Immunological abnormalities in juvenile rheumatoid arthritis. Scand. J. Rheumatol., Suppl. *66*:107, 1987.

Midtvedt, T.: Intestinal bacteria and rheumatic disease. Scand. J. Rheumatol., Suppl. *64*:49, 1986.

Miller, L. C., and Dinarello, C. A.: Biological activation of interleukin-1 relevant to rheumatic diseases. Pathol. Immunopathol. Res., *6*:22, 1987.

Miossec, P.: The role of interleukin 1 in the pathogenesis of rheumatoid arthritis. Clin. Exp. Rheumatol., *5*:305, 1987.

Moll, J. M. H.: Inflammatory bowel diesease. Clin. Rheum. Dis., *11*:87, 1985.

Moll, J. M. H.: New criteria for the diagnosis of ankylosing spondylitis. Scand. J. Rheumatol., Suppl. *65*:12, 1987.

Moskowitz, R. W.: Primary osteoarthritis: epidemiology, clinical aspects and general management. Am. J. Med., *83*(5A):5, 1987.

Murnaghan, J. P.: Adhesive capsulitis of the shoulder. Orthopedics, *1*:153, 1988.

Møller, P.: Seronegative arthritis. Scand. J. Rheumatol., Suppl. *66*:119, 1987.

Nakad, A., et al.: Nodular regenerative hyperplasia of the liver and esophageal varices in Felty's syndrome. Acta Clin. Belg., *43*:45, 1988.

Nixon, J.: Intervertebral disc mechanics. J. R. Soc. Med., *79*:100, 1986.

Ohta, A., et al.: Adult Still's disease. J. Rheumatol., *14*:1139-1146, 1987.

Padula, S. J., Clark, R. B., and Korn, J. H.: Cell-mediated immunity in rheumatic disease. Hum. Pathol., *17*:254, 1986.

Panush, R. S., and Borwn, D. G.: Exercise and arthritis. Sports Med., *4*:54, 1987.

Partsch, G.: Laboratory features of psoriatic arthritis. Z. Rheumatol., *46*:220, 1987.

Perlman, S. G.: Psoriatic arthritis in children. Pediatr.

Dermatol., *1*:283, 1984.

Petersen, J.: B lymphocyte function in patients with rheumatoid arthritis. Dan. Med. Bull., 35:140, 1988.

Petty, R. E., and Malleson, P.: Spondyloarthropathies of children. Pediatr. Clin. North Am., 33:1079, 1986.

Petty, R. E.: Current knowledge of the etiology and pathogenesis of chronic uveitis accompanying juvenile rheumatoid arthritis. Rheum. Dis. Clin. North Am., 13:19, 1987.

Peyron, J. G.: Osteoarthritis. The epidemiologic viewpoint. Clin. Orthop., 213:13, 1986.

Phillips, B. M., and David, T. J.: Pathogenesis and management of arthropathy in cystic fibrosis. J. R. Soc. Med., 79(Suppl. 12):44, 1986.

Phillips, P. E.: Infectious agents in the pathogenesis of rheumatoid arthritis. Semin. Arthritis Rheum., 16:1, 1986.

Phillips, P. E.: Evidence involving infectious agents in rheumatoid arthritis and juvenile rheumatoid arthritis. Clin. Exp. Rheumatol., 6:87, 1988.

Pisetsky, D. S., and Snyderman, R. (Eds.): Immunology of the rheumatic diseases. Rheum. Dis. Clin. North Am., 13:411, 1987.

Pope, R. M., and Talal, N.: Autoimmunity in rheumatoid arthritis. Concepts Immunopathol., 1:219, 1985.

Pujol, J. P., and Loyau, G.: Interleukin-1 and osteoarthritis. Life Sci., 41:1187, 1987.

Reginato, A. J., and Schumacher, H. R., Jr.: Crystal-associated arthropathies. Clin. Geriatr. Med., 4:295, 1988.

Reginato, A. J., et al.: Adult onset Still's disease. Semin. Arthritis Rheum., 17:39, 1987.

Revell, P. A.: Examination of synovial fluid. Curr. Top. Pathol., 71:1, 1982.

Revell, P. A.: Tissue reactions to joint prostheses and the products of wear and corrosion. Curr. Top. Pathol., 71:73, 1982.

Richardson, B., and Stobo, J. D.: The major histocompatibility complex antigens in rheumatoid arthritis and juvenile arthritis. Bull. Rheum. Dis., 31:21, 1981.

Roschman, R. A., and Rothenberg, R. J.: Palmonary fibrosis in rheumatoid arthritis. Semin. Arthritis Rheum., 16:174, 1987.

Rosenberg, A. M.: Uveitis associated with juvenile rheumatoid arthritis. Semin. Arthritis Rheum., 16:158, 1987.

Roudier, J., et al.: The Epstein-Barr virus glycoprotein gp 110, a molecular link between HLA DR4, HLA DR1, and rheumatoid arthritis. Scand. J. Immunol., 27:367, 1988.

Saag, M. S., and Bennett, J. C.: The infectious etiology of chronic rheumatic diseases. Semin. Arthritis Rheum., 17:1, 1987.

Sambrook, P. N., and Reeve, J.: Bone disease in rheumatoid arthritis. Clin. Sci., 74:225, 1988.

Sany, J.: Prospects in the immunological treatment of rheumatoid arthritis. Scand. J. Rheumatol., Suppl. 66:129, 1987.

Schiffenbauer, J., and Schwartz, B. D.: The HLA complex and its relationship to rheumatic disease. Rheum. Dis. Clin. North Am., 13:463, 1987.

Schneider, H. A., et al.: Rheumatoid vasculitis. Semin. Arthritis Rheum., 14:280, 1985.

Schorr-Lesnick, B., and Brandt, L. J.: Selected rheuma-

tologic and dermatologic manifestations of inflammatory bowel disease. Am. J. Gastroenterol., 83:216, 1988.

Schumacher, H. R., and Gall, E. P. (Eds.): Rheumatoid Arthritis: An Illustrated Guide to Pathology, Diagnosis and Management. Philadelpia, J. B. Lippincott, 1988.

Scott, J. T.: Gout. Baillière's Clin. Rheumatol., 1:525, 1987.

Sequeira, W.: Diseases of the pubic symphysis. Semin. Arthritis Rheum., 16:11, 1986.

Shah, B. C., and Khan, M. A.: Review of ankylosing spondylitis. Compr. Ther., 13:52, 1987.

Sheppeard, H.: An update on mechanisms of cartilage destruction in rheumatoid arthritis. Aust. N. Z. J. Med., 13:195, 1983.

Shumacher, H. R., Jr.: Crystals, inflammation, and osteoarthritis. Am. J. Med., 83(5A):11, 1987.

Sigal, L. H.: The neurological presentation of vasculitis and rheumatologic syndromes. Medicine, 6:157. 1987.

Sigal, L. H., Johnston, S. L., and Phillips, P. E.: Cellular immune responses to cartilage components in rheumatoid arthritis and osteoarthritis. Clin. Exp. Rheumatol., 6:59, 1988.

Silman, A. J.: Musculo-skeletal disorders in childhood. Br. Med. Bull., 42:196, 1986.

Sinico, R. A., Fornasieri, A., and D'Amico, G.: Role and clinical significance of rheumatoid factors in glomerulonephritis. Contrib. Nephrol., 61:149, 1988.

Smiley, J. D., Hoffman, W. L., Moore, S. E., and Paradies, L. H.: The humoral response of the rheumatoid synovium. Semin. Arthritis Rheum., 14:151, 1985.

Snyderman, R.: Mechanisms of inflammation and leukocyte chemotaxis in the rheumatic diseases. Med. Clin. North Am., 70:217, 1986.

Sokoloff, L.: Animal models of rheumatoid arthritis. Int. Rev. Exp. Pathol., 26:107, 1984.

Sokoloff, L.: Endemic forms of osteoarthritis. Clin. Rheum. Dis., 11:187, 1985.

Sokoloff, L.: Kashin-Beck disease. Rheum. Dis. Clin. North Am., 13:101, 1987.

Stanescu, V., Stanescu, R., and Maroteaux, P.: Articular degeneration as a sequella of osteochrondrodysplasias. Clin. Rheum. Dis., 11:239, 1985.

Stevens, M. B. and Hahn, B. H.: Reiter's syndrome. Bull. Rheum. Dis., 32:31, 1982.

Stuart, J. M., and Kang, A. H.: Monkeying around with collagen autoimmunity and arthritis. Lab. Invest., 54:1, 1986.

Stuart, J. M., Townes, A. S., and Kang, A. H.: Collagen autoimmune arthritis. Annu. Rev. Immunol., 2:199, 1984.

Sturge, R. A.: The remote effects of rheumatic diseases on the hand. Clin. Rheum. Dis., 10:449, 1984.

Suteanu, S., Gabrielescu, E., and Stoicescu, M.: Advances in the physiochemical, immunologic and cytologic investigation of the synovial fluid. Med. Interne, 25:3, 1987.

Swanson, A. B., and de Groot-Swanson, G.: Osteoarthritis in the hand. Clin. Rheum. Dis., 1:393, 1985.

Symmons, D. P.: Mortality in rheumatoid arthritis. Br. J. Rheumatol., 27(Suppl. 1):44, 1988.

Talal, N.: Interleukins, interferons and rheumatic

disease. Clin. Rheum. Dis., *11*: 633, 1985.

Terkeltaub, R., and Ginsberg, M. H.: Molecular mechanisms of gouty arthritis, Surv. Synth. Pathol. Res., 3:386, 1984.

Thompson, G. H. (Ed.): Arthrogryphosis multiplex congenita. Clin. Orthop., *194*:2, 1985.

Threlkeld, A. J., and Currier, D. P.: Osteoarthritis: effects on synovial joint tissues. Phys. Ther., *68*:364, 1988.

Toivanen, A.: Reactive Arthritis. Boca Raton, CRC Press, 1988.

Trentham, D. E.: The immunopathogenesis of rheumatoid arthritis. J. Rheumatol., *12*(Suppl. 12):7, 1985.

Typpö, T.: Osteoarthritis of the hip. Radiologic findings and etiology. Ann. Chir. Gynaecol., *74*(Suppl. 201):1, 1985.

Utsinger, P. D., Zvaifler, N. J., and Ehrlich, G. E.: Rheumatoid Arthritis: Etiology, Diagnosis and Treatment. Philadelphia, J. B. Lippincott, 1985.

Varga, J., Giampaolo, C., and Goldenberg, D. L.: Tophaceous gout of the spine. Arthritis Rheum., *28*:1312, 1985.

Venables, P.: Epstein-Barr virus infection and autoimmunity in rheumatoid arthritis. Ann. Rheum. Dis., *47*: 265, 1988.

Wallace, D. J.: The role of stress and trauma in rheumatoid arthritis and systemic lupus erythematosus. Semin. Arthritis Rheum., *16*:153, 1987.

Weinblatt, M. E.: Toxicity of low dose methotrexate in rheumatoid arthritis. J. Rheumatol., *12*(Suppl. 12): 35, 1985.

Weissmann, G., and Korchak, H.: Rheumatoid arthritis: the role of neutrophil suppression. Inflammation, *8* (Suppl.):S3, 1984.

Wengrower, D., Pollak, A., Okon, E., and Stalnikowicz, R.: Collagenous colitis and rheumatoid arthritis with response to sulfasalazine. J. Clin. Gastroenterol., *9*:456, 1987.

Wilder, R. L.: Proinflammatory microbial products as etiologic agents of inflammatory arthritis. Rheum. Dis. Clin. North Am., *13*:293, 1987.

Wilson, R. L.: Rheumatoid arthritis of the hand. Orthop. Clin. North Am., *17*:313, 1986.

Wise, C. M., White, R. E., and Agudelo, C. A.: Synovial fluid abnormalities in various states. Semin. Arthritis Rheum., *16*:322, 1987.

Woodrow, J. C.: Genetic aspects of spondyloarthropathies. Clin. Rheum. Dis., *11*:1, 1985.

Wooley, P. H., and Chapedelaine, J. M.: Immunogenetics of collagen-induced arthritis. CRC Crit. Rev. Immunol., 8:1, 1987.

Woolf, A. D., and Dieppe, P. A.: Mediators of crystal-induced inflammation in the joint. Br. Med. Bull., *43*:429, 1987.

Zarins, B., and McInerney, D. K.: Calcium pyrophosphate and pseudogout. Arthroscopy, *1*:8, 1985.

Zatourian, J., Finelli, L. J., and Blumenthal, D.: Reiter's syndrome. J. Am. Podiatr., Assoc., 77:653, 1987.

Ziff, M.: Autoimmune aspects of rheumatoid arthritis. *In* The Autoimmune Diseases. Edited by Rose, N. R., and Mackay, I. R. Orlando, FL., Academic Press, 1985.

Ziff, M., Cavender, D., and Haskard, D.: Pathogenetic

factors in rheumatoid synovitis. Br. J. Rheumatol., *27* (Suppl. II):153, 1988.

Zvaifler, N. J. (Ed.): Pathogenesis of chronic inflammatory arthritis. Rheum. Clin. North Am., *13*:179, 1987.

Tendons and Aponeuroses

Hueston, J.: The role of the skin in Dupuytren's contracture. Ann. R. Col. Surg. Engl., 67:372, 1985.

Hunter, S. C., and Poole, R. M.: The chronically inflamed tendon. Clin. Sports Med., 6:371, 1987.

Koss, P. G.: Disseminated gonococcal infection. The tenosynovitis-dermatitis and suppurative arthritis syndromes. Cleve. Clin. Q., 52:161, 1985.

Leach, R. E., and Miller, J. K.: Lateral and medial epicondylitis of the elbow. Clin. Sports Med., 6:259, 1987.

Taylor, L. J.: Musculoaponeurotic fibromatosis. Clin. Orthop., 224:294, 1987.

Trauma

Banks, A. S., and McGlamry, E. D.: Tibialis posterior tendon rupture. J. Am. Podiatr. Med. Assoc., 77:170, 1987.

Hattrup, S. J., and Johnson, K. A.: A review of ruptures of the Achilles tendon. Foot Ankle, 6:34, 1986.

Cysts

Ho, G., Jr., and Mikolich, D. J.: Bacterial infection of the superficial bursae. Clin. Rheum. Dis., *12*:437, 1986.

Patel, S. C., and Sanders, W. P.: Synovial cyst of the cervical spine. Am. J. Neuroradiol., 9:602, 1988.

Reilly, J. P., and Nicholas, J. A.: The chronically inflamed bursa. Clin. Sports Med., 6:345, 1987.

Young, L., Bartell, T., and Logan, S. E.: Ganglions of the hand and wrist. South. Med. J., *81*:751, 1988.

Tumors

Dabska, M., and Koszarowski, T.: Clinical and pathologic study of aponeurotic (epithelioid) sarcoma. Pathol. Annu., 17(Pt. 1):129, 1982.

Dreyfuss, U. Y., Boome, R. S., and Kranold, D. H.: Synovial sarcoma of the hand. J. hand Surg. (Br.), 11:471, 1986.

Duvall, E., Small, M., Al-Muhanna, A. H., and Marin, A. D. G.: Synovial sarcoma of the hypopharynx. J. Laryngol. Otol., 101:1203, 1987.

Enzinger, F. M., and Weiss, S. W.: Soft Tissue Tumors. 2nd Ed. St Louis, The C. V. Mosby Company, 1988.

Evans, H. L.: Synovial sarcoma. Pathol. Annu., 15(Pt. 2):309, 1980.

Fletcher, C. D., and McKee, P. H.: Sarcomas: a clinicopathological guide with particular reference to cutaneous manifestations. III. Angiosarcoma, malignant haemangiopericytoma, fibrosarcoma and synovial sarcoma. Clin. Exp. Dermatol., *10*:332, 1985.

Hajdu, S. I.: Pathology of Soft Tissue Tumors. Philadelphia, Lea & Febiger, 1979.

Schajowicz, F.: Tumors and tumorlike lesions of bone and joints. New York, Springer-Verlag, 1981.

Soule, E. H.: Synovial sarcoma. Am. J. Surg. Pathol., *10* (Suppl. 1):78, 1986.

61

Soft Tissues

THIS chapter considers the diseases that affect principally the adipose and collagenous tissues. The non-neoplastic disorders of the adipose tissues will be considered first, then the non-neoplastic disorders of the collagenous tissues, and the tumors of the fatty and fibrous tissues.

ADIPOSE TISSUE

The principal non-neoplastic diseases of the adipose tissues are obesity, fatty infiltration, lipodystrophy, Weber-Christian disease, fat necrosis, sclerema neonatorum, and subcutaneous fat necrosis of the newborn.

OBESITY. An excess of adipose tissue in the body is called obesity. Any person who weighs 20% more than the desirable weight for a person of that age and build as shown in actuarial tables is considered to be obese. Another definition states that any person who has a body mass index (weight in kg divided by height in m) greater than the 85th percentile for young adults is obese. By these definitions, 30% of men and 40% of women in the United States are obese. Obesity is more than unsightly. It can cause major complications and shorten life.

Lesions. Normally, the number of adipocytes in the body increases until a person is 20 years old and then remains constant for the rest of that person's life. If obesity develops in childhood, the number of adipocytes formed is greater than normal, and usually each adipocyte contains more fat than normal. If mild or moderate obesity develops during adult life, the number of adipocytes in the body is normal, but each cell contains more fat than usual. Only when obesity that develops during adult life is severe is there increase in the number of adipocytes as well as increase in the quantity of fat stored in each cell. If a person loses weight, the quantity of fat in each adipocyte falls, but the number of adipocytes does not alter.

In some obese people, the activity of the adipose tissue lipoprotein lipase attached to the endothelium increases. The enzyme hydrolyzes circulating triglycerides, releasing free fatty acids that are taken up by the adipocytes.

Complications. Many obese people are resistant to insulin. The resistance is caused in part by a reduction in the number of insulin receptors on their cells, often more importantly by a fault in the intracellular metabolism of glucose. Only a minority of obese people have non-insulin-dependent diabetes mellitus, but 85% of patients with non-insulin-dependent diabetes are obese.

In many obese people, increased production of very low density lipoproteins in the liver causes hypertriglyceridemia. The increase is due in part to hyperinsulinemia, in part to the increased turnover of free fatty acids common in obesity.

Hypertension is common in obese people. It is due mainly to hypervolemia without increase in the peripheral resistance. Atherosclerosis is often extensive and severe. Gallstones are common in the obese. The urinary excretion of 17-hydroxycorticosteroids is frequently increased. Occasionally the concentration of cortisol in the plasma rises. Secretion of the growth hormone is impaired.

Pathogenesis. In most fat people, obesity is caused by overeating. In some, the hypothalamic centers that regulate eating are abnormal. More often the overeating is caused by psychologic or social factors. Lack of exercise makes it easier to gain weight, but is not usually a major factor. Obesity is more likely to cause indolence than lack of exercise is to cause obesity.

Obesity is one feature of Cushing's syndrome. It occurs in Fröhlich's syndrome and occasionally in other forms of hypopituitarism. Hypothryoidism sometimes causes obesity, though only a minority of patients with hypothyroidism are obese, and few obese people have hypothyroidism. A minority of patients with hyperinsulinism caused by an islet cell tumor become obese. In some kindred, genetic factors favor the development of obesity.

Treatment and Prognosis. Reduction in quantity of food eaten is the best treatment for obesity. Drugs that reduce the appetite are of limited value. If other methods fail, a jejunoileal shunt or a gastroplasty is sometimes beneficial.

Pickwickian Syndrome. The Pickwickian syndrome develops in some obese people who weigh over 130 kg. It is called after fat Joe in Dickens' Pickwick Papers. During the day, the patients are somnolent and frequently doze off. In most of them, the sleepiness is caused by episodes of apnea that wake the patient at night. The weight of the fat and the relaxation of the pharynx that occurs during sleep cause obstruction of the upper part of the airway. Hypercapnia and hypoxia follow and wake the patient. Occasionally cardiac arrythmia causes sudden death. In many of the patients, a reduced response to hypercapnia and hypoxia causes hypoventilation during the day. The chest wall moves little. The P_{CO_2} in arterial blood rises to over 50 mm Hg before the respiratory center responds. The P_{O_2} falls. Some develop secondary polycythemia or pulmonary hypertension. Loss of weight restores normal respiratory function.

FATTY INFILTRATION. The term *fatty infiltration* is occasionally used to describe the intracellular accumulation of fat usually called steatosis or fatty change. More often it is used to describe the presence of adipose tissue in an organ in which it is not usually present or is normally present only in small quantity.

Fatty infiltration is common in the pancreas and heart, but can occur in other organs. It is common in older people of normal weight, as well as in the obese. In the heart, columns of adipocytes lie among the muscle fibers of the ventricles; in the pancreas, much of the organ is replaced by adipose tissue. The replacement of skeletal muscles by adipose tissue that occurs in some forms of muscular dystrophy and myopathy is similar.

LIPODYSTROPHY. The lipodystrophies are a group of conditions in which there is loss or excess of adipose tissue in part or all the body. They are divided into generalized and partial forms. Each is subdivided into congenital and acquired types. The types of lipodystrophy associated with the injection of insulin are considered separately.

Partial Lipodystrophy. Acquired partial lipodystrophy, sometimes called partial lipoatrophy, is the commonest of the lipodystrophies. The patients are adult. Most are women. In most, adipose tissue is slowly lost from the face and upper part of the trunk. The limbs and lower part of the trunk are unaffected. Less often only the lower part of the body is affected, or the disease is confined to one side of the body. Many of the patients have proteinuria or the nephrotic syndrome. Some have the dense deposit type of membranoproliferative glomerulonephritis. The nephritic factor is often present in the plasma. The activity of C3 is low. Some patients have insulin resistance, hyperglycemia, hypertriglyceridema, or acanthosis nigricans.

The congenital form of partial lipodystrophy is inherited as an autosomal dominant character. Most of the patients are women. Adipose tissue is lost from the trunk and limbs, but the face and sometimes the neck are spared. In most patients, the loss of adipose tissue does not begin until adult life. Many of the patients have insulin resistance and hyperglycemia; some have hypertriglyceridemia or develop xanthomata. Acanthosis nigricans is common. Some patients have hypertrophied labia majora and polycystic ovaries. Some have malformed eyes or teeth.

Generalized Lipodystrophy. The acquired form of generalized lipodystrophy, sometimes called total lipodystrophy, usually follows some other disease, often measles, chickenpox, whooping cough, or infectious mononucleosis, less often hypothyroidism, hyperthyroidism, or pregnancy. Men and women are affected equally. In some patients, painful, subcutaneous nodules precede the disappearance of the adipose tissue.

The congenital form of the disease is inherited as an autosomal recessive character. In some patients, the atrophy of the adipose tissue is evident at birth. In some, it does not appear until adult life. Men and women are affected equally. The external genitalia are often hypertrophied. In women, the ovaries are frequently polycystic. Mental retardation and dilation of the third ventricle develop in 50% of the patients.

In both types of generalized lipodystrophy, the adipose tissue throughout the body slowly atrophies. The number of adipocytes does not change, but they become small, with little or no fat, resembling fibocytes. The liver is enlarged, with severe fatty change and sometimes cirrhosis. Some of the patients have proteinuria or the nephrotic syndrome. Most have acanthosis nigricans. Hypertrichosis of the face, neck, trunk, and limbs is common. Some have cardiomegaly or a goiter.

In congential generalized lipodystrophy and in acquired generalized lipodystrophy that begins in childhood, growth is accelerated, but the epiphyses close early and stature is normal. Often the face is large and coarse, and the hands and feet are big. The viscera are enlarged. Often there is widespread enlargement of lymph nodes. The changes are like those of acromegaly, but the concentration of growth hormone in the plasma is normal or low.

In both types of generalized lipodystrophy insulin resistance is common. Insulin receptors are reduced or abnormal, and the intercellular metabolism of glucose is deranged. Glucagon levels are high and the concentration of free fatty acids in the plasma is increased. The activity of endothelial lipoprotein lipase is low. Many of the patients have hypertriglyceridemia caused by increase in both chylomicrons and very low density lipoproteins. Some have a hypermetabolic state, though thyroid function is normal.

Most patients with generalized lipodystrophy die within a few years, most often from hepatic or renal failure. No treatment is known to benefit the disorder.

Insulin Lipodystrophy. Insulin lipodystrophy is the name given to the atrophy or hypertrophy of the adipose tissue that sometimes occurs at the site of injection of insulin. Its cause is unknown.

WEBER-CHRISITIAN   DISEASE. Weber-Christian disease is named after the British physician Weber who reported it in 1925, and the American physician Christian who described it in 1928. It is uncommon.

Weber-Christian disease is usually confined to the subcutaneous adipose tissue. The most common form of the disease is called relapsing febrile nodular panniculitis. The subcutaneous tissue is called the panniculus adiposus, and inflammation of the subcutaneous tissue is called panniculitis. The patient is usually a woman. Multiple tender nodules 0.5 to 10 cm across develop in the skin, most often in the thighs or lower part of the trunk. Usually the overlying skin is red and inflamed. Occasionally one of the lesions ulcerates through the skin, draining oily material. Many of the patients have low fever, leukocytosis, or eosinophilia. Less often there is only a single lesion, the disease is confined to the mesentery, or it involves adipose tissue throughout the body.

At first, the lesions show acute inflammation. Many of the adipocytes in the affected region rupture. The exudate is predominantly of neutrophils, which are soon replaced by macrophages, smaller numbers of lymphocytes, and plasma cells. The macrophages take up the fat from the ruptured adipocytes. Their cytoplasm becomes finely vacuolated. Some of them are multinucleated. At this stage, the mass consists principally of closely packed macrophages. Occasionally the core of a lesion becomes necrotic, forming a fat-filled cyst. Occasionally some of the macrophages form ill-defined granulomata. As time passes, collagen is deposited among the macrophages and the lesion becomes increasingly fibrotic. The fat-filled macrophages become less numerous. Eventually all that remains is a collagenous scar.

The lesions of Weber-Christian disease last from one week to two months, then shrink and disappear. Sometimes a scar remains at the site of a lesion. Most patients have recurrent attacks, but in most the disease becomes quiescent after months or years. The pathogenesis of Weber-Christian disease is unknown. Adrenocortical steroids or immunosuppressive drugs are sometimes beneficial.

FAT NECROSIS. Trauma to adipose tissues frequently causes localized fat necrosis. Cold causes similar lesions. The fat released from the ruptured adipocytes excites short-lived acute inflammation. The fat is then taken up by macrophages. Clumps and sheets of finely vacuolated, fat-filled macrophages accumulate in the injured region. Collagen is laid down among the macrophages, and a scar forms as the macrophages gradually disappear.

Traumatic fat necrosis is common in the breasts and is discussed in Chapter 43. The fat necrosis caused by release of enzymes from the pancreas is discussed in Chapter 38.

SCLEREMA NEONATORUM. Sclerema neonatorum, from the Greek for hard and the Latin for newborn, is an unusual condition in which hard, waxy nodules develop in the subcutaneous adipose tissue a few days after birth and extend to involve much of the subcutaneous tissue and sometimes other adipose tissues. On section, the affected skin is thick and hard, like lard. Microscopically, many of the adipocytes in the affected regions are large and filled by fine, needle-shaped crystals of triglyceride. The proportion of saturated fatty acids in the crystals is higher than in normal subcutaneous fat. Similar crystals are present in macrophages. Sometimes there are foci of necrosis with an exudate of neutrophils and eosinophils or foci of calcification. Sclerema neonatorum develops in infants who have some other severe and often fatal disease. Many of the children die shortly after birth. The disorder probably results from failure to develop the enzymes that desaturate palmitic and stearic acids.

SUBCUTANEOUS FAT NECROSIS OF THE NEWBORN. Subcutaneous fat necrosis of the newborn is caused by trauma or cold. Multiple nodules of fat necrosis develop in the subcutaneous tissue in otherwise healthy infants. Frequently some of the nodules become necrotic or drain oily fluid, Microscopically, the lesions are like other forms of traumatic fat necrosis, except that some of the adipocytes contain crystals like those of sclerema neonatorum and the inflammatory reaction is often granulomatous, with many multinucleate macrophages. The lesions heal by scarring within two months, leaving no permanent deformity. Rarely, similar lesions develop in a child in whom adrenocortical steroids are suddenly withdrawn after having been given in high dose, a condition called poststeroid panniculitis.

COLLAGENOUS TISSUE

The non-neoplastic diseases of the collagenous and elastic tissues are caused by abnormalities in the collagen fibers, elastic fibers, or both. Scurvy is discussed in Chapter 22. This section considers Marfan's syndrome, homocystinuria, the Ehlers-Danlos syndrome, and pseudoxanthoma elasticum.

MARFAN'S SYNDROME. Marfan's syndrome is named after the French pediatrician who described it in 1896. It is inherited as an autosomal dominant character of variable expressivity. In 20% of the patients, it results from a new mutation. About 1 person in 7000 has the disease. Men and women are equally affected. Many of the patients show only some of the features of the syndrome. In some kindred, only the skeletal changes occur, in some only the lesions in the eyes, and in some only the disease of the aorta.

People with Marfan's syndrome are tall and thin. They have long limbs and long, thin fingers. The elongation of the fingers is called arachnodactyly, from the Greek for spider and finger. The chest is often malformed, bulging outward, a condition called pigeon breast or pectus carinatum, from the Latin for breast and keel; or it is hollowed, a condition called funnel breast or pectus excavatum, from the Latin for to hollow out. Scoliosis and kyphosis are common. The palate is usually high and arched. The joints are often abnormally mobile, but occasionally are stiff, with contractures in the hands. Cutaneous striae are common over the shoulders and buttocks.

Dislocation of the lenses in the eyes occurs in most of the patients. Usually the dislocation is upward. Glaucoma and detachment of the retina are less frequent.

Medionecrosis of the media of the aorta begins during the first years of life and is often severe. It may involve the great arteries or the pulmonary arteries. Dilatation of the aorta is common, especially in its upper part. Many of the patients develop a dissecting aneurysm. Enlargement of the aortic valve ring frequently causes aortic incompetence.

Less often the aortic valve is stenotic. Myxomatous degeneration of the mitral valve sometimes causes the floppy valve syndrome and mitral incompetence.

The lesions of Marfan's syndrome are treated as they arise. No treatment can alter the underlying abnormality in the collagenous and elastic tissues.

HOMOCYSTINURIA. An excess of homocystine in the plasma and urine is most often caused by deficiency of cystathionine β-synthetase inherited as an autosomal recessive character. Rarely, it results from deficiency of 5, 10-methylenetetrahydrofolate reductase or cobalamin reductase. In Ireland, 1 person in 40,000 lacks cystathionine synthetase. In other parts of the world, 1 person in 200,000 lacks the enzyme. Homocystine and methionine accumulate in the tissues. The concentrations of cystine and cysteine are low.

Over 80% of children with cystathionine synthetase deficiency have dislocation of the lenses of the eyes, usually downward, often with glaucoma. Often the body habitus resembles that of Marfan's syndrome. Osteoporosis is severe in 60% of the patients. Nearly 50% of them are mentally retarded. Thrombosis of a coronary, renal, or cerebral artery often develops during childhood. Medionecrosis of the aorta begins in childhood. The risk of dissecting aneurysm is increased. Over 30% of the patients die of cardiovascular disease, usually thrombosis, before the age of 30 years. If begun in infancy, a diet low in methionine and supplemented with cystine and pyridoxine prevents or ameliorates the disease.

The other forms of homocystinuria cause mental retardation and sometimes megaloblastic anemia.

EHLERS-DANLOS SYNDROME. The Ehlers-Danlos syndrome is named after the Danish dermatologist Ehlers who described it in 1901 and the French dermatologist Danlos who reported it in 1908. More than nine types of the syndrome have been distinguished. All are uncommon. Some of the patients fit into none of the categories. The collagen is abnormal in all forms of the disease, but in most the nature of the defect is unknown.

Type I is the most severe form of the disease. It is inherited as an autosomal dominant character. When the patients are young, the skin feels soft and velvety. It is abnormally distensible. Large folds of skin can be pulled out, but snap back when released. As the patient ages, the skin is still easily distensible, becomes less elastic, and often hangs in redundant folds, especially around the elbows, palms, and soles. The skin is fragile and easily injured. Wounds in the skin gape open and heal with large, thin scars like cigarette paper. The patients bruise easily, often with hemorrhages 1 to 2 cm across in the skin. Sometimes the hemorrhages calcify. The joints are hyperextensible and easily subluxated or dislocated. The repeated injuries to the joints often cause osteoarthritis. Hernias and varicose veins are common. The mitral valve is sometimes myxomatous and incompetent. Early rupture of the membranes often causes premature birth.

Type II is inherited as an autosomal dominant character. It is similar to type I, but milder. The skin is moderately extensible and easily bruised, but is not abnormally fragile. The joints are less severely affected than in type I.

Type III is inherited as an autosomal dominant character. The joints are severely affected, but the skin is little involved. Some of the patients work as contortionists. Repeated dislocations are common. Osteoarthritis develops as the patients age.

Type IV may be inherited as an autosomal dominant or as an autosomal recessive character. The skin is thin and fragile. The cutaneous veins are prominent. Bruising is easy, often with considerable hemorrhage. Only the joints of the digits are abnormally motile. Massive bleeding from large vessels in the colon is common. Spontaneous rupture of the intestine, aorta, an intracranial blood vessel, or some other blood vessels may occur. Collagen III is defective in these people. In some of the patients, the pro-α(III) chains are abnormal. In other patients, the secretion of type III procollagen is impaired.

Type V is inherited as an X-linked recessive character. The skin and joints are moderately affected, though the skin is not unduly fragile. Some of the patients have a floppy mitral valve and mitral prolapse.

Type VI is inherited as an X-linked recessive character. The skin and joints are moderately involved. Intramuscular bleeding sometimes occurs. The eyes are easily ruptured by minor trauma. The sclerae are sometimes blue. Kyphoscoliosis is frequent. In some patients with type VI, lysyl oxidase is deficient and the quantity of hydroxylysine in the collagen is low.

Type VII can be inherited as an autosomal dominant or an autosomal recessive character. The joints are severely affected. Multiple dislocations are common and may occur in utero. The skin is less severely involved. The conversion of procollagen to collagen is defective. In some of the patients, procollagen-N-proteinase is deficient, preventing the cleavage of the N terminal end from type I procollagen. In others the structure of the procollagen is abnormal and it cannot be cleaved by the proteinase.

Type VIII is inherited as an autosomal dominant character. The patients have periodontitis in addition to moderate involvement of the joints and skin.

Type IX is inherited as an X-linked recessive character. The skin is moderately distensible, but not fragile and does not bruise easily. The joints are little affected. Diverticula in the urinary bladder are common and may rupture spontaneously. Hernias are frequent. Skeletal abnormalities are common. Most patients with type IX have a defect in copper metabolism. The concentration of copper in the cells is high, but the concentrations of copper and ceruloplasmin in the plasma are low.

Patients with Ehlers-Danlos syndrome are treated symptomatically. No treatment modifies the defect in the formation of collagen.

PSEUDOXANTHOMA ELASTICUM. Pseudoxanthoma elasticum develops in 1 person in 100,000. It may be inherited as an autosomal dominant or an autosomal recessive character. Men and women are affected equally. Not all patients show all features of the disease.

In 70% of the patients, lesions develop in the skin, usually when the patient is 20 to 50 years old. The neck, axillae, and groins are the regions most often involved. In the affected region, the skin becomes loose, inelastic, and wrinkled, with yellowish papules that tend to become confluent. Microscopically, the epidermis and upper dermis are normal. Thick, irregular fibers that stain for elastica and calcium are numerous in the deeper part of the dermis. Electron microscopy shows that these fibers are degenerate elastica, with deposits of calcium in and adjacent to them. Some of the collagen fibers in the regions involved are irregularly twisted.

Vascular changes are present in 80% of the patients. Calcification of the elastica in the media of large and small arteries is prominent, often with atherosclerosis or thickening of the intima of the vessel and severe narrowing of the lumen. The vascular changes can cause intermittent claudication, angina pectoris, cardiac arrhythmias, a cerebrovascular accident, or mental deterioration. Hypertension develops in 50% of the patients. Some have congestive heart failure. In 10% of the patients bleeding from superficial vessels in the intestinal tract or elsewhere is severe and may cause death.

In 90% of patients with pseudoxanthoma elasticum, angioid streaks develop in the retinae. Degeneration and calcification of the elastica in Bruch's membrane cause it to crack. At retinoscopy, the cracks appear as red, gray, or black streaks two or three times the diameter of a retinal vein. Foci of hemorrhage or fibrosis are often associated with the streaks. Often the choroidal vessels are affected. Occasionally blindness results.

The defect in pseudoxanthoma elasticum is in the elastica. No way of arresting or reversing the defect is known.

TUMORS

A wide variety of benign and malignant tumors arise from the adipose and collagenous tissues. Some of them are restricted to one part of the body. Some can arise wherever adipose or collagenous tissue occurs. The tumors largely confined to one organ are described with the diseases of that organ. The tumors that involve the adipose and collagenous tissues throughout the body are described in this chapter.

Particularly with the tumors of the collagenous tissues, the distinction between tumor-like lesions of the soft tissues, benign tumors, and malignant tumors is often obscure. Some inflammatory, tumor-like conditions infiltrate the surrounding tissues. Some of the benign tumors of the collagenous tis-

TABLE 61-1.   FIBROMATOSES

Keloid
Nodular fasciitis

Dupuytren's contracture
Juvenile aponeurotic fibroma
Peyronie's disease

Proliferative myositis
Myositis ossificans
Congenital torticollis

Retroperitoneal fibrosis
Mediastinal fibrosis

Nasopharangeal angiofibroma
Desmoid tumor

sues invade to a limited degree, but do not metastasize. Some tumors of low grade malignancy invade, but metastasize only late and infrequently.

Fibromatosis. The term *fibromatosis* is used to describe a group of tumors and tumor-like lesions of fibrocytes in which a proliferation of fibrocytes tends to invade the adjacent tissues to a limited extent but which rarely metastasize. Table 61-1 lists these conditions. Many of them are not neoplastic. Some are benign tumors. The desmoid tumor is a low grade malignancy.

Benign

The adipose tissues give rise to four types of benign tumor; lipoma, adiposis dolorosa, hibernoma, and lipoblastomatosis. The benign tumors and tumor-like conditions of the collagenous tissues include nodular fasciitis, eosinophilic fasciitis, retroperitoneal fibrosis, mediastinal fibrosis, fibroma, myxoma, elastofibroma, and juvenile hyaline fibromatosis. The benign mesenchymoma and fibrous hamartoma of infancy are tumors or tumor-like lesions that contain both adipose and collagenous tissue, often together with abnormal blood vessels.

LIPOMA. The benign tumor of adipose tissue called a lipoma is one of the most common tumors. Most of the patients are over 40 years old. Over 70% of them are women.

Lipomata are most common in the subcu-
taneous fat of the shoulders, back, chest, neck, and thighs. They occur wherever there is adipose tissue, but are uncommon on the face, scalp, feet, and hands. Usually there is only one lipoma, but sometimes there are several. In some patients with multiple lipomata, the lesions are symmetrical or unilateral. In some the distribution of the lesions is similar in other members of the patient's family.

Most subcutaneous lipomata form a well-circumscribed mass that is clearly demarcated from the surrounding adipose tissue. The lesion usually has a thin, collagenous capsule. When it is removed and sectioned, it is often hard to distinguish from the surrounding adipose tissue. Most are from 2 to 10 cm across. A few have weighed more than 30 kg. Most lipomata arising in other tissues are similar. A lipoma of the retroperitoneal tissue is often large. A lipoma of the bowel is frequently pedunculated. Lipomata that arise in muscle and occasionally a lipoma in the subcutaneous tissue are less well demarcated and appear to infiltrate the surrounding tissues.

Microscopically, 85% of lipomata consist of normal looking adipose tissue. In the larger tumors, the mass is divided into lobules by fine collagenous septa.

In less than 10% of the lipomata, the tumor consists in part of normal looking adipocytes, in part of bands of fine collagenous tissue that lie among the adipocytes. Such a lesion is called a fibrolipoma. In 5% of the tumors, small blood vessels are numerous in the lesion, often lying in fine collagenous septa. Angiolipomata of this sort are often less well demarcated than the tumors that consist entirely of well-differentiated adipose tissue. In less than 1% of lipomata, part of the tumor, usually the central part, consists of myxomatous tissue like that of a myxoma. Some of these tumors infiltrate the adjacent tissues.

Most lipomata are cured by excision. The infiltrating tumors sometimes recur if not completely excised.

ADIPOSIS DOLOROSA. Adiposis dolorosa, called Dercum's disease after the American neurologist who described it in 1892, is a rare condition in which the patient develops painful or tender masses of adipose tissue.

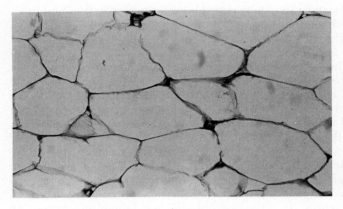

Fig. 61-1. Lipoma. The adipose tissue that constitutes most of these tumors appears normal.

Most of the patients are over 50 years old. Over 95% of them are women. The lesions are most common around the knees, ankles, and elbows. Most are between 0.5 and 5 cm across. The patients are often obese and have emotional instability or dementia. Some have an adenoma of the pituitary, thyroid, or an adrenal gland. The cause of the pain is unknown. Local anesthesia is sometimes helpful.

HIBERNOMA. A hibernoma is a rare tumor so called because microscopically it resembles the hibernating organ of animals. Most of the patients are young adults. The tumor is most common in the neck and upper part of the trunk. It forms a well-defined, lobulated mass that is usually brown. Microscopically, it consists of nodules of tumor cells separated by collagenous septa. The tumor cells have abundant, well-defined, vacuolated or granular cytoplasm and small, spheroidal, pyknotic nuclei. They closely resemble the cells of the brown fat common around the adrenal glands in children. The vacuoles contain lipid. Lipochromes are abundant in the cells. The tumor grows slowly. Excision cures.

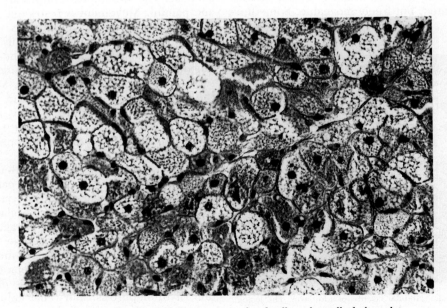

Fig. 61-2. A hibernoma showing its vacuolated cells with small, dark nuclei.

LIPOBLASTOMATOSIS. Lipoblastomatosis is an uncommon condition in which one or several fatty masses develop in the subcutaneous tissue in a child, usually in a limb. Most of the patients are under three years old. Nearly 70% of them are boys. Microscopically, a lipoblastoma consists of lobules of tumor cells separated by vascular septa. In the lobules, adipocytes are mixed with lipoblasts and spindle-shaped or stellate cells. The lipoblasts have fine droplets of lipid in their abundant cytoplasm. The spindle-shaped and stellate cells often are widely separated by an abundant, myxoid stroma. In 90% of the patients, excision cures. In 10%, the lesion recurs. The tumors do not metastasize.

NODULAR FASCIITIS. Nodular fasciitis, also called infiltrative fasciitis, proliferative fasciitis, and pseudosarcomatous fasciitis, is the most common of the tumors and tumor-like lesions of the collagenous tissues. Most of the patients are between 20 and 35 years old. Men and women are affected equally.

The lesion is most often in the subcutaneous tissue, less often in relation to a deeper fascial plane or intramuscular. In 50% of the patients, the lesion is in an upper limb, most often in a forearm; in 20% in the trunk; in 20% in a lower limb; and in 10% in the head or neck. The lesion is ovoid, not encapsulated, but freely moveable. Sometimes

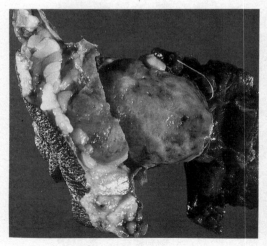

Fig. 61-3. Nodular fasciitis of a forearm. The lesion has been bisected.

it is mucoid; sometimes it is firm and gray. Most lesions are between 0.5 and 4 cm across.

Microscopically, the lesion consists of plump spindle-shaped or stellate fibrocytes in a mucinous stroma. The cells show little atypicality. By electron microscopy, most are myofibrocytes. Mitoses are often present but are never atypical. Usually reticulin fibers are abundant, but collagen is sparse. Most of the lesions contain many small, thin-walled blood vessels. Almost always, lymphocytes, macrophages, and other inflammatory cells are scattered throughout the lesion. Some of the macrophages may be multinucleated. At its margin, the lesion invades the surrounding tissues. Old lesions occasionally become hyalinized.

The lesion usually enlarges rapidly for one or two weeks. Less often, it develops more slowly. In 50% of the patients, it is tender.

Nodular fasciitis is probably inflammatory, not neoplastic. Its cause is unknown. Less than 10% of patients give a history of trauma. Excision nearly always cures. Less than 1% of the lesions recur.

EOSINOPHILIC FASCIITIS. Eosinophilic fasciitis causes swelling of the distal part of the upper and lower limbs. Occasionally it involves the trunk or the neck. It often follows exercise. The swollen extremities are tender and painful. Movement is restricted. Biopsy shows an exudate of lymphocytes, plasma cells, macrophages, and eosinophils in the dermis and collagenous septa of the subcutaneous tissues. IgG and complement are sometimes present in the lesions. Many of the patients have eosinophilia and hypergammaglobulinemia. Some have aplastic anemia. The disorder sometimes resolves spontaneously. Adrenocortical steroids are usually beneficial.

RETROPERITONEAL FIBROSIS. Retroperitoneal fibrosis is uncommon. The patient is usually a man between 40 and 60 years old. An ill-defined plaque of dense collagenous tissue develops in the retroperitoneal tissues, usually over the lumbar vertebrae or the sacrum. Commonly the fibrosis surrounds one or both ureters, less often the vena cava or aorta. It frequently causes ureteric obstruction, hydronephrosis, and renal failure and sometimes narrowing of the vena cava or aorta. Microscopically, the lesion consists of well-differentiated collagenous tissue. Broad bundles of collagen lie between normal-looking fibrocytes. Clumps of lymphocytes and macrophages are usually present in the lesion. Foci of calcification are common.

The cause of retroperitoneal fibrosis is unknown. In 15% of the patients, it follows methysergide therapy, less often treatment with methyldopa. In 10%, the patient has a carcinoid tumor or some other malignancy. Some 3% of the patients have also mediastinal fibrosis. Another 3% have also another form of fibromatosis. A few have hypoglycemia, probably caused by the great demand for glucose by the tumor.

Complete removal of the abnormal collagenous tissue is usually impossible. Surgical relief of ureteric or vascular obstruction is often needed. Partial resection of the mass relieves the hypoglycemia. Adrenocortical steroids may be of help. Less than 10% of the patients die of the disease.

MEDIASTINAL FIBROSIS. Mediastinal fibrosis is similar to retroperitoneal fibrosis. A mass of collagenous tissue like that in retroperitoneal fibrosis develops in the mediastinum, usually around the great vessels.

Compression of the superior vena cava is often the first sign of the disease.

FIBROMA. A circumscribed nodule consisting of fibrocytes and the collagen they produce is called a fibroma. Such lesions are not common. Most are not neoplastic. The nodule forms when a pyogenic granuloma or some other small inflammatory lesion heals by scarring.

MYXOMA. A myxoma is rare. Myxomatous regions in other tumors of the adipose and collagenous tissues are common. The patient is usually an adult. The tumor usually arises in the subcutaneous tissue, sometimes in a muscle or the retroperitoneal space. Most myxomata are from 0.5 to 5.0 cm across, but especially in the retroperitoneum the tumor sometimes weighs more than 1 kg. Macroscopically, it is ill-defined, soft, and slimy. Microscopically, it consists of stellate or rounded myofibrocytes separated by abundant, mucoid intercellular substance. At its margins, the tumor usually infiltrates a short way into the adjacent tissues. Excision usually cures. A few of the tumors recur.

ELASTOFIBROMA. An elastofibroma is an uncommon tumor that almost always arises in relation to the inferior angle of a scapula.

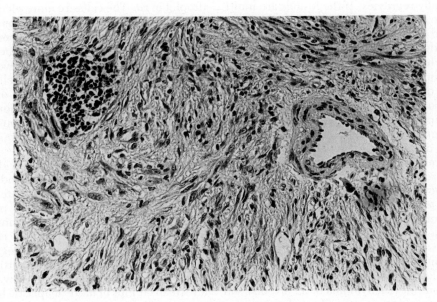

Fig. 61-4. Retroperitoneal fibrosis, showing the well-differentiated fibrocytes that make up the lesion and one of the clumps of inflammatory cells often present.

Most of the patients are over 50 years old. The tumor forms an ill-defined mass 5 to 10 cm across that is usually attached both to the scapula and the underlying chest wall. Microscopically, it consists of hyalinized collagenous tissue in which there are large numbers of coarse, branching elastic fibers. Probably the lesion is a response to injury rather than a neoplasm. Excision cures.

JUVENILE HYALINE FIBROMATOSIS. Juvenile hyaline fibromatosis is an uncommon condition inherited as an autosomal recessive character. Multiple, ill-defined masses develop in the skin during childhood and occasionally continue to appear during adult life. The masses are 0.1 to 5 cm across. They consist of hyalinized collagenous tissue. Some children have more than 100 of them.

BENIGN MESENCHYMOMA. A benign mesenchymoma is an uncommon malformation consisting of a disorderly mixture of well-formed adipose and collagenous tissue together with thick-walled blood vessels and sometimes smooth muscle, cartilage, or bone. The lesion is most often in the neck or mediastinum. It is present at birth. The lesion frequently grows disproportionately as the child grows, compressing adjacent structures. Usually growth of the lesion ceases when the patient is about 20 years old. Often it partially regresses. If the lesions are multiple, the child is said to have congenital generalized fibromatosis.

FIBROUS HAMARTOMA OF INFANCY. A fibrous hamartoma of infancy is an uncommon condition most frequent in boys. A small nodule develops in the skin during infancy or childhood. Occasionally more than one lesion is present. Microscopically, the lesion consists of a mixture of adipose and collagenous tissue, often with many blood vessels and sometimes bundles of smooth muscle. Excision cures.

MALIGNANT. Less than 1% of malignant tumors arise in the soft tissues. The malignant tumor of the adipose tissue is called a liposarcoma. The collagenous tissues give rise to a tumor of low malignancy called a desmoid tumor and to the more malignant fibrosarcoma and malignant fibrous histiocytoma. Rarely, a malignant mesenchymoma or an alveolar soft part sarcoma arises in the fibroadipose tissue.

Metastases to the adipose and collagenous tissues are rare.

LIPOSARCOMA. About 15% of malignant tumors of the soft tissues are liposarcomata. Most of the patients are between 40 and 70 years old. Nearly 70% of them are men.

Lesions. In men, nearly 40% of liposarcomata arise in a thigh, 15% in the back, 10% in a groin, 5% in an arm, and 5% in a buttock. In women, 40% of them are in a thigh, 15% in the retroperitoneum, 10% in a lower leg, 5% in an arm, and 5% in a buttock. The tumor is usually well demarcated. On section, some liposarcomata resemble a lipoma. Some are largely or partially myxomatous. Some show foci of necrosis or hemorrhage. Most are 10 to 20 cm across. Especially in the retroperitoneum, some liposarcomata become enormous, weighing more than 5 kg.

Microscopically, liposarcomata are divided into five types; well-differentiated, myxoid, fibroblastic, lipoblastic, and pleomorphic. Often a tumor shows more than one of these patterns of growth. Intermediate forms occur. About 3% of the tumors are well differentiated, 25% are mainly myxoid, 10% principally fibroblastic, 10% largely lipoblastic, and 20% predominantly pleomorphic.

Well-differentiated liposarcomata consist principally of adipocytes with a single large droplet of fat. The cells are more pleomorphic than those of a lipoma. The pleomorphism is most evident in the nuclei. Some of the nuclei are notched. In part of much of the tumor, preadipocytes containing several large droplets of fat and rounded or stellate lipoblasts with many small droplets of fat are mixed with the adipocytes. The more primitive cells are particularly numerous around blood vessels and at the margins of the tumor.

A myxoid liposarcoma is divided into lobules by a network of small blood vessels. Much of the tumor consists of stellate or ovoid cells separated by an abundant mucinous stroma. Small vacuoles of fat are numerous in the cells. Part of the tumor may consist of closely packed, larger preadipocytes containing large vacuoles of fat with little or no mucinous stroma. Mitoses are few. Only a few small clumps of more anaplastic lipoblasts are present.

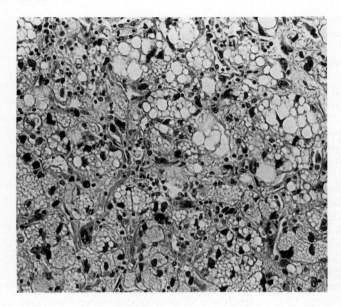

Fig. 61-5. A liposarcoma showing tumor cells filled with many small droplets of fat.

In a fibroblastic liposarcoma, the vascular network is like that of a myxoid sarcoma, but in most parts of the sarcoma the tumor cells are elongated, with glycogen and fine droplets of fat in their cytoplasm.

A lipoblastic liposarcoma is also called a round cell or epithelioid liposarcoma. It consists principally of rounded lipoblasts and preadipocytes. The lipoblasts have abundant, ill-defined cytoplasm that is granular and eosinophilic and contains fine vacuoles of fat. Their nuclei are rounded with prominent nucleoli. The preadipocytes contain a few larger vacuoles. Mitoses are sometimes frequent. In some tumors, the lipoblasts are closely packed. More often they are separated by a moderate quantity of mucoid or fibrillar intercellular substance.

The cells of a pleomorphic liposarcoma differ greatly in size and shape. Some are small and spindle-shaped. Some are larger with eosinophilic, granular cytoplasm. Often the tumor contains bizarre giant cells with more than one nucleus. In some of the tumors, the tumor cells contain little or no lipid. In some, they contain only a few small droplets of fat. In some, many of the tumor cells have large vacuoles filled with fat. The nuclei of the tumor cells are hyperchromatic, with nucleoli. Mitoses are common and some-times abnormal. Some of the tumors contain occasional well-differentiated preadipocytes with several large droplets of fat or occasional adipocytes with a single, large vacuole.

Behavior. The better differentiated liposarcomata grow slowly and extend only a short distance into the surrounding tissues. The pleomorphic tumors often grow rapidly and invade more extensively. The myxoid and fibroblastic forms of liposarcoma tend to occur at an earlier age than do other types of liposarcoma.

About 30% of the well-differentiated tumors recur after resection. About 50% of myxoid sarcomata recur and 60% of fibroblastic tumors. Nearly 70% of lipoblastic liposarcomata and 60% of the pleomorphic tumors recur.

In 25% of liposarcomata, the tumor progresses to a more anaplastic form, usually after several years. Most often a myxoid sarcoma becomes lipoblastic or pleomorphic, sometimes after it has recurred more than once. Less often a lipoblastic tumor becomes pleomorphic.

Over 50% of liposarcomata metastasize. The more anaplastic the sarcoma, the greater the risk of metastasis. Less than 5% of well-differentiated tumors metastasize; the majority are of the pleomorphic form. Metastases are common in the liver and intestinal tract, less frequent in the lungs, brain, and bones.

Clinical Presentation. A liposarcoma is usually first discovered when the patient detects a mass. The retroperitoneal tumors are detected when they compress some adjacent structure.

Treatment and Prognosis. A liposarcoma is treated by radical excision followed by irradiation. The value of chemotherapy is uncertain.

Few patients with a well-differentiated liposarcoma die of the tumor. Nearly all patients with a myxoid liposarcoma are alive five years after diagnosis. Over 80% of them are alive 10 years later. About 60% of patients with a fibroblastic or lipoblastic tumor survive five years. Nearly 50% survive 10 years. About 40% of patients with a pleomorphic tumor survive five years, and 30% survive 10 years.

DESMOID TUMOR. A desmoid tumor takes its name from the Greek for a band or tendon. About 5% of malignant tumors' soft tissues are desmoids. The patients are usually 20 to 40 years old. Men and women are affected equally. A desmoid tumor is classed with the fibromatoses. Some consider it benign. Some consider it a well-differentiated form of fibrosarcoma.

Desmoid tumors are most common in the shoulders, chest wall, mesentery, thighs, knees, neck, and pelvis. In women, a desmoid tumor sometimes develops in the rectus abdominis after pregnancy. Occasionally there is more than one tumor. Macroscopically, the tumor is usually fairly well defined, though it invades the surrounding tissues. Most are 5 to 10 cm across. On section, the tumor is firm and gray. Microscopically, it consists of plump fibrocytes separated by well-formed collagen bundles. Mitoses are few. The tumor cells and the collagen they form often form intertwining bands. At its margin, the tumor invades the neighboring structures.

A desmoid tumor grows slowly. Some are painful. Over 40% of desmoid tumors recur after excision, some more than once. The recurrence usually is evident within a year. Less than 3% metastasize, usually to the lungs, usually after several recurrences. Rarely, a desmoid progresses to a more dangerous malignancy. Some of the patients die of the tumor.

FIBROSARCOMA. About 10% of malignant tumors of the soft tissues are fibrosarcomata. Most occur in people between 35 and 55 years old. Over 60% of the patients are men.

Nearly 40% of fibrosarcomata arise in a thigh, 30% in an upper limb, 15% in a lower limb, 10% in the trunk, and 10% in the head or neck. The tumor forms a firm, well-defined mass in the deeper tissues. Most are 2 to 10 cm across. On section, the tumor is gray and firm.

Microscopically, most fibrosarcomata are well differentiated, consisting of uniform, spindle-shaped cells separated by the collagen they form. The cells are more pleomorphic than those of a desmoid tumor. Electron microscopy shows that most are myofibrocytes. Mitoses are present. Occasionally part or much of a fibrosarcoma is myxoid and consists of spindle-shaped or stellate cells separated by mucinous intercellular substance. Occasionally a fibrosarcoma is more anaplastic and has bizarre, pleomorphic cells that are sometimes multinucleated in addition to the spindle-shaped cells and the collagen they form.

A fibrosarcoma grows slowly. Some tumors are present for many years before the patient seeks treatment. Some are induced by irradiation.

A fibrosarcoma is treated by radical excision. Nearly 50% recur, sometimes repeatedly. Over 60% metastasize, most often to the lungs, bones, and liver. Less than 3% spread to lymph nodes. Less than 50% of the patients live five years.

MALIGNANT FIBROUS HISTIOCYTOMA. Over 15% of malignant tumors of the soft tissues are malignant fibrous histiocytomata. Most of the patients are over 50 years old. Nearly 70% of them are men. In the United States, the tumor is more common in white than in black or oriental people.

Malignant fibrous histiocytomata are most common in the limbs and retroperitoneum. The tumor forms a bosselated mass. It is usually 5 to 10 cm across. On section, the tumor is fleshy; gray, white or yellowish; often with foci of hemorrhage and necrosis.

Microscopically, many malignant fibrous histiocytomata grow in a storiform pattern,

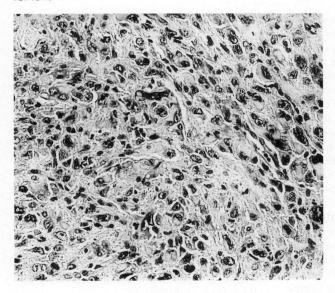

Fig. 61-6. A malignant fibrous histiocytoma showing pleomorphic tumor cells, some of which are multinucleate.

with elongated, spindle-shaped tumor cells radiating from a central focus. Often many of the tumor cells are pleomorphic and atypical. Mitoses are usually numerous. Some are abnormal. Foci of chronic inflammation with lymphocytes, plasma cells, and macrophages are often present. The macrophages sometimes contain lipid or hemosiderin. Inflammation is more extensive in 20% of the tumors. It is usually most marked at the margin of the tumor. Some tumors have myxoid regions, in which the tumor cells are separated by mucoid intercellular substance. In these regions, the tumor cells contain vacuoles filled with mucin. Some of the tumors contain giant cells that resemble osteoclasts or the multinucleated cells seen in xanthomata. Some are highly vascular. Some consist mainly of large, anaplastic cells.

Electron microscopy shows that the tumor cells in a malignant fibrous histiocytoma are myofibrocytes. They usually express HLA-DR antigens, but do not take the immunofluorescent stains for macrophages. The macrophages present are a reaction to the tumor and are not neoplastic.

Some malignant fibrous histiocytomata grow slowly. The tumor has often been present for some months before the patient seeks advice. Some enlarge rapidly. Some of the patients have fever, neutrophilia, or eosinophilia. A few develop hypoglycemia. In a few the tumor is induced by radiation.

A malignant fibrous histiocytoma is treated by radical excision. It recurs after excision in 40% of the patients. It metastasizes in 60%, to the lungs in 80% of those with metastases, to the lymph nodes in 30%, the liver in 15%, and the bones in 15%. Over 50% of the patients die of the tumor, most within five years.

MALIGNANT MESENCHYMOMA. A malignant mesenchymoma is rare. Most of the patients are adults. It arises most often in the muscles of a limb or in the retroperitoneum. The tumor is large and infiltrates the surrounding structures. Microscopically, it shows a mixture of mesenchymal tissues, some well differentiated, some anaplastic and sarcomatous. Sometimes one element in the mesenchymoma overgrows the rest and makes up much of the tumor. A malignant mesenchymoma often recurs after local excision. Metastases are uncommon.

ALVEOLAR SOFT PART SARCOMA. Alveolar soft part sarcomata make up 2% of malignant tumors of the soft tissues. Most of the patients are between 20 and 40 years old. Nearly 70% of the patients are women.

The tumor is most common in the limbs, but sometimes arises in the abdominal wall or retroperitoneum. Macroscopically, it is often adjacent to a muscle, well demarcated, and 5 to 10 cm across. On section, it is yellowish and firm, often with foci of hemorrhage or necrosis. Microscopically, the tumor consists of lobules—the alveoli of the name—separated by fine, vascular septa. Each lobule contains from 5 to 50 tumor cells. The tumor cells are large and regular, with abundant granular cytoplasm. They are weakly eosinophilic. Their nuclei are eccentric, with one or two nucleoli. A few mitoses are present. The tumor cells line the walls of the lobules, but are arranged at haphazard in the center of the lobules.

Most alveolar soft part sarcomata grow slowly; some enlarge rapidly. The tumor tends to recur after local removal. Metastases develop in 50% of the patients, most often to the lungs, brain, or bone, sometimes several years after the removal of the primary tumor. Nearly 60% of the patients survive for more than five years; over 40% for 10 years.

BIBLIOGRAPHY

Adipose Tissue

Adachi, Y., et al. Mesenteric panniculitis of the colon. Dis. Colon Rectum, 30:962, 1987.

Alexander, J. K.: The cardiomyopathy of obesity. Prog. Cardiovasc. Dis., 27:325, 1985.

Berchtold, P., Sims, E. A., Horton, E. S., and Berger, M.: Obesity and hypertension. Biomed. Pharmacother., 37:251, 1983.

Björntrop, P.: Morphological classification of obesity. Int. J. Obesity, 8:525, 1984.

Björntorp, P.: Obesity and the risk of cardiovascular disease. J. Cardiovasc. Surg., 17:3, 1985.

Björntorp, P.: Hypertension and other complications of human obesity. J. Clin. Hypertens., 2:163, 1986.

Brone, R. J., and Fisher, C. B.: Determinants of adolescent obesity. Adolescence, 23:155, 1988.

Cohen, J.: Obesity. J. R. Coll. Gen. Prac., 35:435, 1985.

Dornfeld, L. P., Maxwell, M. H., Waks, A., and Tuck, M.: Mechanisms of hypertension in obesity. Kidney Int. (Suppl.), 22:S254, 1987.

Editorial: Sudden cardiac death in obesity. Lancet, 1:628, 1988.

Fitzgerald, F. T.: The problem of obesity. Annu. Rev. Med., 32:221, 1985.

Fretzin, D. F., and Arias, D. M.: Scleroderma and subcutaneous fat necrosis of the newborn. Pediatr. Dermatol., 4:112, 1987.

Krieger, D. R., and Landsberg, L.: Mechanisms in obesity-related hypertension. Am. J. Hypertens., 1:84, 1988.

Maxwell, M. H., and Waks, A. U.: Obesity and hypertension. Bibl. Cardiol., 41:29, 1987.

Osler, M.: Obesity and cancer. Dan. Med. Bull., 34:267, 1987.

Patterson, J. W.: Panniculitis. Arch. Dermatol., 123:1615, 1987.

Rimon, D., et al.: Cardiomyopathy and multiple myeloma. Complications of scleredema adultorum. Ann. Intern. Med., 148:551, 1988.

Rothwell, N. J., and Stock, M. J.: Whither brown fat? Biosci. Rep., 6:3, 1986.

Schmieder, R. E., and Messerli, F. H.: Obesity hypertension. Med. Clin. North Am., 71:991, 1987.

Simopoulos, A. P.: Characteristics of obesity. Ann. N. Y. Acad. Sci., 499:4, 1987.

Sugerman, H. J.: Pulmonary function in morbid obesity. Gastroenterol. Clin. North Am., 16:225, 1987.

Wexner, S. D., and Attiyeh, F. F.: Mesenteric panniculitis of the sigmoid colon. Dis. Colon Rectum, 30:812, 1987.

Collagenous Tissue

Pyeritz, R. E.: Inheritable defects in connective tissue. Hosp. Pract., 22(2):153, 1987.

Sykes, B., and Smith, R.: Collagen and collagen gene disorders. Q. J. Med., 56:533, 1986.

Tumors

Allen, P. W.: Myxoid tumors of soft tissues. Pathol. Annu., 15(Pt. 1):133, 1980.

Altmannsberger, W., and Osborn, M.: Mesenchymal tumor markers: intermediate filaments. Curr. Top. Pathol., 77:155, 1987.

Angervall, L. (Ed.): Soft tissue tumors. Semin. Diagn. Pathol., 3:239, 1986.

Angervall, L., Kindblom, L. G., Rydholm, A., and Stener, B.: The diagnosis and prognosis of soft tissue tumors. Semin. Daign. Pathol., 3:240, 1986.

Antman, K. H., and Elias, A. D.; Chemotheraphy of advanced soft-tissue sarcomas. Semin. Surg. Oncol., 4:53, 1988.

Ariel, I. M.: Incidence of metastases to lymph nodes from soft-tissue sarcomas. Semin. Surg. Oncol., 4:27, 1988.

Batsakis, J. G., and Manning, J. T.: Soft tissue tumors. Otolaryngol. Clin. North Am., 19:659, 1986.

Bennett, K. G., Organ, C. H., Jr., Cook, S., and Pitha, J.: Bilateral elastofibroma dorsi. Surgery, 103:605, 1988.

Bramwell, V. H., et al.: Review of the clinical trials activity of the soft tissue and bone sarcoma group of the European Organization for Research and Treatment of Cancer. Semin. Surg. Oncol., 4:45, 1988.

Chung, E. B.: Pitfalls in diagnosing benign soft tissue tumors in infancy and childhood. Pathol. Annu., 20(Pt. 2):323, 1985.

Davis, A. D., and Dunham, W. K.: Soft tissue sarcomas. Ala. J. Med. Sci., 25:21, 1988.

Dehner, L. P.: Mesenchymal neoplasms in childhood. Am. J. Surg. Pathol., 10(Suppl. 1):32, 1986.

Dieste, M. C., et al.: Malignant fibrous histiocytoma of the broad ligament. Gynecol. Oncol., 20:225, 1987.

Eilber, F. R.: Soft tissue sarcomas of the extremity. Curr. Probl. Surg., 8(9):1, 1984.

Enzinger, F. M.: Malignant fibrous histiocytoma 20 years after Stout. Am. J. Surg. Pathol., 10(Suppl. 1):43, 1986.

Enzinger, F. M., and Weiss, S. W.: Soft Tissue Tumors. 2nd Ed. St Louis, The C. V. Mosby Company, 1988.

Fayad, M. N., et al.: Juvenile hyaline fibromatosis. Am. J. Med. Genet., 26:123, 1987.

Fletcher, C. D., and Krausz, T.: Cartilagenous tumors of soft tissue. Appl. Pathol., 3:208, 1988.

Fletcher, C. D., and McKee, P. H.: Sarcomas: a clinico-pathological guide with particular reference to cutaneous manifestations. I. Dermatofibrosarcoma protuberans, malignant fibrous histiocytoma and the epithelioid sarcoma of Enzinger. Clin. Exp. Dermatol., 9:451, 1984.

Fletcher, C. D., and McKee, P. H.: Sarcomas: a clinico-pathological guide with particular reference to cutaneous manifetations. II. Malignant nerve sheath tumour, leiomyosarcoma and rhabdomyosarcoma. Clin. Exp. Dermatol., 10:201, 1985.

Fletcher, C. D., and McKee, P. H., Sarcomas: a clinico-pathological guide with particular reference to cutaneous manifestations. III. Angiosarcoma, malignant haemangiopericytoma, fibrosarcoma and synovial sarcoma. Clin. Exp. Dermatol., 10:332, 1985.

Fletcher, C. D., and McKee, P. H.: Sarcomas: a clinico-pathological guide with particular reference to cutaneous manifestations. IV. Extraskeletal osteosarcoma, extraskeletal chrondrosarcoma, alveolar soft part sarcoma, clear cell sarcoma. Clin. Exp. Dermatol., 10:523, 1985.

Fu, Y. S., Parker, F. G., Kaye, G. I., and Lattes, R.: Ultrastructure of benign and malignant adipose tissue tumors. Pathol. Annu., 15(Pt. 1):67, 1980.

Fukuda, Y., Miyake, H., Masuda, Y., and Masugi, Y.: Histogenesis of unique elastinophilic fibers of elastofibroma. Hum. Pathol., 18:424, 1987.

Fuselier, C. O., et al. Selected soft tissue malignancies of the foot. J. Foot Surg., 24:162, 1985.

Greager, J. A., and Das Gupta, T. K.: Adult head and neck soft tissue sarcomas. Otolaryngol. Clin. North Am., 19:565, 1986.

Hajdu, S. I.: Pathology of Soft Tissue Tumors. Philadelphia, Lea & Febiger, 1979.

Hajdu, S. I.: Differential Diagnosis of Soft Tissue and Bone Tumors. Philadelphia, Lea & Febiger, 1986.

Hancock, B. J., and Vajcner, A.: Lipoma of the colon. Can. J. Surg., 31:178, 1988.

Hays, D. M.: Malignant solid tumors of childhood. Curr. Probl. Surg., 23:161, 1986.

Hertler, A. A., and Moore, J. O.: Sarcomas in the elderly. Clin. Geriatr. Med., 3:781, 1987.

Itoh, H., et al.: Treatment of desmoid tumors in Gardner's syndrome. Dis. Colon Rectum, 31:459, 1988.

Juettner, F. M., et al. Malignant fibrous histiocytoma of the lung. Thorac. Cardiovasc. Surg., 35:226, 1987.

Lattes, R.: Tumors of the Soft Tissues. Washington D. C., Armed Forces Institute of Pathology, 1981.

Lattes, R.: Pseudosarcomatous lesions and borderline tumors of soft tissues. Appl. Pathol., 6:154, 1988.

Mazeron, J. -J., and Suit, H. D.: Lymph nodes as site of metastasis from sarcomas of the soft tissue. Cancer, 60:1800, 1987.

McDonnell, T., Kyriakos, M., Roper, C., and Mazoujian, G.: Malignant fibrous histiocytoma of the lung. Cancer, 61:137, 1988.

Meister, P.: Malignant fibrous histocytoma. Pathol. Res. Pract., 183:1, 1988.

Mullen, B., and Richardson, J. D.: Primary anterior mediastinal tumors in children and adults. Ann. Thorac. Surg., 42:338, 1986.

Otto, H. F., Berndt, R., Schwechheimer, K., and Möller, P.: Mesenchymal tumor markers: special proteins and enzymes. Curr. Top. Pathol. 77:179, 1987.

Porter, K. M., Porter, S. R., and Scully, C.: Lingual metastasis of alveolar soft part sarcoma. Oral Surg. 65:742, 1988.

Reiman, H. M., and Dahlin, H. C.: Cartilage- and bone-forming tumors of the soft tissues. Diagn. Pathol., 3:288, 1986.

Robinson, E., Neugut, A. I., and Wylie, P.: Clinical aspects of postirradiation sarcoma. J. Natl. Cancer Inst., 80:233, 1988.

Rosen, G.: Bone and soft part sarcomas. Surg. Annu., 20:121, 1988.

Rosenberg, S. A.: Combined treatment approaches to soft tissue sarcomas. Hosp. Pract., 22(7):151, 1987.

Ruzicka, T., Vieluf, D., Landthaler, M., and Braun-Falco, O.: Benign symmetric lipomatosis Launois-Bensaude. J. Am., Acad. Dermatol., 17:663, 1987.

Scott, J., Foster, R., and Moore, A.: Retroperitoneal fibrosis and nonmalignant carcinoid. J. Urol., 138:1435, 1987.

Scougall, P., et al.: Desmoid tumors in childhood, Orthop. Rev., 16:481, 1987.

Seifert, G. (Ed.): Morphological tumor markers. Curr. Top. Pathol., 77:1, 1987.

Shenaq, S. M.: Benign skin and soft tissue tumors of the hand. Clin. Plast. Surg. 14:403, 1987.

Stal, S., Hamilton, S., and Spira, M.: Hemangiomas, lymphangiomas and vascular malformations of the head and neck. Otolaryngol. Clin. North Am., 19:769, 1986.

Suarez, V., and Hall, C.: Mesenteric fibromatosis. Br. J. Surg., 72:976, 1985.

Suehiro, S., and Inai, K.: Mesenteric fibromatosis in familial polyposis. Acta Pathol. Jpn., 37:1837, 1987.

Sykes, J. M., and Ossoff, R.H.: Paragangliomas of the head and neck. Otolaryngol. Clin. North Am., 19:755, 1986.

Taylor, L. J.: Musculoaponeurotic fibromatosis. Clin. Orthop., 224:294, 1987.

Torosian, M. H., and Wein, A. J.: Liposarcoma of the spermatic cord. J. Surg. Oncol., 34:179, 1987.

Visoná, A., et al.: Juvenile hyaline fibromatosis. pathologica, 79:357, 1987.

Weiss, S.W.: Proliferative fibroblastic lesions. Am. J. Surg. Pathol., 10(Suppl. 1):14, 1986.

Wick, M. R., Swanson, P. A., and Manivel, J. C.: Immunohistochemical analysis of soft tissue sarcomas. Appl. Pathol., 6:169, 1988.

Wright, J. R. Jr., Kyriakos, M., and DeSchryver-Kecskemeti, K.: Malignant fibrous histiocytoma of the stomach. Arch. Pathol. Lab. Med., 112:251, 1988.

Yousem, S. A., and Hochholzer, L.: Malignant fibrous histiocytoma of the lung. Cancer, 60:2532, 1987.

62

Skin

MANY inflammatory and neoplastic disorders involve the skin. This chapter considers the conditions that affect principally or only the skin. The secondary changes that occur in the skin in diseases that involve primarily some other organ are discussed in the chapter that considers the diseases of that organ. The infections of the skin will be considered first, then the conditions that cause bullae or vesicles, the diseases in which macules or papules are prominent, the disorders of pigmentation, the conditions that affect principally the epidermis, cutaneous appendages, cutaneous vessels, dermis, or subcutaneous tissue, the collagen diseases, and tumors. This subdivision is often arbitrary. Many of the diseases of the skin affect all the cutaneous structures.

INFECTION

Only the bacterial infections that involve principally or only the skin—impetigo, erysipelas, folliculitis, cutaneous adenitis, the form of tuberculosis called lupus vulgaris, and the tuberculids—are discussed in this section. The lesions caused by the human papillomaviruses are considered with tumors and tumor-like lesions of the skin later in the chapter. The many other infections that involve the skin are discussed in Chapters 16 to 21.

Bacterial infections confined to the skin are most often caused by the entry of organisms through a breach in the epidermis. Minor infections of this sort caused by the bacterial flora normally present on the skin are frequent, but usually heal within a few days and often pass unnoticed. Less often infection apparently confined to the skin is caused by entry of a more virulent organism through a defect in the epidermis or by hematogenous extension from a lesion in some other part of the body.

IMPETIGO. Impetigo, from the Latin for to assail, is a superficial infection of the skin. It is most common in infants and children, but can occur in adults, especially under the breasts and in other moist regions, and in people with immunodeficiency. Three kinds of impetigo are distinguished, impetigo contagiosa, bullous impetigo, and ecthyma. All are controlled by local or systemic antibiotic therapy.

Impetigo Contagiosa. Impetigo contagiosa is the common type of impetigo. It is most frequently caused by group A streptococci. Superinfection with staphylococci is common. Less frequently impetigo contagiosa is caused by staphylococci. The lesions are infectious, and the disease is easily spread to other parts of the skin by fingers or fomites. Epidemics of the disease sometimes develop in children.

The lesions of impetigo contagiosa are usually less than 2 cm across. They are frequently multiple. A pustule develops in the skin and soon ruptures, releasing yellowish fluid. A crust forms over the lesion. If the crust is removed, a raw, weeping area is exposed. Microscopically, the pustule develops between the keratinized and spinous layers of the epidermis. The epidermal cells separate, forming a vesicle that is filled with neutrophils. The deeper layers of the epidermis are edematous. Neutrophils penetrate between the epidermal cells. The underlying dermis is congested and edematous with an exudate principally of neutrophils and lymphocytes.

Bullous Impetigo. Bullous impetigo is caused by phage group II staphylococci. Vesicles develop between the spinous and keratinized layers of the epidermis and rapidly enlarge to form large bullae. At first the bullae contain clear fluid. Inflammation in the epidermis and dermis is less marked than in impetigo contagiosa.

The vesicles are caused by the toxin exfoliatin secreted by the organisms, as are the lesions in the scalded skin syndrome discussed in Chapter 16. The staphylococci can be isolated from the bullae in bullous impetigo, but they cannot be isolated in the scalded skin syndrome.

Ecthyma. Ecthyma, from the Greek for pustule, is usually caused by group A streptococci, usually with staphylococcal superinfection. It is most common in the lower limbs. The lesions resemble those of impetigo but ulcerate. The underlying dermis is acutely inflamed.

ERYSIPELAS. Erysipelas takes its name from the Greek for red and skin. It is nearly always caused by group A streptococci. In most patients, the streptococci come from the throat and infect the skin of the face by penetrating a minor injury in the epidermis. Less often, the infection complicates surgery.

Erysipelas often begins on the nose and over several days spreads onto the face. The inflamed skin is dusky red and indurated. The margin of the lesion is sharp and usually palpable. Microscopically, the lesion shows acute inflammation of the dermis, with congestion, edema, and an exudate predominantly of neutrophils. Streptococci are numerous. The patients have chills, fever, and other signs of infection. Untreated, erysipelas of the face often subsides after one or two weeks. In some patients, it recurs. In other parts of the body, it persists longer. Antibiotics control the infection.

FOLLICULITIS. Infection of a hair follicle is called folliculitis. Superficial folliculitis involves principally the skin around the hair follicles. Deep folliculitis affects mainly the deeper part of the follicles. Deep folliculitis is divided into two acute forms, furuncle and carbuncle, and several chronic types.

Superficial Folliculitis. Acute superficial folliculitis is a form of impetigo contagiosa with lesions centered around the hair follicles. Chronic superficial folliculitis is similar but more persistent. Acute inflammation continues in the epidermis, but superficial abscesses and scarring develop in the dermis.

Furuncle. A boil or furuncle, from the diminutive of the Latin for thief, is common. A staphylococcal infection of a hair follicle develops into an abscess that destroys the follicle. The lesion is usually 1 or 2 cm across, painful, itchy, and tender. It has a core filled with thick, yellow pus rich in fibrin. The wall of the abscess is acutely inflamed, with an exudate principally of neutrophils. Occasionally a boil points spontaneously. If not, incision and antibiotic therapy may be needed. A small scar is left when the lesion heals. A patient who develops multiple boils is said to have furunculosis.

Carbuncle. A carbuncle, from the diminutive of the Latin for coal, results from the coalescence of several furuncles. The lesion is most common on the back of the neck. Sometimes it is more than 10 cm across. Channels beneath the skin link the adjacent furuncles together. Often multiple sinuses drain onto the surface of the skin. The lesions cause pain, fever, and other signs of infection. Antibiotics and, when necessary, surgical drainage bring cure.

Chronic Deep Folliculitis. Chronic deep folliculitis can develop in any part of the body that bears hairs. It is given a name that indicates the site of the lesion. Sycosis barbae, from the Greek for fig and beard, is an infection of the bearded region; folliculitis decalvans, of the skull; folliculitis nuchae, of the neck. The lesion begins with acute inflammation around the deep part of one or more hair follicles. Often an abscess destroys the follicle. The inflammation fails to resolve. Plasma cells and lymphocyte become mixed with the neutrophils in the exudate. Fragments of hair often excite a foreign body reaction. Healing causes scarring and permanent loss of the hair.

CUTANEOUS ADENITIS. Bacterial infection of the glands of the skin is uncommon. The condition called hidradenitis suppurativa, from the Greek for sweat and a gland, involves the apocrine glands of the axillae and groins. An abscess develops in the gland or glands affected. The lesions discharge pus onto the skin and heal by scarring. The infection begins in a neighboring hair follicle obstructed by a plug of keratin and involves the glands secondarily.

TUBERCULOSIS. Tuberculosis of the skin is uncommon. Five kinds of tuberculous skin disease are distinguished. Lupus vulgaris is a primary infection of the skin. Scrofuloderma is caused by extension of the infection from underlying tuberculous lymphadenitis. Tuberculosis orificialis is caused by an escape of tubercle bacilli from the mouth or some other orifice. Miliary tuberculosis sometimes involves the skin. Tuberculids are a rare manifestation of tuberculosis. The cutaneous lesions of scrofuloderma, tuberculosis orificialis, and miliary tuberculosis are like those of tuberculous infection in other parts of the body. Only lupus vulgaris and tuberculids are considered here.

Lupus Vulgaris. Lupus vulgaris, from the Latin words for wolf and common, is a secondary infection of the skin in a person previously sensitized to tubercle bacilli. In 90% of the patients, it involves the head or neck. One or more reddish brown patches develop in the skin. They contain pale yellow nodules 0.1 cm in diameter called apple jelly nodules. Microscopically, the lesions show granulomatous inflammation of the type usual in tuberculosis. Organisms can usually be cultured from the lesions, but are hard to demonstrate in sections. The epidermis at the margin of the lesions often has long extensions that extend deep into the dermis, a condition called pseudoepitheliomatous hyperplasia. If untreated, the lesions enlarge sluggishly. They heal with scarring in the dermis and thinning of the epidermis.

Tuberculids. Tuberculids are rare. They occur in people sensitized to tubercle bacilli. Two kinds are distinguished. A papulonecrotic tuberculid is a form of leukoclastic vasculitis with a perivascular exudate of mononuclear cells. In lichen scrofulosorum, brown papules less than 0.5 cm across show microscopically noncaseating granulomata around hair follicles and sweat glands. The pathogenesis of the lesions is uncertain. Tubercle bacilli cannot be isolated from them. An immunologic mechanism is probably involved.

BULLOUS AND VESICULAR DISEASES

Blisters are a prominent feature of the bullous and vesicular diseases. Among the noninfectious conditions discussed are ecze-

ma, pemphigus, pemphigoid, dermatitis herpetiformis, erythema multiforme, Darier's disease, benign familial pemphigus, epidermolysis bullosa, miliaria, erythema toxicum neonatorum, herpes gestationalis, subcorneal pustular dermatosis, transient acantholytic dermatosis, and trauma.

ECZEMA. Eczema, from the Greek for to boil over, is one of the most common skin diseases. About 30% of patients consulting a dermatologist have eczema. Often the term *dermatitis*, from the Greek for skin, is used to describe some or all the forms of eczema.

Among the several different kinds of eczema are contact dermatitis, atopic dermatitis, stasis dermatitis, nummular dermatitis, lichen simplex chronicus, seborrheic dermatitis and generalized exfoliative dermatitis. The lesions in the skin are similar in all.

Lesions. Eczema begins with papules, macules, or vesicles that enlarge and merge to form ill-defined, erythematous, edematous lesions. In the regions involved, the skin is thickened, crusted, fissured, or scaly.

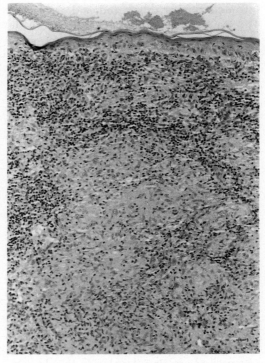

Fig. 62-1. Lupus vulgaris. The dermis shows the granulomatous reaction usual in tuberculosis.

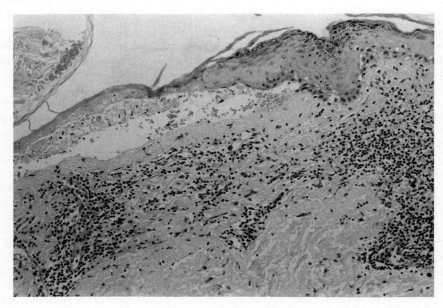

Fig. 62-2. Acute eczema. A vesicle is present between the epidermis and the dermis, and the dermis shows a perivascular inflammatory exudate.

Frequently plasma oozes from the lesions. The lesions may be few and small or multiple and widespread. Nearly always they are itchy. Microscopically, acute, subacute, and chronic forms of the disease are described.

Acute eczema affects principally the epidermis. Fluid accumulates in and between the epidermal cells. Vesicles form in the epidermis as the intercellular edema grows more severe and separates the epidermal cells more widely. Often some of the vesicles fuse to form bullae. Sometimes all that remains between the vesicles are the thin walls of greatly distended epidermal cells. Often parakeratosis or a scab of clotted plasma overlies the lesion. Occasionally a few lymphocytes or plasma cells are present in the epidermis or in a vesicle. Less often, neutrophils are present in the superficial part of the lesion. The underlying dermis is congested and edematous, with an exudate mainly of lymphocytes and macrophages around the blood vessels.

In subacute eczema, the epidermis is less edematous. Vesicles are still present, but are less numerous and are usually small. The epidermis is thickened. Usually parakeratosis overlies the lesion. Often a scab is present over the lesion. The inflammation in the epidermis and dermis persists.

In chronic eczema, the epidermis is no longer edematous. Vesicles are no longer present. The epidermis is thickened. Often a thick layer of keratin or parakeratosis overlies the lesion. Long rete pegs extend down into the dermis. The blood vessels in the dermis are prominent, but there is no longer congestion or edema. Inflammatory cells are few.

In all kinds of eczema, the lesions are often complicated by trauma resulting from scratching to relieve the itching. Secondary infection is common and adds changes like those of impetigo to the lesions of eczema.

Contact Dermatitis. Contact dermatitis is common. A great many agents cause eczema when applied to the skin. Cosmetics, hair dyes, metal buttons, and clips, nickel and other metals, plastics, synthetic rubber, rosin, poison ivy and other plants, drugs, solvents, and pesticides are among its many causes.

Contact dermatitis can be caused in two ways. Some substances are toxic and damage the skin when applied to it. They cause eczema in everyone who suffers sufficient exposure. Other agents cause eczema only when applied to the skin of a person sensitized to the agent. In nonsensitized people, they cause no injury.

Substances that damage the skin directly, usually produce erythema within a few minutes. If the injury is mild and the injurious agent is promptly withdrawn, the edema and erythema subside with a few hours or days. If the injury is more severe, acute eczema develops, often with many neutrophils. If the injurious agent is withdrawn, the lesion resolves after two or three weeks, leaving no residual injury. If exposure to the injurious agent continues, the lesion in the skin changes from acute to subacute and then to chronic eczema. If the agent is withdrawn, the lesion resolves, but often the epidermis in the region affected is thin and the dermis is scarred.

The agents that cause contact dermatitis only in people sensitized to the agent do so by a delayed hypersensitivity reaction. Usually erythema becomes evident 24 to 48 hours after the substance has been applied to the skin. If the reaction is mild, only transient congestion and edema develop. If it is more severe, it causes acute, subacute, or chronic eczema.

Usually the hypersensitivity or allergic type of contact dermatitis occurs only in the region in which the causative agent is applied. Occasionally if the dose of the agent is large or the patient is highly sensitive, the reaction becomes widespread. Occasionally the reaction occurs at the site of a previous reaction, though the causative agent is applied to some other part of the body.

In most people the sensitization in allergic type of contact dermatitis is caused by a previous application of the substance involved. The agent serves as a hapten. The hapten is conjugated with a protein carrier and is processed in part by the Langerhans cells in the skin. When the agent is again applied, a delayed hypersensitivity reaction follows.

Phototoxicity and photoallergy are discussed in Chapter 23. In phototoxicity, the substance that causes injury directly is harmful only if the part involved is exposed to light. In photoallergy, a substance that induces allergic contact dermatitis does so only if the region involved is exposed to light.

Atopic Dermatitis.   Atopic dermatitis de-velops in 2% of the population. In 70% of the patients it is familial. In 90% of the patients, the disease begins in infancy or childhood; in 10% of the patients, in adult life. Boys and girls are affected equally. Over 30% of the patients have hay fever or asthma.

Atopic dermatitis often begins with acute eczema on the cheeks and scalp. When the child begins to crawl, the flexures are frequently involved. Itching is severe. Even minor irritation of the skin causes itching. Scratching adds to the injury. The eczema persists for years with exacerbations and remissions. It gradually becomes chronic and in most children less severe. The uninvolved skin is usually dry and lined.

The immune system is abnormal in patients with atopic dermatitis. In most, the eczema is caused by an abnormal delayed hypersensitivity reaction to antigens in food or dust. In over 80% of the patients, depressed suppressor activity causes an increased concentration of IgE in the plasma. The concentration of IgE does not correlate with the severity of the eczema. Over 90% of the patients fail to respond to agents that cause delayed hypersensitivity in normal people. Most are more susceptible to cutaneous viral, bacterial, and fungal infections than are normal people. The ratio of alpha to beta adrenergic receptors in their tissues is high.

In over 50% of the patients, atopic dermatitis resolves during childhood. In some, it persists into adult life, usually in the flexures. About 10% develop cataracts in their eyes.

Stasis Dermatitis.   Stasis dermatitis is a form of subacute or chronic dermatitis caused by venous stasis in the lower legs. The region affected is erythematous and edematous and often shows scaling, oozing, or crusting. Frequently the lesions are stained brown. Often an indolent stasis ulcer develops in the hypoxic tissue. Microscopically, the lesions are like those of other forms of subacute and chronic eczema, except that they contain many macrophages filled with hemosiderin. Old lesions become scarred and fibrotic.

Nummular Dermatitis.   Nummular dermatitis, from the Latin for money, is a form of subacute eczema in which the lesions are round and fairly well demarcated and are studded with small vesicles or erosions.

Lichen Simplex Chronicus.   Lichen simplex chronicus is a form of chronic eczema in which there are thick, scaling, erythematous patches in the skin. Sometimes it is called neurodermatitis. It has no relation to nerves.

Seborrheic Dermatitis. Seborrheic dermatitis is a form of chronic eczema that looks macroscopically and microscopically like psoriasis. The lesions are reddish brown, well demarcated, and scaling. Microscopically, the epidermis is slightly thickened, with focal parakeratosis, lengthening of the rete ridges, and occasionally, clumps of neutrophils in the horny layer.

Generalized Exfoliative Dermatitis. Eczema involving much of the skin is called generalized exfoliative dermatitis, from the Latin to strip of leaves, or generalized erythroderma, from the Greek for red and skin. The patient develops a scaling, oozing, erythematous rash over much or all of the body. Microscopically, the skin shows acute, subacute, or chronic eczema.

Generalized exfoliative dermatitis is sometimes an extreme form of contact or atopic dermatitis. It is sometimes a reaction to a drug. About 20% of the patients have lymphoma. The dermatitis sometimes develops before the lymphoma is recognized.

PEMPHIGUS. Pemphigus takes its name from the Greek for a blister. The patients develop bullae in the skin and often in the mucous membranes. Pemphigus is uncommon. Most of the patients are between 40 and 60 years old when the disease begins. Men and women are affected equally. Pemphigus is more frequent in Jews than in other races. Four types of pemphigus are distinguished, pemphigus vulgaris, pemphigus vegetans, pemphigus foliaceus, and pemphigus erythematosus. About 80% of the patients have pemphigus vulgaris.

Pemphigus Vulgaris. In pemphigus vulgaris, the patients develop bullae in the skin and mucous membranes. Often the disease is at first localized, most frequently to the face, trunk, or oral mucosa. In 50% of the patients, oral lesions precede the involvement of the skin by up to a year. Sometimes there are recurrent crops of bullae that resolve completely between attacks. Eventually, the disease becomes generalized, involving much of the skin, the oral mucosa, and sometimes other mucous membranes.

The bullae are often several centimeters across. As the disease worsens, they grow larger and often fuse. Most are flaccid; some are tense. Most contain serous fluid. Often the superficial part of a bulla is lost, leaving a painful, red, weeping surface. In the later stages of pemphigus vulgaris, when the disease has become widespread, much of the superficial part of the epidermis is lost. The loss of fluid, electrolytes, and protein from the raw surface is great. Infection of the lesions is likely. The pain, bleeding, and hypersalivation caused by the erosions in the mouth frequently make eating impossible.

Pemphigus vulgaris begins with intercellular edema in the lower part of the epidermis or mucosal epithelium. The connections between the basal cells and between the basal cells and the cells of the layer immediately above them are weakened and lost, a process called acantholysis, from the Greek for thorn and loosening. The intercellular cement between the cells is destroyed. The desomosomes between the cells separate and disappear. The intercellular bridges between one basal cell and another and between the basal cells and the cells above them are no longer evident.

The overlying epidermis or epithelium separates from the basal cells. A ragged, linear slit forms between the basal cells and the overlying epidermis or epithelium. Sometimes the slit extends into a hair follicle or forms in a hair follicle. Often pressure on the lesion causes the slit to enlarge, or a shearing force applied to apparently normal epidermis or mucosal epithelium causes a slit to form.

The slit extends laterally and becomes filled with fluid to form a bulla. The basal cells remain attached to the basement membrane, though separated from one another. The overlying epidermis or epithelium is at first well preserved. Later, it is often lost, leaving only the layer of basal cells. Often clumps of epidermal or epithelial cells and isolated epidermal or epithelial cells lie free within a bulla. The isolated cells become spheroidal, with large, hyperchromatic nuclei and homogeneous cytoplasm. Often the dermis forms broad villi lined by a single layer of loosened basal cells that bulge into the basal part of the bullae. Often projections from

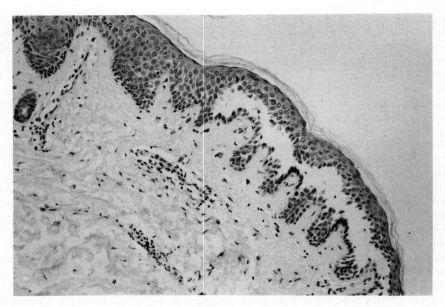

Fig. 62-3. Pemphigus vulgaris, showing the intraepidermal slit that forms between the basal layer of the epidermis and its overlying part.

the overlying epidermis or epithelium extend down into the bullae.

Many of the lesions of pemphigus vulgaris heal without residual injury. The basal cells proliferate, forming projections that extend into the bullae and meet cords of cells extending downwards from the overlying epidermis or epithelium. The basal and more superficial cells unite, restoring the integrity of the epidermis or epithelium.

In the early stages of pemphigus vulgaris, the dermis shows little inflammation, though a few eosinophils are often present in the dermis or in the bullae. If the superficial part of a bulla is lost, inflammation is often severe, with eosinophils and plasma cells.

If pemphigus vulgaris is extensive, the loss of albumin from the lesions reduces the concentration of protein in the plasma to as little as 35 g/L (3.5 mg/100 mL). Usually the concentration of immunoglobulins is increased. The concentrations of sodium chloride and calcium in the plasma fall, but the concentration of potassium is often normal. Anemia and leukocytosis are usual.

Pemphigus vulgaris is caused by antibodies against the cement substance of the epidermis and mucosal epithelium. Antibodies against

the cement substance are present in the plasma in 90% of patients with pemphigus vulgaris. The titer of the antibodies corresponds well with the severity of the disease. The antibodies bind to the cement between the cells of the epidermis or mucosal epithelium and fix complement. IgG antibodies can be demonstrated in the epidermis or epithelium by immunofluorescence in almost all patients. In 50% of the patients IgA, IgM, or complement are also present in the skin or mucosa. If normal epidermis is cultured with anticement antibodies, it undergoes acantholysis.

Untreated, 90% of patients with pemphigus vulgaris die, usually of infection, toxemia, or shock. Adrenocortical steroids in high dosage suppress the disease. The dosage can then be reduced or supplemented with immunosuppressive drugs such as azathioprine or methotrexate. In some patients, the immunosuppressive agent can be withdrawn after one or two years without causing relapse.

Pemphigus Vegetans. Pemphigus vegetans is a type of pemphigus vulgaris. Two kinds of pemphigus vegetans are distinguished.

In the more common form of pemphigus

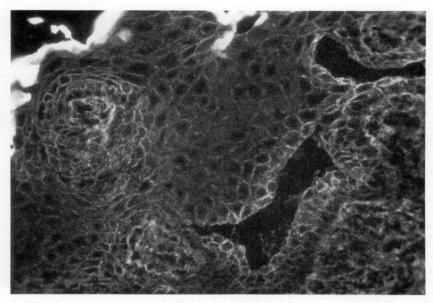

Fig. 62-4. Immunofluorescent staining showing the distribution of anticement antibodies in the epidermis in pemphigus vulgaris. (Courtesy of Dr. S. Ritchie)

vegetans, the disease begins like pemphigus vulgaris. As the lesions heal, the upgrowth of dermal papillae and the downgrowths from the overlying epidermis or epithelium are more extensive than in pemphigus vulgaris. Normal epidermis or epithelium is not restored. Instead, warty lesions form. Microscopically, they show thickened, hyperkeratotic epidermis or epithelium that extends down into the dermis or underlying collagenous tissue and sometimes forms warty excrescences. Abscesses filled with eosinophils are present in the epidermis or epithelium.

In the less common type of pemphigus vegetans, the slits and bullae that develop in the early stages of the disease are filled with eosinophils. An exudate containing many eosinophils is present in the dermis and epidermis. As the lesions heal, they become warty with intraepidermal or intraepithelial abscesses filled with eosinophils, as in the more common form of pemphigus vegetans. This form of the disease has a more benign course than the usual form of pemphigus vulgaris.

Pemphigus Foliaceus. Pemphigus foliaceus tends to occur in people 10 to 30 years old. It is fairly common in parts of Brazil, where it is called fogo selvagem, the Portuguese for wildfire, but is uncommon in other parts of the world.

Bullae form in the skin, but the mucous membranes are not usually involved. The superficial wall of the bullae is thin and is soon shed, leaving a red, rough, weeping surface that becomes crusted and often is secondarily infected. The epidermis in the eroded regions becomes thick and hyperkeratotic, with large greasy scales. Eventually much of the skin is involved, with an erythematous, scaling rash in which bullae may no longer be evident and that is indistinguishable from generalized exfoliative dermatitis.

Microscopically, the bullae form by acantholysis immediately under the horny layer of the epidermis. The superficial wall of the bullae consists of little but keratin. Bullae also arise deeper in the epidermis, but are less common. Particularly in the later stages of the disease, the acantholysis sometimes causes loss of the superficial part of the epidermis, without forming a bulla.

As weeks and months pass, the eroded epidermis becomes thickened and hyperkeratotic, with prominent elongation and fusion of its rete ridges. Often the cells of the granular layer of the epidermis become shrunken and basophilic. The underlying dermis is inflamed, with an exudate of macrophages and lymphocytes, sometimes neutrophils, or numerous eosinophils.

Antibodies against the intercellular cement substance of the epidermis are present in the plasma and in the epidermis in pemphigus foliaceus. They bind principally to the superficial part of the epidermis, rather than to its deeper part, as in pemphigus vulgaris.

Without treatment, pemphigus foliaceus is usually milder and advances more slowly than does pemphigus vulgaris. Not uncommonly, there is complete remission, even spontaneous cure. Treatment is with adrenocortical steroids and immunosuppressive agents, as for pemphigus vulgaris.

Pemphigus Erythematosus. Pemphigus erythematosus is a form of pemphigus foliaceus that remains localized in one part of the skin, often the face. Macroscopically, the lesions resemble those of seborrheic dermatitis or the facial lesion of systemic lupus erythematosus. Microscopically, they are indistinguishable from pemphigus foliaceus.

Anticement antibodies are present in the epidermis and in the plasma. In addition, 80% of the patients have antibodies deposited in the superficial part of the dermis, as in disseminated lupus erythematosus. They show no other evidence of lupus erythematosus.

Pemphigus erythematosus often persists for years, with exacerbations and remissions, but without extension to other parts of the body. In some patients, the disease eventually resolves without teatment. In some, it progresses to generalized pemphigus foliaceus.

PEMPHIGOID. Patients with pemphigoid develop bullae like those of pemphigus, but the bullae develop between the basal cells of the epidermis or the epithelium of a mucous membrane and their basement membrane. There is no acantholysis. Nearly 80% of the patients are over 60 years old, though occasionally pemphigoid develops in a young adult or a child. Two kinds of pemphigoid are distinguished: bullous pemphigoid and cicatricial pemphigoid.

Bullous Pemphigoid. Bullous pemphi-

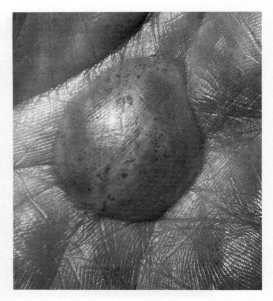

Fig. 62-5. A vesicle in the skin of a patient with bullous pemphigoid. (Courtesy of St. Michael's Hospital, Toronto, Department of Medical Art and Photography)

goid is occasionally confined to one part of the body, most often the lower limbs. More often, it involves much of the body. The groins, axillae, and flexor surfaces of the arms are usually the regions most severely affected. Irregular erythematous lesions with a pale center appear in the skin. Large, tense bullae develop both in the erythematous regions and in the skin between them. In 30% of the patients, a few small lesions are present in the mouth.

Bullous pemphigoid begins with edema in the basal part of the epidermis or epithelium. the anchoring filaments that bind the basal cells to their basement membrane are lost. The hemidesmosomes in the basal part of the basal cells disappear. The basal cells separate from the basement membrane. Fluid accumulates, forming a bulla between the basal cells and the basement membrane.

After two days, epidermal or epithelial cells from the margins of the bullae begin to slide across the exposed basement membrane. In a few days more, the base of the bulla is covered by a layer of epidermal or epithelial cells. The bullae now lie within the epidermis or epithelium, between the newly formed epidermal or epithelial cells

In 50% of the patients, the cause of erythema multiforme is unknown. In the others, it develops one to three weeks after herpes, a mycoplasmal infection, or less often some other kind of infection, or one to three weeks after the administration of a sulfonamide or some other drug. The nature of the lesions and the delay in their appearance suggest that the disease is caused by an immunologic reaction of the immune complex type.

In most patients, erythema multiforme is mild, and the lesions resolve without permanent injury. In some, the disease recurs, often only at long intervals. If it is severe, adrenocortical steroids usually control the condition. Without treatment, 30% of patients with the Stevens-Johnson syndrome or the subepidermal type of toxic epidermal necrolysis die.

DARIER'S DISEASE. Darier's disease, or keratosis follicularis, is named after the French dermatologist who described it in 1898. It is not common. Darier's disease is inherited as an autosomal dominant character. New mutations occur. It has two forms, a severe type which becomes evident in childhood and worsens as the patient ages, and a mild type, which appears only in adult life and is limited to regions exposed to light.

Scaling papules develop, often in relation to hair follicles, and slowly extend to involve more and more of the skin. The papules may coalesce to form warty, crusted plaques. Occasionally vesicles are evident in the lesions. The papules usually appear first on the face or trunk, but as the disease grows more extensive, considerable areas of the skin or the nails may be involved. Occasionally there are lesions in the oral mucosa.

Microscopically, the epidermis is thickened and hyperkeratotic. Keratin plugs often occlude hair follicles. Sometimes the epidermis extends irregularly downwards into the dermis.

Clefts that form by acantholysis appear between the basal layer and the remainder of the epidermis. They often have irregular walls. Acantholytic cells are usually free in the clefts. Often villi project from the dermis up into them. The villi are lined by a single layer of basal cells. The dermis shows chronic inflammation, with an exudate predominantly of lymphocytes.

Corps ronds are scattered in the granular and horny layers of the epidermis. They take

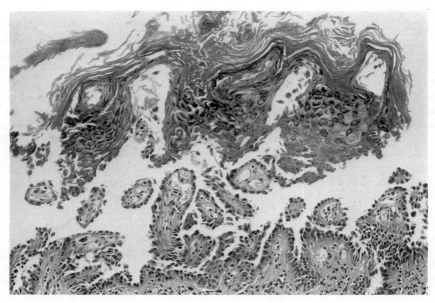

Fig. 62-10. Darier's disease. Dermal villi project into the cleft. Occasional corps ronds are present in the epidermis overlying the cleft.

their name from the French for body and round. A corps rond is a large cell, with a central, spheroidal, pyknotic nucleeus surrounded by a clear halo. The peripheral part of the cytoplasm is basophilic. Grains, named from the Latin for a grain, as of wheat, are present in the horny layer and sometimes within the clefts. They have grain-shaped nuclei and homogeneous basophilic or eosinophilic cytoplasm.

The tonofibrils and desmosomes of the epidermal cells are abnormal in Darier's disease. The tonofilaments become detached from the desmosomes and accumulate in tangled masses, together with large keratohyaline granules. In the corps ronds, they are compacted together at the periphery of the cells. In the grains, they fill the cytoplasm. The desmosomes separate and disappear.

Small doses of retinoic acid usually control the lesions in Darier's disease.

BENIGN FAMILIAL PEMPHIGUS. Benign familial pemphigus is called Hailey-Hailey disease, after the American dermatologists who described it in 1939. It is inherited as an autosomal dominant character. About 30% of the cases are due to a new mutation.

Benign familial pemphigus is usually confined to intertriginous areas, especially the axillae and groins and to regions like the sides of the neck where the skin is rubbed. Flaccid bullae appear in the affected regions. They tend to heal in the center, with hyperpigmentation, while new lesions develop at the periphery of the original bullae. The lesions are often itchy and may be painful.

Microscopically, the epidermis overlying the lesions shows moderate hyperkeratosis. Often narrow downgrowths of epidermis extend into the dermis. Clefts form by acantholysis immediately above the basal cells of the epidermis. They enlarge to form bullae. Dermal villi lined by a single layer of basal cells project into the clefts and bullae. Single acantholytic cells and small clumps of cells are numerous in the clefts. The epidermal cells overlying the clefts and bullae become partially separated from one another, looking like a dilapidated brick wall. A few corps ronds or grains like those of Darier's disease are often present in the epidermis, but they are never numerous.

The defect in Hailey-Hailey disease affects principally the tonofilaments and desmo-

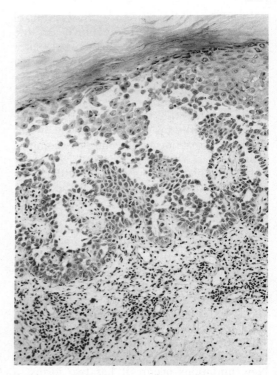

Fig. 62-11. The suprabasal cleft in a patient with benign familial pemphigus, showing acantholytic cells free in the cleft and the loosening of the overlying epidermal cells.

somes. The tonofilaments in the epidermal cells become detached from the desmosomes. Tangled masses of tonofilaments and keratohyaline granules accumulate in the cells. The desmosomes degenerate and disappear. Often complex microvilli develop on the abnormal keratinocytes.

The lesions of benign familial pemphigus tend to regress after some months. They often recur at the same location after a remission that sometimes lasts for several years. Little can be done to alter the course of the disease.

EPIDERMOLYSIS BULLOSA. A number of diseases of the skin that cause bullae are grouped together under the term *epidermolysis bullosa.* Most are genetically determined. They vary from mild and trivial conditions, to disabling and even fatal disorders. In all, minor trauma causes blisters to develop in the skin. No treatment is known, other than local measures.

Epidermolysis Bullosa Simplex. Epidermolysis bullosa simplex is inherited as an autosomal dominant character. Minor trauma to the skin causes bullae that heal without scarring. Often the bullae become less frequent or cease as the patient grows into adult life. The bullae result from degeneration of the basal cells of the epidermis. They form between the epidermis and its basement membrane, but gradually move towards the surface of the epidermis as the epidermis regenerates from below.

EPIDERMOLYSIS BULLOSA OF THE HANDS AND FEET. Epidermolysis bullosa of the hands and feet is inherited as an autosomal dominant character. Bullae develop following trauma, but only on the hands and feet. The bullae result from degeneration of the basal cells of the epidermis and form between the epidermis and its basement membrane.

Dystrophic Epidermolysis Bullosa. Two kinds of dystrophic epidermolysis bullosa occur: a milder form inherited as an autosomal dominant character and a more severe form inherited as an autosomal recessive trait. Bullae that are present at birth and involve much of the skin develop between the dermis and the epidermal basement membrane, presumably because of destruction of the anchoring fibrils. The nails are frequently involved. The recessive form of the disease usually has similar lesions in the oral mucosa and esophagus. The dominant form occasionally involves the oral mucosa. Especially in the recessive form, the lesions heal with scarring. Occasionally a squamous cell carcinoma develops in one of the scarred lesions.

Epidermolysis Bullosa Letalis. Epidermolysis bullosa letalis is inherited as an autosomal recessive character. Blistering is widespread at birth and usually brings death within a year or so. The bullae have little tendency to heal. Oral and esophageal lesions and malformation of the nails are usual. Occasionally the respiratory tract is involved. The bullae develop between the basal cells of the epidermis and the basement membrane. The hemidesmosomes of the basal cells of the epidermis or epithelium are few and small, allowing the basal cells to separate from the basement membrane.

Generalized Atrophic Benign Epidermolysis Bullosa. Generalized atrophic benign epidermolysis bullosa is inherited as an autosomal recessive character. The lesions are similar to those of epidermolysis bullosa letalis, but are less severe. Malformation of the hemidesmosomes of the basal cells of the epidermis allows bullae to form between the epidermal cells and their basement membrane.

Epidermolysis Bullosa Acquisita. Epidermolysis bullosa acquisita is not genetically determined. Usually it begins in adult life. Mild trauma causes blisters between the dermis and the epidermal basement membrane. Deposits of immunoglobulin and complement can usually be demonstrated on the dermal side of the basement membrane, suggesting that this disorder is immunologically mediated. No such deposits are found in the genetically determined forms of epidermolysis bullosa.

MILIARIA. In miliaria, obstruction of sweat ducts causes small vesicles in the skin. It takes its name from the Latin for millet. Two types of miliaria are distinguished: miliaria crystallina and miliaria rubra.

Miliaria crystallina occurs in regions in which the skin is slightly damaged by sunburn or in some other way and when sweating is excessive. Swollen epidermal cells in the horny layer obstruct the mouth of the sweat ducts. Small droplets of sweat accumulate beneath the horny layer, forming a small vesicle, like a dewdrop. The vesicles soon dry out and disappear.

Miliaria rubra, or prickly heat, occurs when there is excessive sweating in regions covered by clothing. The sweat ducts are obstructed in the deeper part of the epidermis, usually by infection with Staphylococcus aureus. Often a plug of amorphous material that stains with the periodic acid-Schiff reaction is present in the duct. Sweat leaks from the obstructed ducts into the deeper part of the epithelium to form small vesicles. The vesicles are itchy and have an erythematous rim. Lymphocytes and macrophages accumulate in and around the vesicles.

ERYTHEMA TOXICUM NEONATORUM. Erythema toxicum neonatorum develops in 40% of the newborn. Tiny macules, papules, and pustules appear in the skin within 48 hours of birth, sometimes with an erythematous rash, but disappear spontaneously after a few days or weeks. The cause of the rash is unknown.

The macules show only a little edema in the dermis, with a few eosinophils around blood vessels. The papules show more severe edema, with many eosinophils and some neutrophils in the upper dermis, particularly around the upper part of the hair follicles. The pustules result from the migration of the eosinophils with a few neutrophils into the epidermis around the hair follicles and usually form immediately below the horny layer of the epidermis.

HERPES GESTATIONIS. Herpes gestationis is an uncommon condition that develops during pregnancy. Its etiology is not known.

Itchy vesicles like those of bullous pemphigoid develop in the skin and sometimes in the oral mucosa. With them comes a patchy, erythematous rash. The vesicles are caused by degeneration of the basal cells of the epidermis and develop between the basal cells and their basement membrane.

In all patients, there is a linear deposit of C3 along the basement membrane. A linear deposit of IgG is present in similar distribution in 50% of the patients. Rarely, IgM or IgA is also present. Most patients have in their blood the HG factor and IgG able to fix to the basement membrane of normal skin and to activate complement.

PYODERMA GANGRENOSUM. In pyoderma gangrenosum, one or more ulcers appear in the skin. A pustule develops in the dermis and breaks down forming an ulcer that gradually enlarges, sometimes becoming 10 cm across. The ulcers have a purple, undermined edge. Bullae are sometimes present at their margin. Microscopically, the bed of the ulcer is acutely inflamed, often with chronic inflammation in the deeper part of the dermis and in the subcutaneous tissue. Often intraepidermal or subepidermal bullae are present at the margin of the ulcers. Necrotizing vasculitis is evident in the dermal blood vessels in early lesions and is commonly present at the margin of the ulcers. In some patients, perivascular accumulations predominantly of lymphocytes are present at the margins of the ulcers. The cause of pyoderma gangrenosum is uncertain. In 50% of the patients, it complicates another disease, most often ulcerative colitis, less frequently Crohn's disease, rheumatoid arthritis, chronic active hepatitis, or myeloid leukemia. Some of the patients have a monoclonal gammopathy, most often with an excess of IgA.

Adrenocortical steroids usually cause the lesions to resolve.

SUBCORNEAL PUSTULAR DERMATOSIS. In subcorneal pustular dermatosis, pustules develop in the skin, usually on the trunk in middle-aged women, and persist for a long time. Degeneration of the cells in the superficial part of the epidermis results in the formation of vesicles just beneath the horny layer of the epidermis. The vesicles become filled with neutrophils with a few eosinophils. A few leukocytes and a little edema may be present in the underlying epidermis. A mild, perivascular exudate of neutrophils with a few eosinophils, lymphocytes, and macrophages is present in the dermis.

The cause of subcorneal pustular dermatosis is unknown. No infectious agent has been identified. The condition responds to sulfapyridine and sulfones.

TRANSIENT ACANTHOLYTIC DERMATOSIS. In transient acantholytic dermatosis, itchy vesicles and papules develop, most often on the skin of the chest, back, and thighs. In most patients, the lesions disappear after two weeks to three months. In a few, they persist for years. Most of the patients are elderly men. The vesicles are caused by acantholysis. Microscopically, the lesions may resemble those of pemphigus vulgaris, pemphigus foliaceus, Darier's disease, or Hailey-Hailey disease or may show some combination of these appearances.

TRAUMATIC BLISTERS. Friction causes blisters in the epidermis by damaging the keratinized cells in the midpart of the epidermis. A cleft appears in the epidermis and fills with serous fluid to form the blister.

An electric burn can cause blistering in the skin by separating the epidermis from the dermis. Often the basal cells of the overlying epidermis are elongated at right angles to the blister, and long cytoplasmic projections extend down from the cells into the blister. The underlying dermis often shows coagulation necrosis.

MACULAR AND PAPULAR DISEASES

Among the conditions in which cutaneous macules or papules are the major feature of the disease are psoriasis, parapsoriasis, pityriasis rosea, lichen planus, lichen nitidus, lichen striatus, lichen sclerosus, pityriasis rubra pilaris, acrodermatitis papulosa infantum, erythema dyschromicum perstans, urticaria, angioedema, urticaria pigmentosa, and lipoid proteinosis.

PSORIASIS. Patients with psoriasis develop well-defined, scaling plaques in the skin. The name is from the Greek word used to describe itchy, scaly, scabby diseases of the skin. In temperate countries such as the United States or the United Kingdom, 2% of the population has psoriasis. It is uncommon in black people and in the tropics. Most of the patients are young adults when the disease begins. Psoriasis is uncommon in children and rarely begins in people over 45 years old. Men and women are affected equally.

The lesions of psoriasis are roughly symmetrical. They are most common on the extensor surfaces of the limbs and on the scalp, though if the disease is extensive, much of the skin can be involved. The mucous membranes are not affected. New lesions are likely to appear in any region in which the skin is irritated or traumatized.

Psoriasis usually begins with appearance of a few small round lesions that are flat, sharply defined, and slightly elevated above the surrounding skin. They are covered by fine, silvery scales. If the scales are rubbed off, small bleeding points are revealed. The disease may remain confined to one or a few regions for months or years, but usually becomes more extensive as new crops of lesions appear. In most patients, the extension is slow. Occasionally many new lesions appear within a few days.

As months pass, the lesions tend to enlarge and fuse, forming plaques from 1 to 10 cm across. The plaques are sharply demarcated. Their margins are hard and elevated. Often the scales are evident only at the margin of a lesion, and the center is thin and pigmented. Less often a patient has many small, erythematous lesions that are less well defined or has extensive lesions that are red and erythematous, with little scaling. In 25% of the patients, the nails are pitted or ridged.

In the early stages of psoriasis, the capillaries in the superficial part of the dermis are dilated, with edema and a perivascular exudate of lymphocytes and macrophages that extends into the basal part of the epidermis. In foci, the granular cells of the epidermis

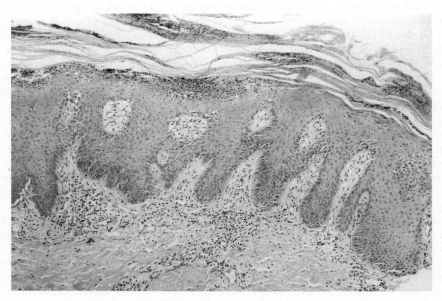

Fig. 62-12. Psoriasis. The rete pegs are elongated and fuse. Pustules of Kogoj are present in the upper part of the epidermis and Munro microabscesses are present in the overlying parakeratosis.

become vacuolated and disappear, and a thick layer of parakeratosis forms over the epidermis. Neutrophils accumulate among the parakeratotic cells. As the lesion ages, the foci of parakeratosis become more extensive and merge. Occasionally neutrophils form microabscesses in the superficial part of the epidermis.

When the lesions are fully developed, the rete ridges elongate, extending deep into the dermis and often fuse. The superficial part of the rete ridges is usually thin, and their ends are broad and bulbous. The dermal papillae are also long and bulbous. They are edematous with widely dilated capillaries and a slight exudate of lymphocytes and macrophages, sometimes with a few neutrophils. The surface epithelium is thin, especially over the dermal papillae. It lacks granular cells. Instead of orthokeratin, a thick layer of parakeratosis covers the lesion. Neutrophils are often present in the superficial part of the epidermis. Electron microscopy shows that many of them are within the epidermal cells. Sometimes the neutrophils within the cells form microabscesses called spongiform pustules of Kogoj after a Yugoslavian physician born in 1895. Larger microabscesses filled with neutrophils called Munro microabscesses after the British physician who described them in 1898 are often present in the overlying parakeratosis.

Many of the lesions in psoriasis show only some of the features seen in a fully developed lesion. As the lesions age, the inflammation wanes. Microabscesses of Kogoj and Munro become few. The elongation of the rete ridges persists, but the surface epidermis becomes thicker and granular cells often reappear. Some lesions show foci of orthokeratosis with underlying granular cells mixed with regions that lack granular cells and show parakeratosis. The erythematous lesions often are indistinguishable from eczema. A biopsy is most likely to establish the diagnosis if taken from a young, scaling lesion or from the margin of an older lesion.

In active lesions of psoriasis, the rate of replication of the epidermal cells is increased. Normally, it takes 13 days for a newly formed basal cell in the epidermis to differentiate and travel to the surface, where it is shed; in active psoriasis, it takes 5 days. In the basal cells of normal epidermis, a cell cycle takes 200 hours; in psoriasis, it takes 100 hours. In psoriasis, the proportion of basal cells that divide is increased. The high mitotic rate in active lesions of psoriasis with prominent parakeratosis reflects the increase in the rate of replication of the epidermal cells.

Electron microscopy shows that the epidermal cells are abnormal in active psoriasis. Tonofilaments and keratohylaine granules are reduced in number and are malformed. The glycoprotein cement between the epidermal cells is deficient.

Antibodies against the corneal layer of the epidermis are detectable in the plasma in 90% of normal people. They are demonstrable in the epidermis in 30% of normal people. These antibodies are demonstrable in the parakeratotic layer in most lesions of psoriasis, usually together with other immunoglobulins and complement. Their presence is probably due to insudation of plasma, not to an immunologic reaction.

Nearly 10% of patients with psoriasis have arthritis. About 50% of these people have rheumatoid arthritis, with rheumatoid factors in their plasma. The other 50% have psoriatic arthritis, discussed in Chapter 60.

Psoriasis is usually treated by topical application of adrenal corticosteroids, preparations of tar, or other drugs. Ultraviolet light given after sensitization of the lesions by oral psoralen is usually effective if the disease is severe, though the ultraviolet light may induce carcinoma of the skin. Systemic therapy with methotrexate is sometimes helpful.

Pustular Psoriasis. Pustular psoriasis is uncommon. A number of different types of the disorder have been distinguished. It may develop in a patient with pre-existing psoriasis or may be the first sign of psoriasis. It may involve much of the body or be confined to the hands and feet. Crops of pustules with surrounding erythema develop in the skin. They may appear in psoriatic lesions or in otherwise normal skin. Often the oral mucosa is involved. The pustules resolve after some weeks, but are likely to recur.

The pustules form in the upper part of the epidermis as do the microabscesses of Kogoj, but are larger, often replacing much of the epidermis. The lesions are sterile. As the underlying epidermal cells proliferate, the pustule moves into the horny layer, forming a large abscess of Munro. Usually the lesions show also other features of psoriasis.

PARAPSORIASIS. In parapsoriasis, reddish brown, scaling papules or macules appear, most often in the skin of the trunk or limbs. The lesions may appear quickly but usually develop gradually over the course of months and persist for a long time. Sometimes they form a network on the skin or enlarge to form plaques. Eventually the lesions heal, with thinning of the skin and telangiectasia.

At first, the lesions of parapsoriasis show only chronic inflammation in the dermis, with a sparse exudate of lymphocytes and macrophages. As they age, the exudate tends to form a band immediately beneath the epidermis. Often the basal cells of the epidermis become swollen, and a few of the inflammatory cells penetrate between them. The epidermis is a little thickened and shows patchy parakeratosis.

In 50% of patients with large plaques or a reticular network on the skin, the lesions contain atypical cells like those of mycosis fungoides. In less than 10% of the patients, the lesion develops into mycosis fungoides.

PITYRIASIS ROSEA. Pityriasis rosea is not uncommon, especially in the spring and fall. It usually affects young adults. Ovoid, pinkish-brown macules develop on the trunk, less often on the limbs or oral mucosa. The macules have fine scales at the periphery and a paler center. They are often itchy. They resolve after four to seven weeks. The name *pityriasis* is derived from the Greek for bran, and rosea is from the Latin for rose-colored.

In the lesions, the dermis shows an exudate of lymphocytes and macrophages, sometimes with a few eosinophils or neutrophils. The exudate may extend into the epidermis. The epidermis is thickened and edematous. Sometimes the edema is sufficient to form small, intraepidermal vesicles.

LICHEN PLANUS. Lichen planus takes its name from the plants called lichens and the Latin for flat. The patients usually develop flat plaques in the skin or mucous membranes. Most of the patients are between 30 and 60 years old. Men and women are affected equally.

The lesions usually affect only a small part of the skin or mucous membrane. They are most common on the flexor surface of the forearms, calves, glans penis, and oral mucosa. Most often the lesions in the skin are flat, violaceous, and shiny. Frequently they are polygonal. Usually they are itchy. Most are 0.2 to 0.3 cm across. Less often the cutaneous lesions are warty, ulcerated, pigmented, or vesicular. In the scalp and other hairy regions, the lesions sometimes develop around hair follicles and cause alopecia. The nails are involved in 10% of the patients. In the mouth, the lesions are usually white and lacy. Occasionally they are vesicular or ulcerated.

Microscopically, the lesions show irregular thickening of the epidermis, with hyperkeratosis and thickening of the granular layer. The rete ridges of the epidermis are long and pointed, like the teeth of a saw. The basal cells of the epidermis are swollen and degenerate. The epidermal basement membrane is often frayed or ruptured. A dense exudate, mainly of lymphocytes, but with some macrophages and sometimes a few neutrophils, lies in the upper dermis and is closely applied to the epidermis. Most of the lymphocytes are helper T cells. Often the inflammatory cells extend into the epidermis, obscuring the epidermodermal junction. A few of the macrophages in the exudate may contain melanin from the injured epidermis.

In 40% of the patients, spheroidal, homogeneous, eosinophilic bodies about 20 μm in diameter are present in the basal layer of the epidermis or in the exudate. These bodies are degenerate basal cells. They stain with the periodic acid-Schiff reaction and for cytokeratin.

Occasionally a cleft develops between the basal cells and their basement membrane. In the vesicular forms of lichen planus, this cleft enlarges to form the vesicles.

The mucosal lesions of lichen planus are similar, with a dense band of exudate hugging the epithelium, but the epithelium is often thinned rather than thickened, and there is parakeratosis as well as hyperkeratosis.

In the scalp, the hair follicles become filled with keratin. The hair follicles and sebaceous glands disappear, bringing permanent baldness in the affected part of the scalp.

Patients with lichen planus develop bul-

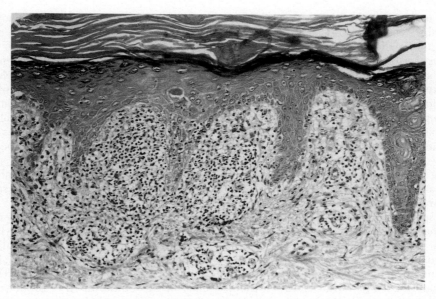

Fig. 62-13. Lichen planus, showing hyperkeratosis, elongation of the rete ridges, and a colloid body within the epidermis. The inflammation is usually more severe than in this picture.

lous pemphigoid more frequently than would be expected. Patients with both diseases are said to have lichen planus pemphigoides. Other patients have both lichen planus and lichen nitidus.

Lichen planus is probably caused by injury to the basal cells of the epidermis, and the inflammatory reaction follows. It is less probable that it is a form of delayed hypersensitivity reaction. Fibrin is abundant in the upper dermis. Occasionally granular IgM is deposited along the basement membrane. The dead basal cells that form the hyaline bodies adsorb immunoglobulins and stain strongly for IgA, IgG, IgM, and complement.

In 85% of the patients, lichen planus resolves within 18 months. In some, it persists for years. Topical steroids ease the itching, but do little to change the course of the disease. Rarely a squamous cell carcinoma develops in a hyperkeratotic lesion on a leg or from an ulcerated lesion in the mouth.

LICHEN NITIDUS. Lichen nitidus takes its name from the Latin for shining or glittering. It is not common. It can occur at any age. Flesh-colored, smooth-surfaced papules, 2 or 3 mm across, develop in some part of the skin or on a mucous membrane. Common sites are the penis, arms, and abdomen. The nodules remain discrete and do not fuse.

Microscopically, a discrete nodule of lymphocytes and macrophages, often with a few multinucleated macrophages, in the upper dermis closely applied to the epidermis. The overlying epidermis is thin, with hydropic degeneration of its basal cells. Parakeratosis is prominent. Often the epidermis extends down into the dermis at the margin of the exudate, as if to grasp the nodule of inflammatory cells. Occasionally the basal cells are entirely destroyed, and the epidermis separates from the dermis.

The lesions of lichen nitidus persist for a long time, but eventually resolve. Some consider lichen nitidus a form of lichen planus, but most think it a separate disease.

LICHEN STRIATUS. Lichen striatus is an uncommon condition most often seen in children. A longitudinal band of papules appears suddenly on a limb. The papules are not itchy and disappear within a year. Microscopically, lymphocytes, plasma cells, and macrophages can be seen around vessels in the dermis. The overlying epidermis is edematous, with foci of parakeratosis.

LICHEN SCLEROSUS. Lichen sclerosus, formerly called lichen sclerosus et atrophicus, is most common in the vulva, where it is sometimes called kraurosis vulvae. It also occurs on the glans penis, where it is known as balanitis xerotica obliterans, and occasionally elsewhere on the skin, where it forms sharply demarcated, flat, white plaques, with or without lesions on the genitalia. Microscopically, the lesions in other parts of the skin resemble those on the vulva, described in Chapter 41.

PITYRIASIS RUBRA PILARIS. Pityriasis rubra pilaris is rare. Red, hyperkeratotic papules develop in and around hair follicles and coalesce into lesions like those of psoriasis. The word *pilaris* is from the Latin for hair. The lesions sometimes extend to involve much of the skin. Microscopically, the hair follicles are plugged with keratin. As the disease extends, the surrounding epidermis becomes slightly thickened, with hyperkeratosis and foci of parakeratosis. The dermis shows mild, chronic inflammation.

ACRODERMATITIS PAPULOSA INFANTUM. Acrodermatitis papulosa infantum, or the Gianotti-Crosti syndrome as it is called after the Italian physicians who reported it in 1930 and 1955, is caused by infection with the hepatitis B virus, nearly always of subtype ayw. The patients are usually children, but occasionally adults are affected. After the prodromal signs of hepatitis, papules and an erythematous rash develop on the face, limbs, and buttocks. Lymphadenopathy and mild hepatitis are usual. Lymphocytes and macrophages are present in the upper dermis, mainly around blood vessels. The epidermis may be edematous and thickened. The rash subsides within two months.

ERYTHEMA DYSCHROMICUM PERSTANS. Most patients with erythema dyschromicum perstans are Latin Americans from Central or North America. The disease can develop at any age. Erythematous nodules develop in some part of the skin, most often on the trunk, arms, or face, and gradually become gray as they become increasingly pigmented. The nodules slowly enlarge and coalesce to form lesions several centimeters across with a gray center and an erythematous edge. They persist indefinitely.

Microscopically, active lesions show hydropic vacuolization and degeneration of the basal and lower keratinized cells of the epidermis, with an exudate of lymphocytes and macrophages in the upper dermis. Many of the macrophages contain melanin from the damaged epidermis. In quiescent lesions, only the melanin in the dermis remains.

URTICARIA. Urticaria, from the Latin for a nettle, is a condition in which transient wheals appear in the skin. Contact with a stinging nettle produces typical urticaria. A wheal is a well-demarcated swelling in the skin with a blanched center and erythematous margin. It is nearly always intensely itchy. Most wheals persist for a few hours or days and then disappear, leaving no residual injury. The swelling is caused by edema of the dermis, usually with a sparse exudate predominantly of lymphocytes. Occasionally the exudate is more severe and contains eosinophils as well as lymphocytes. Sometimes the overlying epidermis is also edematous.

The edema is caused by increased vascular permeability. In many patients with urticaria, the cause of the increased permeability is unknown. Some of these people have repeated attacks of urticaria, a disease called hives. In other people, urticaria is caused immunologically. In some, it results from injury to the skin. The list of agents that can cause urticaria is long.

In some patients, urticaria is caused by an antigen in food or dust that reacts with IgE bound to mast cells in the skin, releasing histamine and other vasoactive substances from the mast cells. The antigen may be ingested or applied directly to the skin. If it is applied to the skin, the urticaria is usually confined to the region exposed to the antigen. Some drugs cause urticaria by a similar mechanism. Occasionally urticaria is caused when IgG or IgM bound to mast cells reacts with its antigen.

In penicillin sensitivity, other forms of drug sensitivity, serum sickness, viral, bacterial, and parasitic infections, and other conditions, urticaria is caused by immune complexes deposited or formed in the dermis. The complexes activate complement, releasing its vasoactive products.

Insects, plants, and stinging animals sometimes cause urticaria by introducing histamine or another vasoactive substance directly into the skin. Nonsteroidal anti-inflammatory drugs, bee venom, and other drugs and toxins potentiate stimuli that might otherwise be unable to cause urticaria. In some people, morphine, codeine, curare, and other drugs damage the mast cells directly and cause urticaria when injected into the skin. Some people are abnormally sensitive to histamine or methacholine and develop urticaria when a dose too small to affect a normal person is injected into the skin.

In some people, exposure to cold causes urticaria. In some of these people, the sensitivity to cold is inherited. In others, it is secondary to multiple myeloma, cryoglobulinemia, or syphilis. In other people, exposure to sunlight is the cause. Some of these people are sensitive to rays between 310 and 370 nm in length, some to rays of between 400 and 500 nm. Some people are abnormally sensitive to mechanical trauma. Firm pressure on the skin causes a wheal, a phenomenon called dermatographism.

Urticaria is managed by avoiding its cause, when this is possible, and avoiding aspirin and other drugs that facilitate its development. Often antihistamines prove of great value.

ANGIOEDEMA. Similar localized edema of the deeper part of the skin and internal organs is called angioedema. Angioedema may be produced by external factors as in urticaria or may result from the inherited deficiency of the inhibitor of the esterase Cls of complement discussed in Chapter 29.

URTICARIA PIGMENTOSA. Urticaria pigmentosa is the name given to a group of uncommon disorders in which there is an excess of mast cells. Sometimes the term *mastocytosis* is used to describe these conditions. Urticaria pigmentosa is occasionally inherited as an autosomal dominant character, but in most patients no hereditary predisposition can be demonstrated.

Urticaria pigmentosa usually begins in infancy. One or many lesions appear in the skin. Usually the lesions are small reddish-brown macules. Sometimes they are larger brown plaques. Occasionally the greater part of the skin is involved. When a lesion is stroked, erythema and edema develop in the surrounding skin, often with itching, less often with vesiculation. Some of the patients suffer episodes of flushing of the skin, itching, hypotension, nausea, vomiting, or diarrhea. The lesions usually regress during adole-

scence, but occasionally persist into adult life.

Less often, urticaria pigmentosa first becomes evident in adolescence or adult life, with papules and plaques like those of the infantile form of the disease. In some of the patients, the lesions become telangiectatic. Pruritus may be troublesome. Generalized symptoms like those of the infantile form of urticaria pigmentosa are common. The frequency of peptic ulcer is increased.

Microscopically, the papular lesions show increased numbers of mast cells in the upper part of the dermis, especially around capillaries. The mast cells are easily missed unless special stains are used to demonstrate their granules. In the nodular and generalized forms of urticaria pigmentosa, the mast cells are more numerous and form tumor-like masses. The mast cells in the masses are large and cuboidal. They are often closely applied to the epidermis. Less often they extend into the subcutaneous fat. The pigmentation of the lesions is due to increase in melanin in the epidermis. Often melanin is present in macrophages in the dermis. If vesicles develop, they are at first subepidermal, but may move nearer the surface of the epidermis as healing brings re-epithelization at the base of the vesicles. A few eosinophils are present in the lesions. They become more numerous if urticaria is induced by stroking the lesions.

In both kinds of urticaria pigmentosa, there is some increase in mast cells in the internal organs. In the infantile form of the disease, it is usually slight and of little note. In the adult form, it is greater. The number of mast cells in the bone marrow is increased in 75% of adults with urticaria pigmentosa.

The wheals, erythema, and itching caused by stroking the lesions of urticaria pigmentosa result from the release of histamine from the mast cells. The eosinophils usually present in the lesions may be attracted by histamine. The general symptoms in patients with mastocytosis are due principally to the release of large quantities of histamine into the blood. The excretion of histamine in the urine is greatly increased. Heparin released from the mast cells may contribute to the bleeding tendency occasionally seen in these patients.

Little can be done to alter the course of

urticaria pigmentosa. Antihistamine drugs may ease some of the symptoms. H_1 and H_2 antagonists are often of benefit. Drugs like aspirin and codeine that release histamine from mast cells must be avoided.

Systemic Mastocytosis. In 10% of adults with mast cell disease, one or more of the internal organs is severely involved. Such people are said to have systemic mastocytosis. Most of the patients have increasingly severe urticaria pigmentosa, first with papules and macules, later with larger and more numerous lesions. Occasionally the disease is confined to the internal organs, sparing the skin.

The bones are the internal organ most often involved. The increase in mast cells in the bone marrow sometimes causes lytic lesions, sometimes new bone formation and osteosclerosis. The liver, spleen, and lymph nodes are less often seriously affected. Occasionally the intestines, lungs, meninges, or some other organs are involved.

In most patients with systemic mastocytosis, the disease worsens slowly. The mast cells in the skin and internal organs are increased in number, but appear to be normal.

In a few patients, systemic mastocytosis progresses rapidly, with increasing lymphadenopathy, hepatomegaly, splenomegaly, loss of weight, malaise, nausea, vomiting, and diarrhea. Many of the patients have anemia, leukopenia, thrombocytopenia, hepatic dysfunction, or malabsorption. Bleeding may result from thrombocytopenia, lack of prothrombin, or a circulating anticoagulant like heparin. The organs are heavily infiltrated by atypical, probably neoplastic mast cells. Some patients develop mast cell leukemia. This form of the disorder is treated by chemotherapy, as is a lymphoma.

LIPOID PROTEINOSIS. Lipoid proteinosis, or hyalinosis cutis et mucosae, is a rare condition inherited as an autosomal recessive character. The children affected are usually hoarse at birth, with yellowish plaques and nodules in the larynx and in other mucosae. The tongue is often enlarged. Yellowish or white nodules and papules in the skin become evident later. They are most common on the face and hands. Sometimes a line of small nodules develops along the edge of the eyelids. The nodules may become warty or

may resolve leaving pitted scars. Eventually patchy alopecia develops.

Some of the children have other congenital defects. Mental retardation or epilepsy are common. Occasionally calcification of the hippocampal gyri becomes evident. The teeth may be hypoplastic or absent.

Microscopically, the lesions in the skin and mucosae show a prominent accumulation of hyaline material around blood vessels, within and around their basement membrane. Similar hyaline material accumulates around the sweat glands, which become small and shrunken. In the older lesions, the dermis is considerably thickened by bundles of hyaline material that are particularly prominent in its upper part and often run perpendicular to the surface. Droplets of lipid are usually scattered in the hyaline material. Similar hyaline material accumulates around small blood vessels in other parts of the body. In the brain, it may calcify.

The hyaline material consists largely of glycoprotein and stains strongly with the periodic acid-Schiff reaction. It consists of a mesh of wavy, branching fibrils 1 to 2 or 5 to 10 nm in diameter, set in amorphous material, together with fine collagen fibers. The hyaline material contains predominantly type IV collagen, like basement membranes, though some type III collagen is present. The basement membrane of the affected vessels is reduplicated, with several layers of basement membrane enmeshed in the fibrillar material. Immunoglobulins are present in the hyaline material, probably because of leakage of plasma from the affected vessels rather than because of an immunologic reaction. Fibrocytes, endothelial cells, and smooth muscle cells in the affected regions have abundant, dilated, rough endoplasmic reticulum, containing both fibrillar and amorphous material.

Lipoid proteinosis is probably an inborn error of metabolism. The similarity of its lesions to the cutaneous lesions of prophyria is striking.

DISORDERS OF PIGMENTATION

The color of the skin depends principally on the quantity of melanin present in the

epidermis. In many conditions, the quantity
of melanin is changed, causing increase or
decrease in the pigmentation of the skin. The
alteration in pigmentation may involve much
or all of the skin or may be confined to
some part of it. In some conditions, there is
also abnormal pigmentation of the mucous
membranes.

Hyperpigmentation

The most common cause of hyperpigmentation of the skin is exposure to ultraviolet
light, to get a highly prized suntan. Ultraviolet light increases the production of melanin by the melanocytes in the epidermis and
darkens the melanin previously formed. It
does not increase the number of melanocytes
in the skin.

Endocrine disorders cause increased pigmentation of the skin by increasing the
production of melanin without increase in
the number of melanocytes. The increased
secretion of the melanocyte-stimulating hormone and adrenocorticotrophic hormone in
Addison's disease causes widespread pigmentation of the skin and oral mucosa.
Pituitary tumors that secrete these hormones
cause a similar darkening of the skin. Estrogens cause increased pigmentation, especially
of the nipples and genitalia. In pregnancy a
blotchy pigmentation, called a pregnancy
mask, chloasma, or melasma, may develop
on the face. Similar pigmentation of the face
sometimes develops in women taking contraceptive pills containing estrogens.

Some metabolic and nutritional disorders,
such as hemochromatosis, Wilson's disease,
and the cutaneous forms of porphyria, cause
increased pigmentation of the skin. Especially
in hemochromatosis, some of the excess of
melanin escapes from the epidermis and is
phagocytosed by macrophages in the dermis.
Gaucher's disease, Niemann-Pick disease,
vitamin B_{12} deficiency, and vitamin A deficiency cause generalized hyperpigmentation
of the skin. Sprue, Whipple's disease, and
hyperthyroidism can cause generalized or
patchy hyperpigmentation in the skin. Pel-
lagra causes hyperpigmentation in regions
exposed to light. Liver failure and cachexia
sometimes increase the production of melanin
in the skin.

Arsenical poisoning and chemotherapeutic
drugs such as busulfan can cause melanosis of
the skin. Sulfonamides, antibiotics such as
tetracycline, tranquilizers like chlorpromazine, and other drugs can sensitize the skin to
sunlight, causing increased pigmentation of
the skin.

The café au lait spots of neurofibromatosis
and fibrous dysplasia and the pigmented
spots of the Peutz-Jeghers syndrome are
caused by a localized overproduction of
melanin in the epidermis, without increase
in the number of melanocytes. Especially
in neurofibromatosis, the melanosomes are
sometimes larger than normal. Scleroderma
sometimes causes generalized hyperpigmentation. Many of the diseases discussed in
other parts of this chapter cause local hyperpigmentation of the skin.

POIKILODERMA CONGENITALE. Poikiloderma congenitale, from the Greek for spotted,
is a rare condition inherited as an autosomal
recessive character. When the affected child
is a few months old, an erythematous rash
appears on the face and limbs. As the rash
fades, a reticulated pattern develops in the
affected regions of the skin. Atrophic, hypo-
pigmented regions are bordered by hyperpigmented, telangiectatic zones. This reticulated pattern persists throughout life.

The patients are often short. Cataracts
develop during childhood in 30% of them.
Hypogonadism is common. Some patients
have retinal atrophy, deafness, loss of subcutaneous fat, photosensitivity, deficiency of
immunoglobulins, malformation of the nails,
or pancytopenia.

In the early stages of the disorder, the
dermis shows moderate chronic inflammation. The basal cells of the epidermis release
pigment that accumulates in macrophages in
the dermis. The dermal vessels are dilated.

POIKILODERMA ATROPHICANS VASCULARE.
Patients with poikiloderma atrophicans vasculare develop ill-defined areas of erythema
and scaling, with mottled pigmentation and
telangiectasia. As time passes, the erythema
fades, and the affected skin becomes atrophic,
with patchy pigmentation and prominent
telangiectasia.

Microscopically, early lesions show thinning of the epidermis, with loss of rete ridges
and hydropic degeneration of the basal cells
of the epidermis. The dermis shows a band of

exudate mainly of lymphocytes and macrophages closely applied to the epidermis and extending into it. Often a few macrophages in the exudate contain melanin. The dermis is edematous, and its vessels are dilated. In late lesions, the exudate is reduced, though the atrophy of the epidermis, the hydropic degeneration of its basal cells, the dermal edema, and the ectasia of the dermal blood vessels persist.

Most patients with poikiloderma atrophicans vasculare have systemic lupus erythematosus, dermatomyositis, lymphoma, or mycosis fungoides. Some have poikiloderma congenitale or a related disorder. Occasionally no underlying disease can be discovered.

Hypopigmentation

Hypopigmentation of the skin is less common than hyperpigmentation. It can be striking, especially when foci of hypopigmentation develop in people with dark skin.

Endocrine disorders can reduce the production of melanin in the skin. In hypopituitarism, the skin often becomes pale. Sometimes foci of depigmentation are present in the darkened skin of patients with Addison's disease.

The production of melanin in the skin is often reduced in African children with kwashiorkor. Loss of melanin from their hair gives it its characteristic red color. In phenylketonuria, the synthesis of melanin is impaired, changing black hair to brown and reducing the color of the skin.

When applied topically, hydroquinone and other drugs cause local depigmentation by reducing the number of melanocytes in the epidermis. The loss of pigment is sometimes permanent. Flecks of depigmentation like raindrops are often seen in the pigmentation caused by arsenic.

Leprosy, pinta, and other diseases cause foci of depigmentation in the skin. Burns and ionizing radiation can either increase or decrease the pigmentation of the skin. Pigmentation is much reduced in the Chédiak-Higashi syndrome, with only a few, abnormal melanosomes in the melanocytes. Hyperthyroidism can cause depigmentation as well as hyperpigmentation. Many skin diseases cause localized depigmentation of the skin.

ALBINISM. Albinism takes its name from the Latin for white. In albinos, almost no melanin is formed. The skin is pink and cannot tan. The eyes are pink because of lack of melanin in the irides. The hair is colorless.

There are two kinds of albinism. Each is inherited as an autosomal recessive character. In both, melanocytes are present in the epidermis, but cannot produce melanin normally.

In one form of albinism, the melanocytes lack tyrosinase. They contain melanosomes, but cannot form melanin. In the other form of the disease, the defect in the melanocytes is unknown. They contain tyrosinase and form melanosomes. They make a little melanin, but not enough.

PIEBALDISM. Piebaldism is inherited as an autosomal dominant character. The patients have patches of skin in which the melanocytes are absent. About 85% of them have a white forelock arising from a unpigmented zone in the forehead. Often there are spots of hyperpigmentation in the unpigmented regions. Occasionally, the people affected have other congenital abnormalities, most often in the eyes or ears.

VITILIGO. In vitiligo, pigment is lost from well-defined, irregularly shaped patches of skin as the melanocytes in the lesions degenerate and disappear. Often there is hyperpigmentation at the margins of the lesions. As time passes, the lesions tend to enlarge. In some patients, aseptic meningitis precedes the loss of pigment. The cause of vitiligo is unknown. It has been suggested that immunologic mechanisms may be involved.

EPIDERMAL DISEASES

Among the disorders that involve principally the epidermis are ichthyosis, xeroderma pigmentosum, incontinentia pigmenti, keratosis palmaris et plantaris, porokeratosis, acrokeratosis verruciformis and the perforating dermatoses, Kryle's disease, perforating folliculitis, elastosis perforans serpiginosa, and reactive perforating collaginosis.

ICHTHYOSIS. Ichthyosis takes its name from the Greek for a fish, because in these disorders the skin often shows coarse scales like the scales of a fish. Ichthyosis vulgaris, sex-linked ichthyosis, lamellar ichthyosis, and epidermolytic hyperkeratosis are the more common forms of the disease. Erythrokeratodermia variabilis and ichthyosis linearis circumflex are rare, as are Sjögren-Larsson, Refsum's, Rud's, and Netherton's syndromes in which the patients have other disorders as well as ichthyosis.

Ichthyosis Vulgaris. Ichthyosis vulgaris affects 1 person in 100. It is inherited as an autosomal dominant character. The disease becomes evident during childhood, with dryness of the skin and accentuation of hair follicles. Coarse or branny scales develop, particularly on the trunk and legs, but sparing the flexures. The palmar creases are abnormally marked. Particularly in cold, dry weather there is often hyperkeratosis of the heels, with increased scaling in the legs. Often people with ichthyosis vulgaris have some atopic disorder such as hay fever, asthma, or eczema.

Microscopically, the skin shows hyperkeratosis, often with plugs of keratin in the hair follicles. The granular layer of the epidermis is thin or absent. The dermis is normal.

In ichthyosis vulgaris, the synthesis of keratin is abnormal. The keratohyaline granules are small and crumble. The cells of the horny layer of the epidermis are less flexible than normal. They remain bound together to form the scales because their desmosomes fail to degenerate in the normal way.

No cure of ichthyosis vulgaris is possible, but local measures preserve comfort.

Sex-Linked Ichthyosis. Sex-linked ichthyosis is inherited as a sex-linked recessive character. The disease is most severe in boys, though girls bearing the abnormal gene are sometimes affected. One boy in 6000 has the disease.

The scaling is evident at birth or soon after. It involves most of the body, including the flexures, but sparing the palms. There are often small opacities in the cornea, but they do not interfere with sight. The skin shows hyperkeratosis, but has a normal granular layer.

The enzyme steroid sulfatase, which helps dissolve the intercellular cement in the epidermis, is deficient. The cement persists, binding the superficial epidermal cells together to form the scales. The synthesis of keratin is normal, but the desmosomes in the horny layer of the epidermis fail to disappear.

Lamellar Ichthyosis. Lamellar ichthyosis is inherited as an autosomal recessive character. In its most severe form, an infant with lamellar ichthyosis is born covered with thick, horny plaques separated by deep fissures. Death comes within a few days. Such an infant is called a harlequin fetus, from the resemblance of the plaques to the diamonds of harlequin's costume.

More often, an infant with lamellar ichthyosis is born a collodion baby, with a thick horny layer like collodion over much or all the body. The thick horny layer is tight. It pulls down the eyelids and pulls open the mouth. The collodion layer is shed after a few days, leaving large, coarse scales, widely separated, which cover much of the body and persist throughout life. The face is often less affected, though ectropion persists. To add to the patient's discomfort, the lesions sometimes develop a strong odor.

In lamellar ichthyosis, the epidermis is moderately hyperkeratosic and sometimes parakeratosic. The granular layer is present. Sometimes the epidermis is thickened. Sometimes there is chronic inflammation of the upper dermis.

The skin of people with lamellar ichthyosis shows two abnormalities. The proportion of basal cells actively synthesizing nucleic acid is increased. The quantity of cement between the epidermal cells is increased and binds the superficial cells of the epidermis together.

Lamellar ichthyosis must be distinguished from lamellar exfoliation of the newborn, in which the collodion membrane is shed a few days after birth, leaving normal skin.

Epidermolytic Hyperkeratosis. Epidermolytic hyperkeratosis is inherited as an autosomal dominant character. The affected infants are born with red, tender, weeping skin, often with blisters or bullae. Within a few days, the skin becomes covered by thick, warty scales, and the infant becomes more comfortable. Superficial bullae, often large, painful, and easily infected, continue to appear during childhood, but thereafter only the scaling remains. In contrast to other kinds of ichthyosis, the scaling is greatest in the flexures, though any part of the skin can be affected.

In some kindred, epidermolytic hyperkeratosis is confined to the palms and soles. In other patients, the lesions involve only part of the body or are arranged in linear fashion, with regular lines of hyperkeratotic scales. Other members of the same kindred often have epidermolytic hyperkeratosis of the usual generalized sort.

Microscopically, the epidermis of patients with epidermolytic hyperkeratosis shows moderate hyperkeratosis and moderate thickening of the granular layer. The granular and upper spinous layers appear vacuolated because of the accumulation of fluid between the cells.

Electron microscopy shows that excessive quantities of tonofibrils and keratohyaline granules are formed in the epidermal cells. The desmosomes are defective. Often only hemidesmosomes are formed. The failure to form normal desmosomes allows the separation of the epidermal cells to give the prominent vacuolation of the epidermis. If bullae develop, they result from separation of the epidermal cells in the midpart of the epidermis. The mitotic rate in the epidermis is as much as 5 times the normal rate.

Erythrokeratodermia Variabilis. Erythrokeratodermia variabilis is a rare form of ichthyosis. Transient, erythematous, irregularly shaped, scaly lesions develop, together with persistent scaly plaques that show hyperkeratosis and thickening of the epidermis. It is inherited as an autosomal dominant or an autosomal recessive character.

Ichthyosis Linearis Circumflex. Ichthyosis linearis circumflex is a rare condition inherited as an autosomal recessive character. Migrating, irregular, erythematous, scaly lesions occur with malformation of the hairs in the affected regions. Microscopically, there is thickening of the epidermis with elongation of the rete ridges, with parakeratosis at the margins of the lesions but hyperkeratosis in their centers.

Syndromes Including Ichthyosis. Four rare syndromes including ichthyosis are inherited as autosomal recessive characters. In the Sjögren-Larsson syndrome, described by the Swedish physicians in 1957, there is lamellar ichthyosis with mental retardation and spastic paralysis. In Refsum's syndrome, named after the Norwegian physician who described it in 1946, the patients have mild ichthyosis vulgaris, with severe peripheral neuropathy, which causes muscular weakness, cerebellar ataxia, and retinitis pigmentosa. It results from inability to metabolize phytanic acid taken in the diet. The basal cells of the epidermis contain vacuoles of lipid. In Rud's syndrome, reported by the Danish physician in 1927, the patients have ichthyosis vulgaris, mental retardation, epilepsy, and hypogonadism. In Netherton's syndrome, described by the American physician in 1958, the patients have lamellar ichthyosis and trichorrhexis invaginata.

XERODERMA PIGMENTOSUM. Xeroderma pigmentosum is a rare condition, inherited as an autosomal recessive character. In some patients, congenital defects in the nervous system cause mental retardation or other neurologic deficiencies. The name comes from the Greek for dry.

In xeroderma pigmentosum, the skin is excessively sensitive to light of wavelengths 280 to 310 nm. Erythema and scaling, like sunburn, develop in regions exposed to light, usually during the first year of life. A multitude of freckles develop in the exposed skin. Within a few years, the exposed skin becomes thin and atrophic, with more freckles and usually telangiectases. Often retraction of the skin drags on the eyelids or mouth, and the skin over the nose becomes tight and shrunken. Similar changes occur in the eyes, with conjunctivitis and pigmentation of the conjunctivae, sometimes keratitis and impairment of vision.

Beginning in adolescence, malignant tumors appear in the damaged skin. Multiple squamous cell carcinomata are the most common. Some patients develop basal cell carcinomata. About 3% of the patients develop a malignant melanoma. Rarely, there is a fibrosarcoma or some other mesenchymal malignancy.

Microscopically, in the early stages of xeroderma pigmentosum the epidermis in the affected regions shows hyperkeratosis and thinning, with a patchy increase of melanin in its basal layers. The dermis shows mild, chronic inflammation, with an exudate principally of lymphocytes. Later, the damaged skin shows more clear evidence of solar injury, with solar keratoses and basophilic degeneration of the collagen in the dermis.

The fault in xeroderma pigmentosum is in the repair of deoxyribonucleic acid. The deoxyribonucleic acid in the skin of the patients is normal, but they cannot repair the injury to the deoxyribonucleic acid caused by ultraviolet light. In most patients, the enzyme deoxyribonucleic acid endonuclease needed for the repair of the deoxyribonucleic acid is deficient. In a few, this enzyme is intact. New deoxyribonucleic acid to repair the damage is synthesized, but it cannot be incorporated into the chromosomes.

Patients with xeroderma pigmentosum must be protected from exposure to sunlight by every means possible. Even so, most of the patients develop a malignant tumor early in adult life.

INCONTINENTIA PIGMENTI. Incontinentia pigmenti is an uncommon disorder inherited as an X-linked dominant character. Nearly 95% of the patients with incontinentia pigmenti are heterozygous girls. Presumably in boys with their single, unopposed X chromosome and in girls who are homozygous for the gene that causes incontinentia pigmenti, the disease is so severe that death comes in utero.

Incontinentia pigmenti is usually evident at birth or becomes evident soon after. At first, erythema with lines of bullae is most evident on the limbs. After two months or so, the bullae are gradually replaced by warty lesions. These persist for another two months or more and are gradually replaced by irregular, brown or slate-colored patches most prominent on the trunk. As years pass, the discolorations slowly fade until by the time the patient is 20 years old the skin is normal or nearly so. Eosinophilia is often pronounced in the early stages of the disease.

In 80% of patients with incontinentia pigmenti, there are serious congenital defects in the brain, teeth, eyes, heart, or other organs. In 25%, there is patchy alopecia.

Microscopically, the early erythematous, vesicular lesions show edema of the epidermis, which separates the epidermal cells, to cause vesicles like those of eczema. Eosinophils are numerous in the vesicles, in the adjacent epidermis, and together with lymphocytes and macrophages in the underlying dermis. The warty lesions have irregular, hyperkeratotic fronds, often with intraepidermal keratin pearls or other evidence of irregular keratinization. The underlying dermis shows chronic inflammation, with a few macrophages containing melanin. In the pigmented regions of the final stage of the disease, large numbers of macrophages filled with melanin are seen in the upper dermis, usually with reduction in the melanin content of the overlying epidermis. Often the basal cells of the epidermis are swollen or degenerate, explaining the release of the melanin.

The disease called incontinentia pigmenti must not be confused with the incontinence of pigment common in many conditions in which the basal cells of the epidermis are injured, releasing melanin, which is taken up by macrophages in the upper dermis.

KERATOSIS PALMARIS ET PLANTARIS. Hyperkeratosis of the palms of the hands and the soles of the feet is not uncommon. The disease may be inherited as an autosomal dominant or an autosomal recessive character. Most often the patients have localized or widespread hyperkeratosis of the palms and soles that tends to extend onto the dorsa of the hands and feet and sometimes to the wrists and elbows, ankles, and knees. Some kindred in which the disease is inherited as an autosomal recessive character have also periodontosis. In some in which the disease is inherited as an autosomal dominant character, the hyperkeratosis is confined to small, sharply demarcated foci in the palms and soles. Some of the lesions develop into squamous cell carcinoma.

In most of the patients, the epidermis is thickened, with a thick granular layer and severe hyperkeratosis. The upper dermis often shows a mild, chronic inflammatory exudate. In some kindred in which the disease is inherited as an autosomal dominant character, the epidermis shows changes like those of epidermolytic hyperkeratosis.

POROKERATOSIS. Porokeratosis is inherited as an autosomal dominant character. It takes its name from the Greek for a ford or way through. The patients may have only one or a few large lesions or many small lesions most common on the trunk, palms, and soles. Sometimes the lesions are confined to the regions exposed to sunlight or are linear, sometimes limited to one part of the skin. The lesions have a depressed center and a furrow filled with keratin at their raised margin.

Microscopically, the furrow at the margin of the lesions is V-shaped and oblique, with its apex pointing away from the lesion. In the center of the furrow, rising up from its base, is a column of parakeratotic cells, with considerable hyperkeratosis above and around them. The granular layer of the epidermis is lacking at the base of the furrow, but is well marked elsewhere in the wall of the furrow and in the surrounding epidermis. The epidermis in the center of the lesion is normal or thinned. The dermis may show mild, chronic inflammation.

ACROKERATOSIS VERRUCIFORMIS. Acrokeratosis verruciformis is inherited as an autosomal dominant character. It often occurs in patients who have Darier's disease or who subsequently develop Darier's disease. Flat, hyperkeratotic, sometimes warty papules develop mainly on the dorsal surfaces of the hands and feet. The papules show hyperkeratosis and thickening of the epidermis. Often the epidermis projects up into the overlying hyperkeratosis in a sharp peak, like a church spire.

PERFORATING DERMATOSES. Four unrelated conditions cause perforation of the epidermis: Kryle's disease, perforating folliculitis, elastosis perforans serpiginosa, and reactive perforating collagenosis.

Kryle's Disease. Kryle's disease, named after the Austrian physician who described it in 1916, is rare. The patients develop papules up to 1 cm across with a central, conical core of keratin. The papules are most common on the extensor surfaces of the limbs. Microscopically, a pit lined by epidermis and filled with keratin and debris extends down into the dermis. In foci in the deeper part of the pit, the granular layer is often absent and parakeratotic cells overlie the epidermis. In some patients, the epidermal cells in the deeper part of the pit degenerate and disappear, allowing the keratin plug to come in contact with the dermis. A granulomatous reaction develops in the dermis at the site of the perforation.

Perforating Folliculitis. Perforating folliculitis was more common than Kryle's disease but has become rare. Papules like those of Kryle's disease develop on the limbs and buttocks. Microscopically, the lesions develop in hair follicles. The affected follicles are distended with keratin, parakeratin, and debris, including degenerate elastic fibers. Usually a curled up hair is present in the follicle. The follicle perforates, with inflammation and degeneration of elastica in the dermis at the site of perforation.

Elastosis Perforans Serpiginosa. Elastosis perforans serpiginosa is uncommon. Hyperkeratotic papules up to 5 mm in diameter form rings in the skin. Microscopically, the lesions show a proliferation of elastica in the upper part of the dermis. The overlying epidermis is thick and hyperkeratotic and extends down into the abnormal dermis. Narrow, winding channels perforate the thickened epidermis. Fragments of degenerate elastica are extruded through them.

Reactive Perforating Collagenosis. Reactive perforating collagenosis is rare. The lesions begin in childhood. Papules up to 1 cm across, with a central core of keratin, develop in regions that have suffered some mild injury. Early lesions show necrosis of a dermal papilla, with thinning of the overlying epidermis. Lymphocytes and macrophages accumulate around the necrotic tissue, which is extruded through the epidermis. A plug of keratin and debris fills the gap, and the epidermis regenerates beneath it.

DISEASES OF THE EPIDERMAL APPENDAGES

Among the noninfectious, non-neoplastic diseases that involve principally the epidermal appendages are acne vulgaris, acne conglobata, rosacea, alopecia, epidermal dysplasia, trichostasis spinulosa, Fox-Fordyce disease, and the malformations of the hair.

ACNE VULGARIS. Acne vulgaris is common in adolescents and young adults, less so in children. Almost all teenagers have a few of its whiteheads and blackheads. Both boys and girls are affected, but acne tends to be more severe and to persist longer in boys. The word *acne* probably comes from the Greek for a point. *Vulgaris* is the Latin word meaning common.

Acne occurs on the face, neck, upper part of the trunk, and upper part of the arms. Rarely, other parts of the skin are affected. Usually, acne begins and is most severe on the face. Small plugs obstruct the mouths of hair follicles and sebaceous glands. If the plugs are white, they are called whiteheads; if black, they are called blackheads. In most people this is the extent of the disease. Only if acne is unusually severe do papules, pustules, nodules, and cysts develop in and around some of the obstructed follicles. In a minority of the patients, the lesions become large and unsightly, causing considerable distress to the patient. Often acne is episodic, with periods of activity separated by intervals of remission and quiescence.

Two kinds of acne vulgaris are distinguished, inflammatory and noninflammatory. In the noninflammatory lesions, the affected follicles are plugged by keratinized cells mixed with sebum. The plug is called a comedo, from the Latin for a glutton. If a comedo forms deep in a follicle where the follicular epithelium is not pigmented, its keratinized cells contain no melanin, and a whitehead results. If it develops near the opening of a follicle where the follicular epithelium is heavily pigmented, its cells are heavily pigmented with melanin, and a blackhead results. Usually the mouth of a follicle containing a whitehead is small, so that the comedo feels deep set. The mouth of a follicle containing a blackhead is widely dilated, and the comedo projects above the surface of the skin.

The inflammatory lesions of acne vulgaris develop when the dermis around a follicle or follicles becomes inflamed. If the inflammation is minor, only a few lymphocytes and macrophages accumulate around the follicle or follicles. If it is more severe but is superficial, neutrophils form a pustule around the follicle affected. If it is still more severe and deeper, the lesion is larger and is called a nodule. Often the follicle or follicles affected rupture, releasing comedones and keratin into the nodule. Neutrophils are abundant in the exudate, but are mixed with lymphocytes and macrophages. Often multinucleated macrophages phagocytose fragments of keratin extruded into the dermis.

Secondary infection with bacteria and fungi is common in acne vulgaris. The lesions are often heavily infected with Proprionibacterium acnes, a diphtheroid commonly present around the hairs in normal people.

Acne vulgaris is caused by increased proliferation of the epithelial cells in the lower part of the hair follicles. Increased numbers of keratinocytes are shed into the lumen of the follicle and adhere together more firmly than is normal. They are bound together by the sebum to form a comedo.

Androgens increase the rate of cellular proliferation in the hair follicles and the secretion of sebum. Probably dihydrotestosterone, not testosterone, is the principal cause of the increased activity. The secretion of androgens is normal in boys with acne vulgaris, but testosterone is converted to dihydrotestosterone more rapidly in skin with acne than in normal skin. In girls, premenstrual exacerbation of acne is common.

Several factors cause inflammation in acne vulgaris. Rupture of the follicles releasing sebum and keratin into the dermis causes acute and granulomatous inflammation. The bacteria in the lesions break down the lipids in sebum to irritant fatty acids that may escape into the dermis. A cell-mediated immunologic reaction against Proprionibacterium acnes probably adds to the inflammation.

In most people, acne vulgaris resolves when the patient is between 20 and 30 years old, leaving no residual injury. If the lesions are large and inflammation is severe, local or more widespread scarring is likely. Occasionally a keloid develops in a lesion. Sunlight and applications that cause desquamation in the skin open the follicles and speed healing. Tetracycline and other antibiotics control the infection and help resolve the more serious lesions. Cosmetics, cutting oils, and chlorinated hydrocarbons increase the risk of developing acne by increasing the likelihood of follicular obstruction.

Acne Conglobata. Acne conglobata is a severe form of acne vulgaris. The patients are nearly all men. Large cystic lesions form, sometimes involving the buttocks or legs. Often they develop into foul, interconnecting abscesses. Treatment is difficult. Scarring often is extensive.

ROSACEA. Rosacea, from the Latin for rose-colored, used to be called acne rosacea.

Rosacea is common. It may occur at any age. It is most frequent in women 30 to 50 years old, although the more serious forms of rosacea are more frequent in men.

A persistent erythema develops in the skin of the nose and cheeks, often with telangiectasia. Exacerbations and remissions are common. As the disease worsens, papules, pustules, and nodules like those of acne vulgaris develop in the affected region, but comedones are not found. The inflammatory lesions can become extensive and disfiguring and lead to scarring. Occasionally the eyes are involved, with blepharitis, conjunctivitis, iritis, and sometimes keratitis. In men, but rarely in women, hyperplasia of the sebaceous glands and the surrounding connective tissue sometimes causes the enlargement of the lower part of the nose called rhinophyma, from the Greek for the nose and a tumor, sometimes without other evidence of rosacea.

The erythematous skin shows only a moderate exudate of lymphocytes and macrophages in the dermis, often more marked around dilated, telangiectatic vessels. The papules, pustules, and nodules are microscopically like those of the inflammatory form of acne vulgaris. In over 10% of patients with rosacea, granulomata are found in the dermis. The granulomata consist of clumps of the large macrophages with abundant, eosinophilic cytoplasm called epithelioid cells. Often some of the macrophages are multinucleated, or a rind of lymphocytes surrounds the clump of macrophages. Sometimes the center of the granulomata is necrotic.

In rhinophyma, the sebaceous glands are increased in size and number, with dilated ducts sometimes containing keratinous debris. The surrounding connective tissue is often congested with a moderate exudate of lymphocytes and macrophages.

The cause of rosacea is unknown. The granulomata present in the skin in some patients with rosacea are probably a reaction to keratin and other foreign material extruded into the dermis. It is no longer believed that the lesion is a tuberculid. The parasite Demodex folliculorum is common in rosacea, but is probably a secondary infection, not the cause of the disease. Alcohol and overeating worsen rosacea by causing flushing of the face, but do not initiate the disease.

ALOPECIA. Alopecia, from the Greek for a mange of foxes that causes loss of hair, is a term used to describe loss of hair, localized or generalized. Baldness, alopecia areata, alopecia cicatrisata, alopecia mucinosa, and secondary alopecia are its principal forms.

Baldness. Loss of hair from the scalp is called baldness. The recession of hair from the temples that is the mildest form of baldness occurs in 90% of men and 80% of women. In 60% of men and in 25% of women, thinning of the hair on the crown of the head is evident by the time the person is 50 years old. By the age of 80 years, almost all men are partially bald, and in most women the hair on the head is thin and sparse.

At first the hairs lost are apparently normal, but later most of them are of less than the normal diameter. The vascular sheath around the hair follicles degenerates. The follicles atrophy and disappear. The sebaceous and sweat glands persist. The failure of the hair follicles in the scalp is related to the concentration of androgens in the plasma, though it is not clear why some men become bald and others do not. Hereditary factors are sometimes important, as shown by the frequency and severity of baldness in some families.

Alopecia Areata. In alopecia areata, there is rapid and usually complete loss of hair from one or more sharply circumscribed areas in the scalp or elsewhere in the skin. If all the hair is lost from the scalp, the condition is called alopecia totalis. If all the hair on the body is lost, it is called alopecia totalis.

In the regions involved, the hair follicles are small. They resemble the anagen or telogen stages of developing hair follicles. They contain only fine, ill-formed hairs or no hair at all. The sebaceous glands are sometimes normal, sometimes atrophic. A moderate exudate of lymphocytes and macrophages often surrounds the abnormal follicles.

In some patients, alopecia areata may be due to a cell-mediated immunologic response. In some, it is precipitated by stress or infection. If the area affected is small, the hair usually returns spontaneously within nine months. More extensive loss of hair is usually permanent.

Alopecia Cicatrisata. In alopecia cicatrisata, small, irregular foci of alopecia develop in the scalp and slowly enlarge as years pass. The hairless skin is thin, white, and atrophic. Usually a few normal hairs remain in the hairless regions. Early in the disease, a moderately severe exudate of lymphocytes and macrophages develops around the upper part of the hair follicles and the sebaceous glands in the affected regions. The inflammatory cells extend into the follicles and the sebaceous glands. The sweat glands are not affected. Eventually, most of the hair follicles and sebaceous glands degenerate and disappear. The inflammation wanes. Collagenous bundles containing many elastic fibers replace the lost follicles. The dermis becomes increasingly fibrotic. The cause of alopecia cicatrisata is unknown. Some think it a form of lichen pilopilaris.

Alopecia Mucinosa. In alopecia mucinosa, papules or red, raised plaques develop in the skin. The lesions are devoid of hair, though this may not be obvious except in the scalp. In the affected regions, the epithelial cells of the sebaceous glands and hair follicles become swollen and degenerate. Large amounts of mucopolysaccharide accumulate in the damaged glands and follicles and may form small cysts. The surrounding dermis often shows an exudate of lymphocytes, macrophages, and sometimes eosinophils. The lesions usually resolve within two years. Sometimes new lesions appear long after the earlier ones. About 20% of patients have mycosis fungoides or some other form of lymphoma.

Secondary Alopecia. Many forms of injury cause alopecia by damaging the hair follicles. Sometimes a person compulsively pulls out his or her own hair, a disorder called trichotillomania, from the Greek words for hair, pull, and frenzy. Continued traction on the hair with rollers damages the hair follicles. Some of the chemicals used in shampoos and dyes do so. Radiation often causes temporary or permanent alopecia by damaging the follicles. Thallium causes alopecia by inhibiting the growth of hair, most obviously in the scalp. Heparin and similar compounds have a similar though milder effect. Antimitotic drugs often cause serious alopecia, though the loss of hair is temporary, and withdrawal of the drug allows regrowth

of the hair. Large doses of vitamin A cause alopecia. Occasionally quinine, thiouracil, allopurinol, or some other drug does so.

Injury to the hairs is called trichorrexus nodosa, from the Greek for hair and breaking. Nodules on the damaged hairs mark regions in which they are frayed and easily broken. Shampoos and hair dyes sometimes cause this sort of injury. It is common in agininosuccinicaciduria.

ECTODERMAL DYSPLASIA. Two forms of ectodermal dysplasia are distinguished. The hidrotic form is inherited as an autosomal dominant character. Sweating is normal. The patients have alopecia and often malformation of the nails, but the teeth are usually normal. Some of the patients are mentally deficient. The anhidrotic form is inherited as an X-linked recessive character. Boys have a severe form of the disease. In girls, it is mild. The patients cannot sweat and so are intolerant of heat. They have alopecia or fine, sparse hair. The teeth develop late and are malformed. Some patients develop cataracts or corneal opacities. The mucous glands of the respiratory tract are sometimes deficient. Most of the patients have a bossed forehead, saddle nose, and pointed chin.

In both types of ectodermal dysplasia, the hair follicles and sebaceous glands are small, malformed, and less numerous than is normal. In the hidrotic form, the eccrine and apocrine glands are normal. In the anhidrotic form, the eccrine glands are few or absent. The apocrine glands are present in some patients, absent or hypoplastic in others.

TRICHOSTASIS SPINULOSA. In elderly people, spikelike comedones sometimes project from the hair follicles in the face or less often some other part of the skin. The spikes develop because the follicles fail to shed their hairs and come to contain 10 to 20 hairs surrounded by a keratinous sheath.

FOX-FORDYCE DISEASE. Fox-Fordyce disease is named after the American dermatologists who reported it in 1902. The patients are almost all women. Rounded, itchy papules develop in the axillae and groins and in other regions where there are apocrine glands. As the papules become numerous, there is loss of apocrine sweating. The mouths of the ducts of the affected glands are obstructed by a plug of keratin. The ducts rupture. Apocrine sweat escapes into the epidermis and upper dermis, often causing tiny cysts. An inflammatory exudate mainly of lymphocytes develops around the cysts. The cause of Fox-Fordyce diease is unknown. It tends to persist indefinitely, in spite of treatment.

MALFORMED HAIR. Patients with monilethrix, from the Latin for a necklace and the Greek for hair, are born with normal hair, but after a few months some of the hairs become beaded by regularly spaced constrictions and easily break, causing alopecia. Often hair follicles become plugged with keratin.

Pilus tortus is an uncommon hereditary disorder in which some of the hairs become twisted and break, causing patchy alopecia. Some of the patients show mental retardation. The name is from the Latin for hair and twisted.

In pilus annulatus, from the Latin for ringed, the hairs are of normal diameter, but contain air-filled cavities.

Trichorrhexis invaginata occurs almost exclusively in women, usually in association with ichthyosis linearis circumflexa, but sometimes with lamellar ichthyosis. The hair of the scalp is short and fragile. The hairs resemble bamboo, with the distal end of the hair invaginated into the proximal part, to form the joint.

VASCULAR DISEASES

The conditions that affect primarily the vessels in the skin are the different types of purpura and vasculitis. The changes in the blood vessels common in other diseases of the skin are secondary to the underlying disorder.

PURPURA. The hemorrhages into the skin and other tissues called purpura, from the Latin for purple, are common and occur in many conditions. If the hemorrhages are less than 3 mm across, they are called petechiae, a term of unknown origin adopted in modern Latin. Larger hemorrhages are called ecchymoses, from the Greek for an extravasation of blood.

Purpura has many causes. In most patients it results from disease of the platelets, especially thrombocytopenia, discussed in Chapter 52, or from one of the diseases of the blood vessels that result in vascular purpura, discussed in Chapter 25.

Recent purpuric lesions in the skin show only hemorrhage into the dermis, with little or no inflammatory response unless the underlying disease causes other changes. The extravasated red cells are at first well preserved. In the course of some days they break up, releasing hemosiderin, and are removed by macrophages.

VASCULITIS. Many of the forms of vasculitis that involve the body as a whole affect the skin. Some are most obvious in the skin or are confined to the skin. The conditions that involve principally the skin include leukoclastic vasculitis, polyarteritis nodosa, cryoglobulinemia, pityriasis lichenoides; lymphoid papillomatosis, purpura pigmentosa chronica, malignant atrophic papulosis, granuloma faciale, erythema elevatum diutinum, acute febrile neutrophilic dermatosis, and livedo reticularis-atrophi blanche. Erythema induratum and erythema nodosum are discussed later in the chapter in the section on diseases of the subcutaneous tissue.

Leukoclastic Vasculitis. Allergic vasculitis, or anaphylactoid purpura, commonly involves the skin. Because debris from the fragmented nuclei of dead neutrophils is usually prominent in the lesions in the skin, this kind of vasculitis is often called leukoclastic vasculitis, from the Greek for broken into pieces.

Leukoclastic vasculitis of the skin may develop acutely, especially when it is associated with vasculitis of other organs, as in the Henoch-Schönlein syndrome. The lesions in the skin persist for about four weeks and then resolve. In 50% of the patients, they recur. In other patients, leukoclastic vasculitis of the skin is more chronic and persists longer. In many of the patients with the chronic form of the condition, the disease is confined to the skin.

Purpura and ecchymoses are usual in the acute form of leukoclastic vasculitis of the skin. Some of the patients have also urticaria, an erythematous rash, papules, vesicles, or bullae. Some of the lesions may ulcerate. In the more chronic form of leukoclastic vasculitis, petechiae are often confined to the lower

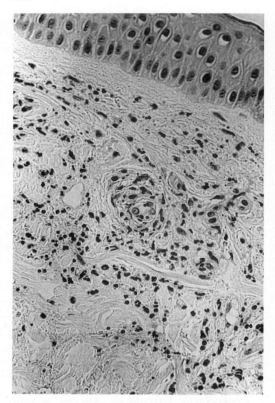

Fig. 62-14. Leukoclastic vasculitis. The inflammation is centered around a small blood vessel in the dermis. Many of the nuclei of the neutrophils are fragmented.

legs. Often the severity of the disease waxes and wanes. Sometimes there are papules, blisters, or ulcers in addition to the petechiae, or instead of them.

In both types of leukoclastic vasculitis of the skin, the lesions are largely confined to the small blood vessels in the dermis. The endothelial cells in the affected vessels are swollen and often separated one from another. Their basement membrane may be breached. Neutrophils are numerous in the walls of the affected vessels and extend into the adjacent tissue. Fibrin and red cells are often admixed with the exudate. In older lesions, hemosiderin is present in macrophages. Debris from the nuclei of dead neutrophils is often prominent.

Leukoclastic vasculitis is caused by the deposition or formation of immune complexes in the walls of the dermal vessels and the activation of complement by the complexes. C3 is usually demonstrable in lesions less than 24 hours old, and often IgM or IgA is also demonstrable. In older lesions, complement and immunoglobulins are rarely found, presumably because the complexes are phagocytosed by the neutrophils and destroyed.

Polyarteritis Nodosa. The skin is involved in 25% of the patients with polyarteritis nodosa. Usually tender, erythematous nodules show the position of the involved arteries, though sometimes there is instead an erythematous, urticarial, or purpuric rash. The lesions in the arteries are like those in other parts of the body.

Cryoglobulinemia. Patients with one of the forms of cryoglobulinemia described in Chapter 55 sometimes develop purpura or ulceration of the skin. The blood vessels in the dermis of the affected regions are filled with a homogeneous precipitate of cyroglobulins, which stains brightly with the periodic acid-Schiff reaction. In monoclonal cryoglobulinemia, a sparse exudate of lymphocytes sometimes surrounds the affected vessels. In mixed cryoglobulinemia, the involved vessels show leukoclastic vasculitis.

Pityriasis Lichenoides. Pityriasis lichenoides is divided into two forms: the more active pityriasis lichenoides et varioliformis acuta and the more sluggish pityriasis lichenoides chronica. Both are most common in children and young adults.

In pityriasis lichenoides et varioliformis acuta, erythematous papules 2 to 4 mm across appear principally on the trunk. After a few days, the papules become hemorrhagic, sometimes vesicular or crusted. They heal in about two weeks, often leaving a little scar or a hyperpigmentation. As one crop of papules heals, others appear. The disease usually continues for months or years before it resolves.

In pityriasis lichenoides chronica, repeated crops of similar papules appear mainly on the trunk, but develop more slowly, are more scaly, often up to 10 mm across, and take four weeks or more to disappear. Usually the disease continues for six months or more.

Microscopically, the acute type of pityriasis lichenoides shows a prominent exudate of lymphocytes and macrophages around small blood vessels in the dermis. The exudate and the accompanying edema may extend into the epidermis. Often red cells are mixed with the exudate and may be present in the epidermis. The overlying epidermal cells are swollen and degenerate or necrotic. In the chronic form of the disease, a similar exudate of lymphocytes and macrophages surrounds small blood vessels in the dermis, but changes in the epidermis are less prominent. In recent lesions of pityriasis lichenoides, IgM and C3 can sometimes be found in the walls of the more severely affected vessels, suggesting that the disease may be immunologically mediated.

Lymphomatoid Papillomatosis. In lymphomatoid papillomatosis, the clinical presentation and lesions are like those of pityriasis lichenoides et varioliformis acuta, except that mixed with the cells of the exudate are large, atypical lymphocytes, like those seen in mycosis fungoides. In most patients, the course of lymphomatoid papillomatosis is like that of pityriasis lichenoides. A few patients have developed a non-Hodgkin's lymphoma. Some consider that lymphomatoid papillomatosis is a form of pityriasis lichenoides; some prefer to consider it a form of mycosis fungoides.

Purpura Pigmentosa Chronica. Purpura pigmentosa chronica is sometimes called Majocchi-Schamberg disease after an Italian (1849–1929) and an American (1870–1934) dermatologist. It is a group of conditions of unknown etiology that show some combination of groups of petechial spots in the skin with surrounding telangiectasia and macules of brownish pigmentation. Occasionally the lesions are itchy, scaly, or thickened. Often the disease remains localized to the lower limbs, but it can become extensive, as the lesions slowly extend as months and years pass. Purpura pigmentosa chronica may eventually resolve. Sometimes adrenocortical steroids induce regression of the lesions.

Microscopically, there is an exudate of lymphocytes and macrophages, perhaps with a few neutrophils, in the upper dermis, mainly around the vessels. The endothelium of the vessels is swollen, and the small vessels in the upper dermis are dilated. The exudate may extend into the epidermis. Sometimes there is patchy parakeratosis. In new lesions, there are a few red cells in the exudate. In older lesions, hemosiderin is evident in macrophages, and the vasculitis is less severe.

Malignant Atrophic Papulosis. Malignant atrophic papulosis, or Degos' syndrome, named after the French physician who described it in 1942, is a rare condition that usually presents first in the skin. Thickening of the intima narrows or occludes small arteries and arterioles in the deeper part of the dermis or in the subcutaneous tissue, resulting in small foci of infarction. The infarcts in the skin are first erythematous papules up to 5 mm across, but gradually become white like porcelain in the center of the lesions. In the majority of the patients, other organs are sooner or later involved, though perhaps not for months or years. Involvement of the arteries and sometimes the veins of the gut brings nausea, abdominal pain, perhaps melena or vomiting, and not uncommonly death from hemorrhage or perforation. Less often, the brain, heart, kidneys, or some other organ is involved. The cause of the intimal thickening in malignant atrophic papulosis is unknown. IgM, IgG, or C3 is often demonstrable in the vessels, but it is not clear that the disease is mediated immunologically.

Granuloma Faciale. Granuloma faciale is an uncommon disorder in which one or more erythematous macules develop on the face or occasionally in another part of the skin. The macule gradually enlarges and may become several centimeters across. The lesions persist indefinitely. Microscopically, there is a dense exudate, particularly in the upper part of the dermis, though a narrow band of normal collagen separates the exudate from the epidermis. The exudate consists largely of neutrophils and eosinophils, with lesser numbers of lymphocytes, plasma cells, macrophages, and mast cells. The vessels in the exudate are dilated, with fibrin in and around their walls. Debris of the nuclei of dead granulocytes is evident especially around the vessels. Sometimes a few red cells are present in the exudate, or there is hemosiderin in macrophages. Granuloma faciale is believed to be a form of vasculitis, though its etiology is unknown. IgG, IgM, IgA, and complement are present in the basement membrane of the epidermis and around the dermal vessels.

Erythema Elevatum Diutinum. Erythema elevatum diutinum is a rare condition, that takes its name from the Latin for elevated and long lasting. Nodules and plaques appear in the skin, most often over joints. They enlarge slowly, often with scaling or purpura. Sometimes the lesions ulcerate, discharging fatty material. The size of a nodule may change in the course of a day. Occasionally a nodule will disappear spontaneously, only to recur. Usually the disease progresses slowly for five to ten years, but then regresses spontaneously.

Microscopically, vasculitis in the dermis causes swelling of the endothelium in the dermal vessels and deposition of fibrin in and around their walls. There is a dense perivascular exudate mainly of neutrophils, though with some lymphocytes and macrophages and sometimes eosinophils or plasma cells. Often nuclear debris from dead neutrophils is evident. Sometimes there are a few red cells in the exudate, or some of the macrophages contain hemosiderin. In the late stages, the exudate is less severe, though still predominantly neutrophilic. Sometimes there are many foam cells, as macrophages take up lipid from destroyed cells, or some degree of fibrosis. Immunoglobulins and other plasma proteins are present in the lesions. It is not clear whether they have leaked from the damaged blood vessels or are due in part to an immunologic reaction.

Acute Febrile Neutrophilic Dermatosis. In acute febrile neutrophilic dermatosis, called Sweet's syndrome after the British dermatologist who described in 1964, tender, raised, erythematous plaques up to 2.0 cm across develop on the face and limbs. They appear suddenly, and persist for one to eight months. Most of the patients are women. Some have myeloid leukemia. Microscopically, a dense infiltrate of neutrophils with a few lymphocytes, macrophages, and eosinophils surrounds blood vessels in the dermis. The walls of the blood vessels show little abnormality. The upper part of the dermis is edematous, sometimes sufficiently severely to cause vesiculation.

Livedo Reticularis-Atrophie Blanche. Livedo reticularis, from the Latin for lead-colored, is a persistent bluish reticulation or mottling of the skin, seen particularly on the lower part of the legs, most commonly in women. Painful ulcers that develop in the affected skin leave a white, atrophic scar when they heal. This stage of the disorder is called atrophie blanche, the French for white atrophy. In the early stages of the disease, the vessels in the dermis show a leukoclastic vasculitis. Often they are occluded, and the overlying skin is infarcted and ulcerated. In the later stages, the vessel walls are thickened and hyaline. Often their lumen is obliterated or recanalized. The epidermis is thin. The dermis is sclerotic. Only a sparse exudate of lymphocytes and plasma cells remains. Usually livedo reticularis-atrophie blanche is idiopathic. Occasionally it complicates a collagen disease, infection, or tumor.

DERMAL DISEASES

In several of the noninfectious disorders that involve principally the dermis, granulomata are the dominant feature of the disease. Granuloma annulare, necrobiosis lipoidica, foreign body granulomatosis, and the lesions caused by the bites of arthropods are disorders of this type. Sarcoidosis, rheumatoid arthritis, rheumatic fever, and rosacea are among other conditions that cause noninfectious granulomata in the skin. Focal dermal hypoplasia, acrodermatitis chronica atrophicus, and scleredema are also considered in this section.

GRANULOMA ANNULARE. Granuloma annulare is not common. It occurs most frequently in women and girls. Some 70% of the patients are under 30 years of age; 40% are less than 15 years old. Diabetes mellitus is unduly common in patients with granuloma annulare.

Papules appear in the skin, most often in the hands or feet. Usually the papules are arranged to form a ring, 1 to 5 cm in diameter, as the name *annulare*, from the Latin for a ring, suggests. Less often the papules become confluent to form a plaque or are umbilicated. Occasionally granuloma annulare develops more deeply, with lesions similar to rheumatoid nodules. Occasionally it is widespread, involving much of the skin.

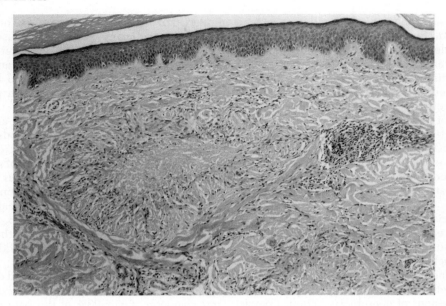

Fig. 62-15. Granuloma annulare. A palisade of macrophages surrounds a necrotic focus in the dermis.

Rarely, the core of a lesion drains onto the surface of the epidermis through a narrow sinus.

Microscopically, the lesions of granuloma annulare are usually in the dermis. The overlying epidermis may be normal or thinned. Occasionally a lesion develops in the subcutaneous tissue. A fully developed lesion shows one or more foci of degeneration in which the collagen bundles become blurred, homogeneous, and hyaline. The nuclei between the bundles of collagen disappear, leaving only fine, nuclear debris. The quantity of mucopolysaccharide in the degenerate foci increases, so that the lesions stain metachromatically with toluidine blue. A prominent palisade of macrophages forms around the foci of degeneration, often with a moderate exudate of lymphocytes more peripherally. Sometimes a few of the macrophages are multinucleated.

The foci of degeneration in the dermis in granuloma annulare are not always complete. Often degenerate bundles of collagen are mixed with normal ones. Instead of the prominent palisade of macrophages, an exudate of lymphocytes and macrophages is intermixed with the degenerate collagen bundles.

The lesions of granuloma annulare persist for a long time with little change, but may resolve after several years. The cause of granuloma annulare is unknown.

NECROBIOSIS LIPOIDICA. Necrobiosis lipoidica can occur at any age, but is most frequent in young adults. More than 70% of the patients are women. Nearly 70% of them have diabetes mellitus.

One or more irregular, sharply defined patches with a yellowish center and violaceous periphery develop on the shins. The center of the lesion gradually becomes thin, white, and atrophic, often with telangiectasia, and may ulcerate. In 15% of the patients, lesions like those of granuloma annulare are present elsewhere on the skin, nearly always in addition to lesions on the shins.

Microscopically, the lesions of necrobiosis lipoidica usually show scattered foci of degeneration of collagen in the dermis. The foci are ill-defined and can be large. In the affected parts of the dermis, the collagen bundles are fragmented, blurred, often eosinophilic, and hyaline. Fine bundles of new collagen are mixed with the degenerating collagen. Frequently, the quantity of mucopolysaccharide is increased in the foci of degeneration, which often contain fine droplets of fat. An exudate of lymphocytes and macrophages surrounds the foci and may extend into them. Sometimes the macrophages form a palisade that partially surrounds a focus of degeneration. Often some of the macrophages are multinucleated.

In some patients, well-defined granulomata are scattered in the dermis. The granulomata consist of large macrophages, some of which are multinucleate. Asteroids are sometimes present. A mild or moderate exudate predominantly of lymphocytes is present in the dermis between the granulomata. In some of these patients, foci of necrosis are few or absent.

Especially in lesions on the shins that show extensive degeneration of collagen, the blood vessels in the deeper part of the dermis often have thickened walls that stain strongly with the periodic acid-Schiff reaction. The vessels are sometimes partly or completely occluded.

The lesions of necrobiosis lipoidica persist for many years, but sometimes resolve, leaving a scar. Control of the accompanying diabetes mellitus usually brings improvement. The cause of necrobiosis lipoidica is unknown. Some think it secondary to diabetic disease of the vessels, but it is at least as likely that the changes in the vessels are secondary to the disease.

FOREIGN BODY GRANULOMATA. A wide variety of foreign materials induce a foreign body reaction in the skin if they gain entry to the dermis. The foreign material first induces acute inflammation. By the time a biopsy of the lesion is taken, this has usually been replaced by an exudate predominantly of macrophages and lymphocytes. If the foreign material is particulate, the macrophages form multinucleated giant cells. They often accumulate around the foreign material or phagocytose it. If the inflammation persists, fibrosis develops around the lesion.

Among the materials that induce a foreign body reaction in the skin are oils such as paraffin, silicaceous dust, asbestos, and beryllium. Splinters of wood and fragments of sutures do so. Contamination with the powder from a surgeon's glove excites a brisk foreign body reaction. The zirconium in some deodorants causes granulomata like those of sarcoidosis in people sensitive to it. Endogenous substances such as keratin excite a foreign body reaction if they gain entry to the dermis.

ARTHROPOD BITES AND STINGS. The bites and stings of many arthropods cause only fleeting acute inflammation. The bite of a mosquito is an example. Some cause an urticarial reaction of the sort caused by the sting of a bee or wasp, especially in people sensitive to these insects.

Sometimes the bite of a tick or another arthropod causes a persistent nodule in the dermis. A dense exudate mainly of lymphocytes but with smaller numbers of macrophages, plasma cells, and sometimes eosinophils develops in the dermis. Often some of the macrophages are multinucleated or have hyperchromatic, atypical nuclei. Sometimes germinal centers develop in the exudate. Occasionally the mouth parts of the tick can be identified.

FOCAL DERMAL HYPOPLASIA. Focal dermal hypoplasia is inherited as an X-linked dominant character. Over 90% of the patients are girls, probably because the unopposed X chromosome bearing this character is usually lethal in boys. In foci that are frequently linear, the dermis is greatly thinned, causing lesions that resemble striae gravidarum. The subcutaneous fat sometimes herniates through the weakened dermis, forming fatty bulges beneath the epidermis. In places, the skin may be absent, forming an ulcer that slowly granulates and heals. The nails are poorly formed or absent. Often there is partial alopecia. Malformed teeth and skeletal deformities are common. The eyes may be malformed. Often there is mental retardation or seizures.

ACRODERMATITIS CHRONICA ATROPHICANS. Acrodermatitis chronica atrophicans is almost confined to northern, central, and eastern Europe. It develops in people 40 to 50 years old. The skin on a limb becomes itchy and then erythematous. As months pass, it gradually atrophies. Fibrous bands and nodules sometimes develop in the atrophic skin or around joints. Sometimes the sclerotic bands and nodules calcify. Sometimes a squamous cell carcinoma or a basal cell carcinoma develops in the abnormal skin.

At first, the dermis is edematous, with an exudate of lymphocytes and macrophages around dermal vessels and beneath the epidermis. The epidermis becomes atrophic. The rete ridges are lost. As time passes, the dermis atrophies, until it is less than half its normal thickness, with loss of both collagen and elastica. Except for the sweat glands, the epidermal appendages atrophy and disappear. The subcutaneous tissue grows thin. The fibrous bands and nodules consist of hyalinized collagen.

Acrodermatitis chronica atrophicans is probably caused by infection with an arbovirus, with the wood tick Ixodes ricinus serving as the vector. Large doses of penicillin given early in the course of the disease cure.

SCLEREDEMA. Scleredema, sometimes called scleredema adultorum, takes its name from the Greek for hard. It usually develops in an adult, though children can be affected. Often it begins after an infection.

Scleredema causes widespread thickening and stiffening of the skin. Usually it begins in the face and spreads to involve the arms and trunk. Occasionally, the tongue or skeletal muscles are swollen and stiffened.

In 80% of the patients, the process continues to worsen for one to two weeks and then slowly resolves in the course of months. In the other 20%, the lesions persist for as long as 40 years. Many of the patients with the persistent form of the disease have diabetes mellitus. Others have a monoclonal gammopathy.

In the regions involved, the superficial part of the subcutaneous tissue is replaced by coarse bundles of dermal collagen. Microscopically, the dermis seems to be up to 3 times its normal thickness. The sweat glands are in its upper part. Often the bundles of collagen are separated by abundant intercellular substance.

DISEASES OF THE SUBCUTANEOUS TISSUE

This section considers erythema nodosum and erythema induratum. Weber-Christian disease, sclerema neonatorum, and subcutaneous fat necrosis of the newborn are discussed in Chapter 61.

ERYTHEMA NODOSUM. Erythema nodosum has become less common. The patients are usually 20 to 35 years old. About 75% of them are women.

After prodromal symptoms of fever, malaise, and arthralgia, discrete, erythematous, tender nodules 1 to 5 cm in diameter appear on the anterior surface of the lower legs and occasionally in other parts of the skin. There may be only a few nodules, or there may be dozens. Occasionally, they become confluent. As they age, the nodules become bluish or greenish. They resolve in three to six weeks without leaving a scar. Often new

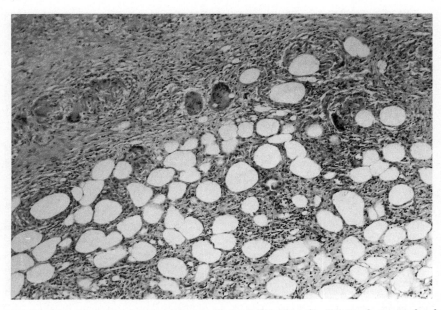

Fig. 62-16. Erythema nodosum showing inflammation and fibrosis at the junction between the dermis and subcutaneous tissue.

lesions appear as old lesions regress, so that the disease continues for months and in exceptional cases for years.

Microscopically, the early lesions of erythema nodosum show an exudate of lymphocytes and neutrophils with a few macrophages and perhaps eosinophils in the fibrous septa of the subcutaneous fat. In places, the exudate extends between the fat cells and becomes more extensive. Often the exudate is prominent around small vessels in the subcutaneous tissue and occasionally around medium-sized veins. The exudate extends into the media of the vessels affected, which often have a thickened intima. Thrombosis does not occur. The dermis is little affected, though it may show a mild, mainly perivascular exudate predominantly of lymphocytes.

As the lesions age, the neutrophils disappear, so that the exudate consists of lymphocytes and macrophages. Often multinucleated giant cells formed from the macrophages become prominent, but granulomata are rarely seen. Lipophages are numerous in regions where fat cells are ruptured.

Erythema nodosum is probably caused by a cell-mediated immunologic reaction, though its presumed cause is identified in only 30% of the patients. It most frequently follows streptococcal pharyngitis, less often tuberculosis, leprosy, a yersinial infection, coccidioidomycosis, histoplasmosis, lymphogranuloma venereum, or some other infection. It develops in 30% of patients with sarcoidosis. Sometimes it complicates ulcerative colitis, Crohn's disease, or Beçhet's disease, lymphoma, or leukemia. Drugs such as sulfonamides, gold salts, bromides, and oral contraceptives can precipitate an attack.

ERYTHEMA INDURATUM. Erythema induratum is uncommon. One or more tender nodules up to 3 cm in diameter develop in the subcutaneous tissue of the calves, usually in girls 10 to 20 years old, often in winter. As months pass, the nodules become purplish red and closer to the surface. Often they ulcerate, forming indolent ulcers, which eventually heal leaving an atrophic scar.

Microscopically, early lesions of erythema induratum show only chronic inflammation of the subcutaneous tissue, with an exudate of lymphocytes, plasma cells, and macrophages greatest in the fibrous septa between the lobules of fat. After a few weeks, granulomata develop in the exudate. They consist of a loose aggregate of large macrophages, some of which are multinucleated.

Vasculitis is usually severe. Small and

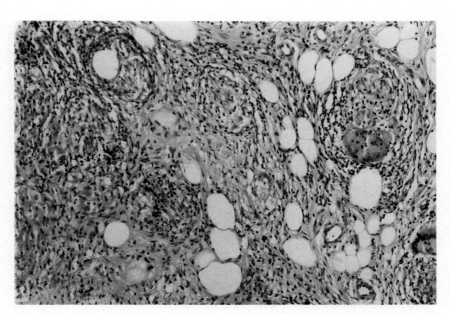

Fig. 62-17.   Granulomata in the subcutaneous tissue in a patient with erythema induratum.

medium-sized arteries and veins in the subcutaneous tissue have a prominent exudate of lymphocytes, plasma cells, and macrophages in their walls. The endothelium of the vessels becomes swollen. Often there is thrombosis, with obliteration of the lumen. Occasionally, vasculitis is the principal feature of the lesion.

As the lesions age, the inflammation extends into the dermis. Often necrosis becomes extensive in the lesions. The necrotic tissue is finely granular, much as in tuberculosis. Destruction of fat often causes an accumulation of lipophages.

The lesions heal with scarring and the restoration of a thin, atrophic epidermis.

Erythema induratum has long been considered due to tuberculosis, perhaps a tuberculous infection of the skin, but more probably a tuberculid, an allergic response to tuberculosis elsewhere in the body. There is little reason to think that this is the case. Tubercle bacilli cannot be cultured from the lesions; the patients with erythema induratum do not have tuberculosis more frequently than does the population at large; antituberculous therapy does not benefit the lesions of erythema induratum. It seems likely that erythema nodosum is a form of angiitis.

Nodular Vasculitis. Nodular vasculitis is now considered a form of erythema induratum. It is most common in women 30 to 50 years old. Recurrent, tender nodules develop in the subcutaneous tissue of the legs. The lesions resolve after some months and usually do not ulcerate.

Biopsy shows inflammation of arteries and veins in the subcutaneous tissue, much as in erythema induratum, with an exudate of lymphocytes, plasma cells, and macrophages in and around the affected vessels, sometimes with partial necrosis of the vessel wall or thrombosis. The inflammation is confined to the region of the vessels and does not spread as widely as in the usual type of erythema induratum. Granulomata are not usually present.

COLLAGEN DISEASES

Several of the collagen diseases affect the skin. The lesions of cutaneous lupus erythe-matosus and scleroderma are considered here. Dermatomyositis is discussed in Chapter 58. The other collagen diseases are described in Chapter 10.

Lupus Erythematosus. Two kinds of lupus erythematosus of the skin are distinguished. In systemic lupus erythematosus the skin lesions are only one feature of a disease that involves other organs as well. Serologic abnormalities are usually prominent. In discoid lupus erythematosus, the disease is confined largely or entirely to the skin. No lesions are present in internal organs. Serologic changes are present in only 50% of the patients. When antinuclear and other abnormal antibodies are present, they are never in high titer.

Some have suggested that discoid lupus erythematosus and systemic lupus erythematosus are different diseases, but the similarity of their lesions and the observation that 5% of patients with discoid lupus erythematosus eventually progress to systemic lupus erythematosus make it clear that the two are variants of a single disease process.

Discoid Lupus Erythematosus. In discoid lupus erythematosus, the lesions are most common on the nose and cheeks, but can occur on the scalp, ears, arms, upper chest, or in the oral cavity. Most patients have one or more well-defined, erythematous, edematous plaques in the skin, often with thick scales overlying and with keratin plugs in the hair follicles. As the years pass, the lesions often become scarred, with thin, atrophic skin, sometimes with warty hyperkeratoses at the margins of the lesions. Sometimes scarring is extensive enough to cause deformity. Sometimes the nose or ears are partially destroyed.

About 10% of patients with cutaneous lupus erythematosus have a form of discoid lupus erythematosus called subacute cutaneous lupus erythematosus. The patients have extensive erythematous lesions on the face, neck, upper trunk, arms, and hands. People with this kind of rash are more likely to have or to develop mild systemic lupus erythematosus than are patients with the usual form of discoid lupus erythematosus.

In both forms of discoid lupus erythematosus, the epidermis over the lesions is usually thinned, though at the margins of the

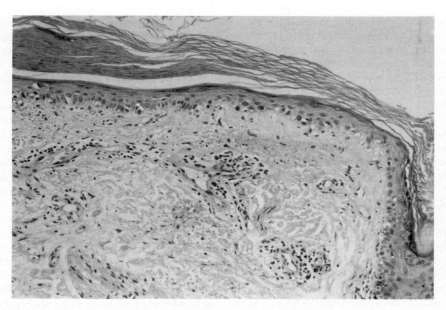

Fig. 62-18.   Discoid lupus erythematosus. Hyperkeratosis and parakeratosis are evident. A keratin plug obstructs a hair follicle at the right of the picture. The epidermis is thin with degeneration of its basal cells. A mild, patchy exudate is present in the dermis.

lesions it may be thick and warty. Hyperkeratosis is usually marked, with hair follicles and other depressions in the epidermis filled with keratin plugs. Foci of hydropic swelling and degeneration are usually prominent in the basal cells of the epidermis. Often degenerate basal cells in the lower part of the epidermis form homogeneous, eosinophilic, hyaline bodies about 10 μm across. Sometimes the basal cells contain tubuloreticular structures resembling paramyxoviruses. The inclusions are not caused by viral infection, but result from the deranged metabolism of the damaged basal cells.

The epidermal basement membrane is often thick and irregular. In regions where the degeneration of the basal cells is severe, it may be fragmented. Often long, thin extensions of the basal cells extend into the dermis and are surrounded by basement membrane. If the cells die, the extensions of basement membrane into the dermis remain.

The dermis shows a patchy exudate of lymphocytes with a few plasma cells and macrophages most prominent around the appendages. The patches of exudate are usually dense and well demarcated. The intervening dermis is edematous, with dilated vessels. Often there are a few extravasated red cells in the upper dermis or a few macrophages containing melanin.

Except in lesions less than two months old, granular deposits of IgG or IgM, less often of IgA, are present in the lesions in over 90% of people with discoid lupus erythematosus. The deposits form an irregular band along the epidermodermal junction, often with extension into the upper part of the dermis. C3 and the later components of the complement sequence are present in similar distribution. Often fibrin is also demonstrable. Electron microscopy shows that the deposits are in the upper part of the dermis beneath the basement membrane. No such deposits are present in the uninvolved skin in people with discoid lupus erythematosus.

Local application of adrenocortical steroids and the administration of antimalarial drugs such as chloroquine and hydroxychloroquine can usually control discoid lupus erythematosus.

Systemic Lupus Erythematosus.   The skin is involved at some time during the disease in 80% of patients with systemic lupus erythe-

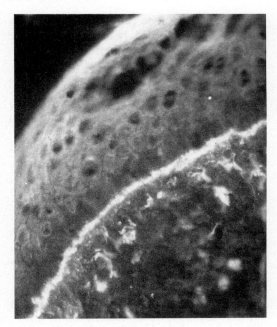

Fig. 62-19. IgG deposited along the epidermodermal junction in discoid lupus erythematosus. (Courtesy of Dr. S. Ritchie)

matosus. An erythematous, ill-defined butterfly rash develops on the nose and cheeks in 40% of the patients. The rash does not cause scaling, atrophy, or scarring. Occasionally it is petechial or vesicular or ulcerates. About 30% of patients with systemic lupus erythematosus become sensitive to sunlight and develop an erythematous rash, sometimes with blistering or purpura, in the parts exposed to the sun. In 30%, involvement of the scalp causes alopecia. Less than 20% have lesions like those of discoid lupus erythematosus. About 20% develop Raynaud's phenomenon, sometimes with ulceration of the fingers or painful ulcers elsewhere in the skin. In 10%, the mucous membranes are involved. About 10% have urticaria. Rarely, a patient with systemic lupus erythematosus develops subcutaneous nodules like those of rheumatoid arthritis.

The erythematous lesions of systemic lupus erythematosus show microscopically only edema of the dermis, perhaps with a few lymphocytes or macrophages. The more developed lesions show changes like those of discoid lupus erythematosus. The dermis

often shows deposits of a structureless, eosinophilic material called fibrinoid, which stains strongly with the periodic acid-Schiff reaction. The fibrinoid consists of fibrin and of other proteinaceous material. It is most abundant in the upper dermis, where it collects between collagen bundles and around blood vessels, especially close under the epidermis. Vasculitis in the skin may result in focal necrosis and ulceration.

In the subcutaneous fat, the adipose tissue atrophies. Mucinous ground substance accumulates between the adipocytes. Usually there is a lymphocytic exudate, sometimes foci of fibrinoid change.

Granular deposits of IgG, IgM, or less often IgA, together with complement and sometimes fibrin, are present on the dermal side of the basement membrane in over 90% of patients with systemic lupus erythematosus. Similar deposits of immunoglobulins, but not of complement, are present along the basement membrane in apparently normal skin in regions exposed to sunlight in over 80% of people with untreated systemic lupus erythematosus. Deposits of immunoglobulins are found in normal skin of regions not exposed to sunlight in only 50% of people with untreated systemic lupus erythematosus.

The presence of deposits in regions not exposed to sunlight suggests that there is serious injury to the kidneys. Over 80% of people with systemic lupus erythematosus who have serious renal injury have deposits of immunoglobulin in apparently normal skin not exposed to sulight, but only 20% of those without clinical evidence of renal injury.

The lesions in the internal organs and the serologic changes in the plasma in systemic lupus erythematosus are discussed in Chapter 10 and in the chapters describing the disorders of the organs principally affected.

SCLERODERMA. Two kinds of cutaneous scleroderma are distinguished. In systemic scleroderma, the lesions in the skin are only one feature of a generalized disease. In morphea, or circumscribed scleroderma, the disease is confined to the skin.

Morphea. The term *morphea* comes from the Greek for shape or form. The patients are usually young adults or children. About 70% of them are women or girls.

Most patients with morphea have one or

more erythematous plaques with a smooth, ivory-colored surface and a thin, lilac border. The plaques are round or oval but sometimes coalesce to form lesions up to 15 cm across. They tend slowly to enlarge. Some of the patients have small, superficial lesions called guttae, from the Latin for a drop, as well as the plaques.

Less often a patient has a line of firm, ivory-colored lesions on a limb or the scalp. The lesions are sometimes associated with atrophy and scarring of the underlying muscles that cause a contracture or ankylosis. Occasionally the lesions are confined to one side of the face, and the muscles on that side of the face are atrophic. In a few patients, the disease involves much of the skin and shows some combination of these types of lesion.

Microscopically, early lesions or biopsies from the lilac border of an enlarging plaque show thickening of the dermis by thick, closely packed bundles of collagen. A moderate exudate mainly of lymphocytes is present between the collagen bundles and around blood vessels. The exudate is more prominent in the subcutaneous tissue, particularly in its fibrous septa. New collagen is laid down in the subcutaneous tissue and gradually replaces the subcutaneous fat. The new collagen is at first fine and delicate, but as the lesions age, the collagen matures into thick, coarse bundles. Only in the linear type of morphea do the inflammation and fibrosis extend into the underlying muscles.

In old lesions, the inflammatory exudate has almost entirely disappeared, except perhaps deep in the subcutaneous tissue. The epidermis is normal, but the dermis consists of coarse, crowded bundles of collagen that are often hyalinized. The dermis seems thick, because of the replacement of much of the subcutaneous fat by similar coarse collagen. The eccrine glands are atrophic and seem squeezed by the collagen. Instead of being near the junction between the dermis and the subcutaneous fat, they seem to be in the middle of the dermis, because of the replacement of the subcutaneous tissue by collagen. In the linear, unilateral and generalized forms of morphea, the fibrosis extends into the underlying muscles.

The lesions of morphea persist for years, but may then resolve, leaving a pigmented area in the skin. The cause of the disease is unknown. It does not progress to systemic scleroderma. Rarely, a patient has both morphea and systemic scleroderma.

Systemic Scleroderma. The skin is always involved sooner or later in systemic scleroderma. Raynaud's phenomenon is the first sign of the disease in 50% of the patients and develops in 95%.

In more than 90% of the patients, the skin of the fingers becomes shrunken, taut, thick, and firmly bound to the underlying tissues. In 5% of the patients, the sclerosis begins on the trunk. There may be ulceration, hyperpigmentation, hypopigmentation, or telangiectasia in the sclerotic skin. The joints in the fingers become fixed by contractures in the shrunken muscles and in the tendons, as well as by the tight, thick skin.

In most patients, the sclerosis slowly extends proximally. Occasionally it advances rapidly. The skin of the face becomes tense, shrunken, and thickened so that all expression is lost. Sometimes the sclerotic skin becomes calcified. Occasionally a calcified lesion ulcerates, or sclerotic nodules like those of morphea are present.

Microscopically, the thick skin in systemic scleroderma is similar to that in the lesions of morphea. There is little inflammation. The dermis and subcutaneous tissue are replaced by coarse, sometimes hyaline bundles of collagen. The sweat glands are compressed and atrophic. Often the hair follicles are lost, bringing alopecia. Especially if the patient shows Raynaud's phenomenon, the intima of the digital arteries is greatly thickened, narrowing the lumen, in the same way as thickening of the intima narrows the arterial lumen in lesions of scleroderma in other parts of the body.

TUMORS

The tumors and tumor-like lesions of the skin are divided into cysts, tumors of the epidermis, tumors of the cutaneous appendages, tumors of the melanocytes, tumors of the dermis, and metastases. Table 62-1 lists the different tumors and tumor-like lesions of the skin.

TABLE 62-1.   TUMORS AND TUMOR-LIKE CONDITIONS OF THE SKIN

Cysts
  Bronchogenic cyst
  Cutaneous ciliated cyst
  Dermoid cyst
  Epidermal cyst
  Eruptive vellus hair cyst
  Median raphe cyst of the penis
  Milium
  Pilar cyst
  Steatocystoma
  Thyroglossal cyst

Benign epidermal tumors
  Acanthosis nigricans
  Arsenical keratosis
  Clear cell acanthoma
  Condyloma accuminatum
  Epidermal nevus
  Epidermodysplasia verruciformis
  Keratoacanthoma
  Molluscum contagiosum
  Seborrheic keratosis
  Solar keratosis
  Verruca palmoplantaris
  Verruca plana
  Verruca vulgaris
  Warty dyskeratoma

Malignant epidermal tumors
  Basal cell carcinoma
    Basal cell nevus
    Basosquamous carcinoma
    Fibroepithelioma
    Fibrosing basal cell carcinoma
    Nevoid basal cell carcinoma syndrome
    Superficial basal cell carcinoma
    Usual type

  Bowen's disease
  Erythroplasia of Queyrat
  Merkel cell carcinoma
  Squamous cell carcinoma

Appendage tumors
  Apocrine tumors
    Apocrine carcinoma
    Apocrine hidrocystoma
    Cylindroma
    Hidradenoma papilliferum
    Syringocystoma papilliferum

  Eccrine tumors
    Chondroid syringoma
    Clear cell hidradenoma
    Eccrine carcinoma
    Eccrine hidrocystoma
    Eccrine poroma
    Eccrine spiradenoma
    Syringoma

  Sebaceous tumors
    Nevus sebaceous
    Sebaceous adenoma
    Sebaceous carcinoma

    Sebaceous epithelioma
    Senile sebaceous hyperplasia

  Tumors of hair follicles
    Calcifying epithelioma
    Pilar tumor
    Trichoepithelioma
    Trichofolliculoma
    Tricholemmoma

Melanocytic tumors
  Pigmented nevi
    Balloon cell nevus
    Compound nevus
    Congenital pigmented nevus
    Dysplastic nevus
    Halo nevus
    Intradermal nevus
    Junctional nevus
    Spitz nevus

  Benign epidermal lesions
    Becker's melanosis
    Freckles
    Lentigo senilis
    Lentigo simplex

  Benign dermal lesions
    Blue nevus
    Cellular blue nevus
    Mongolian spot
    Nevus of Ito
    Nevus of Ota

  Malignant melanoma in situ
    Acral lentiginous melanoma in situ
    Lentigo maligna
    Superficial spreading melanoma

  Malignant melanoma

  Malignant blue nevus

Dermal tumors
  Atypical fibroxanthoma
  Connective tissue nevus
  Dermatofibroma
  Dermatofibrosarcoma protruberans
  Digital fibrokeratoma
  Digital mucous cyst
  Fibrous papule of the face
  Focal mucinosis
  Infantile digital fibromatosis
  Nevus lipomatosus
  Soft fibroma
  Tuberous sclerosis

Vascular tumors
  Angiokeratoma
  Angioma serpiginosum
  Angiosarcoma
  Capillary hemangioma
  Cavernous hemangioma
  Cherry hemangioma
  Kaposi's sarcoma
  Nevus flammeus

TABLE 62-1. CONT'D

Papular angioplasia	Xanthelasma
Pyogenic granuloma	Xanthogranuloma
Venous lake	
	Lymphoid tumors
Tumors of smooth muscle	Lymphocytoma cutis
Leiomyoma	Lymphocytic infiltration of the skin
Leiomyosarcoma	Mycosis fungoides
Smooth muscle hamartoma	Sézary's syndrome
Tumors of macrophages	
Eruptive xanthoma	Secondary tumors
Histiocytosis X	Leukemia
Plane xanthoma	Lymphoma
Reticulohistiocytosis	Metastatic carcinoma
Tuberous xanthoma	Metastatic melanoma

Cysts

Epidermal cysts, milia, and pilar cysts are common in the skin. Less often a patient has a steatocystoma, cutaneous dermoid cyst, or eruptive vellus hair cysts. Occasionally a woman has on a leg a cyst several centimeters in diameter lined by ciliated epithelium like that of the fallopian tubes, or a man has a cyst lined by pseudostratified epithelium in the median raphe of the penis. Rarely, a bronchogenic cyst or thyroglossal cyst develops in the skin.

EPIDERMAL CYST. An epidermal cyst can develop at any age. It is common in both men and women. Usually there is only one cyst, but occasionally there are several. The cysts are most common on the face, scalp, neck, and trunk. In Gardner's syndrome, discussed in Chapter 35, the patient has numerous epidermal cysts, multiple adenomata of the colon, multiple fibromata of the skin, and multiple osteomata.

An epidermal cyst forms a spheroidal mass in the skin. It is usually 1 to 5 cm in diameter when the patient consults a physician. The cyst enlarges slowly.

Microscopically, an epidermal cyst lies in the dermis. It is lined by epidermis that differentiates normally. If the patient's skin is pigmented, the epidermis lining the cyst is pigmented. No epidermal appendages are present in the wall of the cyst. Keratin is shed from the surface of the epidermis into the lumen of the cyst, where it forms a laminated mass. Usually the dermis around the cyst shows no reaction. If the cyst ruptures and keratin escapes into the dermis, a brisk, foreign body giant cell reaction often with acute and chronic inflammation occurs.

Most epidermal cysts arise from hair follicles, which lose continuity with the surface

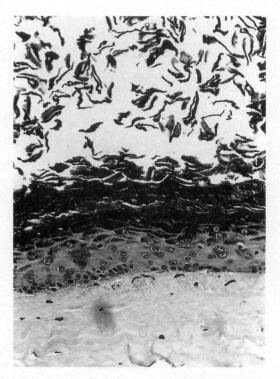

Fig. 62-20. The wall of an epidermoid cyst. Keratin shed from the surface of the keratinizing epithelium fills the cavity.

and dilate as the cyst develops. A few are due to the implantation of a fragment of epidermis into the dermis.

Most epidermal cysts are benign. Rarely, one gives rise to a squamous cell carcinoma, Bowen's disease, or a basal cell carcinoma.

MILIUM. A milium, from the Latin for a millet seed, is a tiny epidermal cyst, 1 to 2 mm in diameter. Milia are common, especially on the face. They may be primary, arising from an otherwise normal hair follicle, or secondary to obstruction of a sweat duct, sebaceous duct, or hair follicle.

PILAR CYST. A pilar cyst, from the Latin for a hair, used to be called a sebaceous cyst. Some prefer to name it a tricholemmal cyst, from the Greek for hair and rind. Pilar cysts are less common than epidermal cysts. If epidermal and pilar cysts are grouped together, only 25% of them are pilar. Over 90% of pilar cysts arise in the scalp. Over 70% of the patients have more than one cyst. About 10% of them have more than 10 cysts. In many of the patients, the tendency to develop pilar cysts is inherited as an autosomal dominant character.

Macroscopically, a pilar cyst is indistinguishable from an epidermal cyst. It forms in the dermis but is lined by stratified squamous epithelium with no intercellular bridges between the cells and no granular layer. As they move to the surface of the epithelium, the cells become large and pale and merge gradually with the structureless, eosinophilic material that fills the cyst. Electron microscopy shows that the cells contain parallel tonofibrils but no keratohyaline granules. The structureless material in the cyst is amorphous keratin. In 25% of the patients, the cyst is partially calcified. Usually the dermis around the cyst shows no reaction. If a pilar cyst ruptures, its content excites acute, chronic, and granulomatous inflammation.

Pilar cysts arise from hair follicles. The epithelium that lines the cyst is similar to that in the outer root sheath or tricholemma of the follicles.

STEATOCYSTOMA. Steatocystoma multiplex is a rare condition inherited as an autosomal dominant character. Multiple cysts usually 1 to 3 cm across develop in the skin. They may be present at birth or may not become evi-

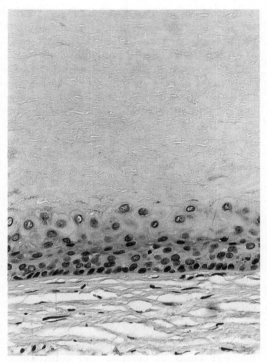

Fig. 62-21. A pilar cyst. The epithelium lining the cyst gradually merges with the structureless material that fills the cavity.

dent until after puberty. The cysts are most numerous over the trunk and proximal part of the limbs. If incised, they release an oily fluid. Occasionally a similar lesion, called a steatocystoma simplex, develops in a person who has no genetic predisposition to this sort of disease.

The cysts form in the dermis from hair follicles. The wall of the cyst is thrown into complex folds and is lined by stratified squamous epithelium without intercellular bridges or keratohyaline granules. The cells at the surface of the epithelium are large and eosinophilic, like those in a pilar cyst. In most lesions, flattened sebaceous glands are numerous in the wall of the cyst. Sometimes hair follicles extend into the dermis from a cyst, or hairs are present in its lumen.

DERMOID CYST. A dermoid cyst of the skin is uncommon. Usually there is only one. It develops most frequently in the face along a line of embryonic closure. The cyst is present at birth or appears soon after birth. Most are 1 to 5 cm across. The cyst forms in the dermis from fragments of epidermis included during organogenesis. It is lined by epidermis and filled with keratin. Hair follicles extend from the cyst wall into the surrounding dermis. Their hairs project into the cyst. Sebaceous glands are usually present in relation to the hair follicles. Less often eccrine or apocrine glands arise from the wall of the cyst. Dermoid cysts of the skin bear no relation to the benign teratomata of the ovaries also called dermoid cysts.

ERUPTIVE VELLUS HAIR CYSTS. Eruptive vellus hair cysts arise in children or young adults, most often on the trunk. The cysts are 0.1 to 0.2 cm across, and usually disappear after a few years. The cysts are in the dermis. They are lined by epidermis. Hair follicles in the cyst wall form vellus hairs that lie within the cyst.

Benign Epidermal Tumors

Seborrheic keratosis, solar keratosis, the different kinds of verruca and condyloma, keratoacanthoma, and molluscum contagiosum are common benign tumors and tumor-like conditions of the skin. Clear cell acanthoma, warty dyskeratoma, acanthosis nigricans, epidermal nevi, and arsenical keratoses are less frequent.

SEBORRHEIC KERATOSIS. Seborrheic kera-

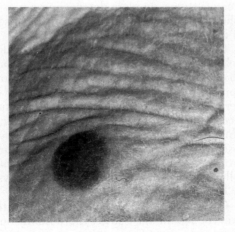

Fig. 62-22. A seborrheic keratosis on the cheek of an elderly patient. (Courtesy of St. Michael's Hospital, Toronto, Department of Medical Art and Photography)

toses rarely appear before the patient is 40 to 50 years old. They grow increasingly common as age increases. Often there are several, sometimes a large number. The lesions are common on the trunk, face, and limbs, but spare the palms and soles. Small seborrheic keratoses are present on the face in 30% of adult black people, a condition called dermatosis papulosa nigra.

A seborrheic keratosis is usually less than 1 cm across, but can be much larger. It is sharply demarcated, dark brown or black. The lesion is usually elevated above the surrounding skin. Often it looks as if it were stuck onto the skin. The surface of the lesion may be soft and warty, covered by greasy scales, or smooth with keratotic plugs.

Microscopically, a seborrheic keratosis stands above the surface of the skin. A line drawn from the intact epidermis at one side of the lesion to the intact epidermis on the other passes beneath the lesion. A number of different types of seborrheic keratosis have been distinguished. Often a single lesion shows more than one of these patterns.

In a hyperkeratotic seborrheic keratosis, a thick layer of keratin overlies the lesion. The epidermis is slightly thickened. It is usually thrown into papillomatous folds. Sometimes a spike of epidermis like a church spire sticks up into the overlying keratin. The epidermis consists mainly of squamous cells, though clumps of basal cells are present. Sometimes keratin pearls are present within the epidermis.

More common is the acanthotic type of seborrheic keratosis, in which the lesion consists of a sponge work of thick plates of basal cells, supported by a corresponding mesh of dermal papillae. On section, the plates of basal cells form a network, with islands of dermis between them. Foci of sudden keratinization in the plates of basal cells form the spheroidal clumps of keratin called keratin pearls. Cells with intercellular prickles are few.

The adenoid or reticulated type of seborrheic keratosis is similar, except that the plates of basal cells are thin and on section form a delicate meshwork. In the clonal type, clumps of basal or larger cells with intercellular bridges are present within the epidermis.

The quantity of melanin present in seborrheic keratoses varies greatly. Melanin is usually abundant in the adenoid lesions and sparse in the hyperkeratotic ones. In the acanthotic lesions there may be much or little. About 50% of acanthotic lesions show an excess of melanin.

If a seborrheic keratosis is irritated by chemical or mechanical trauma, many of its basal cells differentiate into squamous cells, often arranged in whorls, with ill-formed keratin pearls. At times it may be difficult to distinguish such a lesion from a squamous cell carcinoma.

Seborrheic keratoses are benign. They do not develop into basal cell carcinomata, in spite of the similarity of the microscopic appearance of an acanthotic or adenoid seborrheic keratosis to a basal cell carcinoma. Superficial excision or desiccation cures.

SOLAR KERATOSIS. Solar keratoses, also called actinic keratoses from the Greek for a ray of light, are common in middle-aged or elderly people who have been much exposed to sunlight. They are particularly common in people with a fair skin. The greater the exposure to sunlight, the greater the risk of developing solar keratoses. The lesions are usually multiple. They are most common in men on the face, hands, and bald spots on the head. The other cutaneous lesions caused by sunlight are discussed in Chapter 23.

A solar keratosis is usually less than 1 cm across. The lesion is most often erythematous and scaling. Occasionally it is pigmented or hyperkeratotic. Sometimes a cutaneous horn forms over the lesion.

A hypertrophic solar keratosis shows an excess of keratin overlying the lesion. Often the epidermis is thickened. It may be flat or form papillomatous projections. In an atrophic solar keratosis, the epidermis is thin and has lost its rete ridges. In an acantholytic solar keratosis, acantholysis forms a cleft immediately above the basal layer of the epidermis, like that of Darier's disease. Occasionally a solar keratosis is pigmented, with increase in melanocytes and increased storage of melanin in the keratinocytes.

Solar keratoses usually show mild to moderate dysplasia. The cells in basal layers of the epidermis are atypical and disordered. Regular differentiation occurs more superficially. Occasionally the dysplasia extends through

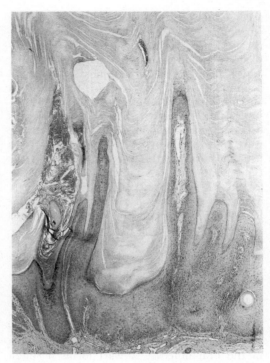

Fig. 62-23. A solar keratosis forming a cutaneous horn.

the whole thickness of the epidermis as in Bowen's disease.

The underlying dermis usually shows chronic inflammation with an exudate principally of lymphocytes and plasma cells. The collagen in the dermis often shows the degeneration common in people excessively exposed to sunlight.

Over 20% of patients with solar keratoses develop a squamous cell carcinoma in one of the lesions. The carcinomata do not differ from other squamous cell carcinomata of the skin, except that the risk of metastases is low.

ARSENICAL KERATOSIS. Arsenical keratoses are discussed in Chapter 24. Warty lesions develop on the palms and soles in people who have taken small quantities of arsenic for many years. Microscopically, the lesions are similar to solar keratoses and show similar dysplasia. Some of them develop into squamous cell carcinoma.

VERRUCA. A tumor-like wart caused by infection with a human papillomavirus is called a verruca, from the Latin for wart, or a condyloma, from the Greek for a knuckle or a knob. Five types are distinguished: verruca vulgaris, verruca plana, verruca palmoplantaris, epidermodysplasia verruciformis, and condyloma acuminatum. Condylomata acuminata usually develop on the genitalia and are discussed in Chapters 40 and 41.

Verruca Vulgaris. The common wart is called a verruca vulgaris, the Latin words for wart and common. A verruca vulgaris is usually caused by the human papilloma virus type 2, though types 1, 2, 3, 4, 7, 10, 13, 26, 27, 28, 29, and 32 can cause cutaneous warts. The virus replicates in the nucleus of the infected epidermal cells, where it sometimes forms crystalline arrays. By electron microscopy, viral particles are often numerous, sometimes few. Their presence can be demonstrated by nuclear hybridization.

Verrucae vulgares are common, especially in children. Immunodeficiency increases the risk of developing warts. They are most frequent on the fingers, but can occur in any part of the skin. Occasionally a wart develops in the oral mucosa. A wart forms a rough nodule, usually less than 0.5 cm across, that stands above the surface of the skin. In the face and scalp, a thin, horny thread occasionally projects from the surface of the wart, a variety of verruca vulgaris called a filiform wart.

Microscopically, a verruca vulgaris is a papilloma. It has spiky fronds with a fine, fibrovascular core covered by thick, stratified, squamous epithelium. Large quantities of keratin overlie the fronds and partially conceal them. In a young wart, many of the superficial cells in the upper part of the epidermis are vacuolated. They have a pyknotic nucleus surrounded by a clear halo and pale cytoplasm without keratohyaline granules. Layers of parakeratotic cells overlie the tips of the papillae. In the superficial epithelial cells in the troughs between the papillae, coarse keratohyaline granules are prominent. Occasionally eosinophilic inclusions are present in the nuclei or less often in the cytoplasm of some of the epithelial cells. They are an abnormal product formed by the cells, not viral bodies.

A verruca vulgaris usually persists for weeks or months, then regresses. As it ages,

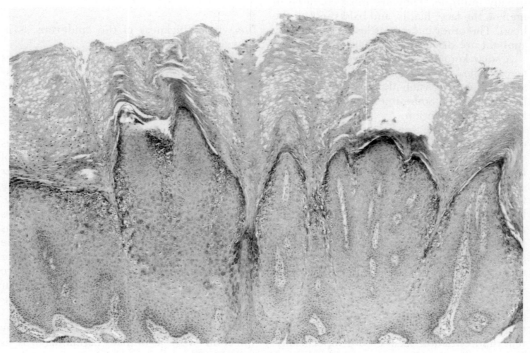

Fig. 62-24. A verruca vulgaris.

the vacuolated cells, layered parakeratin, and prominent keratohyaline granules become less prominent and may disappear. The infected epidermal cells are shed and are replaced by normal epidermis. An exudate mainly of lymphocytes accumulates in the underlying dermis. If a verruca vulgaris is removed, it often recurs in the same or some other place, probably because of reinfection.

Verruca Plana. Verrucae planae, from the Latin for wart and flat, are most common on the face and dorsum of the hands. Most are caused by the human papilloma virus type 3. The lesion is usually less than 0.5 cm across. It forms a brownish plaque that is slightly raised above the surrounding epidermis. Microscopically, the epidermis is thickened and hyperkeratotic. Many of the superficial epidermal cells are large, with pale cytoplasm and pyknotic nuclei. Parakeratosis and keratohyaline granules are not prominent. The lesions persist for some weeks and then regress. Local removal of a lesion is often followed by recurrence at the same or another site.

Verruca Palmoplantaris. Palmoplantar warts are most common on the soles of the feet, but sometimes develop on the palms, fingers, or toes. Two kinds of verruca palmoplantaris occur. Superficial or mosaic palmoplantar warts are similar to verrucae vulgares. They are usually caused by human papilloma viruses of types 2 or 3. A deep plantar wart, sometimes called a myrmecia, from the Greek for anthill, is most often caused by a virus of type 1.

A deep plantar wart is often painful or inflamed. It is covered by thick callus that pushes the lesion below the surrounding epidermis. Microscopically, eosinophilic, cytoplasmic material is present in the cells in the basal layer of the epidermis and grows more abundant as the cells near the surface. In many of the cells in the superficial part of the epidermis, it forms large, irregular inclusions that merge with the overlying parakeratosis and hyperkeratosis. Other superficial epidermal cells are vacuolated, with small pykotic nuclei. Some have a small, eosinophilic inclusion in the nucleus.

Epidermodysplasia Verruciformis. In epidermodysplasia verruciformis, the patients have T-cell dysfunction inherited as an autosomal recessive character that makes them unable to overcome cutaneous infection with a human papilloma virus. The human papilloma viruses 3, 5, 8, 9, 12, 14, 15, 17, 19, 20, 21, 22, 23, 24, 25, 26, 27, 28, 30, 32, 36, 39, and 40 can all cause the disease. Two forms of epidermodysplasia verruciformis occur. Both begin in childhood.

In one form, caused most frequently by the human papilloma virus type 3, the patients have numerous verrucae planae. All parts of the skin are involved. The risk of malignancy is not increased.

The other form of epidermodysplasia verruciformis is most often caused by the human papilloma virus type 5. The patients have red or brown scaly lesions in the skin as well as numerous verrucae planae. The epidermal cells in the scaly lesions are often irregularly shaped. Many are swollen with foamy cytoplasm. Some of their nuclei are pyknotic. Some are empty with their nucleoplasm pressed against the nuclear membrane. When this type of epidermodysplasia verruciform is caused by the human papilloma virus type 5 or 8, some of the lesions develop into Bowen's disease or less often a squamous cell carcinoma.

EPIDERMAL NEVUS. Epidermal nevi are uncommon. The nevi are congenital malformations present at birth or appearing soon after. Occasionally there is only a single lesion. More often there are many, often arranged in linear fashion and confined to one side of the body. Occasionally the lesions are widespread and bilateral, a condition called ichthyosis hystrix, from the Greek for a hedgehog. The individual lesions are usually warty, but may be red, scaling, and itchy. Other congenital malformations are often present.

Microscopically, most epidermal nevi are hyperkeratotic. The underlying epidermis is thickened. Often the epidermis is thrown into papillomatous folds, like those of a verruca vulgaris. The rete ridges often are elongated and extend down into the dermis. If the lesions are inflamed and scaling, the skin shows in addition changes like those of eczema.

In the patients with widespread, bilateral epidermal nevi and occasionally in people with unilateral or solitary lesions, the microscopic appearance is indistinguishable from that of epidermolytic hyperkeratosis. Epidermal nevi do not become malignant. Only cosmetic treatment is needed.

ACANTHOSIS NIGRICANS. In acanthosis nigricans, brownish, warty lesions develop in the skin, most often in the axillae, neck, genital regions, or beneath the breasts. Microscopic examination reveals hyperkeratosis. The epidermis is slightly and irregularly thickened. Often its lower margin is ridged, like the teeth of a saw. In spite of the name *nigricans*, there is little or no increase in melanin in the lesions.

Some patients with acanthosis nigricans have a tumor of an internal organ, most often an adenocarcinoma. Some have an endocrine disorder, most commonly a pituitary adenoma that causes acromegaly. In some, acanthosis nigricans is familial. The lesions may appear during childhood, or not until adult life. In most, no predisposing condition is evident.

KERATOACANTHOMA. A keratoacanthoma is less common than a squamous cell carcinoma of the skin. If squamous cell carcinomata and keratoacanthomata are grouped together, 40% of the lesions are keratoacanthomata. Most of the patients are over 45 years old. About 70% of them are men. Nearly all patients are white. Immunosuppression increases the incidence of keratoacanthomata.

Almost 95% of keratoacanthomata arise on the face, hands, or other regions exposed to sunlight. In most patients, they do not occur on the palms or soles and do not involve the mucous membranes of the month and larynx. Most patients have only a single lesion, but some have several. The lesions may arise simultaneously or one after another. Rarely, lesions begin to appear in childhood. They regress in the usual way, but new lesions appear so that the patient has usually several keratoacanthomata in different stages of evolution. Rarely, an adult develops hundreds of keratoacanthomata 0.2 to 0.3 cm across.

A keratoacanthoma lesion begins as an erythematous plaque. In most patients it enlarges rapidly for two weeks to two months to form a shiny, dome-shaped nodule 1 to 2 cm across. A plug of keratin protrudes from the center of the lesion. The lesion then becomes quiescent and persists with little change for two weeks to two months. It then begins to resolve, the

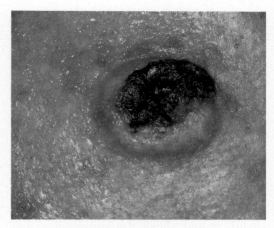

Fig. 62-25. A keratoacanthoma on a cheek, showing the elevated lesion with a central plug of keratin. (Courtesy of St. Michael's Hospital, Toronto, Department of Medical Art and Photography)

mass shrinks, and the keratin plug is extruded. After a few months, nothing remains but a small scar.

Especially on the nose and eyelids, a keratoacanthoma occasionally becomes 5 cm or more across. It damages the underlying tissues, but regresses in the usual way. Rarely, a keratoacanthoma on a hand or leg fails to regress, becoming as much as 20 cm across. Rarely, a keratoacanthoma develops beneath a nail, forming a tender mass that fails to regress and may erode the phalanx.

Microscopically, a keratoacanthoma is shaped like a volcano. The mouth of the crater is small, so that the lesion bulges beneath the surrounding epidermis. The surrounding epidermis remains normal until it joins the abnormal epithelium of the lesion at the mouth of the crater. The sides of the dome-shaped lesion seen macroscopically are covered by normal epidermis.

The crater is lined by thick, irregular squamous epithelium and is filled with keratin. The epithelium lining the crater projects irregularly into both the crater and the surrounding dermis. Often it is slightly atypical, especially in its basal part where it extends into the dermis. Often glassy epithelial cells prematurely filled with keratin or keratin pearls are present within the epithelium lining the cavity. The dermis around the lesion is usually inflamed, with an exudate mainly of lymphocytes and macrophages, with a few neutrophils, eosinophils, and plasma cells.

Most keratoacanthomata arise in a hair follicle. Only in the patients with hundreds of tiny lesions, some of them on the palms, soles, and on mucous membrane, do keratoacanthomata arise elsewhere. The cause of the disease is unknown. It is often suggested that keratocanthomata are caused by a viral infection, but it has not proved possible to establish this theory.

Probably keratoacanthomata never become malignant. The few lesions thought to have turned into a squamous cell carcinoma were probably carcinoma from the outset. Excision cures.

Molluscum Contagiosum. Molluscum contagiosum takes its name from the Latin words for soft and touch. It is caused by a poxvirus, which is brick-shaped, 300 nm by 230 nm. It is abundant in the cytoplasmic inclusions prominent in the lesions.

Molluscum contagiosum is common, especially in children. The lesions are often multiple. They can appear anywhere in the skin and on the conjunctiva. A dome-shaped, waxy nodule usually less than 0.5 cm across develops in the skin. It often has an umbilicated center from which a little cheesy material can be expressed.

Microscopically, the lesion is bowl-shaped with a lining of thick epidermis. Its deep surface has broad, rounded projections that bulge into the dermis. The normal, orderly differentiation of the epidermis is preserved. In its more superficial part, eosinophilic inclusions are present in most of the epidermal cells. They grow larger as the cells near the surface. In the horny layer, the inclusions are up to 35 μm in diameter and compress the nucleus into a crescent at the margin of the cell. Inclusions sometimes lie free in the keratin overlying the lesion.

The lesions in molluscum contagiosum persist for weeks or months and then resolve. The epidermal cells degenerate and are shed. An exudate mainly of lymphocytes appears in the dermis. Curettage or excision gives a more rapid cure.

Warty Dyskeratoma. A warty dyskeratoma is an uncommon lesion that occurs in people over 45 years old, most often on the

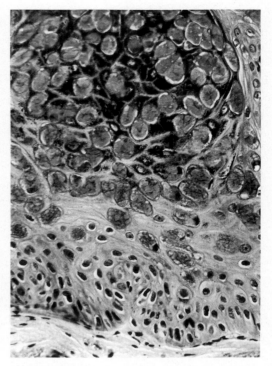

Fig. 62-26. The large viral inclusions of molluscum contagiosum.

face, scalp, or neck, occasionally in the oral mucosa. A single papule less than 1 cm in diameter develops, with an umbilicated center containing a plug of keratin.

Microscopically, the lesion is flask-shaped, with the plug of keratin filling an invagination leading to a cleft above the basal cells of the epidermis, like the clefts of Darier's disease. Acantholytic epidermal cells lie free in the cleft. Dermal papillae lined by a single layer of basal cells grow into it from its dermal aspect. Corps ronds are usually present in the epidermis near the mouth of the lesion. The patients do not develop Darier's disease. Untreated, the lesion persists indefinitely. Excision cures.

Clear Cell Acanthoma. A clear cell acanthoma is an uncommon lesion usually found in people over 45 years old, most often on a leg. A sharply defined, red nodule grows slowly to form a dome-shaped mass, 1 to 2 cm in diameter, which appears to be stuck on the surface of the skin. Often the periphery of the tumor is covered by fine scales.

Microscopically, the lesion consists of a sponge work of broad plates of epidermal cells. The cells are large and pale, with large quantities of glycogen in their cytoplasm. They stain strongly with the periodic acid-Schiff reaction. Neutrophils are scattered in the tumor and may form microabscesses in the epithelium. The dermal papillae that fill the spaces between the plates of epidermal cells reach close to the surface. Their blood vessels are dilated and congested. A perivascular exudate mainly of lymphocytes is present.

A clear cell acanthoma is benign. Excision cures.

Malignant Epidermal Tumors

Malignant tumors of the epidermis are the most common of malignant neoplasms. In white people, over 20% of malignant tumors arise from the epidermis. Both squamous cell carcinoma and basal cell carcinoma of the skin

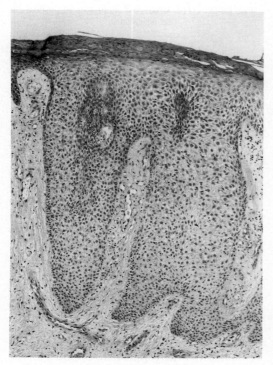

Fig. 62-27. A clear cell acanthoma, showing the clear cells that make up the tumor.

are common. Bowen's disease and Merkel cell carcinoma are less frequent.

SQUAMOUS CELL CARCINOMA. In white people, 3% of malignant tumors are squamous cell carcinomata of the skin. In black people, less than 1% of malignant tumors are of this sort. People who have fair skins, live in sunny parts of the world, and work out of doors are especially likely to develop a squamous cell carcinoma of the skin. The patients are usually over 50 years old, often older. About 60% of them are men.

Over 95% of squamous cell carcinomata of the skin arise in a region exposed to sunlight. About 25% of them arise on an ear, 15% on a cheek, and 15% on the dorsum of the hands. About 20% of people with a squamous cell carcinoma of the skin sooner or later develop a second squamous cell carcinoma in the skin. In men, 15% of the patients develop a second squamous cell carcinoma within four years. In women, less than 5% of the patients do so.

A squamous cell carcinoma of the skin usually begins as an indurated papule, which enlarges slowly as months pass to form an ulcer 1 to 2 cm in diameter, with an indurated base and a firm, slightly raised margin. If neglected, the carcinoma continues to grow slowly and may eventually form an ulcer several centimeters across. It invades and erodes the underlying structures. Less often, a squamous cell carcinoma of the skin forms a warty growth, an indurated plaque, or a cutaneous horn like those of solar keratoses.

Irregular columns of neoplastic squamous cells grow down from the epidermis into the underlying dermis. In microscopic sections cut in cross section, the downgrowths form the islands of malignant cells seen in the dermis.

Most squamous cell carcinomata of the skin are well differentiated. The tumor cells keratinize in fairly normal fashion. Basal cells are at the periphery of the invading columns and gradually differentiate into the keratinized cells present in the center of the columns. Keratin pearls are often present within the columns. Usually some of the tumor cells show premature keratinization. They have homogeneous, eosinophilic cytoplasm and a pyknotic nucleus.

Occasionally a squamous cell carcinoma of

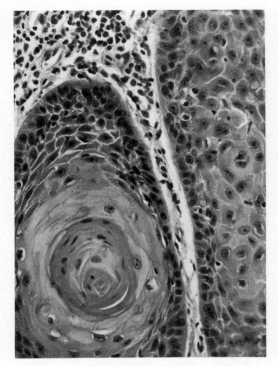

Fig. 62-28. A squamous cell carcinoma of the skin, showing the atypicality of the tumor cells and their gradual differentiation towards the center of the invading columns.

the skin is anaplastic and consists of large, pleomorphic cells with little evidence of squamous differentiation. Occasionally the tumor consists of spindle-shaped cells that can be mistaken for those of a poorly differentiated fibrosarcoma. Sometimes the cells of a squamous cell carcinoma contain so much glycogen that their cytoplasm is clear and watery. Sometimes acantholysis in the invading columns gives the tumor a pseudoglandular appearance. Acantholytic cells are usually free in the clefts that form within the columns.

There are often wide gaps in the basement membrane around the invading columns of a squamous cell carcinoma of the skin. The abnormal keratinization in the tumor cells is shown by an aggregation and condensation of tonofilaments, especially around the nucleus. The number of desmosomes between the tumor cells is less than in normal epidermis. Microvilli project into the wide spaces be-

tween the tumor cells. Sometimes desmosomes, perhaps with tonofilaments attached, are present within the cytoplasm of the carcinoma cells.

In white people, most squamous cell carcinomata of the skin are caused by ultraviolet radiation. They can readily be produced experimentally in animals exposed to ultraviolet irradiation. In white people, all other causes of squamous cell carcinoma of the skin are uncommon. Sunlight is less dangerous to black people. Some cause other than sunlight can be found in 25% of black patients who develop a squamous cell carcinoma of the skin.

Ionizing radiation is a potent cause of squamous cell carcinoma of the skin. Chronic arsenical poisoning causes squamous cell carcinoma. Oils and other substances containing carcinogens can cause squamous cell carcinoma of the skin, as in mule spinners and chimney sweeps. The risk of squamous cell carcinoma of the skin is great in people with xeroderma pigmentosum. Rarely, a squamous cell carcinoma arises in an old, draining sinus or in psoriasis, lichen planus, discoid lupus erythematosus, or some other chronic skin disease.

Overall, 2% of squamous cell carcinomata of the skin metastasize, usually only to the regional lymph nodes. Squamous cell carcinomata of the skin induced by ionizing radiation are more dangerous than those induced by sunlight. Only 0.5% of squamous cell carcinomata arising in a solar keratosis metastasize, but over 25% of those induced by ionizing radiation do so. Squamous cell carcinomata arising in apparently normal skin are more dangerous than those arising in solar keratoses. Nearly 20% of squamous cell carcinomata arising in normal skin metastasize. The risk of metastasis increases if the carcinoma is allowed to grow large or if it is unusually anaplastic.

Provided metastases have not developed, any form of local eradication of the tumor cures: surgical excision, irradiation, desiccation, or chemical destruction by zinc chloride.

BOWEN'S DISEASE. Carcinoma in situ of the epidermis is called Bowen's disease, after the American dermatologist who described it in 1912. The similar lesion on the glans penis described in Chapter 40 is called erythroplasia of Queyrat. Patients with Bowen's disease are usually over 50 years old. Men with fair skin are especially likely to develop the condition.

The patient develops a well-defined, irregularly shaped lesion from 1 to 5 cm across. Usually the lesion is erythematous. Often it is scaly or crusted. Nearly 30% of the patients have more than one lesion. The disease is no more common in regions exposed to sunlight than in other parts of the skin.

Microscopically, the epidermis is thickened, with elongation and thickening of the rete ridges. Atypical, disorderly epidermal cells occupy the whole thickness of the epidermis, often with a layer of parakeratosis on the surface. The cells are usually large and may be multinucleated. Often some of them keratinize prematurely, with homogeneous, eosinophilic cytoplasm and a pyknotic nucleus. Occasionally the cells in the upper part of the epidermis become vacuolated. Usually the dermis shows a moderate exudate of lymphocytes, plasma cells, and macrophages.

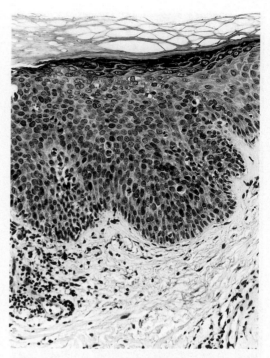

Fig. 62-30. Bowen's disease, showing the sudden transition between the normal epidermis on the right and the lesion.

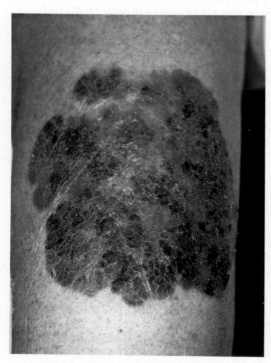

Fig. 62-29. Bowen's disease. (Courtesy of St. Michael's Hospital, Toronto, Department of Medical Art and Photography)

The etiology of Bowen's disease is rarely apparent. No doubt some of the lesions result from injury by ultraviolet light. Only rarely is there a history of exposure to arsenic. A few of the patients have epidermodysplasia verruciformis. Occasionally an internal carcinoma coexists with Bowen's disease.

The lesions of Bowen's disease tend to enlarge slowly as years pass. Less than 10% of them eventually develop into an invasive squamous cell carcinoma, though usually not for many years, sometimes only after 20 or 30 years. Excision or some other kind of local destruction cures.

BASAL CELL CARCINOMA. In white people, basal cell carcinoma is the most common of malignant tumors. At least 15% of malignant neoplasms in white people are basal cell carcinomata. Probably the percentage is higher because many of these tumors are removed in a doctor's office and never recorded in cancer statistics. In black people, less than 0.2% of malignant tumors are basal carcinomata. A black person is more likely to have a squamous cell carcinoma of the skin than a basal cell carcinoma. Most of the patients are over 40 years old. People who are fair-skinned, who live in sunny climates, and who work out of doors are especially likely to develop a basal cell carcinoma.

Usual Type. Nearly 90% of the usual type of basal cell carcinomata arise on the head or neck, 75% of them on the nose or cheeks. They are rare on the palms and soles.

A basal cell carcinoma usually begins as a waxy papule with a few telangiectatic vessels on its surface. The lesion slowly enlarges as months pass, more slowly than does a squamous cell carcinoma. Eventually, the nodule forms a small ulcer, 1 to 2 cm across, with a firm, raised edge. If not removed, the carcinoma continues to grow, slowly enlarging, slowly extending deeper into the underlying tissue, and forming a larger ulcer. After many years, the lesion can become enormous, a huge ulcer destroying half the face and exposing the meninges. These enormous lesions that slowly erode the tissues gave the basal cell carcinoma its name of rodent ulcer, a term still often used to describe the more modest basal cell carcinomata commonly seen.

Microscopically, a basal cell carcinoma consists of broad columns of epithelial cells that invade the dermis in tortuous fashion.

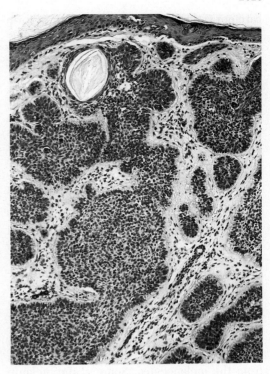

Fig. 62-32. A basal cell carcinoma. The columns of invading tumor cells have a palisaded periphery. One contains a keratin pearl.

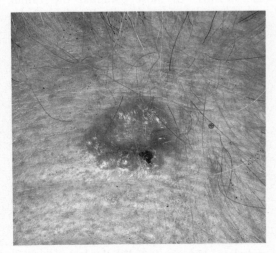

Fig. 62-31. A basal cell carcinoma of the forehead. (Courtesy of St. Michael's Hospital, Toronto, Department of Medical Art and Photography)

When cut in cross section, the columns appear as clumps of tumor cells separated by the tumor's stroma. The clumps are often large and irregularly shaped. Most of the tumors arise from the epidermis. A few originate from a hair follicle.

The tumor cells are all much alike. They have regular, spheroidal or ovoid nuclei, and a moderate quantity of basophilic cytoplasm. The cells are ill-defined and do not show intercellular bridges. Often the tumor cells at the margin of the invading columns are elongated at right angles to the margin of the column to form a palisade, while the tumor cells within the column are arranged in a disorderly jumble. Mitoses may be many or few. Rarely, a few large, atypical tumor cells are scattered among the smaller, more regular cells.

Often sudden keratinization within the columns of tumor cells forms keratin pearls. Sometimes the keratin pearls in a basal cell carcinoma become so large that they form small cysts filled with keratin. In some tumors, the tumor cells in the center of the columns of tumor cells degenerate, forming cystic spaces.

Occasionally, a basal cell carcinoma has fine, anastomosing plates of tumor cells, which microscopically resemble a carcinoma adenoides cysticum. Sometimes the columns of a basal cell carcinoma contain glandular spaces. Rarely, these glandular acini resemble those of a sweat gland.

Melanocytes can be demonstrated among the tumor cells in 70% of basal cell carcinomata. The melanocytes are not neoplastic, but are normal cells that have proliferated together with the tumor. Usually they are few, and the tumor is not obviously pigmented. Occasionally the melanocytes are more numerous and contain large quantities of melanin. Rarely, there is so much melanin in a basal cell carcinoma that it can be mistaken for a malignant melanoma. The tumor cells contain little melanin, apparently because they are unable to accept melanosomes from the melanocytes. Some of the melanin escapes into the adjacent dermis and is taken up by macrophages.

The stroma around the columns of a basal cell carcinoma consists of fine collagen, with abundant intercellular substance. There may be a slight exudate mainly of lymphocytes in the stroma. The overlying epidermis is often normal, though in places the continuity of the tumor with the epidermis or with a hair follicle is evident.

Many writers have suggested that basal cell carcinomata arise from epidermal cells of the type that form cutaneous appendages or from cells that have begun to differentiate into an appendage. Some prefer to consider the basal cell carcinoma a form of poorly differentiated appendage tumor. In support of this view, it is noted that by electron microscopy, the cells in a basal cell carcinoma look more like cells in the hair follicles than normal basal cells of the epidermis. The keratin pearls common in the tumors have been considered an attempt to form hairs. Occasionally a basal cell carcinoma forms structures like a sweat gland. Tumors intermediate between a basal cell carcinoma and a tumor of a cutaneous appendage occur.

Almost all basal cell carcinomata are caused by ultraviolet irradiation. Because of their sensitivity to sunlight, patients with xeroderma pigmentosum are likely to develop multiple basal cell carcinomata. Occasionally a basal cell carcinoma is caused by ionizing radiation or arsenical poisoning or develops in the scar of a burn.

Basal cell carcinomata invade slowly but inexorably. If allowed to grow unchecked, they eventually bring death by eroding a vital structure or by opening a route for infection. Metastases have occurred in less than 100 patients. In half of these, they were confined to the regional lymph nodes. In some, there were hematogenous metastases in the lungs, bones, liver, or other organs.

Because of the rarity of metastases, some do not consider that basal cell carcinomata are malignant. They prefer to call the tumor a basal cell epithelioma.

Superficial Basal Cell Carcinoma. A superficial basal cell carcinoma is most common on the chest. One or more erythematous, scaling patches with a fine, pearly border slowly enlarge. Small ulcers are usually present within the lesions. Sometimes the center of a lesion becomes atrophic and scarred. Microscopically, the epidermis is usually thin but otherwise is normal. Multiple small nodules of basal cell carcinoma extend down from the epidermis into the upper third of the dermis. In most patients, the tumor never invades more deeply. In a few, it develops into an invasive basal cell carcinoma of the usual type.

In a section, a superficial basal cell carcinoma appears to be multicentric. Each of the nodules of tumor seems to be a separate neoplasm. A three-dimensional reconstruction shows that the nodules of tumor are interconnected. The carcinoma probably arises from a single focus and forms radiating columns of tumor cells that remain immediately beneath the epidermis or attached to it.

Fibrosing Basal Cell Carcinoma. A fibrosing basal cell carcinoma is an unusual form of basal cell carcinoma most common on the trunk. The tumor forms an ill-defined, indurated, yellowish plaque. Ulceration occurs only late. Macroscopically. the lesion is more like morphea than a carcinoma. Microscopically, narrow cords of tumor cells like those of other basal cell carcinomata are widely separated by an abundant stroma with well-formed bundles of collagen. Often the cords of tumor cells are only one cell thick. Foci of more typical basal cell carcinoma are few. The lesion may be hard to distinguish from metastatic carcinoma of the breast. The carcinoma enlarges slowly. As time passes, it often becomes sclerotic in the center. It rarely extends beyond the dermis.

Fibroepithelioma. A fibroepithelioma is an uncommon lesion most often found on the back. The patient has one or more pedunculated or erythematous nodules that often are more like a fibroma than a carcinoma. Microscopically, fine, anastomosing strands of tumor cells like those in other basal cell carcinomata extend down from the epidermis. The strands are usually only one or two cells thick. They are separated by a fine, loose collagenous stroma. In occasional foci, the strands become thicker and more like the columns of tumor cells in the usual form of basal cell carcinoma. Most fibroepithelioma remain confined to the dermis and grow slowly. Occasionally one becomes an invasive basal cell carcinoma of the usual type.

Nevoid Basal Cell Carcinoma Syndrome. The rare nevoid basal cell carcinoma syndrome is inherited as an autosomal dominant character of variable expression. Hundreds or thousands of tiny basal cell carcinomata appear during childhood. All parts of the skin are affected. Many of the tumors remain quiescent as the years pass, but after puberty some of them are likely to grow, invading and ulcerating like ordinary basal cell carcinomata. New lesions continue to appear. About 50% of adults with the syndrome have small pits, 1 to 3 mm in diameter, in the palms and soles. The pits in the palms and soles are caused by tiny basal cell carcinomata, which cause thinning of the overlying keratin. Often, there are odontogenic cysts and other congenital malformations. Microscopically, the tumors are like other basal cell carcinomata.

Basal Cell Nevus. Basal cell nevi are rare. Multiple, small basal cell carcinomata arising from hair follicles are present at birth or appear soon after. In some patients, most parts of the skin are involved. In some, the lesions are confined to linear bands on one side of the body. The tumors often obstruct the hair follicles, causing comedones or epidermal cysts. Some of the lesions may resemble a trichoepithelioma or eccrine spiradenoma. The damage to the follicles causes patchy alopecia. The lesions persist as the patient ages, but do not grow larger.

Basosquamous Carcinoma. Occasionally a carcinoma of the skin shows microscopically features of both basal cell carcinoma and squamous cell carcinoma. In a few of these tumors, two carcinomata, one squamous, one basal, happen to lie adjacent to one another. In most, the squamous and basal elements are intermixed, and there is only one tumor. Some think that such basosquamous carcinomata are intermediate between a basal cell carcinoma and a squamous cell carcinoma; others deny that such a hybrid could exist. Whatever the nature of these unusual tumors, it is wise to treat them as the more dangerous squamous cell carcinoma.

MERKEL CELL CARCINOMA. Merkel cells are neuroendocrine cells in the epidermis. They are named after the German anatomist who described them in 1880. Rarely, a Merkel cell carcinoma, sometimes called a trabecular carcinoma, arises from the Merkel cells.

About 50% of the tumors arise in skin of the head and neck. There is usually a solitary nodule. Occasionally the tumors are multiple. Microscopically, anastomosing bands and clumps of uniform, cuboidal tumor cells are present in the dermis. They sometimes invade the subcutaneous fat, but do not usually reach the epidermis. The tumor cells contain neurosecretory granules 120 to 210 nm in diameter. By the time the tumor is removed, 50% of the patients have metastases in the regional lymph nodes. More widespread metastases develop in 20% of the patients.

Appendage Tumors

A variety of tumors arise from the cutaneous appendages. Some of them are hamartomata, many are benign neoplasms, and a few are malignant. Most are uncommon. They occur with much the same frequency in all races.

Many types of appendage tumor have been described, often with only minor differences between different types. Only the main forms of appendage tumor are described here. The appendage tumors are divided into four groups, those that resemble a hair follicle, those that resemble a sebaceous gland, those that resemble an apocrine gland, and those that resemble an eccrine gland.

It is often assumed that an appendage tumor arises from the structure it resembles. Many of them do. Some arise from one appendage and differentiate to resemble another. Some arise from the epidermis and differentiate into an appendage tumor.

TUMORS OF HAIR FOLLICLES. The tumors of the hair follicles resemble some part of a hair follicle, though often imperfectly. The principal types are trichofolliculoma, trichoepithelioma, calcifying epithelioma, pilar tumor, and tricholemmoma.

Trichofolliculoma. A trichofolliculoma, from the Greek for hair and the Latin for a small bag, is a benign neoplasm. A solitary nodule develops in an adult, most often on the face. Often the lesion has a central pore from which projects a clump of white, woolly hairs. Microscopically, a trichofolliculoma has a central cavity lined by stratified squamous epithelium. The cavity is filled with keratin, often with fragments of hair. Follicles bud into the dermis from the cavity. Many are well-formed and contain hairs. Some are malformed and become little cysts filled with keratin. A loose, collagenous stroma surrounds the lesion. Excision cures.

Trichoepithelioma. A trichoepithelioma is a benign neoplasm. In most patients, a single lesion appears in childhood or early adult life, most often on the face. It grows to be an elevated, flesh-colored nodule 1 to 2 cm across. Less often, a patient has a form of the disease inherited as an autosomal dominant character. Multiple lesions appear in childhood and gradually increase in number. They begin as papules, enlarge for a few years, then become stationary. Most are less than 1 cm across, flesh colored, often with telangiectasia. Some of the patients with multiple trichoepitheliomatosis have also multiple cylindromatosis.

Microscopically, the tumor consists of columns of epithelial cells extending down into the dermis. The cells in these columns are like those of a basal cell carcinoma. Large

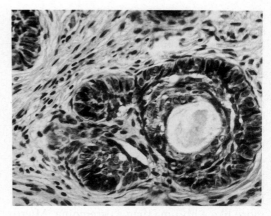

Fig. 62-33. A trichoepithelioma. A keratin cyst is present within the column of invading tumor cells.

cysts filled with keratin are prominent in the columns of tumor cells. Occasionally abortive hairs can be found within the tumor. Often the lesions are pigmented with melanin. A fine collagenous stroma surrounds the tumor and shows a foreign body giant cell reaction if rupture of the cysts releases keratin into the stroma. Microscopically, it is not possible always to distinguish clearly between a trichoepithelioma and a basal cell carcinoma. If the lesion is solitary, it should be considered to be a basal cell carcinoma unless there is clear evidence of pilar differentiation. If the lesions are multiple, the familial history and the course and distribution of the lesions indicate the diagnosis.

In the solitary form of trichoepithelioma, excision curses. In multiple trichoepitheliomatosis, complete eradication of all the tumors is difficult. Incomplete removal may be followed by recurrence.

Calcifying Epithelioma. A calcifying epithelioma, often called a calcifying epithelioma of Malherbe, after the French dermatologist who described it in 1880, or sometimes a pilomatricoma, from the Latin for a hair and the parent stem of a plant, is the most common of pilar tumors. A single, firm nodule, usually 0.5 to 3 cm in diameter, occasionally larger, develops deep in the skin, most often on the face or arms. Calcifying epitheliomata can arise at any age, but 40% of them are in children under 10 years old, and 60% of them develop before the age of 20 years.

Microscopically, a calcifying epithelioma is well-defined and often encapsulated. It lies deep in the dermis, often extending into the subcutaneous fat. The tumor consists of irregular sheets of epithelial cells. Usually the cells at one margin of a sheet or around its periphery stain darkly, while the remainder are pale. The pale cells are called shadow cells. In young lesions, the dark cells are numerous. In old lesions, they are few or absent. The dark cells are small. Their cytoplasm is scant, ill-defined, and basophilic. Their nuclei are round or ovoid and stain deeply. The pale cells are clearly demarcated, with weakly acidophilic cytoplasm. They have no nuclei. The transition between the two types of cell is sometimes sudden, sometimes gradual. Occasionally keratin pearls are present in the sheets of epithelial cells. A few melanocytes are often present among the epithelial cells. Occasionally the epithelial cells contain melanin. Filaments of cytokeratin are present in the dark cells and are abundant in the pale cells. Keratohyaline granules are not present. The epithelial cells usually contain citrulline, a substance present in the epithelium of the hair follicles but not in the epidermis.

A calcifying epithelioma has a collagenous stroma that often shows a prominent, foreign body granulomatous reaction to keratin released by the pale cells. Calcification is evident in 75% of the tumors. In most, it is extensive. Most often the calcification is in the sheets of pale cells. Occasionally it is in the stroma. Foci of ossification are present in 20% of the tumors.

Many think that a calcifying epithelioma is a benign neoplasm derived from the hair follicles. Others consider that at least some of the tumors are ruptured pilar cysts. Almost all calcifying epitheliomata are benign. Excision cures. Rarely, the lesion is locally invasive and may recur if not completely removed.

Pilar Tumor. Pilar tumors, also called proliferating tricholemmal tumors, are uncommon. They take their name from the Latin for hair. Over 90% of them develop in the scalp, the rest on the back. Nearly 80% of the patients are elderly women. Some of the patients have also one or more pilar cysts. The tumor forms a nodule that slowly enlarges

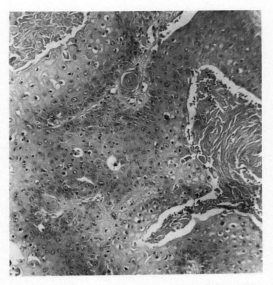

Fig. 62-34. A pilar tumor. The well-differentiated tumor cells differentiate suddenly into structureless material that fills the cavities within the columns of tumor cells.

and often ulcerates. Microscopically, it is a sharply defined mass, consisting of clumps of slightly atypical squamous cells separated by a collagenous stroma. In the center of the clumps, the tumor cells differentiate suddenly into structureless, amorphous keratin like that in a pilar cyst. Often small foci of calcification are present in the tumor. Occasionally some of the tumor cells contain large quantities of glycogen and so have clear cytoplasm.

In most patients, a pilar tumor remains localized and is cured by excision. Only in 2 patients, has a pilar tumor metastasized to a lymph node.

Tricholemmoma. A tricholemmoma takes its name from the Greek words for hair and the skin of a fruit. Most patients have only a single tumor. A few have Cowden's syndrome, named after the first patient reported in 1963, a condition inherited as an autosomal dominant character in which the patients have multiple tricholemmomata, fibrous hamartomata in the breasts, intestines, thyroid gland, and other organs, and an increased incidence of carcinoma of the breast and other malignant tumors.

Tricholemmomata are most common on the face. The tumor forms a small nodule usually less than 1 cm across. In most of the tumors, one or several downgrowths bulge from the epidermis into the dermis. Some of them surround a hair follicle. The cells at the periphery of the extensions often form a palisade. Some of those within the downgrowths contain sufficient glycogen to have a clear cytoplasm. Often a mass of keratin overlies the lesion. Less often, a plate of similar cells forms parallel to the epidermis with many connections to it, a lesion called a tumor of the follicular infundibulum. Small hair follicles are present in the plate. Both types of tumor are benign. Excision cures.

SEBACEOUS TUMORS. Sebaceous tumors form structures that resemble sebaceous glands. They include the nevus sebaceous, senile sebaceous hyperplasia, sebaceous adenoma, sebaceous epithelioma, and sebaceous carcinoma.

Nevus Sebaceus. A nevus sebaceus is a hamartoma present at birth or developing soon after. Usually there is only one lesion, most often on the scalp or face. During childhood, the lesion forms a soft, hairless plaque. At puberty, it becomes warty and thickened. Less often, a patient has multiple sebaceous nevi. Usually some of the lesions are arranged in lines. Some of these patients have epilepsy, are mentally retarded, or have skeletal deformities. Some of them have both sebaceous nevi and epidermal nevi.

Microscopically, during childhood a nevus sebaceus shows only dilated hair follicles filled with keratin and epithelial buds projecting from these follicles into the dermis. At puberty, the epithelial buds develop into sebaceous glands of almost normal appearance, but more numerous and closer together than is normal. The hair follicles within the lesion remain small, atrophy, and may disappear. The overlying epithelium is thick and thrown into warty folds. In 70% of sebaceous nevi, ectopic but well-formed apocrine glands develop in the dermis deep to the lesion.

If left untreated, a syringocystadenoma papilliferum or some other kind of appendage tumor develops in the nevus in 15% of the patients. A basal cell carcinoma takes origin in the lesion in over 5% of the patients, but is usually small. Rarely, a squamous cell carcinoma arises in the lesion. A sebaceous nevus is benign, but should be excised to avoid these complications.

Senile Sebaceous Hyperplasia. In senile sebaceous hyperplasia, one or more soft, yellowish, slightly elevated lesions, 0.2 to 0.3 cm across, develop in people over 50 years old. They are most common on the forehead and cheeks. Microscopically, the lesions consist of a single, well-circumscribed, but greatly enlarged sebaceous gland, with many lobules draining into a dilated central duct. Apart from its size, the gland is normal. The hyperplastic glands can be eradicated for cosmetic reasons.

Sebaceous Adenoma. A sebaceous adenoma is a rare tumor. In most patients, a solitary nodule less than 1 cm in diameter appears on the face or scalp. A few have multiple sebaceous adenomata and malignant tumors of internal organs.

Microscopically, a sebaceous adenoma is well-defined and consists of irregular lobules like those of a sebaceous gland. Two kinds of cells are present in the lobules. At the margin are small dark cells like the germinal cells of normal sebaceous glands. Within the lobules the cells are larger and show the usual sebaceous differentiation. Most lobules contain both types of cell, but some consist almost entirely of one or the other. Occasionally there are foci of keratinization in some of the lobules. Sometimes the lobules become cystic. Excision cures.

Sebaceous Epithelioma. A sebaceous epithelioma is most common on the face or scalp. It resembles a basal cell carcinoma both macroscopically and microscopically. Columns of tumor cells invade the dermis. Many of the columns have a peripheral palisade of cells like those of a basal cell carcinoma and a disorderly arrangement of similar cells centrally. The tumor differs from a basal cell carcinoma in that some of the tumor cells show clear sebaceous differentiation. The lesion is treated as is a basal cell carcinoma.

Sebaceous Carcinoma. A sebaceous carcinoma is rare. Most arise from the meibomian glands of the eyelids. Usually, the tumor forms an ulcerated nodule. Microscopically, irregular columns of tumor invade the underlying tissues. In most of the columns, the cells in the center of the column show sebaceous differentiation and those at the periphery are pleomorphic and atypical. Often parts of the tumor show atypical squamous differentiation, with keratinization, as in a squamous cell carcinoma. Differentiation like that of a basal cell carcinoma does not occur. Widespread metastases are common in sebaceous carcinomata arising from meibomian glands, but sebaceous carcinomata arising elsewhere rarely metastasize.

APOCRINE TUMORS. The more common tumors that resemble apocrine glands are the apocrine hidrocystoma, hidradenoma papilliferum, syringocystoma papilliferum, cylindroma, and apocrine carcinoma.

Apocrine Hidrocystoma. An apocrine hidrocystoma is a benign neoplasm that takes its name from the Greek for sweat. It forms a nodule up to 1.5 cm across, usually on the face. Often the tumor is bluish. Microscopically, cystic spaces are present in the dermis. The spaces are lined by columnar or cuboidal apocrine cells. Myoepithelial cells are often present between the lumenal cells and the basement membrane. Occasionally some of the spaces are lined by a double layer of cells like those seen in a duct. Excision cures.

Hidradenoma Papilliferum. A hidradenoma papilliferum is an uncommon tumor, found almost always on the labia majora, though it can arise from the apocrine glands in the perianal region or from those in the nipple. It is described with the tumors of the vulva in Chapter 41.

Syringocystadenoma Papilliferum. A syringocystadenoma papilliferum is a benign neoplasm that takes its name from the Greek words for Pan's pipe, pouch, and gland, and the Latin words for nipple and to bear. In 75% of the patients, the tumor develops on the face or scalp. In 30% of the patients, it arises at puberty in a sebaceous nevus; in 10% of the patients, together with a basal cell carcinoma. In the other patients, a papule or line of papules appears in early childhood. The lesions increase in size at puberty and often become crusted.

Microscopically, the epidermis over the lesion is thick and often forms warty folds. One or more cystic spaces extend down from the epidermis. The superficial part of the cyst is lined by keratinized epidermis. The lower part is filled by large papillary infoldings lined by a double layer of epithelial cells. The lumenal cells are columnar or cuboidal and sometimes show apocrine secretion. The deeper cells are small and cuboidal. Often large acini lined by a single layer of apocrine cells extend from the deeper part of cystic space into the dermis. The stroma of the tumor nearly always shows a dense inflammatory exudate mainly of plasma cells most severe in the papillary projections into the cyst. Excision cures.

The origin of the syringocystadenomata papillifera is debated. Of the few tumors fully studied, some have shown apocrine differentiation in the tumor cells, but others have shown eccrine differentiation. Probably most syringocystadenomata papillifera arise from apocrine glands, but a few take origin in eccrine sweat glands.

Cylindroma. Cylindromata of the skin are neoplasms. They must not be confused with the carcinoma adenoides cysticum of the salivary glands that is also called a cylindroma.

In the solitary form of the disease, a single tumor appears during adult life, most often on the scalp or face. The tumor forms a smooth, dome-shaped mass, usually between 0.5 and 5.0 cm across.

Multiple cylindromatosis is a condition inherited as an autosomal dominant character. Lesions like those of the solitary form of the disease begin to appear in adult life and grow increasingly numerous. They are most common on the scalp but also occur on the face, trunk, and limbs. Sometimes they cover the entire scalp like a turban, a condition called a turban tumor. Many of the patients have also multiple trichoepitheliomata.

Microscopically, a cylindroma consists of intertwining columns of tumor cells. In section, the columns are irregularly shaped, vary considerably in size, and are packed close together. Most of the tumor cells are small, with spheroidal, dark staining nuclei. Often the tumor cells form a palisade at the margin of the columns of tumor. Glandular spaces or ducts are present within some of the columns of tumor cells. Often they are numerous. Occasionally they are few. The acini are lined by tall, secretory cells; the ducts, by cuboidal ductular cells. A thick, hyaline membrane surrounding the columns of tumor cells consists in large part of a greatly

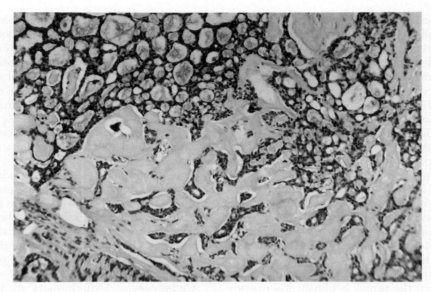

Fig. 62-35. A cylindroma of the skin, showing columns of tumor cells containing many ductlike spaces.

thickened basement membrane. Fragments of similar hyaline material are sometimes present within the columns of tumor cells.

The origin of cylindromata of the skin is uncertain. Both enzymatically and structurally, they show features of both apocrine and eccrine glands. The evidence slightly favors apocrine differentiation.

Most cylindromata of the skin are benign. Local excision cures. Rarely, a cylindroma of the skin becomes malignant and its cells become anaplastic and pleomorphic. The tumor invades the surrounding tissues and may metastasize widely.

Apocrine Carcinoma. Carcinomata of the apocrine glands are rare. They arise most often in an axilla and form acini lined by tall, eosinophilic cells, like those of an apocrine gland. The tumor cells contain the enzymes of an apocrine gland. Some apocrine carcinomata invade only locally. Others metastasize widely.

Eccrine Tumors. The principal tumors of the eccrine sweat glands are the eccrine hidrocystoma, syringoma, clear cell hidradenoma, eccrine poroma, eccrine spiradenoma, chondroid syringoma, and eccrine carcinoma.

Eccrine Hidrocystoma. An eccrine hidrocystoma is caused by temporary obstruction of an eccrine duct. It is not a neoplasm. One or more bluish, translucent, cystic nodules 0.1 to 0.3 cm across develop on the face. Microscopically, a small cyst in the dermis is lined by two layers of cuboidal cells like those of eccrine glands. Occasionally an eccrine gland is in continuity with the cyst. The cyst does not communicate with the surface of the skin.

Syringoma. A syringoma is a benign neoplasm of the duct of an eccrine gland. There are usually several lesions, sometimes a large number. The disease is most common in adolescents and young adults. Many of the patients are girls. The lesions are most numerous on the lower lids, but are also common on the cheeks, abdomen, vulva, and in the axillae.

Numerous small ducts lined by two layers of flattened cells are present in the dermis, widely separated by a collagenous stroma. The cells lining the ducts have the fine structure of eccrine ductular cells and contain similar enzymes. Near the epidermis, some of the ducts are lined by stratified epithelium and contain keratin. If one of these ducts ruptures, a foreign body reaction to the keratin develops in the dermis. Occasionally solid strands of epithelium like that lining the ducts are present in the tumor. The lesions

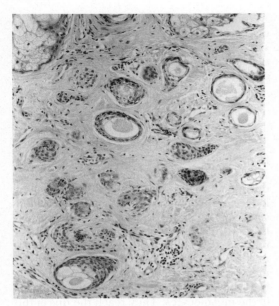

Fig. 62-36. A syringoma, showing small ducts, some of which are becoming keratinized.

do not enlarge but can be removed for cosmetic reasons.

Clear Cell Hidradenoma. A clear cell hidradenoma is a neoplasm also called a clear cell myoblastoma, a nodular hidradenoma, and other names. The patient is usually adult. One or occasionally more nodules 0.5 to 2 cm across arise in the skin. The lesion may ulcerate.

Microscopically, the tumor is well-circumscribed or encapsulated. Usually it lies in the dermis without connection to the epidermis. The tumor consists of large lobules of tumor cells supported by a collagenous stroma. Within the lobules are two kinds of tumor cell. Some are polygonal with spheroidal nuclei, clear cytoplasm containing much glycogen, and prominent cell walls. Others are elongated with ovoid nuclei and dark basophilic cytoplasm containing tonofibrils. Both types of tumor cell are always present. Either may be predominant. Clear cell hidradenomata are not always predominantly of clear cells.

Often there are branching ducts within the lobules of tumor cells. The ducts may be lined by cuboidal cells like those of an eccrine duct or by columnar, secretory cells like those of an eccrine gland. Often degeneration within the lobules of tumor cells leads to cystic spaces. Sometimes foci of keratinization are present.

Most clear cell adenomata are benign. Excision cures. A few are malignant. The malignant tumors are more anaplastic and have a high mitotic rate. The tumor invades the surrounding tissues and metastasizes to the regional lymph nodes and more distantly.

Eccrine Poroma. An eccrine poroma is a neoplasm that takes its name from the English word pore. Most patients have only one lesion. A few have hundreds. In 70% of the patients, the lesion or lesions are on the soles of the feet. Less often a lesion is found on the hands or fingers, the neck, chest, or nose. Most of the patients are between 40 and 60 years old. The tumor forms a firm, raised nodule, usually less than 2 cm across. Rarely the lesion is linear, or warty.

Microscopically, the tumor usually replaces the basal part of the epidermis and forms broad, anastomosing columns that extend into the dermis. Less often it consists of islands of tumor cells within the epidermis, is confined to the dermis, or forms fine strands that ramify in the dermis. The tumor cells are smaller than the prickle cells of the epidermis and are sharply demarcated from them. They are cuboidal, with uniform, dark, spheroidal nuclei. Intercellular bridges join the tumor cells. In most eccrine poromata, ducts like these of eccrine sweat glands are present within some of the clumps of tumor cells. Especially in people with pigmented skin, melanocytes are sometimes present in the tumor.

The fine structure of the tumor cells is like that of the outer layer of the intraepithelial part of the eccrine ducts. They contain tonofilaments and are joined by desmosomes, but they do not keratinize. They contain enzymes like those of the eccrine ducts. Glycogen is abundant in some of the cells.

Most eccrine poromata are benign. Excision cures. Occasionally a benign eccrine poroma becomes malignant, or a poroma is malignant from the outset. The malignant tumors have larger, more irregular nuclei that are sometimes multinucleate. Often the surrounding epidermal cells are hyperplastic and hyperkeratotic. The malignant tumors metastasize to the skin, the regional lymph nodes, and to internal organs. In the skin, the metastases form islands of tumor cells in the epidermis and dermis. Often the tumor is present in dermal lymphatics.

Eccrine Spiradenoma. An eccrine spiradenoma is a neoplasm that takes its name from the Greek for a coil. Usually a single tumor 1 to 2 cm across appears in a young adult. Any part of the skin may be involved. Often the tumor is tender or painful. Less often there are several tumors, rarely a large number of them.

Microscopically, there are one or more sharply defined nodules of tumor in the dermis, without connection to the epidermis. The nodules of tumor consist of closely packed cells with little cytoplasm. Most of the tumor cells have small, darkly staining, spheroidal nuclei. Some of the cells within the nodules, have large, pale nuclei and often surround small lumina. Sometimes hyaline material is present in the stroma of the tumor or between the tumor cells. The enzymes present in the tumor cells and their fine structure both suggest that the eccrine spiradenoma originates from an eccrine gland.

Most eccrine spiradenomata are benign. Excision cures. Rarely, one has become malignant.

Chondroid Syringoma. A chondroid syringoma is a neoplasm formerly called a mixed tumor of the skin. It forms a firm nodule 0.5 to 3 cm across, most often on the head. Microscopically, the tumor resembles a pleomorphic adenoma of a salivary gland. It is benign. Excision cures.

Eccrine Carcinoma. Eccrine carcinomata are rare. The tumor can arise in any part of the skin. Macroscopically it is indistinguishable from other carcinomata of the skin. Microscopically, most of the tumors consist of tubular lumina lined by one or two layers of cells. The tumor cells often contain the enzymes present in eccrine glands. Less often an eccrine carcinoma secretes large quantities of mucus that escapes into the stroma. Small clumps of carcinoma cells float in the mucus, as in other types of colloid carcinoma. Rarely, an eccrine carcinoma resembles an adenoid cystic carcinoma of a salivary gland. It forms solid masses of cells in which there are numerous small lumina.

All types of eccrine carcinoma are difficult to distinguish from carcinoma metastatic to the skin. Metastases to the regional lymph nodes develop in 50% of the patients. Internal organs are involved in 40%.

Melanocytic Tumors

The melanocytes in the skin are derived from the neural crest and migrate into the skin together with the peripheral nerves during fetal life. Most of the melanocytes lodge in the basal layer of the epidermis, but some remain in the dermis. In the epidermis, the melanocytes develop long tentacles, which ramify between the basal cells of the epidermis. The melanocytes synthesize melanin in membrane-bound melanosomes. As they mature, the melanosomes pass into the tentacles of the melanocytes. They reach the tips of the tentacles, which are pinched off and phagocytosed by the epidermal cells. The melanosomes come to lie within the phagosomes of the epidermal cells, where they are degraded by the lysosomal enzymes. In normal skin, most of the melanin is within the epidermal cells, with little remaining within the melanocytes that make it.

The tumors and tumor-like proliferations of melanocytes that occur in the skin are divided into six groups: pigmented nevi, benign epidermal lesions, benign dermal lesions, melanoma in situ, malignant melanoma, and malignant blue nevus.

Non-neoplastic melanocytes are often present in nonmelanocytic skin tumors, notably in seborrhoeic keratoses and basal cell carcinomata. They form melanin in the normal way, but often are unable to transmit it to the tumor cells. The melanin accumulates in the melanocytes or escapes to be phagocytosed by macrophages in the stroma of the tumor or in the dermis.

PIGMENTED NEVUS. Pigmented nevi, often called moles or nevocellular nevi, are malformations, not neoplasms. They are the most common of all tumor-like lesions. Moles begin to appear soon after birth, are most numerous in young adults, and then gradually disappear. On the average, a young adult has 40 pigmented nevi.

A pigmented nevus begins as a multifocal

proliferation of melanocytes in the basal part of the epidermis. The proliferating melanocytes form small clumps of cells at the epidermodermal junction. As the nevus ages, some of the melanocytes move from the clumps into the dermis. The melanocytes in the dermis do not proliferate. At this stage, the lesion has clumps of proliferating melanocytes at the epidermodermal junction and groups of nonproliferating melanocytes in the dermis. After some years, the proliferation of melanocytes at the epidermodermal junction stops. The clumps of melanocytes at the epidermodermal junction disappear, leaving only the quiescent melanocytes in the dermis. In many moles, the melanocytes in the dermis eventually atrophy and disappear. The melanocytes normally present in the dermis and the Schwann cells surrounding the dermal nerves play no part in the formation of a pigmented nevus.

The formation of clumps of melanocytes at the epidermodermal junction is called junctional activity. Pigmented nevi that show junctional activity but no extension into the dermis are called junctional nevi. When both junctional activity and dermal nevus cells are present, the lesion is called a compound nevus. When nevus cells are present in the dermis but there is no junctional activity, the lesion is called an intradermal nevus.

Most pigmented nevi in children are junctional or compound nevi. Usually junctional activity is prominent. About 50% of moles in young adults are compound nevi that show some junctional activity, though it is not usually extensive. In older people, over 90% of nevi are intradermal. Junctional activity persists most often in lesions on the genitalia, palms, and soles.

The junctional, compound, and intradermal stages of the ordinary kind of pigmented nevus are most common. Uncommon variants that are present in a small minority of people include the balloon cell nevus, halo nevus, Spitz nevus, dysplastic nevus, and congenital pigmented nevus.

Most pigmented nevi are benign. A few progress to malignant melanoma. The risk of malignant change is highest in patients with the dysplastic nevus syndrome or a giant congenital pigmented nevus.

Junctional Nevus. Most junctional nevi

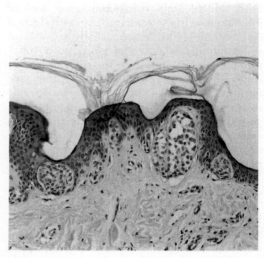

Fig. 62-37. A junctional nevus. Well-demarcated clumps of melanocytes at the epidermodermal junction.

are flat, pigmented lesions less than 0.5 cm across. The clumps of proliferating melanocytes are sharply demarcated from the adjacent epidermis. Some lie within the epidermis, separated from the dermis by a thin layer of epidermal cells. Others appear to be partially separated from the epidermis, lying between the epidermis and the dermis.

The melanocytes in the clumps are called nevus cells. They are usually rounded or polygonal, less often spindle shaped and arranged in a swirling pattern. The cells resemble normal cutaneous melanocytes except that they have no tentacles. The nevus cells form melanin but are not usually heavily pigmented. In adults and in most children, they are regular, with no atypicality and no mitoses. In some children, they are moderately atypical and show occasional mitoses.

The epidermis overlying the clumps of melanocytes at the epidermodermal junction is normal. The underlying dermis is normal unless the lesion is injured or inflamed.

Compound Nevus. Compound nevi are usually pigmented lesions slightly elevated above the surrounding skin. Less often a compound nevus is papillomatous. Microscopically, the lesions show junctional activity like that in a junctional nevus, together with nevus cells in the dermis. In children, the junctional activity is usually prominent. In most adults, only occasional small foci of junctional activity remain. The intradermal component of the lesion usually consists of small clumps of cuboidal cells, with spheroidal nuclei. In children, the cells are sometimes slightly atypical. In adults, they are uniform and regular. Mitoses may be present in children. They are not found in adults. In young compound nevi, the intradermal nevus cells are confined to the upper part of the dermis. As the lesions age, the nevus cells penetrate into the deeper parts of the dermis.

Intradermal Nevus. Intradermal nevi are often dome shaped and about 0.5 cm across. The lesion is usually brown, but is sometimes little darker than the surrounding skin. Often a few coarse hairs grow from the lesion. Less often an intradermal nevus is pedunculated or papillomatous. It is not always pigmented.

In most intradermal nevi, the nevus cells form small clumps in the dermis, which often are arranged in rows perpendicular to the epidermis. The nevus cells are cuboidal, with regular, spheroidal nuclei, and are all much alike. Frequently a few of them are multinucleate, with several nuclei in the center of the cell. Usually the nevus cells near the surface of the skin are larger than those deeper in the dermis. Melanin is sometimes abundant in the more superficial nevus cells, but is nearly always sparse or absent in the deeper part of the lesion. If melanin is abundant, some of it escapes into the dermis and is taken up by macrophages. Mitoses and other evidence of cell division are never present.

In the deeper part of an intradermal nevus, the nevus cells sometimes become spindle shaped and may be arranged in loose bundles. Occasionally the spindle-shaped nevus cells are wound into an onion-like body resembling a Meissner's corpuscle. Such a nevus is called a neuronevus because of its resemblance to neural structures and to a neurofibroma. Occasionally only the spindle-shaped cells deep in the dermis are present without cuboidal cells in the upper dermis. Occasionally adipocytes are present among the nevus cells.

The overlying epidermis is usually normal. Often the nevus cells are separated from it by a band of uninvolved dermis. Occasionally the epidermis is thickened, hyperkeratotic, and

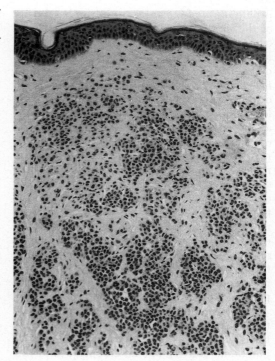

Fig. 62-38. An intradermal nevus. Clumps of nevus cells are present in the dermis, but there is no junctional activity.

warty. In pedunculated nevi, fine plates of epidermis one or two cells thick often extend into the dermis between the clumps of nevus cells and anastomose to form a reticular pattern. Often large keratin pearls develop in these extensions into the dermis. Occasionally a hair follicle within the lesion is dilated and filled with keratin.

Balloon Cell Nevus. Balloon cell nevi are uncommon. They can occur in any part of the body. The nevus is usually less than 0.5 cm across, brown, and slightly raised. Microscopically, the lesion is a compound or intradermal nevus in which many of the nevus cells are 20 to 40 µm across and have clear, empty cytoplasm. Their small, homogeneous, and dark nuclei are in the center of the ballooned cells. Often some of the balloon cells are multinucleate. The ballooning is caused by degeneration and swelling of the melanosomes, which fail to produce melanin. The term *balloon cell nevus* is not used unless the majority of the nevus cells are of this type. A few balloon cells are present in 2% of pigmented nevi.

Halo Nevus. Halo nevi are most common on the back in young adults. Often there is more than one. The lesion shows a depigmented halo 0.1 to 0.5 cm wide around a pigmented nevus. In most of the lesions, the nevus in the center of the lesion gradually regresses over the course of several months. The halo persists longer, but usually disappears after months or years.

Halo nevi are compound or intradermal nevi. In the lesions that regress, a dense exudate mainly of lymphocytes and macrophages is present in the nevus. It surrounds the clumps of nevus cells and penetrates into them. Often it extends into the basal part of the epidermis, but its deep margin is usually sharp. The nevus cells slowly degenerate and disappear. After the nevus has been destroyed, the inflammation wanes and disappears. In the lesions that do not regress, no inflammatory infiltrate is present.

In the surrounding halo the melanocytes degenerate and are lost. The production of melanin ceases. Dopa oxidase and other melanocytic enzymes can no longer be detected. In the lesions in which the central nevus regresses, the melanocytes overlying the nevus also degenerate, though they persist longer than those in the halo.

During the disappearance of a halo nevus, the patients have in the plasma antibodies against cytoplasmic antigens of malignant melanoma cells. The antibodies react with nevus cells and melanocytes in the halo, but not with melanocytes or nevus cells in other parts of the body. Presumably the nevus cells in the halo nevi regress, and the melanocytes in the halo are a clone that differs antigenically from melanocytes and nevus cells in other parts of the body. The abnormal clone excites an autoimmune reaction that leads to the destruction of the nevus. The dense inflammatory infiltrate suggests that the destruction of the nevus is a cell-mediated rather than a humoral reaction. When the destruction of the nevus is complete, the antibodies disappear from the plasma.

Spitz Nevus. A Spitz nevus is named after the American pathologist who described it in 1948. Formerly, it was called a juvenile melanoma. Spitz nevi are most common on the face and limbs. Occasionally there is more than one. The lesion is usually a flesh-colored, dome-shaped, hairless nodule less than 1 cm across. A Spitz nevus can develop at any age. Less than 50% of them occur in children under 14 years old. Over 25% of the patients are over 30 years old.

Most Spitz nevi are compound nevi, usually with prominent junctional activity. A few are junctional or intradermal nevi. The clumps of nevus cells at the epidermodermal junction and the groups of nervus cells in the dermis are usually sharply demarcated. Two kinds of nevus cells are present, spindle cells and epithelioid cells. In 50% of Spitz nevi, spindle cells predominate; in 20%, the epithelial cells are predominant. The spindle cells are elongated and usually arranged in whorls. The epithelioid cells are large with abundant, well-defined, often eosinophilic cytoplasm. Frequently some of the epithelioid cells are multinucleate. Their nuclei are often large, hyperchromatic, and irregular. Mitoses are present in 50% of the lesions. In the deeper parts of the lesion, the nevus cells are usually smaller and better differentiated. In 90% of the lesions, little or no melanin is produced. Less than 5% are heavily pigmented.

In 50% of Spitz nevi, the papillary dermis is edematous with widely dilated blood vessels. Often the dermis shows an exudate predominantly of lymphocytes. The exudate is perivascular or forms a band at the deep margin of the lesion. The overlying epidermis is often hyperplastic with long rete ridges, but may be thin or ulcerated. Eosinophilic globules that stain strongly with the periodic acid-Schiff reaction are present in the epidermis in 60% of Spitz nevi. Similar globules present in the epidermis in 2% of malignant melanomata and 1% of other pigmented nevi do not stain with the periodic acid-Schiff reaction.

The plemorphism and atypicality of the nevus cells in a Spitz nevus often make it hard to distinguish from a malignant melanoma. The lesion is benign. Excision cures.

Dysplastic Nevus. Some kindred develop multiple dysplastic nevi as well as the ordinary type of pigmented nevi and often multiple malignant melanomata, a disorder called the dysplastic nevus syndrome. Sometimes one or a few dysplastic nevi develop in a patient without a genetic predisposition to develop this kind of lesion. Dysplastic nevi are usually 0.5 to 1.5 cm across, irregularly shaped, and mottled brown, black, and pink. Often the center of the lesion is nodular. New lesions appear during adult life.

Microscopically, dysplastic nevi are compound nevi. Often junctional activity extends laterally beyond the limit of the dermal part of the nevus. The cells in the clumps at the epidermodermal junction and in the upper dermis are moderately atypical. Frequently the nevus cells in the upper dermis are elongated and lie parallel to the epidermis. Mitoses are few or absent. Usually an exudate principally of lymphocytes is present at the deep margin of the lesion.

Dysplastic nevi are benign, but some of them develop into malignant melanomata. Because of this danger, all lesions that might be dysplastic nevi should be removed from a patient found to have one of these lesions.

Congenital Pigmented Nevus.   About 1% of newborn infants have one or more congenital pigmented nevi. Most of the lesions are more than 1.5 cm across. Some have the distribution of bathing trunks, cover much of a limb, or form a cap on the head. The smaller lesions are raised, pigmented, and often hairy. Occasionally a lesion is pale and cerebriform or shows irregular, spotty pigmentation. The giant congenital pigmented nevi are usually warty, deeply pigmented, and hairy. Some of the infants with a giant congenital pigmented nevus have pigmentation of the meninges, hydrocephalus, mental retardation, or epilepsy. Other congenital malformations may be present.

The smaller congenital pigmented nevi are junctional or compound nevi. Often isolated nevus cells are present in the epidermis in addition to the clumps of nevus cells at the epidermodermal junction. The intraepidermal nevus cells frequently extend into the hair follicles and eccrine glands. Usually, some of them are atypical. In the dermis, the nevus cells tend to arise from the appendages and to be concentrated around them. They often form columns one or two cells thick between collagen bundles. In 50% of the lesions, they extend into the subcutaneous fat.

The cerebriform and spotted congenital lesions are intradermal nevi. The cerebriform lesions often show neuroid differentiation. The spotted lesions are largely confined to the regions around the eccrine glands or are concentrated around the hair follicles.

The giant congenital pigmented nevi show some combination of compound nevus, intradermal nevus, and blue nevus. Often neuroid differentiation is extensive.

Over 10% of people with a giant congenital pigmented nevus develop malignant melanoma, some in childhood, some not until adult life. The melanoma may arise in the giant nevus or from a smaller lesion in some other part of the skin. Most of the malignant melanomata begin with neoplastic junctional activity at the epidermodermal junction. A few arise within the dermis. Only 1% of people with no lesion greater than 20 cm across develop melanoma.

BENIGN EPITHELIAL LESIONS.   In the benign, tumor-like lesions of epidermal melanocytes, overproduction of melanin or proliferation of melanocytes produces focal lesions in the epidermis. The disorders to be considered include freckles, lentigo simplex, lentigo senilis, and Becker's melanosis.

Freckles.   Freckles, called ephelides from the Greek for freckle, are common in people with fair skin. They appear in regions exposed to light during childhood, darken on exposure to sunlight, and tend to disappear in adult life. In an ephelis the quantity of melanin in the basal cells of the epidermis is increased, but there is no increase in the number of melanocytes. The melanocytes in the lesions are larger than usual and have longer tentacles. They produce larger and more heavily melanized melanosomes than do the melanocytes in the surrounding skin.

Lentigo Simplex.   Lentigo simplex takes its name from the Latin words for lentil and plain. In most patients a few lesions appear in childhood or later in life. Any part of the skin can be involved. The lesions are brown or black, not raised above the surrounding skin or indurated and are usually less than 0.5 cm across. Rarely, a child has hundreds or thousands of lentigines. In some of the children with numerous lentigines, the condition is inherited as an autosomal dominant character, and other congenital anomalies are present.

The number of melanocytes is increased in lentigo simplex. Occasionally small clumps of melanocytes are present at the epidermodermal junction. The quantity of melanin in the melanocytes and in the basal keratinocytes is greater than normal. Some of the melanosomes are larger and more heavily pigmented than is normal. The length of the rete ridges is usually increased. Often melanin escapes into the dermis where it is phagocytosed by macrophages. Frequently the dermis shows mild, chronic inflammation.

The lesions of lentigo simplex persist but do not enlarge. They do not become malignant. No treatment is needed.

Lentigo Senilis. More than 90% of white people over 70 years old have one or more lentigines seniles in regions exposed to sunlight. The condition is sometimes called solar lentigo. The lesions are flat, brown, and irregularly shaped. Most are less than 1 cm across. They are most common on the backs of the hands.

The rete ridges of the epidermis are elongated in the lesions and become club-shaped. Small epithelial buds sometimes extend from the ridges into the dermis. Occasionally the ridges anastomose, forming a reticular network in the dermis. The epidermis between the ridges is often thin. The quantity of melanin in the melanocytes and basal keratinocytes is greatly increased in the rete ridges. The melanin in the keratinocytes often persists into the upper layers of the epidermis. The melanocytes are larger than normal and have more extensive processes. In some patients the number of melanocytes increases. In some it is normal. Melanin is often present in macrophages in the dermis. Often the dermis shows mild, chronic inflammation.

Lentigines seniles tend become more numerous as years pass. They slowly enlarge and sometimes coalesce. They do not become malignant.

Becker's Melanosis. Becker's melanosis is named after the American dermatologist who described it in 1949. The patient is usually a man about 20 years old. A large, sharply demarcated patch of pigmentation appears, most often on one shoulder or on the chest. Occasionally there is more than one lesion. Often the lesion is hairy. In the lesion, the epidermis is thickened and the rete ridges are elongated. The basal keratinocytes and the melanocytes are heavily pigmented. The number of melanocytes increases. The hair follicles are normal. Macrophages in the dermis contain melanin. Some patients have a smooth muscle hamartoma in the dermis.

BENIGN DERMAL LESIONS. The benign, tumor-like proliferations of dermal melanocytes are the blue nevus, cellular blue nevus, Mongolian spot, and nevi of Ota and Ito.

Blue Nevus. A blue nevus is usually a solitary lesion. Occasionally a patient has more than one. The nevus usually develops during childhood. In 50% of the patients, it is on the dorsum of a hand or foot. The lesion is firm, well-defined, and blue or black. Most are less than 1 cm across.

Long, slender, wavy melanocytes with long branching processes form bundles between the collagen fibers of the dermis. Usually the melanocytes lie parallel to the epidermis. Occasionally the lesion extends into the subcutaneous fat or reaches the epidermis. Laterally the lesion merges with the dermis without a clear margin. Most of the melanocytes are filled with fine granules of melanin. Macrophages containing melanin are often present in the lesion. The melanocytes stain for dopa oxidase. The macrophages do not. Occasionally a patient has a pigmented nevus overlying a blue nevus.

Blue nevi are benign. They do not become malignant. Excision cures.

Cellular Blue Nevus. Cellular blue nevi are less frequent than the ordinary type of blue nevus. The nevus forms a bluish nodule usually 1 to 3 cm across. Its surface may be smooth or irregular. Often the lesion involves the subcutaneous tissue. More than 50% of cellular blue nevi develop on the buttocks.

In cellular blue nevi, two types of tumor cell are present. Some are elongated, pigmented melanocytes like those of the usual form of blue nevus. Others are larger, spindle-shaped cells with ovoid nuclei and abundant cytoplasm. The larger cells are often arranged in a storiform pattern. They contain little or no melanin. Occasionally a pigmented nevus overlies the lesion. Electron microscopy shows that both types of cell are melanocytes.

Most cellular blue nevi are benign. Complete excision cures. In a few patients, tumor cells like those of the nevus have been found in regional lymph nodes, though there was no other evidence of extension of the tumor. In a few, the nevus has become malignant.

Mongolian Spot. Mongolian spots are common in Oriental and black infants and sometimes in Caucasians. They are present at birth, but usually fade and disappear after three or four years. A mongolian spot usually occurs in the lumbosacral region and looks like a bluish bruise. Occasionally one occurs in some other part of the skin. Microscopically, a mongolian spot is similar to a blue nevus, though the dermal melanocytes are less numerous.

Nevi of Ota and Ito. The nevus of Ota is named after the Japanese physician who described it in 1939. An extensive discoloration of the skin of the face is present at birth or appears in childhood. The lesion is unilateral in 90% of the patients. It is most common around the orbit. Most patients are Japanese. Some 80% are women. The nevus of Ito, called after the Japanese physician who reported it in 1954, is similar, but affects the skin about one shoulder. Occasionally a similar lesion develops in some other part of the body. Microscopically, the lesions show in part changes like those of an ordinary blue nevus, in part the less marked concentration of dermal melanocytes seen in a mongolian

spot. Rarely, a nevus of Ota becomes malignant.

Malignant Melanoma in Situ. Lesions in which a proliferation of malignant melanocytes is confined to the epidermis are called malignant melanoma in situ. Three kinds of malignant melanoma in situ are distinguished: lentigo maligna, superficial spreading melanoma, and acral lentiginous melanoma in situ. All tend to progress to invasive malignant melanoma. Early excision of the lesions is needed to avoid the development of an invasive melanoma.

Lentigo Maligna. Lentigo maligna is also called Hutchinson's freckle, after the English surgeon Sir Jonathan Hutchinson who described it in 1890. The patient is nearly always over 50 years old. Most are about 70 years old. In 80% of the patients, the lesion is on the face, less often in other regions exposed to sunlight, and rarely in other parts of the skin. A small, brown patch appears. It enlarges slowly as years pass, becoming irregularly shaped and irregularly pigmented. Sometimes part of a lesion heals or becomes depigmented. After 10 or 20 years, the lentigo is often about 10 cm^2 in area, but can be much smaller or considerably larger.

In the early stages of a lentigo maligna, the epidermis is thin. Its basal layers are strongly pigmented. Often melanin is present in the more superficial epidermal cells. The number of melanocytes is a little increased and their

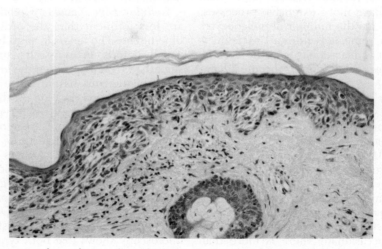

Fig. 62-39.   Lentigo maligna, showing the proliferation of atypical melanocytes in the basal part of the epidermis.

arrangement is slightly disordered. Occasionally a few macrophages containing melanin or mild chronic inflammation are present in the dermis.

In more advanced lesions, the number of melanocytes in the basal part of the epidermis is greatly increased. They sometimes outnumber the basal keratinocytes. In many regions, the arrangement of the melanocytes is disorderly. Occasionally, some of them form small clumps at the epidermodermal junction. Their nuclei are large, hyperchromatic, and pleomorphic. The cytoplasm of some of the tumor cells may be vacuolated. Frequently the atypical melanocytes extend into the hair follicles. Occasionally they are present in the more superficial part of the epidermis.

The abnormal melanocytes contain many melanosomes. The cells in the clumps at the epidermodermal junction lose their processes, but the other tumor cells have long processes that extend between the keratinocytes and pass melanosomes to them. Often both the melanosomes and the keratinocytes are heavily pigmented.

The dermis under the lesion contains many macrophages filled with melanin. Usually it shows chronic inflammation, often with a band predominantly of lymphocytes beneath the epidermis. Frequently the inflammation extends beyond the lesion in the epidermis.

In 30% of the patients, the lesion becomes an invasive melanoma. Usually invasion does not occur until the lentigo has been present for 5 or 10 years, and has become more than 5 cm across. Occasionally it develops rapidly in a small lesion.

When a lentigo maligna becomes an invasive melanoma, one or more nodules appear within the lesion. They enlarge rapidly. Sometimes the nodules become warty, heavily pigmented, or ulcerated or bleed. Microscopically, the nodules show junctional activity with malignant melanocytes in the clumps of cells at the epidermodermal junction. The malignant melanocytes in the clumps invade the dermis. The other parts of the lentigo remain in situ.

Superficial Spreading Melanoma. A superficial spreading melanoma is often called a pagetoid melanoma in situ, because of the similarity of the lesion to Paget's disease of the nipple or sometimes precancerous melanosis. The patients are usually 40 to 50 years old. Nearly 70% of superficial spreading melanomata arise on the head, neck, trunk, or lower leg. The lesion forms an irregularly shaped, irregularly pigmented, slightly raised plaque, usually less than 2.5 cm across. It enlarges slowly.

Microscopically, the epidermis is usually slightly thickened. Large, pale cells, like those of Paget's disease of the nipple, are scattered in the epidermis. Near the epidermodermal junction, the tumor cells usually form small clumps, but in the superficial part of the epidermis they lie singly. The cells have atypical nuclei and often contain melanin. The tumor cells have lost almost all their tentacles, but contain large numbers of melanosomes in their cytoplasm. The melanosomes are abnormal, without the cross-linking of their filaments normally seen, and form little melanin. A exudate of lymphocytes, plasma cells, and macrophages is present in the upper dermis. Some of the macrophages contain melanin. Often the inflammation extends beyond the epidermal lesion.

Progression to an invasive melanoma often occurs within a year. A focus of induration, ulceration, or bleeding develops in the lesion. Microscopically, the invasive region shows junctional activity and malignant melanocytes invading the dermis. The remainder of the lesion shows only pagetoid melanoma in situ.

Acral Lentiginous Melanoma in Situ. Acral lentiginous melanomata in situ develop in the palms of the hands, soles of the feet, and under or around the nails. The term *acral* comes from the Greek for terminal. The tumor forms an ill-defined zone of increased pigmentation or, if it develops under a nail, a longitudinal band of increased pigmentation.

Microscopically, early lesions show an increase in the quantity of melanin in the epidermis and in the number of melanocytes. A few of the melanocytes are slightly atypical. Older lesions show some combination of lentigo maligna and pagetoid melanoma in situ. Often the lesion is deeply pigmented, with large quantities of melanin throughout the epidermis and in macrophages in the dermis.

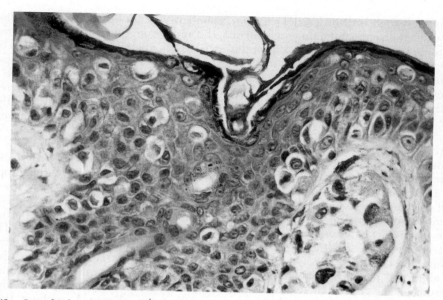

Fig. 62-40. Superficial spreading melanoma, showing the proliferation of large, pale melanocytes in the epidermis.

Invasion usually develops within a few months. Junctional activity begins at the site of invasion, and malignant melanocytes invade the dermis.

MALIGNANT MELANOMA. Invasive malignant melanomata of the epidermis is usually called malignant melanoma without further qualification. Some prefer the term *melanocarcinoma*. This term became popular when it was thought that malignant melanomata of the epidermis arose from altered keratinocytes. This is not the case. Malignant melanomata arise from the epidermal melanocytes. The old term *melanosarcoma* is no longer used.

About 2% of malignant tumors in the United States are malignant melanomata of the epidermis. Some 55% of the patients are women. Most are over 40 years old. More than 3% of the patients sooner or later develop a second primary melanoma.

Malignant melanomata are rare in children. When a malignant melanoma does arise in a child, it is like the lesions in adults and behaves similarly. In children, care must be taken not to mistake an active compound nevus for a malignant melanoma.

Most malignant melanomata of the epidermis arise in white people. They are most common in those with fair skin and in those who live in sunny climates. In the United States and the United Kingdom, 2 white people in every 100,000 develop a malignant melanoma. In Queensland in Australia, 16 white people in every 100,000 develop a malignant melanoma. Malignant melanomata are uncommon in black people and in oriental people. When a malignant melanoma does occur in a black person, it usually arises in an unpigmented region, such as a palm or sole, often from an acral lentiginous melanoma in situ.

The incidence of malignant melanoma is increasing. In Norway, the United States, and the United Kingdom, the incidence of malignant melanoma more than doubled between 1950 and 1970. The data suggest that some new factor causing the increase began to act about 1900.

About 70% of invasive malignant melanomata of the epidermis arise in a superficial spreading melanoma. Some 10% arise in an acral lentiginous melanoma in situ; 5% in a lentigo maligna. The remaining 15% arise without preceding melanoma in situ. Such lesions are called nodular melanomata.

Lesions. The macroscopic appearence of a pigmented lesion is not a reliable guide to its nature. Without biopsy, only 50% of malignant melanomata of the skin are diagnosed correctly. A benign pigmented lesion sometimes strongly suggests malignant melanoma. Some malignant melanomata masquerade as benign pigmented or unpigmented lesions.

The changes in the melanomata in situ that suggest progression to invasive melanoma have been described. In the early stages of invasive melanoma, the changes in the melanoma in situ are not always striking. Any change in a pigmented lesion that could be melanoma in situ should suggest the possibility of invasive melanoma.

Nodular melanomata are invasive from the outset. About 70% of them arise on the face or neck. The lower leg, trunk, and arms are other common sites. Occasionally a nodular melanoma arises in the vulva, or mouth, or conjunctiva. A second nodular melanoma develops in 1% of the patients.

Most nodular melanomata form a deeply pigmented nodule that bulges above the surface of the skin as it enlarges rapidly. Often the nodule is surrounded by an irregular zone of pigmentation or erythema. Sometimes satellite lesions surround the main mass. Often the nodule is ulcerated or bleeds. Less often a nodular melanoma mimics some other pigmented lesion or is manifest only by itching, enlargement, ulceration, or bleeding in a mole.

Almost all invasive melanomata of the skin begin with junctional activity, with clumps of malignant melanocytes at the epidermodermal junction, much as in a junctional nevus. Exceptions are the malignant blue nevi, the few malignant melanomata that develop deep within a giant congenital pigmented nevus, and the rare malignant melanomata that seem to arise from the intradermal part of an intradermal nevus.

In most invasive melanomata, junctional activity involves a large proportion of the epidermodermal junction. Usually, large numbers of melanoma cells stream down into the dermis from the clumps of malignant melanocytes at the epidermodermal junction. In many lesions, a continuous sheet of tumor cells extends from the epidermis into the dermis. Often the rete pegs of the epidermis are elongated as if they were drawn down by the invading melanoma cells.

In most malignant melanomata, malignant melanocytes from the clumps at the epidermodermal junction invade the overlying epidermis. Isolated tumor cells or small clumps of tumor cells lie between the keratinocytes in the upper part of the epidermis.

Most malignant melanomata have both large, polygonal cells and elongated, spindle-shaped cells. Usually the polygonal cells are predominant. Only when a malignant melanoma arises from an acral lentiginous melanoma in situ or a lentigo maligna are spindle cells likely to be predominant. There is no tendency to improved differentiation in the deeper part of the tumor.

Usually the polygonal cells form clumps or sheets separated by a scanty collagenous stroma. Rarely, the stroma is extensive, with only small, widely separated clumps of melanoma cells. In most malignant melanomata

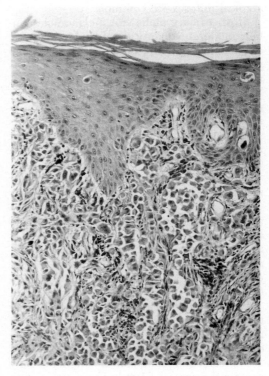

Fig. 62-41. Malignant melanoma. Large, polygonal tumor cells invade the dermis.

the polygonal tumor cells are anaplastic and pleomorphic, with irregular, hyperchromatic nuclei. Sometimes bizarre, multinucleated giant cells are present. Less often the malignant cells are better differentiated and more like the cells of a compound nevus. In these tumors the malignant cells often form clumps and columns like those of a pigmented nevus. Rarely, some of the tumor cells in the dermis are like those of a balloon cell nevus. They have abundant, pale cytoplasm and small, regular, central nuclei.

The spindle cells tend to grow in swirling bundles. At times the dermal part of a spindle-cell melanoma resembles a fibrosarcoma. Occasionally the spindle-shaped tumor cells are widely separated by an abundant collagenous stroma, and the lesion resembles a blue nevus.

Mitoses are nearly always present in invasive melanomata. They are often few, but are sometimes numerous. The mitoses are present both in the clumps of cells at the epidermodermal junction and in the cells in the dermis. In the more anaplastic tumors, atypical mitoses are common.

Most primary malignant melanomata contain moderate quantities of melanin. Some are heavily pigmented, and some contain no melanin. A malignant melanoma that contains no melanin is called an amelanotic melanoma. If a melanoma is moderately or heavily pigmented, melanin is usually present both in the tumor cells and in macrophages in its stroma. The deeper part of a malignant melanoma usually contains as much melanin as does its superficial portion.

An exudate of lymphocytes with smaller numbers of plasma cells and macrophages is usually prominent at the deep margin of a melanoma that extends only a short way into the dermis. The majority of the lymphocytes in the exudate are activated T cells. Inflammation is usually scant or absent at the margin of a melanoma that extends deep into the dermis or into the subcutaneous tissue.

If an invasive melanoma arises from one of the forms of melanoma in situ, the changes of melanoma in situ are usually evident in the epidermis around the invasive lesion.

The cells of a malignant melanoma usually contain the protein S100 and sometimes stain for vimentin. They do not stain for cytokeratins. Some stain with antibodies against the cells of other malignant melanomata. Electron microscopy sometimes can demonstrate melanosomes in the cells of an anaplastic tumor, proving it to be a melanoma.

Behavior. Malignant melanomata of the epidermis first invade the underlying dermis. Many of them remain confined to the dermis long enough to allow complete excision. Some invade more deeply, extending into the subcutaneous tissues.

Metastases usually appear first in the regional lymph nodes. In some patients, they are present before the primary tumor is detected. Occasionally the metastases remain confined to the regional lymph nodes, but often they extend to more distant nodes. Not uncommonly, a malignant melanoma causes extensive involvement of lymph nodes as the tumor spreads from one group of lymph nodes to the next.

Blood-borne metastases are common, unless the primary tumor is promptly eradicated. The lungs are involved in 90% of people dying of melanoma, the central nervous system in 80%, the gastrointestinal tract in 70%, the liver in 70%, the heart in 70%, the peritoneum in 60%, the skin in 60%, and the adrenal glands in 50%. Metastases sometimes occur in the mucosa of the bowel and in other unusual sites.

Malignant melanomata are unpredictable. Some grow sluggishly for years and then suddenly metastasize widely. Some spread widely and then become arrested. Some patients with widespread metastatic melanoma remain in good health. Many of the malignant tumors that have regressed spontaneously have been malignant melanomata.

Occasionally a patient with widespread metastatic melanoma has melanuria. Products of tyrosine metabolism escape from the tumor cells into the plasma and are excreted in the urine. They darken when exposed to air.

Rarely, a malignant melanoma causes generalized melanosis. Melanin escapes from the tumor cells into the blood and is taken up by macrophages in such quantity that the skin, mucous membranes, and conjunctivae turn black. The intima of the blood vessels and some of the internal organs are similarly pigmented.

In 5% of patients with metastatic melanoma, no primary tumor is evident. In most of these patients, the primary tumor was probably removed months or years earlier and discarded in the belief that it was a harmless, pigmented nevus. In some, the primary tumor may have regressed and disappeared. In a few, a primary melanoma arising in an internal organ is mistaken for a metastasis.

Metastatic Melanoma. In most patients, the metastases of a malignant melanoma are similar to the primary tumor. In some, the metastases are more anaplastic or occasionally are better differentiated. In many metastatic melanomata, the tumor forms large sheets with little stroma between them. The tumor cells are large and clearly demarcated. They are slightly separated from one another. Their cytoplasm is eosinophilic and abundant. The nuclei have large nucleoli.

Frequently some of metastases are more heavily pigmented than are others. Occasionally an amelanotic or slightly pigmented primary tumor gives rise to deeply pigmented metastases, or some of the metastases from a deeply pigmented primary melanoma contain little or no pigment.

Secondary melanoma in the skin forms a nodule in the dermis. Unless the lesion ulcerates, the overlying epidermis is intact. The junctional activity nearly always demonstrable in a primary malignant melanoma is not present.

Immunologic Abnormalities. About 40% of patients with invasive malignant melanoma have in their plasma antibodies against cytoplasmic antigens in the melanoma cells. These antibodies are not specific for the patient's melanoma, but react with the cells of any melanoma. They seem identical with the antibodies in people with a halo nevus. Similar antibodies can sometimes be found in the blood of people with other kinds of tumor, even occasionally in normal people.

Antibodies against antigens in the cell membrane of the cells of the patient's own melanoma can be demonstrated in 40% of people with malignant melanoma. This kind of antibody does not occur in people without a melanoma. About 20% of people with a malignant melanoma that has not extended far have in their blood antibodies that damage

the cells of the melanoma when cultured with them in vitro. Usually the antibodies do not react with the cells of other melanomata.

All these antibodies against melanoma cells are most common in the early stages of the disease. They tend to disappear as the tumor becomes widespread.

Nearly 60% of patients with invasive melanoma develop a delayed hypersensitivity reaction when melanoma cells or an extract of melanoma cells is injected into the skin. A similar reaction develops in 20% of normal people when melanoma cells are injected in similar fashion.

In more than 60% of patients with malignant melanoma, antigens from the melanoma cells can cause transformation of the patient's lymphocytes. In more than 50% of the patients, antigens from the melanoma cells cause the release of lymphokines from the lymphocytes.

In more than 70% of patients with malignant melanoma, the patient's lymphocytes kill melanoma cells in vitro or inhibit their growth. The lymphocytes of many normal people are able to injure melanoma cells in vitro in similar fashion. T cells, B cells, and null cells all show this sort of cytotoxicity, though the B cells often require a factor present in the serum of people with melanoma, perhaps an antibody. Immunization with the bacillus of Calmette and Guérin sometimes slightly increases the ability of lymphocytes to damage melanoma cells.

The sera of many patients with malignant melanoma contain a factor that impairs the cytotoxic reaction of the lymphocytes. The nature of this blocking factor is uncertain. Many patients with widespread malignant melanoma react poorly to agents unrelated to the melanoma that normally stimulate cellular or humoral immunity.

Whether these immunologic changes are a valuable defense against malignant melanoma or a response to it that is of little benefit to the patient is uncertain. There is a strong suggestion that activated lymphocytes attack the melanoma cells early in the course of the disease. Both the presence of activated lymphocytes in the blood and the lymphocytic exudate at the base of the tumor suggest that this may well be so. If so, this defense fails as the tumor extends.

Pathogenesis. The relationship between pigmented nevi and malignant melanoma is uncertain. Patients often say that a malignancy developed at the site of a mole, but it is hard to evaluate these accounts. Remnants of a pigmented nevus are present beside or deep within the malignant lesion in more than 10% of invasive melanomata, suggesting strongly that in some patients a malignant melanoma does arise from recrudescence of junctional activity in a previously benign lesion.

Ultraviolet radiation is of major importance in the causation of malignant melanoma. Malignant melanomata develop predominantly in fair-skinned people. They are more common in sunny countries. Malignant melanomata of the lower leg are more common in women, perhaps because they wear skirts, exposing their legs to the sun.

The role of trauma is controversial. The possible danger of injuring or irritating moles has long been discussed, without clear evidence that injury does cause malignant transformation of the lesion. Malignant melanomata of the sole of the foot are more common in people who walk barefoot, perhaps because of repeated injuries to the sole.

The suggestion that malignant melanomata are likely to develop during pregnancy has not been substantiated, but sometimes a malignant melanoma grows more aggressively during pregnancy. Rarely, a malignant melanoma regresses during pregnancy, only to recur after it.

Picornaviruses like those that cause tumors in animals have been found in human malignant melanomata. Reverse transcriptase has been identified in human melanoma cells, suggesting that such viruses might cause the melanoma.

Genetic factors may be involved. People from Scandinavia are particularly likely to develop malignant melanomata. In some families, there is an inherited predisposition to develop malignant melanomata. About 3% of patients with malignant melanoma show a familial predisposition of this sort. Malignant melanomata are twice as common in close relatives of patients with a malignant melanoma as in the general population. People with xeroderma pigmentosum have a greatly increased risk of developing lentigo senilis and malignant melanoma.

Treatment and Prognosis. A malignant melanoma of the skin is treated by excision with an ample margin around and deep to the tumor. Some remove the regional lymph nodes even if there is no evidence that they are involved, but most think that this does not improve the prognosis. If metastases develop, radiotherapy, chemotherapy, and attempts to excite an immunologic reaction against the melanoma by giving the bacillus of Calmette-Guérin or a similar agent are of limited value.

The prognosis is good in elderly people who develop an invasive melanoma in lentigo maligna. Excision of the tumor brings cure in over 90% of the patients. The prognosis is gloomy in people with an invasive melanoma arising in acral lentiginous melanoma in situ. Nearly 90% of the patients die within four years.

With invasive melanomata arising in a superficial spreading melanoma or as a nodular melanoma, the prognosis depends on the depth of the invasion of the dermis. Because nodular melanomata tend to grow more rapidly than do invasive melanomata arising in superficial spreading melanoma, they are more dangerous, but if the depth of invasion of the skin is the same, the prognosis is the same in the two types of invasive melanoma.

In one system for measuring the depth of invasion of the skin, melanomata of the epidermis are divided into five groups. In level I, the tumor is confined to the epidermis and its appendages, that is to say, it is a melanoma in situ. In level II, the tumor has invaded the fine, papillary dermis immediately below the epidermis, but has not reached the coarser reticular dermis. In level III, the melanoma has filled the papillary dermis and impinges on the reticular dermis without invading it. In level IV, the tumor invades the reticular dermis. In level V, the tumor invades the subcutaneous fat.

If this system is used, all melanomata confined to level I are cured by local excision. If a nodular melanoma or an invasive melanoma arising in superficial spreading melanoma in situ is at level II when it is excised, over 90% of the patients are alive five years later. If it is at level III, 65% of the patients survive five years; if at level IV, 55%; and if at level V, 45%.

Another system for measuring the depth of invasion of the skin measures the distance from the top of the granular layer of the epidermis to the deepest extension of the tumor in lesions in which the epidermis is intact and from the base of ulcer to the deepest part of the tumor in lesions that are ulcerated. Only tumor invading from the epidermis itself is measured. Melanoma invading the dermis from a skin appendage may be further from the granular layer of base of the ulcer, but is not considered.

With this system, almost all melanomata less than 0.76 mm thick are cured by local excision. Over 75% of patients with a tumor 0.77 to 1.5 mm thick are alive five years later. Over 60% of those with tumors more than 1.5 mm thick survive five years.

Other factors are of less importance in determining the prognosis of a malignant melanoma. Women do better than men. In one series, 53% of men and 67% of women survived five years. The prognosis is better when a melanoma arises in the hairy part of the limbs than when it is on the face, neck, or trunk. Large lesions do worse than small lesions. Ulceration worsens the prognosis. Anaplastic lesions are more dangerous than well-differentiated tumors. An abundance of melanin makes the melanoma more easily detected and improves the prognosis. A prominent lymphocytic exudate at the base of the lesion is a good sign.

If the regional lymph nodes are involved, the prognosis depends on the number of lymph nodes affected. In one series, 45% of the patients with only one node involved but less than 10% of those with four nodes affected, were alive five years later. Few patients with hematogenous metastases live long.

MALIGNANT BLUE NEVUS. Malignant blue nevi are rare. The tumor resembles a cellular blue nevus, but the tumor cells are more atypical and often pleomorphic. Mitoses are present and are occasionally abnormal. Foci of necrosis are not uncommon. The tumor may ulcerate through the epidermis or extend into the subcutaneous tissue. In some pa-

tients, the tumor metastasizes to the regional lymph nodes. In a few, widespread hematogenous metastases develop.

Dermal Tumors

The tumors and tumor-like lesions that involve principally the dermis are divided into five groups: collagenous tumors, vascular tumors, tumors of smooth muscle, tumors of macrophages, and lymphoid tumors.

COLLAGENOUS TUMORS. The collagenous tumors and tumor-like conditions of the dermis include the dermatofibroma, dermatofibrosarcoma protruberans, atypical fibroxanthoma, tuberous sclerosis, soft fibroma, digital fibrokeratoma, fibrous papule of the face, focal mucinosis, digital mucinous cyst, infantile digital fibromatosis, connective tissue nevus, and nevus lipomatosus.

Dermatofibroma. A dermatofibroma is a common neoplasm sometimes called a sclerosing hemangioma, fibrous histiocytoma, or histiocytoma. Some 80% of dermatofibromata arise on a limb. Women are affected more often than men. Most of the patients are between 20 and 50 years old. Occasionally there is a history of minor injury at the site of the lesion. Most patients have only a single lesion, but some have two or three.

A round or ovoid lesion appears in the skin. Most dermatofibromata are less than 0.5 cm across. A few are 2 or 3 cm in diameter. The lesion is usually dome-shaped, but sometimes is depressed. Most dermatofibromata are brown. Some are bluish, reddish, or yellowish. The lesion persists indefinitely, but does not enlarge.

Microscopically, the majority of dermatofibromata consist of intertwining bundles of spindle-shaped fibrocytes separated by collagen. In some tumors, the collagen is abundant and the fibrocytes are small and inconspicuous. In others, the fibrocytes are more numerous and larger, with only fine collagen fibers between the tumor cells. Many of the tumors have a storiform pattern. The fibrocytes show little atypicality. Mitoses are rare or absent.

In many dermatofibromata, some or many of the tumor cells resemble macrophages.

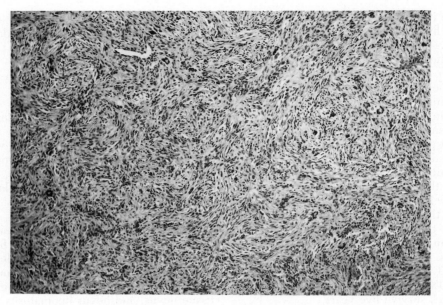

Fig. 62-42. A dermatofibroma showing the bundles of well-differentiated fibrocytes that make up the tumor.

They are roughly ovoid, well-defined, and have abundant cytoplasm. Their nuclei are round or ovoid and vesicular. Only a few fine collagen fibers separate the cells. In 30% of the tumors, some of the macrophage-like cells contain droplets of fat or granules of hemosiderin. Occasionally some of them are distended by fat. Often some of the macrophage-like cells are multinucleate. If a multinucleate cell contains fat, the nuclei are at the margin of the cell.

Small blood vessels with thick endothelium are scattered throughout a dermatofibroma. In some lesions, they are numerous. Sometimes the fibrocytes swirl around the vessels. Occasionally there are small hemorrhages adjacent to the vessels.

In 80% of dermatofibromata, the overlying epidermis is thickened, and its rete ridges are elongated. Often the quantity of melanin in the basal part of the epidermis is considerably increased. Occasionally the rete ridges interconnect as they do in a seborrheic keratosis. In 2% of the lesions, downgrowths from the epidermis like those of a superficial basal cell carcinoma are present over the lesion.

Dermatofibromata are not well-defined. They are often separated from the epidermis by a band of dermis with fine collagen fibers, but merge vaguely with the dermis at their lateral margins. Occasionally a dermatofibroma extends irregularly into the subcutaneous tissue.

Electron microscopy leaves little doubt that dermatofibromata are tumors of fibrocytes. Some macrophages are present in the lesions, but even the macrophage-like tumor cells have the fine structure of a fibrocyte or myofibrocyte. If it is necessary to remove the tumor for diagnostic or cosmetic reasons, excision cures.

Dermatofibrosarcoma Protruberans. A dermatofibrosarcoma protruberans is a malignant neoplasm. It is not common. A firm, brownish or reddish plaque develops in the skin, most often on the trunk, occasionally on the proximal part of a limb, or elsewhere. The patient is usually an adult, more often a man than a woman. As the years pass, the tumor enlarges slowly and may become irregular and nodular. It may ulcerate. After 10 years or more, it may grow to be over 10 cm across.

Microscopically, a dermatofibrosarcoma protruberans shows intertwining bundles of fibrocytes, much as in a desmoid tumor. Often parts of the tumor show a storiform

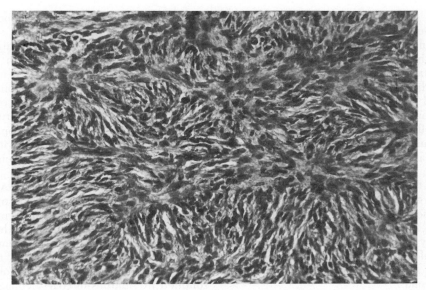

Fig. 62-43. A dermatofibrosarcoma protruberans, showing the storiform pattern and mild atypicality usual in these tumors.

pattern, with the nuclei of the tumor cells radiating as from the hub of a wheel. The tumor cells are mildly atypical and show occasional mitoses. Often there are fragments of basement membrane between them. The tumor merges vaguely with the surrounding dermis. It may extend into the subcutaneous tissue or more deeply. The overlying epidermis may be slightly thickened or may be thin, even invaded by the tumor with ulceration.

A dermatofibrosarcoma protruberans invades slowly but persistently. Complete excision cures. Incomplete excision is often followed by recurrence. Metastases occur in only 5% of the patients after many years and often after several unsuccessful attempts to eradicate the tumor surgically. They are most common in the regional lymph nodes and the lungs.

Atypical Fibroxanthoma. Atypical fibroxanthomata are common. A tumor appears in skin exposed to sunlight in an elderly person or on the trunk or limbs in a younger person, sometimes in a region previously irradiated. The tumor forms a nodule usually less than 3 cm across. Sometimes it ulcerates. The lesion often enlarges progressively, but may become stationary and persist with little change for years.

Microscopically, the tumor is highly cellular. It extends to the epidermis and often invades the subcutaneous tissue. Some of the tumor cells are small and resemble fibrocytes. Others are larger, polygonal, with abundant cytoplasm that sometimes is foamy or vacuolated. The nuclei of the tumor cells are hyperchromatic and irregular. Mitoses are numerous and often atypical. Bizarre, multinucleated giant cells are often present. Only occasional strands of collagen separate the tumor cells.

An atypical fibroxanthoma is believed to be a form of the malignant fibrous histiocytoma of deeper tissues described in Chapter 61. Like the malignant fibrous histiocytoma, it is probably derived from fibrocytes. The prognosis is better than that of a malignant fibrous histiocytoma. Most atypical fibroxanthomata are cured by excision, perhaps because the tumor is discovered while it is still small. A few metastasize to the regional lymph nodes.

Tuberous Sclerosis. Tuberous sclerosis is a disease inherited as an autosomal dominant character that causes lesions in many organs, most notably in the central nervous system, kidneys, and heart. It is discussed in Chapter 57. In the skin, it causes angiofibromata on the face, larger fibromata on the face and scalp, subungual fibromata, shagreen patches, and foci of depigmentation.

Angiofibromata used to be called sebaceous adenomata. They develop in childhood. Multiple reddish papules appear on the cheeks, nasolabial folds, and chin. Microscopically, the lesions show an ill-defined proliferation of fine collagenous tissue in which there are many small blood vessels. Intercellular substance is abundant in the lesions. The fibrocytes are usually stellate. The sebaceous glands in the lesions are atrophic.

The larger fibromata that develop on the face and scalp in some of the patients consist of coarse, sclerotic collagen arranged concentrically around atrophic hair follicles. The subungual fibromata are sometimes similar, but often show the loose fibrosis seen in an angiofibroma.

Shagreen patches, named after a coarse kind of leather, are most common in the lumbosacral region. They are slightly raised lesions that resemble pigskin. Microscopically, most patches show replacement of the deeper part of the dermis by dense, hyalinized collagen. Less often, the roughly parallel bundles of collagen in the dermis are replaced by interwoven bundles of similar collagen.

Small, leaflike patches of depigmentation are present in the skin in many people with tuberous sclerosis. They are present at birth or appear soon after, before other manifestations of the disorder are evident. In the depigmented regions, the melanocytes are small and produce little melanin.

Soft Fibroma. A soft fibroma, often called a skin tag, sometimes an acrochordon from the Greek words for end and sausage, is probably a malformation rather than a neoplasm. Soft fibromata are common in middle-aged people especially in women. Some of the patients develop multiple papillae less than 0.3 cm across, most frequently on the neck and in the axillae. Some develop a single filiform lesion about 0.5 cm long. Others develop a more broadly based, soft, pedunculated lesion often more than 1 cm long, most commonly on the lower part of the trunk. Microscopically, the lesion consists of unremarkable dermis covered by normal epidermis. In 30% of filiform lesions, remnants of a pigmented nevus are demonstrable.

In some of the larger lesions, adipocytes are present within the lesion.

Digital Fibrokeratoma. A digital fibrokeratoma is an uncommon growth that develops in adult life. An elongated or dome-shaped mass extends from near one of the interphalangeal joints of a finger or toe or from a palm or sole. Sometimes it resembles a supernumerary digit. Microscopically, a thick, hyperkeratotic epidermis with thick, branching rete ridges covers unremarkable dermis.

Fibrous Papule of the Face. A fibrous papule of the face is common. A firm, dome-shaped nodule less than 0.5 cm across develops, most frequently on the nose. Microscopically, the lesions resemble the angiofibromata that develop in tuberous sclerosis. Vellus hair follicles are often surrounded by bundles of coarse collagen. The overlying epidermis is sometimes pigmented, or melanophores are present in the dermis.

Focal Mucinosis. In focal mucinosis, also called cutaneous myxoma, a solitary nodule about 1 cm across develops on the face, trunk, or a limb. The lesion is sometimes erythematous or fluctuant. Microscopically, it shows replacement of the dermis by myxomatous tissue. Intercellular material is abundant in the lesion and surrounds stellate myofibrocytes. Excision cures.

Digital Mucous Cyst. A digital mucous cyst forms an often cystic lesion less than 1 cm across at the base of a fingernail or toenail. Young lesions are like those of focal mucinosis. Older lesions tend to become a cyst filled with mucus. Some think the disease a form of focal mucinosis. Others think it is caused by leakage of joint fluid into the tissues. The lesions sometimes recur after excision.

Infantile Digital Fibromatosis. In infantile digital fibromatosis, also called recurrent digital fibroma, one or more fibromata are present on the fingers at birth or appear during childhood. In 75% of the children, the lesions recur if removal is attempted. Microscopically, the lesions consist of interlacing bundles of collagen and myofibrocytes. The lesion often extends into the subcutaneous tissue. Many of the myofibrocytes contain granular inclusions 3 to 10 μm in diameter without a limiting membrane. The inclusions are formed by malformation and aggregation of the myofilaments in the tumor cells. As the child ages, the lesions disappear, leaving a scar.

Connective Tissue Nevus. Connective tissue nevi are hamartomata present at birth or that appear soon after. In some patients, the disorder is inherited as an autosomal dominant character. Some have osteopoikilosis as well as connective tissue nevi, a condition called dermatofibrosis lenticularis. Slightly elevated, indurated plaques develop in the skin. Microscopically, the dermis is thickened. Occasionally its collagen bundles are hyalinized. Elastic fibers are sometimes increased, sometimes normal, sometimes reduced.

Nevus Lipomatosus. A nevus lipomatosus is an uncommon malformation most often found on a buttock. Occasionally the lesion does not develop until adult life. The patient develops a group of flat, wrinkled, yellowish papules. In the lesions, the dermis is partly replaced by adipose tissue. The adipocytes form small clumps among the collagen bundles of the dermis. Occasionally a pigmented nevus develops in a nevus lipomatosus.

VASCULAR TUMORS. Vascular tumors and tumor-like conditions of the skin are common. Among them are the nevus flammeus, capillary hemangioma, cavernous hemangioma, pyogenic granuloma, angiokeratoma, angioma serpiginosum, cherry hemangioma, papular angioplasia, venous lake, Kaposi's sarcoma, and angiosarcoma.

Nevus Flammeus. A nevus flammeus, from the Latin for flaming, is a malformation often called a port wine mark. Up to 75% of infants have a lesion of this sort in the midline of the head, most often in the occipital region. Most of these lesions fade and disappear within a year. Some persist as discolored patches that do not become raised or nodular. Less frequently a nevus flammeus is on the lateral side of the head. Occasionally it is bilateral or involves other parts of the body. On the face, a lateral lesion darkens and often becomes raised and nodular as the child ages. It persists throughout life.

Some of the patients with a lateral nevus flammeus on the face have the Sturge-Weber syndrome discussed in Chapter 57. Patients with a nevus flammeus on a limb sometimes have the Klippel-Trenaunay syndrome named after the French physicians who described it in 1900. The limb or limbs affected is hypertrophied. It often has arteriovenous fistulae or develops varicose veins.

In children with the midline type of nevus flammeus, the dermis shows little abnormality. If the lesions persist into adult life, the blood vessels in the upper dermis are dilated.

The lateral lesions show little abnormality until the patient is over 10 years old, but the blood vessels in the dermis then grow increasingly ectatic. The superficial vessels are most affected, but vessels deep in the dermis are also dilated. Loose collagenous tissue surrounds the ectatic vessels. In patients with the Klippel-Trenaunay syndrome, capillaries and fibrocytes proliferate around the arteriovenous anastomoses. Red cells lie free of proliferating tissue and hemosiderin accumulates. The proliferation is benign but can resemble Kaposi's sarcoma.

Capillary Hemangioma. A capillary hemangioma, or strawberry mark, of the skin is a common malformation. One or a few lesions are present at birth or become evident soon after. Rarely, large areas of skin are involved. The lesions are most common on the face and are more common in girls than in boys. Capillary hemangiomata grow rapidly for three to six months, becoming bright red, tense, and often several centimeters across. When the child is a few years old, the lesions begin to regress. In 90% of the patients, they disappear completely, leaving no disfigurement.

In its early stages, a capillary hemangioma of the skin consists of clumps and cords of endothelial cells set in a collagenous stroma, with little or no canalization. Later, lumina appear, and the mass becomes a typical capillary hemangioma. As the lesions regress, the vessels become hyalinized and are replaced by collagenous tissue.

Cavernous Hemangioma. Cavernous hemangiomata are malformations that appear in the skin during the first months of life, most often on the face, more often in girls than in boys. There may be one or several of them. Often a strawberry hemangioma overlies a cavernous lesion. Occasionally large

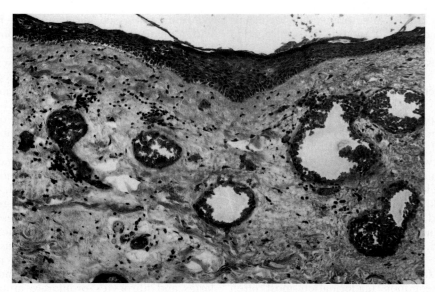

Fig. 62-44. A nevus flammeus, showing widely dilated blood vessels in the dermis.

cavernous hemangiomas of the skin cause considerable deformity. Cavernous hemangiomata enlarge slowly for some years and then partially regress. Usually part of the lesion persists into adult life.

Occasionally a child with a cavernous hemangioma develops thrombocytopenia. A few have Maffucci's syndrome of enchondromatosis and cavernous hemangiomata in the skin and other organs. Occassionally a child has the blue rubber bleb syndrome, so called because of the appearance of the lesions. Most of these children have also hemangiomata in the gut and other internal organs.

Cavernous hemangiomata of the skin are in the deeper part of the dermis and the subcutaneous tissue. They have large blood spaces supported by collagenous tissue. Occasionally muscle is present in the wall of some of the vessels.

Pyogenic Granuloma. A pyogenic granuloma of the skin is similar to the pyogenic granulomata that arise in other organs. It is probably a response to injury, not a neoplasm. The lesion can develop in any part of the skin at any age. A small, erythematous papule enlarges rapidly to form a pedunculated mass rarely more than 1 cm across. Microscopically, the lesion consists of proliferating capil-

laries set in a edematous stroma. In most lesions, neutrophils are numerous. If untreated, a pyogenic granuloma resolves, leaving a small scar.

Angiokeratoma. Five kinds of angiokeratoma are distinguished. Fabry's disease, angiokeratoma corporis diffusum, is described in Chapter 27. In angiokeratoma of Mibelli, named after an Italian dermatologist (1860–1910), lesions appear on the dorsum of the fingers and toes in childhood or adolescence. In scrotal angiokeratoma, multiple lesions appear on the scrotum in adults. In papular angiokeratoma, one or a few lesions develop in young adults, usually on a lower limb. In angiokeratoma circumscriptum, one or more lesions develop in infants or children.

In most forms of angiokeratoma, the lesions are dark red papules less that 0.5 cm across. In angiokeratoma circuscriptum, the lesions coalesce into plaques sometimes more than 5 cm across. Sometimes a nevus flammeus or cavernous hemangioma is present beneath a plaque of angiokeratoma circumscriptum.

Microscopically, the lesions are similar in all types of angiokeratoma. Widely dilated blood vessels are present in the papillary dermis and sometimes extend into the upper part of the reticular dermis. Only in angiokeratoma circumscriptum do the ectatic

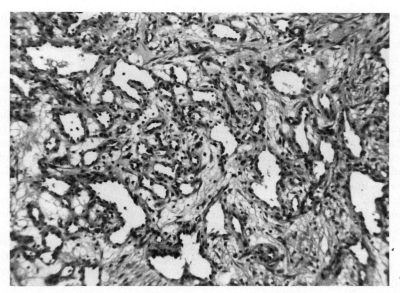

Fig. 62-45. A pyogenic granuloma showing the numerous, irregularly shaped capillaries usual in these lesions.

vessels extend deep into the dermis or into the subcutaneous tissue. The overlying epidermis is often thickened and hyperkeratotic. Often a dilated vessel is surrounded by rete ridges and appears to be within the epidermis. Frequently some of the ectatic blood vessels are thrombosed in people with papular angiokeratoma or angiokeratoma circumscriptum.

Angioma Serpiginosum. In angioma serpiginosum, punctate, red dots form irregular mottled, linear, or reticular patterns, most often on the legs in women. As years pass, the lesions slowly extend. Biopsy shows only ectasia of the blood vessels in the dermal papillae.

Cherry Hemangioma. Cherry hemangiomata are bright red lesions a few millimeters in diameter that begin to appear in the skin early in adult life and become increasingly numerous as age increases. They are especially common on the trunk. At first the lesions resemble a capillary hemangiomata, but as they grow older, the blood vessels gradually dilate. The overlying epidermis is usually thin.

Papular Angioplasia. In papular angioplasia, multiple purplish papules a few millimeters across develop on the face in old people. Microscopically, they show a pro-liferation of blood vessels with extravasation of red cells much as in Kaposi's sarcoma.

Venous Lake. Venous lakes are soft, blue lesions, which develop in the skin in old people, usually on the face, and which are often multiple. They result from dilatation of a single vein.

Kaposi's Sarcoma. The classic form of Kaposi's sarcoma involves principally the skin. It is described together with the other types of Kaposi's sarcoma with the tumors of blood vessels in Chapter 25.

Angiosarcoma. Malignant tumors of blood vessels are rare, but when they do occur they often involve the skin. They are described in Chapter 25.

Proliferating Angioendotheliomatosis. Proliferating angioendotheliomatosis is an uncommon condition. Purple plaques and nodules develop in the skin and may ulcerate. In the lesions, the blood vessels in the dermis are filled by a proliferation of endothelial cells. In some patients, the proliferating endothelial cells are atypical, with hyperchromatic nuclei and mitoses. In these people the disease usually extends to vessels throughout the body and brings death within a year. In other patients, the endothelial cells show little atypicality, and the lesions resolve, usually within 6 to 12 months.

TUMORS OF SMOOTH MUSCLE. Three tumor-like lesions of smooth muscle arise in the skin; smooth muscle hamartoma, leiomyoma, and leiomyosarcoma. All are uncommon.

Smooth Muscle Hamartoma. Smooth muscle hamartomata of the skin are rare. In the part of the skin affected, a group of nodules develop in childhood or early adult life. Sometimes the region is hyperpigmented or hairy. Microscopically, the lesions show bundles of well-differentiated smooth muscle running randomly through the dermis.

Leiomyoma. Four types of leiomyomata arise in the skin. The most common are multiple tumors that arise from the arrector pili muscles. Less often a single tumor arises from an arretor pili, a blood vessel, or on the genitalia.

Multiple leiomyomata arising from the arrectores pilorum begin to appear in adolescence and become increasingly numerous on the face, trunk, and limbs. They form smooth, round nodules, not often more than 1 cm across. At times, the lesions become confluent. Some lesions regress while others enlarge. Often the tumors are both painful and tender. Sometimes the disease is familial.

A solitary leiomyoma arising from an arrector pili muscle appears during adult life and may be up to 2 cm across. It is often tender and painful. A solitary leiomyoma that arises from a blood vessel, usually takes origin from a vein in the subcutaneous tissue. The lesion is usually less than 4 cm in diameter and often is tender or painful. A solitary leiomyoma arising from the dartos muscle of the scrotum, a labium majus, or the nipple, forms a similar nodule but is rarely painful or tender.

The leiomyomata arising from the arectores pilorum and those developing in the scrotum, labium, or nipple form ill-defined masses in the dermis. The lesions consist of interwoven bundles of well-differentiated smooth muscle cells, each surrounded by its basement membrane. More or less collagen is present between the muscle bundles.

The angioleiomyomata arising from blood vessels in the skin are spheroidal and well demarcated. They consist of interwoven bundles of smooth muscle, with little or no collagen between the muscle bundles. Usually large veins are present in the lesion, with the muscular wall of the vein merging with the muscle of the tumor.

Why many of the leiomyomata of the skin are painful or tender is not clear. Some may compress or distort small nerves. Some of the tumors lack cholinesterase, suggesting that the pain may be caused by increased cholinergic activity. At times the pain is caused by contraction of the muscle in the tumors.

Leiomyosarcoma. Leiomyosarcomata of the skin are rare. They are similar to leiomyosarcomata of other parts of the body.

TUMORS OF MACROPHAGES. Tumor-like lesions that consist mainly of macrophages are common in the skin. They include eruptive xanthoma, tuberous xanthoma, plane xanthoma, xanthelasma, reticulohistiocytosis, xanthogranuloma and histiocytosis X. In many of these conditions, the macrophages are called histiocytes. The term *xanthoma*, from the Greek for yellow, is used to describe conditions in which lipid accumulates in macrophages in the skin or other organs.

Eruptive Xanthoma. Eruptive xanthomata develop in patients with an excess of triglyceride in the blood. They are common in people with the genetically determined hyperlipidemias of types I, IIB, III, IV, and V, with their excess of chylomicra, lipoproteins that migrate in the pre-β range, or both. They are less common in other kinds of hypertriglyceridemia, such as that in uncontrolled diabetes mellitus.

When the concentration of triglyceride in the plasma grows high, crops of itchy nodules develop, particularly on the extensor surfaces of the limbs of the buttocks. They are often erythematous or yellow with an erythematous margin. Most are less than 0.5 cm across. If the concentration of lipid in the blood falls, the lesions disappear. Microscopically, eruptive xanthomata show a mixture of macrophages filled with fat, lymphocytes, and neutrophils. Most of the fat in the lesions is triglyceride.

Tuberous Xanthoma. Tuberous xanthomata develop in people with an excess of β-lipoproteins in the blood. They are particularly common in people with hereditary hyperlipemia of type IIA, but also occur in people with hyperlipemia of type III and less often in people with types IIB and IV.

Large, yellow or orange masses develop over the elbows, knuckles, knees, ankles, or on the buttocks, often in regions subject to trauma. They are often irregularly shaped and may be as much as 5 cm across. Tuberous xanthomata do not regress if the hyperlipemia is controlled. Microscopically, they consist of macrophages filled with fat, with an admixture of inflammatory cells in the early stages and increasing fibrosis in the late stages. Some of the fat-filled macrophages are multinucleated. Some of the multinucleated cells have randomly distributed nuclei like those of a foreign body giant cell. Some have the nuclei arranged around the margin of the cell to give what is called a Touton giant cell, after the German dermatologist born in 1858.

Tendon xanthomata are similar to tuberous xanthomata, except that they occur in tendons, most often the Achilles tendons or the extensor tendons of the fingers. Tendon xanthomata occur in people with hereditary hyperlipemia of types IIA and III, less often type IIB.

Plane Xanthoma. Plane xanthomata are most common in people with type III hyperlipidemia and in patients with liver disease. Occasionally they develop in a person with type IV hyperlipidemia, normal plasma lipids, myeloma, lymphoma, or widespread dermatitis.

Plane xanthomata are flat, yellow, or brown macules from 1 to 5 cm across. They tend to occur in skin folds, especially in the palmar creases. In type III hyperlipidemia, they are common on the palms and fingertips. In liver disease, they are most frequent on the palms and dorsa of the hands. Microscopically, the lesions are similar to tuberous xanthomata, though they do not become fibrotic.

Xanthelasma. When a plane xanthoma develops on an eyelid, it is called a xanthelasma, from the Greek for yellow and metal plate. More than 70% of them occur in people with normal concentrations of lipid in the blood. Most of the rest develop in people with hyperlipidemia of Type IIA or Type III.

Reticulohistiocytosis. Reticulohistiocytosis occurs in adults. Over 70% of the patients are women, most about 40 years old. Some have only one or a few rounded nodules up to 2 cm across on the head and neck. Others have numerous lesions in many parts of the skin. Over 70% of the people with multiple lesions develop polyarthritis before the skin lesions appear. The arthritis is often severe. The interphalangeal joints are particularly affected. Almost all other patients develop arthritis subsequently. In more than 50% of the people with multiple lesions, the mucous membranes of the mouth and nose are involved. Rarely, there is infiltration of a lung or another internal organ.

Microscopically, the lesions show an accumulation of macrophages, with abundant, clearly defined eosinophilic cytoplasm that looks like ground glass. The cytoplasm stains strongly with the periodic acid-Schiff reaction and resists digestion with diastase. Occasionally there is a little lipid in the macrophages. Many of the macrophages are mononuclear, but multinucleated macrophages are always present and often are numerous. In early lesions, many lymphocytes and plasma cells are intermixed with the macrophages. In older lesions, lymphocytes and plasma cells are few, and strands of collagen wind between the macrophages, usually isolating each of the large, multinucleated cells. The macrophages contain many lysosomes, but Langerhans inclusions have not been identified. The involved joints show a similar infiltration with macrophages, at first in the synovium, later in the ends of the bones.

In the patients with only a few lesions, the disease usually resolves after some years, and the lesions disappear. In patients with numerous lesions, some regress while others enlarge and new lesions appear. After seven or eight years, the disease gradually becomes quiescent in most patients, and the lesions heal. Both the lesions in the skin and the destruction of the joints often leave permanent disability.

Xanthogranuloma. Xanthogranulomata usually appear in infants during the first six months of life, though occasionally they develop in older children or aults. One, a few, or as many as 100 reddish or yellowish papules develop in the skin, most often on the face or scalp. Usually the lesions regress and disappear within a year. Rarely in adults, repeated crops of lesions develop and regress more quickly, a condition called generalized eruptive histiocytosis. The concentration of lipids in the blood is normal. Rarely, infiltrations of similar character develop in the lungs, liver, spleen, testes, or heart. Rarely, xanthogranulomata involve an eye.

Microscopically, early lesions show an accumulation of macrophages in the dermis, together with a few lymphocytes and eosinophils. Some of the macrophages contain fat; most do not. In older lesions some of the macrophages are multinucleated and the exudate of lymphocytes and eosinophils is more severe. Touton giant cells like those in xanthomata are common. Finally, the macrophages disappear, leaving some fibrosis.

Most think that the xanthogranulomata are a response to injury. Some think the disease a form of histiocytosis X, but the macrophages in xanthogranuloma do not contain the Langerhans inculsions found in histiocytosis X.

Histiocytosis X. Letterer-Siwe disease and other forms of histiocytosis X often affect the skin. They are described in Chapter 51.

LYMPHOID TUMORS. The skin is often involved by tumors of the hematopoietic system, both lymphoma and leukemia. T-cell neoplasms are especially likely to involve the skin. Mycosis fungoides is often confined to the skin. These and other neoplasms of the hematopoietic system that affect the skin are described in earlier chapters. There remain non-neoplastic lesions of the skin that can mimic lymphoma or leukemia; lymphocytoma cutis and lymphocytic infiltration of the skin.

Lymphocytoma Cutis. Lymphocytoma cutis is a nonneoplastic accumulation of lymphocytes in the skin. It is sometimes called Spiegler-Fendt sarcoid, after the Austrian dermatologists Spiegler who described it in 1894 and Fendt who reported it in 1900, or pseudolymphoma. About 70% of the patients are women. Most of them are 15 to 30 years old.

About 75% of the patients have a single lesion, most often on the face. The others have several lesions, sometimes in different parts of the skin. The lesions range from nodules less than 1 cm in diameter to plaques more than 5 cm across. They may be skin colored, purple, or red.

Microscopically, the lesions show a dense exudate in the dermis. The larger lesions extend into the subcutaneous tissue. Usually the exudate is separated from the epidermis by a narrow band of uninvolved dermis. The exudate consists principally of a mixture of lymphocytes and macrophages, though there are usually a few plasma cells and sometimes a few eosinophils. The lymphocytes and macrophages are well differentiated and mixed at random. In many patients, there are germinal centers in the exudate. If germinal centers are present, most of the lymphocytes are B cells, which are polyclonal. If they are not, the majority are T cells.

Lymphocytoma cutis is believed to be a reaction to injury. The localized form of the disease usually resolves spontaneously after persisting for months or years. The disseminated form may also resolve, though only after many years. Local irradiation or local injection of adrenocorticosteroids usually causes the lesions to regress.

Lymphocytic Infiltration of the Skin. Lymphocytic infiltration of the skin occurs most often in men 20 to 40 years old. One or more reddish brown papules appear, most often on the face, neck, or trunk. The lesions extend peripherally. Some become several centimeters across. Some heal in the center but extend at the periphery. The lesions persist for months or years, but then regress leaving no scarring. They often recur later, at the same or another site.

Microscopically, there is a dense exudate in the dermis, predominantly of lymphocytes, though usually with a few macrophages and plasma cells. Often the exudate is concentrated around appendages or blood vessels. Sometimes, but not always, the lesions respond to drugs like chloroquine, as do the lesions of discoid lupus erythematosus.

Some think that lymphocytic infiltration of the skin is a form of discoid lupus erythematosis. More probably it is a response that can be initiated in more than one way.

SECONDARY TUMORS. A variety of tumors can metastasize to the skin, but except in leukemia involvement of the skin is not common.

Metastatic Carcinoma. Carcinomata of internal organs metastasize to the skin in less than 5% of patients with an internal carcinoma. When cutaneous metastases do appear, they are usually late in the course of the disease.

In men, metastatic carcinomata reach the skin in the blood and form spheroidal nodules of tumor. The primary tumor is in a lung in 25% of men with carcinoma metastatic to the skin; in the colon in 20%; the mouth in 15%; a kidney in 7%; and in the stomach in 7%.

In women, metastatic carcinoma in the skin is more common, because of the frequency with which carcinoma of the breast metastasizes to the skin. In 70% of women with metastatic carcinoma in the skin, the primary tumor is in the breast. Usually the involvement of the skin results from lymphatic extension from the breast and begins in the mammary region with nodules or indurated plaques. Sometimes the tumor cells in these lesions form inconspicuous columns between the collagen bundles of the dermis and can easily be overlooked. Hematogenous metastases from the breast to the skin also occur, sometimes causing focal areas of alopecia in the scalp. Internal carcinomata can also metastasize to the skin in women. In 10% of women with metastatic carcinoma in the skin, the primary tumor is in the colon; in 5% it is in a lung; and in 5% it is in an ovary.

Metastatic Melanoma. The skin is a common site for metastases of malignant melanoma. The melanoma can spread in the lymphatics, perhaps with chains of metastases along the course of a lymphatic, or can spread by the blood stream. Metastatic melanoma in the skin forms nodules, sometimes pigmented, sometimes not. Microscopically, the metastases are like a primary malignant melanoma, except that there is no junctional activity and usually no lymphatic exudate at the base of the tumor. If carcinomata and melanomata metastatic to the skin are grouped together, the metastases in the skin are from a melanoma in 10% of men and in 5% of women.

LEUKEMIA AND LYMPHOMA. The skin is involved in 5% of patients with Hodgkin's disease, though only late in the disease. Nodules or plaques appear in the skin and may ulcerate. Microscopically, the lesions show infiltration of the dermis by Hodgkin's disease. In the non-Hodgkin's lymphomata, skin lesions are more common and often appear early in the disease. About 5% of patients with a non-Hodgkin's lymphoma have skin lesions when the diagnosis is made. Over 15% develop them sooner or later. The lesions show infiltration of the dermis by the lymphoma. About 10% of patients with lymphatic or myeloid leukemia develop focal lesions in the skin, usually late in the disease. The lesions are often red or purple and dome-shaped. They show infiltration of the dermis by the leukemic cells. Patients with a non-Hodgkin's lymphoma or lymphatic leukemia sometimes develop eczema or generalized erythroderma.

BIBLIOGRAPHY

General

Ackerman, A. B.: Histologic Diagnosis of Inflammatory Skin Diseases. Philadelphia, Lea & Febiger, 1978.

Ackermann, A. B., et al.: Differential Diagnosis in Dermatopathology II. Philadelphia, Lea & Febiger, 1988.

Beutner, E. H., Chorzelski, T. P., and Kumar, V.: Immunopathology of the Skin. New York, John Wiley & Sons, 1987.

Daróczy, J., & Rácz, I.: Diagnostic Electron Microscopy in Practical Dermatology. Budapest, Akadémiai Kiadó, 1987.

Lever, W. F., and Schaumburg-Lever, G.: Histopathology of the Skin. 6th Ed. Philadelphia, J. B. Lippincott Co., 1983.

Maize, J. C., and Ackerman, A. B.: Pigmented Lesions of the Skin. Philadelphia. Lea & Febiger, 1987.

Mehregan, A. H.: Pinkus' Guide to Dermatohistopathology. 4th Ed. East Norwalk, Appleton & Lange, 1986.

Okun, M. R., Edelstein, L. M., and Fisher, B. K.: Gross and Microscopic Pathology of the Skin. 2nd Ed. Canton, Dermatopathology Foundation Press, 1987.

Schaumberg-Lever, G., and Lever, W. F.: Color Atlas of Histopathology of the Skin. Philadelphia, J. B. Lippincott Co., 1988.

Infection

Bailie, F. B., et al.: Infectious cutaneous gangrene. Ann. Plastic Surg., 19:238, 1987.

Binassi, M.: Profile of cutaneous toxoplasmosis. J. Dermatol., 25:357, 1986.

Dinning, W. J., and Marston, S.: Cutaneous and ocular tuberculosis. J. R. Soc. Med., 78:576, 1985.

Hurwitz, R. M., and Ackerman, A. B.: Cutaneous pathology of the toxic shock syndrome. Am. J. Dermatopathol., 7:563, 1985.

Paletta, C., and Jurkiewicz, M. J.: Hidradenitis suprativa. Clin. Plast. Surg., 14:383, 1987.

Reyes-Flores, O.: Granulomas induced by living agents. Int. J. Dermatol., 25:158, 1986.

Sheagren, J. N.: Staphylococcal infections of the skin and of skin structures. Cutis, 36(5A):2, 1985.

Tuazon, C. V.: Skin and skin structure infections in the patient at risk. Am. J. Med., 76(5A):166, 1984.

Wickboldt, L. G., and Fenske, N. A.: Streptococcal and staphylococcal infections of the skin. Hosp. Pract., 21(3A):41, 1986.

Bullous and Vesicular Diseases

Abel, E.A., and Wood, G. S.: Mechanisms in contact dermatitis. Clin. Rev. Allergy, 4:339, 1986.

Adams, R. M.: Dermatitis in the microelectronics industry. State Art Rev. Occup. Med., 1:155, 1986.

Ahmed, A. R. (ed.): Bullous pemphigoid. Clin. Dermatol., 59(1):1 1987.

Ahrens, E. M.: Cutaneous reactions to neurologic drugs. Neurol. Clin., 5:499, 1987.

Andersen, K. E., et al.: Contact dermatitis. Contact Dermatitis, 16:55, 1987.

Arbesfeld, S. J., and Kurban, A. K.: Behçet's disease. J. Am. Acad. Dermatol., 19:767, 1988.

Atherton, D. J.: Diet and atopic eczema. Clin. Allergy, 18:215, 1988.

Basset, F., Soler, P., and Hance, A. J.: The Langerhans' cell in human pathology. Ann. N. Y. Acad. Sci., 465:324, 1986.

Beutner, E. H., Chorzelski, T. P., and Jablonska, S.: Immunofluorescence tests. Int. J. Dermatol., 24:405, 1985.

Birmingham, D. J.: Contact dermatitis and related dermatoses associated with petroleum recovery and use. State Art Rev. Occup. Med, 3:511, 1988.

Breathnach, S. M., and Katz, S. I.: Cell-mediated immunity in cutaneous disease. Hum. Pathol., 17: 161, 1986.

Breathnach, S. M.: Immunologic aspects of contact dermatitis. Dermatol. Clin., 4:5, 1986.

Briggaman, R. A., Gammon, W. R., and Woodley, D. T.: Epidermolysis bullosa acquisata of the immunopathologic type (dermatolytic phemphigoid). J. Invest. Dermatol., 85(1 Suppl.):79s, 1985.

Bruynzeel-Koomen, C. A., and Bruynzeel, B. L.: Inhalant allergens as contactants in patients with atopic dermatitis. J. Dermatol. (Tokyo), 14:524, 1987.

Camp, R. D. R., and Greaves, M. W.: Inflammatory mediators in the skin. Br. Med. Bull., 43:401, 1987.

Campbell, J. A.: Diet therapy of celiac disease and dermatitis herpetiformis. World Rev. Nutr. Diet., 51:189, 1987.

Castro, R. M., Roscoe, J. T., and Sampaio, S. A.: Brazilian pemphigus foliaceus. Clin. Dermatol. 1(2): 22, 1983.

Chu, A. C.: Bullous dermatoses. Curr. Top. Pathol., 74:225, 1985.

Craighead, J. E. (ed.): Pathogenesis, clinical features, and management of the non-dermatological complications of epidermolysis bullosa. Arch. Dermatol, 124:705, 1988.

DeSwarte, R. D.: Drug allergy. Clin. Rev. Allergy, 4:143, 1986.

Diaz, L. A., Anhalt, G. J., Patel, H. P., and Provost, T. T.: Autoimmune cutaneous diseases. In The Autoim-

mune Diseases. Edited by Rose, N. R., and Mackay, I. R. Orlando, FL, Academic Press, 1985.

Editorial: Cutaneous photosensitivity. Lancet, 1:1317, 1988.

Epstein, W. L.: Plant-induced dermatitis. Ann. Emerg. Med., 16:950, 1987.

Espinoza, C. G., and Fenske, N. A.: Dermatological manifestations of toxic agents. Ann. Clin. Lab. Sci., 18:148, 1988.

Fabbri, P., Lotti, T., and Paconesi, E.: Pathogenesis of pemphigus. The role of epidermal plasminogen activators in acantholysis. Int. J. Dermatol., 24:422, 1985.

Fine, J. -D.: Monoclonal antibodies and the skin biopsy. Am. J. Med. Sci., 290:143, 1985.

Fine, J. -D.: Epidermolysis bullosa. Int. J. Dermatol., 25:143, 1986.

Fine, J. -D.: Changing clinical and laboratory concepts in inherited epidermolysis bullosa. Arch. Dermatol., 124:523, 1988.

Fineman, S. M.: Urticara and angioneurotic edema. Prim. Care, 14:503, 1987.

Fiore, P. M., Jacobs, I. H. and Goldberg, D. B.: Drug-induced pemphigoid. Arch. Ophthalmol., 105:1660, 1987.

Fisher, A. A.: Reactions of the mucous membranes to contactants. Clin. Dermatol. 5(2):123, 1987.

Fisher, G. B., Jr., Greer, K. E., and Cooper, P. H.: Congenital self healing (transient) mechanobullous dermatosis. Arch. Dermatol., 124:240, 1988.

Fitzmaurice, M.: The immunopathology of pemphigus vulgaris. Cleve. Clin. Q., 53:283, 1986.

Goodman, R. M. (Ed.): Genodermatoses. Clin. Dermatol., 3(1):1, 1985.

Greaves, M. W., and Camp, R. D.: Prostaglandins, leukotrienes, phospholipase, platelet activating factor, and cytokines: an integrated approach to inflammation Dermatol. Rev. 280 (Suppl):533, 1988.

Guin, J. D., and Beaman, J. H. (eds.): Plant dermatitis. Clin. Dermatol., 4(2):1, 1986.

Haber, R. M., Hanna, W., Ramsay, C. A., and Boxall, L. B. H.: Hereditary epidermolysis bullosa. J. Am. Acad. Dermatol., 13:252, 1985.

Hall, R. P.: The pathogenesis of dermatitis herpetiformis. J. Am. Acad. Dermatol., 16: 1129, 1987.

Halpern, G. M., and Scott, J. R.: Non-IgE antibody mediated mechanisms in food allergy. Ann. Allergy, 58:14, 1987.

Hanifin, J. M.: Atopic dermatitis. Monogr. Allergy, 21:116, 1987.

Hickman, J. G.: Pyoderma gangrenosum. Clin. Dermatol. 1(1):102, 1983.

Ho, V. C., Stein, H. B., Ongley, R. C., and McLeod, W. A.: Penicillamine induced pemphigus. J. Rheumatol., 12:583, 1985.

Holgate, S. T., Robinson, C., and Church, M. K.: The contribution of mast cell mediators to acute allergic reactions in human skin and airways. Allergy, 43 (Suppl. 5):22, 1988.

Huff, J. C.: Erythema multiforme. Dermatol. Clin., 3:141, 1985.

Ikai, K., and Imamura, S.: Prostaglandin D2 in the skin. Int. J. Dermatol., 18:619, 1988.

Izuno, G. T.: Cutaneous immunofluorescence. Clin. Lab. Med., 6:85, 1986.

Jordon, R. E., Kawana, S., and Fritz, K. A.: Immunopathologic mechanisms in pemphigus and pemphigoid. J. Invest. Dermatol., 85(1 Suppl.)72s, 1985.

Kahn, G.: Photosensitivity and photodermatitis in children. Dermatol. Clin., 4:107, 1986.

Kaplan, A. P., Buckley, R. H., and Mathews, K. P.: Allergic skin disorders. J. A. M. A., 258:2900, 1987.

Kaplan, R. P., and Callen, J. P.: Pemphigus associated diseases and induced pemphigus. Clin. Dermatol. 1(2):42, 1983.

Kegel, M. F.: Dominant disorders with multiple organ involvement. Dermatol. Clin., 5:205, 1987.

Korman, N.: Pemphigus. J. Am. Acad. Dermatol., 18:1219, 1988.

Kumar, V., Beutner, E. H., and Chorzelski, T. P.: Autoimmunity and the skin. Concepts Immunopathol., 1:318, 1985.

Labib, R. S., Patel, H., Anhalt, G. J., and Diaz, L. A.: The pemphigus antigens. Clin. Dermatol., 1(2):82, 1983.

Ledesma, G. N., and McCormack, P. C.: Erythema multiforme. Clin. Dermatol., 4(1):70, 1986.

Leung, D. Y., and Geha, R. S.: Immunoregulatory abnormalities in atopic dermatitis. Clin. Rev. Allergy, 4:67, 1986.

Liu, H. N., Su, W. P., and Rogers, R. S., III: Clinical variants of pemphagoid. Int. J. Dermatol., 25:17, 1986.

Ljunggren, B., and Bjellerup, M.: Systemic drug photosensitivity. Photodermatol., 3:26, 1986.

Malkinson, F. D.: Pyoderma gangrenosum v malignant pyoderma. Arch. Dermatol., 123:333, 1987.

Martin, J. E., and Harkless, L. B.: Pyoderma gangrenosum. J. Am. Podiatr. Med. Assoc., 76:416, 1986.

Maurer, T.: Skin as a target organ of immunotoxicity reactions. Dev. Toxicol. Environ. Sci., 12:147, 1986.

Menné, T., and Christophersen, J.: Epidemiology of allergic contact sensitization. Curr. Probl. Dermatol., 14:1–30, 1985.

Menné, T., Christophersen, J., and Maibach, H. I.: Epidemiology of allergic contact sensitization. Monogr. Allergy, 21:132, 1987.

Meyrick Thomas, R. H., Black, M. M., and Bhogal, B.: The value of immunofluorescence techniques in the diagnosis of skin disorders. Rec. Adv. Histopathol., 12:69, 1984.

Millikan, L. E.: Vesciculobullous skin disease with prominent immunologic feature. J. A. M. A., 258: 2910, 1988.

Morlière, P.: Drug-induced photosensitivity. Biochemie, 68:849, 1986.

Paller, A. S.: Allergy in atopic dermatitis. Prim. Care, 14:491, 1987.

Picut, C. A., et al.: Pemphigus research. Immunol. Invest., 15:689, 1986.

Pyeritz, R. E.: Inheritable defects in connective tissue. Hosp. Pract., 2(2):153, 1987.

Rehman, R. S.: Histology of adverse cutaneous drug reactions. Clin. Dermatol., 4(1):23, 1986.

Roth, H. L.: Atopic dermatitis revisited. Int. J. Dermatol., 26:139, 1987.

Rystedt, I.: Hand eczema and long-term prognosis in atopic dermatitis. Acta Derm. Venereol. (Suppl.), 117:1, 1985.

Sampson, H. A.: The role of 'allergy' in atopic dermatitis. Clin. Rev. Allergy, 4:125, 1986.

Sampson, H. A.: Late-phase response to food in atopic dermatitis. Host. Pract., 22(12):111, 1987.

Schlumberger, H. D. (ed.): Epidemiology of allergic diseases. Monogr. Allerg., 21:1, 1987.

Schorr-Lesnick, B., and Brandt, L. J.: Selected rheumatologic and dermatologic manifestations of inflammatory bowel disease. Am. J. Gastroenterol., 83:216, 1988.

Schwaegerle, S. M., Bergfeld, W. F., Senitzer, D., and Tridrick, R. T.: Pyoderma gangrenosum. J. Am. Acad. Dermatol., 18:559, 1988.

Shimada, S., and Katz, S. I.: The skin as an immunologic organ. Arch. Pathol. Lab. Med., 112:231, 1988.

Shmunes, E.: The role of atopy in occupational skin diseases. State Art Rev. Occup. Med., 1:219, 1986.

Shornick, J. K.: Herpes gestationalis. J. Am. Acad. Dermatol., 17:539, 1987.

Silverman, A. K., Fairly, J., and Wong, R. C.: Cutaneous and immunological reactions to phenytoin. J. Am. Acad. Dermatol., 18:721, 1988.

Singer, K. H., and Hashimoto, K.: Pathogenesis of autoimmunity in pemphigus. Annu. Rev. Immunol., 3:87, 1985.

Sodhi, V. K., and Sausker, W. F.: Dermatoses of pregnancy. Am. Fam. Physician, 37:131, 1988.

Sternbach, G., and Callen, J. P.: Dermatitis. Emerg. Med. Clin. North Am., 3:677, 1985.

Tabas, M., Gibbons, S., and Bauer, E. A.: The mechanobullous diseases. Dermatol. Clin., 5:123, 1987.

Taylor, J. S. (ed.): Occupational dermatoses. Dermatol. Clin., 6:1, 1988.

Thivolet, J.: The role of MCA in dermatology: monoclonal antibodies in cutaneous immunohistochemistry. J. Dermatol. (Tokyo), 13:313, 1986.

Wintroub, B. U., and Stern, R.: Cutaneous drug reactions. J. Am. Acad. Dermatol., 13:167, 1985.

Young, E. M., Jr., and Barr, R. J.: Sclerosing dermatoses. J. Cutan. Pathol., 12:426, 1985.

Macular and Papular Diseases

Bos, J. D.: The pathomechanisms of psoriasis. Br. J. Dermatol., 118:141, 1988.

Brenner, S., and Horwitz, C.: Possible nutrient mediators in psoriasis and seborrheic dermatitis. World Rev. Nutr. Diet., 5:133, 1988.

Burrall, B. A., and Huntley, A. C.: Urticaria and angioedema. Clin. Rev. Allergy, 3:95, 1985.

DiCicco, L. M., Fraki, J. E., and Mansbridge, J. N.: The plasma membrane in psoriasis. J. Dermatol., 26:631, 1987.

Farnham, J., and Grant, J. A.: Angioedema. Dermatol. Clin., 3:85, 1985.

Gottlieb, A. B.: Immunologic mechanisms in psoriasis. J. Am. Acad. Dermatol., 18:1379, 1988.

Jorizzo, J. L. (ed.): Urticaria. Dermatol. Clin., 3(1):1, 1985.

Juhlin, L.: Additives and chronic urticaria. Ann. Allergy, 59 (5 Pt. 2):119, 1987.

Lambert, W. C.: Premycotic eruptions. Dermatol. Clin., 3:629, 1985.

Laurent, M. R.: Psoriatic arthritis. Clin. Rheum. Dis.,

11:61, 1985.

Lyons, J. H., 3rd: Generalized pustular psoriasis. Int. J. Dermatol., *26*:409, 1987.

Novick, N. L., and Phelps, R.: Erythema dyschromicum perstans. Int. J. Dermatol., *24*:630, 1985.

Olafsson, J. H.: Cutaneous and systemic mastocytosis in adults. Acta Derm. Venereol. (Suppl.), *115*:1, 1985.

Partsch, G.: Laboratory features of psoriatic arthritis. Z. Rheumatol., *46*:220, 1987.

Paul, E., Grelich, K. D., and Dominante, G.: Epidemiology of urticaria. Monogr. Allergy, *21*:87, 1987.

Perlman, S. G.: Psoriatic arthritis in children. Pediatr. Dermatol., *1*:283, 1984.

Rasmussen, J. E.: Psoriasis in children. Dermatol. Clin., *4*:99, 1986.

Ridley, C. M.: Lichen sclerosus et atrophicus. Br. Med. J., *295*:1295, 1987.

Ros, A. M.: Photosensitive psoriasis. Acta Derm. Venereol. (Suppl.), *131*:1, 1987.

Rowland Payne, C. M.: Psoriatic science. Br. Med. J., *295*:1158, 1987.

Stein, D. H.: Mastocytosis. Pediatr. Dermatol., *3*:365, 1986.

Wright, N. A.: Changes in epidermal cell proliferation in proliferative skin disease. Curr. Top. Pathol., *74*:141, 1985.

Disorders of Pigmentation

Barnes, L.: Vitiligo and the Vogt-Koyanagi-Harada syndrome. Dermatol. Clin., *6*:229, 1988.

Bolognia, J. L., and Pawelek, J. M.: Biology of hypopigmentation. J. Am. Acad. Dermatol., *19*:217, 1988.

Bystryn, J. -C., and Pfeffer, S.: Vitiligo and antibodies to melanocytes. Prog. Clin. Biol. Res. *256*:195, 1988.

Falabella, R.: Idiopathic guttate hypomelanosis. Dermatol. Clin., *6*:241, 1988.

Goudie, R. B., Jack, A. S., and Goudie, B. M.: Genetic and developmental aspects of pathological pigmentation patterns. Curr. Top. Pathol., *74*:103, 1985.

Grimes, P. E., and Stockton, T. Pigmentary disorders in blacks. Dermatol. Clin., *6*:271, 1988.

King, R. A., Olds, D. P., and Townsend, D.: Mechanisms of depigmentation in human occulocutaneous albinism. Prog. Clin. Biol. Res., *256*:183, 1988.

King, R. A., and Summers, C. G.: Albinism. Dermatol. Clin., *6*:217, 1988.

Kinnear, P. E., Jay, B., and Witkop, C. J., Jr.: Albinism. Surv. Ophthalmol., *30*:75, 1985.

Lucky, P. A., and Nordlund, J. J.: The biology of the pigmentary system and its disorders. Dermatol. Clin., *3*:197, 1985.

McGavran, M. H.: Cutaneous pigmentation. Clin. Plast. Surg., *14*:301, 1987.

Nordlund, J. J. (ed.): Pigmentation disorders. Dermatol. Clin., *6*:161, 1988.

Ortonne, J. -P.: Piebaldism, Waardenburg's syndrome and related disorders. Dematol. Clin., *6*:205, 1988.

Epidermal Diseases

Baden, H. P., and Bronstein, B. R.: Ichthyosiform dermatosis and deafness. Arch. Dermatol., *124*:102, 1988.

Cohen, B. A.: Incontinentia pigmenti. Neurol. Clin., *5*:361, 1987.

El-Benhawi, M. O., and George, W. M.: Incontinentia pigmenti. Cutis, *41*:259, 1988.

Feingold, K. R., and Elias, P. M.: Endocrine skin interactions. J. Am. Acad. Dermatol., *19*:1, 1988.

Goodman, R. M. (ed.): Genodermatoses. Clin. Dermatol., *3*(1):1, 1985.

Hori, Y., and Takayama, O.: Circumscribed dermal melanoses. Dermatol. Clin., *6*:315, 1988.

Johnson, R. T., and Squires, S.: Defects in the early and late stages of nucleotide excision repair and the origins of cancer. Prog. Clin. Biol. Res., *259*:1, 1988.

Jung, E. G.: Xeroderma pigmentosum. Int. J. Dermatol., *25*:629, 1986.

Kanitakis, J., Tsoitis, G., and Kanitakis, C.: Hereditary epidermolytic palmoplantar keratoderma (Vörner type). J. Am. Acad. Dermatol., *17*:414, 1987.

Kegel, M. F.: Dominant disorders with multiple organ involvement. Dermatol. Clin., *5*:205, 1987.

Kraemer, K. H., and Slor, H.: Xeroderma pigmentosum. Clin. Dermatol., *3*(1):33, 1985.

Lambert, C. W.: Genetic diseases associated with DNA and chromosomal instability. Dermatol. Clin., *5*:85, 1987.

McGuire, J.: The biologic basis of the ichthyoses. Dermatol. Clin., *4*:67, 1986.

Mallory, S. B., and Stough, D. B., IV: Genodermatoses with malignant potential. Dermatol. Clin., *5*:221, 1987.

Neilsen, P. G.: Herditary palmoplantar keratoderma and dermatophytosis. Int. J. Dermatol., *27*:223, 1988.

Pallotta, R., and Dalprá, L.: Chromosomal instability in incontinentia pigmenti. Ann. Génét., *31*:27, 1988.

Strauss, B. S.: Cellular aspects of DNA repair. Adv. Cancer Res., *45*:45, 1985.

Takebe, H., Nishigori, C., and Satoh, Y.: Genetics and skin cancer of xeroderma pigmentosum in Japan. Jpn. J. Cancer Res., *78*:1135, 1987.

Timme, T. L., and Moses, R. E.: Diseases with DNA damage-processing defects. Am. J. Med. Sci., *295*:40, 1988.

Williams, M. L.: A new look at the ichthyoses. Pediatr. Dermatol., *3*:476, 1986.

Williams, M. L., and Elias, P. M.: Genetically transmitted, generalized disorders of cornification. The ichthyoses. Dermatol. Clin., *5*:155, 1987.

Diseases of the Epidermal Appendages

Ancona, A. A.: Occupational acne. State Art Rev. Occup. Med., *1*:229, 1986.

Bergfeld, W. F., and Redmond, G. P.: Androgenic alopecia. Dermatol. Clin., *5*:491, 1987.

Birnbaum, P. S., and Baden, H. P.: Heritable disorders of hair. Dermatol. Clin., *5*:137, 1987.

Borodin, M. B.: Drug-related alopecia. Dermatol. Clin., *5*:571, 1987.

Camacho-Martinez, F.: Eosinophilic pustular folliculitis. J. Am. Acad. Dermatol., *17*:686, 1987.

Camacho-Martinez, F., and Ferrando, J.: Hair shaft dysplasia. Int. J. Dermatol., *27*:71, 1988.

Cline, D. J.: Changes in hair color. Dermatol. Clin., *6*:295, 1988.

Dawber, R. P.: Aetiology and pathogenesis of hair loss. Dematologica, 175(Suppl. 2):23, 1987.

DeVillez, R. L. (ed.): Androgenic alopecia. Clin. Dermatol., 6(4):1, 1988.

Hall, J. R., et al.: Familial dyskeratotic comedones. J. Am. Acad. Dermatol., 17:808, 1987.

Mitchell, A. J., and Balle, M. R.: Alopecia areata. Dermatol. Clin., 5:553, 1987.

Morris, D. V.: Hirsutism. Clin. Obstet. Gynaecol., 12:649, 1985.

Muller, S. A.: Trichotillomania. Dermatol. Clin., 5:595, 1987.

Murphy, G. M., and Greaves, M. W.: Acne and psoriasis. Br. Med. J., 296:546, 1988.

Newton, R. C., Hebert, A. A., Freese, T. W., and Solomon, A. R.: Scarring alopecia. Dermatol. Clin., 5:603, 1987.

Parsons, J. M.: Pityriasis rosea update: 1986. J. Am. Acad. Dermatol., 15:159, 1986.

Rebora, A.: Rosacea. J. Invest. Dermatol., 88 (3 Suppl.):56s, 1987.

Reid, R. L., and van Vugt, D. A.: Hair loss in the female. Obstet. Gynec. Surv., 43:135, 1988.

Rittmaster, R. S., and Loriaux, D. L.: Hirsutism. Ann. Intern. Med., 106:95, 1987.

Salinas, C. F., Opitz, J. M., and Paul, N. W.: Recent advances in ectodermal dysplasias. Birth Defects, 24(2):1, 1988.

Solomon, L. M., Cook, B., and Klippel, W.: The ectodermal dysplasias. Dermatol. Clin., 5:231, 1987.

Spencer, L. V., and Callen, J. P.: Hair loss in systemic disease. Dermatol. Clin., 5:565, 1987.

Stroud, J. D.: Hair-shaft anomalies. Dermatol. Clin., 5:581, 1987.

Whipp, M. J., Harrington, C. I., and Dundas, S.: Fatal Squamous cell carcinoma associated with acne conglobata in a father and daughter. Br. J. Dermatol., 117:389, 1987.

Wiemer, D. R.: Rhinophyma. Clin. Plast. Surg., 14:357, 1987.

Yonkosky, D. M., and Pochi, P. E.: Acne vulgaris in childhood. Dermatol. Clin., 4:127, 1986.

Vascular Diseases

Burton, J. L.: Livedo reticularis, porcelain-white scars, and cerebral thrombosis. Lancet, 1:1263, 1988.

Cohen, P. R., and Kurzrock, R.: Sweet's syndrome and malignancy. Am. J. Med., 82:1220, 1987.

Gibson, L. E., and Winkleman, R. K.: Cutaneous granulomatous vasculitis. J. Am. Acad. Dermatol., 14:492, 1986.

Jegasothy, B. V.: Immune complexes in the reactive inflammatory vascular dermatoses. Dermatol. Clin., 3:185, 1985.

Jorizzo, J. L., Solomon, A. R., Zanolli, A. R., and Leshin, B.: Neutrophilic vascular reactions. J. Am. Acad. Dermatol., 19:983, 1988.

Kaudewitz, P., et al.: Monoclonal antibody pattern in lymphoid papulosis. Dermatol. Clin., 3:749, 1985.

Kitchens, C. S.: The purpuric disorders. Semin. Thromb. Hemostat., 10:173, 1984.

Mor, F., Leibovici, L., and Wysenbeek, A. J.: Leukocytoclastic vasculitis in malignant lymphoma. Isr. J. Med. Sci., 23:829, 1987.

Paller, A. S.: Vascular disorders. Dermatol. Clin., 5:239, 1987.

Patterson, J. W., and White, R. M.: Lymphoid papulosis South. Med. J., 79:850, 1986.

Rehman, R. S.: Histology of adverse cutaneous drug reactions. Clin. Dermatol., 4(1):23, 1986.

Ryan, T. J., and Burge, S. M.: Cutaneous vasculitis. Curr. Top. Pathol., 74:57, 1985.

Sams, W. M., Jr.: Human hypersensitivity vasculitis. J. Invest. Dermatol., 85(1 Suppl.):144s, 1985.

Solomon, A. R.: The histologic spectrum of the reactive inflammatory vascular dermatoses. Dermatol. Clin., 3:171, 1985.

Spraker, M. K.: The vascular lesions of childhood. Dermatol. Clin., 4:79, 1986.

Tosca, N., and Stratigos, J. D.: Possible pathogenetic mechanisms in allergic cutaneous vasculitis. Int. J. Dermatol., 27:291, 1988.

Visani, G., et al.: Sweet's syndrome with accelerated stage chronic myeloid leukemia. Acta Hematol., 79:207, 1988.

White, J. W., Jr.: Gyrate erythema. Dermatol. Clin., 3:129, 1985.

Willemze, R.: Lymphoid papillomatosis. Dermatol. Clin., 3:735, 1985.

Dermal Diseases

Braverman, I. M.: Elastic fiber and microvascular abnormalities in aging skin. Dermatol. Clin., 4:391, 1986.

Brien, J. P.,: Acinic granuloma. Int. J. Dermatol., 24:473, 1986.

Fenske, N. A., and Conrad, C. B.: Aging skin. Am. Fam. Physician, 37:219, 1988.

Frieden, I. J.: Aplasia cutis congenita. J. Am. Acad. Dermatol., 14:646, 1986.

Krinsky, W. L.: Dermatoses associated with the bites of mites and ticks. Int. J. Dermatol., 22:75, 1983.

Reyes-Flores, O.: Granulomas induced by living agents. Int. J. Dermatol., 25:158, 1986.

Richey, M. L., Richey, H. K., and Fenske, N. A.: Age-related skin changes. Geriatrics, 43(4):49, 1988.

Rimon, D., et al.: Cardiomyopathy and multiple myeloma. Complications of scleredema adultorum. Arch. Intern. Med., 148:551, 1988.

Truhan, A. P., and Roenigk, H. H., Jr.: The cutaneous mucinoses. J. Am. Acad. Dermatol., 14:1, 1986.

Young, E. M., Jr., and Barr, R. J.: Sclerosing dermatoses. J. Cutan. Pathol., 12:426, 1985.

Diseases of the Subcutaneous Tissue

Fretzin, D. F., and Arias, D. M.: Scleroderma and subcutaneous fat necrosis of the newborn. Pediatr. Dermatol., 4:112, 1987.

Hannuksela, M.: Erythema nodosum. Dermatol. Clin., 4:88, 1986.

Patterson, J.W.: Panniculitis. Arch. Dermatol., 123: 1615, 1987.

White, J. W.: Erythema nodosum. Dermatol. Clin., 3:119, 1985.

Collagen Diseases

Arnett, F. C.: HLA and genetic predisposition to lupus erythematosus and other dermatologic disorders. J. Am. Acad. Dermatol., 13:472, 1985.

Callen, J. P. (ed.): Lupus erythematosus. Clin. Dermatol., 3(3):1, 1985.

Mimori, T.: Scleroderma-polymyositis overlap syndrome. Int. J. Dermatol., 26:419, 1987.

Serup, J.: Localized scleroderma (morphoea). Acta Derm. Venereol. Scand. (Suppl.), 122:3, 1986.

Young, E. M., Jr., and Barr, R. J.: Sclerosing dermatoses. J. Cutan. Pathol., 12:426, 1985.

Tumors

Abel, E. A.: Clinical features of cutaneous T-cell lymphoma. Dermatol. Clin., 3:647, 1985.

Ackerman, A. B., and Mihara, I.: Dysplasia, dysplastic melanocytes, dysplastic nevi, the dysplastic nevus syndrome, and the relation between dysplastic nevi and malignant melanoma. Hum. Pathol., 16:87, 1985.

Albino, A. P.: Status of oncogenes in malignant melanoma. Prog. Clin. Biol. Res., 256:361, 1988.

Armstrong, B. K., and Holman, C. D.: Malignant melanoma of the skin. Bull. W. H. O., 65:245, 1987.

Audisio, R. A., Lodeville, D., Quagliuolo, V., and Clemente, C.: Sebaceous carcinoma arising from the eyelid and from extra-ocular sites. Tumori, 73:531, 1987.

Basset, F., Nezelof, C., and Ferrans V. J.: The histiocytoses. Pathol. Annu., 18 (Pt. 2):27, 1983.

Batsakis, J. G., Regezi, J. A., Soloman, A. R., and Rice D. H.: Mucosal melanomas. Head Neck Surg., 4:404, 1982.

Beck, D. E., Fazio, V. W., Jugelman, D. G., and Lavery, I. C.: Perianal Bowen's disease. Dis. Colon Rectum, 31:419, 1988.

Becker, Y.: Dose radiation-induced abrogation of skin Langerhans cell functions lead to enhanced incidence of skin tumors in patients with genet Cancer Invest., 5:507, 1987.

Bender, B. L., and Yunis, E. J.: The pathology of tuberous sclerosis. Pathol. Annu., 17(Pt. 1):339, 1982.

Berger, T. G., and Dawson, N. A.: Angioendotheliomatosis. J. Am. Acad. Dermatol., 18:407, 1988.

Beutner, K. R.: Human papillomavirus infection. J. Am. Acad. Dermatol., 20:114, 1989.

Bhawan, J.: Angioendotheliomatosis proliferans systemisata. Semin. Diagn. Pathol., 4:18, 1987.

Bickers, D. R.: Sun-induced disorders. Emerg. Med. Clin. North Am., 3:659, 1985.

Breslow, A.: Prognosis in cutaneous melanoma. Pathol. Annu., 15(Pt. 1):1, 1980.

Briggs, J. C.: Melanoma precursor lesions and borderline melanomas. Histopathology, 9:1251, 1985.

Brodell, R. T., and Santa Cruz, D. J.: Cutaneous pseudolymphoma. Dermatol. Clin., 3:719, 1985.

Broder, E.: Ataxia-telangiectasia. KROC Found. Ser., 19:1, 1985.

Burke, J. S.: Malignant lymphomas of the skin. Semin. Diagn. Pathol., 2:169, 1985.

Bystryn, J. C.: Immunology and immunotherapy of human malignant melanoma. Dermatol. Clin., 3:327, 1985.

Cann, C. I., Fried, M. P., and Rothman, K. J.: Epidemiology of squamous cell carcinoma of the head and neck. Otolaryngol. Clin. North Am., 18:367, 1985.

Cerio, R., and McDonald, D.M.: Benign cutaneous lymphoid infiltrates. J. Cutan. Pathol., 12:442, 1985.

Chandra, J. J.: The clinical recognition and prognostic factors of primary cutaneous malignant melanoma. Med. Clin. North Am., 70:39, 1986.

Chyu, J., Medenica, M., and Whitney, D. H.: Verruciform xanthoma of the lower extremity. J. Am. Acad. Dermatol., 17:695, 1987.

Clark, W. H., Jr.: The dysplastic nevus syndrome. Arch. Dermatol., 124:1207, 1988.

Clendenning, W. E.: Perpectives on cutaneous T cell lymphoma. Clin. Exp. Dermatol., 11:109. 1986.

Cohen, P. R.: Becker's nevus. Am. Fam. Physician, 37:221, 1988.

Cooper, P. H.: Angiosarcoma of the skin. Semin. Diagn. Pathol., 4:2, 1987.

Cordon-Cardo, C.: Biochemical and immunologic diagnosis of cancer. Tumour Biol., 82:151, 1987.

Cruz, D. J.: Sweat gland carcinoma. Semin. Diagn. Pathol., 4:38, 1987.

Cruz, P. D., Jr., East, C., and Bergstresser, P. R.: Dermal, subcutaneous, and tendon xanthomas. J. Am. Acad. Dermatol., 19:95, 1988.

Dorfman, R. F.: Kaposi's sarcoma. Am. J. Surg. Pathol., 10(Suppl. 1):68, 1986.

Dorfman, R. F.: Kaposi's sarcoma: evidence supporting its origin from the lymphatic system. Lymphology, 21:45, 1988.

Dufresne, C. R., and Hoopes, J. E.: Pseudomalignancies. Clin. Plast. Surg., 14:367, 1987.

Dyall-Smith, D., and Varigos, G.: Human papillomaviruses and cancer. Australas. J. Dermatol., 26:102, 1985.

Edelson, R. L.: Cutaneous T cell lymphoma. J. Dermatol. (Tokyo), 14:397, 1987.

Elder, D. E.: Dysplastic nevi. Dermatol. Clin., 6:257, 1988.

Emmett, E. A.: Occupational skin cancers. State Art Occup. Med., 2:165, 1987.

Esterly, N. B.: Cutaneous hemangiomas. Curr. Probl. Pediatr., 17(1):1, 1987.

Evans, R. D., et al.: Risk factors for development of malignant melanoma. J. Dermatol. Surg. Oncol., 14:393, 1988.

Fidler, I. J.: The biology of melanoma metastasis. J. Dermatol. Surg. Oncol., 14:875, 1988.

Fletcher, C. D., and McKee, P. H.: Sarcomas: a clincopathological guide with particular reference to cutaneous manifestations. I. Dermatofibrosarcoma protuberans, malignant fibrous histiocytoma and the epithelioid sarcoma of Enzinger. Clin. Exp. Dermatol., 9:451, 1984.

Fossati, G., et al.: Immune response to autologous human melanoma. Biochem. Biophys. Acta, 865:235, 1986.

Friedman, R. J., Heilman, E. R., Rigel, D. S., and Kopf, A. W.: The dysplastic nevus. Clinical and pathologic features. Dermatol. Clin., 3:239, 1985.

Friedman, R. J., Rigel, D. S., and Heilman, E. R.: The relationship between melanocytic nevi and malignant melanoma. Dermatol. Clin., 6:249, 1988.

Gard, D.: Nonpigmented premalignant lesions of the skin. Clin. Plast. Surg., 14:413, 1987.

Garvin, A. J.: A histopathologic classification of cutaneous lymphomas. Dermatol. Clin., 3:587, 1985.

Gianotti, F., and Caputo, R.: Histiocytic syndromes. J. Am. Acad. Dermatol., 13:383, 1985.

Gill, P. G.: Malignant melanoma: a clinical perspective. Med. J. Aust., 148:638, 1988.

Goldenhersh, M. A., Savin, R. C., Barnhill, R. L., and Stenn, K. S.: Malignant blue nevus. J. Am. Acad. Dermatol., 19:712, 1988.

Gorlin, R. J.: Nevoid basal-cell carcinoma syndrome. Medicine, 66:98, 1987.

Gottlieb, G. J., and Ackerman, A. B. (eds.): Kaposi's Sarcoma. Philadelphia. Lea & Febiger, 1987.

Greene, M. H.: The dysplastic nevus syndrome. Important Adv. Oncol., 173, 1986 (Review).

Gupta, A. K., Lipa, M., and Haberman, H. F.: Proliferating endotheliomatosis. Arch. Dermatol., 122:314, 1986.

Gupta, R. K.: Circulating immune complexes in malignant melanoma. Dis. Markers, 6:81, 1988. .

Gutierrez, M. M., and Mora, R. G.: Nevoid basal cell carcinoma syndrome. J. Am. Acad. Dermatol., 15:1023, 1986.

Hamm, H., Happle, R., and Bröker, E. B.: Multiple agminate Spitz naevi. Br. J. Dermatol., 117:511, 1987.

Hashimoto, K., et al.: Congenital self-healing reticulohistiocytosis (Hashimoto-Pritzker type). Int. J. Dermatol., 25:516, 1986.

Hashimoto, K., Mehregan, A. H., and Kumakiri, M.: Tumors of Skin Appendages. Stoneham, MA, Butterworths, 1987.

Headington, J. T., Roth, M. S., and Schnitzer, B.: Regressing atypical histiocytosis. Semin. Diagn. Pathol., 4:28, 1987.

Heathcote, J. G., Guenther, L. C. and Wallace, A. C.: Multicentric reticulohistiocytosis. Pathology, 17:601, 1985.

Herlyn, M., et al.: Biology of tumor progression in human melanocytes. Lab. Invest., 56:461, 1987.

Herlyn, M., and Koprowski, H.: Melanoma antigens. Am. Rev. Immunol., 6:283, 1988.

Hoss, D. M., and Grant-Kels, J. M.: Significant melanotic lesions in infancy, childhood and adolescence. Dermatol. Clin., 4:29, 1986.

Houghten, A. N., Cordon-Cardo, C., and Eisinger, M.: Differentiation antigens of melanoma and melanocytes. Int. Rev. Exp. Pathol., 28:217, 1986.

Howley, P. M.: The role of papillomaviruses in human cancer. Important Adv. Oncol., i 55, 1987 (Review).

Howley, P. M., and Schlegal, R.: The human papillomaviruses. Am. J. Med., 85(2A):155, 1988.

Hutchinson, B. L.: Malignant melanoma of the lower extremity. Clin. Podiatr. Med. Surg., 3:533, 1986.

Illig, L.: Epidemiologic aspects of malignant melanoma. Anticancer Res., 7:1309, 1987.

Jablonska, S., and Orth, G.: Warts/human papillomaviruses. Clin. Dermatol., 3(4):1, 1985.

Jurecka, W.: Neurogenic tumors of the skin. Wein. Wochenschr. (Suppl.), 176:3, 1987.

Kanitakis, J., et al.: Congenital self-healing histiocytosis (Hashimoto-Pritzker). Cancer, 61:508, 1988.

Kaplan, E., and Nickoloff, B. J.: Clinical and histologic features of nevi with emphasis on treatment approaches. Clin. Plast. Surg., 14:277, 1987.

Kaplan, E., and Nickoloff, B. J.: Clinical and histological features of nevi with emphasis on treatment approaches. Dermatol. Clin., 6:131, 1988.

Kathuria, S., Rieker, J., Jablokow, V. R., and van den Broek, H.: Plantar verrucous carcinoma (epithelioma cuniculatum). J. Surg. Oncol., 31:71, 1986.

Keeney, G. L., Banks, P. M., and Linscheid, R. L.: Subungual keratoacanthoma. Arch. Dermatol., 124:1074, 1988.

Kitagawa, M., et al.: Angiosarcoma of the scalp. Virchow's Arch. (A), 412:83, 1987.

Klinesmith, D'A.M., and Perricone, N.V.: Common skin problems in the elderly. Dermatol. Clin., 4:485, 1986.

Kraemer, K. H., and Greene, M. H.: Dysplastic nevus syndrome. Dermatol. Clin., 3:225, 1985.

Kripkie, M. L.: Impact of ozone depletion on skin cancers. J. Dermatol. Surg. Oncol., 14:835, 1988.

van der Kwast, Th. H., et al.: Primary cutaneous adenoid cystic carcinoma. Br. J. Dermatol., 118:567, 1988.

Kwittken, J.: Dysplasia in dermatology. Mt. Sinai J. Med., 55:176, 1988.

Lambert, W.C., et al.: Melanoacanthoma and related disorders. Int. J. Dermatol., 26:508, 1987.

Leader, M., Patel, J., Collins, M., and Henry, K.: Antialpha 1-antichymotrypsin staining of 194 sarcomas, 38 carcinomas and 17 malignant melanomas. Am. J. Surg. Pathol., 11:133, 1987.

Lee, J. A.: Melanoma and exposure to sunlight. Epidemiol. Rev., 4:110, 1982.

Lee, Y. T.: Loco-regional primary and recurrent melanoma. Cancer Treat. Rev., 15:135, 1988.

Lejeune, F. J.: Epidemiology and etiology of malignant melanoma. Biomed. Pharmacother., 40:91, 1986.

Lew, R. A., Koh, H. K., and Sober, A. J.: Epidemiology of cutaneous melanoma. Dermatol. Clin., 3:257, 1985.

Lin, A. N., and Carter, D. M.: Skin cancer in the elderly. Dermatol. Clin., 4:467, 1986.

Lineaweaver, W. C., Wang, T. -N., and Leboit, P.L.: Pilomatrix carcinoma. J. Surg. Oncol., 37:171, 1988.

McCance, D. J.: Human papillomaviruses and cancer. Biochim. Biophys. Acta, 823:195, 1986.

McGovern, V. J.: Melanoma. New York, Raven Press, 1983.

McMeekin, T. W., Baerg, R. H., Snyder, A. J., and Ishibashi, P. L.: Eccrine poroma. J. Am. Podiatr. Med. Ass., 78:43, 1988.

McMillan, E. M.: Monoclonal antibody patterns in cutaneous lymphoid infiltrates. Dermatol. Clin., 3:593, 1987.

Mallory, S. B., and Stough, D. B., IV: Genodermatoses with malignant potential. Dermatol. Clin., 5:221, 1987.

Marks, R.: Nonmelanotic skin cancer and solar keratosis. Int. J. Dermatol., 26:201, 1987.

Massa, M. C., and Medenica, M.: Cutaneous adnexal tumors and cysts. Pathol. Annu., 20 (Pt. 2):189, 1985; 22(Pt. 1):225, 1987.

Matloub, H. S., et al.: Eccrine porocarcinoma. Ann. Plast. Surg., 20:351, 1988.

Metcalf, J. S., and Maize, J. C.: Melanocytic nevi and malignant melanoma. Dermatol. Clin., 3:217, 1985.

Mihm, M. C., Jr., Murphy, G. F., and Kaufman, N.: Pathobiology and Recognition of Malignant Melanoma. Baltimore, Williams & Wilkins, 1988.

Morag, C., and Metzker, A.: Inflammatory linear verrucous epidermal nevus. Pediatr. Dermatol., 3:15, 1985.

Moreno, A., et al.: Porokeratotic eccrine osteal and dermal duct nevus. J. Cutan. Pathol., 15:43, 1988.

Morris, B. T.: Cutaneous malignant melanoma in the elderly. Dermatol. Clin., 4:473, 1986.

Morris, D. M., Sansui, I. D., and Lanehart, W. H.: Carcinoma of eccrine sweat glands. J. Surg. Oncol., 31:26, 1986.

Muggia, F. M., and Lonberg, M.: Kaposi's sarcoma and AIDS. Med. Clin. North Am., 70:139, 1986.

Murphy, G. F.: Cutaneous T cell lymphoma. Adv. Pathol., 1:131, 1988.

Murphy, G. F., and Mihm, M. C.: Lymphoproliferative Diseases of the Skin. Stoneham, MA, Butterworths, 1986.

Nanus, D. M., Kelsen, D., and Clark, D. G. C.: Radiation-induced angiosarcoma. Cancer, 60:777, 1987.

Novick, N. L., Kest, E., and Gordon, M.: Advances in the biology and carcinogenesis of basal cell carcinoma. N. Y. State J. Med., 88:367, 1988.

O'Brien, P. C., Denham, J. W., and Leong, A. S. -Y.: Merkel cell carcinoma. Aust. N. Z. J. Surg., 57:847, 1987.

Paller, A. S.: Metabolic disorders characterized by angiokeratomas and neurologic dysfunction. Neurol. Clin., 5:444, 1987.

Paller, A. S.: Ataxia-telangiectasia. Neurol. Clin., 5:447, 1987.

Paller, A. S.: Epidermal nevus syndrome. Neurol. Clin., 5:451, 1987.

Paller, A. S.: The Sturge-Weber syndrome. Pediatr. Dermatol., 4:300, 1987.

Paller, A. S.: Vascular disorders. Dermatol. Clin., 5:239, 1987.

Panizzon, R., and Schnyder, U. W.: Familial Becker's nevus. Dermatologica, 176:275, 1988.

Pasyk, K. A., Argenta, L. C., and Schelbert, E. B.: Angiokeratoma circumscriptum. Ann. Plast. Surg., 20:183, 1988.

Picascia, D. D., and Robinson, J. K.: Actinic cheilitis. J. Am. Acad. Dermatol., 17:255, 1987.

Piette, W. W.: Myeloma, paraproteinemias, and the skin. Med. Clin. North Am., 70:155, 1986.

Rabinowitz, A. D., and Silvers, D. N.: Pathology of melanoma. Dermatol. Clin., 3:285, 1985.

Ragi, G., Turner, M. S., Klein. L. E., and Stoll, H. L., Jr.: Pigmented Bowen's disease and review of 420 Bowen's disease lesions. J. Dermatol. Surg. Oncol., 14:765, 1988.

Reifer, D. M., and Hornblass, A.: Squamous cell carcinoma of the eyelid. Surv. Ophthalmol., 30:349, 1986.

Rhodes, A. R.: Melanocytic precursors of cutaneous melanoma. Med. Clin. North Am., 70:3, 1986.

Rhodes, A. R., et al.: Risk factors for cutaneous melanoma. J. Am. Med. Ass., 258:3145, 1987.

Rigel, D. S., et al.: Precursors of malignant melanoma. Dermatol. Clin., 3:361, 1985.

Rigel, D. S., Rogers, G. S., and Friedman, R. J.: Prognosis of malignant melanoma. Dermatol. Clin., 3:309, 1985.

Rilke, F., Giardini, R., and Lombardi, L.: Recurrent atypical cutaneous histiocytosis. Pathol. Annu., 20 (Pt. 2):29, 1985.

Ringel, E., and Moschella, S.: Primary histiocytic dermatoses. Arch. Dermatol., 121:1531, 1985.

Rogozinski, T. T., and Janniger, C. K.: Bowenoid papillomatosis. Am. Fam. Physician, 38:161, 1988.

Romerdahl, C. A., and Kripke, M. L.: Advances in the immunobiology of the skin. Implications for cutaneous malignancies. Cancer Metastasis Rev., 5:167, 1986.

Roper, S. S., and Spraker, M. K.: Cutaneous histiocytosis syndromes. Pediatr. Dermatol., 3:19, 1985.

Rosenthal, J. R., and Koh, M. K.: Malignant melanoma and pigmented lesions. Compr. Ther., 14:16, 1988.

Rubenstein, D., Shanker, D.B., Boxall, L., and Krafchik, B.: Multiple cutaneous granular cell tumors in children. Pediatr. Dermatol., 4:94, 1987.

Safai, B.: Pathophysiology and epidemiology of epidemic Kaposi's sarcoma. Semin. Oncol., 14(2 Suppl. 3):7, 1987.

Salinas, F. A., and Wee, K. H.: Prognostic and pathogenic implications of immune complexes in human cancer. Adv. Immun. Cancer Ther., 2:189, 1986.

Sedano, H. O., and Gorlin, R. J.: Acanthosis nigricans. Oral Surg., 63:462, 1987.

Shapiro, S. D., Lambert, W. C., and Schwatz, R. A.: Cowden's disease. Int. J. Dermatol., 27:232, 1988.

Shenaq, S. M.: Benign skin and soft tissue tumors of the hand. Clin. Plast. Surg., 14:403, 1987.

Silva, E. G., et al.: Endocrine carcinoma of the skin (Merkel cell carcinoma). Pathol. Annu., 19 (Pt. 2):1, 1984.

Silvers, D. N.: On the subject of primary cutaneous melanoma. Progr. Surg. Pathol., 4:277, 1982.

Slater, D. N.: Lymphoproliferative conditions of the skin. Rec. Adv. Histopathol., 12:83, 1984.

Slater, D. N.: Recent developments in cutaneous lymphoproliferative disorders. J. Pathol., 153:5, 1987.

Sober, A. J.: Solar exposure in the etiology of cutaneous melanoma. Photodermatol., 4:23, 1987.

Stal, S.: Keratoacanthoma. Clin. Plast. Surg., 14:425, 1987.

Stal, S., Hamilton, S., and Spira, M.: Hemangiomas, lymphangiomas and vascular malformations of the head and neck. Otolaryngol. Clin. North Am., 19:769, 1986.

Stal, S., Loeb, T., and Spira, M.: Melanoma of the head and neck. Otolaryngol. Clin. North Am., 19:549, 1986.

Stegman, S. J.: Basal cell carcinona and squamous cell carcinoma. Med. Clin. North Am., 70:95, 1986.

Suchi, T., et al.: Histopathology and immunohistochemistry of peripheral T cell lymphomas. J. Clin. Pathol., 40:995, 1987.

Swerdlow, A. J., and Green, A.: Melanocytic naevi and melanoma. Br. J. Dermatol., 117:137, 1987.

Syrjänen, K. J.: Human papillomavirus (HPV) infections and their associations with squamous cell neoplasia.

Arch. Gewulstforsch., *57*:417, 1987.

Syrjänen, K. J.: Biology of human papillomavirus (HPV) infections and their role in squamous carcinogenesis. Med. Biol., *65*:21, 1987.

Syrjänen, K., Gissman, L., and Kos, L. G.: Papillomaviruses and Human Disease. New York, Springer-Verlag, 1987.

Takebe, H., Nishigori, C., and Satoh, Y.: Genetics and skin cancer of xeroderma pigmentosum in Japan. Jpn. J. Cancer Res., *78*:1135, 1987.

Thaller, S. R., and Bauer, B. S.: Cysts and cyst-like lesions of the skin and subcutaneous tissues. Clin. Plast. Surg., *14*:327, 1987.

Thomson, H.: Cutaneous hemangiomas and lymphangiomas. Clin. Plast. Surg., *14*:341, 1987.

Toback, A. C., and Edelson, R. L.: Pathogenesis of cutaneous T-cell lymphoma. Dermatol. Clin., *3*:605, 1985.

van der Valk, P., and Meijer, C. J. L. M.: Cutaneous histiocytic proliferations. Dermatol. Clin., *3*:705, 1985.

Wade, T. R., and White, C. R.: The histology of malignant melanoma. Med. Clin. North Am., *70*:57, 1986.

Wagner, R. F., Jr., and Nathanson, L.: Paraneoplastic syndromes, tumor markers, and other unusual features of malignant melanoma. J. Am. Acad. Dermatol., *14*:249, 1986.

Weedon, D.: Melanoma and other melanocytic skin lesions. Curr. Top. Pathol., *74*:1, 1985.

Weiss, L. M., Crabtree, G. S., Rouse, R. V., and Warnike, R. A.: Morphologic and immunologic characterization of 50 peripheral T cell lymphomas. Am. J. Pathol., *118*:316, 1985.

Wick, M. R. (ed.): Pathology of unusual malignant cutaneous tumours. Clin. Biochem. Analysis., *20*:1, 1985.

Index

Page numbers in *italics* refers to illustrations; numbers followed by the letter "t" refer to tables.